MYLES
TEXTBOOK
for
MIDWIVES

V. Ruth Bennett BA MEd RN RM MTD is a midwifery lecturer at the University of Surrey's European Institute of Health and Medical Sciences. She worked previously at the Royal College of Midwives where she was instrumental in developing advanced courses for midwives, including the first Masters Degree in midwifery in the UK, in which she still participates at Surrey. She has had extensive experience at home and overseas, including 10 years at the Nazareth Hospital in Israel and 7 years at the Princess Margaret Hospital in Swindon. She gained much insight into midwifery education and other issues through membership of the English National Board Midwifery Committee and other bodies.

Linda K. Brown BA MEd RN RSCN RM MTD worked for 5 years as the Course Director for Midwifery Courses by Distance Learning at the South Bank University in London. She was responsible, during that time, for developing the acclaimed Diploma into a Degree course for midwives. This built on her previous involvement in the development of the MSc in Advanced Midwifery Practice at the University of Surrey and teaching midwives on the PGCEA course. She has been able to contribute to midwifery on a national basis through her former membership of the Council of the Royal College of Midwives and of the Professional Midwifery Advisory Network of the English National Board for Nursing, Midwifery and Health Visiting.

For Churchill Livingstone

Commissioning Editor: Mary Law, Ellen Green, Inta Ozols
Project Manager: Valerie Burgess
Project Development Editor: Mairi McCubbin
Designer: Judith Wright
Marketing Manager: Hilary Brown

MYLES TEXTBOOK *for* MIDWIVES

Thirteenth Edition

Edited by

V. Ruth Bennett BA MEd RN RM MTD

Linda K. Brown BA MEd RN RSCN RM MTD

Foreword by

Mary E. Uprichard DBE RGN RSCN RM MTD
Formerly President, UKCC, and Director of Midwifery Education,
Northern Ireland College of Midwifery, Belfast

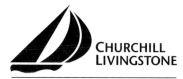

CHURCHILL
LIVINGSTONE

EDINBURGH LONDON NEW YORK PHILADELPHIA SYDNEY TORONTO 1999

CHURCHILL LIVINGSTONE
An imprint of Harcourt Brace and Company Limited

© E. & S. Livingstone Limited 1953, 1956, 1958, 1961, 1964, 1968
© Longman Group Limited 1971, 1975, 1981, 1985
© Longman Group UK Limited 1989, 1993
© Harcourt Brace and Company Limited 1999

First edition 1953   Eighth edition 1975
Second edition 1956   Ninth edition 1981
Third edition 1958   Tenth edition 1985
Fourth edition 1961   Eleventh edition 1989
Fifth edition 1964   Twelfth edition 1993
Sixth edition 1968   Thirteenth edition 1999
Seventh edition 1971

Standard Edition ISBN 0 443 05586 6
International Edition ISBN 0 443 06392 3

British Library of Cataloguing in Publication Data
A catalogue record for this book is available from the British Library.

Library of Congress Cataloging in Publication Data
A catalogue record for this book is available from the Library of Congress

Medical knowledge is constantly changing. As new information becomes
available, changes in treatment, procedures, equipment and the use of
drugs become necessary. The editors and contributors and the publishers
have, as far as it is possible, taken care to ensure that the information given
in this text is accurate and up to date. However, readers are strongly
advised to confirm that the information, especially with regard to drug
usage, complies with latest legislation and standards of practice.

The
publisher's
policy is to use
**paper manufactured
from sustainable forests**

Printed in China
GCC/01

Contents

Contributors

Jean Evelyn Bain BN DipN RN Neonatal Cert
Practice Development/Research Nurse, Ninewells
Hospital, Dundee, UK

Greta Beresford BA MA RGN RM ADM MTD
PGCEA FPCert
Self-employed Midwife, Almeley, UK

V. Ruth Bennett BA MEd RN RM MTD
Lecturer, European Institute of Health and
Medical Sciences, University of Surrey, UK

Ruth Bevis MA RGN RM RHV ADM
Senior Midwife, Ealing Maternity Unit,
Southall, UK

Eileen M. Brayshaw MSc MCSP SRP FETC
Physiotherapy Manager, St James's University
Hospital, Leeds, UK

Linda K. Brown BA MEd RN RSCN RM MTD
Formerly Course Director for Midwifery Courses
by Distance Learning, South Bank University,
London, UK

Patricia Cassidy BA RGN RM DipN(Lond) MTD
Lecturer (Midwifery), University of Paisley,
Paisley, UK

Terri Coates MSc RN RM ADM DipEd ENB901, 932
Distance Learning Tutor, Distance Learning
Centre, South Bank University, London;
Clinical Midwife, Salisbury District Hospital,
Salisbury, UK

Helen Crafter MSc RGN RM FPCert ADM PGCEA
Senior Lecturer in Midwifery, Thames Valley
University, Wolfson Institute of Health Sciences,
London, UK

Sarah Das BSc(Hons) RM RGN DipM
Project Co-ordinator, National Maternity Record
Project, London, UK

Margie Davies RGN RM
Midwifery Liaison Officer, Multiple Births
Foundation, Queen Charlotte's and Chelsea
Hospital, London, UK

Chloe Fisher MBE MNEB SRN SCM MTD
Honorary Clinical Specialist (Infant Feeding),
Women's Centre, Oxford Radcliffe Hospital,
Oxford, UK
36 Feeding

Liz Floyd BN MSc RN RM ADM
Research Midwife, University of Leeds, Leeds, UK
3 Community midwifery

Jocelyn Franey BSc(Hons) RM RN ADM PGCEA
ENB901
Part-time Lecturer, University of Portsmouth;
part-time Family Planning Practitioner,
Portsmouth Health Care Trust, Portsmouth, UK
32 Family planning

Claire Greig BN MSc RGN SCM ADM MTD Neonatal
Cert
Lecturer (Midwifery), Napier University,
Edinburgh, UK
40 Trauma during birth, haemorrhage and convulsions

Annie C. Halliday RN RM RCT RMT
Midwife Teacher, Glasgow Caledonian
University, Glasgow, UK
37 The healthy low birth weight baby
41 Congenital abnormalities

Edith M. Hillan MSc MPhil PhD DipLSc RGN RSCN RM
Professor of Midwifery, Nursing and Midwifery
School, University of Glasgow, Glasgow, UK
24 Physiology and management of the second stage of labour

Liz Hynes (née Spruce) MSc PGCEA ADM SCM SRN
Senior Lecturer in Midwifery, University College
of Suffolk, Great Yarmouth, UK
2 The midwife's client
30 Physiology, complications and management of the puerperium
31 The postnatal emotional and psychological response

Lea Jamieson BEd(Hons) MSc RGN RM MTD
Midwifery Education Consultant (Midwifery
Education Adviser KCL), London, UK
12 Preparing for parenthood: daily life in pregnancy

Rosemary Jenkins RGN RM MTD DMS MBIM MSc
Nursing Officer, Department of Health,
London, UK
47 Organisation of health care in the United Kingdom

Victoria Margaret Lewis BSc(Hons) ADM RM
RGN PGCEA
Freelance Consultant Midwife, Swansea, UK
16 Common medical disorders associated with pregnancy
17 Hypertensive disorders of pregnancy

Alison Livingston RGN RM CertEd(FE) ENB402/904
Community Neonatal Sister, St Peter's Hospital,
Chertsey, UK
39 Respiratory problems
43 Metabolic and endocrine disorders and drug withdrawal

Carmel Lloyd PGDip(Ed) RGN RM ADM PGCEA
ENB901
Lecturer, Midwifery and Women's Health
Studies, Nightingale Institute, King's College
London, London, UK
16 Common medical disorders associated with pregnancy
17 Hypertensive disorders of pregnancy

Rosemary Mander MSc PhD RGN SCM MTD
Senior Lecturer, University of Edinburgh,
Edinburgh, UK
6 Research in midwifery
33 Bereavement and loss in maternity care

Christine McCourt BA PhD
Senior Lecturer in Health Services Research,
Thames Valley University, London, UK
46 Community health and social services

Sue McDonald BAppSc PhD RN RM CHN FACM
Senior Health Researcher for Midwifery and
Nursing, King Edward Memorial Hospital,
Centre for Women's Health, Perth, Australia
25 Physiology and management of the third stage of labour

Mary McGowan
Registrar of Births, Deaths and Marriages,
Hatfield Register Office, Hatfield, UK
48 Vital Statistics

Sinead McNally BA MSc SCM SRN MTD
Midwifery Lecturer, Faculty of Health Studies,
Napier University, Edinburgh, UK
10 Preparing for pregnancy

Maureen M. Michie MEd RGN RM RSCN MTD
Midwifery Lecturer, Glasgow, UK
34 The baby at birth
35 The normal baby

Irene D. Murray BSc(Hons) RN RM MTD
Teaching Fellow (Midwifery), Department of
Nursing and Midwifery, University of Stirling,
Inverness, UK
11 Change and adaptation in pregnancy

Pat Percival BAppSc MAppSc PhD RN RM CHN
FRCNA
Postgraduate Coordinator, School of Nursing,
Edith Cowan University, Perth, Australia
42 Jaundice and infection

Jean Proud BA MSc RM RGN MTD
Part-time Lecturer, University College of St
Martin, Lancaster, UK
20 Specialised antenatal investigations

Carolyn Roth BA MSc SRN SCM ADM PGCEA
Senior Lecturer, South Bank University, London,
UK
*18 Sexually transmissible and reproductive tract
infection in pregnancy*

Della Sherratt BEd(Hons) MA RN RM MTD
NDNCert FETCert
Director of International Developments,
University of the West of England,
Bristol, UK
4 International midwifery

Christine V. Shiers RGN RM ADM PGCEA
Senior Lecturer, Course Leader, University of
Brighton, Brighton, UK
14 Abnormalities of early pregnancy
*26 Prolonged pregnancy and disorders of uterine
action*
29 Midwifery and obstetric emergencies

Helen Stapleton RM MSc MNIMH
Research Midwife, University of Sheffield,
Sheffield, UK
44 Complementary therapies in midwifery

Anne Thompson BEd(Hons) RM RN MTD
Technical Officer, World Health Organization,
Geneva, Switzerland
5 Ethics in midwifery

Josephine Williams RGN RM DipN(Lond) ADM
AIRM
Consultant, Healthcare Risk Resources
International Ltd, Brighton, UK
7 Risk management in midwifery

Jane Winship DipN(Lond) PostgradDip RN RM MTD
Formerly Professional Officer, Midwifery and
European Affairs, UKCC, London, UK
9 The regulation of midwifery

Foreword

The Forewords in the two previous editions of this textbook make reference to the major changes in health care and in education provision that have impinged in so many ways on the delivery of maternity care and the practice of the midwife. Indeed, since the first edition of *Myles Textbook for Midwives* in 1953, there have been changes and developments. What is different, even since the publication of the 12th edition, is the pace and profundity of change influenced by major changes in society, changes in health need, the location of health care, incredible advances in technology and the Human Genome Project. These last two, together with consumerism, perhaps more than any other factors, are likely to have the greatest impact on future health provision. Alongside these developments and of major importance is the full integration of midwifery within the higher education sector.

Never in the history of midwifery could it be more obligatory that the midwife practises from a sound knowledge base rooted in research, ensuring evidence-based practice, with each midwife being fully accountable and answerable for her/his practice. This new edition of *Myles Textbook for Midwives* is most timely and Ruth Bennett and Linda Brown, as joint editors, have again most effectively provided an up-to-date multi-author text of major repute. There are many new authors in this edition contributing from their own expertise and knowledge, bringing new dimensions and new thinking. While the fifty-three chapters largely retain similar subject headings, there has been significant re-arranging of the chapters which enhances the integration of the text, retaining a good balance between the scientific basis of midwifery practice and the importance of meeting the emotional and psychological needs of the family, within a framework of personalised and individualised care. The stated aims at the commencement of each chapter are a helpful addition and the ever-increasing amount of recommended quality reading at the end of each chapter is an important feature of the book. As midwifery education and practice move forward within the influence of higher education, this new edition should ensure that *Myles Textbook for Midwives* remains an authoritative and major text for all students of midwifery and internationally.

Mary E. Uprichard DBE

Preface

Midwives, as never before, are writing, publishing and reading a vastly extended literature. Nevertheless, there is a need for a midwifery textbook which collects together the essence of the knowledge that contributes to the practice of midwifery. The 13th edition of *Myles Textbook for Midwives* draws on the expertise of a host of writers, most of them midwives, who have diligently researched and distilled their knowledge and presented it in an accessible form for students and practitioners alike. We are grateful to the many eminent midwives who have continued to add to the value of this text and to those who have joined their number in this edition.

The importance of the woman as client remains the chief focus of the book and, in order to enhance that emphasis, the order of material has been completely revised. The midwife as practitioner introduces the book and the section on midwifery practice includes a chapter on the women who make up the midwife's clientele. No longer is it appropriate to include a chapter introducing sociology, as students now make a much more extended study of this field, but an awareness of the background and circumstances of the women who seek care at the hands of the midwife is still essential. Importantly, a chapter on international midwifery widens the field for those who may travel to other countries or who practise elsewhere than in the United Kingdom.

The material that concerns the childbearing continuum is no longer divided into a 'normal' section and an 'abnormal' section but is integrated according to the chronology of pregnancy, labour and the puerperium, followed by the baby, in order to reduce the false impression that women's experiences fall into either one category or the other. The midwife is, after all, the person who safeguards the normality of the childbearing experience, whatever events occur.

The material concerning the new-born baby has been reorganised in order to shift the focus onto the baby and the midwife's role rather than the environment of intensive care. Chapters on healthy low birthweight babies and on recognising the ill baby will be helpful to midwives and a chapter exclusively discussing respiratory problems has been added. The chapters on the various conditions that a midwife needs to understand in caring for babies with specific problems have been retained and thoroughly revised.

A number of matters follow the clinical material, including a discussion of complementary therapies and their origins, intended not to enable the midwife to apply them, for that requires a specialised text, but to understand their contribution to practice. Here, too, are found chapters which overarch the whole spectrum of practice, such as exercises, community practice, the organisation of health care and vital statistics. The book concludes with a section on anatomy and physiology, which traditionally was presented first; following a perceptive comment by a reviewer of an earlier edition it has been placed last in order that the pre-eminence of the woman as a person is not overshadowed by the examination of her inner parts. In spite of the much extended knowledge that students now need, it was felt apposite to retain these chapters in order to met the needs of midwives who want a reminder of their knowledge or those who are in isolated situations and have recourse to few textbooks.

References are used extensively throughout the book in order to ground the material in research and authoritative opinion, and further reading is offered at the end of the chapters in the expectation that readers will seek more knowledge and discussion than can be contained in a single text.

We hope that you enjoy using the 13th edition and find it as useful and practical as midwives have the past editions. Women deserve the best care that midwives can give and we are delighted that this book has made its contribution to enhancing that care.

Godalming 1998

V. Ruth Bennett
Linda K. Brown

Acknowledgements

The volume editors wish to record their thanks to those authors who originated some of the chapters in earlier editions and whose work has provided the foundation for the current volume. These include:

Jo Alexander
Jean Ball
Thelma Bamfield
Anne Bent
Tricia Murphy-Black
Deborah Hughes
Sarah Kelly
Margaret Lang

Anne Matthew
Sarah Rankin
Sarah Roch
Jennifer Sleep
Elizabeth Thomson
Valerie Thomson
Valerie Tickner
Elizabeth Torley

They also wish to thank those critics and correspondents who wrote with constructive suggestions and ideas, without whose contributions this edition would be the poorer. They warmly acknowledge the encouragement and support of friends, colleagues and well-wishers as well as the unstinting work of the chapter authors, the quality of whose work has eased the job of editing considerably.

Midwifery

SECTION CONTENTS

The midwife

V. Ruth Bennett   Linda K. Brown

The midwife has one of the most rewarding jobs one can imagine. Worldwide her role is to be alongside women giving birth and to share in their joy – and pain. It is work that carries great responsibilities and demands skills and knowledge of a high order, necessitating a thorough education and sound learning. The midwife is proud of her distinctive role and feels humble in being privileged to be 'with woman'.

The chapter aims to:

- define the midwife in terms both of her relationship with women and the formal definitions of the World Health Organization and the European Community

- describe the skills of the midwife

- consider the responsibilities and rewards of being a midwife

- discuss the continuing education and development of practising midwives

- identify the chapters of the book that cover the different aspects of midwifery practice.

MIDWIVES AND WOMEN

Women throughout the ages have depended upon a skilled person, usually another woman, to be with them during childbirth. That person is the midwife, literally 'with woman'. Her* skill is based on a mixture of art and science, art because it requires her to be able to understand the woman's needs, to encourage her and build her confidence, science because it demands a high degree of knowledge and decision-making ability. It is this

* Wherever the female gender is used, the male is also implied, where appropriate, and vice versa.

thorough grounding in knowledge and experience that allows the midwife to refrain from taking control away from the mother while being at hand to step in where assistance is needed. Commitment to caring for the woman will lead the midwife to offer continuity wherever this is possible and to see through her responsibility to the individual mother.

An investigation into the maternity services in the UK (House of Commons 1992) established that women place a high premium on continuity, control and choice. This was followed by *Changing Childbirth*, the Report of the Expert Maternity Group (DH 1993) under the chairmanship of Baroness Cumberlege. *Changing Childbirth* set standards and targets for health care providers which focused on the woman and her needs and promoted the concepts outlined above.

Midwives see birth as a social event as opposed to a medical one and it is part of their remit to preserve this normal family context for women even when there are deviations from physiological expectations. Developments in patterns of the provision of care have led to schemes such as team midwifery and a renewal of interest in community-based practice (Hughes 1992, Melia et al 1991). Midwifery teams have evolved in many ways including hospital teams, community teams and teams providing both hospital and community care. These were reviewed and evaluated for the Department of Health in an Institute of Manpower Studies report (Wraight et al 1993). Later developments have included group practice midwifery and one-to-one care (Page 1995). One key difference between these new initiatives and team midwifery is that in the one-to-one scheme midwives have an identified caseload and manage their own time and resources. Under these arrangements midwives work in pairs within a group of six and this means that mothers get to know both partners well and the team in addition. This helps to ensure that women are delivered by midwives known to them and to advance the ethic of continuity of carer (Page 1995).

The UK Labour Government elected in 1997 declared its intention to move to an overall pattern of health care which is focused on primary care and the community base (DH 1997), a pattern which already predominates in the developing world and which harmonises with the trends in maternity care in Britain.

Definition of the midwife (Box 1.1)

In 1972 a definition of the midwife was developed by the International Confederation of Midwives (ICM) and a year later it was adopted by the International Federation of Gynaecology and Obstetrics (FIGO) followed by the World Health Organization (WHO). In 1990 at the Kobe Council meeting, ICM amended the definition which was later ratified by FIGO (in 1991) and by WHO (in 1992).

The concept of the midwife as an independent practitioner in her own right is one that is precious to those within the profession but not always fully understood. The midwife may diagnose pregnancy and various conditions related to it, give certain drugs without prescription, especially during labour and the postnatal period, and retain responsibility for the total care of a childbearing woman as long as events remain within the range of normality. She is entitled to call upon medical assistance if it is required but is also empowered

---

Box 1.1 International definition of the midwife (ICM 1992)

A midwife is a person who, having been regularly admitted to a midwifery educational programme, duly recognised in the country in which it is located, has successfully completed the prescribed course of studies in midwifery and has acquired the requisite qualifications to be registered and/or legally licensed to practise midwifery.

She must be able to give the necessary supervision, care and advice to women during pregnancy, labour and the postpartum period, to conduct deliveries on her own responsibility and to care for the newborn and the infant. This care includes preventative measures, the detection of abnormal conditions in mother and child, the procurement of medical assistance and the execution of emergency measures in the absence of medical help. She has an important task in health counselling and education, not only for the women, but also within the family and the community. The work should involve antenatal education and preparation for parenthood and extends to certain areas of gynaecology, family planning and child care. She may practise in hospitals, clinics, health units, domiciliary conditions or in any other service.

to undertake emergency measures pending the doctor's arrival.

European Community Midwives' Directive

In spite of variety within the European Union (EU), a common Directive (80/155/EEC Article 4) defines the activities of the midwife (Box 1.2).

AN INDEPENDENT PRACTITIONER

The competent midwife is able to carry out a wide range of skills. Some of her tasks overlap with those of the nurse, while others are similar to those of the obstetrician and paediatrician.

Skills of the midwife

The Midwives Rules (UKCC 1993) detail the outcomes which programmes of midwifery education must achieve (Rule 33(3)). They encompass not only skills and duties but ability to appreciate the woman's background and the effect this may have on her well-being and that of her own baby. The midwife takes responsibility for her own actions but also may initiate care by others and is able to function in a multiprofessional team. Keeping up to date is an essential aspect of practice and she must work within legislation governing the profession. Her wise judgement is applied to decisions for care and also takes into account ethical principles (see Ch. 5).

Promotion of health. The midwife has an excellent opportunity to teach families about healthy living through parent education (see Ch. 12) both before and after the birth of the baby. Advice about health care needs to take into account the influence of social factors and to be given in the context of a political awareness and cultural understanding regarding her clients. Society is today composed of people from many religious and cultural backgrounds, some of whom may speak languages which are not the native tongue of the midwife. The use of link workers and interpreters may help to bridge the gap and to make health education accessible to all without offending sensibilities.

Assessment. Health is not simply an absence of disease and especially not a judgement about the 'normality' of a person. Health is not an impossible ideal nor even a potential that a person could reach if she followed a healthy lifestyle. It depends on context and on relationships and on the trust that a person can place in her body and herself (Benner & Wrubel 1989). The midwife needs a deep perception of the influence of emotions and of the meaning of events for an individual in the light of that person's understanding and the priorities which emanate from her experience. Physical factors are obviously important but other dimensions

---

Box 1.2 Activities of a midwife: the European Directive (UKCC 1994)

Member states shall ensure that midwives are at least entitled to take up and pursue the following activities:

- to provide sound family planning information and advice;
- to diagnose pregnancies and monitor normal pregnancies; to carry out examinations necessary for the monitoring of the development of normal pregnancies;
- to prescribe or advise on the examinations necessary for the earliest possible diagnosis of pregnancies at risk;
- to provide a programme of parenthood preparation and a complete preparation for childbirth including advice on hygiene and nutrition;
- to care for and assist the mother during labour and to monitor the condition of the fetus in utero by the appropriate clinical and technical means;
- to conduct spontaneous deliveries including where required an episiotomy and in urgent cases a breech delivery;
- to recognise the warning signs of abnormality in the mother or infant which necessitate referral to a doctor and to assist the latter where appropriate; to take the necessary emergency measures in the doctor's absence, in particular the manual removal of the placenta, possibly followed by manual examination of the uterus;
- to examine and care for the new-born infant; to take all initiatives which are necessary in case of need and to carry out where necessary immediate resuscitation;
- to care for and monitor the progress of the mother in the postnatal period and to give all necessary advice to the mother on infant care to enable her to ensure the optimum progress of the new-born infant;
- to carry out the treatment prescribed by a doctor;
- to maintain all necessary records.

are equally essential to consider when assessing the well-being of a mother and her child.

Managing care.   Midwifery is a balance between giving care and affirming the woman's ability to care for herself. The midwife must be competent to diagnose pregnancy and carry out examinations of the woman and her baby in order to assess their condition. She plans whatever care is necessary and sees that it is implemented. Very often, it will be the woman herself who will administer the care and the midwife treats her as an equal, if not the senior partner (Ashton 1992), in planning. The midwife's responsibility continues as she evaluates the effectiveness of the plan which has been carried out and changes it as necessary. The care has implications for the whole family and all aspects of their situation must be considered.

Independent action.   The midwife is the expert in normal midwifery and has an obligation to care for mothers and babies. In emergency situations she is trained, while summoning medical aid, to take immediate steps to treat mother or baby and to continue to give care while help is on the way and indeed after help arrives.

Initiating the action of others.   The midwife is never in a position to relinquish care of a mother and baby (except to another midwife or in order to transfer care at the end of the postnatal period). She may, however, have need of the expertise and intervention of other disciplines. The obstetrician and general practitioner (GP) should be her closest allies and may be called upon to give aid when deviations from normal arise. Similarly the paediatrician is available for the care of the baby. Dietitians, physiotherapists, social workers and health visitors are among other professionals to whom the midwife may refer in appropriate circumstances.

Undertaking care prescribed by a doctor.   The duty to administer care and treatment prescribed by a registered medical practitioner goes beyond simply following instructions. The midwife is expected to interpret orders and, if necessary, question or challenge. There may be circumstances in which she has to urge the doctor to take action and others in which she may caution restraint. When a midwife has called in a doctor, the respon-

sibility for the problem becomes that of the doctor, and she must follow medical orders, but there remains a duty to continue caring for the mother and baby even when the doctor has taken charge.

Communication.   The skilled midwife develops effective communication with her clients, her colleagues and those in other disciplines. This will involve enabling them to express their wishes and views and exercising empathy towards them. On occasion this will mean consciously setting aside personal views to listen carefully to the client (or fellow professional) to understand a different viewpoint and to accept that the other person has a right to make a different choice. Effective listening skills are essential and support of the individual will build the trust needed to allow expression of her feelings (UKCC 1996). Other circumstances may demand that the midwife expresses her own viewpoint and supports it with clear reasons.

Research awareness.   As midwifery research grows year by year, it becomes increasingly important for the competent midwife to be alert to new knowledge that has been established by research and to develop a questioning and reflective attitude towards her own practice. There is a wealth of literature and resources now available to help midwives to know what has been established by systematic enquiry. More and more midwives are ready to investigate questions by undertaking their own local studies and audit procedures. Chapter 6 will help midwives to understand the research process and to evaluate research reports, while Chapter 8 gives a guide to quality control and audit.

Evidence-based   practice.   The use of the term 'evidence-based' rather than 'research-based' practice has been growing (Renfrew 1997). It is intended to foster the use of systematic reviews such as *Effective Care in Pregnancy & Childbirth* (Chalmers et al 1989) and the *Guide to Effective Care in Pregnancy and Childbirth* (Enkin et al 1995) as well as, more recently, the Cochrane Collaboration reviews and those of the National Health Service (NHS) Centre for Reviews and Dissemination in York now brought together in the Cochrane Library (BMJ Publishing Group). The midwife has a responsibility to make use of these resources to inform her practice. It is recognised that some areas of practice are still under-researched and evidence is unavailable.

The midwife will never be absolved from the duty to weigh up the clinical evidence elicited by her personal observation and to take account of her experience, nor should the individual preferences of the client be overlooked.

A team member. Being an independent practitioner goes hand in hand with membership of the multiprofessional team which exists to care for mothers and babies and their families. The midwife must take the trouble to understand the roles of her colleagues and to develop harmonious relationships with them.

Keeping the law. The practice of a midwife is controlled by law. Midwives must have an understanding of the requirements of the legislation relevant to the practice of midwifery. In the UK the Nurses, Midwives and Health Visitors Acts 1979, 1992 and 1997 are the basis of this legislation (see Ch. 9); other Acts of Parliament that are relevant include the Congenital Disabilities (Civil Liabilities) Act 1976, the Data Protection Act 1984, the Births and Deaths Registration Acts and Public Health Acts (see Ch. 44) and the Acts regulating the prescription and use of drugs. Dimond has written extensively on the interpretation and application of law in midwifery, particularly in the journal *Modern Midwife* (now *The Practising Midwife*) and in her own book on *Legal Aspects of Midwifery* (Dimond 1994).

Ethical issues. Certain codes and standards are agreed by the profession and midwives, like nurses and health visitors, are bound by the *Code of Professional Conduct* (UKCC 1992b). This includes matters such as maintaining confidentiality, maintaining and improving one's own professional competence, while acknowledging any limitations and working with clients in such a way as to foster their independence and respect them as unique individuals. The practitioner is enjoined to report circumstances which would jeopardise standards of practice or which would endanger the safe and appropriate care of clients or the health and safety of colleagues. The midwife may find herself in a situation where her own values are challenged and she has to assist parents in choices which involve moral judgements. Chapter 5 provides a framework in which she may consider such difficult decisions.

Assignment of duties to others. The midwife may not delegate any of her midwifery responsibilities to a non-midwife (although a registered medical practitioner may appropriately give midwifery care). She will often, however, have need of the assistance of other staff such as nurses, health care assistants and auxiliaries and perhaps of family members, especially the partner or mother of her client. She may assign appropriate duties to such helpers but retains the responsibility to supervise and monitor any tasks that she has asked them to undertake.

Responsibilities of the midwife

The unique status of the midwife brings tremendous satisfaction and reward; it also demands that she is accountable for her actions and it lays upon her great responsibility.

Competence. Each midwife has a responsibility to maintain professional competence. The sphere of her practice is clearly laid down in the *Midwives Rules* (UKCC 1993) and *The Midwife's Code of Practice* (UKCC 1994) and is subject to the principles of the *Code of Professional Conduct* (UKCC 1992b). As midwifery practice develops, there may be occasion to integrate new skills into the range of those that midwives use in order to meet the needs of mothers and babies. Some of these will be required by all midwives and in due course will become part of the normal preparation of midwives during their basic training programmes in the way that perineal repair has done in recent years; others will be specific to midwives practising in certain settings, for example a midwife may (with appropriate study and experience) add ultrasonography to her skills in order to provide an additional service to women attending antenatal clinics. The UKCC (1992a) publishes a booklet entitled *The Scope of Professional Practice* to guide practitioners in judging when this scope may appropriately be adjusted.

The supervisor of midwives has a special responsibility in regard to maintaining standards of midwifery practice (see Ch. 9). Part of her responsibility is to ensure that all midwives are fully competent and that they notify their intention to practise year by year. If any midwife lacks appropriate education, the supervisor has a duty to ensure that this is arranged in order to maintain the midwife's skills and to protect the public. The role of the supervisor has received a good deal of attention in recent years with the development of new programmes of preparation for supervisors (Thomas & Mayes 1996) and a move to separate management from supervision in understanding at least. In some areas different individuals exercise the roles to avoid confusion. There is a desire to move towards fostering good practice rather than simply looking out for bad practice and towards leading and encouraging autonomy rather than seeking to control (Kirkham 1996).

Responsibility to keep records. Rule 42 (UKCC 1993) requires the midwife to keep detailed records which must be made 'as contemporaneously as is reasonable', in other words as near the event as possible. Records must be in a form acceptable to the employer and approved by the local supervising authority. A midwife in independent practice will discuss the format of her records with her supervisor of midwives.

The midwife's record is distinct from that of the doctor although she may contribute to the medical record, especially during pregnancy. She must keep records of the midwifery history (see Ch. 13) and of all antenatal examinations which she makes. During labour, records of observations, examinations and care are essential and it is here that it is particularly important to enter details promptly, because events move on so rapidly (see Chs 21 and 22). A register of controlled drugs is kept for the purpose of monitoring the issue and use of drugs of addiction. The midwife's register of births is usually kept communally by hospital midwives but individually by a community midwife. The fact that several midwives may make entries in a shared record does not absolve the individual midwife from entering all details of her own observation and care personally. Postnatal

records are equally important and must be made at the time of each attendance (UKCC 1994 Section 7.1; see also Ch. 30).

Maternity units use a wide variety of records and notes, including those which are designed to be entered into a computer and others which are appropriate to the midwifery process or to varying styles of individualised care.

All records that are made by a midwife must be preserved for a period of not less than 25 years. The reason for this is that the record may be needed for the midwife's protection in cases of litigation or allegations of professional misconduct. Under the Congenital Disabilities (Civil Liabilities) Act 1976, a child may sue for damages where he has suffered as a result of negligence during his mother's pregnancy or labour and this litigation may be delayed as long as 21 years after the events involved. Scottish law makes similar provisions.

Responsibility to the family. As midwives are involved with very intimate aspects of the life of a family, they have a special duty to practise with absolute integrity. Confidentiality is of prime importance. Sensitive, private matters must be handled with delicacy and the midwife should value each individual without censure for beliefs or standards which may be at variance with her own. This does not mean that she does not use her judgement; she should constantly assess the needs of the mother and child within the family and may perceive a need for education or for warning of danger or for intervention on behalf of an unprotected member such as a child at risk of abuse.

In order to offer the best care possible, the midwife needs to keep her knowledge and skills up to date. She may tap resources beyond her own if the family requires other support such as that of a social worker.

Society is subject to constant change and the midwife is challenged to be flexible in order to adapt to change as it occurs. Whatever the circumstances, 'a woman will need to be physically safe, psychologically satisfied and morally unoffended during pregnancy and childbirth' (RCM 1987).

Responsibility to the profession. Midwives have a responsibility for the image of their profession. For all to keep moving forward, each individual must be sufficiently committed to play an active role in order to preserve standards and improve care. For some this will mean initiating change or trying experiments, for others it will mean following in the footsteps of the innovators.

Professional involvement includes awareness of the activities of professional organisations and statutory bodies. Current journals should be read as a matter of course; discussion documents are often circulated for consultation and comment and it is vital that midwives respond to requests for their opinions. All should become members of professional organisations; some must be ready to accept office locally and nationally. Every midwife should use her vote in statutory body elections; a few are needed who have developed the knowledge and expertise to stand for election or accept appointment to a national board or committee.

Drawing midwifery issues to the attention of the public may necessitate use of the media and midwives should be ready to write to the newspapers or to take part in broadcast features when appropriate. There are some occasions when the best course of action is to lobby Members of Parliament and midwives made good use of the opportunity to do this during the hearings of the Select Committee of Health which culminated in the Winterton report (House of Commons 1992). However, they need to understand that neither the media nor the politicians are waiting to take up their causes, since midwifery is but one of a huge range of interest groups who want their particular issue forwarded. Declercq (1994) stresses that midwives need to learn to communicate in ways that policy makers understand, that it is easier to defend the status quo than to drive a new policy through, that the media care for but a short time and that coalition building is essential. He also urges midwives to understand that research matters and that it is important to clarify who is a midwife without wasting resources on debates over who is a 'real' midwife.

Midwives need not be afraid of making their voices heard. Responsible exercise of the means of activating those in power has in the past helped to achieve a better service for mothers and babies.

Responsibility to society. The midwife needs to act as a responsible citizen. She may be in a position to highlight areas of concern such as social deprivation, poor housing, racial prejudice, the effects of violence or the progress of epidemics or prevalent infections such as AIDS or tuberculosis. Her response in such circumstances may be to warn, to mobilise resources or to offer active care.

Midwives enjoy the trust of the public. Each midwife should value that trust and earn its continuation.

The rewards of being a midwife

The birth of an individual baby is unique and unrepeatable. The midwife is enormously privileged to share that event and contribute her skill to its accomplishment. If she has been fortunate enough to have known and worked with the family throughout pregnancy, or even before, she will derive great satisfaction from the continuity of care, especially if she can also assist with the integration of the baby into the family. Continuity is also much appreciated by the mother and adds to her feeling of security (Audit Commission 1997).

Sometimes things do not go so well and the baby dies before birth or soon after. At these times the midwife is treading on delicate ground as she shares the pain of the parents' loss but she may earn their gratitude for her support if she has been able to use her skills to comfort them and accept their feelings of grief (see Ch. 33).

There is a delight for the midwife in developing and perfecting the skills of her art and in preparing her mind in the science of midwifery for possible contingencies. Many of her skills are gained through experience and adapted to individual mothers and babies through her judgement of circumstances. There are few instances where she is not working as a partner with the mother and helping her to achieve competence in her own abilities. On occasion the midwife is in the position of acting to avert disaster and when life is saved, the relief is overwhelming. Nowhere is this more evident than in the developing world where childbirth is still the cause of a high number of maternal deaths and the midwife plays a key role in the community to further and promote health (see Ch. 4).

AN EDUCATED PRACTITIONER

Since the middle of the 20th century midwives in the UK have enjoyed the privilege of statutory periodic refreshment and have attended approved courses every 5 years. In recent times the scope and range of refresher courses has widened and various alternatives are available such as 1-week residential courses, 2-week practical courses and single study days which can be accumulated. Equally important, however, is the need to read and reflect on a continuous basis, to use books and journals, discuss cases with peers, encourage colleagues (Hunt 1991) and implement changes that are tested by the use of research (Downe 1991). The range of advanced courses is growing each year, many midwives are acquiring Bachelors' and Masters' degrees and some earn doctorates through high quality research.

The UKCC, by means of PREP (post-registration education and practice), has indicated that all practitioners must in future demonstrate their continuing education by keeping a professional profile of learning throughout their careers; the renewal of registration depends on being able to demonstrate that they have been developing their knowledge during the previous 3 years and have completed at least 5 days (or 35 hours) of study during that time. This will be fully operational from April 2001 (UKCC 1997a). Meanwhile midwives continue to attend 5-yearly statutory refresher courses which are considered fully to meet the requirements (UKCC 1997b). All practitioners should be keeping personal profiles of their professional development and the reader is advised to consult one of the many guides (e.g. Hull & Redfern 1996, RCM Trust 1995).

Advanced practice. The concept of advanced practice has been the subject of professional debate for some time. There is no doubt that midwifery needs good leadership in the clinical setting as well as in education and management. Sisto & Hillier (1996) suggest that this may have two aspects. The first is *mastery*, meaning the skill of the clinical expert who appraises and utilises research knowledge, developing a high level of competence, and the second is that of an *advanced practitioner* who is more future-oriented with an overview of practice and an influence on policy. Both act as role models and consultants to other midwives and act as change agents and educators. Other writers (e.g. Charlton 1996) have postulated that midwives should take on more medical tasks and Warwick (1996) stresses the importance of leadership with a breadth of vision of maternity service and health care as a whole. Undoubtedly midwives do practise across the boundaries of normal and complicated care (Sisto & Hillier 1996) and the trends in professional development now demand that experienced midwives seek opportunities to advance through scholarship and theory building (Bryar 1995). Midwives also need to look at their philosophies of care and determine how their practice needs to develop.

The UKCC's Code of Professional Conduct (1992b) states, 'As a registered … midwife … you are personally accountable for your practice and, in the exercise of your professional accountability, must: (…) maintain and improve your professional knowledge and competence'. The midwife who takes this statement seriously will become the skilled person on whom a mother depends and she will take joy in providing a service which will satisfy her clients. Now, more than ever, the woman should be the focal point of care, listened to and involved in decisions (Audit Commission 1997); the next chapter considers the woman as the midwife's client.

REFERENCES

Ashton R 1992 Who can speak for women? Nursing Times 88(29): 70
Audit Commission 1997 First class delivery. Audit Commission, London
Benner P, Wrubel J 1989 The primacy of caring. Addison-Wesley, California

Bryar R M 1995 Theory for midwifery practice. Macmillan, Basingstoke
Chalmers I, Enkin M, Keirse M J N C 1989 Effective care in pregnancy and childbirth. Oxford University Press, Oxford, vols 1, 2
Charlton D 1996 What constitutes an advanced practising

midwife? British Journal of Midwifery 4(4): 174–175

Congenital Disabilities (Civil Liabilities) Act 1976 HMSO, London

Declercq E R 1994 A cross-national analysis of midwifery politics: six lessons for midwives. Midwifery 10(4): 232–237

Department of Health (DH) 1993 Changing childbirth part 1: report of the expert maternity group. HMSO, London

Department of Health (DH) 1997 The New NHS: modern, dependable. Cm 3807 The Stationery Office, London

Dimond B 1994 Legal aspects of midwifery. Books for Midwives Press, Hale

Downe S 1991 The midwife as practitioner: midwifery standards – uniformity or quality? Midwives Chronicle 104(1236): 2–3

Enkin M, Keirse M, Renfrew M, Neilson J 1995 A guide to effective care in pregnancy and childbirth. Oxford University Press, Oxford

House of Commons 1992 Health Committee, second report: maternity services. HMSO, London

Hughes 1992 Midwifery care for the poor. MIDIRS Midwifery Digest 2(1): 23–25

Hull C, Redfern E 1996 Profiles and portfolios: a guide for nurses and midwives. Macmillan, Basingstoke

Hunt S 1991 Continuing education for midwives – a woman's right. Midwives Chronicle 104(1236): 6–7

International Confederation of Midwives (ICM) 1992 Definition of the midwife. ICM, London

Kirkham M (ed) 1996 Supervision of midwives. Books for Midwives Press, Hale

Melia R J et al 1991 Consumers' views of the maternity services: implications for change and quality assurance. Journal of Public Health Medicine 13(2): 120–126

Page L (ed) 1995 Effective group practice in midwifery. Blackwell, Oxford

Renfrew M J 1997 Influencing the development of evidence-based practice. British Journal of Midwifery 5(3): 131–134

Sisto S, Hillier D 1996 Advanced midwifery practice: myth and reality. British Journal of Midwifery 4(4): 179–203

Royal College of Midwives (RCM) 1987 Towards a healthy nation. RCM, London

Royal College of Midwives (RCM) Trust 1995 Portfolio development series 1–9. RCM, London

Thomas M, Mayes G 1996 The ENB perspective: preparation of midwives for their rôle. In: Kirkham M (ed) Supervision of midwives. Books for Midwives Press, Hale

United Kingdom Central Council for Nursing, Midwifery & Health Visiting (UKCC) 1992a The scope of professional practice. UKCC, London

United Kingdom Central Council for Nursing, Midwifery & Health Visiting (UKCC) 1992b Code of professional conduct, 3rd edn. UKCC, London

United Kingdom Central Council for Nursing, Midwifery & Health Visiting (UKCC) 1993 Midwives rules. UKCC, London

United Kingdom Central Council for Nursing, Midwifery & Health Visiting (UKCC) 1994 The midwife's code of practice. UKCC, London

United Kingdom Central Council for Nursing, Midwifery & Health Visiting (UKCC) 1996 Guidelines for professional practice. UKCC, London

United Kingdom Central Council for Nursing, Midwifery & Health Visiting (UKCC) 1997a PREP and you. UKCC, London

United Kingdom Central Council for Nursing, Midwifery & Health Visiting (UKCC) 1997b Midwives' refresher courses and PREP. UKCC, London

Warwick C 1996 Leadership in midwifery care. British Journal of Midwifery 4(5): 229

Wraight A, Ball J, Seccombe I, Stock J 1993 Mapping team midwifery. Institute of Manpower Studies, Brighton

FURTHER READING

Alexander J, Levy V, Roch S E G 1990, 1993, 1995, 1996 Midwifery Practice series. Macmillan, Basingstoke

Alexander J, Levy V, Roth C 1997 Midwifery Practice series. Macmillan, Basingstoke

Cross R E 1996 Midwives and management: a handbook. Books for Midwives Press, Hale

Hunt S, Symonds A 1995 The social meaning of midwifery. Macmillan, Basingstoke

Kargar I, Hunt S C (eds) 1997 Challenges in midwifery care. Macmillan, Basingstoke

Kirkham M J, Perkins E R (eds) 1997 Reflections on midwifery. Baillière Tindall, London

Murphy-Black T 1995 Issues in midwifery. Churchill Livingstone, Edinburgh

Robinson S, Thomson A 1989, 1991, 1994, 1996 Midwives, research and childbirth. Chapman & Hall, London, vols 1–4

Symonds A, Hunt S C 1996 The midwife and society: perspectives, policies and practice. Macmillan, Basingstoke

The midwife's client

Liz Hynes (née Spruce)

The midwife's direct client is the woman, who, with her developing fetus and then her neonate, should remain the central focus of care. In this introductory chapter, the woman will be viewed as an individual, as part of a family and within the wider social context, as having personal, cultural and religious needs and across the range of ethnicity and equality (Fig. 2.1).

The aim of the chapter is to:

- reflect on the childbearing process from the perception of the woman and to analyse the meaning of 'motherhood' within contemporary society, thus assisting the midwife's understanding of her client

- explore emotional issues evoked before, during and after pregnancy with reference to the roots of knowledge and response

- discuss the relationship between the midwife and the woman's partner and family.

The chapter will initiate discussion of a range of issues and use a system of cross referencing to subsequent chapters for further information. The intention is to provoke original thought whilst standing as an introduction to the whole.

> Pregnancy is a long and very special journey for a woman. It is a journey of dramatic physical, psychological and social change; of becoming a mother, of redefining family relationships and taking on the long-term responsibility for caring and cherishing a new born child. Generations of women have travelled the same route, but each journey is unique (DH 1993).

MOTHERHOOD THROUGH THE AGES

It is only relatively recently that motherhood as a unique concept has been researched, despite the

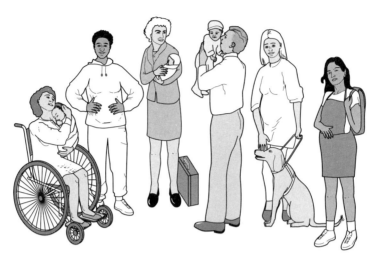

Fig. 2.1 The potential client group.

fact that the woman's role as a mother has provided a literary cornerstone for centuries. The 'mother' has usually been represented in three ways, historically, psychoanalytically and fictionally. A fourth dimension is currently under scrutiny by contemporary social scientists such as Oakley, that of the real-life mother (Kaplan 1992).

Archaeological evidence throughout the world demonstrates the underlying power of matriarchy, with women venerated as goddesses. In art, the female figure was often depicted as the bearer and nourisher with a 'primal power' (Rich 1986). The historical perception of women as secondary beings probably stems from Biblical times and the belief that: 'Adam was first formed, then Eve. And Adam was not deceived, but the woman being deceived was in the transgression. Notwithstanding she shall be saved in childbearing, if they continue in faith and charity and holiness with sobriety' (I Timothy 2: 13–15). The introduction of the then named 'sins of the flesh' is attributed to Eve, and for women to atone for this sin, the agonies of childbirth were to be endured.

During the middle ages, virginity was viewed as the 'ideal' state for women, with menstruation linked to the power of demons. Women experiencing labour were considered to be in 'an unclean state spiritually' (Carter & Duriez 1986). Whilst the production of a child was paramount, motherhood itself appeared irrelevant, with the life of the woman viewed as secondary. The designated 'midwives' were advised to favour the infant in situations threatening life and if a woman died during childbirth, burial on sacred ground was forbidden. Women were not permitted entry to the Church until around 6–8 weeks after the birth and then were required to undergo a purification ceremony. Motherhood was seen by women as a burden to be endured with the knowledge that death was a likely outcome. Prolonged labour often resulted in maternal demise; this was contributed to by pelvic anomalies resulting from rickets due to inadequate dietary intake of vitamin D, calcium and phosphorus.

The 1914–18 World War brought about some change in attitude and women became seen as: 'saviours of the race … moulding future generations on whom society's hopes rested' (Richardson 1993). In the original preface to *Maternity Letters from Working Women* first published in 1915, the Right Honourable Herbert Samuel wrote of the importance of forging improvements to help women during pregnancy and childbirth. The motivation behind this was to eradicate widespread suffering and to boost the population, in the belief that: 'The ideas for which Britain stands can only prevail so long as they are backed by a sufficient mass of numbers' (Llewellyn Davies 1978). In 1917, formation of The Woman's Guild led to the demand that: 'the care of the mother should have equal consideration with the care of the infant' (Carter & Duriez 1986). Sylvia Pankhurst, the daughter of Emmeline, who went on to develop the women's suffragette movement, published *Save The Mothers* in 1930. She was appalled by the neglect of mothers' needs and called for a national maternity service (Carter & Duriez 1986).

The 20th century has seen western women evolve from the confines of a paternalistic society, where restriction of the power of the mother was seen as a way of assuring the maintenance of patriarchy. The inception of the feminist movement led toward equality of opportunity, giving women the right to control their own destiny. With respect to pregnancy, this freedom was partly initiated by the introduction of maternity clothes in 1905 (Simkin 1996). Women no longer needed to remain 'confined' out of sight. Artificial feeding shortly followed, heralded as 'the thing to do' but also offering women the ability to delegate some of the responsibilities associated with motherhood. Maternal and perinatal mortality rates remained high with the associated fear of labour and birth. The introduction, therefore, of methods for limiting the pain of labour motivated some women to take the lead and refuse to be attended by a doctor unless he offered the pain-free option. This coincided with the inception of the suffrage movement with women seeking education and individual status. However, motherhood and mothering remained primarily under the control of men such as Truby King, who wrote advice on childrearing during the 1920s. Later, amongst others, Dr Benjamin Spock published his user-friendly advice on *Baby and Child Care* in 1946: revised editions of this remain a popular choice with some mothers today.

The 1939–45 World War expedited the process of change and was followed by rapid technological advancement. By the 1960s, developments such as electronic fetal heart rate monitoring were deemed to improve safety for both mothers and babies and the British Government led the move toward 100% hospital births. However, some women soon felt that they had become 'just a body, a defective machine that needed a good mechanic' (Simkin 1996). In addition, male doctors increasingly wrote the rules, not only for giving birth but also

for pregnancy. These rules frequently clashed with women's lived experience, resulting in them questioning whether to trust the authority of the doctors or the sensations of their own bodies.

During the 1970s and 1980s a more realistic view of motherhood began to develop and traditional family roles were being challenged. Whilst it was acknowledged that women held the inimitable capacity to achieve motherhood, fathers were being encouraged to take a more active role in parenting by female authors including Dr Miriam Stoppard. There was a move away from Bowlby's (1981) attachment theories of potential adverse long-term effects if bonding did not occur, to the more immediate influence of the mother–baby relationship. By the 1980s women had begun to voice their opinions about the medicalisation of childbirth with its creation of an 'illusion of safety' and the move back toward more natural childbirth followed. Women started seeking to regain control of their own childbirth experience with consumer-led pressure groups such as the National Childbirth Trust (NCT) and through media coverage.

TOWARDS EMPOWERMENT

The idea of maternal power has been domesticated. In transfiguring and enslaving woman, the womb – the ultimate source of this power – has historically been turned against us and itself made into a source of powerlessness (Rich 1986).

In response to women's call for control, the midwifery profession moved toward midwifery-led care with the woman as the central focus; thus challenging the patriarchal medical model of obstetric care. The joint action of women's groups, the midwifery profession and sympathetic others has since been supported by the Government publication *Changing Childbirth* (DH 1993).

Appropriate, non-medicalised language must be used in order to facilitate understanding and enable women to be empowered to make informed choices. Traditionally, the 'power of the profession has dominated that of the woman' (Shirley & Mander 1996) and doctors were seen as holding the supreme power. Many individuals still view a doctor as unapproachable and may have extreme difficulty in asking questions. Even when women do seek answers, the way in which knowledge is imparted can be as important as the content of the information offered and the tone of voice must be such that it avoids expression of an overt bias.

In order to break down potential barriers, to empower and offer informed choice to women and their partners, balance is required with full liaison between concerned individuals, both professional and lay people. Groups such as maternity service liaison committees (see Ch. 47) provide a forum to work toward this, often sponsored by local purchasers on behalf of the client population. The philosophy of contemporary maternity services is to be 'woman centred' and for the midwife to work in partnership with the client; it is necessary to appreciate the multifaceted needs of individual women. Refer to Figure 2.2 for a diagrammatic representation of 'the ripple effect on the woman towards empowerment'.

The majority of human females are still nurtured with the inherent knowledge that their ultimate purpose is to become mothers, and at some stage in their reproductive lives the desire to achieve this can become overwhelming. Whilst a woman will seek and achieve other goals in her journey through life, she may still see motherhood as a pivotal point, believing that to remain childless somehow signifies failure at womanhood. A feminist viewpoint is that it is male dominance which has led to many women being convinced that unless motherhood is achieved, they are not truly women (Tong 1989).

The meaning of motherhood in contemporary society remains a contentious issue. Individual interpretation may include the nature or nurture debate and technological advances have raised further issues relating to the definition of a mother. Is the mother the woman who produces the egg which becomes fertilised or the woman who becomes pregnant by artificial implantation of the embryo and who subsequently gives birth to the infant? Is the woman who adopts a baby the mother? Is there a difference between the ability and function of a natural mother and receiving mother? Research is exploring some of these issues

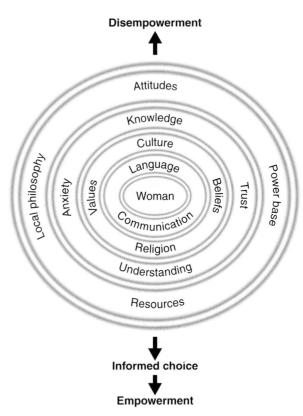

Fig. 2.2 The potential ripple effect on the woman during the childbearing experience leading toward empowerment.

and no doubt the debate will continue. From the midwife's perspective, a mother is a woman who requires her care under the Midwives' Rules (UKCC 1993) and Code of Practice (UKCC 1994) pertaining to her professional role. The means by which an individual woman achieved the status is secondary.

THE WOMAN AS THE MIDWIFE'S CLIENT

Many different women seek motherhood and may become the midwife's client, including:

- women in stable partnerships
- women following treatment for infertility
- women following previous loss of a baby at any

stage during pregnancy, at birth or in the neonatal period

- women with special needs
- women with chronic health problems
- women with learning difficulties
- physically or sensory disabled women
- lesbian couples
- adoptive mothers
- the relinquishing mother
- surrogate mothers
- teenagers and those whose life options may appear otherwise restricted
- single women either through choice, separation or bereavement
- older women who may have waited for financial stability or the right partner.

This list is not intended to be exhaustive and each 'category' should not be seen in isolation. All women with whom the midwife comes into contact should be viewed holistically and it is important to develop a partnership based on mutual trust and understanding.

Individual women will vary in their expectations and needs during the childbearing process. Women are becoming more informed and able to access information. Promotion of informed choice is an essential element of contemporary midwifery care but 'Choice is not a very meaningful word unless it is used in relation to the circumstances in which people live their lives' (Richardson 1993). It should be remembered that for some women, their choice is to relinquish control and it should not be assumed that all women desire or are capable of taking decisions about their care. They are, however, all entitled to information given in such a way as to assist their comprehension.

The ability to communicate effectively may need assistance and not all clients of the midwife will have English as their first language. In order to facilitate understanding of information given to or asked of a woman, strategies may need to be developed such as the use of interpreters or phrase cards. A woman may wish to have a relative or friend with her who is able to translate on her behalf and it is important that this is not obstructed due to inflexibility of any unit protocols. Language can be used as an instrument of power and it is important that any lack of understanding is recognised to avoid the induction of fear and anxiety. Even where the midwife and her client both speak the same language, certain words or terms may be used which are unfamiliar to the woman. One example of this is use of the expression 'flat baby' for a neonate requiring resuscitation. The new parents, hearing such a reference to their baby, may imagine some gross abnormality and become extremely alarmed. It is vital to reflect upon the words used in front of women and their partners and ensure that appropriate language is used, thereby avoiding potential misunderstanding.

Expectations and emotional response during the childbearing process stem from a combination of several factors including theoretical knowledge, values and beliefs and the accumulation of past experiences. This may also be affected by a woman's relationship with her own mother and her experience of being 'mothered'. The requirement to make public any pre-existing medical or physical conditions or elements of personal past history for the 'good' of this pregnancy and future infant will influence the woman's response and needs, as will the support and care she receives once pregnancy is confirmed.

Previous birth experiences tend to remain as deep memories which often become more vivid in subsequent pregnancies. Simkin (1992) reflects that women with positive long-term memories of their birth experiences tend to remember that they felt in control. But are memories accurate? From her small longitudinal study of 20 women who were interviewed in 1988–1989, having given birth and completed questionnaires in 1968–1974, Simkin found that a lot of detail was lost over the time gap but specific incidents were clearly remembered, such as timing of onset of labour, interventions and certain significant information or actions. The significance attached to negative events tended to be intensified whereas positive memories remained more static and accurate.

It is important, therefore, that each woman is given the opportunity to discuss any past experiences which she feels may affect the way she develops her current expectations. There is, arguably, no other single life event that has such a profound effect as giving birth and as an event it is unsurpassed for the ripple effect which it, in turn, has upon society. The childbearing process may 'carry the potential for immense positive or negative impact on [the individual's] development as woman and mother and on the future of the children she brings into our world' (Simkin 1996).

Preconception and conception

Many women become pregnant by design but do not necessarily prepare themselves in order to achieve optimum health prior to conception. For other women, conception remains unplanned, so their health status for the very early stages of pregnancy is dependent on their existing lifestyles and the level of education and application of knowledge attained to date. The male partner, whilst possibly anticipating fatherhood, rarely considers his preconceptual health. A number of couples will consciously prepare themselves in order to increase the likelihood of conceiving and also to ensure that the resultant embryo has the best possible start to life. It should be remembered that unless a couple seeks such advice, the very early and most important stages of embryonic and fetal development will have passed prior to the usual first point of contact with a health professional between 8 and 12 weeks' gestation. Specific information related to physical preparation, dietary advice and health education for pregnancy can be found in Chapter 10. Aspects relating to positive health promotion are considered in Chapter 12.

Whilst physical preparation is given ample consideration, emotional readiness for potential disappointments which may befall attempts to conceive or readiness for pregnancy itself is often given scant attention. Psychological status may provoke a physiological response which can sometimes interfere with fertility, the ability to achieve the desired pregnancy or maintenance of a successful pregnancy (see Chs 14 and 32).

Making a conscious decision to 'try for a pregnancy', particularly if following previous loss of a baby either during or after pregnancy, can itself create anxieties. The resultant stress can sometimes lead to difficulties between a couple if either one of them starts to focus too profoundly on ovulation and the most likely time to conceive.

The desire to achieve a successful pregnancy can take over and a woman's whole life may appear to revolve around her menstrual cycle. In some couples this may lead to sexual difficulties due to the pressure to 'perform' at certain times or the loss of the spontaneity previously enjoyed in their sexual relationship (see Ch. 10). Refer to Chapter 45 for stress management strategies.

The media generally paint a picture of pregnancy as being easy to achieve. Publication of unplanned pregnancies and abortion rates in addition to strong advertising campaigns relating to how to avoid pregnancy add fuel to this belief. Indeed, for many women, conception may be a very simple process, occurring either by 'accident' or design. However, the reality of planning a pregnancy is not always straightforward and many couples may wait months before conceiving. During this time they may develop varying degrees of anxiety about one or other's fertility; this may be complicated further, depending on age or pre-existing medical conditions. For instance, a woman who has rheumatoid arthritis may need to discontinue potential teratogenic medication which controls her condition while trying to conceive. If this becomes protracted, her arthritis may deteriorate. Inevitable anxiety will develop related to balancing her desire for a pregnancy and the knowledge that often progress of the disease is suppressed during pregnancy (Richardson 1992), against the risk of further decline of her medical condition while waiting to conceive. The consequential stress may also adversely affect the odds of conceiving.

The practicalities and range of infertility treatments are discussed in Chapter 10. A couple undergoing treatment for infertility will often be subjected to a regimen which removes the freedom of control over their lifestyle. Although they will have entered into this voluntarily, even eagerly, and be fully informed of the process, it is inevitable that psychological strain will develop. When the desire for a baby is so great, it becomes impossible to detach emotionally from pursuit of the goal. It is well known that a couple who have been through a range of options in search of parenthood, even going as far as adoption, may then find that pregnancy occurs naturally. It would seem that once all hope of achieving pregnancy has been dashed and disappointment psychologically accepted, relaxation of the quest leads in some cases to removal of some hidden barrier within. Tong (1989) cites several radical feminists who 'believe that reproductive technology poses an enormous threat to whatever powers women still possess and that biological motherhood ought not to be forsaken in favor of artificial motherhood'.

Some couples may be referred for genetic screening before trying for a baby. This may be due to a known familial risk or due to a chromosomal abnormality identified during a previous pregnancy. A woman who suffers from a disability such as spina bifida may wish to determine the risk of this being reproduced in her child. Calculation of risk is a recurring theme throughout the childbearing process. What constitutes high risk is often subject to debate and may vary with differing interpretation. The knowledge that there cannot be confirmation of no risk may cause extreme distress for some couples where others may consider odds of 1 : 50 to be of low risk. James (1988) defined an 'at-risk pregnancy' as one 'in which there is a risk of an adverse outcome in the mother and/or baby that is greater than the incidence of that outcome in the general population'. Preconception counselling is essential for couples who are determined as being 'at risk', with ongoing support once a pregnancy is achieved. Further information related to genetic screening can be found in Chapter 10.

Although midwives may not come into contact with women while in pursuit of conception, it is important that they are aware of the psychological complexities which the woman may have experienced prior to that first point of contact with her midwife. An effective booking interview (see Ch. 13) should facilitate such discussion and enable the development of an individual plan for pregnancy care which will assist the recognition of potential psychological deviation from normal.

Pregnancy

Many women instinctively 'know' when they are pregnant, even before they have missed a period. Altered taste or 'pica' may be a very early sign noticed by the woman. This is something not widely discussed in the literature and may contribute to the apparent cravings which some women report. There is a tendency within the medical profession not to believe that a woman is pregnant until confirmed by some form of testing. This may make the woman feel that she is inadequate from the outset, in that she is not capable of interpreting signs within her own body. Women now have access to self-testing kits which can confirm their intuition in the privacy of their own homes but these tend to be expensive and therefore an unrealistic option for some women. Tests can be obtained via family planning clinics or general practitioners and the majority of women can now have pregnancy confirmed shortly after the first missed menses. Conversely, some women may not know when they are pregnant. This may be a subconscious desire not to be pregnant, the belief that they are unable to conceive or, perhaps owing to a poor obstetric history, they may be unable to interpret or believe the signs. Refer to Chapters 11 and 12 for full information on diagnosis, the physiological changes which occur during pregnancy and further discussion of psychological response.

The emotional response to the news of potential or confirmed pregnancy will vary depending on numerous factors such as whether it is a planned event or following a lengthy period of infertility and the mood may swing between excitement and anxiety. Some women may want to retain the knowledge privately as a self-protective instinct or to enable personal adjustment to the knowledge: others may want to share the news far and wide immediately.

The numerous physiological and psychological changes which occur during pregnancy can sometimes provoke an unanticipated emotional reaction and the revival of past conflicts. If these have not been successfully resolved, they may colour emotional progression throughout the childbearing process. Women who have had a stable and secure childhood, who have been allowed to traverse the stages toward adulthood with support, who have negotiated social and personal relationships and who have achieved the 'cutting of the parental cord' may enter pregnancy in a very different way from those who have experienced growing up as a traumatic event fraught by unresolved crises.

Rutter (1981) published work which does not appear to have been refuted to date. He discussed adverse effects in child development which may extend into adulthood when maternal deprivation has occurred over any prolonged period. Unresolved psychologically traumatic events such as physical or sexual abuse, or grief which has been repressed, may come to the surface during pregnancy. If such issues are not worked through effectively during the transition through pregnancy, they can lead to psychological sequelae and may adversely affect the maternal–infant relationship (Raphael-Leff 1991) and/or maternal emotional morbidity.

Other stressful conditions which may affect psychological adaptation during pregnancy include the rather inadequately named 'minor disorders' such as nausea and constipation (see Ch. 12). Constant nausea can be extremely debilitating and may not appear at all minor to the woman and, whilst well-meaning advice may be adhered to, the reality is often that nothing works for long and the woman may feel that she is viewed as making a fuss or exaggerating. The concept of pregnancy being heralded as a normal life event may, to the woman, appear discordant depending on her life experience. In a woman who has rarely been ill, the discomfort of heartburn, intestinal pains due to constipation and the constant desire to vomit can indeed be perceived as more akin to an illness than anything previously experienced. Fortunately, not all women develop the unpleasant side-effects of pregnancy but, for those who do, the opportunity to be listened to and to be taken seriously is important, as in some women these 'minor disorders' last well into the second trimester or beyond. As most women tend to appear more anxious during pregnancy, it is important that they receive adequate explanation and reassurance that any symptoms developed are not potentially harmful to the developing fetus. Without such support, some women may become distressed, which can lead to an antenatal depressive condition.

The first scan can be a joyous experience and reassuring; conversely, it may be a stressful event, depending on a woman's past and current obstetric history, her expectations and the subsequent findings. The woman may be content to accept that her baby is an integral part of her own body and therefore 'hers' and the invasion of technology with its ability to 'show' the baby to the mother may in fact be a dismembering experience. Katz Rothman (1996) discusses this and comments that the use of technology in this way may result in removal of control from the mother.

Pregnancy, though not an illness, does imply dangers and risks to both the woman and her child. Technological advances are aimed to determine levels of risk. Women have to face numerous decisions during pregnancy and it has become a very stressful time, particularly in relation to screening choices for fetal abnormality. A study designed to evaluate the opinions of two groups (one health professionals, the other non-health professionals) related to women's choice and information and screening for Down syndrome, found that both groups made value judgements about the role of the mother and the birth of an infant with a disability (Marteau & Drake 1995). This study consisted of the analysis of responses to a series of scenarios and was undertaken in the UK, Portugal and Germany. Findings indicate an expectation within western society that because of the availability of effective screening technologies, a positive result should lead to a termination of the pregnancy, with the aim of eradication of individuals with the disorder. This view, whilst not held by all and subject to continual debate, may lead to tremendous stress on a woman faced with such decisions. It is vital that full, unbiased information is available to women and their partners in addition to adequate counselling and ongoing support. If a woman makes the informed decision to continue her pregnancy following diagnosis of an abnormality, then her view must be supported and any contrary opinions withheld. Refer to Chapter 20 for full information on antenatal screening, Chapter 7 for further discussion of risk in pregnancy.

All these factors will affect self-image and self-esteem during pregnancy. Body image is another issue requiring psychological adjustment. Initially, the woman may appear to be gaining weight with no obvious explanation; the basal metabolic rate 'is considerably depressed from early pregnancy' (Hytten 1990). This may produce negative feelings but, as the pregnancy becomes more obvious outwardly, the woman may feel acceptable in that her new body shape epitomises femininity, thus regaining a more positive body image. Any advice offered needs to be sensitive to the individual woman's needs and consider issues such as availability of resources, the pre-existing body/self-image, and idealism versus reality.

For most women the significance of first feeling fetal movement is exciting and may affirm the presence of the baby within; others may feel out of control and that their bodies are being manipulated by this 'parasitic' being. Even when a pregnancy has been planned, the reality of the way in which it appears to take over the body can be an alarming experience.

As pregnancy advances, the woman finds herself subjected to a variety of procedures ranging from abdominal palpation to vaginal examination. 'Periodically, from late teens until old age, women in this society are expected to submit their genitalia and internal reproductive organs to scrutiny by a doctor' (Martin 1989). This invasion of personal space and privacy can be very distressing, particularly for women from cultural backgrounds where feminine privacy is fiercely protected. The required posture could be said to effectively separate the woman from her body and many women talk of their bodies or body parts as separate from themselves, possibly enabling them to deal effectively with such assault, albeit by consent.

The constant physiological changes experienced throughout pregnancy may each bring an associated psychological response. Deviation from the physiologically normal does not necessarily lead to emotional imbalance. Many women will adapt appropriately to events during pregnancy, but for some it can become a period of increasing stress which, if not managed effectively, may provoke deviation from psychological health.

Labour

Interpretation of the definition of the onset of labour may differ between the 'obstetric' terminology and the woman's perception. Pain for the woman may be profound but she may still find herself informed that she is not in established labour. This may make the woman feel distressed or out of control.

Empowering the woman during labour means enabling her to believe in herself and her ability to cope, utilising her strength and determination. Immediately offering her a way out, such as with an epidural anaesthetic, can for some women signify failure and despair.

A small Swedish study examined the experience of the encounter with the midwife during labour and delivery from the woman's perspective. It demonstrated that for some women to retain control, it was necessary for them to feel secure, safe and that the relationship with the midwife was one of trust in which a rapport had been established based on empathy. The women wanted guidance as opposed to dictation or direction, they needed encouragement to listen to their own intuitive responses and they needed a sense of peace, with periods of quietness permitting contemplation. Whilst a relatively small study, based on a group of middle-class women, the qualitative nature of the research design lends validity to the conclusion that the key issue for the woman was 'to be seen as an individual, to have a trusting relationship and to be supported and guided on one's own terms' and above all be assured of the presence of a midwife (Berg et al 1992).

Control during labour may also be affected by the environment. Hospitals, for some women, can be fearful and alien places in which they feel disempowered. Remaining within the home environment can be the equivalent for women of 'becoming your own boss ... when they give birth at home they own the whole shop and can be in charge of the entire enterprise' (Martin 1989). Such issues and feelings require discussion to alleviate potential sources of anxiety and facilitate retention of self-esteem wherever labour occurs.

Cultural variations between individual needs should be acknowledged. Whilst choice and greater flexibility are becoming more commonplace during the management of labour, it is important that particular religious or cultural needs are met wherever possible. This may require facilitation and adaptation by the midwife. If valued rituals are not adhered to, some women may experience extreme distress and possible admonishment from their family and peers. One example of this in Jewish law is that certain activities are forbidden during the Sabbath, known as Shabbos. If caesarean section is required, the couple are not permitted to sign consent forms and the husband may seek advice from the Rabbi. However, if undertaken as a life-saving operation, Jewish law will not be broken (Waterhouse 1994). It is advisable that a woman with particular cultural or religious needs is encouraged to discuss these with midwives antenatally and that details of her requests are clearly documented so that appropriate strategies may be developed. This principle also applies to any woman with physical or sensory disability (see p. 11) or any special needs.

> Birth can be medical, sexual, empowering, belittling, spiritual, humiliating, joyous, painful, terrifying, routine. Often it is all these things at once (Katz Rothman 1996).

Each stage of labour brings its own challenges. Effective support and communication with full unbiased information are the basic ingredients for women to retain their sense of self and the degree of control they desire.

Refer to Chapters 22 and 23 for full discussion of the importance of psychological support during labour, and Chapters 21, 22 and 24 for the physiological processes of labour.

Postnatal period

The normal emotional transition to motherhood inevitably involves some degree of stress. A combination of feelings will present. A woman may feel a sense of loss: loss of her independent former self, loss of expectations, loss of unrealised hopes. She will be aware of the absence of the internal presence of her baby and a shift in the focus of attention. Some women may need a period of time during which they re-embody before being fully able to relate to their newborn and behave as required in their new role. Intermingled with such thoughts will be feelings of relief, joy and a sense of achievement, accompanied by the likely additional sensations of exhaustion and overwhelming tiredness. Caring for a totally dependent and demanding baby, coming to terms with tech-

niques for feeding and changing and the natural fears related to the health of the infant will produce stress. All of this is part of the normal process of adjustment occurring during the early puerperium and it is only when disruption occurs and the stress changes to distress, that deviation from psychological health may occur.

Several non-western cultures allow women a defined period for recovery of between 20 and 40 days postpartum during which they are often only cared for by other women of their family or village. This may include specific diets and certain taboos or rituals such as that of some Chinese women who may believe that bathing or showering during the first postnatal month could be detrimental to their subsequent health (Schott & Henley 1996). In the western world we have generally moved away from the 'lying-in period' owing to increased understanding of the importance of early mobility and promotion of self-care. Whilst health education is vital, this needs to be handled sensitively and with respect.

With regard to certain issues, perhaps much could be learned from other cultural groups who still treat the new mother as 'special'. Early discharge from hospital may mean some women being expected to resume normal household duties in addition to caring for their babies. This is likely to exacerbate tiredness and create distress which may lead to psychological morbidity. The opportunity for adequate sleep coupled with good support are important factors for a normal transition to motherhood.

Another valuable aid to healthy postnatal adjustment is the opportunity to discuss the birth experience. Where possible, this needs to be with the midwife or professional most closely involved in the care around the birth and occur within 48 hours. In addition to this, some units are now offering the opportunity to attend an interview up to a year or more after delivery in order to debrief and discuss unresolved anxieties (Charles 1994, Friend 1996). The routine adoption of debriefing following childbirth has yet to be scientifically evaluated but if found to be beneficial it may help to create positive memories and to promote long-term psychological health.

For further information on these issues and full

discussion of deviation from normal postnatal psychological health, refer to Chapter 31.

THE WOMAN WITH SPECIAL NEEDS

Many women may have specific needs over and above the general needs they have in common with all pregnant women. There can be many categories which may fall under this general heading, but the most important thing is for each woman to be seen as an individual and not labelled by a particular condition or perceived status. This section discusses problems which may be considered under the broad heading of 'special needs', but is not exhaustive. Many of the conditions mentioned will be enlarged on in greater detail, as appropriate, in other chapters.

Chronic health problems

Amongst others these include diabetes, asthma, essential hypertension, epilepsy, multiple sclerosis, haemoglobinopathies, cardiac disease, and renal disease (see Ch. 16). Any woman who has been living with a medical condition is best placed to know her body and its limitations and her strengths and weaknesses and must be given the opportunity to take a lead role in the development of her care. This will usually be in liaison with the appropriate medical and obstetric teams supported by midwives who may have particular specialist knowledge.

Physical or sensory disability

As with chronic disease, the woman will know her own needs and should be closely involved at every step within the partnership of care. Types of physical disability may include artificial limbs, arthritis, hearing or other sensory impairment, cerebral palsy, spinal cord injury or spina bifida. The condition may be separate and distinct from associated medical illness or may be linked to an underlying disorder.

It is vital to enquire as to the nature of the disability and not form assumptions based on visual observation. All too often, people with an obvious disability are treated as of low intelligence or, worse still, ignored. Campion (1990) estimates that there are tens of thousands of women of childbearing age who have a disabling condition. No accurate figures appear to be available as the Department of Health does not currently commission specific data which fit the category. The most recent comparable figures are from a survey (Martin et al 1985) of disabled adults residing in the UK. The closest available breakdown is of women aged 16–59 of which there were 1023 000 with a range of disabilities classified by severity of 1 to 10. The largest group comprises those with locomotion disabilities, which is also true of the total population of the UK with over 4 million adults in this category. Other categories are intellectual functioning, behavioural disturbance and communication difficulties. The next largest group are hearing disabilities at 59 per 1000 adults (Martin et al 1985). The only more recent related figures were collected under the category 'Limiting long-term illness' during the 1991 UK census (OPCS 1993). This did not clearly identify numbers of women of childbearing age who are affected but they appear to number in excess of 500 000. The main conclusion to draw from these limited data is that disability is a real issue for women of childbearing age and must be considered in the planning of maternity services.

When involved with the care of a woman with a disability, it is important not to overlook the fact that no matter what special needs may be apparent, she will also have many of the same concerns regarding pregnancy and childbirth as her able-bodied peers. The health care team must listen to the woman and not merely attend to her perceived different and perhaps 'obvious' needs. Whilst she may be well informed about potential risks to both her own health and that of her growing fetus, it is important to help the woman to see potential additional problems which may arise as pregnancy progresses, particularly where there are mobility issues. The additional weight of the growing uterus and fetus may alter balance and posture and may also give rise to pressure problems for the woman who is wheelchair bound. The normal physiological alterations occurring during pregnancy may give additional problems to the woman who already suffers from constipation and urinary tract infections due to spinal injury. Immobility during pregnancy may increase the incidence of thrombotic complications such as deep vein thrombosis (see Ch. 15), and appropriate preventive measures should be taken.

It is helpful for the focus to be on the positive aspects of both the disability and the pregnancy and health professionals need to be aware of their own opinions related to disability; 'the most damaging barriers are the negative attitudes of other people, particularly amongst health professionals' (Campion 1990). Awareness of body language with simple adaptations to facilitate communication at eye level, can assist greatly in the promotion of self-esteem. Care over language usage is important and conversation should be directed toward the woman, not her companion. If the partner is also disabled, there may be further issues to address; either way it is important to involve the partner in the decision-making process.

Individual concerns could include the woman who has an ostomy bag fitted. Physiological changes and alteration in abdominal shape may cause problems with the site or function during pregnancy. Some women may have distinct fears related to genetic issues and potential risks of passing on a disease or hereditary condition to a baby. Anxiety may be present related to perceived attitudes within society as to the woman's suitability to become a mother and she may fear that the child may be taken away from her on the grounds that it may be considered in the child's best interest. Advice regarding acquiring available benefits should also be offered and at all times the woman should be assured of the professional code of conduct concerning confidentiality (UKCC 1992). Specialist advice and counselling should be sought where necessary with appropriate ongoing support and reassurance.

Later on in the pregnancy, posture and mobility issues may need to be further addressed and also preparations should be made toward labour and birth. A thorough and flexible birth plan is important. Place of birth should be considered carefully and it should not be assumed that the disabled woman is necessarily at high risk in terms of her delivery. Labour and birth at home may well be

the safest option, particularly where the home is adapted to meet the woman's individual mobility needs. A blind or partially sighted woman, for instance, would have many additional hurdles to overcome if admitted to a strange environment. When hospital is considered to be the most appropriate place for the delivery, orientation to the area is vital and also equipment may need to be adjusted or provided, such as cots of suitable height. Choices should not necessarily be limited because of the disability; for instance, labouring in water may be a particularly appropriate option for women with mobility impairment. The obstetric physiotherapist should be involved early and the occupational therapy team may be able to assist with extra equipment or advice. The whole health care team should work together in partnership with the woman in order to provide the best care for the individual whilst maintaining her right to choice and control. 'When control in so many areas of her life may be limited, and many may doubt her ability to be a mother, the disabled woman needs to be involved in all the decisions around the birth of her baby' (Nolan 1994).

Women may be disabled by a medical condition or physically disabled but healthy. The degree of incapacity should be individually determined by assessment of the level at which 'normal' life is affected. Disabled people may find certain tasks difficult and may perform these more slowly than their able-bodied peers, but their independence is important to them and health professionals should enquire as to any help required and not automatically take over from them. Additional equipment such as a flashing monitor to help a deaf woman know when her baby is crying may be required.

Many of the issues discussed under physical disability will be relevant to women who have a mental disability or experience learning difficulties. In addition to these, particular learning needs may need to be addressed. Appreciating the woman's capabilities is essential and generalised assumptions should not be made. Communication and expression difficulties do not mean that feelings are suppressed and fear can be a very real problem. Liaison with other appropriate agencies should be established from an early stage.

While disability itself does not have a direct effect on environmental factors, such as medical systems and professionals, it conditions the way in which medical systems and professionals respond to women (Nosek et al 1995).

Lesbian mothers

Lesbian motherhood may be viewed within society as a contradictory state because of the requirement for the male sperm. Indeed, many lesbian women choose not to become mothers. There is, however, a growing number of women within a secure lesbian relationship who may seek motherhood. The mechanics of achieving this may include self-insemination with donor sperm, artificial reproduction, a form of surrogacy or adoption. Seeking medical assistance to conceive may be hampered owing to homophobic attitudes or prohibitive wording within certain local or national laws.

The midwife may be unaware of the emotional minefield through which the lesbian client may have trod, even if the woman chooses to share the fact of her lesbianism. Information specific to the care needs of lesbian clients is currently scant (Wilton 1996) but physical needs are unlikely to differ from those of any woman. Psychologically, the lesbian client may have additional concerns such as the acceptance of her female partner by health professionals and other women but often she will have developed strategies to overcome potential difficulties. If the client has chosen to share such details with her midwife, it is important that sensitive and appropriate support is offered. As with any woman, deviation from psychological health is only likely when normal adjustment to motherhood is interrupted. Homophobic attitudes are the most likely potential source of disruption of this process.

The British Pregnancy Advisory Service is one organisation which may offer advice to lesbian couples. By law in the UK a single person of either sex may adopt, but not a same-sexed couple, although this view is currently being challenged.

The adoptive mother

'Exclusive mothering is neither inevitable nor biologically determined by pregnancy' (Raphael-Leff 1991). Particular issues for parents adopting a child of whatever age include the complicated process which precedes the arrival of the child. In some ways this could be compared to a pregnancy but one of indeterminate length and of considerable risk due to the uncertainty of its outcome. Sometimes this 'pregnancy' may last for years; there are no outward signs and preparation for prospective parenthood is often limited and somewhat abstract in nature. The eventual 'delivery' can be extremely sudden with perhaps only a few days' notice and the practicalities of preparation for the new arrival have to be dealt with speedily, often with little time for reflection. If the adopting mother is in employment, immediate cessation without the usual notice will be necessary and there is no legal right to 'maternity leave', although certain employers may allow an equivalent paid leave of absence. For the adopting mother, choice and control are not viable concepts and whilst the long wait may have facilitated a degree of psychological preparation, the sudden reality can produce a reaction akin to shock. This is likely to be accompanied by extreme emotions of joy, relief and excitement intermingled with fear and trepidation. New mothers do not normally have to question the permanence of the relationship with their infant, but adoptive mothers may have to face the possibility of this relationship being only temporary until the legal formalities have occurred (see Ch. 46 for description of the law and process relating to adoption). Attendance by a midwife will be dependent on the age of the child, and there is no legal requirement for a midwife to visit unless the baby is less than 10 days old or referral is requested for advice and support with feeding or infant screening. It is important for the midwife to be aware of the potential psychological implications for adopting parents in order to facilitate liaison with other members of the health care team and offer support where required.

The relinquishing mother

The mother surrendering her baby for adoption will experience the physiological alterations which occur during the normal puerperium and require midwifery postnatal care as for any woman following the birth of a baby. The fact that she has chosen to have her baby adopted is sometimes considered in a similar light to women who choose termination of pregnancy, in that this free choice somehow precludes them from feelings. Interpretation may be that once relinquished, this baby is forgotten. Certainly in the past, 'unwanted pregnancy' was hidden away and once the baby was born and given away it was rarely, if ever, mentioned. Fraser (1996) discussed the grief experienced by the 'birth mother' and how such grief can be complicated when the source is not acknowledged. It is important, as with a mother whose baby has been stillborn or died, that the opportunity is offered for the building of appropriate positive memories to facilitate the grief process. Some women may choose to see and hold the baby, some even wish to care for the baby for an initial period, whilst others may prefer not to have any contact with the baby whatsoever. Photographs of the baby should be taken and kept within the mother's case notes if she does not wish to have them at the time. Psychological adjustment to the loss and postnatal recovery will depend greatly upon the nature of the birth experience and the way in which the woman is treated during the puerperium. If the woman's partner is present, it is important that he too is offered the opportunity to see the baby and adjust to the decision of relinquishment. Contemporary society is beginning to recognise the needs of the 'birth mothers' and it is now possible for information to be available to them concerning the future life of the child, whilst maintaining the adoptive family's right to confidentiality of identity.

> Midwives, as a first and important point of contact, need to be aware of the special needs of these vulnerable women and of the impact and long-term implications resulting from the decision that has been made, remembering always that this will be the hardest decision these women will ever make in their lives (Fraser 1996).

Surrogate motherhood

The issues facing the surrogate mother are comparable to those of the relinquishing mother addressed above, with the exception that pregnancy is entered voluntarily with involvement of the prospective adoptive parents. Media attention has focused heavily on the issues of surrogacy because it is a relatively new concept, frequently controversial and therefore strongly newsworthy. This brings the additional complications for the parents of loss of privacy. Numerous ethical issues remain unresolved and the Government has ruled out legislation to control surrogacy agreements and clarify potential rights of prospective parents. Stephen Dorrell, who was Health Secretary in the last Conservative Government, has been quoted as stating that regardless of a birth mother's original intentions 'she should have the full rights of any other mother' (Murphy 1997). The midwife involved in the care must offer support as to any mother, with sensitivity and awareness of the potential psychological response provoked by the situation. It may be advisable for different midwives to provide care of the relinquishing mother and the recipient mother, as this is one case where the prospective adoptive mother may have the baby from birth and midwifery care of the baby is requisite.

Social service departments and adoption agencies are required to provide counselling to all categories of parents affected by the process of adoption. There may also be specific support groups in certain areas.

Other client groups

There are numerous other client groups who may have particular needs during the childbirth process, such as homeless women or travellers who may not be registered with a GP or attend for antenatal care. The younger teenager and the older mother may also have specific additional needs dependent upon a range of factors contributing to their level of risk, including:

- under 16 (see also Chs 3 and 46)
  - physical development and maturity
  - support
  - socioeconomic status of family
- over 40 (see also Ch. 20)
  - obstetric/medical history
  - general health and fitness
  - socioeconomic status.

Both groups of women have increased risk of certain chromosomal abnormalities such as Down syndrome, fetal growth retardation and preterm labour (see Ch. 37).

Recent media attention toward pregnant prisoners has highlighted another client group and advice is now available to assist the midwife to deal effectively with particular issues raised whilst maintaining the principle of the woman as the central focus of care (RCM 1996). In the future the midwife may need to consider her potential role related to a single male or a homosexual couple adopting or parenting a child through surrogacy.

CULTURAL CONCERNS

In a multicultural society it is important for the midwife to be familiar with differing cultural or religious needs of the local client population. Definitions of race which may be used for minority ethnic groups include:

- black – Afro-Caribbean, African and sometimes South Asian
- South Asian – India, Pakistan, Bangladesh, Sri Lanka, i.e. the Indian subcontinent
- others whose first language is not English.

The census of 1991 (OPCS) gave a total population of England and Wales as 49 883 200 of which 6% were of ethnic minority groups. The largest group is of Indian origin, the second largest Afro-Caribbean, with around 43% being born in the UK (Raphael-Leff 1991). Even if born and brought up within Europe or the UK, pregnancy and parenthood may have very different meanings for individuals influenced by language, cultural and religious differences. 'Culture is not genetically inherited. It is acquired during childhood when we absorb the basic values and norms by which our family, our society and community live' (Schott & Henley 1996). The role of the woman or mother may be different and several societies expect men to 'provide for' and 'control' women (Helman 1994). This may present difficulties for some women during the childbirth process, particularly with the current climate favourable towards the empowerment of women, and may lead to cultural conflict, anxiety and even fear.

Poor socioeconomic status accompanied by comprehension difficulties may lead to women failing to attend for antenatal care. It is vital that health professionals develop strategies by which to encourage attendance and that the women are not assumed to be of low education or to have learning difficulties. The NHS Patient's Charter on the Maternity Services states that women have the right to information (DH 1994), but if the language is not compatible this cannot occur. Surveys undertaken during the investigation preceding the publication of the 'Changing Childbirth' report (DH 1993) demonstrated a deficit in knowledge and understanding amongst Bangladeshi, Indian and Pakistani women.

Practices accepted as normal in western society may be abhorrent to other cultural groups. Exposure of the woman's body, especially if to a male doctor, may be humiliating and certain aspects of antenatal care or screening may induce fear and confusion if not fully understood.

Women who are unfamiliar with Western attitudes and patterns of care may sometimes be surprised by the amount of energy and time devoted to clinical care and by the lack of attention paid to the more spiritual and emotional aspects of pregnancy. In many parts of the world it is traditional for women to do everything they can to avoid stress and negative thoughts during pregnancy and to concentrate on positive images. Peace of mind is highly valued and thought to have beneficial effects on the baby (Schott & Henley 1996).

Whilst this emphasis on the woman's psychological health is to be admired, education may be necessary to ensure that it is not to the detriment of physical health or safety of the woman or her baby. There is evidence of a higher rate of perinatal and infant mortality amongst certain cultural groups.

Other culturally specific issues have been discussed under the different headings in this chapter and will also be included, as appropriate, throughout the textbook. The key factor for all women regardless of race, colour or creed is equality of access, the right to information presented in a comprehensible format and holistic individualised care with the woman as the central focus.

CONSUMER INVOLVEMENT IN PLANNING THE PROVISION OF MATERNITY SERVICES

It is important that the client, as consumer of the maternity services, is closely involved in all aspects of development of the service and the provision of woman-centred, community-based care. Within the current climate of health service provision, purchasers are seeking to establish the needs of their local population. It is vital that women have a point of contact in order to influence the purchase of the type of maternity service they desire. Active involvement of consumers in planning, standard setting, the monitoring of standards and auditing of the service is essential for the future of an effective maternity service. Proper lay representation is important on local groups such as the maternity services liaison committees (see above and Ch. 47) and other relevant local forums.

THE WOMAN'S PARTNER

It has already been acknowledged that a woman's partner may not always be a man (see above), but the purpose of this section is briefly to discuss the father of the baby as a secondary client of the midwife.

The 1950s saw the introduction of the concept of mother–child bonding and the father's role was restricted to that of supporter to enable 'the mother to devote herself to the constant care of her child' (Richardson 1993). Contemporary society recognises a more important role for the father and some are now offered 'paternity leave', but the responsibility for child rearing still largely falls to the mother. Motherhood is accepted as a social concept, while fatherhood remains a secondary role (Timpson 1996). It is important, however, that the father is not overlooked and that he be included in decision-making throughout the childbearing process, provided that this is of the woman's choice. Some men may become so involved in fact,

that they may echo some of the symptoms experienced by their partners. A Canadian study found that of 20 couples, 65% of the men reported at least one symptom during their partner's pregnancy. Those most commonly disclosed were an increase in appetite (6), backache (4), feeling depressed (5) and 4 stated that they actually felt better than usual (Drake et al 1988). It is important to acknowledge the psychological adaptations which a man has to cope with, many of which are similar to those of the woman. A man may be less likely to discuss his feelings openly and may have concerns over numerous issues including perhaps the financial burden that a new baby can bring. As with the woman, if such issues are not resolved during the transition through pregnancy, the man may also experience deviation from normal psychological health.

It is now generally expected that the father will be present at delivery, whereas a relatively short time ago, he was barred completely. Some men may feel pressurised to attend and it is important that they are given the opportunity to discuss any fears they may have concerning the birth. However, a Royal College of Midwives' survey involving 441 men in 217 differing areas, found that 88% did not feel 'forced' to attend and 98% actually chose to attend the birth (Reid 1994). The woman may feel empowered by the support of her partner according to the nature of their relationship. If a man feels inadequate observing his partner in pain or disempowered by the process and/or the system, he may become disturbed, which could result in a negative effect upon the actual labour, particularly if there is any dispute between the couple over the nature of pain relief (Hall 1993). A balance is required, permitting flexibility of choice for both partners. If the midwife has been able to develop a positive relationship with the father, preferably in advance of labour, she may be able to help him to explore his feelings.

It should be acknowledged that some cultural groups believe that a man's presence at the birth could actually be dangerous for him. Conversely, in races such as Eskimos and Maoris, the father has a functional and defined role to divert the attention of evil spirits, thereby protecting the fetus in its transition to extrauterine life (Helman 1994).

THE HIDDEN CLIENT – FROM FETUS TO NEONATE

The developing fetus within the woman could be said to be the hidden client of the midwife. Whilst the woman is the central focus and her safety paramount, the entire purpose of midwifery care pivots around the presence of the fetus. As discussed earlier, the value placed on the life of the unborn child has at times during history been placed above that of the woman. Contemporary obstetrics tends to view the mother and fetus as an integral unit with the life of the mother marginally tipping the balance over that of the fetus. When either life is threatened, fetal gestation being at a viable age, the action taken is based on a balance of potential risk to each in association with the wishes of the woman and her partner. In some cases the perceived rights of the fetus may be considered, especially where these appear to be being overridden by the rights of the mother. In legal terms, fetal rights remain a contentious issue but the midwife may need to clarify her role in relation to prime responsibility and bear this in mind when involved in the care of a pregnant woman who may be a drug abuser or heavy smoker. Mair (1992) discussed the potential compensation rights of a child born disabled owing to a negligent act by the mother. Such issues may become more prevalent in the future, and the midwife could become involved in such ethical dilemmas.

Following delivery, 'ownership' of the newborn may appear to be challenged, especially within the hospital where staff appear to 'give' the baby to the mother, and 'offer' it for feeding. Words used around the time of birth can appear contradictory in that at 'the moment of separation, the very moment when one being pulls apart into two, the language that we use is that of bonding, as if two separate things become one … the baby gets presented back to the mother so that she can *form an attachment*' (Katz Rothman 1996). This can be further compounded by the process, albeit necessary, of labelling, weighing and wrapping the baby as a package to be then given to the mother. Women have usually formed a close relationship with their babies long before birth and the neonate appears to recognise the sound of its mother's voice, indicating that it too has formed a unique attachment. Facilitation of total care of the baby by the mother, rather than the midwives, ensures that the woman is empowered to provide a positive contribution to the infant's well-being.

SUMMARY

This chapter has addressed some of the issues relating to the midwife's client group, primarily the woman but also those closely associated with the woman. The emphasis has been on the psychological aspects of the childbearing process and, by referral to appropriate chapters for specific information and reflective analysis, it is hoped that the midwife will develop a broad knowledge base to facilitate efficient, effective and, above all, safe practice, acting always in the best interests of her client.

> For every woman, pregnancy and birth are a unique experience. For some women, supported by family and friends, it will be a time of great happiness and fulfilment. Pregnancy will progress smoothly to the birth of a healthy and much welcomed baby. For others this will not be the case. The pregnancy may not be planned, complications may occur or social circumstances may be adverse. The birth itself may be complicated and the outcome different from the one anticipated or hoped for (DH 1993).

READER ACTIVITIES

1. Find out what resources are available locally to assist women whose first language is not English. You may decide to develop a proposal for action related to the provision of appropriate services such as written, useful phrases or information packs on the more common cultural perspectives in your area.

2. Develop an action plan to assist a couple to make choices, in particular related to the most

appropriate birth companion. Pay attention to the needs of the partner as well as the woman and how the couple may be assisted to discuss potential outcomes of the partner's attendance or non-attendance.

3. The following activities may be undertaken as a timed essay, used as revision notes or as a basis for discussion with a peer group. If you choose to write as a timed essay, allow 1 hour.

   a. Reflect upon the terms 'motherhood', 'fatherhood' and 'parenthood'. List the differing interpretations they may portray. Discuss how these terms are used within contemporary society and how different cultural groups may view them.

   b. Analyse potential communication barriers and how these may be overcome, using appropriate examples.

   c. Explore whether stereotyping is common for certain groups of women and how it may be prevented.

REFERENCES

Berg M, Lundgen I, Hermansson E 1992 Women's experience of the encounter with the midwife during childbirth. Midwifery 12(1): 15

Bowlby J 1981 Attachment and loss 3: loss, sadness and depression. Penguin, Middlesex

Campion M J 1990 The baby challenge – a handbook for women with a physical disability. Routledge, London, pp xiv, 65

Carter J, Duriez T 1986 With child: birth through the ages. Mainstream Publishing, Edinburgh, pp 116, 132, 133

Charles J 1994 Birth afterthoughts. British Journal of Midwifery 2(7): 331–334

Department of Health (DH) 1993 Changing childbirth: report of the expert maternity group. HMSO, London, pp ii, 9

Department of Health (DH) 1994 The patient's charter: the maternity services. HMSO, London

Drake M L, Verhulst D, Fawcett J 1988 Physical and psychological symptoms experienced by Canadian women and their husbands during pregnancy and the postpartum. Journal of Advanced Nursing 13: 436–440

Fraser J 1996 Caring for the woman who relinquishes her baby for adoption. Midwives 109(1303): 222

Friend B 1996 Thoughts after birth. Nursing Times 92(36): 24–25

Hall J 1993 Attendance not compulsory. Nursing Times 89(46): 69, 71

Helman C 1994 Culture, health and illness: introduction for health professionals. Butterworth Heinemann, Oxford, pp 149, 169, 177

Hytten F 1990 Nutritional requirements in pregnancy: what should the pregnant woman be eating? Midwifery 6: 96

James D K 1988 Risk at the booking visit. In: James D K, Stirrat G M (eds) Pregnancy and risk: the basis for rational management. Wiley, Chichester, p 45

Kaplan E A 1992 Motherhood and representation: the mother in popular culture and melodrama. Routledge, New York

Katz Rothman B 1996 Women, providers and control. Journal of Obstetric, Gynecologic and Neonatal Nursing Clinical Issues (March/April): pp 253, 254, 255

Llewellyn Davies M (ed) 1978 Maternity letters from working women: preface. Virago, London

Mair J 1992 Baby v. mother. Journal of the Australian College of Midwives 5(2): 15–20

Marteau T M, Drake H 1995 Attributions for disability: the influence of genetic screening. Social Science & Medicine 40(8): 1127–1132

Martin E 1989 The woman in the body. Open University Press, Buckingham, pp 71, 143

Martin J, Meltzer H, Elliot D 1985 The prevalence of disability among adults. OPCS Social Survey Division surveys of disability in Great Britain. HMSO, London

Murphy J 1997 Surrogate birth laws ruled out by Dorrell. The Mail on Sunday, January 26, p 6

Nolan M 1994 Choice and control for the disabled mother. Modern Midwife 4(4): 10

Nosek M A, Young M E, Howland C A et al 1995 Barriers to reproductive health maintenance among women with physical disabilities. Journal of Women's Health 4(5): 505–518

Office of Population Censuses and Surveys (OPCS) 1991 The preliminary report of the 1991 census for Great Britain. OPCS, London

Office of Population Censuses and Surveys (OPCS) 1993 The 1991 census of limiting long-term illness for Great Britain. OPCS, London

Raphael-Leff J 1991 Psychological processes of childbearing. Chapman & Hall, London, pp 7, 23–25, 68–69

Reid T 1994 Birth rite. Nursing Times 90(50): 16

Rich A 1986 Of woman born – motherhood as experience and institution. Virago Press, London, pp 68, 95

Richardson A 1992 Rheumatoid arthritis in pregnancy. Nursing Standard 6(45): 25–28

Richardson D 1993 Women, motherhood and childrearing. Macmillan Press, London, pp 43, 62

Royal College of Midwives 1996 Pregnant prisoners – RCM recommendations accepted. Midwives 109(1298): 74

Rutter M 1981 Maternal deprivation reassessed, 2nd edn. Penguin, London

Schott J, Henley A 1996 Culture, religion and childbearing in a multiracial society – a handbook for health professionals. Butterworth-Heinemann, Oxford, pp 4, 146, 265

Shirley K E, Mander R 1996 The power of language. British Journal of Midwifery 4(6): 298

Simkin P 1992 Just another day in a woman's life? – Part II: nature and consistency of women's long-term perceptions of their first birth experiences. Birth 19(2): 81

Simkin P 1996 The experience of maternity in a woman's life. Journal of Gynaecological and Neonatal Nursing 25: 249, 252

Timpson J 1996 Abortion: the antithesis of womanhood? Journal of Advanced Nursing 23: 780

Tong R 1989 Feminist thought – a comprehensive introduction. Routledge, London, pp 81, 87

United Kingdom Central Council for Nursing, Midwifery and Health Visiting (UKCC) 1992 Code of professional conduct. UKCC, London

United Kingdom Central Council for Nursing, Midwifery and Health Visiting (UKCC) 1993 Midwives rules. UKCC, London

United Kingdom Central Council for Nursing, Midwifery and Health Visiting (UKCC) 1994 The midwife's code of practice. UKCC, London

Waterhouse C 1994 Midwifery care for orthodox Jewish women. Modern Midwife 4(9): 11–14

Wilton T 1996 Caring for the lesbian client: homophobia and midwifery. British Journal of Midwifery 4(3): 126–131

FURTHER READING

Bowler I M W 1993 Stereotypes of women of Asian descent in midwifery: some evidence. Midwifery 9: 7–16

Cosslett T 1994 Women writing childbirth – modern discourses of motherhood. Manchester University Press, Manchester

Department for Education and Employment 1996 The Disability Discrimination Act 1995. DfEE, London

Frossell S 1996 How to find out what women want. Modern Midwife 6(1): 18–19

Hindley C 1996 Midwifery client vs. public prisoner. British Journal of Midwifery 4(2): 63–64

Katz Rothman B 1988 The tentative pregnancy: prenatal diagnosis and the future of motherhood. Pandora, London

Kelsall J 1994 Maternity care for the deaf: a midwife's mission. Disability, Pregnancy and Parenthood International (January): 4–7

Leap N 1992 The power of words. Nursing Times 88(21): 60–61

Matlin M 1993 The psychology of women 2nd edn. Harcourt Brace Jovanovich College Publishers, Orlando, Florida

Nolan M 1996 The birth of Natasha. One labour: two very different experiences. Modern Midwife 6(2): 6–9

Roberts H (ed) 1992 Women's health matters. Routledge, London

Simkin P 1991 Just another day in a woman's life? Part 1 – women's long-term perceptions of their first birth experiences. Birth 18(4): 203

Spring Rice M 1981 Working class wives – the classic account of women's lives in the 1930's. Virago, London

Wasser A M, Killoran C L, Bansen S S 1993 Pregnancy and disability. Clinical Issues in Perinatal and Women's Health Nursing 4(2): 328–337

Community midwifery

Liz Floyd

In recent years the difference between hospital-based care and community midwifery care has become less distinct as flexible patterns of midwifery care are developed. These patterns of care are focused on the needs of the woman, and so are often community based. Such midwifery care, that reflects the needs of the pregnant woman and takes account of her and her family's personal and social circumstances, is better able to positively influence the health and well-being of her and her baby.

This chapter aims to:

- describe the role of the midwife and the scope of her practice in the community during the antenatal, intrapartum and postnatal periods

- review the skills a midwife requires for home birth, including her responsibility to ensure that women have the necessary information to choose this if they wish

- consider the midwife's relationship with other health care professionals involved in the care of the pregnant woman, especially the GP and the obstetrician.

INTRODUCTION

Community midwifery is one of the functions of community health care. It aims to promote the health and well-being of mothers and babies and to support sound parenting and stable families. It encompasses prepregnancy, pregnancy, birth and the puerperium. Community midwifery has its roots close to the home and in essence is concerned with meeting the health needs of women and their families. It is locally based outside the institution of the hospital, although community midwives sometimes work in hospital, for example supporting women in labour.

The underlying principles that guide community midwifery are the delivery of safe and effective care by supporting the normal processes of pregnancy while detecting the abnormal (Page 1995). These principles act as the goals for all maternity care. However, as the health and well-being of individuals reflect their environment, maternity care that is set within the context of the wider community and environment is able to meet health needs more effectively.

Midwifery care that is provided or based in the community has been undergoing a period of great change. Although systems of care vary widely across the UK, there has historically been a clear distinction between hospital-based care, where the woman is cared for by a team of health professionals with the consultant obstetrician as the lead professional, and care that is provided by members of the primary health care team, namely the community midwife and GP. Since the publication of the Changing Childbirth report (DH 1993), the distinction between midwives who practise in hospital and those who practise in the community is less clear. There have been several new schemes in recent years exploring innovative ways to provide maternity care for women. As a consequence, midwives now work more flexibly, moving between hospital and community to support the woman. With such community schemes, there is a greater chance that the woman and her family will know the midwife who cares for her.

THE ROLE OF THE COMMUNITY MIDWIFE

Care in pregnancy

It is still the norm for a woman to visit her GP to confirm her pregnancy and to discuss options for care, although it is becoming increasingly common for a midwife, often working from a health centre or a GP practice, to fulfil this function. The subsequent booking appointment may be undertaken in the woman's own home at a time convenient to her, although this should of course be by her choice where practicable. Although GPs and obstetricians are often unenthusiastic about domiciliary bookings, these have been shown to improve liaison between the hospital and the GP and to improve women's satisfaction with their care (Sikorski et al 1995). The midwife should always make an appointment before visiting the woman and ensure that the pregnancy remains confidential. Taking a full medical and social history and discussing options for care in the home environment is a highly effective use of time. Options may be discussed in the light of the woman's personal circumstances including her employment, her other children and the support she receives from her partner and her family. It is especially important to ensure that the woman understands the implications of the choices she makes about her pregnancy care. Conducting the interview on the woman's territory helps to facilitate choice and control, including enabling the woman to make informed decisions about any screening tests she is offered. Language difficulties may require that an interpreter is involved.

In the light of the woman's history, a plan can then be made for care during pregnancy and birth. If the woman is considering a home birth the midwife has the ideal opportunity to begin planning with the particular circumstances in mind. If there is no indication of any problems, a plan of visits can be made to suit the woman's individual needs, either at home or at the local clinic. Women receiving antenatal care from general practitioners and midwives have been shown to have fewer nonattendances, fewer hospital admissions and more focused care than women receiving care led by obstetricians (although women tend to be satisfied with whatever form of care they receive) (Tucker et al 1996). There has been criticism of the traditional pattern of antenatal examinations. Although there is support for a reduction in visits, change to long established practices has been slow. Women need to be involved in planning appropriate antenatal care for themselves which encompasses their employment, child care and domestic circumstances as well as their health needs. This concept of partnership is reinforced by women holding their own notes and having full access to their health records.

Whatever the setting, the midwife is responsible for undertaking a thorough examination of the woman so that she can identify any problems and respond to the woman's needs appropriately. She must ensure that all the necessary blood tests and screening tests are carried out and that the results are reported to the woman and recorded in the notes. She needs sufficient skill and experience to practise without the support of an obstetrician immediately available. If a woman does require additional medical care, this must come from either her GP, her obstetrician or another specialist and the midwife must know how to refer the woman to the appropriate person. If ultrasound examination is necessary, the woman will need to make a visit to the hospital. The midwife may continue to be involved in the care of a woman who develops a pregnancy complication and may be able to monitor the condition under the direction of the specialist concerned as well as providing midwifery support for the woman. Fleissig et al (1996) evaluated community-led care for women with complicated pregnancies and showed that it could be successful. For example, a woman who develops diabetes will benefit from close cooperation between the diabetic clinic and the midwife. The community midwife who is able to visit at home and understands the realities of the woman's lifestyle can reinforce the importance of close control of the blood sugar. The midwife can offer practical help tailored to the woman's own needs.

Personalised care may enable a reduction in routine antenatal visits. It is important to recognise, however, that if psychosocial care has benefits, then to reduce antenatal visits will reduce this potential benefit. Other critics, for example Redman (1996), have also argued that reducing the number of antenatal examinations may lead to cases of pre-eclampsia being missed, and thus a rise in mortality and morbidity rates.

Care in pregnancy includes supporting women and their partners in the transition to parenthood and providing an optimum environment for the growth and development of the babies. Social support in pregnancy is of vital importance and has been shown to improve satisfaction with medical care and women's feelings of 'being in control'. It has also been shown to result in higher breastfeeding rates, greater involvement of the father and fewer worrying health problems of the baby

(Oakley 1992). Long-term follow-up studies have shown that 6 years later women reported better relationships with their children, had higher self-esteem and fewer were smoking (Oakley et al 1996).

There is a general view that despite antenatal education many parents feel ill equipped to care for their new babies. Clearly there is a role for health professionals in health education and information giving, both to prevent ill health and to raise the mothers' awareness of health-related behaviours. Although the midwife is the primary carer early in the postnatal period, she is supported by the GP and the health visitor and as time elapses roles and responsibilities become blurred (Robinson et al 1983).

Intrapartum care

Community midwives deliver babies in all settings: at home; in GP- or midwifery-led birthing units; or in consultant units under a variety of different schemes. The opportunity to deliver the baby of a woman who the midwife already knows and has cared for during pregnancy is a highly rewarding experience for many midwives. Practising the full range of midwifery skills outside the institution of the hospital is also very satisfying and fulfilling. However, this experience can also be a daunting one. As well as providing care for planned events, the community midwife is responsible for midwifery support for emergencies that occur outside the hospital or before the woman reaches hospital. She may be required to attend emergencies with the ambulance crew or she may be required to attend by herself. Fulfilling this role requires that the midwife is experienced and skilled and has the support and back-up of the full range of maternity and emergency services.

Many community midwives also deliver babies in hospital, providing continuity of care for the women to whom they have given antenatal care and will care for postnatally. The midwife's skills of communication are as imperative when she is working in a hospital setting, liaising with obstetricians and hospital midwives, as when she is in the woman's home and finds she requires assistance there.

Although home birth is an infrequent event (see below), women and midwives are increasingly aware of it as an option. As so few babies are born at home, students have few opportunities to learn the practical skills required and midwives have little opportunity to develop their experience and confidence. At one time the Association for Improvements in the Maternity Services only received complaints about poor quality of care in hospital but now there is an increasing number of complaints about care at home births. These complaints relate to not carrying essential equipment (Sonicaid, infant resuscitation equipment, nitrous oxide and oxygen), nervous and inexperienced midwives who are probably unused to home births, and to dangerous interventionist practice (Robinson 1997). It is clear that the community midwife needs to be competent and skilful in all areas of her clinical work.

Maintaining the full range of clinical skills poses a unique problem for the midwife working in the community who may undertake very few deliveries either at home or in hospital.

Similarly the midwife who is confident and experienced with home births may not have the same confidence and clinical dexterity when she is working in a hospital. On the delivery suite the midwife is expected to use a range of fetal monitoring equipment, assist with fetal blood sampling, care for women with epidural and spinal analgesia and even assist with caesarean sections. When community midwives are providing care for all women, rather than just for low-risk women, learning and maintaining this array of skills is difficult. This difficulty is felt doubly by midwives who work part time and whose clinical contact time is further reduced.

A study investigating community midwives' experience of home birth found that it was important for them to be able to perform intravenous cannulation, neonatal resuscitation and perineal suturing. Without these skills, the midwives felt anxious and unhappy about booking women to give birth at home (Floyd 1995). Individual performance reviews and assessments of midwives' needs should highlight areas where skills need developing or refreshing. Clinical support for midwives inexperienced with home birth or midwives who are isolated or working alone, is essential to develop and maintain safe practice and expertise. This can take the form of a formalised midwife-to-midwife support system, where an experienced midwife acts as a mentor, or may be achieved through the education system.

The supervisor is crucial in the development of appropriate educational programmes for community midwives which should form part of the midwife's professional portfolio (Macdonald 1996). A clinical skills training scheme, the Maternal and Neonatal Emergencies Training Project (MANET), designed for midwives, GPs and junior obstetric staff is currently under evaluation (Kennedy 1995). Although there is always concern that study leave further depletes the workforce and reduces continuity of care, the importance of well-planned, needs-related, appropriate continuing education for community midwives cannot be overemphasised.

Postnatal care

The postnatal period means a period of not less than 10 and not more than 28 days after the end of labour, during which the continued attendance of a midwife is requisite (UKCC 1993). During this time the aim of care is to promote recovery from birth and the healthy growth and development of the baby, to encourage the independence of the mother in the care of herself and of her baby and to support the family in their new roles in relation to the baby. Some women experience physical or psychological problems as a result of childbirth and postnatal care can alleviate some of this ill health. The mother often wants to talk about her labour and delivery and the community midwife is the ideal person to do the listening. Some women need help to 'debrief' about birth and this can help in the adjustment to becoming a mother.

Each postnatal visit should always have a clear purpose and objective. Problems can be identified by observation and examination of the mother and the baby, as well as by listening to the woman's concerns. The emphasis should always be on the partnership between mother and midwife and so the range of midwifery care including the timing of visits should always be negotiated and discussed first.

If the woman has delivered at home or has been discharged very soon afterwards, the initial emphasis will be on the physical recovery of the mother. Examination will identify satisfactory involution of the uterus and control of bleeding, healing of the perineum, recovery of normal bladder and bowel function, normal blood oxygenation and circulation and the absence of signs of infection. All these will be aided by adequate rest and sleep. The purpose of the physical examination that the midwife undertakes is to assess this recovery and identify any problems. Examination of the temperature, pulse and blood pressure, checking the postpartum haemoglobin, and the examination of the breasts, uterus and perineum form part of the midwife's assessment of the well-being of the mother.

Recent research has shown the extent to which some women suffer long-term health problems as a consequence of childbirth (MacArthur et al 1992). These often go unreported and are often unidentified even by the postnatal examination at 6 weeks (Bick & MacArthur 1995). Backache, pelvic floor injury, including stress incontinence, urinary frequency and haemorrhoids were found to be common and often chronic conditions. Postnatal depression and fatigue were also frequently reported. Altogether, MacArthur et al (1992) reported that 47% of women in their long-term survey had one or more of these health problems. Perineal trauma following episiotomy or laceration may cause discomfort and affect a couple's sexual relationship for several months (Sleep 1991). All these problems are known to affect the ability of the woman to cope with her baby and may cause difficulties with relationships within the family.

The midwife should be able to give practical solutions to specific problems such as a painful perineal laceration but she needs to understand that problems may persist well beyond the scope of her postnatal visiting.

The midwife should support and promote breast feeding where this is appropriate and must observe and monitor changes in the breasts where they affect the health of the mother and baby. Visiting the mother in order to observe a breast feed is essential if the mother is experiencing problems. Planning this requires tact and flexibility if it is to benefit the mother.

The baby should always be observed to identify satisfactory behaviour, including feeding behaviour, breathing and oxygenation, separation of the cord and absence of signs of infection. Monitoring the baby's weight and ensuring that the appropriate screening tests are performed should always be undertaken with the parents' agreement.

The establishment of breast feeding takes far longer than the period that the community midwife is able to visit for and yet it is an integral part of her responsibility. Despite the proven benefits of breast feeding to the baby and mother, it is not widespread. 68% of women in England and Wales started to breast feed in 1995, but only 44% were still feeding at 6 weeks (Foster et al 1997). The main reasons given by women for discontinuation are 'insufficient milk', sore breasts and nipples, and the baby rejecting the breast. The community midwife has a clear responsibility to support breast feeding, but lack of experience or other more urgent demands on her time may leave her feeling unable to continue visiting. Health visitors rarely have sufficient experience or resources to fulfil this essential role. There is therefore little help and support for breast feeding in the community, apart from voluntary groups such as the National Childbirth Trust. Supporting women through these feeding problems requires real commitment and determination, but if the midwife is able to do this it can be a highly effective and worthwhile use of her time in promoting long-term health.

Selective visiting

It is important that the timing as well as the purpose of each postnatal visit is agreed with the mother. If the midwife does not visit each day before day 10, she remains responsible for the care and supervision of the woman and her baby. 'Each midwife remains personally responsible and accountable for the exercise of professional judgement and in determining appropriate practice in relation to the mother and her baby. This, naturally, includes judgements about the number of visits and any additional visits required in the postnatal period' (RCM 1994, p. 231).

She must make it clear how the mother should contact her in the event of any concern arising before the next planned visit. It is possible that overwork could influence some midwives to reduce the frequency and duration of their visits even further. A workload study of community midwives found that an average of only 17 minutes was spent with each client, although this varied with the dependency classification of the woman (Griffin & Hendy 1995). Clearly some women do have ongoing problems and a study by Garcia & Marchant (1996) found that between 10 and 20% of women were still being visited on day 14. Selective visiting can free midwives to concentrate their efforts where they are most needed and has the potential to improve continuity of carer and resolve problems with conflicting advice (Ball 1987). However, it is important to remember that home visiting may bring midwives into contact with some women who find it hard to express their needs and may find it difficult to ask for help.

The community midwife needs clear and effective methods of communication to other health and welfare professionals including the social worker and the health visitor. Although the health visitor usually takes over responsibility after 10 days, if the midwife is continuing to visit because of ongoing problems, effective liaison must take place to ensure that the woman is appropriately supported and does not receive conflicting advice.

There is an argument for extending the statutory scope of the midwife's responsibility to at least 6 weeks, to emphasise the importance of the wider scope of postnatal care. The benefits of social and psychological support have been upheld by research. The midwife may have scope for facilitating women's groups, postnatal support groups, breast-feeding support schemes, family planning services, child care programmes, education schemes in local schools and drop-in centres for teenagers. Some midwives become very involved with such initiatives, acting as much as a community health worker as a midwife. Midwives need to look at these aspects of their work in the light of the evidence and plan what they hope to achieve by the support they offer in order to evaluate the benefits (Garcia & Marchant 1996). Where midwives can become involved in supporting families in such ways the maternity services are able to be more responsive to the specific needs of the population they serve. What is essential is that the midwife endeavours to ensure that the woman has the support networks in place to give her the necessary health surveillance and help that she may continue to require.

HOME BIRTH

Home birth is the birth of a baby in the family home. This usually occurs because the parents believe that birth is a natural process and they want it to take place within the environment of the family home. This is known as planned home birth. If complications arise during pregnancy or labour it may be necessary to transfer the woman to hospital care. Less often, babies are born at home unexpectedly because labour begins prematurely or precipitously. This is usually because a problem develops rapidly in a woman who had planned to deliver in hospital. This is known as an unplanned home birth or sometimes a BBA (born before arrival). Occasionally a baby is born at home because the mother has chosen to avoid any maternity care. Home births are infrequent events and in 1994 represented only 1.8% of all births, although there is some evidence that the rate is increasing. Thirty years ago, one-third of all babies were born at home but the rate fell to an all-time low in 1987 (0.9% of all births). This rate varies and is higher in individual areas, for example in Brighton. Many pressures contributed to this decline and some of these are discussed later in the chapter.

Because so few births take place at home, meaningful and valid investigation is virtually impossible. Nevertheless there is tremendous need for data to evaluate birth at home. A very small pilot study investigated the feasibility of undertaking a randomised controlled trial of hospital versus home birth (Thornton 1996). This showed that although a trial is feasible, it will not provide answers to many of the questions about home birth, especially questions about safety. The Northern Region Perinatal Mortality Survey Coordinating Group (1996) stated that the question about planned home birth was not concerned with whether home birth was safe but whether it was *less* safe than hospital birth. A prospective regional study carried out in the north of England investigated the experiences and outcomes for women who requested home birth (Davies et al 1996). This showed that out of 256 women 43% transferred to hospital, leaving a total of 142 women who planned to and did deliver at home. No stillbirths or neonatal deaths occurred. During the same period a further 182 unplanned home births occurred and at these there were 9 stillbirths and 3 neonatal deaths. Thirty four of these women had received no antenatal care whatsoever. These findings support previous studies that demonstrate the hazards to babies born unexpectedly at home. The National Birthday Trust Survey investigated the outcomes for all women who planned to deliver their babies at home during 1994. This study confirmed that the highest rate of complications occurred amongst women who had unplanned home births, while the overall perinatal outcome for women who planned to and did deliver at home was excellent (Chamberlain et al 1997). Some women will not achieve their desire for a home birth and this study also showed that the transfer rate to hospital delivery was 40% amongst primigravidae although only 10% amongst multigravidae. The main reason for transfer was prolonged labour. Even women who were transferred were glad to have had the opportunity to undertake some of the labour at home.

As perinatal mortality and maternal mortality are infrequent events, other measures, such as satisfaction with care, are required to evaluate the outcome of home birth. These factors are much harder to define and to measure. The Northern Region home birth survey sought women's views on home birth both before the delivery and after. These women reported that they felt more in control and relaxed and that they enjoyed the natural non-clinical environment and the peacefulness and the privacy (Davies et al 1996). As far back as 1978, Kitzinger investigated why women chose to deliver at home and reported that the quality of the experience, a desire to be with their families and the avoidance of unnecessary interventions were important. O'Brien conducted a study published in 1978 when there was strong political pressure for deliveries to take place only in hospital. He demonstrated that the environment in which the baby is born does affect satisfaction and showed that this was greater in deliveries taking place at home.

Carrying out home births enables the midwife to practise her role to the full and helps her to develop her skills and confidence (Davies et al 1996, Floyd 1995). Midwives often have very little home birth experience upon which to develop their skills either as students or in the course of their careers. A study of community midwives' experience of home birth showed that half the midwives had attended fewer than six home births and 9% had never attended any (Floyd 1995). These findings are echoed by the Northern Region survey. In both studies midwives were positive about home birth, and believed it to be important for women to have the option.

Midwives in both studies reported that they had a range of practical concerns and would benefit from better 'on-call' support from colleagues, managers, supervisors and the obstetric team in the event of complications arising, although communication is improving through the use of mobile phones. Midwives also reported that they needed specific clinical skills in suturing, setting up intravenous infusions and in resuscitation of mother and baby. These skills need to be specifically taught and updated in the home rather than in the hospital. Some midwives were anxious about the equipment they carried, in particular adequate and easily portable nitrous oxide and oxygen. Emergency support in the community is now rarely provided by the Emergency Obstetric Unit (or Flying Squad). A well-equipped paramedic service which carries individuals skilled in resuscitation which is able to respond immediately and can transfer women and babies rapidly to a specialist unit is now considered to be more appropriate than a team which attempts to undertake procedures in the home (RCOG 1990).

Care of the woman at home

Preparing for a home birth

Once a woman has indicated that she is considering having her baby at home, the midwife must make time to discuss the advantages and disadvantages in the light of the woman's own individual circumstances. The benefits of delivering in the familiar surroundings of the home must be carefully balanced against the distance from emergency assistance should complications arise. It may be hard for the midwife not to inadvertently convey her own personal feeling and therefore as much unbiased information as possible should be given in order that the woman can make her decision. Discussion should take place early in pregnancy if possible and further preparation when the pregnancy is more advanced, although some women choose a home birth much later in pregnancy. It is important that the midwife is satisfied that she has discussed all the points listed in Box 3.1 with the woman and her partner.

Box 3.2 provides a checklist of requirements in the home in preparation for the birth and Box 3.3 a list of equipment supplied by the midwife.

The midwife is responsible for ensuring that she has the correct equipment with her at all times. She may have her own equipment for her own exclusive use, or it may be stored centrally and collected by her when required. In either case it must be checked scrupulously before and after use because it may be needed in an emergency at any time. Local policy will determine where any drugs she requires will be kept but the midwife must ensure they are always carried and used

> **Box 3.1 Preparation of the woman considering a home birth – points for discussion**
>
> 1. Discuss the advantages and disadvantages of home birth. Try to provide as much factual information as possible including any local statistics.
> 2. Explain the role of the midwife during a home birth including the conduct of labour. Describe what the midwife will do in specific circumstances, e.g. postpartum haemorrhage, asphyxiated baby, shoulder dystocia, transfer to hospital.
> 3. Explain how to contact the midwife when in labour.
> 4. Discuss what the role of the GP is likely to be, depending on whether he wishes to be present at the birth.
> 5. Discuss how often and when the woman will be visited postnatally.
> 6. Talk about how to contact the local home birth support group (if one exists).

> **Box 3.2 Preparing for the birth**
>
> **The mother**
> - Discuss pain relief.
> - Comfort aids for labour; lip balm, massage oils, ice, straws for drinking, cool flannels, clothing.
> - A suitcase packed in case of transfer to hospital. Consider transport to hospital especially any problems with access or any other communication problems.
> - Arrangements for the care and preparation of any other children; ideally another adult should be available to care for the children.
>
> **The baby**
> - Cot, baby clothes, nappies, warm hat, hot water bottle (to warm cot).
>
> **The room**
> - Protection for pillows, mattress and carpet, e.g. polythene covers and old sheets. Spare bed linen.
> - Reliable heating and lighting including an Anglepoise lamp if possible.
> - Clear surfaces.
> - Bathroom or other washing facilities with soap and towels.

in accordance with the Midwives Rules (UKCC 1993) and with due regard to security. A midwife's car will always be a target for theft and so drugs and other equipment should not be left unattended. Sadly it is also possible that a midwife could prove a target for crime and so she should always act to protect her own personal safety. This consideration may mean that during some hours of the night and in some areas, the midwife should not be out alone (see Ch. 7).

Care during labour at home

Unlike hospital where the woman is in unfamiliar surroundings, in her own home she is able to behave spontaneously and normally. A close relationship can develop during the labour but the midwife remains a guest in the home and must respect the family's views and wishes. The midwife should organise the equipment as efficiently but as unobtrusively as possible, while taking great care of furniture and floor coverings. She must not reproduce a delivery room atmosphere, yet must have her equipment rapidly to hand when required. Great skill is needed to rigorously monitor the

Box 3.3 Equipment the midwife requires for a home birth

Maternity pack to be delivered to the woman's home at 37 weeks containing:
- Cotton wool balls, sanitary pads and absorbent pads
- Vaginal examination pack.

Essential equipment in the midwife's delivery bag to be taken to the home during labour:
- Pinard stethoscope and Sonicaid
- Sphygmomanometer
- Urine testing equipment
- Entonox equipment; this must be regularly serviced and should be stored above 10°C (not in the boot of a car) – if the cylinders have been exposed to a low temperature the gases may separate and be dangerous
- Oxygen in small cylinders with apparatus for delivering it to a baby by a face mask
- Portable suction machine
- Intravenous giving set, venflons and fluid such as Hartmann's solution
- Plastic bags for clinical waste
- Sterile gloves, obstetric cream or KY jelly
- Amnihook
- Glycerine suppositories and disposable phosphate enema
- Urethral catheters
- Cotton wool balls
- *Delivery pack*: containing two artery forceps, cord scissors, episiotomy scissors and cord clamp
- *Suture pack*: containing stitch scissors, needle holder, forceps and Spencer Wells forceps plus suture material Vicryl or Dexon, lignocaine 10%, 20 ml syringe and needles
- *Maternal drugs*: Syntometrine 1 ml, ergometrine 0.5 mg plus 2 ml syringes and needles; analgesic drugs such as pethidine 100 mg depending on local policy
- *Baby equipment*: laryngoscope with neonatal blade, baby ambu-bag, endotracheal tubes of different sizes
- *Baby drugs*: Konakion 1 mg and naloxone 400 micrograms/ml (see Ch. 34) 2 ml syringes and small needles
- *Blood bottles*: two small bottles with anticoagulant and one plain bottle for maternal and cord blood samples; 5 ml, 10 ml and 20 ml syringes and needles; tourniquet.

that problems are identified in good time. Accurate and thorough records must be maintained at all times. The classic skills of the community midwife are to monitor, watch, wait and support (Robinson 1997) and therefore the midwife's role is to support the normal processes of labour while monitoring the well-being of the mother and baby throughout. Familiarity with the woman's wishes will determine how the labour and delivery are conducted, where the baby is born and how the third stage of labour is managed. The midwife must be aware of how important it is not to disturb the normal physiological processes by any action or behaviour which could expose the woman to harm.

Throughout the labour, the midwife must be constantly aware that the consequences of any abnormality are more serious at home. She must satisfy herself that she knows how to recognise complications and that she can cope with emergencies when they occur (see Box 3.4). Where two midwives are in attendance, although each remains fully accountable for her actions, there must be agreement over who assumes primary responsibility for decision-making. It has also been reported that where two midwives are in attendance they can spend more time talking to each other than observing the woman. Each situation needs to be assessed sensitively but with due regard for the needs of the woman.

It may be appropriate to inform the delivery suite and the supervisor when a woman is in labour at home, in case a problem occurs and transfer to hospital is necessary. Some midwives may also wish to keep a colleague or manager informed of progress in case they require support. The midwife must ensure that the GP knows that the woman is in labour if he is providing intrapartum care. The midwife must know how to contact the ambulance service and must have an idea how long assistance is likely to take in coming. She must have a clear system of communication with the obstetric unit.

The decisions that a midwife makes during a home birth require the greatest clinical judgements and may be the hardest that a midwife makes in her working life. This sense of responsibility and accountability can make the experience of birth at home as profound for midwives as it is for women.

well-being and condition of the baby and mother effectively and to keep concurrent records yet without disturbing the relaxed atmosphere of the home and the process of labour. Observation of the condition of the mother and baby must be made throughout with sufficient frequency to ensure

Box 3.4 Labour complications arising during a home birth

Prolonged first or second stage
Without fetal distress this is not an acute emergency. The midwife should discuss the likely causes and outcomes with the woman and a member of the obstetric team.

Meconium-stained liquor
In the absence of other complications the midwife must be able to identify how much meconium is present in the liquor and be alert to the potential risk of fetal distress. The causes should be discussed with the woman and a member of the obstetric team.

Fetal heart rate abnormality
The action required depends on the severity.

Antepartum haemorrhage
This is an acute emergency for which it is appropriate to call an ambulance for immediate transfer to hospital.

Shoulder dystocia
This can be an unexpected and acute emergency so the midwife must know how to deal with this situation herself. See Chapter 29.

Postpartum haemorrhage
The midwife must know how to identify the cause of the haemorrhage and to control it. She should know how to insert an intravenous infusion and to suture perineal lacerations.

Retained placenta
The midwife needs to know how to manually remove the placenta in the absence of medical assistance.

Birth asphyxia
The midwife must ensure that she has up-to-date experience of resuscitation. She must have the correct equipment which is checked each time she attends a home birth.

THE PRIMARY HEALTH CARE TEAM

Where the midwife is part of an integrated community and hospital maternity care service, she maintains close clinical and professional links with mainstream maternity care. This ensures that she is not isolated from current professional developments and that she is aware of and involved in the spectrum of maternity practice. However, the disadvantage of her close relationship with the hospital is that she is less closely involved with primary health care. The primary health care team (PHCT) has traditionally consisted of the GP, the health visitor, the midwife and the community nurse and, on occasion, the social worker, counsellor and interpreter. It functions to provide basic front-line health care to the community. Specialist services, when required, are provided by referral to appropriate consultants. However, new patterns are emerging.

In most spheres of primary care the lead professional is usually the GP, but in some maternity schemes the midwife takes the lead. Other professionals may be required to provide essential skills depending on the needs of the local population (Ford & Iliffe 1996). For example, the teamwork required in a deprived, multilingual inner city with a refugee population and experiences of racism and violence is very different from that associated with 'independent midwifery' sought by an educated and affluent population. For the first a culturally attuned translator may be the key worker displacing doctor and midwife, and in the second the midwife is the key worker needing only a distant relationship with the GP.

The role of the GP in maternity care

All women and their families should be registered with a GP who will provide health care and medical services for patients on his list. Homeless people, refugees and other individuals without a permanent place of abode, such as students or seasonal workers, may not be registered. GPs receive a fee for the level of maternity care they provide. Few GPs are interested in providing a total maternity service for their patients and few have maintained their clinical skills in all aspects of maternity care. Only a small proportion of GPs feel sufficiently confident to undertake deliveries in the home and this has led to a general distrust and anxiety with regard to home births. A study investigating GPs' and obstetricians' views on home birth reported that many would try to dissuade women from giving birth at home (Bathgate et al 1995). Some GPs have gone so far as to remove from their list women who insist on this option. This practice has been condemned by the RCGP (1995) who have published a report clarifying the role of the GP. In intrapartum care the role of the GP is to provide midwifery support and his skills should therefore be complementary to those of the midwife. They are not those expected of the specialist. A GP is perfectly entitled not to be personally involved in intrapartum care but he *is* required to respond positively to a woman who requests a home birth. He can either refer the woman to another GP who does provide the care or he can refer her to a community-based midwife. Neither increases his medicolegal responsibility. Midwives remain personally accountable for their actions and decisions even when there is a named GP or consultant in charge. A GP is not obliged to attend the woman at home *unless* the midwife has specifically requested this or the woman summons him in emergency. This requirement is exactly the same for any GP who has not accepted the woman for maternity care. If a midwife is in need of advice or help, she should refer directly to the appropriate professional colleague. For a woman in labour, this will be to an obstetrician or neonatologist. This point was emphasised in a joint statement issued by the RCM and the RCGP (1995) entitled 'Responsibilities in Intrapartum Care'.

Few GPs provide all their antenatal care, as most have shared care arrangements with local trust midwives who attend their clinics to participate in antenatal care. Family doctors are anxious to maintain contact with their patients during pregnancy precisely because it is such an important event for the family. Naturally a woman continues to require medical care while she is pregnant and so it is important that the GP maintains this continuity. The woman also requires a medical examination to ensure that her cardiovascular system is fit for inhalational analgesia. The role of the midwife and the GP should therefore complement each other rather than conflict. A more serious issue concerns the role of practice nurses employed directly by GPs. Tyler (1996) voices the concern that these practice nurses are undertaking a range of midwifery duties. Even where these nurses hold a midwifery qualification, fragmented care and reduced continuity result. It is very difficult to monitor the practice of such nurses and to ensure high-quality care through the supervision system.

DEVELOPMENTS IN THE COMMUNITY MIDWIFERY SERVICE 1900–1997

The history of community midwives this century has reflected the conditions and needs of women and their families. In the early part of the century the high maternal and infant mortality rate was a cause of national concern and this, fuelled by the women's movement, led to increasing pressure on the state to make better provision for childbearing women. Poor general health, unemployment, low wages and poor housing made living conditions difficult for many families. Educating mothers in the care of their babies, better nutrition as well as supervision of pregnancy and labour were the foundation of maternity care. The number of untrained 'handywomen' declined, and most pregnant women received maternity care from qualified doctors and midwives. The domiciliary midwifery service was a popular, efficient and above all a safe service with low rates of mortality and morbidity. Throughout the century maternal mortality and stillbirth rates steadily declined, although this was probably due to improvements in diet and general health, together with better social and health care, rather than specific improvements in maternity care.

From the start of the National Health Service in 1948, district midwives provided a community-based service which functioned within the public health system. The midwife worked from her own home and was accountable only to her supervisor of midwives and to her clients. Domiciliary midwives cared for women booked for home birth, providing all their antenatal, intrapartum and postnatal care. By contrast, women booked for hospital delivery were cared for solely by hospital staff, received all their antenatal care at the hospital antenatal clinic and remained in hospital for the full 'lying-in' period after delivery. Domiciliary midwives' caseloads were heavy with long working and 'on-call' hours (Allison 1995). During the 1950s the serious shortage of hospital beds meant that a woman was unlikely to be able to deliver in hospital unless she had serious problems. Many homes were in very poor condition, and so women often delivered their babies at home in overcrowded and insanitary conditions because there was no alternative. 'In effect district midwives booked women who chose a home birth and all those who could not be fitted in to the system elsewhere.' (Allison 1995, p. 53). The Association for Improvements in the Maternity Services (AIMS) was set up to campaign for more hospital beds. Ironically one of its main functions now is to campaign for women's rights to choose home birth.

During this time it was believed that hospitalisation and intervention in childbirth would improve maternal and neonatal outcomes. During the 1950s and 1960s domiciliary practice declined along with the home birth rate and the trend was to provide hospital care in small cottage-style hospitals or small GP units. In the event of an unexpected home birth, the GP and midwife would attend together and provide whatever expertise they possessed. The district midwife, in contrast with her hospital counterpart, became increasingly isolated from developments within hospital. She became associated with non-interventionist normal practice and her image and authority diminished accordingly.

A review of the maternity services by the Peel Committee (DHSS 1970) recommended an integrated midwifery service which combined domiciliary and hospital maternity care. This review also recommended that all births should take place in hospital despite the lack of evidence to support this. It was not until 1975 that perinatal mortality figures were collected by place of delivery, and these showed that birth at home was associated with higher mortality for babies. These data were not examined closely until the 1980s when more detailed scrutiny showed that a high proportion of these home births were to single young women under 20 and that the higher risks were therefore a result of social factors rather than simply due to the fact that the birth took place at home (Campbell et al 1982, Tew 1995). The Cardiff Births Survey investigated the differences in perinatal mortality between planned and unplanned home births (Murphy et al 1984), and identified the risks to women who planned to deliver in hospital but did not arrive in time (5.4% of the

babies died) and the even more serious risks to women who did not arrange any maternity care whatsoever (20% of these babies died). In contrast only 0.6% of the women who planned to and actually did deliver at home lost their babies. These findings were confirmed by another study of all babies born at home in 1979 (Campbell et al 1984). The findings showed considerable differences between women who planned to and did deliver at home (perinatal mortality rate of 4.1/1000), women who booked to deliver in hospital but delivered at home (perinatal mortality rate of 67.5/1000) and women who were completely unbooked (perinatal mortality rate of 196.6/1000). It remains impossible to assess accurately the relative safety because such studies do not take account of the women who planned to deliver at home, but were transferred to hospital. Any emergency arising during labour is associated with significant risks to the mother and baby.

In the post-war years there was often considerable friction between hospital and community-based midwives. Hospital midwives worked under the obstetrician, who was the dominant partner. By the late 1970s most deliveries occurred in large centralised units. Units with fewer than 500 deliveries per year were considered unable to provide the necessary expertise and resources and so were steadily closed. One of the results of these changes was the development of 'shared care' where antenatal care was shared between the obstetrician and the GP and midwife. The hospital came to be considered as where the important care was carried out, while there was little value seen in the community contribution.

The organisation of community midwifery care

The community midwifery service is organised within a geographically defined area of a health care trust. It aims to provide maternity care that reflects the needs and characteristics of the local population and the social and ethnic backgrounds of individuals. As it is an integrated system, the Head of Midwifery for the trust is responsible for the community service as well as that of the hospital.

Supervisors of midwives are appointed who safeguard and enhance the quality of care, and ensure acceptable standards of practice of all midwives practising in its area. 'Acceptable standards of practice' are defined as care that is sensitive to women's needs and choices, complies with the UKCC Midwives Rules and is based on evidence and contemporary clinical developments (ENB 1996). Supervisors should be available for midwives to discuss their practice and be a source of sound professional advice, as well as monitoring standards and investigating critical incidents. The Midwives Rules (UKCC 1993) are made in accordance with the Midwifery Committee recommendations under the Nurses, Midwives and Health Visitors Act 1979 and define the scope of practice of all midwives while the Midwife's Code of Practice (UKCC 1994) elaborates the rules and acts as a guide.

Midwives practising in the community must ensure that they are fully conversant with these rules as well as with local policies. Midwives who practise outside the organisation of a hospital must ensure that they keep and maintain their records appropriately. Legislation lays down that as records may be required at a later date they must be properly stored either by the midwife herself or in accordance with arrangements made by the supervisor of midwives. Evidence may be required if a case is brought under the Congenital Disabilities (Civil Liabilities) Act 1976 by the child at a later date. The Data Protection Act 1984 and the Access to Health Records Act 1990 both require that midwives keep appropriate records and ensure that confidentiality is maintained throughout. In certain cases individuals are entitled to gain access to the information held about them.

The community midwifery service is responsible for ensuring that midwives are available who can give the necessary high-quality antenatal, intrapartum and postnatal care to meet the needs of the local population. The way that the service is organised will vary between areas to reflect particular local needs. For example, an inner-city area with a large ethnic minority population and a high density of temporary accommodation may require midwives with language skills or who work with a translator. Midwives may need to run a 'drop-in'

centre, or a clinic within a hostel, to ensure that antenatal care is available for women who often have multiple health and social problems. Such women are often not registered with a family doctor and the midwifery service may be able to liaise with a particular GP practice to provide medical care. In contrast, an entirely different service is required in a rural area with a sparsely scattered population at a distance from the maternity unit. Travelling time by midwives may be reduced by a caseload approach to planning care and allocating work. Similarly, the midwifery service could provide midwives able to undertake ultrasound scanning in community clinics. Planned home birth may be more appropriate than the hazards of a lengthy journey to hospital for some multigravid women. Undertaking a profile of the local population and the specific circumstances of women will help in planning an appropriate midwifery service.

Models of community midwifery care

When a woman chooses NHS care she is usually referred to a maternity hospital by her GP. If she is judged to be at low risk, she is usually offered shared care. Women who have complicated pregnancies usually have full hospital care.

Shared care. This is antenatal care shared between the hospital (obstetrician and midwife) and the community (her GP and midwife) with delivery in the hospital under the care of the hospital staff. After discharge, postnatal care is provided at home by the community midwife and GP.

The disadvantage of shared antenatal care is that care is fragmented and women see many different health professionals. It can also lead to interprofessional difficulties if there is no clear pattern of responsibility. Furthermore, midwives working in the community who do not undertake deliveries lose their clinical skills.

Domino service. An extension of shared care is the domino service (domiciliary-midwife-in-and-out) where as well providing antenatal care in the community with the GP, the community midwife also delivers the baby in hospital. If medical assistance is required, it is provided by hospital obstetric staff and the GP has no role in intra-partum care. In some cases there are special informal-style delivery rooms set away from the main delivery suite; in others the community midwives work alongside hospital staff. The midwife then arranges for the woman to be discharged home usually within a few hours of birth. This style of care has proved popular with women but has usually only been available to a few.

Community midwives who frequently deliver babies in hospital maintain their skills and close working relationships with the hospital staff. Providing cover for midwives to undertake the range of duties in the community as well as being on call for deliveries in hospital can be difficult.

GP maternity care.   Rarely, the GP provides GP maternity care for deliveries either at home or in the hospital. The GP provides any necessary obstetric support including instrumental delivery, suturing or resuscitation although he may request an obstetric referral at any time.

Team midwifery.   More recently, schemes have been developed to improve continuity of care for women. Team midwifery consists of teams of midwives who work together to provide care throughout pregnancy, labour and the puerperium to give continuous, coordinated, woman-centred care. The Know Your Midwife scheme showed how continuity could be improved while at the same time radically altering the midwives' working week. Women felt more in control during labour and found it easier being mothers (Flint & Poulengeris 1990). The Kidlington team set up along the same principles provided care for women with both high-risk and low-risk pregnancies. Deliveries were carried out either at home or in the hospital and evaluation showed a greater satisfaction with care and reduction in the use of analgesia (Watson 1990).

The Newcastle Community Midwifery Care Project aimed to develop a preventive community health and social work service, by providing community-based midwifery care within two very deprived areas of the city. The project provided enhanced midwifery care to women during pregnancy, with extended postnatal visits by the project midwives. The midwives were also involved in the running of a neighbourhood centre and facilitating local support groups. The project was shown to reduce smoking and improve the diet of the women and reduced the number of low birthweight babies. It was also very popular with the women. Like other schemes of this type, midwives also report greater job satisfaction (Davies & Evans 1991). Team midwifery can be very popular with women and midwives, but is difficult to implement with midwives who work part time, amongst larger groups of midwives or in hospitals.

Caseload midwifery practice differs fundamentally from team midwifery. Each woman has a 'named midwife' who takes full responsibility for her midwifery care. Each midwife carries a caseload, providing midwifery care for a number of women, throughout pregnancy, birth and the puerperium. Sometimes known as '*one-to-one midwifery practice*', the central aim is to provide an 'individual service to women and their families, respecting their rights, values and beliefs' (Page 1995, p. 176). Within the group practice, midwives manage their own time resources, with no shifts, and no barriers between hospital and community, attending the woman wherever and whenever necessary. Learning to work in this way can be difficult as there is no clear distinction between working time and off-duty time. Midwives with children and other domestic commitments may be unable to accommodate the demands of caseload practice. However, many midwives report more job satisfaction as a result of their increased accountability and responsibility.

Until recently GPs have been unable to purchase maternity provision but in 1996 six practices began to pilot the purchase of maternity care. These pilot projects were specifically charged with the task of providing woman-centred care (Tyler 1996). These six schemes are exploring how GPs can purchase the services of Midwifery Group Practices from trusts. Midwifery group practices are a natural extension of team midwifery whereby midwives work together providing total care to a defined group of women usually based within a geographical location. The midwife acts as the lead professional, providing the majority of the woman's care and liaising with and referring to medical colleagues as appropriate. Caseload midwifery may be particularly suitable for vulnerable women who are not catered for elsewhere. The midwifery group practice at Kings Healthcare in South London aims to provide for such women who want a home birth but special provision is made for women with mental health problems who need particular support from their carers (Warwick 1995). All these systems will require careful evaluation before any conclusions can be drawn about their effectiveness. However, it does mean that health service reform is providing a mechanism for innovation and implementing change in community maternity care.

Since the report of the Expert Maternity Group (DH 1993) there have been many different schemes set up within the community as a result of the Changing Childbirth initiative. Many of these schemes are experimental with fixed-term funding. They require proper evaluation before conclusions can be drawn about their effectiveness.

READER ACTIVITIES

1. Think about what information a woman requires in order to make an informed choice about whether or not to have a home birth. How can she obtain this information?

2. Identify what facilities exist for maternity emergencies in your area and how they operate. What policies or procedures govern their provision?

3. Which of the Midwives Rules apply when a woman who wants a home birth refuses to be transferred during labour? What are the midwife's responsibilities?

4. Find out what community maternity statistics are kept in your area. What records are kept of planned home births, unplanned home births, transfers to hospital of babies planned to be born at home and unbooked deliveries? Who keeps these figures and how are they recorded?

5. Write a community profile for childbearing women in your area. Do they have any particular needs and how could the community midwifery service adapt to meet these needs?

REFERENCES

Access to Health Records Act 1990 HMSO, London

Allison J 1995 Delivered at home. Chapman & Hall, London

Ball J 1987 Reactions to motherhood: the role of postnatal care. Cambridge University Press, Cambridge

Bathgate W, Ryan M, Hall M 1995 Divided views amongst health professionals on place of birth. British Journal of Midwifery 3(11): 583–586

Bick D, MacArthur C 1995 Attendance, content and relevance of the 6 week postnatal examination. Midwifery 11(2): 69–73

Campbell R, Davies I, MacFarlane A 1982 Perinatal mortality and place of delivery. Population Trends 28: 9–12

Campbell R, MacDonald Davies I, MacFarlane A, Berol V 1984 Home Births in England and Wales, 1979: perinatal mortality according to intended place of delivery. British Medical Journal 289: 721–724

Chamberlain G, Wraight A, Crowley P 1997 Home births: the report of the 1994 confidential enquiry by the National Birthday Trust Fund. Parthenon, Carnforth, Lancs

Congenital Disabilities (Civil Liabilities) Act 1976 HMSO, London

Data Protection Act 1984 HMSO, London

Davies J, Evans F 1991 The Newcastle community midwifery care project. Part I The project in action. Part II The evaluation of the project. In: Robinson S, Thomson A (eds) Midwives, research and childbirth. Chapman & Hall, London, vol II

Davies J, Hey E, Reid W, Young G 1996 Prospective regional study of planned home births. British Medical Journal 313: 1302–1306

Department of Health (DH) 1993 Changing childbirth part 1: report of the expert maternity group. HMSO, London

Department of Health and Social Security (DHSS) 1970 Domiciliary midwifery and maternity bed needs. (Chairman Mr J Peel) HMSO, London

English National Board for Nursing, Midwifery and Health Visiting (ENB) 1996 Supervision of midwives: the English National Board's advice and guidance to local supervising authorities and supervisors of midwives. ENB, London

Fleissig A, Kroll D, McCarthy M 1996 Is community led antenatal care a feasible option for women assessed as low risk and those with complicated pregnancies? Midwifery 12: 191–197

Flint C, Poulengeris P 1990 The know your midwife report. South West Thames Regional Health Authority, London

Floyd L 1995 Community midwives views and experience of home birth. Midwifery 11: 3–10

Ford C, Iliffe S 1996 An interprofessional approach to care: lessons from general practice. In: Kroll D (ed) Midwifery care for the future. Baillière Tindall, London

Foster K, Lader D, Cheesbrough S 1997 Infant feeding 1995: a survey carried out by the Office for National Statistics. The Stationery Office, London

Garcia J, Marchant S 1996 The potential of postnatal care. In: Kroll D (ed) Maternity care for the future. Baillière Tindall, London

Griffin B, Hendy M 1995 A community assessment: patient dependency, midwives and mothers needs. Midwives Chronicle 108(1289): 184–187

Kennedy J 1995 The maternal and neonatal emergencies training project. Changing Childbirth Update 4: 15

Kitzinger S 1978 Birth at home. Oxford University Press, Oxford

Kroll D 1996 Working for women: assessing needs, planning care. In: Kroll D (ed) Midwifery care for the future. Baillière Tindall, London

MacArthur C, Lewis M, Knox G 1992 Long term health problems after childbirth: and investigation of 11 701 women delivering in Birmingham. Research and the Midwife Conference Proceedings

Macdonald S 1996 Changing childbirth using supervision to promote change. Changing Childbirth Update 5: 6

Nurses, Midwives and Health Visitors Act 1979 HMSO, London

Murphy J, Dauncey M, Gray D, Chalmers I 1984 Planned and unplanned deliveries at home: implications of a changing ratio. British Medical Journal 288: 1429–1432

Northern Region Perinatal Mortality Survey Coordinating Group 1996 Collaborative survey of perinatal loss in planned and unplanned home births. British Medical Journal 313: 1306–1309

O'Brien M 1978 Home and hospital: a comparison of the experiences of mothers having home and hospital confinements. Journal of the Royal College of General Practitioners 28: 460–466

Oakley A 1992 Social support and motherhood. Blackwell, Oxford

Oakley A, Hicky D, Rajan L, Rigby A 1996 Social support in pregnancy: does it have long term effects? Journal of Reproductive and Infant Psychology 14: 7–22

Page L 1995 Putting principles into practice. In: Page L (ed) Effective group practice in midwifery – working with women. Blackwell Science, Oxford

Redman C 1996 Why antenatal care must not be reduced. Midwives 109(1303): 233

Royal College of General Practitioners (RCGP) 1995 The role of the general practitioner in maternity care. Occasional Paper 72. RCGP, London

Royal College of Midwives Standing Practice Group 1994 Paper 2 – Community postnatal visiting. Midwives Chronicle 107(1277): 231

Royal College of Midwives and Royal College of General Practitioners 1995 Working together – responsibilities in intrapartum care. A joint statement from the RCM and the RCGP, London

Royal College of Obstetricians and Gynaecologists (RCOG) 1990 The future of emergency domiciliary obstetric services (flying squads). RCOG, London

Robinson J 1997 Home birth disasters. British Journal of Midwifery 5(2): 114

Robinson S, Golden J, Bradley S 1983 A study of the role and responsibilities of the midwife. NERU Report no. 1. Kings College, University of London

Sikorski J, Clement S, Wilson J, Das S, Smeeton N 1995 A survey of health professionals' views on possible changes in the provision and organisation of antenatal care. Midwifery 11(2): 61–68

Sleep J 1991 Perineal care: a series of five randomised controlled trials. Robinson S, Thomson A (eds) Midwives research and childbirth. Chapman & Hall, London, vol 2, pp 199–251

Tew M 1995 Safer childbirth. Chapman & Hall, London

Thornton J 1996 Should there be a trial of home versus hospital delivery in the UK? British Medical Journal 312(7033): 753–757

Tucker J, Hall M, Howie P, Reid M, Barbour R, du V Florey C, McIlwaine G 1996 Should obstetricians see women with normal pregnancies? A multicentre randomised controlled trial of routine antenatal care led by GPs and midwives compared with shared care led by obstetricians. British Medical Journal 312: 554–559

Tyler S 1996 Making GP fundholding work for midwives. British Journal of Midwifery 4(8): 431–434

Watson P 1990 Report on the Kidlington Team Midwifery Scheme. Oxford Institute of Nursing, Oxford

Warwick C 1995 Midwifery group practice at Kings Healthcare. Changing Childbirth Update (2): 2

United Kingdom Central Council for Nursing, Midwifery and Health Visiting (UKCC) 1993 Midwives rules. UKCC, London

United Kingdom Central Council for Nursing, Midwifery and Health Visiting (UKCC) 1994 The midwife's code of practice. UKCC, London

International midwifery

4

Della Sherratt

The chapter outlines the issues and agendas facing midwifery from an international perspective. Its focus is on the major events and global issues which have helped raise the profile of midwives and their profession.

The chapter aims to:

- consider the issues facing midwifery in different cultural settings and the practicalities of midwives working outside their own country

- describe the major international events and organisations relevant to midwifery, in particular the International Confederation of Midwives, the global Safe Motherhood Initiative and the Baby Friendly Hospital Initiative

- outline some of the issues facing midwives in other countries, their education, working conditions and the barriers to providing quality midwifery care.

In such a short chapter it is not possible to give an in-depth analysis of the global situation or describe in detail midwifery in every country. When reference is made to the situation in a named country, it is as an example to assist understanding and not to criticise the midwives working there. The aim is to increase understanding and foster a sense of unity and respect for a shared philosophy which underpins the profession, despite the different models, health or education systems in use throughout the world.

INTRODUCTION

Today, globalisation makes it difficult for midwives to concern themselves only with what takes place in their country. The issues and problems of the world increasingly find their way into both the workplace and the home. Technology, the media, ease of travel, all contribute towards this global view of the world as being interrelated parts. Not surprisingly, an increasing number of midwives choose to spend part of their professional career in another country. Often they choose to work in those countries with the greatest need. Increasingly, there are a larger number of midwives from traditionally poor countries seeking employment in another country in order to increase their knowledge. The increased ease of travel makes this possible for more and more midwives. As the more industrialised countries find that they can no longer continue with the high costs of technology and medicalisation of childbirth, they are likely to look towards developing countries for solutions and this in turn will offer more opportunities in the future. Whatever the reason for the increase it is likely that midwives will be working with vastly different cultures, traditions and resources. Not surprisingly, some midwives may find themselves ill at ease and initially overwhelmed by their experience, despite having developed expertise in their own country. It is fair to say that more attention is being given to the adequate preparation of midwives who wish to work in an international field. However, given the diversity of opportunities and experiences that are available today, the rapid pace of change and the polarisation of developed and developing countries, preparation for this area of practice is poor. This chapter will first try to explore some of the issues as well as practicalities of working in an international setting, then will try to outline some of the current international agendas and will be of benefit to those who wish to explore this field of practice, as well those who would just like to know what is happening to midwifery globally.

THE PRACTICALITIES OF WORKING IN ANOTHER COUNTRY

One of the first issues to address is the practical aspects of working in another country. Obtaining permission and ensuring that the correct visa is obtained can be difficult. Many countries require a different visa if the intention is to work rather than visit. If the intention is to work, it may be necessary to provide evidence of the work to be undertaken, often by producing an official letter of invitation from the employing agency or company. Without the correct visa, determining entry into the country and length of stay can be complicated; therefore it is always advisable to check the requirements carefully. Most embassies or consulates will provide the necessary information and documentation to apply for the correct visa.

Attention to health and personal safety is also an essential practicality. It is essential to have adequate medical insurance cover, particularly cover which includes repatriation, as the most common reason for an unscheduled return home is personal ill health. Where possible, insurance cover which will allow an unscheduled return home to deal with personal difficulties is useful, as trying to arrange this very quickly from another country can be traumatic. Many agencies or employers will be sympathetic and this may be covered in the terms of the contract if one exists. When responding to advertisements for a specific post, these details should be clarified before accepting the position. Information on necessary immunisations, health precautions and so on is now readily available and the World Health Organization (WHO) produce data on this for travellers.

However, the issue that is not easy to deal with is the actual feelings and psychological practicalities of working in another culture. Adaptation to working in a different country with different customs, beliefs and traditions can be difficult. A great deal of illness can result from the stress of working in such conditions. Speaking to and if possible spending some time with someone who has worked in the same area can be very helpful and rewarding. However, one difficulty with this is that often one can not tell how well one will cope in a given situation at any given time. The factors which help adaptation are different in every situation. Experience of working in different cultures and countries can help but each situation is new and must be seen as such. Increasingly, organisations are providing courses or workshops for health workers who would like to consider this work, to help explore some of these issues before making a definite decision. The International Health Exchange in the UK and the International Red Cross are two such organisations and they provide excellent courses for those intending to work internationally and those wishing to consider it. Information on such courses is often available in quality primary or international health care journals. Also there is an increase in the number of university programmes that include elective periods where a short time can be spent in another country undertaking a small project or work experience.

One factor which can influence adaptation to working in another country is careful consideration of the motives for undertaking this type of work. More research and study is still required on how and why midwives choose to work in another country, in order to help identify factors which assist with their adequate preparation. On the whole, as with all career choices, there are varied and complex reasons why someone would choose this particular path. Some find themselves in a certain place at a certain time, able and willing to respond to opportunities as they are presented. Others have a burning desire to travel and experience the wider world; that is to say, they have moral, humanitarian, personal or family reasons for choosing this particular professional path. Whatever the reasons, it is the responsibility of each midwife to explore carefully the personal motives for choosing this type of work.

There is no one valid reason, only an issue of individual choice. However, the midwife must apply a certain level of objectivity to ensure the right choice is being made about the suitability, type and place of work that is appropriate. It is all too easy to become quickly disillusioned if the main motive for seeking this type of work was travel, only to find that the project or place chosen makes travel difficult or impossible.

Clarification of motives is also helpful when faced with unfamiliar, frustrating or difficult situations. Working in another country, in a culture that is unfamiliar, is very different from visiting on holiday or for pleasure or interest. However, such work does have its rewards. It can help to develop a wider view of midwifery, motherhood and health. It often assists with reflection by allowing the opportunity to view one's own practice through different eyes. Most midwives who have done such work feel that it allows them to develop greater flexibility, innovations and self-confidence. Of course, much will depend upon the type of work undertaken but the advantages and the friendships that develop whilst undertaking such work often outweigh the difficulties.

Working in a different culture

Changes in midwifery practice may well foster an individual woman-centred approach to care and therefore assist midwives to function in different cultures. As midwives develop models to provide woman-centred care rather than set models of care, women's identity and differences are being acknowledged in both theory and practice. In providing effective woman-centred care, midwives must engage in and develop knowledge of, and respect for, each woman's own cultural identity. Central to all quality care and practice is the need to be culturally appropriate and culturally sensitive.

Providing culturally sensitive care

The requirement to provide culturally sensitive care is embodied in the International Code of Ethics for Midwives (ICM 1993). Midwives know from practice and experience that the women and families they meet are all individuals with individual needs. For convenience, however, they tend to divide them into different groupings such as working class, middle class, northerners, southerners, westerners, white collar workers, rural, urban, city dwellers, travellers, black, Hispanic, Asian or by using some other descriptor. Most of these are labels borrowed from social science and classification of occupations or ethnic origin. However, reference to 'working class', for example, relates not only to occupation, for clearly most people work. These labels usually refer to a set of characteristics and assumptions made about people. These characteristics and assumptions describe a set of stereotyped behaviours associated with certain groups. They really refer more to an individual's culture than to any occupation, economic status or ethnic origin. Whilst labels are useful, they can lead to provision of care being based on the assumptions and stereotyping, which can lead rapidly to either overt or covert discrimination especially where culture becomes confused with ethnicity.

Culture is not static. It cannot be taken out and viewed from all angles. The words or labels needed to describe what is meant by culture simply do not exist. Cultural theorists describe culture as a dynamic process, with families, individuals and events all having an effect and creating a culture (Jenks 1993). Therefore, because it constantly changes, labels are difficult to use. The particular characteristics and assumptions are specific to a given time and place and do not easily translate through history or across countries, continents or even genders. Indeed it would seem that to require such labels is in itself a cultural acquisition. People in the western hemisphere have developed a particularly dualist thought process; they think in terms of opposites and definitives and so are more comfortable with stereotypes and labels. Some other cultures only require notions of lineage or have a more fluid or abstract view of the world, making labels unnecessary or meaningless.

Culturally sensitive care, then, is care which makes a positive acknowledgement that each woman belongs to a family located within a particular society and culture at a particular time. The midwife should not base the provision of care on assumptions of what the woman will want or what information she or her family might require. Neither can assumptions be made about the particular practices, superstitions and beliefs that may be operating in that family. All of these require careful and sensitive exploration with each woman and family.

Development of appropriate culturally sensitive care

The first essential to the development of culturally sensitive care is to listen to women, as often cultural traditions and beliefs are vocalised in particular practices or taboos. Sometimes the reasons for these beliefs or practices are lost in time and history and are too readily dismissed, especially by scientifically minded practitioners with their own professional cultural beliefs. In some countries, particularly in Asia, the cultural beliefs and taboos surrounding pregnancy and birth can make this particularly difficult. Frequently, myths and beliefs are not spoken about directly, for fear of evoking bad spirits or bringing bad luck. Just to

acknowledge the pregnancy, for example, might be viewed as dangerous. This in turn raises obstacles to the receipt of any midwifery care. For example, how can the midwife encourage antenatal care, promote health in pregnancy, or even advise on planned pregnancies in cultures where to do so is unacceptable, unless care is delivered under another guise?

In circumstances outlined above, the only way forward is to work with the local community, especially women's groups and community leaders. Where such leaders are usually men, this can raise other gender-laden issues. For the midwife there may be tensions in how to work with or through male leaders in a way that will empower women. Some gender training or gender sensitivity courses may help and it is essential first to identify, together with the women, any existing strategies. Assisting the male leaders and the community to consider practices and beliefs and the effects that these may have on childbearing women is possible and where this approach has been used it has had positive results.

The important point to remember is that notions of empowerment are also culturally bound. Women from different cultures have different ideas about what they see as empowerment (Chitnis 1988, Collins 1994, Dawit & Busia 1995). Given the opportunity, women from all cultures have clear ideas about what they think would assist them to give birth in a way that is safe and yet culturally sensitive and therefore acceptable to them. The ICM Code of Ethics states that: 'Midwives work with women, supporting their rights to participate actively in decisions about their care, and empowering women to speak for themselves on issues affecting the health of women and their families in their culture or society' (ICM 1993). Adopting a participatory approach to planning, delivering and evaluating care is a powerful tool to assist midwives to provide effective and culturally appropriate care.

Use of appropriate technology

In addition to adopting the right approach, midwives need to concern themselves with the use of appropriate technology. Faced with vast increases in technology, careful consideration is necessary when debating the use of appropriate technology for pregnancy, childbirth and the puerperium. For example, it is at present not considered essential to give iron supplementation routinely to pregnant women in well-nourished populations. However, haemorrhage before, during and after birth remains the major cause of death in countries with poor nutrition, social deprivation and poor health facilities (Royston & Armstrong 1989). In these situations iron supplementation becomes essential. Faced with high maternal mortality and high levels of under-nutrition, it is clearly appropriate to have a protocol that promotes routine iron supplementation to all pregnant women as one of a series of measures to combat high levels of anaemia due to malnutrition.

In more recent years, there is concern about training doctors to undertake surgical procedures such as caesarean sections, without simultaneously providing good anaesthetics and analgesia, hygiene and sanitation for hospitals that offer these facilities. This is not to say such training should not take place. Clearly the facts show that too many women still die because of lack of appropriate emergency obstetric care, lack of equipment or lack of appropriately skilled staff to use the equipment (WHO 1991a). However, importing systems and tools that do not get appropriately adapted can adversely affect the quality of care.

Whilst in themselves the tools may be good, if they are not adapted to meet the cultural complexity of the importing country they may be ineffective or used in an inappropriate way. For example, there is almost universal acceptance that the partograph is a useful and effective tool, yet it is not without its difficulties. For midwives working in a country or a culture where the counting of time is not in units of minutes or hours, the idea of charting events on a graph can be very difficult.

There has been some work in simplifying the partograph for use by traditional birth attendants (TBAs) with limited literacy skills. However, work is ongoing to simplify the tool for use by those who have conceptual difficulty with time or graphic displays of information. Unless local midwives and doctors have culturally appropriate tools to help them understand and interpret the use of the partograph correctly, there may be unnecessary and often unsafe caesarean sections being performed. In this case the tool will not assist women, but in some cases may cause women to face a greater risk than they would have without the technology.

Midwives working in an international arena, therefore, need to ensure that the technology they take with them to other countries is appropriate and that correct training is provided for its implementation and use.

Beware the 'expert'

Finally, it is also important to acknowledge that midwives have their own professional culture that can interfere with the provision of culturally sensitive care, owing to the particular position they hold as professionals or 'experts'. This is problematic for midwives. In an analysis by DeVries (1996), comparing the status of midwives in different countries, the recurrent theme was the attempts to legitimise midwifery through the desire to make the practice of midwifery 'professional' or claims that it is. DeVries argues that this could be disastrous, not only for women but for the survival of the art and science of midwifery. Salvage (1985) makes a similar point when warning all nurses and midwives about the problems of being too 'professionalised'. Salvage alleges that as nurses and midwives become 'professionalised' they are more likely to identify with the doctors than with ancillary staff, patients (women) and relatives. For midwives this means forgetting that they should be 'with' women. For this reason midwives would do well to consider carefully DeVries' warning that: 'in order to survive midwives must ask: survive for whom? For the good of the profession? For their own good as practitioners? Or for the health of the women and babies they serve?' (DeVries 1996, p. 172).

THE ROLE OF THE CONSULTANT MIDWIFE

Whilst the above is an issue of concern for all midwives, for those working as international midwifery consultants or expatriate project workers, trainers or managers, it is particularly problematic. The temptation to allow oneself to be seen as an 'expert' in these situations is even greater. In the eyes of the community, women and other midwives, there is the likelihood of being perceived as identifying with the project managers, donors and politicians, rather than with the local midwives and women. The issue applies to all who work in the field, regardless of cultural or educational background or even of the position and status or experience of the midwife.

It is particularly problematic when working in countries that do not have recent experience of personal autonomy or personal responsibility. Midwives in countries that have a particular political tradition of being controlled from the centre are more familiar at looking towards those in power or to 'experts' to dictate the actual activities of care provided. They are not familiar with democracy or participation in decision-making and may feel slightly afraid and unsure when introduced to such approaches.

It is important for the consultant to avoid falling into the trap of being seen as the person who knows and who will tell them what or how something needs to be done. For the consultant faced with enthusiastic individuals eager for change, tight work schedules, needs that often far outweigh resources and/or expectations that he or she will be able to sort out the problems, it is not always easy to hold firm to facilitation skills and participatory approaches to decision-making. In these situations, advocacy can easily stray into paternalism (or maternalism) and then only the voice of the 'expert' midwife is heard. The midwife's role is always to encourage women to find their own voice and always to ensure that it is the women's voice that is being heard. The key skills for the consultant midwife are listening, supporting and participating in the daily lives of the women they work with.

The midwife working as a consultant in whatever field or country needs patience, humility, a good sense of humour and a great deal of self-determination and self-esteem to carry the role effectively. The role of the consultant can be lonely; therefore anyone taking it on should also ensure that he or she has a good personal support system from family, friends or colleagues back home.

INTERNATIONAL ISSUES

International Confederation of Midwives (ICM)

The International Confederation of Midwives (ICM) is now one of the foremost actors in the global arena working to improve maternity services through the empowering of midwives and promotion of good practice. The ICM, a non-governmental organisation (NGO), came into being in 1919 as the International Midwives' Union. The purpose was 'improving the services available to childbearing women through campaigning for a stronger, better educated and properly regulated midwifery profession' (ICM 1994, p. 1). In the early 1960s the ICM gained accreditation by the United Nations (UN). It has more than 75 member associations that cover approximately 66 countries. However, through its extensive networks, it tries to collect information on and unite midwives from all countries of the world.

The ICM has a small but friendly office situated in London, England, and welcomes both visitors and enquiries from midwives and midwifery organisations from anywhere in the world. Information on the history of the ICM, along with other information and leaflets, is obtainable from ICM, 10 Barley Mow Passage, Chiswick, London W4 4PH. ICM newsletters are free to associations, but available to individuals on payment of a modest subscription.

In recent years, the ICM has been proactive in a variety of global initiatives. By working collaboratively with other agencies it has contributed to the increasing acceptance of the midwife as the key provider of quality maternity care. Working with WHO and the International Federation of Gynaecologists and Obstetricians (FIGO) they developed the International Definition of the Midwife (first devised in 1966, the latest revision being in 1992); see Chapter 1.

ICM accomplishments

Other achievements of the ICM include the development of the International Code of Ethics (ICM 1993) and the instituting and coordination of the International Day of The Midwife (annually on 5 May). Whilst each country and midwifery organisation may choose to devise their own celebrations, ICM Board draw up the major themes. The intention is to assist midwives and midwifery associations to unite under a central banner to promote the role and responsibilities of the midwife under a specific theme. Recent themes have included Safe Motherhood, Equity for Women and The Midwife as the Key Health Promoter.

Perhaps one of the most rewarding accomplishments of the ICM is the bringing together of groups of midwives from different countries for workshops, seminars and the triennial congress. The meetings, particularly the triennial congresses, are valuable not only for allowing midwives internationally to meet, debate and network, but have been a useful vehicle for promoting midwives and midwifery in the host country. The opening ceremony of the Triennial International Congress with midwives dressed in their national costumes remains a favourite and moving spectacle for all who attend.

The pre-Congress workshops have also been extremely beneficial. The action orientation of these workshops has allowed midwives from a variety of countries to develop plans and activities for improving the midwifery services to women nationally and globally. The 1990 Congress in Kobe, Japan took as its theme Midwifery Education for Safe Motherhood and it was at the pre-Congress workshop that the *Midwifery Modules for Safe Motherhood* (WHO 1996a) were first formulated. In 1993, in Vancouver, Canada, the pre-Congress workshop theme was Midwifery Practice: Measuring, Developing and Mobilising Quality Care and in 1996 in Oslo, Norway, preparing National Safe Motherhood plans was the focus of attention. The Oslo pre-Congress workshops offered for the first time a workshop for the preparation of midwifery consultants. This pre-Congress activity ran parallel to and interacted with the national planning workshop. The Oslo Congress was also significant for the launch of the *Midwifery Modules for Safe Motherhood.*

The ICM has been an active participant and influence on the global Safe Motherhood Initiative (SMI) from the outset in Nairobi in 1987. The Confederation endeavours to continue with this important activity by working with WHO, UNICEF and other agencies in addition to many more which seek to promote and assist the development of midwifery and midwifery organisations.

Safe Motherhood Initiative

The global SMI was officially launched in Nairobi in February 1987. The global programme is supported by ICM, WHO, UNICEF, World Bank and many more NGOs, associations and bilateral aid agencies.

The initial aim of SMI was to achieve a reduction in the global number of maternal deaths. The target was to reduce maternal deaths by 50% by the year 2000. A more specific objective was to develop strategies that enable women to have more control over their lives. They should be able to choose if and when they become pregnant. If they choose to become pregnant, there should be easy access to the appropriate support, education, advice and services. The ultimate aim is to enable women and their babies to survive unharmed, both physically and psychologically.

There are various strategies employed. These include ensuring access to safe water, culturally appropriate family planning services, including advice and methods, and free prenatal, intranatal and postnatal care and services. Other strategies include economic support through women's income-generating projects or savings schemes, education of the girl child and women and, increasingly, gender training for both men and women. The latter will help address the inequalities in health and provision. Of equal importance is the access to reliable immunisation programmes, a trained attendant at delivery and emergency obstetric care and services (EOC). Maine (1990) has outlined the need for EOC to be available near to where the birth occurs.

EOC is the term used for the obstetric interventions and services required to meet unpredictable occurrences during pregnancy and labour. The necessity for EOC is demonstrated by the numerous reports which show that such occurrences exist even in groups of persons previously identified as low risk. The previous Risk Approach, whereby

> **Box 4.1** Levels of emergency obstetric care and services (EOC)
>
> **1st level**
> Primary level services based in the community. These should provide for control of haemorrhage, control of sepsis, family planning and intrapartum care which may include vacuum extraction in some countries with very rural peripheral community services.
>
> **2nd level**
> District services. This is the first referral level. Such facilities should be able to offer full prenatal and intra-natal care, control of eclamptic fits, minor obstetric operations, forceps deliveries, vacuum extraction and blood transfusion.
>
> **3rd level**
> Tertiary level or more commonly the second referral level. These facilities offer full comprehensive care to include caesarean sections and blood banking facilities.

pregnant women who were identified as having risk factors and were provided with specialist obstetric care, has received a great deal of criticism in regard to the lack of specificity, sensitivity and predictability and is being replaced by EOC.

WHO define three levels of EOC (Box 4.1).

Although the initial focus of SMI was on maternal mortality, in recent years the focus has shifted slightly and is now on women's health and reproductive health for all, especially adolescents. Today, there is also concern for morbidity as well as mortality. Recent studies in India and Bangladesh give morbidity rates as high as 15 to 16 times that of mortality rates (Goodburn 1995). A great deal of the morbidity was due to unsafe and unhygienic practices based on superstitions and taboos such as putting mustard oil into the vagina to try to hasten cervical dilatation and ensure a speedy exit through the birth canal, or use of excessive fundal pressure to deliver the placenta in the belief that it is the placenta which harbours or attracts the evil spirits.

WHO has established a Safe Motherhood unit to coordinate and evaluate all the Safe Motherhood programmes. The unit does include a midwife. A free newsletter is available containing articles and up-to-date information from around the world on Safe Motherhood programmes, research, events and resources. This, along with other documents

related to Safe Motherhood, is obtainable from WHO in Geneva. Many of the documents and reports are free (no cost), particularly for developing countries. For further information write to Maternal and Newborn Health/Safe Motherhood Unit, Family and Reproductive Health, World Health Organization, 1211 Geneva 27, Switzerland.

Major global actions under the Safe Motherhood banner

• 1987 The Safe Motherhood Initiative was launched in Nairobi.

• 1989 The first global study on maternal mortality was published (Royston & Armstrong 1989) and the World Health Organization's global factbook on maternal mortality (WHO 1991b). The factbook is a compendium of data collected from all over the world. Both are available from WHO, Geneva.

• 1987 The partograph, a tool for effective monitoring of labour, was launched. In 1990 to 1991 a large multicentre trial was undertaken to review the effectiveness of this tool, with reasonably positive results. The report concluded that the tool had potential benefits for the timely management of prolonged labour (WHO 1994a)

• 1990 The ICM Triennial Congress was preceded by a workshop to discuss Midwifery Education For Safe Motherhood. The results of the pre-Congress workshop were recommendations for action to strengthen the curriculum of midwives (WHO/UNICEF/ICM 1991). This report recommended making the curriculum more community-based and including management of selected obstetric emergencies.

• 1994 WHO produced the *Mother–Baby Package: a Practical Guide to Implementing Safe Motherhood in Countries* (WHO 1994b). In this package it is recognised that the key to successful Safe Motherhood is 'appropriately trained midwifery personnel living and working in the community'. The package makes strong recommendations for countries to give priority to developing the midwifery skills of their health personnel, especially those providing community-based care. The recommendations included strengthening of midwifery skills in all aspects of maternity care provision. Importantly these skills must include the immediate management of selected obstetric emergencies such as haemorrhage, prolonged and obstructed labour, puerperal sepsis and hypertension in pregnancy. They also detail the minimum package for basic maternity care, both in terms of what services should be available and the requisite equipment.

• 1996 saw the launch of the WHO *Midwifery Education Modules For Safe Motherhood* (WHO 1996a). There are five modules and these include teachers' and students' notes. Each module deals with a specific aspect of maternal mortality. There is one on the community which discusses how to understand the community, how to measure maternal mortality and how to work with the community to devise culturally and locally applicable solutions to preventing maternal mortality. The other four modules deal with the four major causes of maternal mortality, obstructed labour, pre-eclampsia and eclampsia, postpartum haemorrhage and puerperal sepsis. They are complete training packs and include games, puzzles and quizzes to help both the teacher and the student. They have been thoroughly field tested in more than one country and are available free from WHO, Geneva.

• 1996 WHO held a technical working group on Normal Delivery. This was a working group of internationally credible obstetricians and midwives who together reviewed the evidence for all the current practices and interventions used throughout the world in caring for women having a normal delivery. They have concluded that there are many practices for which there is now sufficient scientific evidence to demonstrate that they are harmful and should be abandoned. These include delivery in the lithotomy position, liberal use of episiotomy, routine perineal shave and enemas and many more. There is also a list of interventions for which scientific evidence is available and supports both the use and promotion of these interventions. These include the provision of continuity of care, making care more humanistic, helping the woman to remain as mobile as possible during labour and allowing the woman to adopt the position of her choice during delivery (WHO 1996b). This document along with other Safe Motherhood documents is available from WHO, Geneva.

Other global events significant to Safe Motherhood

• 1990 saw global action towards improving the health and well-being of children and the international congress, World Summit on the Health of the Child. This summit put the child on the world's agenda (UNICEF 1990). At the UN General Assembly in 1990, the Convention on the Rights of the Child (UN 1990) entered into international law. Both at the World Summit and by signing The Convention on the Rights of the Child, governments agreed that they would take steps to increase the health of children throughout the world. Article 6, which deals with survival and development, lays down the need for effective prenatal care and the right to have the delivery conducted by appropriately trained health personnel. Other articles deal with non-discrimination (effectively outlawing practices such as gender selection, female fetocide and discriminatory feeding practices based on gender), and the best interest of the child, separation from the family and family reunification. By 1997, The Convention on the Rights of the Child had been ratified by all members of the UN, except for Cook Islands, Oman, Somalia, Switzerland, the United Arab Emirates and the United States (UNICEF 1997a).

• 1993 The UNICEF annual report on *The Progress Of Nations* (UNICEF 1993) charting the progress to date of achieving 'Health For All by the Year 2000' reported explicit concern that the targets set in Alma Ata (now Almaty) in 1976 would not be met by the year 2000. Whilst there had been concern from many quarters, this publication did act to prompt some countries like Bangladesh into making different plans.

• 1994 and 1995 Many interesting conferences were held including the International Conference on Population and Developments in Cairo 1994, the World Summit for Social Democracy, Copenhagen 1995 and the Fourth World Conference on Women in Beijing 1995. They all had Safe Motherhood as an integral issue. At all these conferences, governments from all over the world declared an intent to improve the health of women. This included provision for strengthening the health services to women, particularly in and around childbirth.

One recent and important initiative, which has helped focus global attention on the continuing need to develop Safe Motherhood programmes, has been the WHO and UNICEF survey on the 1990 maternal mortality figures (WHO 1996c). The revised estimates for 1990 show the figures for maternal mortality to have been drastically underestimated in some countries. Globally, estimates suggest that there were some 8000 more deaths than was initially thought. Further, it demonstrated that the anticipated decline in maternal mortality was not occurring at the rate required to reach the year 2000 target. In some countries there had been either a levelling off, or even a rise. This is of concern to all involved in Safe Motherhood. It underlines the fact that there is no room for complacency in the attempts to make motherhood safer, if not completely safe. Therefore, the training of health personnel in effective midwifery skills is an urgent, continuing and priority need.

Safe Motherhood, then, is not just about ensuring that women do not die in childbirth. It is about empowering women to take control over their own bodies to enable them to achieve optimum health. This must include being empowered to make effective and informed choices about if and when they will embark upon pregnancy. If they choose to become pregnant, then they should have access to all services, education and support (including community support) needed to achieve a healthy outcome. This includes being assured that the child can reach healthy adult maturity, for without this the pressures on women to conceive many babies will not reduce and family planning strategies will be impeded.

The strategies required to achieve all of these will vary from country to country. The strategies are as much, or more, concerned with the sociological perspectives of women's health, as they are with the provision of effective health services. As Thompson & Bennett (1996) outline in their pre-Congress paper, the provision and access to health care has only a small effect on the overall

determinants for the health of women. It would appear that by far the most important factors for improving women's health are changes in the cultural practices, eliminating gender inequalities and improving the environment in which the woman lives, which includes elimination of poverty and improved nutrition. This inevitably means that in addition to developing appropriate technical midwifery skills, midwives must also involve themselves in political action to address these issues which have a direct effect on improving women's health.

The role of the midwife in Safe Motherhood

There have been many reports, symposia, conferences, events, books and articles on the subject of the Safe Motherhood Initiative and safe motherhood programmes. What all midwives must remember is that safe(r) motherhood, in its broadest and narrowest sense, is still not an option for many thousands of women in the world. Whilst women in highly industrialised countries are subject to a different lack of control over their own bodies than women in developing or transitional market economy countries, both are denied their rights. They are denied the right to choose and denied their right to exercise control over their own birth processes. Some western countries are making progress in this field. New Zealand is perhaps in the forefront of ensuring that women have the right to choose what type of assistance they want during pregnancy and childbirth and where and when they want it. The UK is another, with its Changing Childbirth initiative (DH 1993). Other countries are developing similar initiatives and are trying to give choice to women for care in pregnancy and birth. However, in too many countries the health systems, structures and medicalisation militate against effective implementation of safe motherhood programmes. For this reason, midwives must become more politically active and learn to relate to, work with and seek to influence the leaders and major decision-makers, both at the local and national level.

It is with humility that midwives can boast that throughout the Safe Motherhood Initiative, in many countries they have played and continue to play a pivotal role in helping achieve the goals of SMI; yet more is still required.

Breast feeding and Baby Friendly Hospital Initiative (BFHI)

The Baby Friendly Hospital Initiative (BFHI) is driven by UNICEF and WHO and is now considered to be one of the most effective mechanisms for creating strong political commitment to breast feeding. Unfortunately and despite scientific evidence showing the importance of breast feeding for maternal, infant and child health, global indicators demonstrate that the decline of breast feeding in the 1950s and the trend towards bottle feeding has continued in the 1990s (Saadeh 1993). This is despite the research which supports the promotion of exclusive breast feeding in the first 4–6 months, particularly for the control of diarrhoeal disease and upper respiratory tract infections. Following a review of the then available scientific evidence Saadeh (1993) concludes that: 'the results showed that breastfeeding can save more infant lives and prevent more morbidity than any other intervention strategy' (p. 2).

The BFHI was launched in 1991 following the joint WHO/UNICEF statement on breast feeding in 1989, which outlined the 'Ten Steps to Successful Breastfeeding' (WHO/UNICEF 1989). The 'Ten Steps' (see Ch. 36) have become the management tool and criteria for awarding BFHI status. UNICEF now provides a training package for hospitals who wish to work towards the award of the status 'Baby-Friendly Hospital'. WHO also provides a similar course for breast feeding counselling. Both courses have been implemented in a growing number of countries, with some countries incorporating them into their own national breast feeding programmes.

Difficulties to be overcome

Despite these global initiatives, the lack of exclusive breast feeding for 4–6 months and the practice of discarding the colostrum remain the two major difficulties to be overcome in many countries. Very often such practices, influenced by strong cultural superstitions and belief systems, cannot be overcome by simply presenting mothers with scientific evidence. A recent report suggests that the promotion of exclusive breast feeding is still being hampered by inappropriate advertising and violations of the International Code of Marketing Breast-milk Substitutes (UNICEF 1997b). The aim of the code is to eliminate inappropriate marketing of breast milk substitutes (WHO 1981). Despite almost universal agreement that it is unacceptable and immoral to import and promote formula feed to countries where the water supply is not safe, violations of the code continue. The International Baby Food Action Network (IBFAN) and others seek to promote and protect as well as to identify violations of the International Code of Marketing of Breast-milk Substitutes.

INTERNATIONAL AGENDAS

Midwifery identities

It would appear that the global concerns of midwives and the constraints they face have changed little since Kwast & Bentley's (1991) paper was presented at the ICM pre-Congress workshop in 1990. In their paper they present a view of the constraints and problems facing midwives worldwide, which outlines both the shortage and maldistribution of midwives and the economic and training problems facing midwifery in many countries.

Midwives need specific policies and legislation to practise

One of the most common and urgent needs facing midwives in many countries is the need for specific (if not separate) policies and legislation to enable them to practise. Where separate policies and practices for midwifery are not identified, midwives can be hampered if they have to practise under nursing protocols and legislation. For example, many of the procedures the midwife requires in order to practise essential life-saving skills, as identified in the WHO *Mother–Baby Package* (WHO 1994b), are not always allowed under nursing policies or legislation.

By far the most common and continuing issue that faces midwives internationally is their right to practise. The manifestations of this issue will vary depending on the country concerned. For many, the domination of the medical profession will be the most difficult barrier to overcome. It is heartening to read, for example, that as far back as 1985 WHO and some obstetricians recognised the pivotal role of the midwife in providing quality maternity care (Wagner 1994). However, too often the relationship between the two professions remains contentious and leads to the fragmentation of care and services for women and babies. The principle of providing holistic care to mothers and babies as a unit is still more observed in rhetoric than practice in many countries. For many countries, especially in Russia and the whole eastern bloc, maternity services for pregnancy and childbirth are still dominated by medical practice with almost 100% of all deliveries taking place in a hospital environment under medical supervision. Indeed in some of these countries midwives are faced with falsifying records to indicate that the birth was conducted by a medical officer when in fact it was a midwife who conducted the delivery.

In addition, the unique nature of midwifery practice as separate and distinct from nursing is still not universally accepted. In countries such as many in Africa there are logical and rational reasons for having nurse–midwives and midwifery can appropriately be a qualification obtained after training as a nurse, especially where the nurse–midwife may be the only health care person available in a rural setting. Yet even in these situations there are still issues which must be addressed. The two professions have a distinctive, if overlapping, body of knowledge and practice. They both need valuing for their individual contribution to a nation's health, and legislation and structures must reflect this. The legislation must be sensitive to the particular country situation yet still allow the midwife to undertake all the skills necessary for saving life. Licence to practice is an issue of safeguarding the public and therefore a matter for government concern; so government must ensure that the professional standards remain central. Governance must not be confused with political interference or dominance in the determination of professional standards. It is the responsibility of governments to ensure that frameworks exist

which will ensure that individual health practitioners have appropriate education and supervision to enable them to fulfil their individual functions. For example, where trained TBAs are considered essential to fulfil a need in the country, their role should be regarded as integral to the rest of the maternity service provision and not seen as something outside the formal services or replacing the need for sufficient numbers of appropriately qualified midwives. It is also important to ensure that where TBAs are used they are adequately prepared for their role and are properly supervised and encouraged to work closely with qualified midwives. Without this, the TBA will always remain outside the formal health structures and will be vulnerable and may not be valued for her expertise. More importantly she may feel unable or unwilling to seek appropriate help if and when it is required. Questions such as whether there is a place in modern midwifery for such workers or whether the TBA should be a support worker for the trained midwife, have not yet been resolved in many countries.

Education of midwives

The education of midwives is yet another matter of debate and concern in many countries, for a variety of reasons. As previously stated, in some countries the preparation of midwives may follow on from nursing. There are a number of disadvantages to this, particularly where nursing does not have a sufficiently strong public health basis. The arguments for and against midwifery following nursing will depend on the individual country. However, it is useful to consider one or two of the more common reasons. The midwifery-following-nursing model can result in midwifery being seen as an adjunct to nursing. The consequence in some countries is that midwifery is afforded very little time within the curriculum, as happens in Japan, where the midwifery component only lasts 6 months. It may also lead to fragmentation of care between an institutionalised intrapartum service and separate community-based prenatal care. Role confusion can occur in some countries where the prenatal services are provided by community health workers or public health workers, completely separately from midwives who offer intranatal care. Often these workers have minimal midwifery input into their curriculum, as occurs in the Family Welfare Visitors programme in Bangladesh (M. Leppard, personal communication, 1993).

Training must be skills based. Midwifery is essentially a practical profession where practice is underpinned by evidence and sound practical application. The skills required by the midwife may vary slightly from country to country depending on the specific needs of the country. These skills may include being able to competently undertake a manual removal of the placenta or give intravenous injections of an oxytocic drug for control of postpartum haemorrhage. However, even without drugs, the midwife may find herself in a situation where her knowledge and skills alone can save the woman's life. Faced with a woman having a severe haemorrhage after delivery, the competent midwife, if trained correctly, should be able to apply aortic pressure. This is where the midwife using her clasped hand exerts downward pressure on the abdominal aorta to reduce flow of blood to the uterus (Fig. 4.1). The correct application of aortic pressure may be the only option available for a midwife to stem the flow of the haemorrhage until medical assistance is available. Training for these and other life-saving skills must focus on achieving competence. Very often in some countries, whilst the theoretical knowledge may be taught well in the initial programmes, there is little or no opportunity to practise the skills in the clinical situation. Frequently the trainers themselves may lack confidence and competence in these skills.

Direct entry programmes. With the above in mind, many countries such as the USA and Canada are exploring direct entry into midwifery. Direct entry programmes are established in some countries such as France, the UK and Holland. This, some people feel, would allow more appropriate programmes based on a *fitness for purpose* model. The fitness for purpose approach to curriculum planning (Fig. 4.2) looks at the required competencies of a midwife for that particular situation or country. From this, a programme is then devised which demonstrates how the outcomes and the necessary skills, knowledge and attitudes to practise competently will be met. These should be pertinent to the country in which the training takes place and conform to the international definition

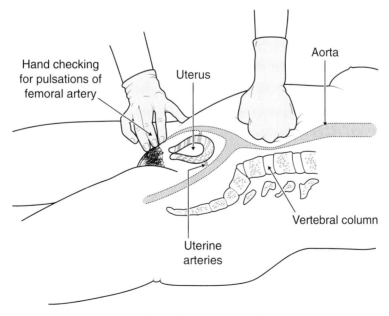

Fig. 4.1 Aortic compression (based on WHO 1996a).

**Factors influencing
the curriculum**

**Outcomes of a
fitness-for-purpose curriculum**

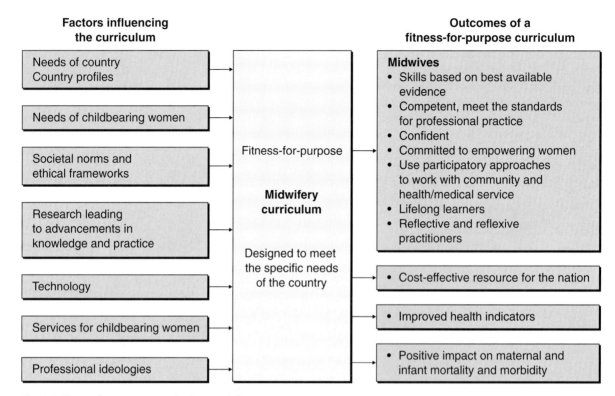

Fig. 4.2 Fitness-for-purpose curriculum model.

of the midwife (WHO/FIGO/ICM 1992). WHO, in the *Mother–Baby Package*, suggests that countries with high maternal and infant mortality rates must look at improving midwifery skills as a matter of urgency (WHO 1994b). Attempts are being made to strengthen the skills of midwives in many countries. However, this is complicated by the fact that identification of who is a midwife is not always easy. In a recent survey, across the 10 countries that make up the WHO South-East Asia Region, there are approximately 18 different categories of worker providing maternity services, of which only seven have midwife in their job title (WHO/ SEARO 1996). Some, such as the border midwives in Bhutan, have only 3 months' training in midwifery and provide delivery-only care.

One of the main difficulties facing the preparation of midwives is the dependence upon the country having sufficient appropriately trained midwife teachers. Many countries, including some European countries such as Germany, are without

a standardised approved preparation for their midwife teachers. It was partly for this reason that the WHO funded the development of the *Midwifery Modules for Safe Motherhood* (WHO 1996a). Also, the omission of research from the curriculum, as has happened in many well-established midwifery programmes, Sweden being one, is detrimental to the preparation of critically thinking midwives. Midwives must be able to be both proactive and responsive to the needs of individual mothers and babies. Many countries are now addressing these deficiencies, but some are being hampered by medical, particularly obstetric and paediatric, domination. Such medical dominance makes undertaking appropriate midwifery research problematic. Without midwives who are active researchers, not simply research assistants or data gatherers for medical research but midwives engaged upon midwifery research, it is difficult to build up sufficient evidence-based practice. Therefore it is essential that some midwives become researchers as well as research users. It is imperative that each country has a mechanism by which some midwives are able to receive adequate preparation as researchers to ensure that country-specific midwifery research is carried out. Such research is not only essential for evidence-based practice but is needed by governments and other decision-makers to allow them to improve their maternity services.

Employment and the working environment

Other problems that face many midwives worldwide include issues surrounding employment and the environments in which they work. Changes such as the rise in human immunodeficiency virus (HIV) and increasing migration to city dwellings (bringing with it the demise of family support networks for childbearing women), will require different approaches to the provision of maternity services. Mass urbanisation, with the results of overcrowding, increased poverty and deprivation often leading to higher crime and violence, has resulted in an increased concern for the safety of midwives at work. Even in some western countries, midwives fear for their own safety and are reluctant to go out to labouring women at night without some form of security cover.

These demographic changes also bring with them an explosion of demands on the health services. The resulting economic burden laid on communities and countries in these circumstances means adequate remuneration is increasingly an issue for many midwives. This is not only in terms of monetary rewards because hospital budgets cannot match the huge demands on the services and sometimes are unable to pay their workers' salaries, but also in terms of reduced opportunities and restrictions on practice. South Africa is only one country faced with such issues. Since the move to free health care following the political changes that marked the end of the apartheid years and coupled with the effects of mass urbanisation, South Africa is facing huge problems in all of its public services. These problems include struggling with an overstretched health service where demand exceeds hospital and district budgets. Therefore midwives are being faced with long periods without a salary and must work in overcrowded and unsatisfactory environments.

Other countries, like Brazil, face similar problems to those in South Africa. In these situations, rural communities also suffer as they too become impoverished. Government services become concentrated on urban populations with rural families being unable to afford private health care. Other issues also face midwives in the rural areas such as inadequate infrastructure, housing, transport and education, which can result in midwives with families not wishing to work in these communities.

Finally, in many countries health service funding often fails to take into account remuneration for community practice, payments being based on formal structured care from hospitals or health centres. In all of these situations, community services and the setting up of independent community practice become difficult and devalued. Even some western countries, such as the UK, some states in the USA and Canada and Norway are facing similar problems with independent midwifery. In the more industrialised countries, however, independent practice is proving difficult due to insurance companies not wishing to pay for this type of service for a variety of reasons. Often the reason relates to the close association with the medical profession who are generally hostile and antagonistic to midwifery-only care. As funding of health care becomes increasingly reliant on insurance schemes, as appears to be happening in many countries, this is likely to become an increasing problem.

The success of the midwives in the Netherlands and the New Zealand midwives' initiatives to have their services recognised as a legitimate option for pregnant women offer hope. However, these successes were as a result of hard-fought battles. In the Netherlands two out of three babies are now born with midwifery-only care (Smulders & Limburg 1995), but the medical profession continues to try to gain control by establishing criteria for women who in their opinion require hospital care for birth. In New Zealand, the midwives' fight to have the Nurses' Amendment Act passed in 1990 was not without fierce opposition (Donley 1995). In each case, although circumstances may be different, the force of medical opposition was enormous and the midwifery profession had to unite and work in partnership with women to achieve success. In both accounts the force of the women's support was paramount. This can only be achieved if women are free and able to offer this support; free in that they are not excessively burdened with malnutrition, ill health and poverty. Unfortunately in some countries many women are still being denied such freedom.

Increasingly, turbulence, war and political upheaval are posing new problems for midwifery. The recent stories that have emerged from Rwanda and former Yugoslavia of the attempts to carry out what has become termed ethnic cleansing give graphic testimony to the impact such upheaval causes to women. Violence against women is more than ever on the international agenda, despite the *UN Convention on the Elimination of All Forms of Discrimination Against Women* (UN 1979) and the *Declaration on Violence Against Women* (UN 1993).

Female genital mutilation is still a concern in many countries, as is the damage inflicted on women as a result of lack of appropriate health care in pregnancy and childbirth. Morbidity, especially pelvic floor problems, incontinence and vesicovaginal fistulae, and the provision of appropriate and safe reproductive health care for refugees and displaced persons are perhaps the most pressing concerns for research and innovations by midwives at the turn of the millennium.

Midwives need to be aware

It is not possible to reflect all the issues or the different approaches being made by midwives in different countries in one short chapter. What is possible, though, is to heighten all midwives' awareness that today, more than ever, globalisation does have an impact on midwifery. As such, midwives from both a theoretical and practical point of view should be aware and keep abreast of what is happening in other countries.

SUMMARY

Globalisation and the impact of technology require midwives in all countries to be aware of just what is going on in the world. In addition, midwives must become more politically active if they are to bring about safe(r) motherhood in their own and other countries. It is clear that what is required to bring about safe motherhood in most countries is sufficient well-trained midwives and the resources to provide holistic quality care, including emergency obstetric care. These must be available close enough for the women to gain access to them. This requires action by community leaders, policy makers and politicians. Therefore midwives must become active in political debate concerning structures of society, but also be able to identify and influence local leaders and key decision-makers in the community. This is more likely to succeed if done through rational considered discussion and community grass roots action.

Awareness of one's own culture, both personal and professional, will help in adopting appropriate and culturally sensitive models for action, including models of care. Midwives must accept that their own cultural baggage will alter their perspective on best practice and fitness for purpose. Therefore, adopting an advocacy role and participatory approaches is not only good practice, but the only way forward. This will require all midwives to ensure that at all times it is the women they serve who are in the front and making the decisions. If midwives are to provide appropriate effective care anywhere in the world, they must always listen to and respect the women they seek to serve.

READER ACTIVITIES

1. Try to obtain a copy of the ICM Code of Ethics and ask yourself how your practice complies with this code.

2. With a colleague consider how you as a

midwife support each individual woman you care for in her right to participate actively in the decisions about her own care.

3. Try to find an opportunity to meet with small

groups of local women and ask them to tell you about the maternity services they receive and the type of maternity services they would like to receive (if possible try to include a small group of women from a minority ethnic group). Ask yourself whether they all have similar experiences. Do they all voice the same concerns? What are the striking similarities and differences?

4. If possible, try to find another midwife who has worked or is working in another country and ask her or him to tell you about the experience.

5. You may like to try to find a midwife in another country with whom you can establish regular correspondence, as a 'pen-friend'. Midwifery journals or midwives' organisations can sometimes help to put midwives in touch with each other in different countries. The ICM would have the contact addresses for many national midwifery associations.

REFERENCES

Chitnis S 1988 Feminism: Indian ethos and Indian convictions. In: Ghandially S (ed) Women in Indian society: a reader. Sage Publications, London

Collins P 1994 Shifting the centre: race, class, and feminist theorizing about motherhood. In: Glenn E, Chang G, Forcey L (eds) Mothering ideology, experience, and agency. Routledge, New York

Dawit S, Busia A 1995 Thinking about culture: some programme pointers. In: Gender development, Oxfam Journal 5(1): 7–11

DeVries R 1996 The midwife's place: an international comparison of the status of midwives. In: Murray S (ed) Midwives and safer motherhood. Mosby, London

Department of Health 1993 Changing childbirth: report of the expert maternity group. HMSO, London

Donley J 1995 Independent midwifery in New Zealand. In: Murphy-Black T (ed) 1995 Issues in midwifery. Churchill Livingstone, Edinburgh

Goodburn E 1995 Maternal morbidity in rural Bangladesh: an investigation into the nature and determinants of maternal morbidity related to delivery and the puerperium. Bangladesh Rural Advancement Committee, Dhaka

International Confederation of Midwives (ICM) 1993 International code of ethics for midwives. ICM, London

International Confederation of Midwives (ICM) 1994 A birthday for midwives: seventy five years of international collaboration. The International Confederation of Midwives 1919–1994. ICM, London

Jenks C 1993 Culture. Routledge, London

Kwast B, Bentley J 1991 Introducing confident midwives: midwifery education – action for safe motherhood. Midwifery 7: 8–19

Maine D 1990 Safe motherhood programmes: options and issues. Centre For Population and Family Health, Columbia University, New York

Royston E, Armstrong S 1989 Preventing maternal deaths. World Health Organization, Geneva

Saadeh R 1993 Breast-feeding: the technical basis and recommendations for action. World Health Organization, Geneva

Salvage J 1985 The politics of nursing. Heinemann, London

Smulders B, Limburg A 1995 Obstetrics and midwifery in the Netherlands. In: Kitzinger S The midwifery challenge, new edn. Pandora, London

Thompson J, Bennett R 1996 Women are dying: midwives in action. ICM/WHO/UNICEF Pre-Congress Workshop, May 1996, Oslo, Norway

United Nations (UN) 1979 Convention on the elimination of all forms of discrimination against women. UN, New York

United Nations (UN) 1990 The convention on the rights of the child. UN, New York

United Nations (UN) 1993 Declaration on violence against women. UN, New York

United Nations Children's Fund (UNICEF) 1990 World summit rights of the child. UNICEF, New York

United Nations Children's Fund (UNICEF) 1993 The progress of nations. UNICEF, New York

United Nations Children's Fund (UNICEF) 1997a The state of the world's children: 1997 summary. UNICEF, New York

United Nations Children's Fund (UNICEF) 1997b Cracking the code (Code No. 16027). UNICEF, Essex

Wagner M 1994 Pursing the birth machine: the search for appropriate birth technology. Ace Graphics, Australia

World Health Organization (WHO) 1981 International code of marketing of breast-milk substitutes. WHO, Geneva

World Health Organization (WHO) 1991a Essential elements of obstetric care at first referral level. WHO, Geneva

World Health Organization (WHO) 1991b Maternal mortality: a global factbook. WHO, Geneva

World Health Organization (WHO) 1994a The application of the WHO partograph in the management of labour. Maternal Health and Safe Motherhood Programme, Division of Family Health, WHO, Geneva

World Health Organization (WHO) 1994b Mother–baby package: a practical guide to implementing safe motherhood in countries. Maternal Health and Safe Motherhood Programme, Division of Family Health, WHO, Geneva

World Health Organization (WHO) 1996a Midwifery modules for safe motherhood. Maternal Health and Safe Motherhood Programme, Division of Family Health, WHO, Geneva

World Health Organization (WHO) 1996b Normal birth. Maternal Health and Safe Motherhood Programme, Division of Family Health, WHO, Geneva

World Health Organization (WHO) 1996c Revised 1990 estimates of maternal mortality: a new approach by WHO and UNICEF. WHO, Geneva

World Health Organization/International Federation of Gynaecologists and Obstetricians/International Confederation of Midwives (WHO/FIGO/ICM) 1992 International definition of a midwife. WHO, Geneva

World Health Organization South-East Asia Regional Office (WHO/SEARO) 1996 Standards for midwifery practice for safe motherhood. Working paper 1 An inter-country consultation November 1996. WHO/SEARO, New Delhi, India

World Health Organization/United Nations Children's Fund (WHO/UNICEF) 1989 Protecting, promoting and supporting breast-feeding: the special role of maternity services. WHO, Geneva

World Health Organization/United Nations Children's Fund/International Confederation of Midwives (WHO/UNICEF/ICM) 1991 Midwifery education action for safe motherhood: report of a collaborative pre-congress workshop, Kobe, Japan 5–6 October 1990. WHO, Geneva

FURTHER READING

Jeffrey P, Jeffrey R, Lyon A 1988 Labour pains and labour power: woman and childbearing in India. Zed Books, London

Koblinsky M, Timyan J, Gay J (eds) 1992 The health of women: global perspective. Westview, Boulder

Murphy-Black T 1995 Issues in midwifery. Churchill Livingstone, Edinburgh

Murray S (ed) 1996 Midwives and safer motherhood. Mosby, London

Murray S (ed) 1996 Baby friendly/mother friendly: international perspectives on midwifery. Mosby, London

Taylor D 1991 The children who sleep by the river. WHO, Geneva

Ethics in midwifery

5

Anne Thompson

The midwife in the course of her work may find herself in situations in which her beliefs and values conflict with those of people whose perspectives are different from her own. She may also be asked for help by parents who are faced by choices that involve moral judgements. This chapter provides a framework within which she may consider such difficult situations and decisions.

The chapter aims to:

- define ethics in terms of a number of key concepts

- examine what is meant by ethics in midwifery practice

- discuss strategies for the constructive resolution of conflict

- review some of the classical moral frameworks for decision-making.

> Professional ethics are among the sinews of a free society; they sustain and extend (when they do not abuse) reliance on trust; they limit coercive regulation and state control where human interests are best served by free, privileged communication. (Dunstan 1987)

FACING UP TO ETHICS

The discussion of ethics in many forms – bioethics, business ethics, the ethics of aid, the ethics of resource allocation, and so on – has become commonplace over the past decade. Media debates have brought key issues before the public and stimulated reflection and controversy. On another level, there has been an explosion of specialised books and journals on the subject, the creation of institutes and the establishment of academic courses – all the paraphernalia of a fully fledged academic discipline. Despite all this, there frequently remains the impression that ethics is not a practical subject or an easy one to tackle. Its acceptance into the curriculum seems to conflict with the commonly accepted view that ethics or morality are personal matters to be determined by the individual alone according to his or her personal lights. This chapter will try to challenge that view and to offer a few tools for grappling with some of the difficult issues which face midwives today.

First of all there is the problem of defining what we mean by 'ethics'. Other words are often used either as synonyms or in close association: morals, rights, law. Although none of them is really synonymous, their use does convey the idea of a framework, of some sort of identifiable system, of order. And this is precisely what the world's thinkers have attempted by 'doing ethics' throughout the centuries. They have tried to articulate human action in terms of such concepts as 'goodness', 'right', 'justice' or 'equity'. The words may sound abstract, but the attempt to express such concepts in a systematic way was an effort to move away from the arbitrary responses of individual thought and emotion and establish some ground rules for an ordered interface between individual and society. In few fields has the tension at this interface

been so strong as in reproductive health. Sophisticated technologies associated with assisted fertilisation, embryo conservation or perinatal problems have raised practical, moral, legal and ethical questions of a complexity for which most people were ill-prepared (Bayertz 1994, Freed & Hageman 1996). Such problems are not limited to industrialised societies – for instance, the use of ultrasound imaging is a clear example of a technology which poses as many questions in developing countries, whether of resource allocation or of inappropriate use, as it does in the West. Three decades of great technological and sociological change have thrown up innumerable questions, posed countless dilemmas (see Fig. 5.1). Improved access to education and increased levels of information and debate through the media have meant that women in many parts of the world are challenging decisions which once they would have accepted simply on the authority of their caregivers. Much current debate in midwifery is stimulated not only by arguments about what constitutes 'right' or 'wrong' but upon issues of power, control, conflict resolution and decision-making as women claim a voice in the decisions which are made about their care.

This chapter is underpinned by these key concepts as it examines what is meant by ethics in

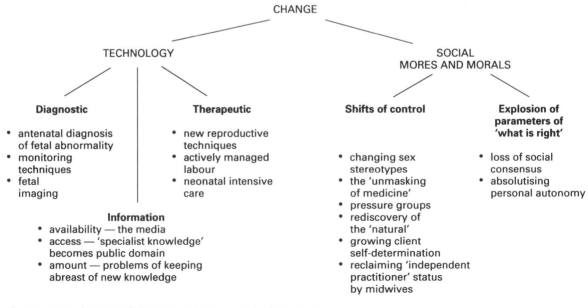

Fig. 5.1 Some elements of change in relation to midwifery practice.

midwifery practice and why it has become an important area for reflection. Since ethics is essentially a very practical matter, the text takes a series of practice issues as its point of departure. The values which underpin many of the decisions and choices in midwifery are frequently a source of conflict, as mothers, midwives and doctors necessarily view childbirth from different perspectives. Strategies for resolving such conflict constructively will be discussed and there will be a brief examination of some of the classical moral frameworks which are used to achieve consistency and coherence in decision-making. The International Code of Ethics for Midwives (ICM 1993) provides a recent and relevant example of such a framework. The emerging concept of 'reproductive rights' as articulated at the United Nations' International Conference on Population and Development (ICPD) in 1994 in Cairo and the Fourth World Conference on Women in Beijing will also be briefly explored (Cook & Fathalla 1996). Above all, this chapter will address the reality of midwifery practice. Ethics may seem abstract, but it determines the quality of the service which is offered – where ethical reflection is absent it is too easy for decisions to be opportunist. Throughout the chapter, readers will be invited to explore their own experience, beliefs and values for, while being an intensely practical discipline in the way that it guides and determines our actions, the root of ethics lies at the core of the individual person. In sharing an honest account of their own values and beliefs while attempting to listen without prejudice to people whose stance is very different, midwives can carry forward the work of the 'reflective community', the development of a social sense of what is right and acceptable for our times and our world, which people have engaged in throughout history (Engelhardt 1986).

What is ethics?

Contemporary concern for ethics in health care has been described as 'a product of the collision of an exquisite technology with an age which has achieved total communication saturation' (Stenberg 1979). While this is partly true it hides the fact that growing awareness of other issues such as

economics, cultural differences, regional inequities, environmental damage and human rights have also stimulated the current wrestling with ethical questions. As awareness grows so the questions multiply, and answers sometimes seem rare. Nonetheless, despite the new technologies' high profile in the media and even in some professionals' minds, it is the ordinary events of daily practice which offer the greatest scope for the exercise of ethical judgements. Schröck (1980) illustrated this very clearly in relation to nursing care, underlining the vital but often overlooked importance of concepts such as trust, honesty and confidentiality.

For the sake of argument the term 'ethics' will be used here in its widest sense, while realising that for many theologians and philosophers there are clear distinctions between ethics and morality. Ethics claims to be a discipline of systematic reflection and analysis designed to enable people to resolve questions about what ought to be done in some sort of consistent and coherent manner. 'Ought' is a value-laden word, heavy with a weight of moral constraint. Kant, an 18th century philosopher who had a great impact on modern thinking, talked about 'imperatives', in the sense that once it is clear what ought to be done one is then compelled to do it (Paton 1947). The criteria by which 'ought' is determined are rooted in systems of moral theory. Whichever of the many theories are chosen as a guide for action, they are all concerned, in one way or another, to identify the 'right' course, the 'good' decision, the 'best' pathway. What form that 'good' or 'best' or 'right' takes depends largely on which of the frameworks one usually chooses to work by.

Examples of such frameworks include those specific to a particular religious tradition and stating rules for right conduct, such as the Ten Commandments or the Koran, or a more universally applicable utilitarian consideration of how to achieve the maximum benefit for the greatest number of people. Ethical frameworks are frequently translated into precepts designed for a group of practitioners, such as the UKCC Code of Professional Conduct (UKCC 1992) or the ICM International Code of Ethics. Some of the more important ethical frameworks will be discussed in more detail towards the end of this chapter. Increasingly over the last half-century the language of human rights has been used in ethical reflection, and more recently it has been directly applied to issues concerning women, health and human reproduction (Tomasevski 1993).

The choice of framework is certain to be coloured by the individual's early experience, upbringing and culture. The fact that ethics claims to be a system of rational enquiry should not disguise the fact that the decisions that the system leads to are made by human beings with hearts that are at least as powerful as their heads (Midgely 1981). Although some philosophers would much prefer ethical reflection to remain uncluttered by messy human emotion, the reality of life in the health care system is that very many of the situations which arise are highly charged with positive or negative feelings which should not be ignored. Childbirth is one of the most significant of human events and as such quite properly engages people's emotions. The process of ethical reflection must take account of this and allow due weight to the fact that we are only able to make decisions as whole people if our hearts are permitted to inform our heads.

Finally, ethics is about the use and abuse of power; the ability of persons, states and systems to change lives and events for good or ill. Sometimes the effect of such power is discreet, almost imperceptible. At other times it is so overwhelming that it tips over into coercion or even violence, verbal, moral or physical. Professionals have a special responsibility to be sensitive to the way in which the power conferred on them by their professional standing is used. Professional codes of ethics are largely designed to protect clients and to ensure that the inherent inequality in the client–caregiver relationship is not abused.

The uses of power – 'controlling the situation'

'Episiotomy will be used for all primigravidae' (delivery suite protocol).
'It would be much better if you let me give him a top-up' (midwife to mother with hungry baby).
'I'm going home anyway' (mother discharging herself against medical advice).

Midwives will not find it difficult to think of examples which illustrate just how much control is exercised over people who make use of the maternity services. On one level this is inevitable. Large institutions need rules and regulations to maintain an acceptable standard of smooth functioning. Protocols, policies and guidelines are developed to ensure some degree of consistency and order in the managing of situations. The difficulty arises when there is conflict between the needs and values of the individual client or practitioner and those of the organisation. The midwife is likely to be as unhappy as the mother with a rigid protocol. The heart of the problem seems to be that an externally determined, formally imposed set of rules is substituted for individual decision-making processes which can take into account the particular features of a given situation. Midwives who are aware of how power hidden in professional status and the health care framework can undermine their clients' ability to express their views will find ways to shift the balance so that the people in their care can have their voices heard (Wagner 1986). The first two articles of the International Code of Ethics for Midwives (Box 5.1) are unambiguous about where power and control should lie and how that shift is achieved.

The ICM Code envisages midwifery care as a partnership. This is a concept which embraces equality and dialogue. Where these characteristics exist there is no inappropriate use of power by one partner over the other. Only then is it possible to establish real trust between them. Most midwives are constantly amazed at the amount of trust shown by the great majority of their clients. To trust renders a person vulnerable and puts the

---

Box 5.1 Articles 1.A and B from the International Code of Ethics for Midwives (ICM 1993)

1. A. Midwives respect a woman's informed right of choice and promote the woman's acceptance of responsibility for the outcomes of her choice.
   B. Midwives work with women, supporting their right to participate actively in decisions about their care, and empowering women to speak for themselves on issues affecting the health of women and their families in their culture/society.

trusted individual in a position of great personal power. Add this to the power midwives already hold by virtue of their professional qualification and status and it is obvious that, unless they take care, the partnership they want to establish with women will be ineffective, because it is unequal.

Nevertheless, it would be both unrealistic and unwise to base all decisions on a case-by-case analysis of particular situations. Formal policies and guidelines, properly established and appropriately used, are critical to effective, safe services. 'Properly established' should mean that midwives are actively involved in designing Unit protocols and that the people to whom policies apply should also be consulted about them. Few people like committee meetings but failure to get involved means that someone else will do the deciding. 'Appropriately used' must mean that, in the ordinary run of day-to-day events, policies do not become a substitute for thought. When, some years ago, the authors of the confidential enquiries on maternal mortality (DH 1989) recommended that each delivery suite in the country develop its own protocols for the management of catastrophic haemorrhage, it was a totally appropriate suggestion. Such situations demand urgent, coordinated and effective action. A team needs to be able to move into action smoothly and swiftly. Debates about values and beliefs must wait. Used in such circumstances, policies like this can save lives. However, this does not dispense health care workers from the duty of identifying clients' wishes. In a case when a team of obstetricians were faced with a Jehovah's Witness giving birth to twins, they respected her request not to have a blood transfusion. They refrained from using their professional power to override her clearly stated, deeply held beliefs. As a consequence the mother died. Many would argue that the doctors' duty was to save her life. The team evidently felt that this duty did not warrant violating the conscience of a self-determining rational adult.

IDENTIFYING THE PROBLEMS

Central issues in caring

When midwives were asked to identify the main sources of moral conflict in their practice, the level of obstetric intervention in the delivery suite accounted for nearly 50% of the items listed (Thompson 1987). 'Bioethical issues' (e.g. termination for fetal abnormality, life support for the very low birthweight or grossly handicapped baby) was the only other category to achieve a two-figure score (14.2%). This perception of unnecessarily high levels of intervention is echoed in a report of a Technical Working Group of the World Health Organization which looked at the whole range of practices commonly used in normal birth (WHO 1996).

Of course it is true that without timely intervention many mothers and babies would have died over recent decades. What is in question is its inappropriate use. There have been successful challenges to intervention levels such as the induction rates of the late 1970s, but it is vital that challenge is well founded, that evidence is clear and that alternative approaches can be demonstrated to be at least as safe as those which are being challenged. The level and quality of collaboration required in modern obstetric care can only be achieved through professional interdisciplinary partnership in a climate of mutual respect and confidence. Midwives are key partners in the obstetric team, well placed to assume the role of advocate and interpreter when needed, to ensure the smooth information flow which enables the whole team to work with the women in their care in a spirit of competent interdependence.

Choice and control

Choice is another issue which has received much attention in recent years. Gilligan (1977) comments that 'the essence of the moral decision is the exercise of choice and the willingness to accept responsibility for that choice'. We have seen how the ICM Code of Ethics stresses this. Women may well, as Gilligan claims, formulate their experience 'in a different voice' from men, with responsibility and caring, rather than justice and 'rationality' as the main motivators of their decisions. Her research demonstrated that 'Women's judgements are tied to feelings of empathy and compassion and are concerned more with the resolution of 'real-life' rather than hypothetical dilemmas'.

The freedom of women to make choices about their childbirth experiences, particularly if the birth itself is to take place in hospital, is largely dependent on the willingness and cooperation of midwives and obstetricians. Many centres, both in the UK and overseas, have taken seriously the challenge of providing women with authentic choice (DH 1993). There can be problems at times when the difference of perception which Gilligan notes comes into play and women's choices do not coincide with the established policies. Wilson (1986) points out that the attempt to provide professional services which respect the autonomy of the client requires the development of strategies which will encourage the free flow of communication. Reorganisation of midwifery care to achieve more continuity, including the use of birth plans and antenatal home visits, could both improve communication and give women a greater sense of control over their birth experience.

Conflicting loyalties

One of the consequences of working in a multidisciplinary team is that the potential for conflict is increased. This is illustrated in the case study in Box 5.2.

This is only one of many possible examples of instances where the individual's professional judgement is in conflict with either her client's or other professionals' views. It is a very painful situation and there are no 'blanket' remedies. The very fact that such a situation can arise between a midwife and her manager or an obstetrician is sufficient for some people to contest the midwife's

---

Box 5.2 Case study: conflict of loyalties

A manager refused to allow a midwife to come in on her day off to deliver a particularly nervous young mother with whom she had built up a good relationship. The woman was tense and anxious throughout a difficult labour, cared for by a midwife she did not know. The outcome was a traumatic instrumental delivery. The couple later tried to book the first midwife privately for the next pregnancy. She declined the request 'reluctantly'.

---

claim to be an autonomous practitioner. Such an argument fails to recognise that all moral decisions are set in a given context, a particular cultural, social or professional framework, and that decisions are not made in some form of neutral, impersonal moral vacuum. Ethics, of its nature, is interpersonal and hence complex. Precisely because 'no man is an island' people are accountable for their actions and professionals are accountable in a public, formal manner, first of all to their clients and then to their profession.

Among the strategies that midwives can develop in order to handle situations of conflict without compromising their own personal integrity is what Joyce Thompson (1984), an American midwife, calls 'professional maturity'. Arguing that to be professional is to be ethical, she describes the characteristics of such maturity as:

- knowledge and acceptance of all the responsibilities inherent in midwifery practice and education
- mutual trust and respect in relationships between clients and different practitioners
- maintenance of competence and ongoing learning
- a knowledge of history, to avoid repeating past mistakes
- risk-taking with responsibility for outcomes
- reasoned decision-making in all domains
- the ability to live with uncertainty.

The recognition of one's personal and professional limitations should be added to complete the list. Although this sounds self-evident, it is frequently as difficult for a practitioner to admit to this as it is to acknowledge uncertainty. Professional training and social expectations combine to put considerable pressure on health care workers to provide answers. In the moral domain, above all, it will usually be quite inappropriate for the midwife to attempt to supply them. The professional's role will be to act as a catalyst to enable clients to reach their own solutions. The response 'if I were you ...' short-circuits the hard work of reflection and analysis in which they will need to engage in order to reach decisions which are truly their own. The midwife's respect for the women's autonomy lies in refraining from bringing the power of professional status to bear on their choice. While doing this the midwife retains responsibility for ensuring that women are in possession of the best possible information before they make their decisions. Professional position gives no automatic right to decide what is best for one's clients.

Values

> Few words have been subjected to such a variety of usage, by economists, philosophers, social scientists of various persuasions and recently by educators at large … there can be no confidence that two authorities who discuss values are referring to the same range of phenomena. (Kitwood 1977)

Despite Kitwood's gloomy account of the uselessness of the word 'values', it is nearly impossible to discuss ethics without it. Here the word will be used in the sense of those action-guiding criteria which people adopt for their standards of performance in relation to other people or situations. Hall (1973) describes a value as a stance that is taken and expressed through behaviours, feelings, imagination, knowledge and actions. Values are inherent in what matters most to individuals, in what has meaning for them and in what they hold most dear. Once this is accepted, it is easy to see that to ignore, dismiss or affront other people's values, even unintentionally, can be an assault on their personal integrity.

Organisations, as well as individuals, function from a chosen set of values which become part of their corporate image. Some, such as the International Confederation of Midwives, externalise and formalise those values in a text which articulates the standards anticipated of their members throughout the world (ICM 1993). In the study mentioned earlier (Thompson 1987), midwives identified five major areas of potential value-conflicts which they experienced (Fig. 5.2). It would be possible to get women and their partners to draw a similar picture from their perspective. Midwives and mothers alike have to develop communication and negotiation skills in order to safeguard their own values to a reasonably satisfactory level.

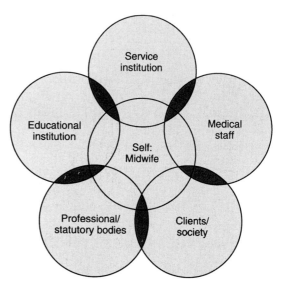

Fig. 5.2 Potential sources of values conflict in midwifery practice.

When midwives were asked what mattered most to them in their practice their replies focused on maintaining a high standard of care with confidence and flexibility, on being able to ensure a satisfactory experience for the women they care for and on achieving a level of personal satisfaction from recognising that their work had been worthwhile. These responses seem concerned with realising a 'best' outcome for midwives and mothers alike. However, constraints imposed by some of the systems noted in Figure 5.2 can alter the picture quite dramatically.

On a more personal level, problems can arise from different interpretations of concepts such as respect for life, fetal or reproductive rights, quality of life and many other controversial issues. The case study in Box 5.3 highlights the difficulties raised by the differing personal stances held by the people involved.

It could be valuable to analyse this case, either alone or with others, suspending personal judgement while trying to understand the thinking of the people involved. Which principles underpinned their choices? Did they clash? On what basis was it decided which should take priority in this situation? Whose decision is it anyway? Who stood to gain from the decisions made? At cost to whom?

> **Box 5.3 Case study: conflict of values**
>
> A midwife took over the care of a woman with a 36-week pregnancy. Labour was being induced at the woman's request. The fetus had recently been diagnosed in her country of origin as suffering from Down syndrome and a cardiac abnormality. The midwife was disturbed to find that none of the customary measures for monitoring fetal well-being were being taken. Discussion with the mother made it clear that she would be happier if the baby did not survive its birth, because her family life would be disrupted and such handicaps were poorly accepted in her country. The midwife was unable to accept what she felt was a level of tacit collusion designed to give the baby minimum chances of survival and, after further discussion, started fetal monitoring and requested the presence of a paediatrician at delivery. The baby responded well to resuscitation and went to the Neonatal Intensive Care Unit. Surgery was later performed successfully. The mother was extremely distressed by the course of events, and the midwife was criticised by the obstetrician, many of her peers and the consultant paediatrician.

Whose rights are respected? How was power used? Is it possible to respect the views of more than one person in the outcome? Indeed, is ethics properly concerned with outcomes only? Does the quality of the process which precedes decision-making have a value in itself?

Questions multiply around a situation like this. If responses are to carry more weight than 'gut feeling' (which should, however, not be ignored), or simple opinion; if the decision is to be based on one principle rather than another; if the choice is to lay claim to being rational and coherent; then the moral frameworks which guide principled thinking will have to be used, even if they are only visible when, as in this case, the situation is examined with hindsight.

STRUCTURES AND STRATEGIES

Moral frameworks

One of the features of the study of ethical theory is that nearly every text will provide a different version of the structure and content of a range of moral frameworks. There is a sense in which this diversity is a healthy and honest reflection of the way human beings are when they come to thinking about the things which matter most to them. If the world's greatest minds, over a period of some 3000 years of documented thought, have failed to agree about what constitutes the 'right' course of action or the 'best' decision in any given set of circumstances, it should be no surprise to us that we find it a challenge to our thinking.

Nevertheless, some general frameworks do exist and they act rather like maps to guide people through the little-known and hazardous terrain of human experience. Like maps, they can be used to identify the features of an unexpected and difficult journey just completed as well as to plan a route through anticipated rough territory. This is important in the professional situation since, so often, events evolve at a speed which leaves little opportunity for planning or reflection. In this case, two things tend to happen. Firstly, people respond using a familiar frame of reference, appealing consciously or otherwise to their usual action-guiding criteria (values). Later, they may review that decision in the light, not only of its outcome, but of the process and the foundations upon which the choice was made. This exercise of reflection, free of the pressures of an emergency, permits the consideration of alternative ethical frameworks and may help people to appreciate and respect other responses than their own.

Ethical frameworks, some of which are briefly sketched here, can broadly be grouped according to whether they are goal based or rule based.

Goal-based theories

These originate from the secular utilitarian tradition associated with the work of Jeremy Bentham and John Stuart Mill. Goal-based theories broadly focus on the degree of benefit to be achieved by any given action. These are sometimes known as *teleological* or *consequentialist* theories and, with their emphasis on the goal to be achieved, on the outcome to be expected from a chosen course of action, they have considerable appeal in a world of practical decision-making such as the NHS, where dilemmas about resource allocation present a permanent challenge.

Rule-based theories

This group of theories stems largely from a range of classical and theological traditions and includes concepts such as natural law, agapeistic theory and deontological ethics.

Natural law has a very long history in European thought and provides the foundation for the legal codes of a number of nations as well as much of the theology of the Roman Catholic Church. It has its roots in belief in a universal rational order written into creation and governing right action between people. This order, supposedly perceivable by all right-minded rational people, is held to be inviolable, for to violate it would be to introduce chaos into society by ignoring divinely instituted moral precepts.

Agapeistic theory comes more directly from the Christian tradition. Downie & Calman (1987) note that the story of the Good Samaritan is one of the most powerful illustrations of the type of love meant by the Greek word *agape*. They describe it as 'an attitude which combines a regard for others as self-governing with a compassion for them in the pursuit of their end'. Agapeistic theory in recent years has been linked with the development of what some have called 'situation ethics', where the central question to be asked in any dilemma is 'what is the most loving thing to do?'. Problems arise when there is failure to reach agreement on what are the criteria by which one can identify the most loving action.

Deontological or duty-based theory is closely linked with the name of Immanuel Kant. Thompson et al (1994) note that Kant maintained that a moral principle must be universal, unconditional and imperative before it can be considered moral and therefore binding. Before an action can be considered good or moral it has to pass the test by which one could will that same action to become universally applicable. A further development of his thinking led him to state that right action never permits the use of people as means to achieve an end, a consideration which has been very influential in deciding what constitutes respect for persons. One clear instance of the application of the rule is seen in the core statement of the Children Act

1976 that all legal decisions must be determined by the child's best interests. Unfortunately there is no space to do justice to his complex theories here.

Rights-based theory has grown in importance as a framework for ethical reflection in recent years. A proper exploration is not possible here, but midwives must be aware of the many tensions experienced by women as a result of gender discrimination which results in their being unable to obtain equitable treatment in many areas of their lives: education, employment, marriage (Coliver 1995). The statements about reproductive rights made at the United Nations' Conferences of Cairo and Beijing are an extension of earlier human rights declarations ratified by the majority of the world, particularly the Convention on the Elimination of All Forms of Discrimination against Women (CEDAW 1979) which asserts (Article 3) that countries are obliged to 'ensure the full development and advancement of women, for the purpose of guaranteeing them the exercise and enjoyment of human rights and fundamental freedoms on a basis of equality with men'. Violence, harmful traditional practices and denied access to health care are aspects of human rights abuse which are immediately relevant to the work of midwives. The recent polarisation described between 'fetal rights' and 'maternal rights' is an area where much reflection and discussion remains to be done (Black 1992). It is well illustrated by the publicity given to a case where one twin of a normal pair was aborted because the mother felt she would be unable to cope. How rights are established, by whom and what their moral weight is lie outside the scope of this text, but the matter deserves much more analytical consideration than it normally receives.

Intuitionism lies somewhere between goal-based and rule-based theories of ethics. Intuitionists not only hold that moral judgements are arrived at by the subjective and personal insights of individuals, by intuition, but they also maintain that there are 'several distinct moral duties that cannot be reduced to one basic duty, in contrast, for example, to utilitarianism' (Pan Dictionary of Philosophy 1979). While intuitionism probably gives more weight to the emotions in the process of forming an ethical judgement than either of the other main systems the rational processes of information gathering, reflection and analysis all have their part in establishing the intuitionist's moral framework.

Principled thinking

All the ethical frameworks which have been considered provide a structure within which ethical principles can be brought to bear on the human situation. These are frequently listed as respect for persons (sometimes discussed as autonomy), benevolence, non-malevolence (the duty to do no harm), justice and utility. Downie & Calman (1987) see respect for persons as the great overarching principle which is served by the four subsidiary principles just mentioned. These are identified as the most 'morally appropriate ways of treating autonomous people'. Engelhardt (1986) sees the principles of respect for autonomy and benevolence (doing what is best for the client) as creating a fundamental tension which health care workers must grapple with in attempting to make moral decisions. He uses the expression 'the morality of mutual respect' to describe the practical

application of the principle of autonomy within the professional situation. There remain a host of other moral principles which play a subsidiary role to the ones we have just mentioned. These include truth-telling, promise-keeping and confidentiality, all of which have obvious application to midwifery practice. The problem with lists of moral principles is that the longer the list gets the greater the potential for conflicting priorities among those principles. Since most people use an amalgam of ethical frameworks in their day-to-day decision-making, what is of more importance, perhaps, than such lists is some way of evaluating the efficacy of the frameworks.

Using the frameworks

Benjamin & Curtis (1992) follow John Rawls in using a method of 'wide reflective equilibrium' in resolving ethical issues. This method uses three elements to construct the 'equilibrium' (Fig. 5.3). They are, firstly, our secure, pretheoretical moral judgements (e.g. causing unnecessary pain to newborn babies is wrong), secondly, our background beliefs and theories (our basic knowledge and beliefs about how the world and people function:

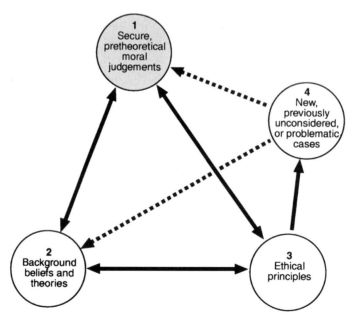

Fig. 5.3 A method of wide reflective equilibrium (after Rawls 1986).

in this example, the negative effects of pain, the vulnerability and lack of autonomy of the newborn) and, thirdly, the ordered sets of moral principles which constitute the framework in question (agapeistic, rule-based, utilitarian, etc.). The appropriateness and validity of the chosen framework are judged by estimating the extent to which the sets of principles do effectively 'give consistent and comprehensive guidance while cohering with two other sets of beliefs'. The three components need to maintain an equilibrium, to be mutually supportive. No one of the elements is permitted to dominate over the others. It may transpire that one form of ethical framework actually maintains this balance better than others. When new situations arise they have to be incorporated into the dynamic which maintains the three main elements in equilibrium. If there is dissonance then some modification of the other elements may need to take place, to accommodate the demands of the new situation. The developments in assisted fertilisation offer good examples of new situations which (a) seem not to be explicitly provided for in any previous code of ethics (unless, in deontological terms, one subscribes to the theories of natural law), (b) require a revision of our previously held background beliefs and theories about the way humans are conceived and (c) put a question mark over our previously secure, pretheoretical moral judgement about what is 'right' or permissible in the field of human reproduction.

This may seem a complex exercise which is for the academics. In reality, much of it is what we do, albeit unconsciously, when we look at a new situation and feel uneasy about it, when we swap ideas about it in the coffee room and try to find out how others react. By those acts we are trying to validate our own response. Where others react differently we may be pushed into looking more closely at why we respond as we do and so become more aware of the origins of our own ethical stance. Sometimes this can be quite disturbing – most of us prefer to have our foundations left unshaken. More frequently, such a process is experienced in the long run as growth and affirmation. The analysis and questioning involved provide an occasion for self-discovery as well as a greater awareness of the perspectives held by others. It is important

that ethical reflection should not be constrained by too limited a use of abstract concepts. It is by the careful analysis of situations and the different approaches which people bring to them that midwives will effectively develop their sense of what constitutes good practice.

This is why this chapter has placed far less emphasis on those concepts which traditionally constitute 'medical ethics' and has focused instead on the use and abuse of power in professional practice, on how midwives can safeguard the autonomy of the women in their care and how they can meet the challenge of maintaining their personal integrity at the heart of a complex network of sometimes conflicting values.

Wilson (1978) claimed that 'reciprocity is the fundamental attribute of a mature moral transaction'. Midwifery is largely based on a continuous dialogue with women and their families. Without such an exchange the service cannot hope to meet their needs, since it will only have its own view of what those needs are. At a much deeper level, that dialogue is the only clear way of honouring the autonomy of the women, giving them a voice which can effect the changes which they see as important. Midwives have spoken a lot in recent years about the duty of 'empowering' women. This cannot be done without the establishment of the trust relationship discussed at the beginning of this chapter.

Covenant

These qualities of reciprocity, mutual respect and dialogue are enshrined in the covenant concept (May 1975, Campbell 1984, 1987, Stenberg 1979). Covenant has its roots in the Judaeo-Christian tradition, where it was frequently used to describe the relationship between God and his people. Writers in the health care field have been attracted to the concept because it has a flexibility and dynamism that is missing from similar structures such as codes and contracts. Covenant partners value each other. There is a mutual commitment, a reciprocal obligation. Both partners give and receive. May argues that the covenant model frees the professional relationship from the one-sided, paternalistic element of philanthropy inherent in models such as codes of conduct or advocacy. It seems a useful framework for the sort of morally responsible professional relationship which midwives and mothers engage in. Its reciprocal nature levels out the inequalities usually present in the client–health care worker relationship. In stressing the self-determination of the client, it reduces the emphasis on the practitioner's role as advocate (cf. UKCC 1989). With its dynamic, reciprocal qualities, which require the establishment of a true partnership, covenant offers potential which midwives may well find corresponds with the demands of their practice. To those who are fearful of the level of commitment required by a professional covenant relationship, May offers the reminder that covenant ethics are realistic in rejecting the idealistic (and arrogant) assumption that professional action should be wholly gratuitous as much as the contractualist precept that every exchange should be governed by self-interest.

Stenberg (1979) offers a seven-point outline of the characteristics of covenant, which have been adapted for midwifery in Box 5.4. Despite its comprehensive nature, Stenberg's account of covenant seems insufficiently to stress the quality of mutuality, the active role of the woman in determining how she wishes to structure this event as a partnership. In midwifery practice where mothers have months to prepare for childbirth, the careful drafting of birth plans can provide a woman with a valuable means of clarifying the 'terms of the covenant' with her midwife.

Box 5.4 Elements of a covenant framework (after Stenberg 1979)

Covenant requires:

- fidelity in both promises and truth-telling
- proficiency – a woman's faith is based on belief in the midwife's competence
- safeguarding the woman's self-concept, her personhood
- care that goes beyond the level of utility to that of ultra-obligation
- control of her person and her environment offered to the woman where possible
- freedom for the woman from fear, pain and the possibility of abandonment
- the encouragement of realistic hope.

The idea of promise-keeping, of fidelity, is central to covenant. The ethical implications of such a stance are evident and widen out from the central commitment to include issues of truthfulness and competence. Midwives, committed to being 'with women', could find this a powerful and relevant model for their practice. Attempts to structure their practice within a covenant relationship could well result in them discovering with May (1975) that 'covenants have a gratuitous, growing edge to them that nourishes rather than limits relationships'.

Making decisions

Whichever ethical framework a midwife chooses to adopt, it will be helpful at times to use some form of systematic approach to decision-analysis. Many are available, but the grid developed by Curtin & Flaherty (1982) and expanded here to incorporate elements such as affective response and reflective process is shown in Figure 5.4. It can be useful as an aid to group discussions and case reviews as well as in personal reflection.

Conclusion

Rebecca Bergman, one of the early writers on nursing ethics, states:

> There is ... a new, evolving ethic ... one of personal responsibility for nursing practice; it is one of social commitment ... to speak up and be counted when an issue is at stake; it is one of accountability ... to take considered action and to present it for scrutiny to those concerned; it is an ethic from dependence to independence to interdependence; from separateness towards togetherness with colleagues and community. A code of ethics should not be a shield, or even a crutch; it should be a firm launching pad from which to project into the future. (Bergman 1976)

The ICM International Code of Ethics for Midwives offers just such a 'launching pad' to midwives worldwide. It will not answer all midwives' questions, but it does provide a framework for reflection on the quality of the professional relationship that is at the heart of midwifery

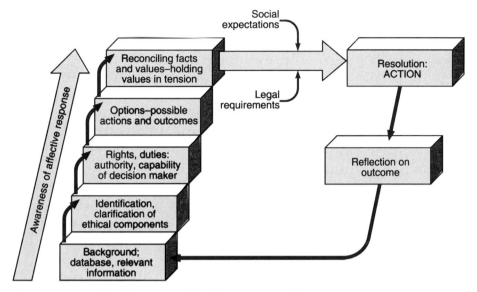

Social
expectations

Reconciling facts
and values–holding
values in tension

Resolution:
ACTION

Legal
requirements

Options–possible
actions and outcomes

Rights, duties:
authority, capability
of decision maker

Reflection on
outcome

Identification,
clarification of
ethical components

Background;
database, relevant
information

Awareness of affective response

Fig. 5.4 Steps in ethical decision-making (after Curtin 1982).

practice, as well as a template for action. It may well be that we constantly raise more questions than we answer, but if the process of careful, honest and painstaking fact-gathering, analysis and reflection gradually creates a climate of confidence, within which midwives and the women they care for can act with greater freedom, integrity and mutual respect, then much will have been achieved.

REFERENCES

Bayertz K 1994 GenETHICS: technological intervention in human reproduction as a philosophical problem. Cambridge University Press, Cambridge

Benjamin M, Curtis J (eds) 1992 Ethics in nursing, 3rd edn. Oxford University Press, Oxford

Bergman R 1976 Evolving ethical concepts for nursing. International Nursing Review 23(4): 116–117

Black R H 1992 Mothers and fetus: changing notions of maternal responsibility. Greenwood Press, London

Campbell A 1984 Moderated love – a theory of professional care. SPCK, London

Campbell A 1987 (ed) A dictionary of professional care. SPCK, London

CEDAW 1979 Convention on the elimination of all forms of discrimination against women. United Nations General Assembly Resolution 34/80 of 18 December. UN, New York

Children Act 1976 HMSO, London

Coliver S (ed) 1995 The right to know; human rights and access to reproductive health information. Article 19 and University of Pennsylvania Press, London

Cook R, Fathalla M 1996 Advancing reproductive rights beyond Cairo and Beijing. International Family Planning Perspectives Alan Guttmacher, New York

Curtin L 1982 In: Curtin L, Flaherty M J (eds) Nursing ethics, theories and pragmatics. Brady Communications, Maryland

Department of Health 1989 Report on confidential enquiries into maternal deaths in England and Wales 1982–84. HMSO, London, p 28

Department of Health 1993 Changing childbirth: report of the expert maternity group. HMSO, London

Downie R S, Calman K C 1987 Healthy respect – ethics in health care. Faber & Faber, London, p 56

Dunstan G R 1987 In: Campbell A (ed) A dictionary of professional care. SPCK, London, p 83

Engelhardt H T 1986 The foundations of bioethics. Oxford University Press, New York

Freed G E, Hageman J R 1996 Ethical dilemmas in the prenatal, perinatal and neonatal periods: Clinics in perinatology. W B Saunders, Philadelphia, vol 23, no 3

Gilligan C 1977 In another voice – women's conceptions of self and of morality. Harvard Education Review 47(4): 487–517

Hall B P 1973 Values clarification as a learning process. Paulist Press, New York

International Confederation of Midwives 1993 International code of ethics for midwives. ICM, London

Kitwood T 1977 What does 'having values' mean? Journal of Moral Education 6: 81–89

May W F 1975 Code, covenant, contract or philanthropy. Hastings Centre Report 5: 29–38

Midgely M 1981 Heart and mind – the varieties of moral experience. Methuen, London

Overall C 1987 Ethics and human reproduction – a feminist analysis. Allen and Unwin, Boston

Paton H J 1947 The moral law. Hutchinson, London. In: Flew A 1989 An introduction to western philosophy. Thames and Hudson, London

Rawls J 1986 In: Benjamin M, Curtis J (eds) Ethics in nursing, 2nd edn. Oxford University Press, Oxford

Schröck R A 1980 A question of honesty in nursing practice. Journal of Advanced Nursing 5: 135–148

Stenberg M S 1979 The search for a conceptual framework as a philosophic basis for nursing ethics: an examination of code, contract, context and covenant. Military Medicine 144: 9–22

Thompson A 1987 Teaching ethics in midwifery education. Unpublished dissertation for BEd (Hons) degree, South Bank Polytechnic, London

Thompson A 1991 Dilemmas in the management of care. Distance Learning Centre, South Bank Polytechnic, London

Thompson I E, Melia K M, Boyd K M 1994 Nursing ethics, 3rd edn. Churchill Livingstone, Edinburgh, p 207

Thompson J 1984 Professional maturity or independence. Journal of Nurse Midwifery 31(2): 92–102

Tomasevski K 1993 Women and human rights. Zed Books, London

United Kingdom Central Council for Nursing, Midwifery and Health Visiting 1989 Exercising accountability. UKCC, London

United Kingdom Central Council for Nursing, Midwifery and Health Visiting 1992 Code of professional conduct. UKCC, London

Wagner M 1986 Birth and power. In: Phaff J M L (ed) Perinatal health services in Europe. Croom Helm, London

Wilson J 1986 Patients' wants versus patients' needs. Journal of Medical Ethics 12: 127–130

Wilson R W 1978 A new direction for the study of moral behaviour. Journal of Moral Education 7(2): 122–129

World Health Organization 1996 Care in normal birth: report of a technical working group. WHO/RHT/MSM 96.9. WHO, Geneva

FURTHER READING

Katz Rothman B 1986 The tentative pregnancy – prenatal diagnosis and the future of motherhood. Pandora, London

Tew M 1990 Safer childbirth? – a critical history of maternity care. Chapman & Hall, London

Research in midwifery

Rosemary Mander

CHAPTER CONTENTS

Research may be regarded by some midwives as an activity which has little relevance to their practice. To correct such misconceptions, this chapter demonstrates the importance of research to *all* midwives, and particularly to those who practise in a clinical setting.

Midwives may be concerned about research because they regard it as an 'ivory tower' activity, that is, undertaken in an academic setting which is alien to their own working environment. Or their concerns may be due to the terminology or the language used. The statistics which feature in some research reports may serve to alarm anxious readers. These are very real concerns which need to be and are being addressed by midwife educators and midwife researchers as well as by writers and publishers.

The chapter aims to:

- consider the significance of research and the extent to which it is utilised

- discuss two main types of research which are likely to be important in midwifery

- suggest how the midwife may best make use of research in her practice

- introduce fundamental ideas which may help the midwife who is considering undertaking a research project.

THE SIGNIFICANCE OF RESEARCH IN MIDWIFERY

Research is fundamentally about asking questions. Such questioning is the basis of the care which we as midwives provide for women and babies. By questioning established or accepted practices, the midwife is in a position to ensure that her care is of an appropriately high standard. In the Briggs report this questioning approach to care was termed 'research-mindedness' and it was recommended as being a characteristic of 'every practising nurse or midwife' (Briggs 1972, p. 109). The Committee suggested that research-mindedness should be fostered during the midwife's basic educational programme, through learning to use a library and learning to utilise research-based material in practice. Research-mindedness does not necessarily involve actually undertaking a research project, but requires the midwife, on the basis of her reading, observation or intuition, to ask whether her practice could be improved and then act on her answer. This is essentially a positive approach to care, which serves to benefit all those who are involved. The Briggs report links the use of research to innovation, which may be introduced at an individual or local level or which may be applied on a larger scale. This report confidently and correctly predicts that through research-mindedness, in both the individual and the wider context, midwifery will be in a strong position to develop as a profession 'by shaping its own future'.

Since the Briggs report, midwifery in the UK has moved in the direction of becoming woman-centred, making research crucial to the woman as well as the midwife. A basic prerequisite if the woman is to make sound decisions relating to her care is accurate research-based information (Mander 1993, p. 24). If such information is not made available to her, either directly or through her midwife, the woman's autonomy becomes meaningless and the system of maternity care has failed this new family.

The fundamental importance of research to all aspects of midwifery, and especially practice, is emphasised by Renfrew (1989, p. 198): 'We cannot do any of these things well if we do not have knowledge about what we are doing. Research is not a separate part of life that you can choose to use or ignore. It is woven into the fabric of good practice …'.

THE REALITY OF THE UTILISATION OF RESEARCH

READER ACTIVITY

Consider what aspects of her working environment make it more likely that the midwife will use research in her practice.

Having established the crucial significance of research to midwifery in general, and especially to midwifery practice, it may be helpful to consider the reality of the midwife's utilisation of research. In the introduction to this chapter suggestions emerged as to why the midwife may be concerned about the relevance of research, making her less likely to utilise it. When this problem was examined among nurses, Hunt (1981) found that their difficulties related largely to their education. She identified the nurses' lack of knowledge about research findings. Even when this difficulty did not apply, the nurse encountered difficulty in, first, understanding and, second, believing the research. Any chance of utilising the research was further hampered by the nurse's ignorance about how it might be applied. An even more sinister phenomenon was also highlighted by this study; this involved the organisational difficulty of the nurse not being allowed to utilise research findings.

The problems identified by Hunt among nurses were endorsed more recently by a study of midwives' attitudes to research utilisation (Meah et al 1996). This study involved 32 midwives taking part in group interviews to elicit the themes which mattered to them. Educational deficits again manifested themselves. The midwives were unable to evaluate research, found difficulty in interpreting statistical material and could not understand research methods. Hunt's sinister organisational impediment was again identified, as Meah and colleagues found that midwives lacked autonomy in implementing research findings and that they had no role models from whom they could learn research-based practice. Clearly, as these researchers correctly observed, many of these faults are at least partly the responsibility of the researchers.

A perplexing phenomenon which also limits the midwife's use of midwifery research was found by Hicks (1992). Using a cross-over technique, 18 midwives were asked to evaluate two research reports. Half were told that the reports were by a midwife and an obstetrician respectively, and the other half were told that they were by an obstetrician and a midwife respectively. The midwives consistently judged the report which they thought to be by the midwife as poorer than the other. Thus, Hicks concludes that midwives have an inappropriately low opinion of other midwives' research; it is likely that this low esteem is another factor serving to inhibit research utilisation.

Another study which further illuminates the problem of midwives' research utilisation was undertaken by Harris (1992). Using research into perineal pain control as her example, she asked 76 staff what research they knew about and what research they utilised. She identified profound ignorance relating to the plentiful and authoritative research on this fundamentally important topic. By way of contrast, though, Harris revealed the staff's better knowledge and enthusiastic implementation of other research which is of questionable authority and relevance. This research recommended the withdrawal of air-rings from frail infirm elderly patients, but the staff were applying it to new mothers.

THE REQUIREMENT TO USE STRONG RESEARCH

It may be that the staff in Harris' (1992) study were confident in their practice because they thought that they were basing their practice on research findings. Unfortunately, their scrutiny of those findings was insufficient for them to identify the findings' questionable standard and their irrelevance to the new mother. Thus, these practitioners' utilisation of research was seriously flawed. This problem is addressed in the paper by Renfrew, mentioned earlier, in which she advocates that midwives should make use of what she calls 'good' research: 'We want to give good care therefore we need to do good research.' (Renfrew 1989, p. 202).

This case is argued at greater length and even more convincingly by Chalmers (1993), who requires the use of, in his words, 'strong evidence' as a prerequisite for safe midwifery practice. By 'safe' Chalmers is referring to the safety of both the client and the practitioner. This indicates the possibility that the midwife whose practice is based on something other than strong research exposes herself to the risk of litigation from a client who has suffered some form of harm as a result of her negligent practice.

Chalmers rehearses some examples of midwifery practice which have been adequately researched and in which the research is well utilised, such as support in labour. He gives other examples in which long-established practice was eventually researched and rejected because it did not stand up to research scrutiny; Chalmers' example is the use of Woolwich breast shells during pregnancy to correct inverted nipples. He provides further examples of practices which have been well researched, but in which the research is sometimes ignored, such as techniques and materials for perineal repair. He continues by drawing our attention to certain interventions which have not been adequately researched and, because they are so widespread, are unlikely to be subjected to research scrutiny: these include routine ultrasound examination in pregnancy and epidural analgesia in uncomplicated labour.

EVIDENCE-BASED PRACTICE

The requirement for midwifery to become a research-based profession has long been recognised, to the extent that this term featured in the Briggs report (1972). Whether this requirement is any nearer to being achieved than it was in 1972 is difficult to assess in view of the research reports, such as that by Meah and colleagues (1996) mentioned above. Since the Briggs committee made its recommendation, however, the knowledge base available to midwives has developed hugely and the research findings on which midwives may draw have become more authoritative. This presents midwives with the requirement of not only choosing research-based practice, but taking the further step of selecting suitably strong research on which to base their practice. In this context what Chalmers termed 'strong research' has become known as evidence, originally as in 'evidence-based medicine' and more recently as 'evidence-based practice'. The development of evidence-based practice was initiated by the observations made by Cochrane (1972), in which he identified the need for scientific rigour in medical clinical decision-making, and later criticised obstetricians mercilessly for their lack of such rigour. A group of obstetricians, with other colleagues practising in the maternity area, responded to this scathing condemnation by attempting to correct the situation. In order to facilitate evidence-based practice for practitioners who lacked the time or the opportunities to search and evaluate the literature, this group set about reviewing the research systematically. This resulted in the publication of two highly significant edited volumes (Chalmers et al 1989) and the ongoing development of the Cochrane Database.

Evidence-based practice has been defined in the following terms: 'the conscientious, explicit and judicious use of current best evidence in making decisions about the care of individual patients' (Sackett et al 1996).

Clearly this definition needs to be modified in the context of midwifery because the 'current best evidence' is also required to be made available to the woman to facilitate her decision-making. This is currently being achieved through a series of 'Informed choice' leaflets (MIDIRS 1996/7). Similarly, the clinical expertise, clinical observations and experience or intuition of the midwife is vital for her to assess what is really the best evidence for the individual woman (Haynes et al 1996). The midwife is crucial, both in providing the research evidence for the mother directly and in informing her about where she can check up on the information which she has been given or further extend her knowledge and understanding, assuming that time permits.

Randomised controlled trials

The strength of the research or quality of the evidence utilised to build evidence-based practice is clearly crucial. For this reason the most powerful research design, the randomised controlled trial (RCT), is the one which is used most frequently in this context.

The RCT overcomes the biases inherent when past experience, single case studies or case series without comparison groups are used as the basis of care (Enkin et al 1990). The reasons for the power of the RCT are found in its objectivity or freedom from bias, which is likely to affect the results when other research designs are utilised. The bias which often materialises, possibly inadvertently, is associated with the sampling or selection of subjects for the experimental treatment or intervention and the control group, who receive either no treatment, a placebo or the standard care. As the name of this design indicates, the allocation of eligible people to either the intervention or the control group is by randomisation, giving them all an equal chance of entering either group and ensuring that there are no systematic differences between the groups. An example of randomisation is in the important RCT on episiotomy (Sleep 1984) in which randomisation was by the opening of an opaque, sealed envelope during the second stage of labour to determine the perineal management. These precautions mean that the findings are relevant or generalisable to a far wider target population than just the sample involved. Enkin and colleagues maintain that the logic underpinning the RCT, if implemented conscientiously, makes this research design 'the gold standard for comparing alternative forms of care' (1990, p. 70). Bias may be further reduced by ensuring that, as far as possible, the woman and baby, those caring for them and those collecting data are 'blind' or unaware of the treatment group to which allocation has been made.

The principles of conducting a randomised controlled trial which justify confidence in the results have been listed by Sleep (1991) (Box 6.1).

After data have been collected to measure the outcomes in both or all treatment groups, these

---

Box 6.1 Principles of conducting a randomised controlled trial (Sleep 1991, p. 201)

1. The number of subjects should be adequate to ensure that differences are not due to chance.
2. Randomisation of the subjects happens before the intervention and there is no withdrawal.
3. The allocation must not be predictable.
4. Compliance with the intervention should be complete.
5. When the data are analysed, each subject is retained in the allocated group, regardless of the actual treatment.

---

data are subjected to demanding statistical tests. Thus, an assessment is made of the possibility that any differences are due to chance rather than the experimental intervention. The application of these tests must be extremely rigorous. When the research report is published a full account of the procedures is included, as well as details of whether there was ever any deviation from this protocol. Because the researcher follows the research protocol in detail, the findings may be checked by other researchers by replicating the study, possibly partially or possibly in its entirety.

Despite the power of the RCT, it is still necessary for the practitioner to scrutinise the research to ensure that the context and intervention are relevant to her situation. This scrutiny is vital in maternity care, where systems of care differ greatly and where cultural values are fundamental to the attitudes of women and staff. Such scrutiny will take account of not only the research findings and the local situation, but also the midwife's observation of the woman and the midwife's personal and professional experience, as well as her intuition.

QUANTITATIVE RESEARCH

The research which has been mentioned up to this point in this chapter has focused on areas of care which are amenable to scientific measurement or quantification. For this reason the methods used are known as quantitative methods (Hicks 1996). In the next section there will be some discussion of another approach, which is known as qualitative. If the researcher's area of interest involves pheno-

mena which may be counted, numbered or otherwise measured then a quantitative approach is appropriate.

When I undertook a study examining student midwives' employment decisions and practice, quantitative methods were appropriate (Mander 1994). These methods permitted counting the number of students and midwives who planned to practise as midwives and the number who had other plans. It was also possible to count the number and to measure the length of time that the midwives practised as such. In this research on employment decisions, as in all quantitative research, it was essential for the researcher to maintain objectivity as far as possible. In this way the researcher tries to remain impartial and to reduce the possibility of bias by avoiding becoming personally involved with the data or the respondents. The researcher must also attempt to limit the scope for personal interpretation of the data, as was described in the account of RCTs (above). This involves the scrupulous pretesting of the research instrument, in the present example a postal questionnaire, to ensure its reliability and validity (see below). A pilot test may be used to test the complete research protocol, rather than a pretest of a particular aspect.

READER ACTIVITY

Suggest three topics in midwifery which have been or could be researched using a quantitative approach.

Quantitative research usually employs quite a structured format, thus giving rise to one of its strengths through being easily replicated. This structure invariably begins with a literature search, on the basis of which the researcher formulates a hypothesis and possibly research questions. The researcher seeks to test the hypothesis and to answer the research questions by using the research approach or design which is most appropriate. Following on from the design are various methods of sampling, data collection and data analysis and the researcher needs to consider a wide range of possibilities before deciding which of them will best answer the research question.

The issues of reliability and validity are crucially

important when considering the methods and the instruments to be used.

• Reliability refers to the constancy or accuracy of a measurement or observation. At a simple level this might refer to ensuring that a sphygmomanometer had been accurately calibrated.
• Validity is the extent to which the research is measuring what it is supposed to be measuring, or whether it is measuring another closely-related phenomenon.

Quantitative research has been criticised on the grounds that it may be reductionist; this is because, in order to make sense of the respondents' behaviour or responses, the researcher must simplify or reduce the events to their most basic component parts. The appropriateness of such a reductionist approach in research into a topic as humanely complex as childbearing is a problem that the researcher must consider carefully when choosing the research approach. It is possible that a quantitative research approach may neglect some important aspect of the phenomenon under study. This may be because the researcher is unaware of its existence or possibly because it is too complex, or otherwise challenging, to cope with.

QUALITATIVE RESEARCH

Qualitative approaches to research may sometimes be more appropriate to help the midwife to find answers to complex and challenging questions (Morse 1992, Morse & Field 1996). While some regard the qualitative research approach as 'soft', it may be more suitable for examining the human situations which are fundamental to childbearing. A crucial feature of all forms of qualitative research lies in their ability to understand the person's experience, which is known by the German term 'verstehen' (Leininger 1985). To achieve this understanding, the researcher must observe, listen to or read the thoughts of the person; thus, the perspective of the person experiencing the phenomenon becomes apparent. This approach has been described as 'emic', and is clearly different from the 'etic' or quantitative approach mentioned above. The qualitative researcher makes no attempt to

achieve objectivity, in fact the reverse applies as the researcher seeks to personally interact with the informant and the data. In this way, the researcher seeks a complete understanding of the phenomenon, event or experience; this is in marked contrast with the likelihood of reductionism in quantitative research.

READER ACTIVITY

Suggest three midwifery topics which have been or could be researched using a qualitative approach.

There are a number of different forms of qualitative research, such as grounded theory and ethnography, which differ in their theoretical basis, the involvement of the researcher and the degree of structure. The qualitative method which is chosen will depend on the extent of existing knowledge about the topic, as determined by the preliminary search of the literature, and the researcher's expertise.

The analysis of qualitative data tends not to use statistical tests, but computer programmes are increasingly frequently used (Dey 1993). As with other stages, the data analysis involves the researcher's profound involvement. This personal input may be challenging, as the topics may be quite emotional, as I found during my study of the midwife's care of the mother who relinquishes her baby for adoption (Mander 1995).

The exploratory nature of qualitative research makes it ideally suited to areas where knowledge is scanty or underdeveloped (Leininger 1985). For this reason this type of research may sometimes be regarded as a basic building brick of midwifery theory. A further strength of qualitative research is that it is able to provide fresh perspectives on phenomena which the 'experts' regard as well understood. Clearly this is important when the midwife needs a comprehensive understanding of the woman's experience of some aspect of childbearing or care.

I have briefly described two different approaches to research which have much to offer midwifery. These two approaches do not need to be regarded as discrete entities, as qualitative and quantitative aspects may be combined in a single research project. This combination may be known as 'triangulation'. While the quantitative approach tends towards the 'scientific' aspects of care, qualitative research tends towards the more human. The exploratory nature of qualitative research means that it has the capacity to 'open up' new areas of knowledge, which is facilitated by its lack of external structure. In the same way, qualitative approaches are likely to provide in-depth detail, rather than large-scale statistically significant evidence which is provided by quantitative studies.

While some researchers regard the gap between these two research approaches as unbridgeable (Carr 1994, Clarke 1995), there are more constructive ways of viewing the situation. Rather than a right or wrong research method, the reader or consumer of research should be thinking in terms of the appropriateness of the research approach for the question which is being asked. It may be that a postal questionnaire and tests of significance are not suitable for studying intimately human problems.

RESEARCH ETHICS

The woman and baby for whom the clinical midwife cares seek her help for precisely that reason, that is, to obtain care. Because of this rather obvious statement, it is necessary to question whether researchers should be able to recruit this woman and baby as research subjects in the course of that care. This question, and others that emerge in using and doing research, raise certain ethical issues which the midwife should consider (Beauchamp & Childress 1989).

Autonomy
Autonomy, or self-rule, is one of the fundamental human rights and means that human beings have the right to decide what does or does not happen to them and to their bodies. As mentioned already, a woman seeking midwifery care has no duty, but is able to choose whether to participate in research associated with that care. Both the researcher and the midwife have a duty to ensure that the woman is aware that she is under no compulsion

to participate in the research and that if she does become involved she is able to withdraw at any point. It may be that pressure on women to be involved in research is subtle, and information about involvement should be provided in writing for her to keep. To enable the woman to make this decision she needs to be informed about the details and implications of the study before agreeing to participate. Researchers are usually required to obtain the woman's consent in writing, but the consent form per se is of little significance compared with the information which allows that consent, if given, to be fully informed. The researcher should also allow the woman sufficient time to consider, and perhaps discuss, whether to be involved; at least 24 hours is recommended. This excludes the possibility of recruiting especially vulnerable women such as those who are in labour or those who have recently given birth to an ill baby. A crucial extension of autonomy is the researcher's responsibility to ensure that the anonymity and confidentiality of each informant or respondent is maintained. This means that not only is the person not named, but also that she is in no way identifiable.

Nonmaleficence
Nonmaleficence, the avoidance of harm, is fundamental to research ethics. Health care providers and some others tend to assume that research is 'a good thing' and the possibility of harm is negligible. It is necessary to remember, though, that the researcher's priority may not always be the welfare of the subject and careful scrutiny of the research protocol is necessary to ascertain whether there are any unforeseen dangers. It is sometimes assumed that, because there is no physical intervention, non-invasive research methods are harmless. This may not be the case, as anxieties and fears may be provoked through interviews or questionnaires, especially when the respondent is unable to follow up any points of concern. Maleficence was raised as a possibility when I interviewed women who had relinquished or were relinquishing a baby for adoption. Far from resurrecting long-forgotten painful sorrows, as had been suggested, these women almost invariably thanked me for allowing them to verbalise unspoken thoughts which were con-

stantly with them. The quantitative researcher may encounter difficulty in trying to achieve nonmaleficence. This difficulty arises out of this researcher's need to avoid involvement in the data collection. Thus, problems emerge when the researcher is aware of a respondent following a course of action which may prove harmful.

Beneficence

Beneficence, or the promotion of good, applies more on a global than individual scale. The subject is informed prior to being recruited that the research may not benefit her as an individual. The midwife needs to consider, though, who will benefit from this woman's participation. Clearly the researcher who is completing a course assignment or a higher degree will benefit, but the midwife should assess whether the benefits extend any further, in terms of contributing to the body of knowledge or improving care.

Ethical issues, such as the three just mentioned, are supposedly the prime concern of research ethics committees (RECs). Protecting the interests of vulnerable groups, such as clients and patients, from harm is the remit of these committees. The functioning of RECs has been the subject of criticism on the grounds of their limited experience, knowledge and outlook (Mander 1992). They may, however, be valuable by providing a forum for peer review of a research project, which may only benefit from an outside opinion. As well as the REC, the researcher planning clinical research must seek the permission of the administration before being allowed access to the women, patients or clients in the research site.

READER ACTIVITY

What ethical issues relating to research have you encountered?

The question that emerges from this discussion of research ethics is how these issues impinge on the clinical midwife's role. The first of the implications relates the effect of a research project on the midwife's usual clinical practice. Because the midwife may be asked to act as a data collector, she should be able to decide whether her existing duties are likely to be jeopardised by accepting this extra workload. She will take this decision having scrutinised the research protocol to evaluate its merits. Second, the midwife may be delegated the role of recruiting suitable women or babies. Again, she should be able to decide whether the study is worthy of her expending her time and effort and that of the women considering participation. To do this, as has been emphasised already, she requires a good understanding of the research. Eventually, the midwife may find herself in the position of considering whether management permission for access is to be given, clearly taking account of the implications for staffing, as well as the research itself. Thus, the need for careful scrutiny of the research project is apparent in all three situations.

As well as these ethical issues for solely clinical midwives, an ethical problem which may be assumed to affect only a small number of midwives was shown by Hicks (1993) to involve a majority. This problem is the failure of midwife researchers to publish their findings. In her sample of 550 randomly selected midwives, 64% had been involved in a research project. Of this number, rather than just collecting data for others, a clear majority (62%) of midwives had experience of doing their own research. In contrast to this large proportion, the small number who had attempted (18%) and the even smaller number (7%) who had succeeded in getting their work into print pales into insignificance.

It is crucial that research findings are shared with practitioners and with other researchers if the two main purposes of midwifery research, the development of knowledge and the improvement of care, are to be achieved. Thus, failure to publish is ethically unjustifiable. Sharing of the findings is fundamental to research and, for this reason, is to be considered as part of the research process itself. This view is advanced by Tierney (1991, p. 318), who states 'the research process is not complete until a written report ... is prepared and disseminated'.

The duty to publish features in many codes of research ethics including the RCN (1977) guidelines: 'The researcher has responsibility ... to publish or make otherwise available the results of the research ... including negative evidence'. This responsibility relates to the researcher's duty to the various groups who have some interest in the research, possibly through their financial or other resources having been utilised, possibly because they invested time and thought in responding or possibly because they may ultimately be the research consumers.

RESEARCH UTILISATION BY THE PRACTITIONER

In this chapter, so far, it has been established that reading research is an essential requirement for safe midwifery practice and that the midwife needs to scrutinise the research reports which have been published to be able to decide whether to use the findings. In this section the scrutiny, critical reading or critique of research reports will be addressed, followed by the use to which the midwife is able to put this information.

Critical reading

The word 'critique' is often used in relation to reading research. This is because its everyday equivalent 'criticism' has too many negative and destructive connotations, which are inappropriate in the context of research. 'Critique', though, carries implications of a rather artificial academic exercise, which are even more inappropriate and, for this reason, this term will be avoided. 'Critical reading' may be a suitable compromise, because the dictionary definition of critical is 'judging well'. This is what reading a research report should involve, in that it should be judged well, in the sense of fairly, rather than harshly or excessively negatively. Similarly, reading research requires an objective examination, in order to identify its strengths and weaknesses. It may be argued that even the best research has some weak points, but the reverse may also be true in that even a weak study is likely to provide some points from which the midwife is able to learn.

As has been mentioned already, asking questions is fundamental to research. This obviously applies to the researcher, but it also applies to the research consumer, the midwife in clinical practice. Many of this midwife's questions will relate to her practice, especially to those routines which may have become established as 'unit policy' and over the use of which she may feel that she has little control. It may be that some of her questions will be answered by the research literature, but whether this is so depends on her critical reading. Thus, the midwife's questioning approach to her practice needs to be extended to her reading of research, in which the following points should be included.

The complete research

The midwife should consider the material in its entirety, rather than taking a piecemeal approach. This complete picture will illuminate points which might otherwise be missed; for example, a small sample might be inappropriate to permit conclusions to be drawn, but if an in-depth qualitative study is being undertaken this would be reasonable. Similarly, in a quantitative study, the tables and statistical tests may appear daunting to some readers, but they are a crucial part of the findings and need to be read in conjunction with the text.

A further advantage of reading the complete report lies in the likelihood of the reader observing any points which may have been neglected or even omitted. In this way the reader would be in a position to question why this information has been neglected or omitted. This may be because of an error or oversight, but may be because the researcher wishes to minimise or disguise some unsatisfactory aspect of the study. An example would be when the response rate to an invitation to participate is not stated. The reader would be justified in being cautious about the quality of this work and may even suspect that this information was omitted because the rate was unacceptably low. The response rate is a good reflection of the suitability of the instrument and may indicate the importance of the research to the sample.

Specific points

While examining the complete report the midwife should question whether the various parts of it form a unified whole, whether they are discrete entities or whether there are gaps in the presentation. A problem which may emerge is that one part does not lead into the next; for example, the research questions may bear little relation to the literature review from which they should have arisen. This would lead the reader to wonder how these questions originated. Another example would be when the conclusions are not clearly derived from the findings, causing the reader to question the possibility of the researcher having decided on the conclusions in advance of doing the research.

The author's name, designation and qualifications may be helpful initially in evaluating the research. This may be because of knowledge of and respect for this researcher's previous work or because an examination of this particular problem from, for example, a midwifery or physiotherapist's point of view is sought. The place where the researcher is based or employed may assist in deciding its relevance if, for example, the report was written in a country where maternity care differs from the reader's.

The introduction should explain the significance of the research topic and allow the reader to decide whether the report is likely to be helpful.

The literature review leads the reader through the development of knowledge about the chosen topic up to the present time to indicate why this current research project was necessary. If recent research is not mentioned, the reader has to question whether the project was undertaken some time previously and is out of date. Additionally, if earlier important research is not mentioned, the question 'Why' must be asked; the omission may have been due to ignorance or perhaps there was another agenda. The literature review should show how the research is based in a relevant theoretical framework.

The hypothesis and/or research questions should emerge inevitably out of the literature review. These statements or questions should be phrased precisely to exclude all possibility of any ambiguity.

The research approach or design should include a discussion of the possibilities which were considered and the reasons why one approach was chosen in preference to another. The researcher should show understanding of the issues relating to the differing approaches and of having read the important literature on research design. The reader must at this point question whether this approach is likely to be able to answer the research questions which are being asked.

The research method describes, with some discussion of the literature and the alternatives which were not selected, the complete research as it was planned. This usually begins with the subjects and the sample; in a quantitative study details of the calculations to produce the number of subjects for findings to be statistically significant would be necessary. The reader would question here whether the subjects in the sample would be able to provide the information to answer the research questions; an example of this not being done is when certain groups, such as children and people with learning difficulties, are not allowed to speak for themselves, but the researcher focuses the project on their parents or carers. Details of how the sample was identified and recruited are also necessary. As mentioned already, a random sample lends strength to a research project, but a convenience sample needs to be identified as such.

The data collection should be detailed in terms of how the research instrument was chosen and how it was designed, tested and applied. This applies particularly to questionnaires, but may also be relevant to interview schedules or observation checklists. The reader must consider whether these aspects are appropriate to answer the research questions, bearing in mind the strengths and weaknesses of the various instruments. Some critical discussion by the researcher of the reliability and validity of the research method would be expected in this section.

The data analysis planned should be explained. This includes a discussion of the relevance of and an explanation of the statistical tests.

Ethical implications of the research should be considered, with some discussion of how any dilemma was resolved. The obtaining of ethical approval is usually reported.

The findings should begin with any aspect of the research which deviated from that described in the method section. Then response rates and other relevant data should be provided. In this section the reader should be aware of any omissions, which might indicate that some aspects of the study were not completed. This section may include some discussion of the findings or the discussion may be in a separate section. This discussion relates the findings to the research questions. The researcher would be expected to identify in this section whether there were any aspects of the research questions which were not answered and the reasons for this. This discussion, hence, may include the researcher's criticism of the research (Benton & Cormack 1991).

The conclusions, as mentioned already, should relate closely to the findings and should be well substantiated. This section may include recommendations which, again, must be well supported by the research.

Using information

In addition to the reasons which have been advanced already for reading research, it is necessary to examine in detail the actions which are likely to follow a midwife's critical reading of a research report. As has been implied already clinical midwives are the research consumers, that is, the people who are in a position to make use of clinical research. They are likely to encounter research reports in a wide range of midwifery, nursing and other journals as well as at meetings and conferences.

Following the midwife's critical reading of a research report in a journal or another publication she has a number of choices open to her (Box 6.2):

• The midwife may be convinced that the research findings are likely to resolve a problem which has been identified in her own clinical

setting. On the basis of this she may seek to implement it in her own clinical area.

• The midwife may decide to reject the study on the grounds that:
    – it does not relate to her working situation
    – the work is too seriously flawed to be of any value
    – the research was undertaken in a country with a different system of maternity care and is not easily transferable.

• Although the research has some weaknesses or was undertaken in a different country, some of the problems identified relate to those in her clinical area. For these reasons, a researcher will be approached to assist the midwifery staff in further investigating this work by replicating this study locally and with a suitably sized sample.

CONCLUSION

In this chapter research has been shown to vary in its quality, its strength and its approach. The midwife who is seeking to practise safely must take the opportunity to ensure that her practice is research-based by reading research critically to ascertain whether it is appropriate and transferable to the context of her own practice or to decide that it is not worthy of implementation. With regular critical reading and application of 'good research' to her own practice the midwife will grow in clinical confidence and eventually may feel ready to undertake research of her own.

Box 6.2 The midwife's actions following reading a research report

• Implementation
• Rejection as inappropriate
• Replication to test appropriateness

READER ACTIVITIES

1. On what basis may a midwife make decisions relating to her practice?

Make a list of the possible bases which she may use.

Think of examples of the decisions which may be made using each basis.

If they have not been, how might these examples be researched?

2. On what 'evidence' is the midwife able to draw when considering whether to rupture the membranes of a woman who is in labour?

REFERENCES

Beauchamp T L, Childress J F 1989 Principles of biomedical ethics, 3rd edn. Oxford University Press, Oxford

Benton D, Cormack D 1991 Reviewing and evaluating the literature. In: Cormack D (ed) The research process in nursing. Blackwell, Oxford, ch 10

Briggs A 1972 Report of the Committee on Nursing. HMSO, London

Carr L T 1994 Strengths and weaknesses of quantitative and qualitative research: what method for nursing? Journal of Advanced Nursing 20(4): 716–721

Chalmers I 1993 Effective care in midwifery: research the professions and the public. Midwives Chronicle 106(1260): 3–12

Chalmers I, Enkin M, Keirse M J N C 1989 Effective care in pregnancy and childbirth. Oxford University Press, Oxford, vols 1, 2

Clarke L 1995 Nursing research: science visions and telling stories. Journal of Advanced Nursing 21(3): 584–593

Cochrane A L 1972 Effectiveness and efficiency. Nuffield Provincial Hospitals Trust, London

Dey I 1993 Qualitative data analysis: a user-friendly guide for social scientists. Routledge, London

Enkin M, Keirse M J N C, Chalmers I 1990 A guide to effective care in pregnancy and childbirth. Oxford University Press, Oxford

Harris M 1992 The impact of research findings on current practice in relieving postpartum perineal pain in a large district general hospital. Midwifery 8(3): 125–131

Haynes R B, Sackett D L, Gray J M A, Cook D J, Guyatt J H 1996 Transferring evidence from research into practice. Evidence-based Medicine 1(7): 196–198

Hicks C 1992 Research in midwifery: are midwives their own worst enemies? Midwifery 8(1): 12–18

Hicks C 1993 A survey of midwives' attitudes to, and involvement in, research: the first stage in identifying needs for a staff development programme. Midwifery 9(2): 51–62

Hicks C 1996 Undertaking midwifery research. Churchill Livingstone, Edinburgh

Hunt J M 1981 Indicators for nursing practice: the use of research findings. Journal of Advanced Nursing 6(4): 189–194

Leininger M M 1985 Nature rationale and importance of qualitative research methods in nursing. In: Leininger M M Qualitative research methods in nursing. Grune & Stratton, Orlando

Mander R 1992 Seeking approval for research access: the gatekeeper's role in facilitating a study of the care of the relinquishing mother. Journal of Advanced Nursing 17(12): 1460–1464

Mander R 1993 Who chooses the choices? Modern Midwife 3(1): 23–25

Mander R 1994 Midwifery training and the years after qualification. In: Robinson S, Thomson A (eds) Midwives, research and childbirth. Routledge, London, vol 3, ch 9

Mander R 1995 The care of the mother grieving a baby relinquished for adoption. Avebury, Aldershot

Meah S, Luker K A, Cullum N A 1996 An exploration of midwives' attitudes to research and perceived barriers to research utilisation. Midwifery 12(2): 73–84

MIDIRS 1996/7 Informed choice for women. (Leaflets 1–10) MIDIRS and the NHS Centre for Reviews and Dissemination, Bristol and York

Morse J M (ed) 1992 Qualitative nursing research: a contemporary dialogue. Sage, London

Morse J M, Field P A 1996 Nursing research: the application of qualitative approaches, 2nd edn. Chapman & Hall, London

RCN 1977 Ethics related to research in nursing. Royal College of Nursing of the United Kingdom, London

Renfrew M J 1989 Ethics and morality in midwifery research. Midwives Chronicle 102(1217): 198–201

Renfrew M J 1997 The development of evidence-based practice. British Journal of Midwifery 5(2): 100–104

Sackett D, Rosenburg W, Gray J A, Haynes B, Richardson W S 1996 Evidence based medicine: what it is and what it isn't. British Medical Journal 312(7023): 71–72

Sleep J 1984 The West Berkshire episiotomy trial. In: Thomson A M, Robinson S (eds) Research and the Midwife Conference Proceedings for 1983. Department of Nursing, Manchester University, Manchester

Sleep J 1991 Perineal care: a series of five randomised controlled trials. In: Robinson S, Thomson A M (eds) Midwives research and childbirth. Chapman & Hall, London, vol 2, pp 199–251

Tierney A 1991 Reporting and disseminating research. In: Cormack D (ed) The Research Process in Nursing. Blackwell Scientific Publications, Oxford

FURTHER READING

Cormack D F S 1996 The research process in nursing, 3rd edn. Blackwell Science, Oxford

Polit-O'Hara D, Hungler B P 1993 Essentials of nursing research: methods appraisal and utilization, 3rd edn. Lippincott, Philadelphia

Rees C 1994 Evaluating a research article. British Journal of Midwifery 2(12): 596–601

Rees C 1997 An introduction to research for midwives. Books for Midwives, Hale

Risk management in midwifery

7

Josephine Williams

This chapter defines the different types of risk and introduces the concept of risk management. The major focus is clinical risk management, particularly in relation to midwifery practice. There is also discussion of the management of non-clinical risks because of their potential effects on both midwifery care and the health and safety of the midwife.

The chapter aims to:

• describe the risk-management process – the identification, analysis and control of risk and, where risk cannot be eliminated, the funding of any resulting loss

• consider risk management in relation to the key risk factors in midwifery practice: staff competence and deployment; communication difficulties and delays; clinical record keeping; maintenance and use of equipment; security; and health and safety regulations

• review systems for reporting and investigating untoward clinical incidents.

Although references are made within the text to specific United Kingdom (UK) legislation and National Health Service (NHS) practices, the basic principles of risk management can be extrapolated and applied universally.

RISK MANAGEMENT

Risk is defined by Collins English Dictionary (1994) as 'the possibility of incurring misfortune or loss; hazard'. Frequently the terms 'risk' and 'hazard' are used interchangeably, the distinction between the two being somewhat blurred. The Health and Safety Commission (HSC) Approved Code of Practice accompanying the Management of Health and Safety Regulations 1992 interprets 'hazard' as 'something with the potential to cause harm', and 'risk' as expressing 'the likelihood that the harm from a particular hazard is realised' (HSC 1992, p. 3). The concept of risk is thus related to probability, with the degree of risk present being affected by the probability of it occurring (see below). Risk is an integral part of daily life and consequently of midwifery practice. It can be divided into two broad categories, clinical risk and non-clinical risk, both of which are pertinent to midwifery care.

Risk management could be described as a systematic, multidisciplinary approach to the management of future uncertainty. It is not about the elimination of all risk, as this would be impracticable. Rather it is a continuous process by which risks are identified, analysed, controlled and funded (Fig. 7.1). This process, although common in industry, was introduced initially into health care in the US in the 1970s, in response to escalating medical negligence litigation and the consequent rise in the cost of premiums for medical malpractice insurance. It has been demonstrated there that over a 10-year period hospitals participating in a 'Risk Modification Triad' of education, consultation and information have experienced an associated reduction in clinical negligence claims (MMI 1996).

In the UK a combination of factors resulted in the recognition of the need for risk management in the health service. In 1990 NHS Indemnity was introduced, which made health authorities and trusts vicariously liable for any harm resulting from the acts and omissions of their employees. In 1991, when the NHS and Community Care Act 1990 was implemented, health authorities and trusts lost Crown Immunity from criminal prosecution. They also became more accountable financially for their services, and assumed liability for any event occurring after 1 April 1991. At the same time, as in the US, the amount and cost of litigation alleging medical negligence was increasing. This coincided with changes in the rules for legal aid assessment in 1990, which allowed minors to be assessed separately from their parents and action to be taken in their own right. This affected obstetric claims in particular, with an estimated trebling of claims alleging negligence in cases of brain-damaged infants over those of the previous year (Acheson 1991, pp. 158–166). This was of concern because of the escalating level of settlements in such cases and the fact that obstetrics, together with gynaecology, is the specialty with the largest proportion of claims settled and the largest proportion of damages paid (James 1991, pp. 36–38).

The loss of Crown Immunity had a particular effect on health and safety issues, with individual trusts being prosecuted by the Health and Safety Executive for breaches of health and safety legislation. The introduction of the Control of Substances Hazardous to Health (COSHH) Regulations (HSC 1988, revised 1994), and a number of new European Community Health and Safety at Work Regulations in 1993 focused attention on the management of non-clinical risk.

The risk management process can be either reactive or proactive. Reactive risk management responds to an untoward incident after it has occurred, with the emphasis being on minimising the effect of any adverse outcomes. An example of this would be the management of claims. Whilst such an approach is sometimes unavoidable, proactive risk management aims to identify risks before any harm has been suffered and to control the risk, thus reducing the likelihood of injury or loss occurring. This approach:

- addresses the various activities of an organisation
- identifies the risks that exist

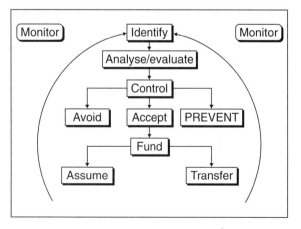

Fig. 7.1 The risk management process (D. Bowden, personal communication, 1996).

- assesses those risks for potential frequency and severity
- eliminates the risks that can be eliminated
- reduces the effect of those that cannot be eliminated
- puts into place financial mechanisms to absorb the financial consequences of the risks that remain.

(NHSME 1993, pp. 1–2)

Proactive risk management is also a quality issue, with the reduction of risk resulting in the provision of higher quality midwifery care. It is closely linked to clinical audit, with risk identification highlighting issues which should be the subject of audit, and audit identifying potential risks.

The risk management process

Risk identification

The key to managing risk is the identification of:

- what could go wrong
- how it could happen
- what the effect would be.

The risk identification process looks at the physical environment, working practices and the organisation as a whole. Whilst this is a continuous process, initially it is best undertaken by a survey of all these areas. This may be performed by the trust risk manager, other suitably trained and experienced staff or external consultants. There are several methods that can be used to identify risk, of which the following are the most appropriate for midwifery practice.

Interviews. A representative cross-section of staff is interviewed individually as to their working practices, their knowledge of and adherence to agreed policies, protocols and guidelines, health and safety requirements and issues such as fire and security. It is essential that the interviewees' confidence is respected, and that no individuals are identified in any report. By giving this assurance, the interviewer is more likely to obtain honest answers to the questions asked. For the same reason interviews should not be conducted by the interviewee's line manager. The interview process will often identify risks which have been overlooked

by those working in the area because of their familiarity with their working practices or because of a lack of appreciation of the risk involved.

Observation and physical inspection. A number of risks can be identified by the assessor walking round a ward or department and questioning staff working there. It is important that the assessor concentrates on the underlying systems in the area being assessed rather than on the detail of one particular issue, so as not to be distracted from the more fundamental problems.

Review of documentation. A review of standards, policies and guidelines demonstrates what documents exist, whether these are current and, where appropriate, research-based, and also, by requesting access to them, whether staff are aware of their existence. An audit of a random selection of case notes is of major importance from the risk management perspective (see below), with high standards of record keeping, as required by the United Kingdom Central Council for Nursing, Midwifery and Health Visiting (UKCC 1993a), contributing to risk reduction.

Analysis of untoward incidents. Such incidents are defined as 'any event which has given or may give rise to actual or possible personal injury, to patient dissatisfaction or to property loss or damage' (NHSME 1993, p. 104). The reporting of untoward incidents is a key part of risk management, and a system should be in place whereby all untoward incidents are reported (see below). From a reactive risk management perspective this allows action to be taken to:

- manage the incident
- correct any errors
- minimise any damage or distress
- manage any consequent claim for damages
- reduce the risk of recurrence.

A more proactive approach, although incorporating these points, places particular emphasis on the management of near misses, which are incidents where the injury, loss or damage was potential rather than actual. Analysis of all untoward incidents reported enables any trends to be identified, so that action can be taken to control the risk.

Questionnaires. Questionnaires can be used to ascertain whether specific working practices are followed, to identify the risk factors present or to assess staff perception of risk. Some respondents may prefer the anonymity of a questionnaire to the perceived potential vulnerability of an interview and thus give more honest answers. However, there is often a low response rate which may affect their validity, and their preparation and analysis can be very time-consuming.

Checklists. These can be used either to identify risks or to check that specific control measures are in place. They are best utilised as an aid to risk identification rather than as an end in themselves, as over-reliance on such lists could cause the assessor to overlook risks which were not included on the list.

Risk analysis

Once risks have been identified it is necessary to analyse their potential outcomes. This is to allow the possible control measures to be prioritised for action. There are two main variables to consider, severity, and probability or likelihood. For the analysis to be truly objective, it would need to be based on hard, statistical data. This is not a practical proposition with clinical risk, where a more subjective approach, based on knowledge and experience, is normally used. A number of techniques exist for prioritisation, which are based on the degree of exposure to risk. Some have originated from industry and are very complex. For practical purposes a basic formula can be used: level of priority = severity of outcome × probability of outcome. The outcomes are broken down into categories, each of which is given a numerical value (Table 7.1). The multiplication of these two values gives the degree of risk exposure, with greater risks having a higher prioritisation rating.

It is important that benchmarks for the various categories of risk are agreed before the exercise is undertaken, so that the analysis is applied consistently. The categories cover several aspects of risk, all of which may affect the prioritisation given. These include:

- personal injury

Table 7.1 Prioritisation of risk outcomes

	Value
Severity rating	
Severe	3
Moderate	2
Low	1
Probability rating	
Probable	3
Possible	2
Remote	1

- cost of staff absence (including use of replacement bank and agency staff)
- damage to or loss of facilities (including replacement costs)
- financial loss
- loss of reputation
- subsequent claims and legal costs.

In addition, there are other factors which need to be considered when finalising an action plan for risk control measures. These are:

- ease of implementation
- cost of implementation
- timescale in which measures are to be implemented.

Risk control

The aim of risk control is to either eliminate the risk or, if this is not possible, to minimise any loss or damage that may result from it. In order to achieve this it is necessary to identify the underlying cause of the risk rather than concentrating on its effects. For example, a delay in performing a caesarean section for severe fetal distress may *result* in a brain-damaged baby, but the risk (i.e. the delay) may be *caused* by one or more factors such as delayed access to an operating theatre, the anaesthetist or obstetrician being in the middle of another case, or lack of recognition of the seriousness of the fetal condition. It is these underlying causes that the risk control measures must address.

If the risk cannot be eliminated, control measures are concentrated on reducing the likelihood and severity of the risk. The methods used will depend on both the category (e.g. clinical, health and safety, security) and nature of the risk. In general terms action is usually taken, where appropriate, in the following order:

- elimination (of the risk)
- substitution (e.g. with a safer method of working)
- use of barriers (e.g. security locks to restrict access)
- safe systems of work (e.g. adherence to agreed policies and guidelines)
- use of warning systems (e.g. hazard warning notices or other signs alerting individuals to risk)
- use of personal protective equipment (PPE) (e.g. eye protection at delivery).

The severity of outcome can be reduced through contingency or disaster planning. This is undertaken by management, in consultation with the relevant staff groups, to identify risks which could have a serious effect on service delivery. Plans are then agreed and rehearsed, so that if that particular event occurs the plan can be put into action, thus reducing the potential disruption. An example of this would be a situation where the delivery suite is affected by fire, with no facilities available for women being admitted in labour. A disaster plan for such a scenario would include the following:

- specific individuals identified as having responsibility for the implementation of the various aspects of the plan
- suitable alternative facilities within the hospital identified to which women in labour on the delivery suite can be evacuated in the short term
- protocols in place whereby neighbouring maternity units, in cooperation with the ambulance service, have agreed to accept transfers of women in early labour from the delivery suite
- procedures in place for the diversion of incoming women in labour to neighbouring maternity units
- the ambulance service being made aware of the plans for transferring and diverting women to neighbouring maternity units
- community midwives or teams having the equipment and resources to provide intrapartum care to additional women at home in the short term

- the operating theatres department having equipment, facilities and staff identified to enable caesarean sections to be performed there, if usually performed on the delivery suite
- a spokesperson (e.g. the public relations manager) ensuring that the general public and the media are aware of the action taken and the reasons for it.

Formal contingency planning is a time-consuming process, and for that reason is confined to the more major risks. Where it is undertaken it is essential that the plan is reviewed regularly, usually not less than annually. However, the same principles are applicable, in a simplified form, to most risk control measures and can thus be utilised as part of a ward or department's approach to risk management.

Risk funding

Where a risk cannot be eliminated, a decision needs to be made regarding the method and level of funding of any loss resulting from the risks that remain. There may be some cost element to the proposed risk control measures, which needs to be considered when deciding what action to take. Considerations are:

- cost
- effectiveness
- practicality
- cost comparison with the consequences of the risk
- associated benefits
- methods of financing
- whether the hospital or trust can afford not to adopt the measure.

Where the potential severity and likelihood are low it may be decided to assume the risk, with any costs being met from departmental budgets. In some cases a contingency fund may be used in which to set aside monies to meet such costs.

Since 1991 trusts have been allowed to purchase commercial insurance to cover most non-clinical risks, with the exception of business interruption relating to NHS activities (i.e. they are not allowed to insure against the loss of NHS revenue from purchasers). The premium charged is related to previous claims history, so there is an incentive to continue to manage risk so as to reduce the likelihood of a claim occurring. It is usual practice for the policy to include an excess, whereby the trust agrees to meet the cost of any claims below a certain figure. Although this reduces the amount of the premium, it must be remembered that the cumulative effect of a number of small losses may be significant.

In the UK when the cost of claims for clinical negligence was transferred to health authorities and trusts in 1990, these costs had to be met from within the overall budget, thus reducing the amount of money available for patient care. In April 1995 the Clinical Negligence Scheme for Trusts (CNST) was established in England. This operates a voluntary scheme of mutual insurance through which trusts can insure against the cost of clinical negligence. The premium has initially been based on trust activity, the number of medical staff and allied health professionals employed and income. In future it will be related more to the claims history. Discounts on the premium payable of up to 25% can be achieved through the trust meeting specific risk management standards (Box 7.1). Because of the potential high cost of obstetric claims, particular emphasis is placed on the key features of standard 11 (see below). A similar system (The All Wales Risk Pool) has been estab-lished in Wales, and although no risk management standards were included when the scheme was first set up, these were introduced in 1997. In Scotland and Northern Ireland no such schemes exist at present.

RISK MANAGEMENT AND MIDWIFERY PRACTICE

Risk assessment is a common occurrence in midwifery practice where it is used to identify the risk factors present in the individual woman's pregnancy. Indeed, various systems of risk scoring have been developed, which demonstrate the degree of risk present in a specific pregnancy (Alexander & Keirse 1989, pp. 345–365). However, this type of risk assessment is focused on the individual woman, whilst risk management, as previously stated, concentrates on the systems in place to minimise the risk to the woman and her family, the midwife and the organisation.

Risk management is both a line management responsibility and the responsibility of the individual midwife. The UKCC Code of Professional Conduct states unequivocally (UKCC 1992a, pp. 11–13) that the midwife is responsible for both the safety and standard of care provided to mother and baby, and for the health and safety of

---

Box 7.1 Clinical Negligence Scheme for Trusts: risk management standards

1. The Board has a written risk management strategy that makes their commitment to managing clinical risk explicit.
2. An Executive Director of the Board is charged with responsibility for clinical risk management throughout the Trust.
3. The responsibility for management and coordination of clinical risk is clear.
4. A Clinical Incident Reporting System is operated in all medical specialties and clinical support departments.
5. There is a policy of rapid follow-up of major clinical incidents.
6. An agreed system of managing complaints is in place.
7. Appropriate information is provided to patients on the risks and benefits of the proposed treatment or investigation, and the alternatives available, before a signature on a Consent Form is sought.

8. A comprehensive system for the completion, use, storage and retrieval of medical records is in place. Record-keeping standards are monitored through the clinical audit process.
9. There is an induction/orientation programme for all new clinical staff.
10. A clinical risk management system is in place.
11. There is a clear documented system for management and communication throughout the key stages of maternity care.

The above is extracted from the CNST Risk Management Standards and Procedures Manual of Guidance which is published by the National Health Service Litigation Authority. © National Health Service Litigation Authority 1996. No part of the above extract may be reproduced, transmitted or stored without the prior written permission of the National Health Service Litigation Authority.

colleagues. These responsibilities are expanded in the UKCC Guidelines for Professional Practice (UKCC 1996, pp. 38–41).

The midwife needs to be aware of both clinical and non-clinical risk. Clinical risk can be defined as being either direct or indirect. Direct risks are those which relate to the actual provision of clinical care. These would include issues such as the standard and timeliness of care provided, consent to treatment, communication, record keeping and infection control. The importance of such risks is reflected in the detailed criteria given by the CNST against which compliance with their standard for management and communication in maternity care can be assessed (Box 7.2). Indirect clinical risks are closely associated with direct risks, and would cover equipment and facilities and contingency planning. Non-clinical risks can also have a considerable effect on client care. This category includes important issues such as security, health and safety, fire and organisational risk.

Risk factors

There are a number of key risk factors in midwifery practice. The midwife needs to be aware of these, as it is often a combination of such factors that results in an untoward incident occurring.

Staffing issues

Midwives are practising today in a culture of continuing change, which results from, in particular, the implementation of the recommendations of 'Changing Childbirth' (DH 1993). The introduction of caseload and team midwifery has led to many midwives being required to practise in all areas of hospital and community midwifery, so as to provide continuity of carer. Whilst, theoretically, all midwives should have acquired the necessary skills as part of their training, in practice this changing pattern of care may result in midwives who have worked in the community for many years being required to provide intrapartum care in a 'high-tech' hospital environment, and midwives with mainly hospital experience having to conduct home births. This scenario highlights the first risk factor, namely competence.

The midwife is personally responsible for maintaining and developing her skills and competence (UKCC 1994), this being of particular importance

---

Box 7.2 Clinical Negligence Scheme for Trusts: management and communication in maternity care

1. The arrangements are clear concerning which professional is responsible for the care at all times.
2. The professional responsible for intrapartum care is clearly identified.
3. There is a detailed multidisciplinary policy for management of the following conditions/situations:
   - Diabetes
   - Major haemoglobinopathy
   - Severe hypertension
   - Multiple pregnancy
   - Vaginal breech delivery
   - Eclampsia
   - Prolapsed cord
   - Antepartum haemorrhage
   - Severe postpartum haemorrhage
   - Shoulder dystocia
   - Failed adult intubation
   - Rupture of the uterus
   - Unexplained intrapartum/postpartum collapse – including amniotic fluid embolism
   - Water birth
   - Anatomical definition and repair of third degree perineal trauma.

4. There is an agreed mechanism for direct referral to a consultant from a midwife.
5. There is personal handover of care when medical or midwifery shifts change.
6. There is a named consultant with designated responsibility for labour ward matters.
7. There is clear guidance on the transfer of care during the intrapartum period.
8. There are fixed consultant sessions on the labour ward of obstetric units for at least 40 hours/week.
9. The delivery interval in caesarean section for fetal distress is subject to a routinely audited standard.
10. There is a personal handover to obstetric locums, either by post-holder, or senior member of the team or vice versa.

The above is extracted from the CNST Risk Management Standards and Procedures Manual of Guidance which is published by the National Health Service Litigation Authority. © National Health Service Litigation Authority 1996. No part of the above extract may be reproduced, transmitted or stored without the prior written permission of the National Health Service Litigation Authority.

when there are changes in the scope of her practice (UKCC 1992b, pp. 8–11). An example of failure to do this is found in the 'Report on Confidential Enquiries into Maternal Deaths in the United Kingdom 1991–1993'. This states 'The midwife was mentioned as contributing to substandard care in only four cases, in each of which she had undertaken work for which she was not appropriately trained' (DH et al 1996, p. 187). Whilst this may be considered an extreme example, it nevertheless emphasises the importance of training.

Although the midwife is accountable for her own practice, her employer is also vicariously liable for any negligence. It is thus part of the employer's responsibility to ensure that training needs are met and that records are kept as proof that such training has been provided. Training needs are best identified on an individual basis through regular performance appraisal. In midwifery, professional training needs are often coordinated by the Supervisor of Midwives. Such training would include the midwife having the opportunity, supervision and support to become familiar with working practices in areas in which she had not recently practised.

It is particularly important that all midwives should participate at least annually in training in neonatal and adult resuscitation, and in the interpretation of cardiotocographs (CTGs). Whilst there is continuing debate regarding the use of CTGs, their interpretation remains a major medico-legal factor. Indeed, the majority of major obstetric claims involving midwives include the failure of midwives to recognise:

- changes in the baseline heart rate leading to bradycardia or tachycardia
- reduced baseline variability, and
- early, variable and late decelerations.

(Mason & Edwards 1993, p. 16)

Deployment is another key staffing issue. This includes not only having a sufficient number of midwives available to deal with the workload, but also the need to ensure that in high-dependency areas, such as the delivery suite or the neonatal unit, staff with the requisite level of experience are on duty at all times. The projected increase in home births in the UK (DoH 1994) has staffing implications, with safe practice requiring two professionals, who may be a midwife and a general practitioner or two midwives, being present at each birth (British Paediatric Association 1993). This is to allow one to be responsible for the mother and the other for the baby, should resuscitation be necessary. It is also important that systems are in place to ensure that midwives do not work excessive hours, thereby putting both their client and themselves at risk through tiredness. This has been historically more of a community issue, but with the introduction of caseload midwifery, the individual midwife may feel obliged to work excessive hours to maintain continuity of carer.

Communication

Communication with the client, midwifery colleagues, and with other professionals providing care is an important, potential area of risk. The midwife is part of a multidisciplinary team, with the roles and responsibilities of each team member being both closely related and complementary to each other. Effective communication within the team is essential for the safe and continuous care of both mother and baby. This can involve communication with obstetric and paediatric medical staff, general practitioners, health visitors and social workers.

Difficulties in communication can arise if there are no clear, agreed protocols or guidelines in place stating under what circumstances assistance should be sought from another professional. Such guidelines should be drafted jointly by representatives of all the professional groups involved, and be reviewed on at least an annual basis. An example of these are delivery suite guidelines, which should be multidisciplinary to ensure continuity of care. Their importance is recognised by the CNST, which lists a number of conditions to be covered in this way (Box 7.2). Whilst communication between midwives and obstetricians is usually good, research has shown that there is sometimes friction present, which can affect the standard of care provided (Green et al 1994). Although the 'Midwives' Rules' require the midwife to report any deviations from the norm to a doctor (UKCC 1993b, rule 40(1)), such friction, where it exists, is clearly a risk to the client and needs to be addressed.

Timeliness of communication is another potential risk issue. In hospital there may be delays in a doctor responding to his or her bleep or protocol may require a midwife to refer initially to a junior doctor, who may not have the requisite knowledge or skills to take any necessary action. It is important that a proactive approach is taken to such situations, with procedures put in place to stop such delays occurring. Communication between staff, both midwives and doctors, when shifts change is also a potential risk factor. The handover should be carried out on a direct one-to-one basis, preferably in the presence of the woman and her partner.

In the community the midwife has to be contactable by her clients and midwifery colleagues at all times. For this purpose she carries a radio pager, and, increasingly, may also be provided with a mobile telephone or personal radio. When commencing each shift, the midwife must check this equipment to ensure that it is operational, and needs to be aware of any 'black spots' where reception of the radio signal is compromised. She should also leave a list of her itinerary, together with any telephone numbers, at her base both as back-up and as a personal security measure (see below).

Midwives exchange information regularly with general practitioners, health visitors and social workers. Agreed mechanisms need to be in place to facilitate this, which take into account the fact that health visitors and social workers (with the exception of the emergency duty team) are only contactable during weekday 'office hours'. Again, an understanding of each other's role and responsibilities ensures that communication issues are given the requisite priority.

Communication is considered by the Expert Maternity Group 'to be of the utmost importance' (DH 1993, p. 3) and is an important part of the midwife's duty of care. It provides the woman with information on which to base her choices with regard to childbirth, thus enabling her to retain control.

It is essential that the information is presented in a form that the client can understand. With women whose first language is not English, this will require the provision of written information in their own language and the use of interpreters. The needs of women who have a hearing impairment or who are blind must be considered and the midwife needs to be aware of the possibility that a woman is unable to read. She must also tailor the information given to meet the needs of the individual client.

From the risk management perspective, communication is particularly important with regard to the obtaining of informed consent. No procedure should be undertaken, except in a dire emergency, without a discussion with the mother regarding the rationale for the procedure and any associated risks and benefits. However, there is a slight degree of risk to many procedures, so it is useful for guidelines to be agreed defining in what circumstances more formal consent should be obtained. A workable guideline would be that 'consent should be obtained for any procedure which is an intervention.' (Beard & O'Connor 1995, p. 357).

When consent is obtained, the discussion regarding the risk of any adverse outcomes should be documented in the case notes. Recall of the information given is sometimes poor (Swan & Borshoff 1994), particularly if the discussion took place in the intrapartum period following the administration of narcotic or inhalational analgesia. Without such documentation, it could be claimed subsequently that such discussion did not take place, and that consent was not truly 'informed'. Where the woman does not speak English, the importance of a full translation being given should be stressed to the interpreter. This is because some individuals, in particular family members, are selective in the information they communicate to the woman.

A woman has the right to refuse to consent to treatment, even though this may result in an adverse outcome for her baby or herself. In such circumstances it is particularly important that this withholding of consent, together with details of the discussion, is documented in the case notes. If practicable, the woman could be asked to countersign the entry as a safeguard against any subsequent disputes. If this is not possible, the entry should be witnessed by a second person. The refusal of Jehovah's Witnesses to consent to any blood transfusion is a situation with which most midwives are familiar. It is usual practice for hospitals to deal with this particular issue proactively in the antenatal period, with specific disclaimer forms being kept for this purpose. An excellent example of a proactive risk management approach to this issue is to be found in the 'Report on Confidential Enquiries into Maternal Deaths in the United Kingdom 1991–1993' (DH et al 1996).

Clinical records

The completion of clear, comprehensive and contemporaneous records is a key part of midwifery practice. The main purpose of clinical records is to be a means of 'organising communication and the dissemination of information among the team providing care for a patient or client' (UKCC 1993b, p. 42). They are also a vital part of the defence case in any litigation alleging negligence, particularly as such cases invariably come to trial some years after the events in question, when memories will have faded. Any decisions made or abnormalities observed, together with the action taken in response, should be noted, even if the management is just to 'wait and see'. Such entries are proof that attention was being paid to the maternal and/or fetal condition. Without such records this would be difficult to prove.

All records should be legible, with each entry dated, timed where appropriate and signed in full. The name and designation of the signatory should be printed after each signature to allow staff who are no longer employed in the trust to be identified. For the same reason a list should be retained of staff signatures and signed initials. Where continuation sheets are used, these should be headed with the client's name and unit number in case the sheet should become detached from the folder. Clinical records are legal documents, and it is important that any additions or alterations are clearly dated and signed. Under no circumstances should correction fluid be used to obliterate any entries.

CTGs are an essential part of the record, and should be securely attached to the folder. Traces should be labelled with the woman's name and unit number, dated, and if the monitor has no clock, have the time recorded at not less than half-hourly intervals. Clocks should be synchronised regularly, particularly where clocks are put backward or forward 1 hour according to season.

The importance of record keeping has been recognised nationally and documented standards exist against which local practice can be measured (Audit Commission 1995, UKCC 1993a). Although many women now carry their own case notes, not infrequently the intrapartum records are retained in file following delivery. It must be remembered that, under the Access to Health Records Act 1990, women have the right to access any records compiled about themselves after 1 November 1991. Particular care therefore needs to be taken that no unprofessional or derogatory comments are made in the case notes which may cause offence to the woman or her family.

Equipment and facilities

Equipment should be regularly maintained, and systems should be in place to ensure that breakdowns are dealt with promptly. Any adverse event associated with the use of medical equipment is investigated by the Medical Devices Agency, which is responsible for monitoring compliance with the European Community Medical Devices Regulations 1994 (SI 1994 No. 3017), which came into effect on 1 January 1995. Items such as resuscitation equipment and blood gas analysers should be checked on a daily basis and records kept of this. It is important that obsolete or unreliable equipment does not continue to be used, as there is a temptation to keep old equipment after its replacement has been acquired, 'in case it is needed in future'. This may be particularly the case where an inadequate number of items such as fetal monitors exists. This is not safe practice, as, if used, there is a risk that any abnormal recordings could be attributed to malfunctioning of the equipment and consequently be ignored.

The midwife must ensure that she has been trained in the use of any equipment that she is required to use. When new items are introduced, all staff required to use them should receive instruction to enable them to do so, with records kept as proof that this has taken place.

Midwives must ensure that the physical environment in which care is provided is safe. This includes monitoring the cleanliness of premises and equipment, so that mother and baby are not put at risk from infection, and also covers the safe disposal of waste, particularly needles and blades. A physical inspection of the premises should note any hazards present, such as unprotected hot radiators or obstructed fire exits.

Security

Although the most common security incident in maternity units is theft and/or vandalism, the threat to which most attention is paid is undoubtedly that of infant abduction. This is understandable, because, despite its rarity, the trauma caused to all involved by such an event is considerable, to which is added the adverse publicity the abduction may attract from the media. The stimulus caused by the risk of an abduction occurring is beneficial to security issues in general, many of the precautions instituted to prevent it having the effect of reducing the risk of other security breaches.

'Risk Management should be at the heart of any security strategy.' (NAHAT 1995, p. 14), and, like risk management, security is the responsibility of everyone. A security strategy therefore should be in place, with the main principles on which it is based including the following:

- raising staff awareness
- raising parents' and visitors' awareness
- use of an identification system
- controlling access and egress
- use of alarm system (e.g. electronic tagging)
- installation of video cameras
- security incident reporting system.

In addition, attention needs to be paid to the personal security of staff. All staff would benefit from training in defusing aggression and breakaway techniques to enable them to cope with any aggressive visitors or members of the public. Midwives working in the community are at particular risk as regards their personal safety. There are a number of precautions that can and should be taken to reduce the level of risk, which should also be incorporated into the security strategy. These include:

- visiting in pairs in areas or at addresses with history of hostility or aggression

- leaving an itinerary of visits at base, together with estimated time of return
- reporting in to base at intervals and at the end of each shift
- carrying personal attack alarms
- provision of mobile telephones or two-way radios
- sonic alarms to repel dogs
- parking car in well-lit area.

Midwives also should be advised to ensure that all equipment carried is kept out of sight in a locked car boot to deter theft. For the same reason, it is inadvisable for a 'Midwife Visiting' badge to be displayed on the car, as this may attract thieves looking for drugs.

Health and safety

There is an increasing number of health and safety and associated regulations of which the midwife needs to be aware. These include:

- Management of Health and Safety at Work Regulations 1992 (SI 2051)
- Provision and Use of Work Equipment Regulations 1992 (SI 2932)
- Manual Handling Operations Regulations 1992 (SI 2793)
- Workplace (Health, Safety and Welfare) Regulations 1992 (SI 3004)
- Personal Protective Equipment at Work Regulations 1992 (SI 2966)
- Health and Safety (Display Screen Equipment) Regulations 1992 (SI 2792)
- Control of Substances Hazardous to Health Regulations 1994 (SI 3246).

All these regulations have major requirements in common, namely:

- to undertake a risk assessment
- to provide information to employees and others
- to provide instruction and training.

These can be applied to midwifery practice by ensuring that the risk identification process includes assessment of any risks to health and safety. Action can then be taken to control the risks identified. Risk factors commonly found in midwifery include exposure to the risk of infection with the hepatitis B or HIV virus through blood splashes at delivery, inhalation of waste anaesthetic gases and the risk of back injury through manual handling activities.

The latter factor is of particular concern because midwives traditionally have not been considered to be at high risk of incurring back injuries, although research has shown that the risk may be greater than had been thought previously. Risk factors that are specific to midwifery include the positions adopted for delivery, particularly when alternative positions or water birth are involved, and assisting with breast feeding (Hignett 1996).

Untoward incident reporting

Although the majority of risk factors can be identified and control measures put in place, incidents will still occur which result in actual or potential harm to clients, staff, the general public or the organisation. As a consequence of this, the untoward incident reporting process lies at the heart of risk management.

It is essential that all such incidents are reported and investigated fully, both to manage any harm suffered and to prevent future recurrence. This includes any feedback received from women about aspects of the care they have received. A debriefing system has been shown to be very beneficial to women by enabling them to question and understand the management of their pregnancy/labour. It has also been shown to reduce the number of complaints made (Smith & Mitchell 1996) (see also Ch. 2). Hospitals and trusts invariably have a centralised system for reporting incidents, which also allows the identification of those which are reportable to the Health and Safety Executive under the Reporting of Injuries, Diseases and Dangerous Occurrences Regulations 1995 (RIDDOR '95) (HSE 1996). This system is ideally linked to the systems for the management of complaints and claims against the trust.

A number of maternity units are now implementing their own clinical incident reporting system for the reporting of specified untoward events. These systems form part of a maternity unit clinical risk management process, which is coordinated by a clinical risk manager, usually a midwife (Dineen 1996, O'Connor & Beard 1996). Whilst there is variation between the systems in use in different trusts, criteria for reporting include events such as low Apgar scores, admission to a neonatal unit, maternal admission to ITU, postpartum haemorrhage in excess of 1 litre and ineffective epidural anaesthesia.

Incidents are usually reported on specially designed forms, but verbal reports, sometimes using an answerphone system, may also be used. For all incidents to be reported, staff (both midwifery and medical) must feel free to do so without fear of disciplinary action being taken against them. This approach may require a culture change within the maternity unit.

All incident reports should be reviewed on a daily basis, with early investigation allowing information to be gathered from the staff involved whilst the incident is still fresh in their minds. The use of a computerised database facilitates the tracking of incidents, thus enabling any patterns to be identified where management action is required. As with the trust-wide system, the incident reporting system should be linked to the complaints management system. This will facilitate the proactive approach to risk, with a prompt and full response to complaints often preventing their subsequent development into a claim for compensation.

READER ACTIVITIES

1. Identify the risks present in your current place of work, and assess what control measures can be put in place to manage them.

2. Review the case notes of three of your recent clients who have been discharged, to audit the standard of record keeping.

3. Draft a leaflet for new parents informing them of what security precautions to take as regards their babies.

REFERENCES

Access to Health Records Act 1990 HMSO, London

Acheson D 1991 Are obstetrics and midwifery doomed? Sir William Power Memorial Lecture, Midwives Chronicle and Nursing Notes (June): 158–166

Alexander S, Keirse M J N C 1989 Formal risk scoring during pregnancy. In: Chalmers I, Enkin M, Keirse M J N C (eds) Effective care in pregnancy and childbirth. Oxford University Press, Oxford, vol 1, pp 345–365

Audit Commission 1995 Setting the records straight: a study of hospital medical records. HMSO, London

Beard R W, O'Connor A M 1995 Implementation of audit and risk management: a protocol. In: Vincent C (ed) Clinical risk management. British Medical Journal, London

British Paediatric Association 1993 Neonatal resuscitation: the report of a British Paediatric Association working party. British Paediatric Association, London

Clinical Negligence Scheme for Trusts 1996 Risk management standards and procedures manual of guidance. CNST, Bristol

Department of Health (DH) 1993 Changing childbirth, Part 1, report of the expert maternity group. HMSO, London

Department of Health (DH) 1994 The challenge of nursing and midwifery in the 21st century: the Heathrow debate, May 1993. Department of Health, London

Department of Health, Welsh Office, Scottish Home and Health Department, Department of Health and Social Services, Northern Ireland 1996 Report on confidential enquiries into maternal deaths in the United Kingdom 1991–1993. HMSO, London, pp 44–47

Dineen M 1996 Clinical risk management – a pragmatic approach. British Journal of Midwifery 4(11): 586–589

Green J, Kitzinger J, Coupland V 1994 Midwives' responsibilities, medical staffing, structures and women's choices in childbirth. In: Robinson S, Thomson A M (eds) Midwives, research and childbirth. Chapman & Hall, London, vol 3, pp 5–29

Health and Safety Executive (HSE) 1996 A guide to the Reporting of Injuries, Diseases and Dangerous Occurrences Regulations 1995. HSE Books, London

Health and Safety Commission (HSC) 1988 The control of substances hazardous to health: approved code of practice. SI 1657. HMSO, London

Health and Safety Commission (HSC) 1992 Management of health and safety at work: approved code of practice. HMSO, London

Hignett S 1996 Manual handling risks in midwifery: identification of risk factors. British Journal of Midwifery 4(11): 590–596

James C 1991 Risk management in obstetrics and gynaecology. Journal of the Medical Defence Union 2: 36–38

Mason D, Edwards P 1993 In: Capstick B (ed) Litigation: a risk management guide for midwives. Capsticks Solicitors/Royal College of Midwives, London

MMI 1996 Monitoring quality, enhancing safety and managing healthcare risks in a time of change. MMI Companies, Deerfield

National Association of Health Authorities and Trusts 1995 Safe and sound: security in NHS maternity units. NAHAT, Birmingham

National Health Service Management Executive 1993 Risk management in the NHS. Department of Health, London

NHS and Community Care Act 1990 HMSO, London

O'Connor A M, Beard R W 1996 Risk management – what is it and how does it work? MIDIRS Midwifery Digest 6(1): 61–64

Smith J A, Mitchell S 1996 Debriefing after childbirth: a tool for effective risk management. British Journal of Midwifery 4(11): 581–586

Statutory Instrument No 2051 1992 Management of Health and Safety at Work Regulations. HMSO, London

Statutory Instrument No 2792 1992 Health and Safety (Display Screen Equipment) Regulations. HMSO, London

Statutory Instrument No 2793 1992 Manual Handling Operations Regulations. HMSO, London

Statutory Instrument No 2932 1992 Provision and Use of Work Equipment Regulations. HMSO, London

Statutory Instrument No 2966 1992 Personal Protective Equipment at Work Regulations. HMSO, London

Statutory Instrument No 3004 1992 Workplace (Health, Safety and Welfare) Regulations. HMSO, London

Statutory Instrument No 3017 1994 European Community Medical Devices Regulations. HMSO, London

Statutory Instrument No 3246 1994 Control of Substances Hazardous to Health Regulations. HMSO, London

Swan H D, Borshoff D C 1994 Informed consent – recall of risk information following epidural analgesia in labour. Anaesthesia and Intensive Care 22: 139–141

United Kingdom Central Council for Nursing, Midwifery and Health Visiting (UKCC) 1992a Code of professional conduct for the nurse, midwife and health visitor. UKCC, London

United Kingdom Central Council for Nursing, Midwifery and Health Visiting (UKCC) 1992b The scope of professional practice. UKCC, London

United Kingdom Central Council for Nursing, Midwifery and Health Visiting (UKCC) 1993a Standards for records and record keeping. UKCC, London

United Kingdom Central Council for Nursing, Midwifery and Health Visiting (UKCC) 1993b Midwives' rules. UKCC, London

United Kingdom Central Council for Nursing, Midwifery and Health Visiting (UKCC) 1994 The midwife's code of practice. UKCC, London, pp 20–23

United Kingdom Central Council for Nursing, Midwifery and Health Visiting (UKCC) 1996 Guidelines for professional practice. UKCC, London

FURTHER READING

Capstick B (ed) 1993 Litigation: a risk management guide for midwives. Capsticks Solicitors/Royal College of Midwives, London

Clements R V (ed) 1994 Safe practice in obstetrics and gynaecology. Churchill Livingstone, Edinburgh

NAHAT 1995 Safe and sound: security in NHS maternity units. NAHAT, Birmingham

Vincent C (ed) Clinical risk management. British Medical Journal, London

Quality assurance in maternity care

Greta Beresford

Midwives acknowledge that they have a professional responsibility to give optimum care to the mothers and babies in the maternity services. But it is not sufficient to claim that, as professionals, they are able to judge quality for themselves. Their assertions must be supported by professionally defined standards, formal assessment of the quality of care they deliver and how change is implemented, if defined standards are to be met.

The chapter aims to:

- describe the process of quality assurance

- assist midwives to establish a systematic review of maternity care

- review the various systems of quality assurance available to assist with the provision of an appropriate quality service

- promote the creation of meaningful quality assurance activities sensitive to the needs of mothers and babies.

DEFINING QUALITY ASSURANCE

Many health care professionals have their own definition of quality assurance. For some it is equated with audit, which implies a scrutiny of activity and may not include a professional commitment to improvement. Others relate it to defining objectives for care, and the process of monitoring the extent to which those objectives are met. Some refer to the very long-running and successful assessment of the clinical outcomes of pregnancy, the Report on Confidential Enquiries into Maternal Deaths in the United Kingdom (DH et al 1996) and the Confidential Enquiry into Stillbirths and Deaths in Infancy (CESDI) (DH 1995) which is a form of nationwide clinical audit into miscarriages, stillbirths and deaths in infancy. These are, however, examples of outcome measurements, rather than quality assurance, which searches for an overall improvement by professionals in the provision of service. The above, and many other definitions, are used to describe quality assurance but may lead to confusion and rejection of the need for such a system if the terms used are not properly understood.

Quality assurance differs from audit in that it encompasses the concepts of the process of evaluating the current level of performance (audit), the process of change and improvement as a result of that evaluation (quality improvement) and an assurance of maintained good quality (quality assurance). The crucial area is an assurance that quality care will be maintained.

Put simply, in the context of health care, quality assurance is an assessment of the effectiveness of health care provision, the efforts made to improve care as a result of assessment, combined with an assurance that quality care will be maintained. This implies an ongoing commitment to review practice.

The basic underpinnings of a system to address quality are in place because registration bodies, including the United Kingdom Central Council for Nursing, Midwifery and Health Visiting, examine and certify the knowledge base of those admitted to professional registers. But knowledge does not remain constant: the knowledge and skills of the experienced midwife differ from those of the midwife recently admitted to the register. Accompanying advances in medical knowledge, the availability of technology and changes in the needs and demands of consumers change and combine to demand constant examination of the appropriateness of care provided by professionals and a commitment to change, as indicated. There is a dearth of information about what quality health care is, how to define it, measure it and consistently achieve and maintain it, particularly when constrained by economic realities and increasingly limited resources. Defining and maintaining high quality is a current concern and there is a need for the efficient and effective use of resources. 'Value for money' has become a byword in health care provision.

As one of the European member states of the World Health Organization, the UK is committed to implementing quality assurance programmes in health care: 'by 1990 all Member States should have built effective mechanisms for ensuring quality of patient care within their health care systems' (WHO 1983).

Quality assurance now has a British Standard to guide it. Since the late 1980s, quality has become an increasingly important factor in the business world. A major impetus has been the success of the Japanese manufacturing companies and these have led the way in implementing quality systems within their businesses. These systems have not been implemented overnight. Japanese companies have taken between 25 and 30 years to fully develop and implement new quality systems.

Quality systems in operation in industry

The British Standard Institution (BSI) and International Standards Organization (ISO) jointly operate a quality assurance standard BSEN ISO 9000 (BS = British Standard, EN = European, ISO = worldwide), originally developed in the UK. To obtain certification that this standard is being met, companies have to meet a number of requirements. They are required to have documents that have been drawn up specifically for the standard under review and maintain an effective and economical quality system that ensures and demonstrates that materials, products or services conform to the specified requirements. Twenty thousand UK firms had achieved certification by the end of 1995.

There is criticism that quality assurance systems developed for industry do not apply to the National Health Service (NHS), but the systematic ways in which these have been implemented and evaluated provide examples to those considering the introduction of quality assessment systems in the NHS.

The NHS is a public service, financed by the public, therefore the public must be assured of quality. The professions aim to be self-regulating, and a concern for quality is fundamental to the caring professions. However, consumers and politicians demand a formal approach to assessing quality and effectiveness of performance. This chapter aims to provide examples of quality assurance systems and presents arguments for stimulating professionals to implement similar systems. If the professionals fail to assess the quality of service they provide, others will do it for them.

BACKGROUND TO THE DEVELOPMENT OF SYSTEMS OF QUALITY ASSURANCE AND AUDIT

In the NHS, in contrast to businesses, systems of audit and quality assurance only gathered momentum during the 1980s with the development of a consumer-centred framework for quality assurance in health care. Various government reports increasingly emphasise the need for professionally led quality health care. One of the earliest was in 1980 when a committee chaired by Mrs Renee Short urged greater concern for the emotional needs of mothers, considered to be neglected in the relentless increase in reliance upon technology in the maternity services (Social Services Committee 1980).

The recommendations contained in the Short Report were encompassed in reports produced by The Maternity Services Advisory Committee (1982, 1984, 1985). These outlined recommendations for optimum care during pregnancy, labour, the postnatal period and neonatal care. Many of those recommendations are still valid and are helpful when midwives are arguing for adequate and appropriate staffing levels to provide care that meets the demands of parents and professionals.

In 1983 the Department of Health and Social Security examined management in the NHS and produced a report entitled: *NHS Management Inquiry* (DHSS 1983). This, the Griffiths Report, was critical of the level of systematic assessment of the quality of care delivered to patients:

> Rarely are precise management objectives set; there is little measurement of health output; clinical evaluation of particular practices is by no means common and economic evaluation is extremely rare. (DHSS 1983, p. 10)

The Report promoted the consumer as the legitimate judge of quality.

NHS and Community Care Act 1990

By far the most sweeping transformation of the NHS occurred in 1990 with the publication of the NHS and Community Care Act, which enabled consumers to select optimum health care treatment alternatives.

The Act introduced the concept of three groups:

- the consumer
- the purchaser
- the provider.

The purchaser

The main purchasers of service were health care trusts whose remit was to assess the health needs of their populations and purchase services to meet those needs. Other purchasers included many (but not all) general practitioners – GP fundholders. They were entitled to purchase care for their clients, as they considered appropriate. The consumer was able to influence the provision of service by accepting or rejecting referral to hospitals, based on his or her assessment of the quality of care provided.

Purchasers drew up a service specification that outlined requirements for a particular service and many were very influential on the type of care offered by providers. Their demands improved standards, while seeking value for money and relevant data in order to compare one provider with another.

The provider

Providers had to demonstrate an ongoing commitment to excellence and develop strategies constantly to examine the care that is offered. They also had to compete with other providers for business. Heightened consumer interest has contributed to the rising concern about quality in health care and providers of services view quality from a client-specific perspective, particularly the quality of technical care provided and its diagnostic and therapeutic components. There is less emphasis on the milieu of care or the manner in which care is given.

A change of government in 1997 shifted the

emphasis of care provision from hospital to primary health care (National Health Service Act (Primary Care) 1997). As the provisions of the Act are implemented, general practitioners will have a major influence on how health care is organised and delivered. Some of the decision-making should be the responsibility of midwives, most of whom are likely to wish to retain the seamless pattern of care between hospital and the community as the most appropriate support for parents during pregnancy, labour and delivery and the postnatal period.

The system of postnatal care provided by midwives in the UK is unique in the world and is of immense benefit to families. However, it is undervalued by those responsible for the allocation of resources, who are looking for higher efficiency and greater productivity at optimum quality. This demands a systematic evaluation of the quality and effectiveness of midwives' work, if they are to influence resource deployment.

Some midwives may argue that although a number of procedures have been shown to be of benefit to the mother or her baby, based on the results of randomised studies such as those described by Chalmers et al (1989), others have not been scrutinised in a similar way, although there is widespread consensus on their value. A temptation may be to reject demands for formal assessment of practice, based on the assumption that improvements in pregnancy outcomes for mothers and babies are self-evident of good practice. This assumption is dangerous; if midwives fail to acknowledge the need for a more systematic evaluation of the quality and effectiveness of the care they provide, others will do it for them and this may be detrimental to the welfare of mothers and babies.

Many techniques may be used, ranging from the simplest form of peer review, in which cases are discussed by colleagues, to randomised controlled trials of procedures designed to test benefits.

Many midwives, possibly without knowing it, evaluate their practice by sharing with groups of colleagues information gained from personal experience and integrating into their own practice the benefits of learning from others. Examples include local branch meetings of the Royal College of Midwives where there is informal discussion on practice, usually local. Speakers who are experts in their particular field are frequently invited to College meetings. Their expertise is not confined to midwifery, but may include areas commensurate with its goals, such as aromatherapy and reflexology, described as alternative therapies aimed at combining psychological support for mothers with non-invasive techniques for pain relief and relieving stress. Another example of examining practice in a relatively informal way is journal clubs where journals are scrutinised and articles assessed for relevance and potential value to practice and credibility of conclusions. Informal meetings and activities such as journal clubs can provide a spur to midwives to review their practice and should not be rejected because they are 'unscientific' – there is room for diversity of approaches if midwives are to set and evaluate standards of midwife-led health care. Most hospitals have regular perinatal audit meetings, designed to review the outcome of clinical care and identify possible areas for improvement. Commendable though these are, they do not meet the requirements of a formal system of audit because of the non-random selection of patients, and because such meetings tend to be biased towards unusual medical conditions. The ruptured uterus (rare) is much more likely to form the basis for discussion than the extent to which women in the postnatal period suffer from depression.

Because the cost of health care has become insupportable, cost-reduction efforts are part of quality assurance, but unless accompanied by knowledge of what constitutes quality health care, providers, whether clinicians providing individual care to mothers and babies or NHS trusts responsible for the care of a geographical population, have difficulty in knowing how to modify or augment services without jeopardising quality. Because the NHS has no universally agreed set of standards to assist purchasers of health care to make decisions based on value for money, there is the danger of a cost-driven service, rather than a quality-driven service.

Chalmers et al (1989) acknowledged the lack of information about the relative effectiveness, safety and long-term benefits of one approach versus another. They embarked upon a systematic review of care during pregnancy and childbirth in 18 countries, scrutinised key journals and many unpublished studies and contacted 40 000 obstetricians and paediatricians. Analysis of practice throughout the world found compelling evidence that many of the practices surrounding childbirth have contributed little to the safety of childbirth and in many instances were actually harmful. The results of their findings have been very influential in prompting doctors and midwives to evaluate the effectiveness and efficiency of various forms of treatment and care.

In spite of the efforts of the professionals to provide care of high quality, the Government felt the need in 1991 to produce a Patient's Charter (DH 1991). The Charter outlined the rights of patients and the standards they have a right to expect as part of the Government's drive to improve and modernise the delivery of the service to the public. The Charter included a commitment to provide a service that is of measurable benefit to people's health. It is important to note that benefits must be measurable and not assessed in an arbitrary or subjective way. Accompanying the Patient's Charter was a White Paper 'Working for Patients' (DH 1989), designed to achieve an efficient service representing good value for money, by introducing a systematic, critical analysis of the quality of medical care, including the procedures used for diagnosis and treatment, the use of resources, and the resulting outcome for the consumer. New rights for consumers were introduced, among them the right to be given detailed information of local health services, including quality standards. The climate of opinion in the NHS that treatment must be dictated by professionals was changed in favour of the right of consumers to make choices, based on knowledge of the quality of care offered.

Nowhere is this more explicit than in the Report of the Expert Maternity Group – *Changing Childbirth* (DH 1993). Each health care trust is required to make quality assurance part of its patient care programme, and to put in place formal complaints procedures for dissatisfied consumers. Money has been allocated by the Government specifically for the purpose of introducing quality assurance packages, and it cannot be used for any other service.

The Report of the Expert Maternity Group reinforces the recommendations of previous government reports that the service should be responsive to the needs of the consumer, that the service should be effective and resources used efficiently. A key objective was that clinical practice should be based on sound evidence and be subject to regular clinical audit.

It is significant that consumers and consumer focus groups, such as the National Childbirth Trust and the Association for Improvements in the Maternity Services were strongly represented on the Expert Maternity Group. This suggests a degree of dissatisfaction with the current provision of maternity services and a view that professionals were not always aware of the needs and wishes of consumers.

Another recommendation was that the views of women who use the service should be regularly monitored and services adjusted to meet their needs (DH 1993, Section 4.2).

Consumer satisfaction surveys

The attempts that are being made to expand consumer choice in the marketplace cannot readily be transferred to the NHS, but steps have to be taken to ensure that the views of consumers are involved when standards for care are being set. A process of evaluation must be included when standards are designed and introduced.

The Audit Commission report on maternity services (1997) collected data from a national representative sample of over 2300 women via a postal questionnaire survey about the care they received. Hospital-based postnatal care attracted the most criticism. Considerable variation between hospitals in the organisation of postnatal care was revealed. Support from staff and the standards of hygiene attracted particular comment. These are areas that lend themselves to peer review and the introduction of quality circles (discussed later in this chapter). Midwives are entirely responsible for postnatal care; it is rare for doctors to be involved in the care of women following delivery where there are no medical complications. The concerns expressed in the Social Services Committee Report (1980) about the lack of psychological support for new mothers and the work of Ball (1994) on the role of postnatal care and its influence on mothers' reactions to motherhood provide abundant evidence of the benefits to the family of high quality postnatal care and demand the attention of all midwives. Postnatal care is unlikely to attract sufficient funding for detailed research into its benefits and problems, but would be an appropriate subject for formal and informal meetings of midwives with consumers and quality circles activities.

The consumers' views of quality

During the 1970s and early 1980s, the use of technology to monitor the progress of labour advanced rapidly in hospitals in the UK. The use of continuous electronic fetal monitoring is an example of technology which was believed to be the answer to detecting the problems of the fetus that occur during labour. As Chalmers et al (1989) discovered when reviewing relevant literature, experience did not live up to expectations. Increasingly, mothers began to reject the blanket use of technology in favour of a less interventionist approach to labour and childbirth. Most of them were probably unaware of the publications of Chalmers and his colleagues, and many probably believed, because they had been told by the professionals caring for them, that continuous electronic fetal monitoring was beneficial to the fetus and to reject such advice was to place the fetus at risk of hypoxia. Chalmers (1989) revealed that although electronic monitoring did reveal fetal heart tracings interpreted as fetal distress, which stimulated an increase in instrumental delivery, perinatal outcome did not improve as a result.

Women wishing to be free to move about in labour consider the technology to be less appropriate than monitoring of the fetus by the midwife using a Pinard stethoscope or simple Sonicaid. Whilst the information obtained will be less specific than that provided by monitoring the fetal heart electronically, it could be argued that it provides a better quality of service for the mother, since it allows her to move about freely in labour, according to her wishes.

The consumer may consider a service to be satisfactory if it meets her stated or implied needs. The midwife knows that women may not always know the options available to them for quality care, or they may choose care that is inappropriate. For the midwife there is no essential conflict between professional excellence and the requirements of the consumer, provided that the former is not too narrowly defined. Professionalism implies a commitment to meeting the requirements of the consumer. An example described later in the chapter is the birth plan that enables the midwife to find out from the mother what her expectations of labour and delivery might be, and to offer advice on the appropriateness of her choice relevant to the safety of her and her baby. If the mother's expectations are fulfilled, according to the birth plan, she is likely to believe that she has received a quality service. Comparing the birth plan with the outcomes of the pregnancy is an example of a low-cost, achievable way of measuring quality and is within the grasp of every midwife.

Another example of improving the consumer's perception of the care provided in hospital was the introduction of a system for women to carry their own notes. The problem of missing records – within the experience of every midwife – was eliminated and women are able to produce their records whenever and wherever they present themselves for maternity care. Frustration at being kept waiting because notes are missing, and lack of confidence in the service because of having to repeat information is eliminated, staff time is saved by not having to search for missing notes and women feel that the service has improved as a result.

Two of the guidelines relating to quality that need to be satisfied according to the Department of Health publication *Working for Patients* (1989) are:

• an attitude which treats patients with dignity and as individuals
• the involvement of patients in their own care.

The use of birth plans and enabling women to hold their own notes contributes to fulfilling these requirements. The delivery of a healthy mother of a healthy baby is not the only criterion of concern for the baby's parents – the mother's experience of birth and the attitude of the staff towards her will leave a lasting impression. It has already been stated that the NHS is more consumer-oriented, and there are greater efforts to obtain consumers' views about what is available to them. However, interpretation of evidence may bring its own problems. National surveys of public satisfaction with the NHS are sometimes conducted. The *Journal of Health Services* (1991) surveyed 2000 people: 75% reported satisfaction with the NHS and 87% of hospital users were satisfied with the treatment they received. General satisfaction with general practitioner services was also reported. However, there was criticism of waiting lists for non-emergency operations and the time it took to obtain a hospital outpatient appointment. It was clear that consumers complained about the system and not about the performance of individual health care providers.

When devising consumer questionnaires, care needs to be taken when formulating questions: is information being sought about the total system or individual performance and personal expectations? In what context are questions being asked: based on personal experience or in relation to current and anticipated government spending? The answers could distort available information and lead to inappropriate adjustments to the service.

OPCS survey manual

Influential in assisting midwives to assess consumers' views of the standard of maternity care was the publication of a manual (Mason 1989) that provided a precisely formulated guide for assessing the impact of the three Maternity Care in Action Reports (Maternity Services Advisory Committee 1982, 1984 and 1985). Acknowledging that many midwives will have little experience of conducting research, the manual assists with the proper use of samples, including analysis techniques and obtaining maximum response rates from consumers. The manual has encouraged midwives to embark on local surveys that yield valid and consistent data on which to assess and improve maternity services locally. A pamphlet assists users of the manual to consider issues such as consumer choice in labour and delivery and assessment of maternity

care policies (Garcia 1989). Repeated use of the survey is encouraged so that a database of the effects of changes in the service would be assembled to provide information on future deployment of resources.

A weakness of consumer satisfaction surveys is that medical outcomes in terms of safety may be underrated in favour of an assessment of the quality of interpersonal care, such as meeting psychological needs and providing adequate pain relief. Surveys need to be accompanied by an assessment of technical quality, and whether the needs of health education, prevention of complications, access to care and effective and efficient use of the service are being addressed.

GOALS AND OBJECTIVES FOR SERVICE

Most NHS health care trusts develop business plans aimed at defining and achieving organisational goals for improving services to consumers, visitors and staff. Budgetary restrictions will inhibit implementation of some objectives, but managers must have a clear vision of the purpose of the organisation and communicate this to staff at all levels if the 'vision', or mission statement, is to become a reality.

Mission statements

The purpose, or vision, of the organisation is usually referred to as a mission statement. A commitment to quality is the cornerstone of mission statements which are short, succinct declarations of intent. An example might be:

> We commit ourselves to providing a professionally led, appropriate, accessible, quality service to each of our clients.

A business plan is a written statement of intent for achieving stated goals. It is designed to identify priorities within the service, longer-term objectives and essential staff education when changes are being considered. Moves towards implementing the recommendations of reports such as that produced by the Expert Maternity Group, *Changing*

Childbirth (DH 1993) must include appropriate education for staff.

Goals are broadly defined and an example might be 'to create a safe, caring and friendly environment for consumers, visitors and staff'.

An objective towards meeting this goal might be to refurbish waiting areas to provide a welcoming environment for consumers and their companions.

Some objectives will have a longer time span than others, for example to develop a unit for the care of mothers with mental illness following childbirth (by 2001 or later); others would be implemented immediately, for example to provide appropriate, consistent advice on infant feeding (ongoing).

Protocols, guidelines and procedures

Many maternity units will have protocols, procedures and guidelines in place to govern the way care should be provided. These terms sometimes lead to confusion and may be used interchangeably. A protocol is a written system for managing care that should include a plan for audit of that care. Most protocols are binding on employees as they usually relate to the management of consumers with urgent, possibly life-threatening, conditions. A protocol may exist for the care of women with antepartum haemorrhage but not for the care of women in labour without complication.

Guidelines or procedures are usually less specific than protocols and may be described as suggestions for criteria or levels of performance which are provided to implement agreed standards.

Whatever system is implemented (if defined standards of practice are to be met), education of staff so that the system is clearly understood and accepted is vital.

Birth plans

From discussion so far it has become clear that quality in health care is being demanded by consumers and that rights have been enshrined in legislation for them to exercise choice in the delivery of care. Birth plans are an example of involving consumers in decision-making about their care. These are usually drawn up during the antenatal period, and are amended as the consumer wishes and as knowledge of the birth process and so on increases.

The mother and midwife together may prepare the birth plan, or the mother may produce a plan that she has prepared.

Birth plans define a standard of practice, and the implications for quality assurance can be assessed when the outcome of the pregnancy is known. Complications may arise that demand changes to the birth plan, but women have the right to expect midwives, as far as possible, to adhere to their valid stated preferences.

Not all countries in the world have the benefit of access to government publications or ready communication with midwives working elsewhere with whom to exchange information based on experience and some will not have access to a variety of textbooks. As professionals, they will be committed to providing care to the best of their ability and seeking ways of improving that care, but may feel overwhelmed by frustration at the lack of opportunity for education and professional development. In St Petersburg in 1997, where midwives and their medical colleagues from the UK had been invited to participate in seminars to enhance safe motherhood, the beginnings of awareness of quality assurance and clinical audit were evident. An exhibition concerned with the tragedy of war was mounted in a large medical institute. Among the exhibits was one dedicated to Florence Nightingale, because of her success in reducing deaths from hospital-acquired infection during the Crimean War. She lacked tools for formal assessment of the outcomes of care, textbooks and role models, but achieved magnificent results by introducing change based on what she observed. Midwives everywhere should be able to adopt the example of Florence Nightingale for measuring and improving quality care.

The exhibition was used by professionals from the West to promote the development of a system of data collection so that the effectiveness of treatment might be measured. The seminar in St Petersburg was aimed at identifying the most cost-effective use of professional skills, particularly those of midwives, and providing them with information on achieving safe motherhood, based on the needs of women.

The development of a professional association for midwives in Russia, with the support of a midwife from the UK, is progressing and should enhance the professional status of midwives. The benefits for the consumer of such an organisation are well known to midwives in the UK, and it is anticipated that, when the Association is established, there will be similar improvements in the quality of care for mothers and babies in Russia. A major benefit will be the development of a system of peer review of midwifery care and the development of a body of midwife-generated knowledge, similar to that achieved in the UK.

Safe Motherhood Indicators have been identified that would be achievable in Russia, and which will be possible to implement within the constraints of the political system and the poverty of the health care system.

A pre-congress workshop was held in Vancouver, Canada, in May 1993 which was part of the Maternal Health and Safe Motherhood Programme (WHO 1994). The workshop related to reducing the appalling total of women who die each year as a result of pregnancy and childbirth. It is estimated that half a million women die each year, and that many of these deaths are avoidable. The workshop focused on measuring and improving midwifery care, and a published report of the results of the workshop contains detailed suggestions for the systematic assessment of practice and improving maternity care. Many of the proposals could be adopted by midwives wherever they work.

EVALUATION OF QUALITY IN HEALTH CARE

A variety of conceptual models of health care evaluation have been published, and it is helpful to be familiar with these before embarking on devising a system of evaluation. Some of the work will already have been done and need not be duplicated, and packages can be purchased.

Measuring the quality of health care is not the same as assembling information on average bed occupancy, perinatal mortality meetings, workload assessment, and so forth, from which to build a picture of the service that is provided. Much of the research on quality of provision has emerged from the USA and Canada. Apart from the concept of professional accountability that urges midwives, and others, to examine the quality of their practice, in the USA funding is related to a predetermined standard of care. If standards fall below an agreed level, funding may be jeopardised.

Rush Medicus System/Monitor. A system widely used in the USA for evaluating the quality of patient care – but not maternity – was the Rush Medicus System. A pioneer in the UK who stimulated the introduction of systems for measuring quality, is Jean Ball. The Rush Medicus System was successfully modified by Goldstone et al in 1983 and the monitoring tool 'Monitor' resulted. Based on questions about patient care, the system stressed the importance of initial assessment of need for individual patients before planning delivery of care, and included a process of evaluation of the delivery and outcome of that care that was unique at the time. The system helped to identify categories of patients, ranging from those requiring minimal care to those needing maximum care accompanied by medical supervision.

Midwifery Monitor. Monitor has since been adapted by Hughes & Goldstone to create Midwifery Monitor, parts I, II and III (Hughes & Goldstone 1990a,b,c). This tool examines antenatal, intrapartum, postnatal and neonatal care respectively, using Maternity Services Advisory Committee recommendations (1982, 1984, 1985). A series of questions obtains client responses to questions, information obtained from records, answers to questions from midwives, and information on research appropriate for midwifery care. A standard of performance is revealed, assessed by the number of defined standards that have been met. This monitoring tool provides a number of answers to questions about the quality of care and helps staff to improve their performance. It is appropriate for use by midwives because it focuses on midwifery care and includes information from consumers.

However, there are some disadvantages: a team of observers is required to monitor staff performance and this not only has implications for human resources (and that can be costly) but also allows intrusion into consumer privacy by those not directly involved in providing care. Extensive training of observers is essential if problems of subjective interpretation are to be avoided.

Quality Patient Care Scale (Qualpacs). Another quality measurement tool that originated in the USA is a Quality Patient Care Scale (Qualpacs). This is the result of a collaboration between two professors, Wandelt & Ager (1974). Qualpacs measures the quality of nursing care at the time it is delivered. It includes obtaining the views of patients and scrutiny of the patients' records and staff interview and observation. A strong point is the emphasis on the importance of patient–staff interaction. Specially trained non-participant nurse observers are used to gather information and evaluate the care that the patient receives. This system of evaluation has been subjected to rigorous assessment in the USA and is used in the UK.

Its advantages include providing staff with an evaluation of their performance, which should lead to improvements in patient care.

The disadvantages of Qualpacs are that it does not readily adapt to assessing midwifery care, it is time consuming and has resource implications because of the training required for observers.

Phaneuf Audit. Another assessment tool is the Phaneuf Audit (Phaneuf 1972). This involves a retrospective audit of outcomes using nursing records to assess the quality of care. Clearly, its effectiveness depends on the quality of the original records and these may not give a comprehensive report of the care that was provided. The Phaneuf Audit enables a 'snapshot' assessment of care, as evaluation can take place over a defined period by selecting a representative sample of records of consumers who have been discharged. The service is assessed against predetermined criteria and responses are either 'yes' or 'no', which are scored 2 and 0 respectively; an 'uncertain' response attracts a score of 1. The combined total yields information about care on a scale from excellent to extremely unsafe. This system of audit enables problems relating to care to be identified and outcomes to be assessed.

Quality circles

Familiar to many midwives are quality circles, often included in quality assurance programmes. Quality circles were invented in the USA in the 1950s as a practical example of a creative autonomous group, based on a belief that several heads are better than one. They were exported to Japan and re-imported to Europe and America 30 years later. It is estimated that one out of every nine Japanese workers is involved in a quality circle.

A quality circle is a voluntary group of workers with a shared area of responsibility. They meet together, usually weekly, in company time on company premises to discuss their quality problems. They analyse causes, suggest solutions and take appropriate action. The process is not automatic. The groups usually have to be helped to learn how to do it. Communication skills, measurement techniques and problem-solving strategies need to be built into a learning programme for them. Quality circles involve multidisciplinary negotiation and encourage understanding of other people's roles.

The positive benefits of quality circles include allowing people to pool their experiences and expertise to examine problems and to offer solutions, which is both good business sense and good motivation. Employees often have a deep understanding of the issues involved in their work and may produce solutions to a range of problems that managers might not have identified. A strategy of seeking continuous improvement has proved to be a great motivator and, being a contributor to success, creates a feeling of personal worth; the more people feel valued, the greater their self-esteem and the greater their contribution. Personal development is encouraged.

Ways of ensuring cooperation in quality circles include valuing people's expertise, involving and consulting them about plans, encouraging openness and honesty and, above all, communicating clearly. Managers have to take their recommendations seriously or explain why not. To ignore a quality circle is to discourage staff in their efforts to improve quality. As with other quality assessment tools, quality circles have cost implications because of the need to train staff and the time that must be allowed for them to meet.

Participation in quality circles may be a logical progression from informal peer group review of performance and journal clubs, especially for those unable to establish or participate in randomised controlled trials or other more formalised methods of assessing quality of midwifery care.

Clinical audit

Clinical audit is about improving practice and providing a better service for consumers, and is widely used. Practitioners are expected to measure and demonstrate the effectiveness of the care they provide and one way of assessing practice is by clinical audit. The NHS Executive (1996) describes clinical audit as a professionally led initiative which serves to improve the quality and output of patient care through clinicians examining their practice and its results and modifying practice where indicated.

Clinical audit is a continuous process that involves identifying an area to be examined, the collection of appropriate data and the introduction of changes in practice as a result of analysis of the data. It is crucial that the effect of the changes is monitored by repeating the audit and introducing further changes, if indicated.

Clinical audit has been criticised because it is based on a medical model and is disease oriented, but it is a valuable tool for evaluating practice and yields better results than counting bed occupancy rates, admissions to hospital and numbers of contacts between consumers and professionals.

Assembling a database enables health care professionals to share knowledge and experience and to network with others who are using and developing clinical audit, so avoiding duplication of effort and resources.

It is important that clinicians audit their own practice, and not somebody else's. It is important to cooperate with others, and a joint audit is possible. The care of a consumer is affected by everyone, not just the doctor, and the most successful audits are those where all disciplines work together to plan them. The impact on others of changes that might be introduced as a result of clinical audit must be considered, as failure to do this may result in a lack of cooperation and a failure to raise standards.

Defining audit terms

Health care professionals are mainly concerned with the outcome of clinical intervention, but there are other aspects of clinical practice that may influence outcome. Audit may influence aspects of service structure and process as well as the outcome of clinical care.

Donabedian (1980, 1986) is a doctor who developed quality assurance methods on the provision of health care in the USA. He distinguished between the effects of the *structure* and of the *process* of service upon its *outcome*. These terms may be defined as follows.

Structure. Structure refers to the availability and organisation of resources against the delivery of a service, and includes human as well as material resources.

An example might be an inventory as to whether each antenatal clinic has an area suitable for use by small children waiting with their parents. Faults and omissions could be promptly and easily corrected.

Process. This refers to the way a consumer is received and managed by the service from the time of admission until the time of discharge.

A review of the case notes would reveal whether the care provided conformed to professional guidelines.

Outcome. This refers to the results of clinical intervention. This includes the appropriateness of diagnosis and treatment and the effect on the consumer's recovery, and the consumer's satisfaction with the care received.

Definition of clinical audit

Clinical audit is an attempt to improve the quality of health care by a systematic, critical analysis of the performance of those providing that care, by comparing the performance against desired standards and improving performance, if indicated, resulting in better services for consumers.

The process of clinical audit

When embarking on a process of clinical audit for the first time, it is better to concentrate on a small area of study, and one that is amenable to change. An example might be to improve breast feeding rates. One must decide what it is necessary to know in order to achieve this. It is extremely important to define objectives at the start of any process of audit and how the results of the process might be used to influence practice.

When an area of study has been chosen, it is vital for there to be clinical consensus on what constitutes good care, that is, what should be happening, a desired level of achievement, a standard. It is likely to be easier to agree any changes as a result of the audit if clinical consensus on good care has been obtained.

Standards should be written statements so that everyone concerned is clear about the objectives of the audit and in agreement that this is the area of audit with which they wish to be concerned.

Definition of a standard

A target standard is an indicator of care defined so precisely that one can say whether it is present or absent. An achieved standard is an indicator of care, together with the observed level of performance. A standard must be achievable, observable and measurable.

A proposed standard relating to breast feeding might be that 80% of women who wish to do so are successfully breast feeding when discharged from the care of midwives. Once a standard has been agreed, it has to be monitored, because only by a process of monitoring will it be known whether care is improving as a result. It is necessary to know what is actually happening, as opposed to what is believed to be happening.

Part of the monitoring process may be the need to look retrospectively at sets of notes, the results of consumer questionnaires, and so on. Audit may also be prospective, observing care as it is delivered.

After data collection, results are analysed and comparison made between what is actually happening and what should be happening.

If the results of analysis reveal that an agreed standard is not being met, there has to be discussion with everyone concerned as to possible reasons why this is so. Changes in practice then need to be agreed. Once these changes have been

implemented, re-audit is indicated to determine whether the defined standard has been reached.

Failure to meet the desired standard may be for a variety of reasons: possibly because guidelines had not been distributed and made clear to those involved in clinical care; possibly because those immediately concerned with the area of care under scrutiny had not been involved in planning the audit or that essential education had not been provided.

Midwives' first experience of quality assurance might be concerned with clinical audit. Breastfeeding rates have been the target of clinical audit and much of the received wisdom in this field has been rejected as a result. Only those practices which have been demonstrated to be effective should be used and policies and procedures must be consistent with available research-based evidence, but audit is not research. Research determines what constitutes good care. Audit determines how well that good care is practised.

Clinical audit is sometimes referred to as the audit cycle. Practitioners:

- agree a standard
- observe practice
- collect data
- analyse the results
- compare with the original standard
- identify opportunity for improving clinical practice
- implement change
- evaluate change and re-audit.

PROFESSIONAL RESPONSIBILITY FOR QUALITY ASSURANCE

The evaluation of professional practice is central to the quality of care. It is difficult to measure 'caring'; it does not easily lend itself to scientific analysis, and the consumer's views of good care may differ from those of the professional. A process of quality assurance can monitor, measure and change practice, but may be less effective in measuring professional competence. Outside the scope of this chapter is the need to find a method of measuring professional performance that combines the properties of acceptability to the professionals with scientific respectability.

The Midwife's Code of Practice (UKCC 1994) and the various documents produced by the United Kingdom Central Council for Nursing, Midwifery and Health Visiting assist practitioners to identify the standards they are expected to achieve. In addition, it is possible to keep up with developments in medicine, assist with research and to generate new knowledge about midwifery.

Evidence-based practice

The results of research should inform our decisions about health care and are an essential ingredient of quality assurance and clinical audit. However, it is evident from the conclusions of Chalmers et al (1989) that research findings appear often to be only slowly and incompletely reflected in practice.

Many journals available to midwives provide a great deal of up-to-date information on research findings relevant to practice but access to information alone does not always influence putting research findings into clinical practice. Research findings have to be relevant to the work of the practitioner, accessible and convincing as a means of influencing behaviour.

Examples of research conducted and published by midwives are that by Romney (1980) and Romney & Gordon (1981) on routine shaving and enemas in labour. Research revealed that these procedures were ineffectual and possibly harmful and they have since been abandoned as part of routine midwifery practice. It is possible that because the research was carried out by midwives for midwives and their practice, change was readily accepted. The results of this research contributed greatly to acknowledgement by doctors of midwifery as a profession and stimulated research by midwives in other areas.

There are various theories on how research gets into practice, and why it may not. Midwives may feel distanced from research projects because their role is confined to collecting data on behalf of the researcher and the final results may not be communicated to them. Research must be approved by the local ethics committee, it may be expensive to implement, and local policies and

protocols may conflict with the results of research, creating dilemmas for midwives because of pressure from employers and the requirements of The Midwife's Code of Practice (UKCC 1994, Par. 2):

> Each midwife as a practitioner of midwifery is accountable for her own practice in whatever environment she practises. The standard of practice in the delivery of midwifery care shall be that which is acceptable in the context of current knowledge and clinical developments. In all circumstances the safety and welfare of the mother and her baby must be of primary importance.

Lomas (1993) identifies three stages of the process by which research gets into practice:

- diffusion – the passive spread of research findings, such as publication in peer review journals
- dissemination – positive distribution of research findings
- implementation – this includes audit of performance, appropriate education, the application of relevant incentives and sanctions and the opinion of respected individuals.

Possession of information alone is unlikely to induce change. Practical teaching, lectures and the introduction of guidelines may be effective (Shaw 1989). These should be evidence-based (Stocking 1992) and those expected to adhere to them should be involved in drawing them up (Dukes & Stewart 1993). Finally, there needs to be management support if change is to be implemented, and the need for resources in monetary terms and time must be acknowledged.

Because mortality rates in the maternity services are commendably low, and randomised controlled trials in maternity not always ethically appropriate, midwives may reject research findings because they are perceived as insufficiently sensitive to the quality of care they wish to provide. Home births for women considered by medical staff to be 'unsuitable' because of actual medical or obstetric problems provide an example. There is intense interest in research and if consumers are to benefit from its findings, it is essential that midwives are aware of their own beliefs about the effectiveness of care and how they may influence changes in practice for the benefit of mothers and babies. However, indiscriminate acceptance of the results of a single piece of research as a basis for modifying practice or introducing new techniques is professionally unacceptable and may harm consumers. Journal clubs may assist midwives to form their own conclusions about the validity of research findings for improving maternity care.

CONCLUSION

A variety of quality related activities exist in the UK and attention has been drawn to some of them in this chapter. Reading associated literature demonstrates a commitment to improving quality and it is possible to extract a minimum standard for quality assurance, education and training that might act as a catalyst for the implementation of assessment tools. Examination of systems of quality assurance in health care provision, including maternity care, shows that no single approach can be wholeheartedly recommended. Three main strands emerge from each of the systems discussed: monitoring care, an assessment of care and improving care which should provide a framework for the introduction of quality assurance programmes.

READER ACTIVITY

Find out:

- if your NHS trust has produced a business plan
- whether it been made available to all staff.

If it has been made available, have you read it? If you have not, obtain a copy to look at.

Does it contain recommendations that have not been implemented during the designated time scale? If so, do you know why implementation has been delayed?

Are you aware of any member of staff who might have contributed to formulating some of the objectives? Discuss with that person how the objectives were arrived at.

REFERENCES

Audit Commission 1997 First class delivery. Audit Commission Publications, London

Ball J A 1994 Reactions to motherhood. Books for Midwives Press, Cheshire

Chalmers I, Enkin M, Keirse M J N C 1989 Effective care in pregnancy and childbirth, Oxford University Press, Oxford

Department of Health (DH) 1989 Working for patients. White Paper, HMSO, London

Department of Health (DH) 1991 The patient's charter. HMSO, London

Department of Health (DH) 1993 Changing childbirth: report of the expert maternity group. HMSO, London

Department of Health (DH) 1995 Confidential enquiry into stillbirths and deaths in infancy. HMSO, London

Department of Health and Social Security (DHSS) 1983 NHS management inquiry. (Chairman: Mr (later Sir) Roy Griffiths) DA (83), HN(86) 34, DHSS, London

Department of Health, Welsh Office, Scottish Home and Health Department, Department of Health and Social Services, Northern Ireland 1996 Report on confidential enquiries into maternal deaths in the United Kingdom 1991–1993. HMSO, London

Donabedian A 1980 The definition of quality assurance and approaches to its measurement. Health Administration Press, Ann Arbor

Donabedian A 1986 Evaluating the quality of medical care. Millband Memorial Quarterly 64(3): 66–206

Dukes J, Stewart R 1993 At the cutting edge. Health Service Journal (22 April): 23

Garcia J 1989 Getting consumers' views of maternity care: examples of how the OPCS survey manual can help. National Perinatal Epidemiology Unit, Oxford

Goldstone L A, Ball J A, Collier M M 1983 Monitor: an index of the quality of nursing care for acute medical and surgical wards. Newcastle-upon-Tyne Polytechnic Products, Newcastle-upon-Tyne

House of Commons Health Committee 1992 Second report: maternity services, volume 1, report together with appendices and the proceedings of the Committee. HMSO, London

Hughes D J F, Goldstone L A 1990a Midwifery monitor I: pregnancy care: an audit of midwifery care in pregnancy. Poly Enterprises, Leeds

Hughes D J F, Goldstone L A 1990b Midwifery monitor II: labour care: an audit of the quality of midwifery care in labour. Poly Enterprises, Leeds

Hughes D J F, Goldstone L A 1990c Midwifery monitor III: care after birth: an audit of the quality of postnatal midwifery care. Poly Enterprises, Leeds

Journal of Health Services 1991 31(4): 625–636

King's Fund 1986 Quality assurance – what the colleges are doing. Project Paper 64. King's Fund, London

Lomas J 1993 Diffusion, dissemination and implementation – who should do what. Annals of the New York Academy of Science 703: 226–235

Mason V 1989 Women's experiences of maternity care: a survey manual. HMSO, London

Maternity Services Advisory Committee 1982 Maternity care in action Part I: antenatal care. HMSO, London

Maternity Services Advisory Committee 1984 Maternity care in action Part II: care during childbirth. HMSO, London

Maternity Services Advisory Committee 1985 Maternity care in action Part III: care of the mother and baby. HMSO, London

National Health Service Act (Primary Care) 1997 HMSO, London

NHS and Community Care Act 1990 HMSO, London

NHS Executive 1996 Promoting clinical effectiveness. NHS Executive, Leeds

Phaneuf M 1972 The nursing audit. Appleton Century Crofts, Detroit

Romney M 1980 Predelivery shaving: an unjustified assault? Journal of Obstetrics and Gynaecology 1: 33–35

Romney M, Gordon H 1981 Is your enema really necessary? British Medical Journal 282: 1269–1271

Shaw C 1989 Medical audit, a hospital handbook. King's Fund Centre, London, p 13

Social Services Committee 1980 Perinatal and neonatal mortality second report, 1979–1980 (Chaired by Mrs Renee Short). HMSO, London

Stocking B 1992 Promoting change in clinical care. Quality in Health Care 1: 56–60

United Kingdom Central Council for Nursing, Midwifery and Health Visiting (UKCC) 1994 The midwife's code of practice. UKCC, London

Wandelt M, Ager J 1974 Quality patient care scale. Appleton-Century-Crofts, New York

World Health Organization (WHO) 1983 The principles of quality assurance. Euro Reports and Studies, 95. WHO, Copenhagen

World Health Organization (WHO) 1994 Midwifery practice: measuring, developing and mobilizing quality care. WHO, Geneva

The regulation of midwifery

E. Jane Winship

Regulation of midwifery relates to the rules under which midwives practise. These rules are enshrined in law – legislation. In order to regulate midwifery practice, midwives, like other practitioners, are required to be registered. This chapter outlines the principles of regulation, registration and legislation in the United Kingdom (UK) but this model can usefully be applied in other countries and situations.

The chapter aims to:

- emphasise that legislation enables midwives to have control of their own practice

- summarise the development and purpose of midwifery regulation

- describe the structure and functions of the regulatory body for midwifery, the UKCC

- discuss the relevance to midwives of the primary legislation in the Nurses, Midwives and Health Visitors Act

- discuss the secondary legislation relating to the practice, education and supervision of midwives drawn up by the UKCC in the form of Midwives Rules

- discuss standards and information necessary for the practice of midwives drawn up by the UKCC in the form of The Midwife's Code of Practice

- outline the European Union and the Midwives Directives

- describe the professional conduct function of the UKCC.

In the text which follows the use of the female gender equally implies the male.

INTRODUCTION

Professional regulation, described simply, 'is the

means by which order, consistency, and control are brought to a profession and its practice.' (ICN 1986).

The world of professional regulation and the law can appear to be threatening and complicated. Many midwives do not think it their business to be involved in creating an adequate system of professional governance or regulation and do not necessarily see the link between their everyday practice of midwifery and their professional legislation. It is hoped that this chapter will provoke reflection on that vital link between legislation and practice. The more midwives learn about and understand how their regulatory systems work, the greater is the chance that these systems will provide the authority and framework necessary for appropriate and safe midwifery care.

Self-regulation is a privilege granted to professions which are capable of taking a lead role in the regulation of their own members.

> All professions that enjoy the privilege through the granting of legal powers to regulate their affairs, need confidence and resolve to stand firm to use that power to develop a high standard of professional practice and integrity for the public good. The use of such legal power in professional practice is not about limiting practice but rather about legitimizing practice and enabling it to grow and develop. (Winship 1996a)

THE PURPOSE OF REGULATION

Why does the regulation of midwifery exist? What are the purposes for which it is designed? Regulation may be devised for a number of purposes but the following are considered to be relevant in the UK:

* to protect the public from unsafe practices
* to ensure quality of care
* to confer accountability, identity and status upon the midwife.

The overriding purpose of the first Midwives Act in 1902 is simple and clear in its aim, and remains exactly the same today as then – *the protection of the public.*

A recent report on the review of the regulation of health professions affirms this purpose. This report (J M Consulting 1996), when considering the purpose of regulation, states that the primary aim of public protection should be paramount and it suggests further that if public protection is not necessary, statutory regulation should not be provided. In considering when regulation is necessary the report suggests that protection of the public is required over occupations which involve either:

* 'invasive procedure or clinical intervention with the potential for harm; or
* 'the exercise of judgement by the unsupervised professional which can substantially impact on patient health or welfare.'

It says that it would also include: 'situations where there is risk to the patient from action or omission, and no other regulations adequately control this risk'.

These important conclusions are very appropriate today in considering why the practice of midwifery and other professions like medicine are regulated. It is suggested that those who question the need for regulation should rethink such questions from the public interest point of view.

Regulation also includes registration and protection of title. What does that mean in terms of public protection? When a midwife qualifies, in order to practise midwifery, she is required by law to register as a midwife with the UKCC, which is the body set up under an Act of Parliament to regulate midwifery and nursing in the UK. This enables legitimate practice as a midwife. The public need to know that they are receiving the services of a suitably qualified person, in this case a midwife, and that that person has not been removed from the register for professional misconduct. Anybody can contact the UKCC and enquire about the registration status of an individual. Confidentiality is maintained about the individual's personal details but confirmation of valid registration is possible.

It is a criminal offence for anyone except a registered midwife or a registered medical practitioner to attend a woman in childbirth (Nurses, Midwives and Health Visitors Act 1997, Section 16(1)), which in essence means that title and function are being regulated by legislation.

As title and function have been mentioned here it may be helpful for you to turn to Chapter 1 and consider the *definition of a midwife* (UKCC 1994a) as adopted by the International Confederation of Midwives (ICM) and the International Federation of Gynaecologists and Obstetricians (FIGO) and later adopted by the World Health Organization (WHO).

Alongside this it is useful and interesting to consider the *activities of a midwife* as defined in the European Union Midwives Directives (UKCC 1994a), also in Chapter 1. It can be seen that the international definition of the midwife and the European Union (EU) activities of the midwife are similar in their descriptions. However, the EU requirements do have some extra and specific activities such as diagnosis of pregnancy, the conduct of episiotomy including repair, the maintenance of records and in emergencies breech delivery and manual removal of the placenta.

THE DEVELOPMENT OF REGULATION IN THE UK

In Britain the first midwifery legislation was introduced in 1902 through private members' bills following prolonged pressure from individuals and organisations. At no time did the Government take the initiative. In some European countries legislation governing the control of midwives had been adopted as early as 1801, having been initiated by their governments, as was the case in Austria, Norway and Sweden. The struggles for legislation to control the practice of midwives in the UK prior to the first Midwives Act and since, have been well documented in recent years, particularly by Cowell & Wainwright (1981), Towler & Bramall (1986), Donnison (1988) and Heagerty (1996). However, it is interesting to note that from 1889 eight Bills were introduced but did not succeed. The reasons for this included:

- opposition from the medical profession as doctors thought that midwives would encroach upon their practice

- opposition from the nursing profession which wanted nurses included in the legislation (the Nurses Registration Act was passed 17 years later in 1919)
- lack of interest by members of parliament
- lack of parliamentary time.

The midwifery statutory bodies

The Midwives Act 1902 established the Central Midwives Board with jurisdiction over midwives in England and Wales. This was followed by the Midwives (Scotland) Act 1915 and the Midwives Act (Ireland) 1918 which established similar bodies in Scotland and Ireland. After the partition of Ireland in 1922 the Republic of Ireland continued with the Central Midwives Board for Ireland until legislation established An Bord Altranais in 1951 which became responsible for the statutory control of both nurses and midwives. In Northern Ireland the Joint Nurses and Midwives Council (Northern Ireland) Act 1922 made provision for a Joint Council to take over responsibility for nurses and midwives and the Nurses and Midwives (Northern Ireland) Act 1970 established the Northern Ireland Council for Nurses and Midwives (NICNM).

It can therefore be seen that prior to 1983 four separate bodies were responsible for the regulation of midwifery in the UK and Republic of Ireland. As there was a generally similar pattern in those regulatory systems and there was reciprocity among them, this section will mainly describe that which applied in England and Wales.

The main provisions of the Midwives Act 1902 were as follows:

1. *Prohibition of unqualified practice.* Unqualified women were prohibited from using any title implying that they were midwives certified under the Act and from attending women in childbirth other than under the direction of a qualified medical practitioner. This was to ensure that a doctor was present when there was an unqualified person in attendance.

2. *The Central Midwives Board* (CMB) was established with the statutory functions of:
   - keeping a register of properly certified midwives
   - framing rules to regulate, supervise and

restrict within due limits the practice of midwives

- arranging for the training of midwives and the conduct of examinations
- setting up professional conduct proceedings with power to remove from the register any midwife found guilty of misconduct and also to restore the name of anyone so removed if judged appropriate.

3. *Rules regulating the practice of midwives*. The Midwives Act 1902 conferred powers on the CMB to make rules regulating practice to keep the public safe. The rules used to be much more detailed, partly because of the then poor educational standards of midwives. As the standard of education and practice of midwives improved, the rules were modified accordingly. In 1947 a Midwife's Code of Practice was introduced to reduce the detail in the rules; however, the Code remained fairly prescriptive even in its last CMB edition in February 1983. The CMB for Scotland and the NICNM, although reducing detail in the midwives' practice rules, did not produce a Code of Practice. The rules have at all times identified the sphere of practice of the midwife as being related to midwifery care of a woman in whom there are no complications.

4. *Local supervising authorities and the supervision of midwives* were also empowered by the Midwives Act 1902. In accordance with the Act, local supervising authorities (LSAs) were appointed to supervise the practice of midwives and ensure that midwives obeyed the midwives' rules. Local government bodies, approved by the CMB, were nominated as LSAs until the reorganisation of the National Health Service in 1974. At that time the regional health authorities in England, area health authorities in Wales, area health boards in Scotland and social services boards in Northern Ireland became the LSAs. The LSAs were given powers to appoint inspectors of midwives. In 1936 the title 'Inspector' was changed to Supervisor of Midwives and a circular from the Ministry of Health in 1937 stated that the supervisor of midwives should be the counsellor and friend of midwives. Practising midwives have been required to give notice of intention to practise to the LSA since the inception of the CMB.

There are some remarkable issues to be noted here and especially for those who would advocate a return to the days of the CMB. 'This powerful body was not, as was the case with other professional statutory bodies, to be largely constituted of members of the occupation to be regulated, but to be in the hands of medical practitioners ...' (RCM 1991, p. 6). What is more the CMB was not required to include even one midwife. At no time did the midwifery statutory bodies have a majority of midwives but they were dominated by doctors who also held the chairmanships until the last decade prior to dissolution in 1983.

In the intervening years the legislation was amended and changed to address the improved education of midwives and differences in health care needs. The midwives involved in the development of this legislation are acknowledged for the great service they have provided for the establishment of safe parameters of care in the midwifery services in the UK.

At the handover of functions of the three existing UK midwifery statutory bodies (England and Wales, Northern Ireland, Scotland) in July 1983 the UKCC took over the three sets of existing rules, and for England and Wales also the Code of Practice.

THE UNITED KINGDOM CENTRAL COUNCIL FOR NURSING, MIDWIFERY AND HEALTH VISITING (UKCC)

Background

On 1 July 1983 the statutory control of the practice, education and supervision of midwives became the responsibility of the UKCC and four National Boards for Nursing, Midwifery and Health Visiting (Boards), one in each of the four countries of the UK. These five bodies are referred to as statutory bodies as they are established with the Nurses, Midwives and Health Visitors Act 1979 which was later amended by the Nurses, Midwives and Health Visitors Act 1992 and consolidated in the Nurses, Midwives and Health Visitors Act 1997.

The UKCC is the regulatory body for nursing,

Box 9.1 The key tasks of the UKCC

- To maintain a register of qualified nurses, midwives and health visitors
- To set standards for nursing, midwifery and health visiting education, practice and conduct
- To provide advice for nurses, midwives and health visitors on professional standards
- To consider allegations of misconduct or unfitness to practise due to ill health.

---

midwifery and health visiting. Its mission is to establish and improve standards of nursing, midwifery and health visiting in order to serve and protect the public. Its key tasks are listed in Box 9.1.

The UKCC promotes safe practice by nurses, midwives and health visitors through the development and promotion of professional standards. In its policy work, health and social trends are identified and strategies are developed for anticipating change in the fields of education and practice, health and social policy. Further public protection is provided through the professional conduct work. Much of the UKCC's effort is put into the development of safe practice. However, when a complaint is made, professional conduct officers investigate it thoroughly and fairly. In this way the UKCC regulates the professions, assisting practitioners to develop and understand their personal and professional accountability (UKCC 1997).

It may be helpful before going further to clarify the difference between *primary* and *secondary legislation* into which all legislation is divided. *Primary legislation is enshrined in Acts of Parliament* which have been debated in the House of Commons and the House of Lords before receiving the Royal Assent. Such legislation is expected to last at least one or two decades before being revised. With the pressure which exists on parliamentary time, Acts of Parliament are frequently designed as *enabling legislation* in that they provide a framework from which statutory rules may be derived, otherwise known as secondary or subordinate legislation. *All secondary legislation is published in statutory instruments (SIs)*. Statutory rules (secondary legislation) do not generally require parliamentary

time as they are, when agreed, endorsed by the Secretary of State and laid before the House of Commons for formal and generally automatic approval. Statutory rules can therefore be implemented or amended much more quickly. (If more information is required about this process, Bent (1992) and Jenkins (1995) both give useful detail on the processing of statutory law.)

The primary legislation in the context of the statutory control of the midwife is the two Nurses, Midwives and Health Visitors Acts 1979 and 1992. These two Acts have now been consolidated in the Nurses, Midwives and Health Visitors Act 1997 which will be referred to in the rest of this chapter as 'the Act'. An example of secondary legislation is the Midwives Rules (UKCC 1993a). Two underlying principles of the Act are the protection of the public and the government *of* the three professions *by* the three professions *for* the three professions.

In order to achieve the latter principle, a majority of the Council and National Board members are nurses, midwives and health visitors. The majority of such members on the Council of the UKCC are elected by the three professions from the four countries of the UK.

In 1992 the UKCC became the elected body, whereas formerly elections had been to the National Boards which then nominated members to the Council. Responsibility for investigation of alleged professional misconduct was transferred from the National Boards to the Council. The National Boards became smaller, executive bodies concerned with the approval and monitoring of education and training and retained responsibility for the supervision of midwives in accordance with UKCC Midwives Rules.

During the passage of the 1979 Act, midwives had determinedly sought for and succeeded in establishing a special clause to be inserted into the Act enshrining in legislation the requirement for a statutory midwifery committee that must be consulted on all midwifery matters. This clause addressed their concerns about retaining control of the practice of midwives and strengthened the Act for midwives. The other strength of the Act is that the supervision of midwives continues to be a statutory requirement for the midwifery profession. This is specified in the primary and in the secondary legislation and it is the UKCC Midwifery Committee that has the responsibility for formulating the rules to control the practice of midwives, which includes the supervision of midwives. More will be said about this when considering the specific aspects of primary and secondary legislation as it relates to midwives.

Membership of the UKCC

The UKCC has a governing Council comprising 40 elected members and 20 members who are appointed by the Secretary of State for Health. The elected members are representative of all parts of the UK and the three professions. Registrants in each of the four countries elect seven nurses, two midwives and one health visitor.

In the 1992 election, as in previous elections, there were separate categories for nurses, midwives and health visitors. Candidates were required to be practising nurses, midwives or health visitors and to declare in which of the three professional categories they wished to be included. Registrants of the three professions were allowed to choose one category in which to vote. This meant that the majority of practising midwives voted for midwives and, similarly, practising nurses for nurses and health visitors for health visitors. Council elections are held every 5 years. The Council meets quarterly. Its committees cover midwifery, nursing and community health care nursing, education, finance and professional conduct. There is a research advisory panel and an ethics advisory panel.

The 60-member Council of the UKCC is supported by an executive team of just over 100 staff. The executive team, led by a Chief Executive/Registrar, is organised into five directorates. These are:

- policy development
- standards promotion
- professional conduct
- business systems (including registration and finance)
- personnel and support services (including communications).

The regulation of midwives and nurses has been a joint process in the UK since 1983 when the UKCC took over the regulatory function from the previous nine statutory and training bodies and this has provided an increased sharing of knowledge and experience between the two professions. However, it was agreed in 1986, in a UKCC report on the future of education, that midwifery is a profession different from, but complementary to, nursing. The UKCC Project 2000 Report stated that:

the role of the midwife is ... substantially different from the nurse in that a midwife potentially has greater professional independence as the decision making is of a different order. The midwife is expected to have diagnostic skills relating to both mother and baby that are similar to the obstetrician, and indeed that there is an overlap of skills between the two. Midwives also have a limited responsibility to prescribe certain scheduled drugs and the right of referral to and discharge from hospitals within limitations. All these, together with the need for manual dexterity and to develop the confidence required to function in this way, point to a potentially special and different preparation for midwifery. (UKCC 1986, p. 50)

PRIMARY LEGISLATION RELATING TO MIDWIFERY

As far as the legal basis for the education, practice and supervision of midwives is concerned, the most important sections of the Act are set out below and listed in Box 9.2. (It should be noted that the Nurses, Midwives and Health Visitors Act 1997 in consolidating the previous 1979 and 1992 Acts of the same name has changed the section numbering, but not the content, of parts of those Acts.)

Section 3 – setting up the UKCC Midwifery Committee

This section directs the UKCC to set up two standing committees, these being a Midwifery Committee and a Finance Committee.

Section 4 – the UKCC Midwifery Committee

The Midwifery Committee *must* have a majority of practising midwives and *must* be consulted by the UKCC on 'all matters relating to midwifery' and 'the Secretary of State shall not approve rules relating to midwifery practice unless satisfied that they are framed in accordance with recommendations of the Council's (the UKCC) Midwifery Committee'.

In legal terms 'shall' is a powerful word and makes it an absolute requirement for the UKCC to satisfy the Secretary of State that the Midwifery Committee is content with all the recommendations for any new or revised rules.

It is expected that all the practising midwife members of the Council will be members of the Midwifery Committee, together with other Council and non-Council members. These will normally include an obstetrician and at least one other medical practitioner who may be a paediatrician or a general practitioner. Persons, including practising midwives, who are not members of the Council are appointed to the Midwifery Committee by the Council from nominations received from the appropriate professional organisations, trade unions and other interested bodies. However, as stated earlier, it is required by the legislation that the majority membership of the UKCC Midwifery Committee are practising midwives.

It is of historical interest here to note that the Nurses, Midwives and Health Visitors Act 1992 changed the functions of the National Boards and included the demise of the Standing Midwifery Committees at all four National Boards. However, it is important to note that at the committee stage of the passage of the Bill that eventually became the 1992 Act, the Secretary of State, in response to a question about the Midwifery Committees, made the following positive statement:

I reiterate the Government's commitment to maintaining the unique and separate nature of the midwifery profession. Midwifery shares, and will continue to share, a common regulatory structure with nursing and health visiting, but its 'special' position will continue to be recognized within that structure, as it has been since 1902. At UKCC level, the powers and responsibilities of the Midwifery Committee will remain as they are now. (Hansard 4 March 1992)

Section 14 – the making of rules regulating the practice of midwives

The UKCC is required in this section of the Act to make rules regulating the practice of midwives. Some important examples are given in this section of the Act and the rules required are presented as secondary legislation and will be considered in detail in the section dealing with the Midwives Rules.

The important issue here is that these rules are drawn up *by midwives for midwives* and this is the basis of professional self-regulation. Self-regulation is not about limiting practice but about enabling its development and providing a framework for accountable decision-making in the interests of public safety.

It is notable that midwifery is the *only* profession enabled by the Act to make rules which are standards for regulating *practice*. However, all three of the professions regulated by the Act are required to make rules relating to their education (see Sections 2(2) and (6) of the Act).

Section 15 – the provision of local supervision of midwifery practice

Section 15(1) designates the bodies who shall be local supervising authorities (LSAs) for midwives in each of the four countries of the UK:

- in England and Wales – Health Authorities
- in Wales – Area Health Authorities
- in Scotland – Health Boards
- in Northern Ireland – Health and Social Services Boards.

Section 15(2) requires the LSA to exercise general supervision over *all* midwives practising within its area in accordance with the UKCC Midwives Rules. This means every practising midwife in whatever environment she practises, whether employed or self-employed. Under this section of the Act the LSA is required to report any alleged misconduct on the part of the midwife to the UKCC and finally it also has power in accordance with the UKCC Midwives Rules to suspend a midwife from practice. This will be discussed in more detail below.

Section 15(3) empowers the UKCC to lay down in rules the qualifications necessary for a person to be appointed as a supervisor of midwives by the LSA.

Section 15(4) gives the National Boards the responsibility for providing advice and guidance to the LSAs in respect of the exercise of their functions as described in Section 15 of the Act.

Section 15(5) was a new section within the amending 1992 Act and empowers the UKCC to make rules prescribing the advice and guidance that is given by the National Boards to LSAs. This is in line with the implementation of the 1992 Act giving the UKCC overall responsibility for the supervision of midwives and empowering it to set standards for the entire UK.

Section 16 – attendance by unqualified persons at childbirth

This is an important section and restricts those who may attend a woman in childbirth.

Sections 16(1) and (2) state that only a registered midwife or registered medical practitioner, or a student midwife or medical student as part of a statutorily recognised course, may attend a woman in childbirth and it therefore makes members of the public liable to prosecution if they intentionally undertake this role.

Section 16(3) lays down a fine not exceeding level 4 on the standard scale to the person who contravenes this part of the Act.

Box 9.2 Most relevant sections of the Nurses, Midwives and Health Visitors Act 1997

Section 3 – setting up the Midwifery Committee
Section 4 – the UKCC Midwifery Committee
Section 14 – the making of rules regulating the practice of midwives
Section 15 – the provision of local supervision of midwifery practice
Section 16 – attendance by unqualified persons at childbirth.

SECONDARY MIDWIFERY LEGISLATION

As discussed earlier, the primary legislation empowers the UKCC to draw up secondary legislation in the form of rules, in this case the Midwives Rules. This is facilitated through the UKCC Midwifery Committee, with its majority membership of practising midwives, and in consultation with the profession. This consultation process is required by the Act in Section 19(3). It should also be appreciated that all practising midwives in the UK have responsibility for the election of practising midwives to the UKCC.

The UKCC constantly reviews its legislation and codes, which set standards to ensure that they are providing an up-to-date foundation and a framework for development, to enable response to the changing needs of client-led care and professional practice. It should be remembered that the Midwives Rules and Midwife's Code of Practice have only applied to the whole UK since 1986. Since 1986 there have been major revisions to both the education and practice rules and the Code of Practice for midwives, the most recent being 1993 (the Rules) and 1994 (the Code of Practice). It should be appreciated that the Midwives Rules are set in legislation and the Code of Practice, whilst not a legislative document, is UKCC policy, which supports and complements the rules, setting out in simple terms the standards and other important requirements and information to assist safe practice.

Legislation should be enabling

It is of paramount importance, when considering the standards set in the Midwives Rules, to understand that such legislation is about *enabling practice* and not about limiting practice.

It can be seen at a glance if one looks at older editions of rules and codes that there has been a concerted move away from prescriptive rules to rules that legally define the sphere of practice of the midwife in the interests of the public, so enabling the midwife to use her clinical judgement. It is also interesting to note here that there are still a number of enquiries from midwives who are actually seeking more prescriptive direction from the UKCC and not less. However, the majority of midwives, who are now practising with greater confidence based on sound knowledge and skills, appreciate the flexibility of rules that are enabling.

Summary of the Midwives Rules

As every midwife practising in the UK must be familiar with and have a copy of these rules they are only summarised below. The UKCC publishes the practice and education rules in a booklet (UKCC 1993a) which is available free of charge from the UKCC. The practice rules only are dealt with in this section.

> Maintenance of standards of practice as set out in the Midwives Rules is in the interest of the public and is the responsibility of any midwife practising in the UK whether employed within or outwith the National Health Service or self-employed. Failure to maintain standards of safety and care is likely to result in an allegation of professional misconduct.

A midwife registered with the UKCC but practising midwifery outside the UK is required to comply with the midwifery legislation in the country in which she is practising.

It should be noted that the Midwives Rules commence with Rule 27, as they are sequential to a whole series of rules made by the UKCC, and end at Rule 45, giving a total of 19 rules for midwives' education and practice.

Interpretation – Rule 27
This section is frequently overlooked but it defines some of the terms used in the rules and must be referred to when reading them. The interpretations avoid the use of lengthy explanations. Three of particular importance are:

• *Mother and baby.* It is necessary to define this because several rules refer to mother and baby when the intent is the pregnant woman and fetus.
• *Postnatal period.* This defines the period for which a midwife is required to attend the mother and baby after the birth of the baby, which is at least 10 days and not more than 28 days. This

means that the law requires each midwife to be personally responsible and accountable for the exercise of professional judgement and in determining appropriate practice in relation to mother and baby. This includes judgements about the number of visits and any additional visits required in the postnatal period. The midwife remains accountable for all such decisions throughout the period of midwifery care (UKCC 1992d). This is an example of enabling legislation as it allows the midwife to use her clinical judgement. It is not dictating how often the midwife should visit or what she should do on such visits, as was the case in older legislation. This enabling of clinical judgement and accountable practice can be applied with the public interest at its root to all the midwives' Practice Rules.

• *Practising midwife.* It is important to note that practising midwife means a midwife who is directly involved in all aspects of clinical midwifery care *and also includes* a midwife who holds a post for which a midwifery qualification is required. Both types of midwife must notify their intention to practise (see Rule 36 below). This is to ensure that those midwives involved in midwifery management and administration and midwifery education are appropriately qualified and kept up to date.

Rule 36 – Notification of intention to practise
Rule 36 enables the supervisor of midwives to identify those midwives whose practice is being supervised and conversely, if used appropriately in a practical sense, equally enables the practising midwife to identify her supervisor of midwives. This rule requires the midwife to 'give notice of her intention to practise to each local supervising authority'. The notice is in a form prescribed by the UKCC and is now sent directly to every practising midwife on the UKCC register in time for such notification to be made by 31 March each year. It is the midwife's responsibility to comply with this rule and the notification is returned to the LSA via the supervisor of midwives for the reason stated above. It should be noted that this annual requirement is quite separate and different from the 'Notification of Practice' introduced with the UKCC Post-Registration Education and Practice

(PREP) requirements which only identifies an area of practice and relates to 3-yearly maintenance of registration requirements (UKCC 1994b).

Rule 37 – Refresher courses

This rule is about the requirement for practising midwives to undertake refresher courses in relation to both on-going maintenance of practice and returning to practice after a break in practice. By 1 April 2001 this rule will be superseded by the UKCC PREP requirements. The changes are being introduced gradually according to the dates when current individual requirements are due, and practising midwives are being notified individually of such requirements in relation to their due renewal of registration. Practising midwives will be required to undertake 5 days of study every 3 years and a theoretical and practical return to practice course after a break in practice of more than 5 years (UKCC 1995b).

There is now a wealth of opportunity for midwives to plan their own personal professional development but assistance will be necessary to make the transition from what has been, for some midwives, a fairly narrow field of opportunity of 'set refresher courses' to a very wide choice governed largely by the innovative ideas of individuals. The important issue here is in relation to supervisors of midwives in the different but equally important role they will need to continue to fulfil and that is the provision of advice and support to midwives relating to the personal review of their competence in order to develop appropriate plans for their own professional development.

Rule 38 – Suspension from practice by a local supervising authority

The power to suspend a midwife from practice is given to the LSA and is allowed in two circumstances:

- for prevention of spread of infection
- when the midwife has been reported to the UKCC for investigation of alleged professional misconduct or has been reported to its Health Committee.

A Registrar's Letter (UKCC 1994d) emphasises the discretionary nature of this rule and says: 'If the LSA chooses to suspend a midwife from practice the decision must be able to be justified as being in the interest of the public or the practitioner'. The letter also re-emphasises the fact that this power cannot be delegated to a supervisor of midwives and that any such decision applies only to the geographical area in which that LSA has jurisdiction. This rule is not there as a threat to practice, it is there to protect the standard of care given to mothers and babies by preventing a midwife who is not able, for a specific reason, to provide a safe standard of care. It is applicable to any practising midwife wherever she is providing care.

Suspension from practice should not be confused with suspension from duty which involves an employer suspending an employee from her place of work in relation to an alleged breach of the terms of a contract of employment and could apply to any health care worker and not only a midwife.

Rule 39 – Duty to be medically examined

The provision to suspend a midwife from practice to prevent the spread of infection may necessitate the midwife undergoing a medical examination. This rule requires the midwife to allow this if the LSA considers it to be necessary.

Rule 40 – Sphere of practice

This is probably the most important of the Practice Rules and defines the parameters within which a midwife may practise. It firstly defines quite clearly that a practising midwife is responsible for providing midwifery care for a mother and baby during the antenatal, intranatal and postnatal periods and for calling in a registered medical practitioner in the presence of any deviation from the normal. Secondly it prohibits a midwife, except in an emergency, from undertaking any treatment which she has not at any time been trained to do or which is outside her sphere of practice.

Rule 41 – Administration of medicines and other forms of pain relief

Practising midwives in the UK are permitted, in

accordance with the Misuse of Drugs Act 1971 and the Medicines Act 1968, to obtain and administer certain medicines, including controlled drugs, on their own responsibility. This rule requires that a midwife does not administer any medicine on her own responsibility unless she has been instructed in its use and is familiar with its dosage and method of administration or application.

The rule also restricts the midwife to using only that equipment for inhalational analgesia or other forms of pain relief which has been approved by the UKCC. A new European Union (EU) Directive relating to medical apparatus (SI 1994 No. 3017) came into force on 1 January 1995. The Directive lays down essential requirements and procedures for checking that apparatus does not compromise the health or safety of patients, clients, users or other people. All apparatus introduced to the market after 13 June 1998 must meet the requirements and will carry a special marking, known as a CE Marking, to confirm this. To apply the CE Marking to a product the manufacturer must have the medical device or apparatus assessed to confirm that it meets the requirements of the EU Directive. Apparatus which is currently approved by the UKCC or receives approval prior to 13 June 1998 for the administration of inhalational analgesia by a practising midwife will not require a CE Marking. After that date the UKCC will only consider for approval for use by a practising midwife, new apparatus for the administration of inhalational analgesia which carries a CE Marking (UKCC 1995c).

Further information about other legislation governing the use of drugs and medicines by the midwife in the UK is included in the section relating to The Midwife's Code of Practice, below.

Rule 42 – Records

The midwife is required by this rule to keep detailed records of observations, care given and medicines or other forms of pain relief administered by her to all mothers and babies. It further specifies the form in which such records must be kept, forbids a midwife to destroy her official records and places a responsibility on her for their safe storage. There is further very useful and detailed information available in a free booklet available from the UKCC entitled *Standards for Records and Record Keeping* (UKCC 1993b).

Rule 43 – Inspection of premises and equipment

In order to ensure that a midwife's methods of practice are satisfactory and her records and equipment are kept in good order, this rule requires her to give every facility for inspection by the supervisor of midwives, the LSA and the UKCC or its designated authority. If necessary, this inspection may be extended to any part of the midwife's residence which she uses for professional purposes.

Rule 44 – Supervisors of midwives

The qualifications of supervisors of midwives appointed by the LSA are laid down in this rule. The supervisor must be experienced and eligible to practise as a midwife and undertake initial and periodic courses of instruction in the duties of a supervisor of midwives to enable preparation for and ongoing maintenance of this key responsibility. The statutory supervision of the practice of midwives is discussed in greater detail below.

Rule 45 – Discharge of statutory functions by a local supervising authority

This rule sets standards for the discharge of LSA functions throughout the UK. The rule helps clarify the standards for LSAs and the supervisors of midwives accountable to them.

THE MIDWIFE'S CODE OF PRACTICE

(UKCC 1994a)

This code is issued by the UKCC to set out standards, other requirements and further information for the professional practice of each midwife practising in the UK. It states that the standard of practice in the delivery of midwifery care shall be that which is acceptable in the context of current knowledge and clinical developments. In all circumstances the safety and welfare of the mother and baby must be of primary importance.

The Midwife's Code of Practice is compiled by the UKCC Midwifery Committee in a similar way to the practice rules to which it is complementary. As this Code of Practice is not set in secondary legislation it can be reviewed and revised as frequently as necessary. It is significant that the Code is not prescriptive in relation to details of midwifery care but rather takes account that the midwife has undertaken a comprehensive course of education and training and is accountable for her own practice. The 1994 edition of The Midwife's Code of Practice was considerably revised to take account of new rules and to make it more 'user friendly' to midwives.

The Code is presented in four main sections:

1. an introduction including the international and European definitions of the activities of the midwife
2. matters directly related to and amplifying the Midwives Practice Rules
3. guidance on other midwifery practice matters not included in the rules, e.g.
   • home births
   • complementary and alternative therapies
4. other legislation relevant to the practice of a midwife, e.g.
   • Congenital Disabilities (Civil Liabilities) Act 1976
   • Data Protection Act 1984
   • Access to Health Records Act 1990
   • relevant parts of Births and Deaths Registration Acts and Public Health Acts
   • exemption from jury service.

From time to time the UKCC also issues short papers in the form of Registrar's Letters relating to practice and/or standards, e.g. a Position Statement on waterbirths (UKCC 1994e)

An important section of The Midwife's Code of Practice is that relating to drugs and the midwife. Whilst the Midwives Rules in Rule 41 refer to medicines including analgesics in relation to the midwife's responsibility, it is the Code that gives reference to the other legislation governing the use of drugs and medicines by the midwife in the UK. All midwives bear a great responsibility when they administer drugs, as substances may act not only upon the mother but also on the fetus

during pregnancy and labour and on the baby in the early days of life.

Legislation and regulations governing the use of drugs and medicines by the midwife in the UK

It is important to appreciate that *midwives do not prescribe drugs* but that *they are exempt from needing a prescription for certain drugs*. This exemption permits the midwife to obtain, possess and administer and, in some cases, destroy controlled drugs and prescription-only medicines.

All midwives must also observe the regulations which govern the giving of drugs prescribed by a medical practitioner and the local policies for administration. It is essential to understand that should a drug error lead to litigation or disciplinary measures, ignorance of the law is no excuse.

Midwives must observe both the statutory Acts and Regulations governing the giving of drugs and the government memoranda concerned with drugs issued by the UK Health Departments (e.g. Department of Health in England, and the Scottish Home and Health Department). These are:

• Misuse of Drugs Act 1971
• Misuse of Drugs Regulations 1985
• Misuse of Drugs Act (1971) Modification Order 1985
• Medicines Act 1968
• Medicines (Products other than Veterinary Drugs) (Prescription Only) Order 1983
• Midwives Rules (UKCC 1993a)
• The Midwife's Code of Practice (UKCC 1994a)
• Standards for the Administration of Medicines (UKCC 1992c).

STATUTORY SUPERVISION OF THE PRACTICE OF MIDWIVES

The statutory basis for the supervision of midwives can be traced through primary legislation from 1902 to the present primary legislation relating to the UKCC. The relevant sections of the Act and the Midwives Rules have been referred to above.

The purpose of supervision of midwives is to protect the public by actively promoting a safe standard of midwifery practice. These standards are agreed by midwives for midwives in the Midwives Rules and Midwife's Code of Practice. Supervision is not about punitive discipline nor is it about establishing only one way of providing safe care to women and babies. It is about quality, about caring and preventing poor practice and also about seeking excellence with midwives supporting midwives in this process. It is about enabling midwives to practise with competence and confidence in a properly resourced work environment (Winship 1996a).

There has been a surge of development in the standards relating to the supervision of midwives over the past few years and the UKCC Midwifery Committee has had a major influence on the way in which the statutory framework and standards have been developed. The UKCC has agreed amendments to Rule 44 to include a set of learning outcomes in the legislation as a method of ensuring a consistent approach to the preparation of supervisors of midwives. It is now required that on completion of a programme of preparation the prospective supervisor of midwives will achieve the following outcomes:

1. an understanding of the way in which supervision of midwives enhances standards of care
2. an understanding of the application of legislation relevant to the supervision of midwives
3. the ability to provide professional support to practising midwives relevant to maintaining and promoting standards of care
4. the ability to encourage midwives to use their experience in practice to enhance their professional development
5. an understanding of accountability and professional responsibility as a supervisor of midwives (SI 1997 No. 1723).

The Midwife's Code of Practice includes amplification of the relevant Rules relating to the supervision of midwives and also two significant UKCC policies in paragraphs 45 and 48, both of which are quoted below:

Paragraph 45

The Council (UKCC) has recommended to LSAs that the LSA function should be discharged by a practising midwife. It is for each LSA to determine its organisational arrangements but the Council considers that this function would best be discharged, and the LSA most appropriately served, by this function being assigned to a practising midwife who is professionally experienced in the supervision of midwives. The Council considers that such a practising midwife should be deployed at LSA level as the designated responsible officer and that the relationship between such a midwife and the Authority's designated chief nursing and midwifery adviser is of particular importance.

Paragraph 48

The Council (UKCC) has recommended to LSAs that for the effective supervision to be achieved, each supervisor should supervise no more than 40 practising midwives. The Council understands that there is variation across the United Kingdom in the supervisor : midwife ratio and that it may take some time for some LSAs to reach the recommended ratio. The Council's annual statistical analysis will enable changes to be monitored. This recommendation is designed to allow both effective supervision and adequate support for midwives practising within and outside the National Health Service.

THE EDUCATION AND TRAINING OF THE MIDWIFE

Midwifery education and training have always been linked with practice and the length of training and its content have increased over the years. In fact it could be said that the statutory control of the practice of midwives starts with the education and training of midwives. The Midwives Education Rules are included as Section A of the UKCC Midwives Rules (1993a). These rules set out requirements relating to the age of entrants and the educational requirements necessary for entry to programmes of education. There are also requirements relating to the length and content of education programmes.

The programmes of midwifery education which are offered by the educational institutions must be approved by the National Boards of the four countries of the UK to meet the kind, standard and content specified by the UKCC Education Rules. Rule 33 of the Midwives Rules sets out the learning outcomes to be met by student midwives by the end of the programme of education. The UKCC has also to ensure that the Education Rules meet the requirements of the EU Midwives Directives. More is said about the European Union below. The Education Rules allow midwives to qualify for registration through a 3-year pre-registration midwifery programme or through an 18-month pre-registration programme (shortened) for first level nurses in general care who have obtained their qualification in accordance with the EU Nursing Directives (UKCC 1995a).

THE PROFESSIONAL REGISTER

The maintenance of the register of nurses, midwives and health visitors is the responsibility of the UKCC. The register has 15 parts: 13 of these relate to nurses of different levels and types, one to health visitors and one to midwives. All midwives are registered on Part 10 of the register, irrespective of length of programme or country of origin.

Registration of qualifications

Midwives who qualify in the UK on successful completion of a programme of midwifery education approved by a National Board, may register with the UKCC on payment of a fee. This is not obligatory but a qualified midwife may not practise unless she is a registered midwife, has notified her intention to practise as a midwife (Rule 36) and has demonstrated that she is up to date in her practice (Rule 37).

Applications for registration from midwives qualified in countries outside the UK are considered by the UKCC on an individual basis except for those midwives who are eligible for registration in accordance with the EU Midwives Directives. Midwives making application for registration are frequently required to obtain further education and training or experience.

Midwives who are nationals of, and undergo midwifery training in, one of the member states of the European Union are registered without further education or experience if they have completed:

- education and training in accordance with the EU Midwives Directives or
- 3 years' practice as a midwife in the 5 years preceding application for registration.

THE EUROPEAN UNION AND THE MIDWIVES DIRECTIVES

Midwives may question whether they need to know about Europe and its implications for midwifery education and training and for midwifery practice. Midwives need to be knowledgeable, politically alert and motivated to providing the best possible standards of care for mothers and babies. The UK is a member of the European Union which enables freedom of movement of qualified Union citizens and therefore midwives do need to be aware of European implications for midwives.

The European Union

There are now 15 countries in full membership of the European Union. These are Austria, Belgium, Denmark, Finland, France, Germany, Greece, Holland, Ireland, Italy, Luxembourg, Portugal, Spain, Sweden and the UK.

The European Economic Area comprises the European Union and three countries which are not full members but are members of the European Free Trade Association (EFTA). Those three countries are Iceland, Liechtenstein and Norway. This is important as these three countries also have freedom of movement of qualified Union citizens, which in the case of midwives means undertaking education and training which complies with the EU Midwives Directives.

The EU Midwives Directives

In EU law Directives are the legal instruments which require member states to bring their national laws into line with EU law within a specified time. Freedom of movement for professionals is enabled in two different ways, by Sectoral Directives and by General Directives. The EU Midwives Directives are Sectoral Directives which are those used in relation to profession- or occupation-specific groups. Sectoral Directives are agreed after national representatives from each of the member states negotiate a detailed agreement on a minimum content and length of training programmes by a process known as harmonisation. When they reach agreement a Directive is produced which has the force of law. The EU Midwives Directives were implemented in 1983 having taken 10 years to be negotiated, partly because of the difference in status and training of midwives in the member states. The important issue is that the EU Midwives Directives are unique among the directives for the professions in that they contain a definition of the sphere of practice of the midwife and an outline of the activities of the midwife (see Ch. 1).

> The EU Midwives Directives are of great importance in indicating that throughout Europe midwifery is a separate and different profession from nursing, whatever route is taken to become a midwife, and that these professionals are serving a clientele with different and specific needs – mothers and babies.
>
> The Midwives Directives lay down the requirements to be met during education and training in order to facilitate freedom of movement of midwives in the European Union, once they are registered midwives.

All pre-registration midwifery programmes (including those programmes that are shortened because applicants hold a qualification that complies with the EU General Nursing Directives) must:

1. prepare the student midwife for her specific role as described in Article 4 of the EU Midwives Directives as the 'activities of the midwife'
2. be consistent with the intent of the Directives with the following principles demonstrably underpinning all pre-registration programmes:
   • midwifery content and application throughout the total duration of the programme
   • midwife teacher input and curriculum management throughout the entire programme
3. enable the student midwife to meet the unique requirements for practical and clinical aspects of midwifery which are listed in Directive 80/155/EEC (UKCC 1990) as follows:
   • advising pregnant women, involving at least 100 prenatal examinations
   • supervision and care of at least 40 women in labour
   • personally carrying out at least 40 deliveries
   • active participation with breech deliveries; where this is not possible because of lack of breech deliveries, practice may be in a simulated situation
   • performance of episiotomy and initiation into suturing; the practice of suturing includes suturing of the wound following an episiotomy and a simple perineal laceration – this may be in a simulated situation if absolutely necessary
   • supervision and care of 40 women at risk in pregnancy or labour or postnatal period
   • supervision and care (including examination) of at least 100 postnatal women and healthy newborn infants
   • observation and care of the newborn requiring special care including those born preterm, post-term, underweight or ill
   • care of women with pathological conditions in the fields of gynaecology and obstetrics
   • initiation into care in the field of medicine and surgery; initiation shall include theoretical instruction and clinical practice.

The EU Advisory Committee on the Training of Midwives (ACTM)

The ACTM is a formal Committee of the EU and was established in 1984 in order to advise the European Commission on matters relating to the training of midwives. The membership consists of three experts from each member country to represent the practising profession, establishments providing training of midwives and the competent authority in the member states. (The competent authority is the authority in a member state responsible for registering qualified midwives. These authorities issue and receive certificates of registration for midwives and investigate disciplinary matters. The competent authority for the UK is the UKCC.)

It is essential if midwives are to exercise influence in the provision of a high standard of care of mothers and babies in the European Union that they should speak with one voice. The ACTM helps in this respect by encouraging midwives to share their knowledge and experiences and to reflect on the different ways of working across the European Union. It also serves to remind midwives to consider all matters in a European perspective (Winship 1996b).

PROFESSIONAL CONDUCT

The UKCC fulfils its functions to establish and improve standards of professional conduct by:

- providing professional advice on standards of conduct
- investigating cases of alleged professional misconduct
- hearing cases of alleged professional misconduct
- dealing with cases of unfitness to practise due to illness.

Advice on standards in addition to the Midwives Rules and The Midwife's Code of Practice is published by the UKCC for the guidance of registered nurses, midwives and health visitors and includes:

- Code of Professional Conduct (UKCC 1992a)
- The Scope of Professional Practice (UKCC 1992b)
- Guidelines for Professional Practice (UKCC 1996)
- Standards for the Administration of Medicines (UKCC 1992c)
- Standards for Records and Record Keeping (UKCC 1993b)

The Code of Professional Conduct is the key document from which the other documents have been developed. This Code was drawn up by the UKCC under the powers of the Act and sets out:

- the value of registered practitioners
- practitioners' responsibilities to represent and protect the interests of patients and clients
- what is expected of practitioners.

This series of booklets issued by the UKCC is reviewed and revised regularly and is likely to be added to in the future. The guidance is applicable to midwives and is complementary to the Midwives Rules and The Midwife's Code of Practice.

Allegations of professional misconduct

The statutory rules of the UKCC (secondary legislation) which govern the Council's professional conduct duties state that the term 'misconduct', which forms part of the measure against which allegations are judged, is defined as 'conduct unworthy of a registered nurse, midwife, or health visitor …' (SI 1993 No. 893). The right to practise is conferred by the UKCC by registration, and this right may be removed only by the UKCC.

In accordance with the Act this is a two-tier procedure. The Council both receives and investigates reports of alleged professional misconduct and conducts hearings. Members of Council who consider the case at the investigation or preliminary proceedings stage may not sit on the Professional Conduct Committee when the case is heard.

The Act requires that membership of committees dealing with alleged professional misconduct should be constituted with due regard to the professional field in which the defendant works. This ensures that when a practising midwife is the subject of an investigation or hearing there will be practising midwives on the relevant committee. Meetings of the investigative Preliminary Proceedings Committee are not open to the public but the public is admitted to Professional Conduct Committee meetings.

The Act empowers the committees dealing with professional conduct proceedings at both levels to include non-Council members as part of the Committee. When this power is used, the majority of members of the Committee must be Council members. Health Committee membership will be composed entirely of Council members.

Preliminary Proceedings Committee

The Preliminary Proceedings Committee considers cases which arise from convictions in Criminal Courts, reports received from public bodies such as Health Authorities, Health Boards or Trusts and complaints made by private individuals or professional colleagues.

The Preliminary Proceedings Committee's powers are to determine whether, following a complaint made against a practitioner, the case of that practitioner should be:

- closed
- referred to a Professional Conduct Committee for hearing
- referred to the Panel of Professional Screeners, with a view to a hearing before the Health Committee, or
- closed by a formal caution as to future conduct.

The process by which an allegation of misconduct is considered by the UKCC Preliminary Proceedings Committee is outlined in Figure 9.1.

The Committee may also consider whether to

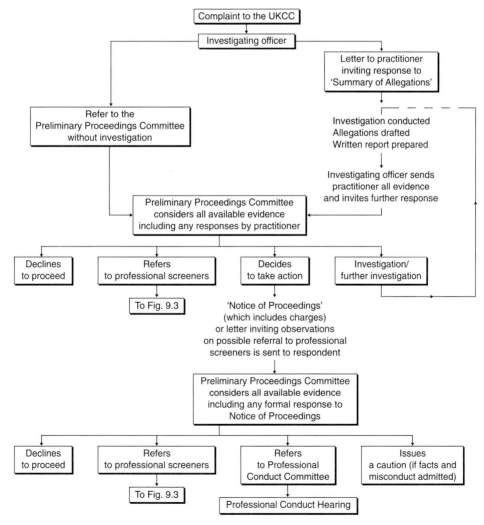

Fig. 9.1 A simplified illustration of the process by which an allegation of misconduct is considered by the Preliminary Proceedings Committee of the UKCC.

impose interim suspension of a practitioner's registration, pending further investigation, and/or early referral to the Professional Conduct or Health Committee. This power will only be used, very occasionally, in circumstances where it is clear that in the interests of public safety, or in the practitioner's own interest, interim suspension should be imposed. If an interim suspension of registration is made, it is applicable across the whole UK and any such suspension must be reviewed every 3 months for as long as the suspension is in force.

The Preliminary Proceedings Committee will not normally meet the practitioner whose case is to be considered and will be basing their judgement upon written reports and evidence. The only exception will be when a Preliminary Proceedings Committee is considering imposing interim suspension of registration, when the practitioner will have the right of audience and representation before the Committee.

Professional Conduct Committee

The role of the Professional Conduct Committee is to consider cases of alleged misconduct which have been referred to it by the Preliminary Proceedings Committee. The Committee also considers applications for restoration to the register from persons whose names have previously been removed.

The Professional Conduct Committee will have in attendance a legal assessor (to advise on admissibility of evidence and points of law) and a Council officer to advise on the Council's procedures and relevant background of the case. Respondents will normally be in attendance (but are not required to attend) at the professional conduct hearing and may be represented. The hearing is held in public. The process by which an allegation of misconduct is considered by the UKCC Professional Conduct Committee is outlined in Figure 9.2.

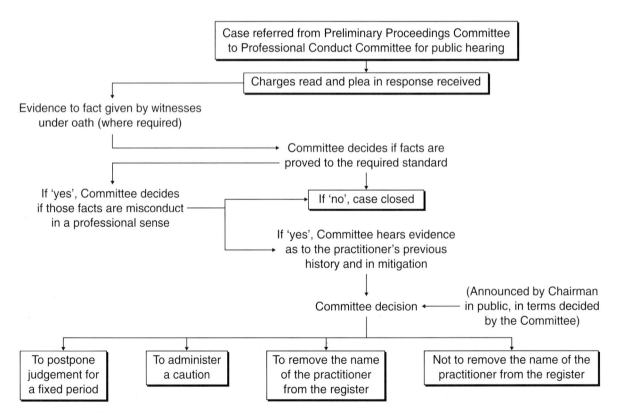

Fig. 9.2 A simplified illustration of the process by which an allegation of misconduct is considered by the Professional Conduct Committee of the UKCC.

If, during the course of a hearing, evidence of possible ill health of the practitioner becomes available, the Professional Conduct Committee can decide to refer a case for consideration by the Health Committee.

Allegations of unfitness to practise due to illness

Experience has demonstrated that many nurses and midwives who have had allegations of professional misconduct against them may be suffering from an underlying health problem which puts the public at risk. In order to deal with such people in a way that will not exacerbate an existing health problem and also be able to minimise risk to the public by consideration of a health problem before professional misconduct has occurred, the UKCC deals with certain cases through its Health Committee. All matters relating to a person who is subject to this procedure are dealt with confidentially and meetings of the Health Committee are held in private. The process by which complaints alleging unfitness to practise are considered is outlined in Figure 9.3.

The Health Committee is not constituted to

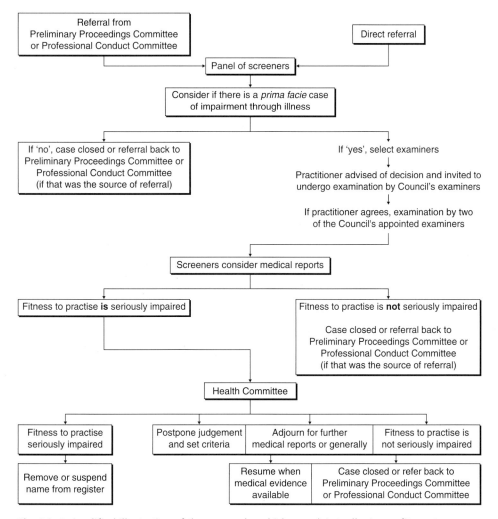

Fig. 9.3 A simplified illustration of the process by which complaints alleging unfitness to practise are considered.

decide whether allegations against, or expressions of concern for, practitioners are proven, but rather to consider the medical evidence and determine whether the practitioner's fitness to practise is seriously impaired by illness and, if so, whether the practitioner is likely to be a danger to the public. The practitioner is normally present (but is not required to be) and may be represented.

There is more detailed and useful information relating to professional conduct in a UKCC booklet entitled *Complaints about Professional Conduct* (UKCC 1993c).

CONCLUSION

This chapter has given an outline of the regulation of the education, practice and supervision of the midwife. Whilst being the responsibility of the UKCC, National Boards and LSAs by virtue of primary and secondary legislation, the regulation of the practice of midwives is also influenced by practising midwives themselves. It is vital that all midwives keep up to date with any proposals for change and participate in elections for, and consultations of, the statutory bodies.

In concluding it is also interesting to consider, in parallel to regulation, *the defining criteria for a profession*. The meaning of the term 'professional' was debated in the House of Lords in July 1992. The following is an extract from Lord Benson's contribution to the discussion (Hansard 8 July 1992). Lord Benson is an accountant by profession.

The nine obligations to the public are these:

First, the profession must be controlled by a governing body which in professional matters directs the behaviour of its members. For their part the members have a responsibility to subordinate their selfish private interests in favour of support for the governing body.

Second, the governing body must set adequate standards of education as a condition of entry and thereafter ensure that students obtain an acceptable standard of professional competence. Training and education do not stop at qualification. They must continue throughout the member's professional life.

Third, the governing body must set the ethical rules and professional standards which are to be observed by the members. They should be higher than those established by the general law.

Fourth, the rules and standards enforced by the governing body should be designed for the benefit of the public and not for the private advantage of members.

Fifth, the governing body must take disciplinary action, if necessary, expulsion from membership should the rules and standards it lays down not be observed or should a member be guilty of bad professional work.

Sixth, work is often reserved to a profession by statute – not because it was for the advantage of the members but because, for the protection of the public, it should be carried out only by persons with requisite training, standards and disciplines.

Seventh, the governing body must satisfy itself that there is fair and open competition in the practice of the profession so that the public are not at risk of being exploited. It follows that members in practice must give information to the public about their experience, competence, capacity to do the work and the fees payable.

Eighth, the members of the profession, whether in practice or in employment, must be independent in thought and outlook. They must be willing to speak their minds without fear or favour. They must not allow themselves to be put under the control or dominance of any person or organisation which could impair that independence.

Ninth, in its specific field of learning a profession must give leadership to the public it serves.

Midwifery is a distinctive profession with a distinctive history and midwives have a contribution to make in ensuring that women and babies continue to receive the safest possible care. Today's midwives are the future of this distinctive profession and must make a positive contribution to the politics of the profession. Midwifery regulation has a future which must be shaped in an accountable and reflective way, remembering that self-regulation is in the public interest and is about enabling safe practice (Winship 1996c).

READER ACTIVITIES

For students and midwives in the UK:

1. Find out which persons are:
   a. the elected practising midwives on the UKCC from the country in which you are working
   b. the members of the UKCC Midwifery Committee
   c. the supervisor(s) of midwives in your locality.

2. Ensure that you have all the up-to-date issues of necessary UKCC guidance documents. Write to the UKCC at 23 Portland Place, London W1N 4JT, and request copies of documents you do not have.

3. Arrange to attend a meeting of the Professional Conduct Committee at the UKCC or one of the UKCC open days or the open session of one of the UKCC Council meetings.

4. Have an in-depth look at the Practice Rules in Section B of the Midwives Rules followed by a group discussion giving practical examples of the application of some of the Practice Rules together with further relevant information from The Midwife's Code of Practice.

5. Find out which drugs your community midwife carries and uses in her practice and how she obtains them, stores them and records them. Find out what standing orders or local policies apply to the administration of drugs by midwives in the hospital in which you work.

For students and midwives working outside the UK:

1. Compare the role of the midwife in your country to that described in this chapter.

2. Find out as much as possible about the statutory (legal) control of the education, training and practice of midwives in your country and compare it with that of the UK, discussing the pros and cons of both systems.

ACKNOWLEDGEMENT

Some sections of this chapter are reproduced from *Supervision of Midwives* (1996), edited by Mavis Kirkham, by permission of Books for Midwives Press, Hale

REFERENCES

Access to Health Records Act 1990 HMSO, London
Bent E A 1992 Module 1 preparation of supervisors of midwives: an open learning programme. English National Board, London
Congenital Disabilities (Civil Liabilities) Act 1976 HMSO, London
Cowell B, Wainwright D 1981 Behind the blue door: the history of the Royal College of Midwives. Baillière Tindall, London
Data Protection Act 1984 HMSO, London
Donnison J 1988 Midwives and medical men, 2nd edn. Historical Publications, London
EEC Midwives Directives 1980 Official Journal of the European Communities No L133 of 11.2.80. HMSO, London
EEC Nursing Directives 1977 Official Journal of the European Communities No 20:176. HMSO, London
Hansard (Commons) 4 March 1992 HMSO, London
Hansard (Lords) 8 July 1992 HMSO, London, pp 1206–1207
Heagerty B V 1996 Reassessing the guilty: the Midwives Act and the control of English midwives in the early 20th century. In: Kirkham M (ed) Supervision of midwives. Books for Midwives Press, England
Health Authorities Act 1995 HMSO, London
International Council of Nurses 1986 Nursing regulation: a report on the present, a position for the future. In: Affara F A, Styles M M (eds) 1993 Nursing regulation guidebook: from principle to power. International Council for Nurses, Geneva
Jenkins R 1995 The law and the midwife. Blackwell Science, Oxford
J M Consulting 1996 The regulation of health professionals. J M Consulting, Bristol
Joint Nurses and Midwives Council (Northern Ireland) Act 1922 HMSO, London
Kirkham M 1996 Supervision of midwives. Books for Midwives Press, England
Midwives Act 1902 HMSO, London
Midwives Act (Ireland) 1918 HMSO, London
Midwives (Scotland) Act 1915 HMSO, London

Ministry of Health 1937 Supervision of midwives. Circular 1620. MoH, London

Misuse of Drugs Act 1971 HMSO, London

Misuse of Drugs Act (1971) Modification Order 1985 HMSO, London

Misuse of Drugs Regulations 1985 HMSO, London

Medicines Act 1968 HMSO, London

Medicines (Products other than Veterinary Drugs) (Prescription Only) Order 1983

Nurses and Midwives (Northern Ireland) Act 1970 HMSO, London

Nurses, Midwives and Health Visitors Act 1979 HMSO, London

Nurses, Midwives and Health Visitors Act 1992 HMSO, London

Nurses, Midwives and Health Visitors Act 1997 HMSO, London

Nurses Registration Act 1919 HMSO, London

Royal College of Midwives (RCM) 1991 Report of the Royal College of Midwives' Commission on legislation relating to midwives. RCM, London

Statutory Instrument No 893 1993 The Nurses, Midwives and Health Visitors (Professional Conduct) Rules 1993. Approval Order 1993. HMSO, London

Statutory Instrument No 3017 1994 European Community Medical Devices Regulations. HMSO, London

Statutory Instrument No 1723 1997 The Nurses, Midwives and Health Visitors (Supervisors of Midwives) Amendment Rules. Approval Order 1997. HMSO, London

Towler J, Bramall J 1986 Midwives in history and society. Croom Helm, England

United Kingdom Central Council for Nursing, Midwifery and Health Visiting (UKCC) 1986 Project 2000: a new preparation for practice. UKCC, London

United Kingdom Central Council for Nursing, Midwifery and Health Visiting (UKCC) 1990 Registrar's Letter 2/1990. Statement of Council's requirements concerning European Community amended requirements for the practical and clinical aspects of midwifery programmes. UKCC, London

United Kingdom Central Council for Nursing, Midwifery and Health Visiting (UKCC) 1992a Code of professional conduct. UKCC, London

United Kingdom Central Council for Nursing, Midwifery and Health Visiting (UKCC) 1992b The scope of professional practice. UKCC, London

United Kingdom Central Council for Nursing, Midwifery and Health Visiting (UKCC) 1992c Standards for the administration of medicines. UKCC, London

United Kingdom Central Council for Nursing, Midwifery and Health Visiting (UKCC) 1992d Registrar's Letter 11/1992. Community postnatal visiting by midwives. UKCC, London

United Kingdom Central Council for Nursing, Midwifery and Health Visiting (UKCC) 1993a Midwives rules. UKCC, London

United Kingdom Central Council for Nursing, Midwifery and Health Visiting (UKCC) 1993b Standards for records and record keeping. UKCC, London

United Kingdom Central Council for Nursing, Midwifery and Health Visiting (UKCC) 1993c Complaints about professional conduct. UKCC, London

United Kingdom Central Council for Nursing, Midwifery and Health Visiting (UKCC) 1994a The midwife's code of practice. UKCC, London

United Kingdom Central Council for Nursing, Midwifery and Health Visiting (UKCC) 1994b The future of professional practice – the Council's standards for education and practice following registration. UKCC, London

United Kingdom Central Council for Nursing, Midwifery and Health Visiting (UKCC) 1994c Registrar's Letter 8/1994. Council's requirements for the content of pre and post registration programmes of education. UKCC, London

United Kingdom Central Council for Nursing, Midwifery and Health Visiting (UKCC) 1994d Registrar's Letter 10/1994. Suspension from practice of midwives and interim suspension of registration for nurses, midwives and health visitors. UKCC, London

United Kingdom Central Council for Nursing, Midwifery and Health Visiting (UKCC) 1994e Registrar's Letter 16/1994. Position statement on waterbirths. UKCC, London

United Kingdom Central Council for Nursing, Midwifery and Health Visiting (UKCC) 1995a Registrar's Letter 2/1995. Midwifery programmes of education – changes in terminology. UKCC, London

United Kingdom Central Council for Nursing, Midwifery and Health Visiting (UKCC) 1995b Registrar's Letter 19/1995. Council's standards for education and practice following registration – return to practice programmes. UKCC, London

United Kingdom Central Council for Nursing, Midwifery and Health Visiting (UKCC) 1995c Registrar's Letter 31/1995. Approval of apparatus for the administration of inhalational analgesia by midwives. UKCC, London

United Kingdom Central Council for Nursing, Midwifery and Health Visiting (UKCC) 1996 Guidelines for professional practice. UKCC, London

United Kingdom Central Council for Nursing, Midwifery and Health Visiting (UKCC) 1997 This is the UKCC. UKCC, London

Winship E J 1996a The UKCC perspective: the statutory basis for the supervision of midwives today. In: Kirkham M (ed) Supervision of midwives. Books for Midwives Press, England, ch 3, pp 38–57

Winship E J 1996b Midwifery in Europe – valuing the European Union Midwives Directives. In: Proceedings. International Confederation of Midwives 24th Triennial Congress, 1996 Oslo, 64: 187–190

Winship E J 1996c The future of midwifery regulation. British Journal of Midwifery 4(12): 653–656

FURTHER READING

Dimond B 1994 The legal aspects of midwifery. Books for Midwives Press, England

Jenkins R 1995 The law and the midwife. Blackwell Science, Oxford

Kirkham M 1996 Supervision of midwives. Books for Midwives Press, England

Pyne R H 1998 Professional discipline in nursing, midwifery and health visiting, 3rd edn. Blackwell Scientific, Oxford

Winship E J 1996 The future of midwifery regulation. British Journal of Midwifery 4(12): 653–656

ESSENTIAL READING

United Kingdom Central Council for Nursing, Midwifery and Health Visiting (UKCC) 1993 Midwives rules. UKCC, London

United Kingdom Central Council for Nursing, Midwifery and Health Visiting (UKCC) 1994 The midwife's code of practice. UKCC, London

Pregnancy

SECTION CONTENTS

Preparing for pregnancy

Sineád McNally

10

Preparing for pregnancy may involve more than the physical preparation of a couple for childbearing. It may involve mental and emotional preparation for pregnancy, labour and the realities of parenting. It may be a time when couples are drawn to reflect on their sexuality, their reproductive potential and the impact of children on their relationship.

The chapter aims to:

- review the environmental and hereditary factors that have an effect on pregnancy outcome and describe methods of preconception screening

- consider the physical, physiological and psychological barriers to conception

- describe the investigation and treatment of male and female infertility

- give an overview of techniques of assisted reproduction together with their legal and ethical implications

- discuss the role of the midwife in the delivery of preconception care.

THE CONCEPT OF PRECONCEPTION CARE

There are many terms used for the care or advice that may be given to a couple planning a pregnancy:

- preconception care
- preconceptual care
- prepregnancy care
- periconceptual care.

The final term 'periconceptual care' refers to the period prior to conception and up to 12–14 weeks of pregnancy. Some believe that the period from conception through to organogenesis should be included in talking about preconception care (Cefalo et al 1995).

Many midwives may see a large component of the mental and physical preparation for pregnancy as belonging to family planning clinics, GPs, infertility clinics and even practice nurses (Pownall 1994). Midwives may not meet a couple until they attend for antenatal care but even the earliest visit rarely occurs before 6 or 8 weeks' gestation. In terms of preconception care, antenatal care is too late. However conscientious antenatal care and attention to health in pregnancy may be, they do not begin until the most vulnerable stages of embryonic development have passed.

Organogenesis is the term given to the period of 60 days after conception, during which time extensive fetal development takes place (Perry 1996, Ward et al 1994). The rapid cell division and differentiation which occurs may be adversely affected by nutritional deficiencies, 'social poisons' or 'risky behaviours' such as smoking and alcohol abuse occurring in the weeks before conception and during organogenesis (Curtis 1996, Shorney 1990).

A midwife's aim thus should be to enhance fetal and maternal health *prior* to conception by utilising the same strategies that she employs as part of antenatal care (Ch. 13).

Many midwives may advise and counsel couples on preconception issues as part of postnatal care, particularly when addressing such matters as resumption of sexual activity and contraception (Ch. 32). Unfortunately, midwives may find it necessary to address preconception issues after a reproductive disaster when a couple will naturally question why it happened and try to prevent the same thing happening again. Hence the interest in health before conception.

There is a plethora of literature, both medical and popular, on advice to ensure an optimal pregnancy outcome (Bradley et al 1995, Brewer 1995, Chamberlain & Lumley 1986, Hajee 1995, Perry 1996). Individuals are becoming increasingly aware of the importance of a healthy lifestyle and would welcome the constructive advice included in this chapter.

Some factors which have an effect on pregnancy

outcome are unalterable, such as parents' relative ages, genetic make-up, intelligence and socio-economic class. Other factors which are addressed here can have an influence and they may have a profound effect on pregnancy outcome.

Diet and nutrition

Gross malnutrition is rare in western society today but suboptimal nutrition is very common, particularly in areas where unemployment and consequent poverty are increasing.

Much of the food consumed today has been processed by techniques which destroy essential nutrients; in addition it is treated with chemicals, preservatives and artificial colouring and flavouring to increase its shelf life and attractiveness to the customer.

Because of soil depletion, the use of artificial fertilisers and intensive farming, even fresh foods may have low nutritional value and contain harmful substances. Organic farming methods use natural fertilisers and avoid chemical pesticides.

For optimal health, processed and refined foods should be avoided altogether. Items from each of the four main food categories should be taken each day (Lashford 1985, Morgan 1994, Steegers-Theunissen 1995).

- *Bread and cereals:*
  - wholegrain cereals provide carbohydrate, fibre, minerals and vitamins.
- *Fresh fruits and vegetables:*
  - either raw or cooked in such a way as to retain nutritional value
  - fruits should be stewed in glass or enamel, not aluminium
  - vegetables should be scrubbed, not peeled, then baked or steamed.
- *Protein foods:*
  - meat, fresh and preferably organically raised
  - fish
  - eggs, preferably free range
  - pulses such as dried peas, beans, lentils.
- *Dairy products:*
  - fresh milk contains vitamins and fatty acids which are destroyed by processes such as drying and sterilisation.

A well-balanced diet should contain sufficient

vitamins and minerals for daily requirements. Some authorities recommend supplements before pregnancy to correct any deficits.

Allergies to foods and food additives appear to be far more prevalent than was previously thought possible. Symptoms are often non-specific and range from the trivial to the disabling. They include hyperactivity and learning difficulties in children. A susceptible child may be sensitised in utero (Bradley et al 1995).

Weight

Prepregnancy weight can have an important bearing on pregnancy outcome. Women whose weight falls outside the optimal range have an increased likelihood of amenorrhoea and infertility. If a woman is underweight, there is evidence of an association with fetal abnormality and low birth-weight. The overweight woman has an increased risk of complications of pregnancy, notably hypertension, in addition to the risk to her own health.

The Quetelet or body-mass index. This is a method of calculating the ideal prepregnancy weight – weight in kilograms is divided by height in metres squared:

• less than 20 (underweight)
• 20–24.9 (desirable)
• 25–29.9 (moderate obesity)
• over 30 (severe obesity).

Advice on diet is given along the lines suggested above. 'Crash dieting' is best avoided as it adversely affects nutritional status. Any woman who does diet rigorously must be strongly advised to use reliable contraception until she is maintaining a desirable weight and a satisfactory intake of nutrients (Dickerson 1995, Wynn 1994).

While women are encouraged to ensure that they are getting enough nutrients, too many may have a detrimental effect. Vitamins A and D, for example, can both be toxic at levels higher than the recommended daily allowance (RDA). Many women take daily vitamin supplementation which they may use instead of following a natural healthy diet. Along with folic acid supplementation, the midwife may need to examine what other vitamins a woman is taking and the amount.

Folic acid supplementation

Recent research has shown that taking extra folic acid preconceptually and during the period of organogenesis can help prevent neural tube defects such as spina bifida (Czeizel 1995, DH 1992, MRC Vitamin Study Group 1991).

Folic acid is the chemical form of folate. Rich sources which contain more than 100 µg (0.1 mg) per serving are Brussels sprouts, spinach, asparagus and black-eye beans. Good sources, such as peas, green beans, broccoli, soya beans, parsnips and iceberg lettuce, provide 51–100 µg (0.051–0.1 mg) per serving. It is unlikely, however, that women will get enough folic acid from food alone. Originally, folic acid supplementation was recommended for women at risk of a recurrence of a neural tube defect (DH 1992).

Folic acid supplements are now widely available 'over the counter' and major pharmaceutical companies advertise brands specifically targeting women of reproductive age. The dose recommended by the Department of Health is 400 micrograms daily until the 12th week of pregnancy (DH 1992). However, the periconceptional supplementation of low-risk women remains controversial.

Exercise and relaxation

Moderate exercise taken regularly in the fresh air improves health, weight and fitness and aids effective relaxation; yoga exercises are an excellent alternative (see also Ch. 45). The contribution of stress to reproductive disaster is only beginning to be appreciated; it is known to predispose to infertility, spontaneous abortion and preterm labour. Taking hot baths, relaxing in a sauna and exercising in hot weather may raise the woman's core temperature. It is thought that this may be associated with congenital abnormalities (Bradley et al 1995).

Avoiding hazards

Smoking. The effects of smoking in pregnancy are well documented. There is a higher rate of spontaneous abortion, congenital abnormalities and fetal and neonatal death associated with smoking. Even if the woman gives up during pregnancy, the risks are still increased above those for the non-smoker.

Men who smoke have lowered testosterone levels; spermatogenesis, sperm morphology and motility are impaired. Intended pregnancy can therefore provide a good incentive for a couple to give up smoking together.

The effects of smoking are potentiated by caffeine and alcohol (McGreal 1995).

Alcohol. It is now recognised that alcohol consumed in pregnancy can damage the fetus but the critical dose and time are still not known. Not only the regular drinker, but also the woman who drinks infrequently with the occasional binge may put her fetus at risk at a very early stage. For this reason, women should be advised to reduce or discontinue alcohol consumption before and during pregnancy (Plant 1990).

Drugs. Many drugs are known to have an adverse effect on pregnancy but for the most part their influences in the period before conception are simply not known.

As none can be entirely free from suspicion of teratogenicity, medication of any kind should be carefully scrutinised. This includes self-medication such as cold cures, painkillers, antacids and laxatives and the use of psychotropic drugs, prescribed or otherwise.

The oral contraceptive pill lowers blood zinc levels and affects liver function. There is resulting interference with vitamin A metabolism, and concentrations which are too high or too low can be teratogenic. The pill also affects folate and vitamin B_{12} metabolism, and lowers levels of other vitamins of the B_{12} complex and of vitamin C (Barnes 1996).

It is therefore advisable for oral contraceptive use to be discontinued at least 3 and preferably 6 months before a woman tries to become pregnant. In the meantime the couple should use some non-invasive method of contraception, and barrier methods have the best safety record. The safe period may be difficult to calculate while steroid hormones are still circulating. A few couples may be able to use coitus interruptus successfully (see Ch. 32).

Infections. In spite of the publicity about rubella and the policy for immunisation of schoolgirls, between 10 and 25% of women of childbearing age lack rubella antibodies. The vaccination is only 95% effective. Any woman planning a pregnancy should have her immune status checked and be given the vaccine if necessary. Stringent contraceptive precautions should of course be taken for 1–3 months.

Pregnancy should be avoided immediately following any immunisation. Gamma globulin may be available for protection during an epidemic if pregnancy is a possibility in a susceptible woman.

Any pre-existing infection, for example of the urinary, reproductive or respiratory tract, or sexually transmitted disease in either partner, should be treated before conception is attempted. The couple should be advised to avoid contact with any infections, particularly viral, as far as possible (Curtis 1996, Shorney 1990).

Noxious substances. The reproductive system, the embryo and the fetus are extremely sensitive to insult; they are vulnerable to levels of environmental pollution much lower than those necessary to affect the general health of an adult.

Lead has been most intensively studied, since it is widely encountered, not just in factories but in traffic exhaust fumes, paints, solder and the domestic water supply. The association with mental retardation and hyperactivity in children is well known; evidence also suggests a link with congenital abnormalities and perinatal death. Other heavy metals such as cadmium and mercury may have the same effect.

Industrial processes. There is reliable evidence of toxic effects from chemicals such as gases (including anaesthetic gases), solvents, dusts, pesticides and from ionising radiation. The effect of prolonged exposure to visual display units (VDUs) is still disputed.

Pollutants may affect the gonads of men and women, causing problems ranging from impotence, menstrual disorders and infertility to spontaneous abortion, congenital abnormalities and cancers in the children.

Employers are obliged by law to tell their employees whether they are working with any chemicals or processes known to be hazardous. A couple planning to start a family should seek this information. If there is a danger, they should avoid exposure to the hazard as far as possible. Midwives may be exposed to substances such as nitrous oxide and other gases or to radiation hazards. Unfortunately, although manufacturers are bound by law to research the effects of their products, few have looked into possible reproductive risks. Statistical proof is indeed hard to collect:

- workers, particularly men, rarely admit to problems related to sexuality unless specifically asked
- doctors investigating fertility problems do not always enquire about work conditions
- the environment is only one of a number of factors which may cause reproductive failure
- experimental work on animals is of limited value, as their susceptibility may be very different from that of humans (Bradley et al 1995).

Medical screening

Some couples may seek more specific attention from a general practitioner or preconception clinic before embarking on a pregnancy. The extent of the tests and examinations which the doctor considers appropriate varies greatly.

Basic check-up

Time is allowed for a relaxed discussion covering dietary habits, lifestyle and possible exposure to hazards. A full medical history is taken from both partners and each has a general examination, including measurement of height, weight and blood pressure. The reproductive history of each is taken, and a menstrual history of the woman. A gynaecological examination is performed, including screening for vaginal infection and a cervical smear. The couple are referred for psychosexual counselling or investigation of subfertility if indicated.

Samples will be obtained for a number of tests:

Urinalysis and investigation for urinary tract infection are carried out.

Blood tests will include haemoglobin estimation, rubella immunity, a test for syphilis, estimation of lead levels and any other investigations indicated, for example screening for sickle cell trait.

Hair analysis is organised by some clinics; it reveals concentrations of up to 18 metals. High levels of toxic metals can be reduced by chelating agents, and low levels of essential trace minerals are corrected by appropriate supplements. The use of hair analysis is controversial because it is retrospective.

Stool samples are analysed in order to detect malabsorption or infestation if indicated.

Semen analysis for abnormal sperm should be done in cases of subfertility, high alcohol intake, coeliac disease or recent debilitating illness.

Drinking water samples from the couple's home may be tested, particularly if the water is known to be soft and acid and if the plumbing includes lead pipes and tanks. The finding of high levels of lead, copper, cadmium or aluminium in the water should be referred to the local Water Board (Wynn & Wynn 1991).

Pre-existing medical conditions

Drug therapy for any pre-existing medical condition should be reduced to the minimum compatible with stabilisation before pregnancy is attempted. A woman receiving long-term medical treatment should be advised to consult her physician before embarking on pregnancy (see Ch. 16). Similarly, a woman who has undergone major surgery or transplant would be wise to consult her doctor. Women with phenylketonuria should reintroduce dietary therapy.

Epilepsy. Anticonvulsants diminish potency and fertility in men and there is a risk of fetal abnormalities if they are taken by either partner. It is not yet clear to what extent this is due to the fact that they induce folate and vitamin D deficiency; supplements of both should be given before pregnancy is attempted. Anticonvulsants should be withdrawn slowly if there have been no attacks for at least 3 years. Otherwise, seizures should be controlled with the single most effective drug. Multiple drugs multiply the risk (Crawford 1997).

Diabetes. The abnormality rate among babies of diabetic mothers is up to five times higher than among those of non-diabetics; if the condition is poorly controlled, damage occurs to the fetus during organogenesis. Oral hypoglycaemic agents are contraindicated in pregnancy and insulin is substituted before conception. Women are taught to use self-testing blood glucose kits and educated to achieve the best possible control before attempting to conceive. In severe cases they may be advised against pregnancy (Elixhauser et al 1996, Parker 1996, Steel et al 1990).

Genetic counselling

Some couples may seek advice because they or a close relative have already produced a child with some anomaly. If it was due to chance or environmental factors, the prospective parents can be reassured and given advice on how to ensure the best possible outcome for their pregnancy. If hereditary factors were involved, the couple are referred to a geneticist who will take an exhaustive family history and carry out any appropriate investigations. They can then be advised about any likelihood of recurrence but must make their own decision about whether or not to take the risk. Other indications for referral to a genetic counselling service are that the woman:

- has had a stillbirth or three or more spontaneous abortions
- is related to her partner (for example first cousins)
- is aged 35 or older and contemplating pregnancy.

It may be possible to offer prenatal diagnosis followed by termination of pregnancy if an anomaly is found. Some couples may opt to avoid pregnancy altogether (Harper 1988).

After the birth of an abnormal baby
Any couple who have an abnormal baby should have the cause explained to them as accurately as may be ascertained. The midwife may be involved in referring such a couple to a genetic counselling service so that individuals at risk may be assisted in understanding the nature of the genetic disorder and possibly be given an estimate of the recurrence risk to the family (Kelly 1986). If their baby dies, the thought of a postmortem is distressing to the parents but they should always be encouraged to give their consent. Determining the exact cause of death may give them peace of mind in the future, even if at the time they cannot imagine ever contemplating another pregnancy. It is the only way that disorders caused by genetic and environmental factors can be distinguished.

Genetically determined disorders

These may be:

- chromosomal disorders
- single gene disorders
  - recessive
  - dominant
  - X-linked
- multifactorial disorders.

Chromosomal disorders
These are usually evident at birth (e.g. trisomies 21, 18 and 13), except in the case of those involving sex chromosomes (e.g. XO – Turner's syndrome; XXY – Klinefelter's syndrome). Habitual abortion may be due to embryos having a severe chromosomal abnormality incompatible with life. Karyotyping of the parents should be carried out if there is a family history of such disorders, after the birth of an affected baby and in cases of habitual abortion. If one of the parents proves to have a translocated chromosome, it should be possible to predict the likelihood of recurrence.

Single gene disorders

Recessive conditions only occur if each chromosome of a pair carries the affected gene. The disorders are usually severe. In the UK the most common is cystic fibrosis; worldwide, the haemoglobinopathies occur most frequently. Inborn errors of metabolism such as phenylketonuria are also transmitted in this way. If the partners are both carriers, their chances of conceiving an affected child are one in four for each pregnancy. The risk of both being carriers is increased in consanguineous marriages, which are common in some cultures.

Dominant conditions occur even if the affected gene is present on only one of a pair of chromosomes. Unless the affected gene is the result of a new mutation, one parent will be affected. The disorders tend to be either mild or of late onset: achondroplasia and Huntington's chorea are examples. If a parent is affected, there is a one-in-two chance of a child being affected.

X-linked conditions may be carried by girls but usually only appear in boys. Examples are haemophilia and Duchenne muscular dystrophy.

Research is proceeding into detection of single gene disorders but at present only a few can be diagnosed in carriers or prenatally and those only in specialised centres.

Multifactorial disorders

It appears that certain combinations of genes, exposed to certain environmental factors, can produce anomalies such as neural tube defects, cleft lip and palate and congenital heart disease. The risk is enhanced if one parent is affected and increases still further after the birth of an affected child.

SEXUALITY

There are few places where couples with psychosexual difficulties may easily find help. This, together with their understandable reticence about such distressing problems, means that the midwife should always be alert for hints that all is not well within a relationship. Teaching pelvic floor exercises and assisting women with breast feeding may lead to a discussion on sexuality. O'Driscoll (1994) refers to the midwife as a 'permission giver' facilitating the woman's desire to talk of her pregnancy and childbirth experience. This may involve the midwife in discussion concerning future pregnancies. However, the midwife needs to be able to identify the psychosexual problems that require more intensive counselling and find out where in her own practice area to refer such a couple.

Sexual difficulties may be the real reason why a couple or individual asks for advice about preconception care or family planning. Problems grave enough to prevent conception are unusual but comparatively minor difficulties may result in considerable unhappiness. Parenthood brings many stresses of its own, so it is important for the long-term future that the couple's relationship is mutually satisfying before conception is attempted (Walton 1994).

Sexual problems are usually caused by emotional factors which are not always consciously recognised. They may result from a traumatic experience in the past or arise from conflicts between particular partners. Untreated, they may manifest themselves in physical or mental illness.

Some difficulties can be alleviated simply by talking them through with an open, caring and accepting listener; others are more deep-seated and need to be referred to an experienced psychosexual counsellor. The aim of treatment is to enable individuals to recognise and overcome the inhibitions which prevent them from trusting and enjoying their own sexuality (O'Driscoll 1994).

Vaginismus

Spasm of the pelvic floor muscles not only forms a physical barrier to intercourse but is also an emotional barrier to the deeper feelings. The woman may have concluded that she has a rigid hymen, that her vagina is too small or that the penis is too big. It is usually sufficient to demonstrate to her that the muscles are under her own control, describing her anatomy in simple terms and stressing the importance of relaxation and arousal before intercourse is attempted. She may take some time to become comfortable with her own body. Some women need to explore real fears about losing control either to another person or to their own sexual feelings (Walton 1994).

'Frigidity'

This imprecise term has been used to cover a whole range of problems, from complete absence of sexual desire to failure to achieve orgasm. The woman may never have found sexual activity pleasurable or satisfying, or the problem may be a feature of a particular relationship, caused by lack of emotional commitment on either side or by poor communication between the partners, which results in inadequate stimulation.

A previously responsive woman may lose interest after a stressful life event. It is not uncommon for this to happen following the birth of a baby. Dyspareunia resulting from a sutured perineum may be a factor, as may tiredness, fear of a further pregnancy and anger with the partner. A woman may find it difficult to combine being a mother with being a lover; she finds the baby so absorbing that any other relationship is an intrusion.

Failure to achieve orgasmic release may result in symptoms of mental or physical ill health. Discussion of technique may help, encouraging the woman to discover what stimulation she needs and to communicate this to her partner. It could be necessary to explore why she is unwilling or unable to give way to her feelings. She may be afraid of emotional commitment or inhibited as a result of a strict upbringing or sexual abuse (Walton 1994).

Impotence

It is rare for a man never to have been able to achieve and maintain an erection long enough for intromission to take place but secondary impotence, after previously satisfactory performance, is not unusual. There may be an organic cause, for example endocrine disorders such as diabetes, or it may be induced by alcohol, barbiturates or antihypertensives. Depression, stress and fatigue can all adversely affect sexual function. A man who experiences an episode of impotence may worry about it so much that he fails again. Impotence is sometimes situational, occurring in a particular relationship as a result of conflict or feelings of guilt, while performance elsewhere is unaffected.

Ejaculatory incompetence

Premature ejaculation is only occasionally severe enough to prevent conception but any degree will reduce the likelihood of both partners obtaining satisfaction. It may be learned behaviour from early hurried sexual experiences or an expression of conflicts within the relationship. Well-motivated men can be taught to postpone ejaculation and ensure that their partners reach orgasm; an understanding of the underlying problems could help the couple to achieve emotional as well as physical satisfaction.

A few men are unable to ejaculate intravaginally. This may be the equivalent of orgasmic dysfunction in the woman, an emotional defence mechanism, perhaps after discovery of the partner's infidelity, or it may be a subconscious refusal to become a father (Mack & Tucker 1996).

INFERTILITY

It has been argued that the biological urge to mate does not imply a desire to be a parent; nonetheless, involuntary childlessness can result in considerable distress.

The World Health Organization (WHO) (1988) has defined subfertility as the inability to achieve a pregnancy after 1 year of unprotected intercourse. According to this criterion, 20% of couples are subfertile, though this falls to 10% after 18 months. The term infertile, strictly speaking, should not be used until it is proved that pregnancy is impossible.

More couples are choosing to start their families later in life but increasing age reduces fertility and the time available for childbearing. Couples over 35 years old should seek help if conception has not occurred within 6 months.

Infertility is said to be *primary* if no conception has ever occurred and *secondary* if there has been a pregnancy, whatever the outcome.

In approximately one-third of cases, male factors are responsible (Box 10.1); in another third, female factors (Box 10.2); in the remainder, a combination of factors is involved, for instance a low sperm count in association with defective ovulation. It is therefore vitally important that subfertility be investigated as a problem of the couple and not of one partner (Hadley 1987, Mack & Tucker 1996).

Preliminary investigations

Before any physical investigations are undertaken, time should be allowed for assessing the quality of the relationship and exploring the reasons behind the request for help. The couple are evidently anxious about their apparent infertility but must be encouraged to talk about whether they really

Box 10.1 Causes of male infertility

Defective spermatogenesis
Endocrine disorders
- Dysfunction of:
  - hypothalamus
  - pituitary
  - adrenals
  - thyroid
- Systemic disease:
  - diabetes mellitus
  - coeliac disease
  - renal failure
Testicular disorders
- Trauma
- Environmental (high temperature):
  - congenital (hydrocele, undescended testes)
  - occupational (furnaceman, long-distance lorry driver)
  - acquired (varicocele, tight clothing)
- Cancer treatment

Defective transport
- Obstruction or absence of seminal ducts:
  - infection
  - congenital anomalies
  - trauma
- Impaired secretions from prostate or seminal vesicles:
  - infection
  - metabolic disorders

Ineffective delivery
- Psychosexual problems (impotence)
- Drug-induced (ejaculatory dysfunction)
- Physical disability
- Physical anomalies:
  - hypospadias
  - epispadias
  - retrograde ejaculation (into bladder)

Box 10.2 Causes of female infertility

Defective ovulation
Endocrine disorders
- Dysfunction of:
  - hypothalamus
  - pituitary
  - adrenals
  - thyroid
- Systemic disease:
  - diabetes mellitus
  - coeliac disease
  - renal failure
Physical disorders
- Obesity
- Anorexia nervosa or strict dieting
- Excessive exercise
Ovarian disorders
- Hormonal
- Ovarian cysts or tumours
- Polycystic ovary disease
- Ovarian endometriosis

Defective transport
Ovum
- Tubal obstruction:
  - infection (gonorrhoea, peritonitis, pelvic inflammatory disease)
  - previous tubal surgery
- Fimbrial adhesions:
  - previous surgery
  - endometriosis
Sperm
- Vagina:
  - psychosexual problems (vaginismus)
  - infection (causing dyspareunia)
  - congenital anomaly
- Cervix:
  - cervical trauma or surgery (cone biopsy)
  - infection
  - hormonal (hostile mucus)
  - antisperm antibodies in mucus

Defective implantation
- Hormonal imbalance
- Congenital anomalies
- Fibroids
- Infection

want children and if they are both equally committed to that goal. There may be pressure from family or friends, an illusion that a baby would improve a deteriorating relationship, even a concern to obtain better housing. Some may be quite happy to remain childless once they know that they could have children if they wanted to.

It is important to establish whether intercourse is taking place and its frequency and timing. It is occasionally discovered that a relationship has not been consummated.

Infrequent intercourse may be due to lack of interest caused by low sexual appetite or excessive

tiredness, or to lack of opportunity. One partner may work away from home for long periods or each may work different shifts. Whatever the reason, the chance of intercourse coinciding with the fertile phase is reduced. Conversely, if ejaculation occurs more than once every other day, sperm count is diminished.

The couple need to understand the female cycle in order that intercourse may be timed to enhance the possibility of conception. Investigations and attempted treatments of subfertility are stressful and may disrupt the delicate hormonal balance necessary for successful conception. In addition, concentrating exclusively on the potentially fertile period puts great strain on a relationship and may result in the man becoming impotent. For these reasons the couple must be encouraged to maintain as much spontaneity as possible in their lovemaking (Mack & Tucker 1996).

General investigations

A full history is obtained from both partners, including occupation, in case it involves contact with industrial pollutants or radioactive materials. Any medical problems are referred to the appropriate specialist for investigation, treatment or stabilisation. Particular attention is paid to a history of sexually transmitted disease which may have resulted in obstruction of the uterine or seminal tubes. In the man, orchitis secondary to mumps after puberty may be significant; in the woman, previous pelvic or abdominal surgery raises the possibility of adhesions.

The couple are asked about fertility to date. Each partner should be given the opportunity to elaborate on this individually, as the other may be unaware of a previous pregnancy.

Approximately 20% of women attending infertility clinics have ovulatory dysfunction. Regular menstruation suggests that ovulation is probably occurring; dysmenorrhoea and 'mittelschmerz' (transient mid-cycle pain in the iliac fossa) reinforce this assumption.

Primary amenorrhoea means that a woman has never menstruated; *secondary amenorrhoea* that periods have ceased. If periods are erratic or infrequent (*oligomenorrhoea*) then even if ovulation is occurring, it will be impossible to predict the date.

Both partners are given a complete medical examination which includes the genitalia. In the man this will disclose conditions such as varicocele and hydrocele which affect fertility and may possibly be treatable. In the woman, hirsutism and obesity may be suggestive of endocrine disorders.

A bimanual and speculum examination will reveal any gross pelvic pathology and a cervical smear can be obtained (Healy 1994).

Specific investigations of male infertility and significance of findings

Semen analysis

This is the basic test for male infertility. It should be carried out before any further investigations on the couple. Average values are assessed on three samples produced over several weeks, as quality is variable. Specimens are produced by masturbation after 2–3 days' abstinence and examined in the laboratory within 1 hour. If satisfactory, the man is assumed to be potentially fertile.

Normal values (WHO 1988):
Volume: 2–6 ml
Total sperm count: more than 40×10^6 per ml
Motility: more than 60% of the sperm moving forward
Morphology: more than 60% of the sperm should appear normal on examination.

Agglutination of sperm in the semen specimen may be due to:

- *Antisperm antibodies*, particularly if the man has had a vasectomy reversal or testicular trauma. Intrauterine insemination with the washed sperm may be successful.
- *Infection*, viral or bacterial. If bacterial, it may respond to appropriate treatment.

Azoospermia (absence of spermatozoa in the semen) is usually untreatable but further investigations may give a clue to the cause.

Biopsy of the testes will show whether sperm are actually being produced. If they are, the problem is presumably one of defective transport.

Chromosome studies from blood or buccal smear may reveal Klinefelter's syndrome (XXY) which always results in sterility.

Oligospermia (oligoasthenoteratozoospermia) (total sperm count less than 20×10^6 per ml) may be improved by attention to diet and general health, particularly reducing smoking and alcohol intake. Reducing the ambient temperature of the testicles may encourage sperm development.

Blood tests for hormone levels may suggest possibilities for treatment. If estimation of gonadotrophin levels reveals reduced amounts of follicle-stimulating hormone (FSH), clomiphene therapy may stimulate the pituitary to produce more FSH to act on the testes. Treatment with testosterone appears to have little value. Abnormally high levels of prolactin may respond to bromocriptine.

Postcoital test

A specimen of aspirated cervical mucus from the female partner is examined, at the fertile time of the cycle, within 6 hours of intercourse. The ability of the sperm to penetrate the mucus can be observed, as can the quality of the mucus, and the test gives confirmation that effective intercourse is taking place.

Research into male factor infertility continues, but at present the prognosis is poor. Treatments such as in vitro fertilisation may succeed in circumventing the problem for some couples.

Specific investigations and treatment of female infertility

Ovulation disorders: tests to establish whether ovulation is occurring

Cervical mucus becomes clear, copious and stretchy at ovulation and shows a ferning pattern when dried on a glass slide.

Ovulation prediction kits can be purchased at a chemist; a simple urine test measures luteinising hormone (LH) levels.

Basal body temperature (BBT) drops slightly before ovulation, then rises by about 0.3°C, remaining at the higher level for the rest of the cycle. This method is now considered cumbersome and inaccurate.

Ultrasound scanning can detect a ripening Graafian follicle (follicle tracking) and thickening of the endometrium.

Hormonal assays. A series of blood tests throughout the menstrual cycle should show fluctuations in circulating oestrogens and progesterone, FSH and LH. The results may suggest possibilities for treatment. Other endocrine disturbances, such as thyroid deficiency, and hyperprolactinaemia, should be excluded.

Stimulation of ovulation

Clomiphene citrate (Clomid) stimulates the hypothalamic–pituitary system, permitting FSH production and so inducing ovulation. 50 micrograms daily are taken in tablet form for 5 days starting within 5 days of the onset of menstruation. Ovulation should occur around day 12–16, and intercourse can be advised on alternate days from days 10–18. Dosage can be increased up to a maximum of 150 mg. Long-term treatment appears to have few benefits.

Human chorionic gonadotrophin (HCG) is identical in action to LH and can be used to trigger ovulation, often in conjunction with clomiphene or some other form of ovulation induction. Intercourse should be advised around the time of administration.

Human menopausal gonadotrophin (HMG) (Pergonal) or pure FSH (Metrodin) may be used if clomiphene has failed or in cases of polycystic ovary disease. It is administered daily by injection from the onset of menstruation until a mature follicle is detected; HCG is then given. Hyperstimulation of the ovaries is a risk. Multiple ovulation can be disastrous if natural conception is intended, though it is necessary for procedures such as in vitro fertilisation (IVF) for which this regimen is also used.

Bromocriptine (Parlodel) is used to inhibit synthesis and release of prolactin by the pituitary. Hyperprolactinaemia may result in low oestrogen and progesterone levels and prevent ovulation. It may be caused by stress or the use of drugs such as tranquillisers.

Ovarian disorders may be discovered at laparoscopy. Cysts or tumours may be removed surgically. Endometriosis may be discovered and can be treated by short-term suppression of ovulation with progestogens.

Ovum transport: investigation of tubal patency

Laparoscopy is carried out under general anaesthetic. Watery dye passed through the cervix can be observed to drip out of the ends of the uterine tubes if they are patent. Additional information can be obtained such as whether the tubes are mobile and free from adhesions and whether there is evidence of pelvic inflammatory disease or endometriosis. The ovaries are examined for abnormalities and evidence of corpora lutea.

Hysterosalpingography is performed during the first 10 days of the menstrual cycle to avoid possible irradiation of an early pregnancy. Radiopaque dye is injected through the cervix; an X-ray will reveal whether the tubes are patent and also the shape of the uterine cavity. The procedure can be painful if there is an obstruction, owing to build-up of pressure inside the tubes. There is also a risk of chemical or allergic reaction to the dye.

The prognosis for treatment of tubal obstruction is poor. There has been some improvement with the development of microsurgical techniques and argon laser surgery, but even if the damage is repaired there remains a risk of ectopic pregnancy. Increasingly, in vitro fertilisation (IVF), which has the effect of bypassing the blocked uterine tubes, is being recommended to women with tubal obstruction.

Sperm transport
Cervical mucus normally changes from a viscid plug to a copious clear fluid under the influence of progesterone at ovulation in order to facilitate the passage of sperm.

The postcoital test has already been described under investigations for male infertility.

The sperm penetration test demonstrates the behaviour of sperm alongside a sample of mucus taken at the fertile time, on a glass slide. It determines whether sperm function or mucus hostility is the problem.

Crossed hostility tests observe the behaviour of the partner's sperm and fresh donor sperm in the woman's cervical mucus.

If the mucus is hostile, or the woman is producing antisperm antibodies to her partner's sperm, intrauterine insemination may be successful (Healy 1994).

ARTIFICIAL REPRODUCTION

Artificial insemination by husband (AIH)

Indications

- Cervical problems (see above).
- Mechanical problems:
  - psychosexual
  - spinal injury
  - other physical disability.
- Antisperm antibodies in the man.
- Mild oligospermia with satisfactory motility.
- Semen stored before commencement of chemo- or radiotherapy.

Procedure

Intrauterine insemination is mostly used in order to enhance the likelihood of success. There should be no tubal pathology and the woman should be ovulating normally, though mild superovulation may be induced. The sperm are separated from the remainder of the ejaculate in the laboratory and, in 0.2 ml of media solution, are flushed into the uterus via the cervix by means of a fine catheter.

Artificial insemination by donor (AID/DI)

Indications

- Azoospermia or oligospermia in male partner.
- Excessive non-motile and/or abnormal sperm.
- Risk of transmission of a hereditary disease.
- Rhesus iso-immunisation; a Rhesus negative donor may be used.
- Lack of a male partner.

Procedure

A vaginal speculum and syringe are used to bathe the cervix in semen. The woman may be asked to lie still for a few minutes afterwards. It is usually carried out 2–3 days before ovulation and may be repeated a couple of days later. Success rates are comparable to those for normal conception.

Donors are carefully selected. They must be of normal intelligence, fit and healthy, with no personal or family history of disease. Each donation is analysed to ensure satisfactory quality. Tests for sexually transmitted diseases, including human immunodeficiency virus (HIV), are repeated at every visit, and the semen is frozen and stored for at least 3 months before use to be sure that tests were negative. Donors are matched as far as possible to the male partner; skin, hair and eye colouring, height and build, and blood group.

Whether the child is told of his origins is for the parents to decide. If they are encouraged to make love around the time of insemination, there will be a possibility, however remote, that the child's social father will be the genetic father.

Some religious groups oppose DI on the grounds that it profanes the sanctity of marriage. Concern has also been expressed at its use by single women, lesbians and virgins who want a child without being involved with a man.

- All clinics offering DI must be licensed by the Human Fertilisation and Embryology Authority.
- If a man consents to his partner receiving DI, he is legally the father of the child.
- The donor is not considered to be the father of the child.
- The Authority will keep a register of donors and resulting births, in order to limit paternities to 10.

People born as a result of DI will be able to obtain information about their origins, and also whether they are related to an intended partner. Whether this will allow the donor to be identified is not yet clear; nor are the implications for recruitment of donors if confidentiality can no longer be guaranteed (Lauritzen 1993).

In vitro fertilisation/embryo transfer (IVF/ET)

Indications

- Tubal damage.
- Oligospermia, poor motility, antisperm antibodies.
- Cervical problems.
- Endometriosis.
- 'Unexplained' infertility.

Procedure

Stage 1. Ovulation induction is performed using drugs to stimulate multiple ovulation. Progress is monitored by ultrasound follicle tracking and serum oestradiol levels.

Stage 2. Ovum recovery is planned when four or more follicles reach 20 mm in size. The ova are harvested using vaginal ultrasound guidance under local anaesthetic or laparoscopy under general anaesthetic. Ova and semen are treated separately before being brought together outside the body.

Stage 3. Embryo transfer is performed 2–3 days later when the zygotes have reached the 4- or 8-cell stage. A maximum of three embryos are placed in the uterus via the cervix to increase the chances of success but reduce the risk of higher multiple pregnancy. Any healthy surplus embryos may be frozen for further attempts if necessary.

Gamete intrafallopian transfer (GIFT)

This may be attempted if there are cervical barriers to conception. At least one uterine (fallopian) tube must be patent and sperm quality must be good. Ova are harvested as for IVF, aspirated into a catheter with the prepared fresh sperm, and placed in the distal end of the uterine tube. Fertilisation should then occur in vivo. The procedure is not covered by the new legislation, so a licence is not required in order to offer it, unless donated gametes are used, and there is no restriction on the number of ova which may be transferred.

Zygote intrafallopian transfer (ZIFT)

Ova are fertilised in vitro, and the embryos are then introduced into the uterine tube.

Intracytoplasmic sperm injection (ICSI)

Intracytoplasmic sperm injection (ICSI) offers new hope to couples where the male partner is diagnosed with very poor semen characteristics and who have undergone one or more cycles of standard IVF procedure (Palermo et al 1992, Van Steirteghem et al 1996).

Oocytes with an intact zona pellucida and clear cytoplasm that have extruded the first polar body are micro-injected. A single, living immobilised spermatozoon is aspirated tail first into the injection pipette. The pipette is pushed through the zona pellucida and into the cytoplasm where the spermatozoon is delivered. After injection the oocytes are washed and stored at 37°C in an incubator. Up to three embryos will be placed into the uterine cavity and pregnancy is confirmed by detecting rising serum HCG concentrations 10 days later.

The potential genetic and other risks should not be neglected. A chromosome analysis should be routinely performed on the male when ICSI is used.

Ovum donation

This is the equivalent of DI for the fertile man whose partner is not ovulating but could carry a pregnancy. Most donations are from women undergoing IVF treatment; ova are fertilised in vitro by sperm from the recipient's partner and placed in the recipient's uterus. Timing is crucial, so either the two women's cycles will be synchronised artificially or the embryos may be frozen before use.

The law regarding ovum donation is the same as that for sperm. All potential donors must be offered counselling about the implications, such as their feelings about the potential child, and the possibility of their own childlessness (Hamberger & Wikland 1992).

Surrogacy

This is the practice whereby one woman carries a child for another with the intention of handing the baby over at birth. It may be seen as the ultimate act of generosity by one woman to another less fortunate than herself, and has probably been going on since time immemorial. However, it arouses considerable public anxiety and, following recommendations by the Warnock report, the Surrogacy Arrangements Act became law in 1985 (Great Britain Committee of Inquiry into Human Fertilisation and Embryology 1984, Kirby 1990). This has since been amended by the Human Fertilisation and Embryology Act 1990.

Surrogacy is legal in the UK as long as no money changes hands (apart from reasonable expenses), but the arrangement is not enforceable in law. The carrying mother is always the legal mother of the child at birth. The commissioning parents, if over 18 years old and married to each other, may apply within 6 months of the birth for a court order making them the legal parents, providing the child was conceived within the law using the gametes of one or both of them and is living with the applicants at the time. The carrying mother cannot agree to the order until 6 weeks after the birth. Both parties are free to change their minds at any time during the pregnancy or until the court order has been made (Mack & Tucker 1996).

Issues raised by artificial reproduction

The birth of the first 'test-tube baby' in July 1978 opened up new possibilities not only in the alleviation of infertility but also for scientific developments. The earliest stages of human development could be observed, raising hopes of detecting and remedying defects, along with anxieties about possible experimentation and manipulation.

The Warnock Report (Great Britain Committee of Inquiry into Human Fertilisation and Embryology 1984) was commissioned in response to public concern. It made an urgent recommendation for the establishment of a statutory licensing authority to regulate research and infertility services. A Voluntary Licensing Authority was set up by the Medical Research Council and the Royal College of Obstetricians and Gynaecologists; the Human Fertilisation and Embryology Act became statute in 1990.

The Human Fertilisation and Embryology Authority (HFEA) was established by the Act 'to regulate, by means of a licensing system, any research or treatment which involves the creation, keeping and using of human embryos outside the body, or the storage or donation of human eggs and sperm. It must also maintain a Code of Practice giving guidance about the proper conduct of the licensed activities.' (HFEA 1991).

The legal implications of the reproductive technologies are now somewhat clearer, but the debate surrounding the introduction of the Act raised many practical and ethical issues which remain controversial. For the couple whose infertility is circumvented by assisted reproduction and who achieve a healthy baby, the benefits are clear, but the techniques are very expensive, and success is limited. Writing about IVF/ET, Wagner & St Clair (1989) argue that 'No new technique should become standard until after rigorous evaluation. Until then, it must remain experimental, guided by the principles covering research on human subjects. Evaluation involves assessment of efficacy, safety and costs. ... IVF/ET and related assisted reproduction technologies have not been scrutinised in this way.' The available evidence is examined regarding the low success rate, the high perinatal mortality and morbidity, the risks to the women, and the financial, psychological and social costs. The authors call for randomised controlled trials to establish the efficacy of treatments, and follow-up studies of the long-term effects. 'With this information, infertile couples can make the best informed choice about their care and countries can make the best informed choice about the appropriate place of IVF/ET in their infertility services.' The debate is far from over (Lauritzen 1993, Mack & Tucker 1996).

CONCLUSION AND THE ROLE OF THE MIDWIFE IN PRECONCEPTION CARE

Preconception care is an ideologically sound concept, but in reality it may be seen as a luxury service only available to a motivated, educated few.

Comprehensive programmes of preconception care that identify and reduce couples' reproductive risks before conception are rare.

Curtis (1996) suggests that while preconception care may be new to some midwives 'the elements are very familiar' to others and can be effectively delivered by them. She further suggests that midwives have 'always provided preconception care outside the domain of a preconception clinic' (p. 16).

With emerging team midwifery and continuity of carer, midwives may have an opportunity to incorporate many elements of preconception care into their daily practice, both prenatal and postnatal. Women may wish to consult their known team for preconception advice before embarking on another pregnancy.

With a greater emphasis on health promotion, midwives are ideally placed to take on this role and participate with other members of the multidisciplinary team in preconception care (Curtis 1996, Pownall 1994).

READER ACTIVITIES

Identify the health services available to well women of childbearing age in your local community. Talk to staff and users of the services. You might consider health centres, general practitioner surgeries, chemist's shops, occupational health departments, family planning and well-woman clinics, psychosexual counselling and genetic counselling services.

1. How accessible are these services (location, hours of opening, 'user-friendliness', ease of referral)?

2. Do they make a positive contribution towards encouraging optimum health before conception?

3. What provision is there in local schools to educate young people about planning for a healthy pregnancy?

4. What services are available for couples concerned about their fertility? What is the pattern of referral for specialist investigation and treatment? How much is available on the National Health Service? What costs might be involved if private treatment is required? How is the money found?

ACKNOWLEDGEMENT

The help of Antigone Sarantaki is acknowledged for information relating to ICSI.

USEFUL ADDRESSES

Association to Aid Sexual and Personal Relationships of People with a Disability (SPOD)
286 Camden Road
London N7 0BJ
Tel: 0171 607 8851

British Agencies for Adoption and Fostering
Skyline House
200 Union Street
Southwark
London SE1 0LX
Tel: 0171 593 2000
Fax: 0171 593 2001

British Diabetic Association
10 Queen Anne Street
London W1M 0BD
Tel: 0171 323 1531
Fax: 0171 637 3644

British Epilepsy Association
Anstey House, 40 Hanover Square
Leeds LS3 1BE
Tel: 0113 243 9393

British Pregnancy Advisory Service (BPAS)
Austy Manor
Wootton Wawen
Solihull
West Midlands B95 6BX
Tel: 01564 793225
Helpline: 0345 304030

Brook Advisory Centres
Central Office
165 Gray's Inn Road
London WC1X 8UD
Tel: 0171 713 9000
Fax: 0171 853 8182

Disability, Pregnancy & Parenthood International
45 Beech Street, 5th Floor
London EC2P 2LX
Tel: 0171 628 2811
E-mail: fad36@dial.pipex.com
(*A move is expected during 1998.*)

Foresight – The Association for the Promotion of Preconceptual Care
28 The Paddock
Godalming
Surrey GU7 1XD
Tel: 01483 427839

Genetic Nurses and Social Workers Association
c/o Ruth Cole
Clinical Genetics Society
Clinical Genetics Unit
Birmingham Maternity Hospital
Edgbaston
Birmingham B12 2TG
Tel: 01216 272634

ISSUE – The National Fertility Association
114 Lichfield Street
Walsall
Birmingham WS1 1SZ
Tel: 01922 722 888

National Endometriosis Society
Suite 50, Westminster Palace Gardens
1–7 Artillery Row
London SW1P 1RL
Tel: 0171 222 2781
Helpline: 0171 222 2776
Fax: 0171 222 2786

Progress
16 Mortimer Street
London W1N 7RD
Tel: 0171 636 5390

Quit
Victory House
170 Tottenham Court Road
London W1P 0HA
Tel: 0171 388 5775
Helpline: 0800 002200
Pregnancy line: 0800 002211

Wellbeing, the Health Research Charity for Women and Babies, formerly Birthright
27 Sussex Place
Regent's Park
London NW1 4SP
Tel: 0171 262 5337
Fax: 0171 724 7725

Women's Health and Reproductive Rights Information Centre (WHRRIC)
52–54 Featherstone Street
London EC1Y 8RT
Tel: 0171 251 6580

REFERENCES

Barnes B 1996 Preparation for pregnancy: the Foresight programme. Health Visitor 69(12): 503–504

Bradley S G, Foresight Organisation, Bennett N 1995 Preparation for pregnancy an essential guide: international research into preconceptual health and pregnancy outcome including the Foresight experience. Glendaruel, Argyll

Brewer S 1995 Planning a baby: a complete guide to preconceptual care. Optima, London

Cefalo R C, Bowes W A, Moos J R, Moos M K 1995 Preconception care: a means of prevention. In: Steegers E A P, Eskes T K A B, Symonds E M (guest eds) Preventive care in obstetrics. Baillière's clinical obstetrics and gynaecology: international practice and research. Baillière Tindall, London, vol 9(3), pp 403–416

Chamberlain G, Lumley J 1986 Prepregnancy care: a manual for practice. John Wiley, Chichester

Crawford P 1997 Epilepsy and pregnancy: good management reduces the risks. Avoiding fetal malformation. Professional Care of Mother and Child 7(1): 17–18

Curtis G 1996 Preconception care. In: Alexander J, Levy V, Roch S (eds) Midwifery practice: core topics I. Macmillan, Basingstoke

Czeizel A E 1995 Primary prevention of birth defects by periconceptional care including multivitamin supplementation. In: Steegers E A P, Eskes T K A B, Symonds E M (guest eds) Preventive care in obstetrics. Baillière's clinical obstetrics and gynaecology: international practice and research. Baillière Tindall, London, vol 9(3)

Department of Health 1992 Folic acid and the prevention of neural tube defects: report from an expert advisory group. Health Publications, Heywood

Dickerson J 1995 Good preconception care starts in school. Modern Midwife 5(11): 15–18

Elixhauser A, Kitzmiller J L, Weschler J M 1996 Short term cost benefit of pre-conception care for diabetes. Diabetes Care 19(4): 384

Great Britain Committee of Inquiry into Human Fertilisation and Embryology 1984 Report of the Committee into Human Fertilisation and Embryology. HMSO, London

Hadley J 1987 Secondary infertility. New Generation 6(2): 46–47

Hajee F 1995 A healthy baby plan … preconceptual care. Practice Nurse 10(3): 193–194, 196

Hamberger L, Wikland M (eds) 1992 Assisted reproduction. Baillière's clinical obstetrics and gynaecology: international practice and research. Baillière Tindall, London

Harper P S 1988 Practical genetic counselling, 3rd edn. John Wright, London

Healy D L 1994 Female infertility: causes and treatment. Lancet 308(6944): 1539–1544

Human Fertilisation and Embryology Act 1990 HMSO, London

Human Fertilisation and Embryology Authority 1991 Code of practice consultation document. HFEA, London

Kelly T E 1986 Clinical genetics and genetic counselling. Year Book Medical Publishers, London

Kirby M 1990 Medical technology and new frontiers of family law. In: McLean S A M (ed) Legal issues in human reproduction. Dartmouth Publishing Company, Aldershot

Lashford S 1985 The twelve month pregnancy: your diet from pre-conception to motherhood. Ashgrove Press, Bath

Lauritzen P 1993 Pursuing parenthood: ethical issues in assisted reproduction. Indiana University Press, Blooming

McGreal I E 1995 Smoking and the pregnant woman. Midwives 108(1290): 218–221

Mack S, Tucker J 1996 Fertility counselling. Baillière Tindall, London

Morgan J 1994 Nutrition and pregnancy: problems and solutions. Nursing Times 90(46): 16–22, 31–33

MRC Vitamin Study Group 1991 Prevention of neural tube defects: results of the medical research council vitamin study. Lancet 338(8760): 131–137

O'Driscoll M 1994 Midwives, childbirth and sexuality (relationships following childbirth). British Journal of Midwifery 2(1): 39–41

Palermo G, Josis H, Devroey P, Van Steirteghem A C 1992 Pregnancies after intracytoplasmic sperm injection of single spermatozoon into an oocyte. Lancet 340: 17–18

Parker C 1996 Pre-pregnancy monitoring for women with diabetes. Professional Care of Mother and Child 6(5): 135, 137–138

Perry L E 1996 Preconception care: a health promotion opportunity. American Journal of Primary Health Care 21(11): 24, 26, 32

Plant M L 1990 Maternal alcohol and tobacco use during pregnancy. In: Alexander J, Levy V, Roch S (eds) Antenatal care: a research based approach. Macmillan Education, London

Pownall G 1994 Preconception care: are midwives in danger of missing the boat? Modern Midwife 4(4): 34–35

Shorney J 1990 Preconception care: the embryo of health promotion. In: Alexander J, Levy V, Roch S (eds) Antenatal care: a research based approach. Macmillan Education, London

Steegers-Theunissen R P M 1995 Maternal nutrition and obstetric outcome. In: Steegers E A P, Eskes T K A B, Symonds E M (guest eds) Preventive care in obstetrics. Baillière's clinical obstetrics and gynaecology: international practice and research. Baillière Tindall, London, vol 9(3), pp 431–443

Steel J M, Johnstone F D, Hepburn D A, Smith A F 1990 Can prepregnancy care of diabetic women reduce the risk of abnormal babies. British Medical Journal 301: 1070–1074

Surrogacy Arrangements Act 1985 HMSO, London

van Steirteghem A C, Nagy P, Josis H, Varheyen G 1996 The development of intracytoplasmic sperm injection. Human reproduction 11: 59–72

Wagner M G, St Clair P A 1989 Are in-vitro fertilisation and embryo transfer benefit to all? Lancet 2(October 28): 1027–1030

Walton I 1994 Sexuality and Motherhood. Books for Midwives, Hale

Ward R H T, Smith S K, Donnai D 1994 Early fetal growth and development. Royal College of Obstetricians and Gynaecologists Press, London

World Health Organization 1988 Laboratory recommendations. WHO, Geneva

Wynn M, Wynn A 1991 The case for preconception care of men and women. AB Academic, Bicester, Oxon

Wynn M 1994 Slimming and fertility. Modern Midwife 4(6): 17–20

FURTHER READING

Bushy A, Craner R 1990 Preconception education: a program for community health nurses. Family and Community Health 13(3): 82–84

Cant S 1992 Infertility: causes and treatment. Nursing Standard 7(13/14): 28–30

Doyle W 1992 Preconceptional care: who needs it? Modern Midwife 2(1): 18–22

Dwinell J 1994 Prepregnancy care: a promising new field or just a fad? Nursing World Journal 20(1): 5–6

Howards S S 1995 Treatment of male infertility. New England Journal of Medicine 332(5): 312–317

Niven C, Walker A 1996 Reproductive potential and fertility control. Butterworth-Heinemann, Oxford

Potrykus C 1992 Stop the cycle of deprivation: improvements in preconceptual care. Health Visitor 65(1): 7–8

11

Change and adaptation in pregnancy

Irene Murray

All changes in a mother's body during pregnancy are associated with, and in some systems caused by, the effects of specific hormones (Case & Waterhouse 1994). These changes enable her to nurture the fetus, prepare her body for labour, develop her breasts and lay down stores of fat to provide calories for production of breast milk during the puerperium. By understanding the numerous physiological changes that occur in a woman's body during pregnancy the midwife is enabled to provide appropriate care and detect abnormality if this should occur (Leader et al 1996).

The chapter aims to:

- give an overview of the changes occurring in different body systems during pregnancy, relating them throughout to the underlying changes in hormone levels

- identify those physiological changes that may mimic or mask disease and those that cause discomfort or inconvenience to the mother

- discuss the diagnosis of pregnancy, distinguishing between possible, probable and positive signs of the condition.

The woman's psychological state is also affected by hormonal changes. These changes are discussed in Chapter 2.

PHYSIOLOGICAL CHANGES IN THE REPRODUCTIVE SYSTEM

The body of the uterus

After conception, the uterus develops to provide a nutritive and protective environment in which the fetus will develop and grow (Nilsson 1990).

Decidua

The decidua is the name given to the endometrium during pregnancy.

Progesterone and oestrogen, initially produced by the enlarged corpus luteum, cause the decidua to become thicker, richer and more vascular at the fundus and in the upper body of the uterus. These areas are the usual sites of implantation, the decidua being thinner and less vascular in the lower pole of the uterus (Chamberlain et al 1991). The decidua provides a glycogen-rich environment for the blastocyst until the trophoblastic cells begin to form the placenta (see Ch. 51). Once the placenta has formed, it is able to produce its own hormones and the corpus luteum is no longer maintained by human chorionic gonadotrophin. After the 13–17th week of pregnancy the corpus luteum atrophies and becomes the corpus albicans (Findlay 1984). Recent studies have shown that decidual cells secrete prolactin and relaxin. Although their function is not yet clear it is thought that relaxin may play a part in the ability of the uterus to distend (Fuchs & Fuchs 1991).

Myometrium

The myometrium consists of bundles of smooth muscle fibres held together by connective tissue. The muscle fibres in pregnancy grow up to 15–20 times their non-pregnant length (Fig. 11.1). This *hypertrophy* (increase in size) and *hyperplasia* (increase in number) of the uterine muscle fibres is due to the effect of oestrogen and progesterone. The uterus continues to grow in this way for the first 3 months, after which its growth is related to distension by the growing fetus and placenta (Llewellyn-Jones 1994).

- *Increase in weight.* From between 50 and 100 g (depending on parity) to 1100 g.
- *Increase in size.* From 7.5 × 5 × 2.5 cm to 30 × 23 × 20 cm (Verralls 1993).

The walls of the myometrium become thicker in the first few months of pregnancy, but as gestation advances, the walls become thinner owing to the gross enlargement of the uterus, being only 1.5 cm thick or less at term (Cunningham et al 1989).

Although progesterone suppresses myometrial activity throughout most of the pregnancy, the uterus begins to generate small waves of irregular and usually painless contractility from the first trimester, known as *Braxton Hicks* contractions. These are infrequent and non-rhythmic and facilitate the formation of the lower uterine segment (McFadyen 1995). They usually increase in frequency and intensity from about the 36th week of pregnancy, causing some discomfort. These 'prelabour' contractions are associated with 'ripening' of the cervix, and eventually become the contractions of labour as the effects of oestrogen supersede those of progesterone (see Ch. 21) (Davey 1995a). Differentiating between Braxton Hicks contractions and the contractions of preterm labour can sometimes be difficult. Diagnosis is made on the presence or absence of cervical dilatation (Coustan 1994).

During pregnancy the muscle layers become more differentiated and organised for their part in expelling the fetus at term (Fig. 11.2).

Muscle layers. The outer longitudinal layer of muscle fibres is thin. It passes longitudinally from the front of the isthmus anteriorly over the fundus and into the vault of the vagina posteriorly, and

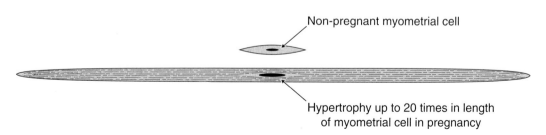
Non-pregnant myometrial cell

Hypertrophy up to 20 times in length of myometrial cell in pregnancy

Fig. 11.1 Increase in length of myometrial cell in pregnancy (adapted from Davey 1995a, p. 90).

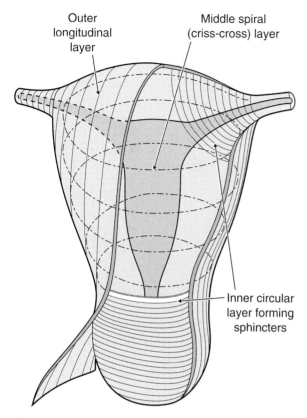

Outer longitudinal layer

Middle spiral (criss-cross) layer

Inner circular layer forming sphincters

Fig. 11.2 Diagrammatic representation of differentiated muscle layers of uterus in pregnancy (adapted from Chamberlain et al 1991, p. 30).

extends into the round and transverse ligaments (McFadyen 1995).

The thick middle layer of spiral myometrial fibres encircles the cavity. During labour the synchronous contraction and retraction of these muscle fibres cause them to become heaped up in the upper uterine segment making it thicker and shorter in length while the lower uterine segment becomes thinner and more stretched (Chamberlain et al 1991).

The thickened upper segment acts as a piston to force the fetus into the receptive, passive lower segment (see Ch. 21) (Symonds 1992). Contraction of these muscle fibres is also necessary to entrap and enmesh bleeding vessels and ligate them after the placenta is delivered (see Ch. 25) (Cunningham et al 1989).

The inner circular layer is thin and forms sphinc-ters around the openings of the uterine tubes at the cornua, and around the lower uterine segment and cervix (McFadyen 1995). During labour the stretching and pulling up of the circular layer of muscles around the cervix into the lower uterine segment causes the cervix to become effaced and dilated (Chamberlain et al 1991).

The perimetrium

This is a layer of peritoneum. It does not totally cover the uterus, being deflected over the bladder anteriorly to form the uterovesical pouch and over the rectum posteriorly to form the pouch of Douglas (see Ch. 49) (de Swiet & Chamberlain 1992). The double folds of perimetrium (broad ligament) hanging from the uterine tubes and extending to the lateral walls of the pelvis become longer and wider as the uterus enlarges. The anterior and posterior folds open out so that they are no longer in apposition and can therefore accommodate the greatly enlarged uterine and ovarian arteries and veins (Davey 1995a).

Spasm of these ligaments can cause sharp groin pain, particularly on the right, because of the dextrorotation of the uterus (Johnson et al 1991).

Blood supply

The blood supply to the uterus through the uterine and ovarian arteries increases to about 750 ml/ minute at term to keep pace with its growth and also to meet the needs of the functioning placenta (Bissonette 1991).

This is made possible by the increase in diameter of uterine blood vessels under the influence of oestrogen and also by the development of new blood vessels (Leader et al 1996). In the first half of the pregnancy the blood vessels form a tortuous network through the uterine walls but as the uterus grows and stretches they become uncoiled, providing the necessary extra length (Llewellyn-Jones 1994).

Changes in uterine shape

Healthy growth of the fetus requires adequate space. After conception the embedded blastocyst demands little space but the upper part of the uterus begins to enlarge as a result of the effects of

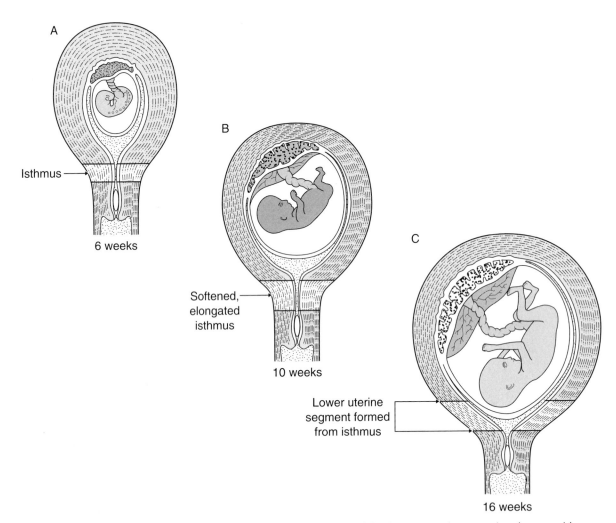

Fig. 11.3 Changes in the uterus between 6 and 16 weeks (not to scale): (A) isthmus 7 mm long, uterine shape ovoid, embryonic sac in upper pole; (B) isthmus long and soft, uterus globular, fetal sac in upper pole; (C) isthmus open to form lower segment, fetal sac occupies both poles.

oestrogen. The uterus changes to a globular shape in early pregnancy to anticipate fetal growth and also to accommodate increasing amounts of liquor and placental tissue (Fig. 11.3). This causes pressure on other pelvic organs (Cunningham et al 1989).

The lower part of the uterus, consisting of the isthmus, softens and elongates to three times its original length during the first trimester, giving the appearance of a stalk below the globular upper segment. This is the beginning of the differentiation between the upper and lower segments of the uterus (Davey 1995a).

12th week of pregnancy

The uterus is no longer anteverted and anteflexed. It has risen out of the pelvis and become upright, although often it inclines and rotates to the right so that the left margin of the uterus faces anteriorly (*dextrorotation*). This is thought to be due to the pressure of the pelvic colon which occupies space in the left part of the pelvis (Cunningham et al 1989). At 12 weeks the uterus is about the size of a grapefruit and the fundus may be palpated abdominally above the symphysis pubis (Leader et al 1996).

16th week of pregnancy

By 16 weeks the conceptus has grown enough to put pressure on the isthmus, causing it to open out so that the uterus becomes more globular in shape (Coustan 1994). The walls of the isthmus become progressively thin as pregnancy advances (Gould 1991).

20th week of pregnancy

The uterus becomes spherical in shape at 20 weeks and has a thicker, more rounded fundus. The shape then continues to elongate until term (McFadyen 1995). The uterine tubes appear to issue from a lower level (Cunningham et al 1989). As the uterus continues to rise in the abdomen, the uterine tubes, being restricted by attachment to the broad ligaments, become progressively more vertical. At 20 weeks the fundus of the uterus may be palpated at or just below the umbilicus (Miller & Hanretty 1997).

30th week of pregnancy

The lower uterine segment can be identified. It is still not complete but can be defined as the portion lying below the reflection of the vesicouterine fold of peritoneum and above the internal os of the cervix (Llewellyn-Jones 1994). At 30 weeks the fundus may be palpated midway between the umbilicus and the xiphisternum (Miller & Hanretty 1997).

38th week of pregnancy

The uterus now reaches the level of the xiphisternum. A reduction in fundal height known as *lightening* may occur at the end of pregnancy when the fetus sinks into the lower pole of the uterus. This is due to softening of the tissues of the pelvic floor together with good uterine tone and further formation of the lower uterine segment (Miller & Hanretty 1997). In the primigravida this also encourages the beginning of a gradual descent of the fetus into the pelvis and the head becomes engaged. In the multiparous woman descent often does not occur until labour aids the process (Chamberlain et al 1991).

The development of the lower uterine segment from the isthmus is finally completed in labour.

It measures approximately one-third of the body of the uterus, is thin, and contains very little smooth muscle. Its contractility is markedly different from that of the fundus and the corpus (Gould 1991).

The cervix

The cervix contains more fibrous tissue and less muscular tissue than the body of the uterus, which explains the fundal dominance of uterine contractions (McFadyen 1995). It acts as an effective barrier against infection during pregnancy. It also is structured to protect the fetus during its development by remaining firmly closed and by providing resistance to pressure from above when the mother is in the upright position (Fuchs & Fuchs 1991).

Under the influence of progesterone, endocervical cells secrete mucus which becomes thicker and more viscous during pregnancy. The thickened mucus forms a cervical plug called the *operculum*, which provides protection from ascending infection (McFadyen 1995).

The cervix remains 2.5 cm long throughout pregnancy, but the hygroscopic properties of oestrogen cause it to increase in width (Llewellyn-Jones 1994). This exposes endocervical cells which can give an appearance of erosion (Cunningham et al 1989). Oestrogen also increases cervical vascularity and, if viewed through a speculum, the cervix looks bluish in colour (Leader et al 1996).

In late pregnancy softening, or *ripening*, of the cervix occurs in response to increasing painless contractions and is under hormonal control. Prostaglandins released from local tissue and reduced collagen concentration within the cervix are also thought to play a part in the cervix becoming softer and more distensible in readiness for the onset of labour (Fuchs & Fuchs 1991). The muscles of the fundus enhance tension in the outer longitudinal layer of muscle of the cervix, leading to a gradual redistribution of cervical tissue which may contribute towards the process of effacement (O'Lah 1996). Effacement or *taking up of the cervix* normally occurs in the primigravida during the last 2 weeks of pregnancy but does not usually take place in the multigravida until labour begins (Verralls 1993).

The vagina

Oestrogen causes changes in the muscle layer and in the epithelium.

The muscle layer hypertrophies and the capacity of the vagina increases (McFadyen 1995). There are also changes in the surrounding connective tissue which allow the vagina to become more elastic (Cunningham et al 1995). These changes enable the vagina to dilate during the second stage of labour to accommodate the passage of the baby. The epithelium becomes thicker and there is marked desquamation of the superficial cells which increases the amount of normal white vaginal discharge known as *leucorrhoea* (Beischer et al 1997).

The epithelial cells also have an increased glycogen content. These cells interact with *Döderlein's bacillus*, a normal commensal of the vagina, and produce a more acid environment (McFadyen 1995). This provides an extra degree of protection against some organisms, but unfortunately an increasing susceptibility to others such as *Candida albicans* (Symonds 1992).

The vagina is more vascular and appears violet in colour, probably because of hyperaemia (Cunningham et al 1989).

CHANGES IN THE CARDIOVASCULAR SYSTEM

Profound changes take place in the cardiovascular system during pregnancy and an understanding of these is important in the care of women with normal pregnancies as well as for the management of women with pre-existing cardiovascular disease.

The heart

Owing to an increase in workload, the heart muscle hypertrophies, particularly in the left ventricle, leading to enlargement of the heart. The growing uterus pushes the heart upwards and to the left. The great vessels are unfolded and so the heart is rotated upwards and outwards, producing electrocardiographic and radiographic changes similar to those in ischaemic heart disease but which are considered normal in pregnancy. Heart sounds

are changed and systolic and other murmurs are common (Chamberlain 1991).

Cardiac output

During pregnancy there is an increase in the heart rate and stroke volume (the amount of blood pumped by the heart with each beat) resulting in a raised cardiac output. This is due to the increased blood volume and the increased oxygen requirements of all maternal tissues as well as the growing fetus (Symonds 1992). The heart rate increases as early as the fourth week of pregnancy by an average of about 15 beats per minute, that is from 70 to 85 beats per minute. The stroke volume rises from about 64 ml to about 71 ml (de Swiet 1991a).

The cardiac output (the rate at which blood is pumped by the heart, expressed as litres per minute) was previously considered to gradually increase by about 40% by late pregnancy (from 5 to 7 litres per minute) in order to perfuse the growing uterus. It subsequently became apparent, however, that cardiac output increases markedly by the end of the first trimester when uterine blood flow has not yet increased significantly (de Swiet 1991a).

This is demonstrated most conclusively by a study by Robson et al (1989) which showed that the cardiac output had risen by 40% above pre-pregnancy values by the 12th week and by 50% by the 34th week. The increase does, however, appear to vary among individuals (Fig. 11.4).

Furthermore, little conclusive evidence exists about cardiac output in the third trimester. A fall in cardiac output was previously considered to be due to compression of the inferior vena cava by the uterus, irrespective of posture, causing reduced venous return and decreased stroke volume. A rise, fall or no change at all has more recently been shown to occur, depending on individual variations (van Oppen et al 1996).

Effects on the blood pressure

Although the cardiac output is increased in pregnancy the blood pressure does not rise because of the reduction in peripheral resistance to about 50% of non-pregnant values. The capacity of veins and venules can increase by a litre. The most obvious cause for this is progesterone which relaxes

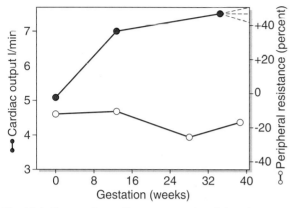

Fig. 11.4 Changes in cardiac output and peripheral vascular resistance during pregnancy. Cardiac output increases by 40% by the 12th week and by 50% by the 34th week of pregnancy. In the last trimester the cardiac output may rise, fall or remain the same, depending on individual variation. (Adapted from Chamberlain et al 1991, p. 35.)

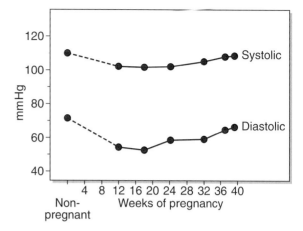

Fig. 11.5 Changes in blood pressure during pregnancy in primigravid women in a sitting position (based on De Swiet 1991a, p. 12).

smooth muscle, causing arterial walls to relax and dilate (Cruikshank & Hays 1991). It may also be due to the increased production of vasodilator prostaglandin (Cunningham et al 1989).

While the systolic pressure remains almost constant, the diastolic pressure drops slightly in the first trimester, reaches its lowest level at 16–20 weeks, and towards term returns to the level of the first trimester (de Swiet 1991a) (Fig. 11.5). During the mid-trimester, changes in blood pressure may cause fainting. In later pregnancy, the unsupported supine position should be avoided as this causes profound hypotension to occur in 10% of pregnant women, known as the *supine hypotensive syndrome*. The pressure of the gravid uterus compresses the vena cava, reducing venous return. Cardiac output is reduced by 25–30% and the blood pressure may fall by 10–15%, which gives rise to feelings of dizziness, nausea and even fainting (Cruikshank & Hays 1991).

Poor venous return in late pregnancy along with increased distensibility and pressure in the veins of the legs, vulva, rectum and pelvis can lead to oedema in the lower leg, varicose veins and haemorrhoids (Case & Waterhouse 1994).

Blood flow

While blood flow increases to the uterus, kidneys,

breasts and skin, there is no increase in blood flow to brain or liver (McFadyen 1995). Much of the increased cardiac output is directed to the utero-placental circulation whose blood flow increases by 10–15% to about 750 ml per minute at term (Bissonette 1991) (Fig. 11.6). This is due to the vascular resistance within the uteroplacental circulation being lower than that of the systemic circulation. In maternal systole, blood flows through the spiral arteries into the choriodecidual space and spurts upwards towards the chorionic plate, allowing exchange of gases, excretion of waste products from the fetus and providing nutrition (Coustan 1994).

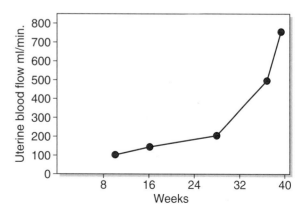

Fig. 11.6 Increase in uterine blood flow in pregnancy (adapted from McFadyen 1995, p. 124).

Regulation of uterine blood flow is of critical importance to the welfare of the fetus. Haemorrhage, uterine contractions, adrenaline and noradrenaline and lying in the supine position in late pregnancy can all reduce uterine blood flow. Chronic impairment can lead to intrauterine growth retardation and ultimately fetal death. Conversely, uterine blood flow is increased physiologically by the effect of angiotensin II on placental tissue, causing local release of vasodilator prostaglandin (Symonds 1992).

Renal blood flow increases by as much as 70–80% by the end of the first trimester, which helps to enhance excretion (Davison & Dunlop 1995). Increased blood flow to the capillaries of the skin and mucous membranes, and in particular to hands and feet, reaches a maximum of 500 ml per minute by the 36th week and is thought to eliminate extra heat generated by fetal metabolism. The associated peripheral vasodilatation explains why pregnant women 'feel the heat' and sweat profusely at times and often suffer from nasal congestion (Llewellyn-Jones 1994).

A greatly increased blood flow to the breasts throughout pregnancy is suggested by the dilated veins on the surface of the breasts as well as enlargement and tingling from early pregnancy (de Swiet 1991a).

The blood volume

The increase in blood volume in pregnancy may be as little as 20% or as much as 100% and varies according to the size of the woman, the number of pregnancies she has had, her parity, and whether the pregnancy is singleton or multiple. The increase begins at about 10 weeks' gestation and is progressive until about 30–34 weeks' gestation, after which a plateau is reached (Cruikshank & Hays 1991). A higher circulating volume is required:

- to provide extra blood flow for placental perfusion at the choriodecidual interface
- to supply the extra metabolic needs of the fetus
- to provide extra perfusion of kidneys and other organs
- to counterbalance the effects of increased arterial and venous capacity
- to compensate for blood loss at delivery.

Raised levels of aldosterone, oestrogen and progesterone during pregnancy are thought to contribute to the increased blood volume (Moore 1994).

The increase in plasma volume corresponds to the increase in blood volume (Cunningham et al 1989) (Fig. 11.7). This helps to compensate for the increased blood flow to the uterus and other organs, reduces the viscosity of the blood, and improves capillary flow. A normal increase in plasma volume is correlated with fetal well-being and birthweight (McFadyen 1995) (see Box 11.1).

The red cell mass, which is defined as the total volume of red cells in the circulation, increases as a result of accelerated production in response to the extra oxygen requirements of maternal and placental tissue. There appears to be a constant increase throughout the pregnancy from about 10 weeks but without the plateau which is seen in plasma volume at 30–34 weeks. This results in a total increase of 18–25%, from a mean non-

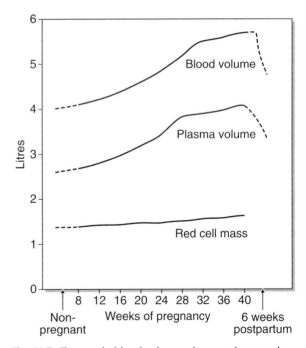

Fig. 11.7 Changes in blood volume, plasma volume and red cell mass during pregnancy; variations depend on size of the woman, her parity and the number of fetuses in utero (based on Llewellyn-Jones 1994 (information from Hytten & Leitch 1971), p. 31).

Box 11.1 Summary of changes caused by increased plasma volume in pregnancy

Haemodilution
- Physiological anaemia
- Decrease in concentration of plasma protein
- Decrease in concentration of immunoglobulins

Increased cardiac output
- Stroke volume increases
- Heart rate increases
- Heart enlarges

pregnant level of 1400 ml up to 1650 ml at term, although the increase may be up to 30% when iron supplementation is given (Cruikshank & Hays 1991).

As the increase in plasma volume is much greater than that of the red cell mass, haemodilution occurs, becoming most apparent at 32–34 weeks' gestation (Letsky 1991) (see Table 11.1). It is characterised by a lowered red cell count and haemoglobin (Hb) level (in spite of the rise in total circulating haemoglobin). The haematocrit concentration, or packed cell volume (PCV) falls from an average non-pregnant figure of 35% to 29% at around 30 weeks. The effect is referred to as *physiological anaemia*. Apparent anaemia can be a sign of excellent physiological adjustment to pregnancy while a high Hb level can be a sign of pathology (McFadyen 1995).

This is supported by a study by Steer et al (1995) which showed that Hb concentrations of 8.6–9.5 g/dl were associated with the highest mean birthweights while levels above 14.5 g/dl were associated with an increase in preterm delivery and low birthweight babies. Failure of the Hb level to fall is also associated with a threefold increase in the incidence of pre-eclampsia.

Most obstetricians have traditionally agreed that the mean minimum acceptable Hb level in pregnancy is 11–12 g/dl. Steer et al (1995) suggest that a mid-trimester fall in Hb concentration to about 10 g/dl appears to be optimal, reflecting good volume expansion. While this may be a valid estimate for women in the western world, Bergsjo et al (1996) regard a Hb level of 9.5 g/dl to be remarkably harmless and levels below this to be a more realistic indicator of pathology in women of different ethnic groups and in developing countries (see also Ch. 16).

Iron metabolism

Iron requirements of pregnancy are about 1000 mg, 500 mg of which is required to increase the red blood cell mass, and 300 mg of which is transported to the fetus, mainly in the last 12 weeks of pregnancy. The remaining 200 mg is needed to compensate for normal daily iron losses by the mother. The normal pregnant woman needs to absorb an average of about 3.5 mg per day of iron, the requirements increasing significantly in the last trimester during which time iron absorption from the gut is enhanced. In normal pregnancy only 20% of ingested iron is absorbed, whereas in the iron-deficient woman as much as 40% may be absorbed by the gut, whereupon it is either incorporated into haemoglobin or stored in the liver (Cruikshank & Hays 1991).

Table 11.1 Falling haemoglobin and haematocrit (PCV) in pregnancy despite rising blood volume and red cell mass

	Non-pregnant	Weeks of pregnancy		
		20	30	40
Plasma volume (ml)	2600	3150	3750	3850
Red cell mass (ml)	1400	1450	1550	1650
Total blood volume (ml)	4000	4600	5300	5500
Haematocrit (PCV) (%)	35.0	32.0	29.0	30.0
Haemoglobin				
Normal (g/dl)	13.9	12.6	12.0	12.2
Lowest acceptable (g/dl)	12.5	11.5	10.5	11.0

The purpose of iron supplementation is to prevent iron deficiency in the mother, not to raise the haemoglobin level. It has been suggested, therefore, that tests for iron stores such as serum ferritin would be a more reliable indicator of iron deficiency than haemoglobin levels, which may lose their value as a result of haemodilution (Montgomery 1990). Steer et al (1995) argue, however, that ferritin is not a useful measure as it falls dramatically in pregnancy regardless of whether iron supplements are given. They suggest that mean corpuscular volume (MCV), which usually remains fairly constant, might prove to be a more robust indicator of iron deficiency unless there is a simultaneous folate deficiency.

Plasma protein

The normal non-pregnant range of total protein is 65–85 g/l. During the first 20 weeks of pregnancy, the plasma protein concentration, and albumin in particular, is reduced from 35 to 25 g/l as a result of the increased plasma volume (Hacker & Moore 1986). This leads to lowered osmotic pressure, contributing to oedema of the lower limbs seen in late pregnancy (Case & Waterhouse 1994). In the absence of disease, moderate oedema is seen as physiological and an indicator of a favourable outcome to pregnancy (Davey 1995b).

Clotting factors

The clotting and fibrinolytic systems undergo major alterations during pregnancy. Plasma fibrinogen (factor 1) increases from the third month of pregnancy progressively until term by 50%. Prothrombin (factor 2) is increased only slightly.

Factors 7, 8, 9 and 10 all increase, as does the manufacture and consumption of platelets, leading to a change in coagulation time from 12 to 8 minutes (Cunningham et al 1989).

The capacity for clotting is thus increased, undoubtedly in preparation for the prevention of haemorrhage at placental separation, but with a resultant higher risk of thrombosis, embolism and, when complications are present, disseminated intravascular coagulation (Letsky 1991) (see also Ch. 15).

White blood cells

White blood cells in pregnancy are slightly increased, reaching levels of $10.0–15.0 \times 10^9/1$ (Table 11.2). While lymphocyte and monocyte numbers remain the same throughout pregnancy, the neutrophils increase, which enhances the blood's phagocytic and bactericidal properties. In the second and third trimesters the action of the polymorphonuclear leucocytes may be depressed, perhaps accounting for the increased susceptibility of pregnant women to infection (Moore 1994).

See Table 11.2 for a summary of changes in blood values in pregnancy.

Immunity

Human chorionic gonadotrophin (HCG) may be responsible for the reduced immune response in pregnancy. Levels of immunoglobulins IgA, IgG and IgM decrease steadily from the 10th to the 30th week and then remain at these levels until term (Llewellyn-Jones 1994). Antibody titres against viruses such as measles, influenza A and herpes

Table 11.2 Summary of common blood values and their changes

	Normal range (non-pregnant)	Change in pregnancy	Timing
Protein (total)	65–85 g/l	↓ 10 g/l	By 20 weeks then stable
Albumin	35–48 g/l	↓ 10 g/l	Most by 20 weeks then gradual
Fibrinogen	15–36 g/l	↑ 10–20 g/l	Progressively from third month
Platelets	$150–400 \times 10^3/mm^3$	Slight decrease	
Clotting time	12 min approx.	↓ to 8 min approx.	
White cell count	$9 \times 10^9/l$	$10–15 \times 10^9/l$	
Red cell count	$4.7 \times 10^{12}/l$	$3.8 \times 10^{12}/l$	Declines progressively to 30–34 weeks

simplex are reduced in proportion to the haemo-dilution effect, therefore viral resistance is un-changed (Cunningham et al 1989).

CHANGES IN THE RESPIRATORY SYSTEM

Pregnancy stresses the respiratory system very little in comparison with the cardiovascular system. The changes occurring, however, can cause some discomfort or inconvenience to the pregnant woman, and disease of the respiratory tract may be more serious during gestation (Cunningham et al 1989).

The mucosa of the respiratory tract becomes hyperaemic and oedematous, with hypersecretion of mucus which can lead to marked stuffiness and epistaxis. As a result many women complain of a chronic cold during pregnancy. Nasal decongestant sprays should be avoided because of their effect on the mucosa when used long term (Cruikshank & Hays 1991).

The shape of the chest changes and the circumference increases early in pregnancy. As the uterus enlarges, the diaphragm is elevated as much as 4 cm, and the rib cage is displaced upwards. The lower ribs flare out and may not always fully recover their original position after pregnancy, which can be a problem to figure-conscious women (de Swiet 1991b) (Fig. 11.8). The total lung capacity is reduced by 5% owing to the elevation of the diaphragm. Respirations remain at the normal frequency of 14–15 breaths per minute but breathing is more diaphragmatic and deeper (Cruikshank & Hays 1991).

There is a progressive increase in oxygen consumption by 15–20% at term, which is caused by the increased metabolic needs of the mother (cardiac and respiratory) and fetus. This is more than compensated for, however, by the 40% rise in tidal volume (amount of air inspired and expired with each breath at rest) and the 20% decrease in residual volume (the amount of air in the lungs after maximum expiration) (Moore 1994). Together these lead to an increase in alveolar ventilation of 5 to 8 l/min which is four times greater

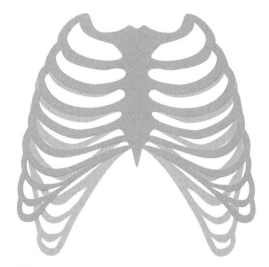

Fig. 11.8 Chest changes in pregnancy. Rib cage in pregnancy (pink) and non-pregnant state (grey) showing elevated diaphragm, increased chest circumference and lower ribs flaring out (based on De Swiet 1991b, p. 88).

than oxygen consumption and results in enhanced gaseous exchange (Davey 1995a).

Since progesterone causes a resetting of the sensitivity of the respiratory centre to CO_2, the amount of air inspired in 1 minute (minute volume) increases by about 26%, resulting in the 'hyperventilation of pregnancy' which causes CO_2 to be washed out of the lungs. Thus alveolar CO_2 concentrations are lower than in the non-pregnant woman, which causes the maternal blood CO_2 tension to be lower, leading to a respiratory alkalosis. Plasma bicarbonate partially compensates for this by decreasing from about 26 to 22 mmol/l. This mild alkalaemia (arterial pH 7.44) facilitates oxygen release to the fetus (Cunningham et al 1989). The maternal PCO_2 is reduced from an average of 5 kPa to 4 kPa or lower while fetal PCO_2 is 6 kPa. This facilitates the transfer of CO_2 from the fetus to the mother. Alveolar O_2 tension remains within normal limits (Case & Waterhouse 1994).

Overbreathing can lead to discomfort, dyspnoea and dizziness. When the need to breathe becomes a conscious one the woman may complain of 'shortness of breath', which is quite common in pregnant women. Care must be taken not to dismiss dyspnoea lightly and miss a warning sign of cardiac or pulmonary disease (Cunningham et al 1989).

CHANGES IN THE URINARY SYSTEM

By the second trimester renal blood flow has increased by as much as 70–80% (Davison & Dunlop 1995). It remains at that level until 30 weeks, after which it declines slowly, although it is still above non-pregnant levels at term (McFadyen 1995). As a result, the kidneys enlarge and glomerular filtration, which is assessed by measuring creatinine clearance, increases by about 45% by 8 weeks. This is maintained throughout the second trimester but decreases significantly during the last weeks of pregnancy (Davison & Dunlop 1995) (Fig. 11.9).

Changes in glomerular filtration are partly responsible for the increased clearance of creatinine, urea and uric acid which are also less efficiently reabsorbed in early pregnancy (Davison & Dunlop 1995). As a result, plasma levels of urea, uric acid and creatinine fall, although uric acid levels return to non-pregnant levels in late pregnancy (Cunningham et al 1989).

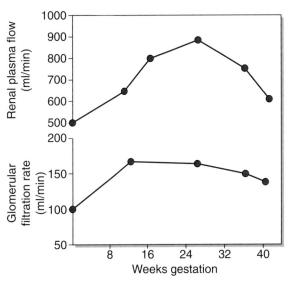

Fig. 11.9 Changes in renal blood flow and glomerular filtration (based on McFadyen 1995, p. 124).

Protein and amino acids are less efficiently reabsorbed, but while amino acids and vitamins are found in much greater amounts in the urine of pregnant women, proteinuria does not usually occur in normal pregnancy (Cunningham et al 1989).

Glucose excretion increases as a result of the increased glomerular filtration rate of glucose rather than diminished reabsorption (Baylis & Davison 1991). Glycosuria is therefore quite common in pregnancy and is not usually related to a high blood sugar level. It should, however, be carefully monitored to exclude diabetes mellitus. Glycosuria can be a cause of urinary tract infection (Moore 1994).

Although 100 extra litres of fluid pass into the renal tubules each day, the urinary output is diminished because of an enhanced tubular reabsorption of water. An accompanying increase in the reabsorption of sodium is promoted, possibly by hormones aldosterone, progesterone, oestrogen and deoxycorticosterone (Miller & Hanretty 1997).

The urine of pregnant women is more alkaline owing to the alkalaemia of pregnancy, which is compensated for by renal bicarbonate excretion (Coustan 1994).

The kidney enzyme renin rises during pregnancy. It acts on angiotensinogen to form angiotensin I and II, which act as a vasoconstrictor, but the blood pressure does not rise because pregnant women are resistant to their effects (Moore 1994).

In early pregnancy increased production of urine causes frequency of micturition, but in later pregnancy frequency is caused by pressure of the growing uterus on the bladder (Chamberlain 1991).

Renal handling of water is more sensitive to maternal posture in pregnancy (McFadyen 1995). Excretion of water is reduced in the upright position or when the woman changes from the recumbent to supine position (particularly in later pregnancy), possibly owing to reduced renal perfusion subsequent to reduced venous return to the heart. Other theories accounting for reduced sodium and water excretion in the supine position relate to the release of ADH and to the elevated pressure in the ureters (Cunningham et al 1989).

Posture also affects the circadian rhythms of

sodium excretion. The woman who rests by day in the recumbent position excretes maximum amounts of urine in the middle of the day. The woman who is active by day, however, accumulates water in the form of dependent oedema. At night this is then mobilised and the increased excretion results in nocturia (McFadyen 1995).

Under the influence of progesterone the ureters become relaxed, and are dilated, elongated and curved above the brim of the pelvis, particularly on the right side because of the dextrorotation of the uterus. This, along with compression of the ureters against the pelvic brim, can result in stasis of urine in the ureters with subsequent bacteriuria and infection of the urinary tract (Moore 1994) (Fig. 11.10). Hydroureter and hydronephrosis may be associated with stasis of urine, pyelonephritis and difficulty in interpreting intravenous pyelography during pregnancy (Coustan 1994). (See also Ch. 16.)

The muscle of the bladder is relaxed owing to raised levels of progesterone (Chamberlain 1991). Bladder vascularity increases and bladder capacity is reduced. To compensate for this, urethral length is increased. Towards the end of pregnancy as the head engages the entire bladder may be displaced upwards (Cunningham et al 1989).

CHANGES IN THE GASTROINTESTINAL SYSTEM

The gums become oedematous, soft and spongy during pregnancy, probably owing to the effect of oestrogen, which can lead to bleeding when mildly traumatised as with a toothbrush (Cunningham et al 1989). There is no good evidence that pregnancy causes tooth decay. Dental problems are more likely to occur because of gingivitis (Hytten 1991b).

Increased salivation, *ptyalism*, is a common complaint in pregnancy, but there is no evidence that more saliva is produced. The problem seems to be associated rather with nausea which prevents women from swallowing their saliva (Hytten 1991b).

Nausea and vomiting complicates about 70% of pregnancies. It usually begins around 4–8 weeks and continues until about 14–16 weeks. Relaxation of the smooth muscle of the stomach and hypomotility in addition to raised levels of oestrogen or human chorionic gonadotrophin (HCG) may all contribute to the problem. Although distressing and at times quite debilitating, and sometimes causing weight loss in early pregnancy, it rarely

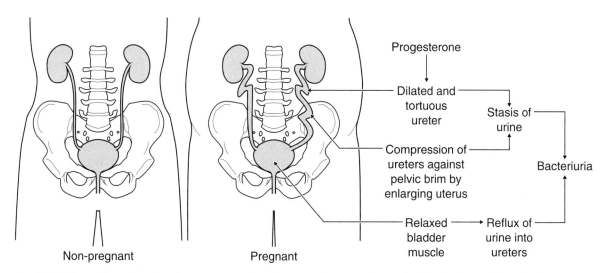

Fig. 11.10 Comparison of ureters in non-pregnant and pregnant women demonstrating factors predisposing to urinary tract infection in pregnancy.

causes nutritional or electrolyte imbalance and is associated with a satisfactory outcome for the pregnancy (Cruikshank & Hays 1991).

Occasionally vomiting may become excessive. Although the cause is still not clear, rising hormone levels are implicated by the fact that the condition is common in multiple pregnancy or hydatidiform mole (Miller & Hanretty 1997).

A change in the sense of taste can occur early in pregnancy. It can be either a metallic taste in the mouth, distaste for something usually enjoyed, or craving for a food not usually eaten. Cravings for coal, wall plaster or mothballs and other bizarre substances (*pica*) are potentially dangerous but will usually be concealed until after delivery (McFadyen 1995). Hytten (1991b) recounts the sense of secrecy which women experience and how they try to keep their cravings a secret even from their partners.

An increase in appetite is also noticed by most women during pregnancy. It is probably related to the resetting by progesterone of the centre in the brain which controls fat storage through energy balance. It may also be due to the fall in plasma glucose and amino acids in early pregnancy. Many women notice an increased thirst in pregnancy. This is probably due to the fall in plasma osmolality, although it may also be related to rising levels of prolactin (Hytten 1990a). Resetting of osmotic thresholds for thirst contributes towards the increased water retention which is a normal physiological alteration of pregnancy (Cunningham et al 1989).

As pregnancy progresses, the stomach and intestines are displaced by the enlarging uterus (Cunningham et al 1989). Raised intragastric pressure without an accompanying increase in tone of the cardiac sphincter causes reflux of acid mouthfuls with epigastric or retrosternal pain. The resulting symptom of heartburn is said to be so common that women do not complain of it (McFadyen 1995). Reduced intraoesophageal pressure and peristalsis with raised intragastric pressure also contribute to the reflux of acid into the oesophagus (Cunningham et al 1989).

Gastric tone and peristalsis are reduced, probably owing to reduced levels of the hormone motilin. Gastric secretion of hydrochloric acid is also reduced, suggesting reduced vagal activity, which may account for the reduced incidence of peptic ulcer (Case & Waterhouse 1994). There are now conflicting opinions about whether pregnancy causes a delay in gastric emptying time, which is of particular relevance if general anaesthesia is required (MacFie et al 1991, Simpson et al 1988). It appears that a glucose meal may cause a delay in stomach emptying related to the greater osmolality of its contents, which explains the nausea often experienced after a glucose tolerance test (Hytten 1991b).

Passage of food through the intestines may be so much slower that there is increased absorption of water from the colon, probably as a result of raised levels of aldosterone and angiotensin, which contributes to the tendency to constipation. A high-residue diet which helps to hold water in its passage through the colon will help to relieve this problem (Hytten 1990a). Constipation may also be caused by mechanical obstruction by the uterus and by the relaxing effect of progesterone on smooth muscle (Cruikshank & Hays 1991). Furthermore, oral iron may contribute to the problem (McFadyen 1995). Constipation may exacerbate haemorrhoids, which are caused by the increased pressure in the veins below the level of the enlarged uterus (Cunningham et al 1989).

The gall bladder increases in size and empties more slowly during pregnancy. Cholestasis which is almost physiological in pregnancy is probably a hormonal effect and can lead to pruritus or gallstone formation (McFadyen 1995). The once widely accepted belief that pregnant women are predisposed to gallstone formation is now considered to be lacking in evidence (Hytten 1991b).

Although hepatic blood flow is unchanged in pregnancy, there are many changes in liver function that mimic liver disease; therefore liver function tests in pregnancy should be interpreted with caution:

- serum albumin levels fall progressively throughout pregnancy and at term are 30% lower than the non-pregnant level
- serum alkaline phosphatase levels rise progressively during pregnancy and at term are two to four times non-pregnant values

- serum cholesterol levels are raised twofold by the end of pregnancy
- many liver proteins are raised in response to oestrogen
- fibrinogen levels are increased 50% by the end of the second trimester (Cruikshank & Hays 1991).

CHANGES IN METABOLISM

The increased dietary intake (calculated as being approximately 200–300 kcal per day) in addition to the gastrointestinal changes of pregnancy are accompanied by characteristic alterations in the metabolism of carbohydrate, protein and fat. These changes, which are brought about by *human placental lactogen,* ensure that glucose is readily available for body and brain growth in the developing fetus, and protect the mother against nutritional deficiencies (Case 1985).

A continuous supply of glucose must be available for transfer to the fetus. Each time the mother eats, the fetus has an enhanced opportunity to acquire glucose. Fasting plasma glucose concentration falls during the first trimester by about 12%, rises between 16 and 32 weeks, then falls again towards term because of the increasing use of maternal glucose to provide the fetus with energy (Cruikshank & Hays 1991).

Insulin secretion correspondingly rises in the second trimester then falls to non-pregnant levels towards term. As HPL levels rise with advancing pregnancy, however, insulin resistance increases, leading to the so-called diabetogenic effect of pregnancy (Cruikshank & Hays 1991). As a result, a glucose load takes a longer time to reach a maximal plasma concentration, but the final plasma concentration is higher than normal and remains elevated for longer, allowing more time for placental exchange (Case & Waterhouse 1994) (Fig. 11.11).

It is therefore most important that pregnant women neither fast nor skip meals because:

- maternal blood glucose levels are critically important for fetal well-being
- fasting in pregnancy produces a more intense ketosis known as 'accelerated starvation' which may be dangerous to fetal health (Cruikshank & Hays 1991).

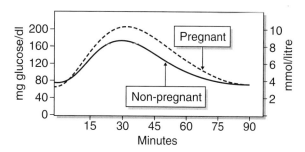

Fig. 11.11 Variations in response to oral glucose tolerance test in pregnant and non-pregnant women (based on Miller & Hanretty 1997, p. 21).

The pregnant woman 'spares' glucose for the fetus in preparation for subsequent fetal demands by using the fat stores laid down in the first half of pregnancy as her primary energy source. As the nutritional demands of the fetus increase in the second half of pregnancy and insulin resistance increases, mobilisation of fat leading to increased concentrations of glucose and fatty acids provides the mother with extra energy supplies (Case & Waterhouse 1994). This process, however, renders her more susceptible to ketosis (Fraser 1991). Even an overnight fast of 12 hours will result in hypoglycaemia and increased production of ketone bodies (Miller & Hanretty 1997) (see also Ch. 16).

Carbohydrate restriction in any diet during pregnancy is therefore not recommended, and there appears to be good justification for the bed-time snack (Metzger et al 1982).

Muslim women who wish to fast during Ramadan may do so under medical supervision if it occurs during the second trimester, but fasting during the first and third trimesters is not recommended, the main danger to the fetus possibly being from dehydration rather than from malnutrition (Athar 1990).

Reduced plasma albumin concentrations due to the increased plasma volume cause the colloid osmotic pressure to be reduced, resulting in limb oedema in late pregnancy. Plasma amino acid concentrations also fall because amino acids are used to make glucose and for fetal energy and protein synthesis (Case & Waterhouse 1994).

Maternal plasma calcium concentrations fall as a result of both fetal needs and the normal haemodilution of pregnancy. If there is enough vitamin D, parathyroid hormone secretion is increased. This doubles the absorption of calcium in the intestine by the end of the second trimester, which provides for fetal needs as well as protecting the mother's skeleton. Pregnant women should, however, be encouraged to increase their calcium intake by about 70% (Case 1985).

MATERNAL WEIGHT

Continuing weight increase in pregnancy is considered to be a favourable indicator of maternal adaptation and fetal growth. Analysis of many studies investigating weight gain in pregnancy demonstrates the wide range that is compatible with normality but suggests the following figures for the primigravida.

Expected increase:

- 4.0 kg in first 20 weeks
- 8.5 kg in second 20 weeks (0.4 kg/week in the last trimester)
- 12.5 kg approximate total.

It is also suggested that the average multigravida gains about 1 kg less than the primigravida (Hytten 1991a).

Many factors influence weight gain. The degree of maternal oedema, maternal metabolic rate, dietary intake, vomiting or diarrhoea, smoking, amount of amniotic fluid and size of the fetus must all be taken into account. A recent study suggests that maternal age, prepregnancy body size, parity, race–ethnicity, hypertension and diabetes also influence the pattern of maternal weight gain (Abrams et al 1995).

See Figure 11.12 for the distribution of the average increase in weight.

Because of the wide range of normality in weight gain, it has been suggested that the routine practice of weighing pregnant women is of doubtful value in the provision of quality antenatal care (Hytten 1990b).

SKELETAL CHANGES

Oestrogen and relaxin encourage relaxation of

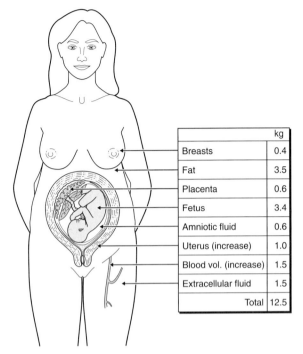

		kg
Breasts		0.4
Fat		3.5
Placenta		0.6
Fetus		3.4
Amniotic fluid		0.6
Uterus (increase)		1.0
Blood vol. (increase)		1.5
Extracellular fluid		1.5
Total		12.5

Fig. 11.12 Disposition of weight gain in pregnancy (data from Hytten 1991c).

pelvic ligaments and muscles, reaching maximum effect during the last weeks of pregnancy (Miller & Hanretty 1997). This relaxation allows the pelvis to increase its capacity in readiness to accommodate the fetal presenting part at the end of pregnancy and in labour.

The ligaments of the symphysis pubis and the sacroiliac joints loosen, as a result of the effects of relaxin and oestrogen (Guyton 1991). Laxity and swelling of connective tissue owing to increased hydration are also responsible for joint changes occurring mainly in the last trimester (McFadyen 1995). The symphysis pubis widens by about 4 mm by 32 weeks' gestation and the sacrococcygeal joint loosens, allowing the coccyx to be displaced backwards. While increased mobility of the pelvic joints facilitates vaginal delivery, it also results in a rolling gait which is likely to be the cause of backache and ligamental pain in late pregnancy (Cruikshank & Hays 1991). Recent research suggests, however, that although relaxin is responsible for relaxation of the pelvic ligaments, it is not associated with symptoms of pain and tenderness (Hansen et al 1996).

Posture usually alters to compensate for the enlarging uterus anteriorly, particularly if abdominal muscle tone is poor. The woman leans backwards, exaggerating the normal lumbar curve and causing a progressive lordosis which shifts her centre of gravity back over her legs. The unfortunate side-effect of this is low back pain which most women suffer during pregnancy, and sometimes shoulder pain. Along with relaxation of the joints, lordosis can lead to unsteadiness of gait and the tendency to fall (Cruikshank & Hays 1991). Chapter 45 gives advice on correct posture.

SKIN CHANGES

From the end of the second month of pregnancy until term, increased activity of the pituitary melanin-stimulating hormone causes varying degrees of pigmentation in almost all pregnant women, although the depth of pigmentation varies according to skin colour and race. A sun tan acquired during pregnancy lasts longer than at any other time (McFadyen 1995).

The areas most commonly affected are the areolae, the abdominal midline, the perineum and the axillae. The face is less frequently involved. It is speculated that these areas become more pigmented than others, either because of increased sensitivity of the melanocytes to the hormone or because of a greater population of melanocytes in these areas (Wade 1984).

The deeper, patchy colouring on the face known as the 'mask of pregnancy' or *chloasma* usually develops in the second half of pregnancy in 50–70% of women. It is commoner in dark-haired, brown-eyed women and is exacerbated by exposure to the sun. It usually regresses completely after delivery (Wade 1984).

In most pregnant women a pigmented line, called the *linea nigra*, runs from the pubis to the umbilicus, and sometimes higher. This line lies over the midline of the rectus muscles which are occasionally unable to withstand the tension of the enlarging uterus and separate, creating a *diastasis recti* (Cunningham et al 1989) (see Ch. 45).

As maternal size increases, stretching occurs in the collagen layer of the skin, particularly over the breasts, abdomen and areas of fat deposition such as the thighs. In some women the areas of maximum stretch become thin and stretch marks, *striae gravidarum*, appear as red stripes during the pregnancy, changing to silvery white lines approximately 6 months after delivery. Stretch marks are considered to be related to the increase in corticosteroids during pregnancy. Scalp, facial and body hair becomes thicker during pregnancy. The excess accumulation of hair is shed postpartum, making some women think that they are going bald, which can be alarming (McFadyen 1995).

A progesterone-induced rise in temperature of 0.5°C together with an increased blood supply to the skin causing vasodilatation makes women feel hotter. Sweating assists in losing extra heat produced by maternal, placental and fetal metabolism (Cunningham et al 1989).

Many women develop *angiomas* during pregnancy, which are minute red elevations on the skin of the face, neck, arms and chest. Reddening of the palms known as *palmar erythema* is also a frequent occurrence. Both are likely to be due to high levels of oestrogen and disappear after the pregnancy (Cunningham et al 1989).

Subcutaneous fat increases but the increase in skin-fold thickness is due to oedema and increased skin vascularity (Hytten 1991a).

THE BREASTS

Owing to the increased blood supply and under the influence of greatly increased hormone activity the glandular tissue of the breast enlarges and the nipple becomes more erectile, although the greatest change in shape takes place around the time of delivery (RCM 1991). Oestrogen causes growth of lactiferous tubules and ducts and also causes deposition of fat. Progesterone causes growth of the lobules, budding of the alveoli and development of their secretory ability (Beischer et al 1997). Growth hormone and glucocorticoids also play a part in their development. Prolactin stimulates the production of colostrum and later milk (Fuchs 1991) (see also Ch. 36).

CHANGES IN THE ENDOCRINE SYSTEM

Placental hormones

Early effects of placental hormones are described in Chapter 51. Later physiological effects caused by oestrogen and progesterone have been highlighted throughout this chapter.

The secretion of HPL and HCG by the feto-placental unit alters the mother's endocrine organs during pregnancy, either directly or indirectly. Raised oestrogen levels increase production of globulins which bind thyroxine and corticosteroids and the sex steroids. As a result the total plasma content of these hormones is increased but the levels of free (and physiologically active) hormones are not necessarily raised (McFadyen 1995).

Pituitary hormones

The weight of the anterior pituitary gland increases by 30–50%, which is why some women suffer from headaches during pregnancy (McFadyen 1995). The secretion of prolactin, adrenocorticotrophic hormone, thyrotrophic hormone and melanocyte-stimulating hormone increases. Follicle-stimulating hormone and luteinising hormone secretion is greatly inhibited by placental progesterone and oestrogen (Case & Waterhouse 1994).

The effects of the increased prolactin secretion are suppressed by oestrogen and progesterone during pregnancy (Howie 1995). Following delivery of the placenta, plasma concentrations of prolactin decrease even in women who are breast feeding, but prolactin is subsequently secreted in pulsatile bursts with suckling to stimulate milk production (Cunningham et al 1989).

The posterior pituitary gland releases oxytocin in low-frequency pulses throughout pregnancy. At term the frequency of these pulses increases, which stimulates uterine contractions. The former theory that contractions only occur on withdrawal of progesterone has still not been proven (Fuchs & Fuchs 1991).

Thyroid function

In normal pregnancy the thyroid gland increases in size by about 13% owing to hyperplasia of glan-dular tissue and increased vascularity (Cunningham et al 1989). There is normally an increased uptake of iodine in pregnancy, which may be to compensate for renal clearance of iodine, which doubles with the increased GFR, leading to a reduced level of plasma iodine (Cunningham et al 1989). Evidence would suggest, however, that the development of a goitre is unlikely in the absence of an iodine deficiency (Rodin et al 1989).

Although pregnancy can give the impression of hyperthyroidism, thyroid function is basically normal. The basal metabolic rate is increased mainly because of increased oxygen consumption by the fetus and the work of the maternal heart and lungs (Ramsay 1991). Rising levels of T_4 (thyroxine) and T_3 (triiodothyronine) and many other hormones do contribute, however, to the increase in basal metabolic rate (Guyton 1991).

Controversy exists as to whether or not levels of thyroid-stimulating hormone rise, remain the same or fall during pregnancy. Likewise there is continuing debate on the postulated thyrotrophic effect of human chorionic gonadotrophin and human chorionic thyrotrophin (Cruikshank & Hays 1991). Nonetheless total thyroxine levels rise sharply from the second month of pregnancy to a plateau which is maintained till term.

T_4 (thyroxine), however, is mainly bound rather than free in the plasma owing to oestrogen-stimulated hepatic production of thyroxine-binding globulin. As a result, the amount of free, unbound (effective) thyroid hormone is not increased in spite of the elevated concentration of total thyroxine (Cunningham et al 1989) (Fig. 11.13).

Adrenal glands

Stimulated by oestrogen, the adrenal gland produces increasing levels of total and free plasma cortisol and other corticosteroids including ACTH from 12 weeks to term (Cruikshank & Hays 1991). Since free cortisol normally suppresses ACTH production, it has been suggested that there may be an alteration in the feedback mechanism (Case & Waterhouse 1994).

It is thought that the raised levels of free cortisol have an antagonistic action to insulin. By raising the levels of glucose in the blood, mobilising maternal fatty acids and amino acids for the pro-

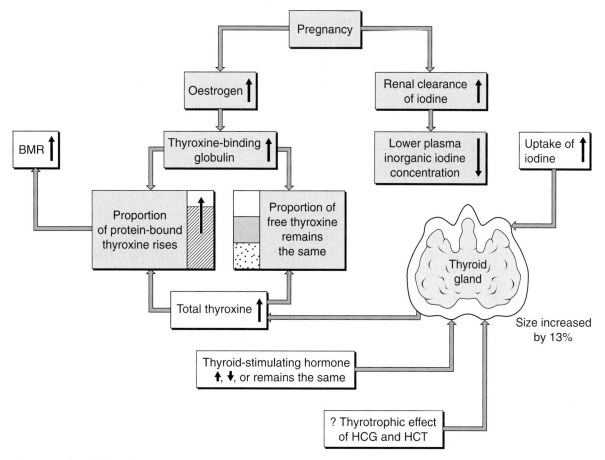

Fig. 11.13 Thyroid function in pregnancy.

duction of glycogen, and decreasing the uptake of glucose by muscle and fat, more glucose is made available for the fetus (de Swiet & Chamberlain 1992). Elevated free cortisol concentrations may also contribute to the characteristic hyperglycaemia after meals during pregnancy (Cruikshank & Hays 1991).

The increase in free plasma cortisol may also be responsible for some of the cushingoid features of normal pregnancy such as fat deposition and striae gravidarum (Davey 1995a).

Because of the stimulus of progesterone and oestrogen, there is a large increase in the concentration of renin by the adrenal cortex in the first 12 weeks of pregnancy in addition to renin produced by the uterus and the chorion (Chamberlain 1991). This activates the renin–angiotensin system, which is associated with maintaining blood pressure and which also balances the salt-losing effect of progesterone by enhancing aldosterone secretion from the adrenal cortex (Cunningham et al 1989). Levels of aldosterone rise from 100–200 ng/l in the non-pregnant state to 200–700 ng/l during late pregnancy. Aldosterone's effect of promoting sodium absorption is most likely to be the key factor in maintaining the delicate balance of salt and water excretion (Cruikshank & Hays 1991) (Fig. 11.14).

Imbalance of these substances can cause pregnant women to reabsorb excess sodium from renal tubules and therefore to retain fluid, which can cause hypertension (Guyton 1991). High levels

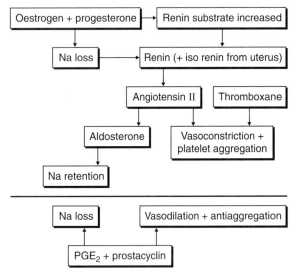

Blood pressure in pregnancy is maintained within the normal range by a balance between mechanisms which affect the circulation.

Fig. 11.14 Maintenance of blood pressure and balance of salt and water excretion by the renin–angiotensin system (based on McFadyen 1995, p. 119).

of angiotensin II would also cause the blood pressure to rise very quickly if it were not for the vasodilator effect of prostaglandin and prostacyclin (McFadyen 1995).

Box 11.2 Breast changes in chronological order (Chamberlain 1989)

3–4 weeks
Prickling, tingling sensation due to increased blood supply particularly around nipple.

6 weeks
Developing ducts and glands cause the breasts to be enlarged, painful and tense, particularly in women who normally experience premenstrual changes.

8 weeks
Bluish surface veins are visible.

8–12 weeks
Montgomery's tubercles become more prominent on the areola. These sebaceous glands secrete sebum which keeps the nipple soft and supple. The pigmented area around the nipple darkens and may enlarge slightly. This area is known as the *primary areola*.

16 weeks
Colostrum can be expressed. Further extension of the pigmented area occurs and is often mottled in appearance, *secondary areola*.

Late pregnancy
Colostrum may leak from the breasts; progesterone causes the nipple to become more prominent and mobile.

DIAGNOSIS OF PREGNANCY

Pregnancy may be diagnosed by the woman herself even before she has missed a period because she feels different. Changes in the breasts can occur as early as 5–6 weeks after conception and may be the first cause for wondering if she is pregnant. Feelings of nausea, changes in food and drink preference and an overwhelming tiredness confirm the belief. There may be frequency of micturition and backache (Chamberlain 1989). The date of *quickening*, the first fetal movement felt by the mother, provides an indicator of gestation. If the date of quickening is recorded, it can be used to check the date of expected confinement. A primigravid woman feels it at 18–20 weeks, the multigravida at 16–18 weeks (Leader et al 1996).

Other methods of ascertaining pregnancy and estimating early gestational age involve the observation of certain characteristics associated with the physiology of pregnancy. Breast changes are listed in Box 11.2.

Hegar's sign. This is the sensation experienced by the fingers when a bimanual vaginal examination is performed. Two fingers are inserted into the anterior fornix of the vagina; the other hand is placed behind the uterus abdominally. Using firm pressure the fingers of both hands almost meet because of the softness of the elongated isthmus, which is marked between the 6th and 12th weeks of pregnancy. The sign is difficult to elicit and is not recommended nowadays because of the risk of inducing miscarriage; it has been superseded by ultrasound examination (Chamberlain 1989).

Jacquemier's sign. A violet-blue discoloration of the vaginal membrane, due to increased vascularity, is observed.

Osiander's sign. This is an increased pulsation felt in the lateral vaginal fornices (Miller & Callender 1989).

These changes cannot in themselves be considered positive signs of pregnancy as they may all be symptoms of other conditions. They have also taken on less importance since the development of quick and sensitive laboratory tests for pregnancy (Miller & Callender 1989). X-rays are also not usually used nowadays in the diagnosis of pregnancy because of the dangers of irradiation. Hearing the fetal heart by Doptone from about 12 weeks' gestation and feeling fetal parts or fetal movement from about 22 weeks of pregnancy are good positive signs of pregnancy. Visualisation of the gestational sac or fetus by ultrasound techniques from 5–6 weeks provides conclusive evidence when early diagnosis is necessary (see Table 11.3) (Chamberlain 1989).

Table 11.3 Signs of pregnancy

Sign	Time of occurrence (gestational age)	Differential diagnosis
Possible (presumptive) signs		
Early breast changes (unreliable in the multigravida)	3–4 weeks +	Contraceptive pill
Amenorrhoea	4 weeks +	Hormonal imbalance
		Emotional stress
		Illness
Morning sickness	4–14 weeks	Gastrointestinal disorders
		Pyrexial illness
		Cerebral irritation, etc.
Bladder irritability	6–12 weeks	Urinary tract infection
		Pelvic tumour
Quickening	16–20 weeks +	Intestinal movement, 'wind'
Probable signs		
Presence of human chorionic gonadotrophin in:		
Blood	4–12 weeks	Hydatidiform mole
Urine	6–12 weeks	Choriocarcinoma
Softened isthmus (Hegar's sign)	6–12 weeks	
Blueing of vagina (Jacquemier's sign)	8 weeks +	} Pelvic congestion
Pulsation of fornices (Osiander's sign)	8 weeks +	
Uterine growth	8 weeks +	Tumours
Braxton Hicks contractions	16 weeks	
Ballottement of fetus	16–28 weeks	
Positive signs		
Visualisation of fetus by:		
Ultrasound	6 weeks +	
X-ray	16 weeks +	
Fetal heart sounds by:		
Ultrasound	6 weeks +	
Fetal stethoscope	20 weeks +	No alternative diagnosis
Fetal movements:		
Palpable	22 weeks +	
Visible	Late pregnancy	
Fetal parts palpated	24 weeks +	

READER ACTIVITIES

1. List all the changes occurring in each system of the body during pregnancy, noting those which the woman will be aware of and those of which she is unlikely to be aware.

2. Where the physiological changes of pregnancy could involve some discomfort, inconvenience or knowledge deficit for the woman, make a plan which will enable her to understand what is taking place within her and how to cope with it.

3. Try to follow your clients through their pregnancies from booking to term and note how the physiological changes of pregnancy affect them all differently. If possible, adapt some of the plans you have already made to their individual needs.

4. Next time you are in contact with women to whom you have offered information or advice, ask them if it helped, and if so in what way.

Remember to record these encounters in your reflective journal.

REFERENCES

Abrams B, Carmichael S, Selvin S 1995 Factors associated with the pattern of maternal weight gain during pregnancy. Obstetrics and Gynaecology 86(2): 170–176

Athar S 1990 Medical aspects of Islamic fasting. Midwives Chronicle 103(1227): 106

Baylis C, Davison J 1991 The urinary system. In: Hytten F, Chamberlain G (eds) Clinical physiology in obstetrics, 2nd edn. Blackwell Scientific Publications, Oxford, ch 11

Beischer N, Mackay E, Colditz P 1997 Obstetrics and the newborn, 3rd British edn. W B Saunders, London

Bergsjo P, Seha H, Ole-King'ori N 1996 Haemoglobin concentration in pregnant women. Acta Obstetrica et Gynecologica Scandinavica 75: 241–244

Bissonette J 1991 Placental and fetal physiology. In: Gabbe S, Niebyl J, Simpson J (eds) Obstetrics – normal and problem pregnancies, 2nd edn. Churchill Livingstone, Edinburgh, ch 4

Case R 1985 Variations in human physiology. Manchester University Press, Manchester, ch 1

Case R, Waterhouse J 1994 Human physiology: age, stress and the environment, 2nd edn. Oxford University Press, Oxford

Chamberlain G 1989 The diagnosis of pregnancy. In: Turnbull A, Chamberlain G (eds) Obstetrics. Churchill Livingstone, London, ch 14

Chamberlain G 1991 The changing body in pregnancy. British Medical Journal 302(23): 719–722

Chamberlain G, Dewhurst J, Harvey D 1991 Obstetrics, 2nd edn. Gower Medical Publishing, London

Coustan D 1994 Maternal physiology. In: Coustan D, Haning R Jr, Singer D (eds) Human reproduction – growth and development. Little, Brown, London, ch 10

Cruikshank D, Hays P 1991 Maternal physiology in pregnancy. In: Gabbe S, Niebyl J, Simpson J (eds) Obstetrics – normal and problem pregnancies, 2nd edn. Churchill Livingstone, Edinburgh, ch 5

Cunningham F, Macdonald P, Gant N (eds) 1989 William's obstetrics, 18th edn. Prentice Hall, London

Davey D 1995a Normal pregnancy: anatomy, endocrinology and physiology. In: Whitfield C (ed) Dewhurst's textbook of obstetrics and gynaecology for postgraduates, 5th edn.

Blackwell Science, Oxford, ch 9

Davey D 1995b Hypertensive disorders of pregnancy. In: Whitfield C (ed) Dewhurst's textbook of obstetrics and gynaecology for postgraduates, 5th edn. Blackwell Science, Oxford, ch 14

Davison J, Dunlop W 1995 Urinary tract in pregnancy. In: Chamberlain G (ed) Turnbull's obstetrics, 2nd edn. Churchill Livingstone, Edinburgh

de Swiet M 1991a The cardiovascular system. In: Hytten F, Chamberlain G (eds) Clinical physiology in obstetrics, 2nd edn. Blackwell Scientific Publications, Oxford, ch 1

de Swiet M 1991b The respiratory system. In: Hytten F, Chamberlain G (eds) Clinical physiology in obstetrics, 2nd edn. Blackwell Scientific Publications, Oxford, ch 3

de Swiet M, Chamberlain G 1992 Basic science in obstetrics and gynaecology, 2nd edn. Churchill Livingstone, London

Findlay A 1984 Reproduction and the fetus. Edward Arnold, London

Fraser R 1991 Carbohydrate metabolism. In: Hytten F, Chamberlain G (eds) Clinical physiology in obstetrics, 2nd edn. Blackwell Scientific Publications, Oxford, ch 8

Fuchs A 1991 Physiology and endocrinology of lactation. In: Gabbe S, Niebyl J, Simpson J (eds) Obstetrics – normal and problem pregnancies, 2nd edn. Churchill Livingstone, Edinburgh, ch 7

Fuchs A, Fuchs F 1991 Physiology of parturition. In: Gabbe S, Niebyl J, Simpson J (eds) Obstetrics – normal and problem pregnancies, 2nd edn. Churchill Livingstone, Edinburgh, ch 6

Gould S 1991 Anatomy. In: Gabbe S, Niebyl J, Simpson J (eds) Obstetrics – normal and problem pregnancies, 2nd edn. Churchill Livingstone, Edinburgh, ch 1

Guyton A 1991 Textbook of medical physiology, 8th edn. Saunders, London

Hacker N, Moore J 1986 Essentials of obstetrics and gynaecology. W B Saunders, London

Hansen A, Jensen D, Larsen E 1996 Relaxin is not related to symptom-giving pelvic girdle relaxation in pregnant women. Acta Obstetrica et Gynecologica Scandinavica 75: 245–248

Howie P 1995 Physiology of the puerperium and lactation.

In: Chamberlain G (ed) Turnbull's obstetrics, 2nd edn. Churchill Livingstone, Edinburgh, ch 42

Hytten F 1990a The alimentary system in pregnancy. Midwifery 6: 201–204

Hytten F 1990b Is it important or even useful to measure weight gain in pregnancy? Midwifery 6: 28–32

Hytten F 1991a Weight gain in pregnancy. In: Hytten F, Chamberlain G (eds) Clinical physiology in obstetrics, 2nd edn. Blackwell Scientific Publications, Oxford, ch 7

Hytten F 1991b The alimentary system. In: Hytten F, Chamberlain G (eds) Clinical physiology in obstetrics, 2nd edn. Blackwell Scientific Publications, Oxford, ch 5

Hytten F 1991c Nutrition. In: Hytten F, Chamberlain G (eds) Clinical physiology in obstetrics, 2nd edn. Blackwell Scientific Publications, Oxford, ch 6

Hytten F, Leitch I 1971 The volume and composition of blood. In: The physiology of human pregnancy, 2nd edn. Blackwell Scientific Publications, Oxford, p 1

Johnson T, Walker M, Niebyl J 1991 Preconception and prenatal care. In: Gabbe S, Niebyl J, Simpson J (eds) Obstetrics – normal and problem pregnancies, 2nd edn. Churchill Livingstone, Edinburgh, ch 8

Leader L, Bennett M, Wong F 1996 Handbook of obstetrics and gynaecology, 4th edn. Chapman Hall Medical, London

Letsky E 1991 The haematological system. In: Hytten F, Chamberlain G (eds) Clinical physiology in obstetrics, 2nd edn. Blackwell Scientific Publications, Oxford, ch 2

Llewellyn-Jones D 1994 Fundamentals in obstetrics and gynaecology, 6th edn. Mosby, St Louis

McFadyen I 1995 Maternal physiology in pregnancy. In: Chamberlain G (ed) Turnbull's obstetrics, 2nd edn. Churchill Livingstone, Edinburgh, ch 7

MacFie A, Magides A, Richmond N, Reilly C 1991 Gastric emptying in pregnancy. British Journal of Anaesthesia 67: 54–57

Metzger B, Vileisis R, Ravnikar V, Freinkel N 1982 'Accelerated starvation' and the skipped breakfast in late normal pregnancy. Lancet 1(March 13): 588–592

Miller A, Callender R 1989 Obstetrics illustrated, 4th edn. Churchill Livingstone, Edinburgh

Miller A, Hanretty K 1997 Obstetrics illustrated, 5th edn.

Churchill Livingstone, Edinburgh

Montgomery E 1990 Iron levels in pregnancy, physiology or pathology? Assessing the need for supplements. Midwifery 6: 205–214

Moore P 1994 Maternal physiology during pregnancy. In: De Cherney A, Pernoll M 1994 Current obstetric and gynaecologic diagnosis and treatment, 8th edn. Prentice-Hall, London

Nilsson L 1990 A child is born. Doubleday, London

O'Lah K 1996 The cervix in pregnancy and labour. In: Studd J (ed) Progress in obstetrics and gynaecology. Churchill Livingstone, London, vol 12, ch 7

Ramsay I 1991 The adrenal gland. In: Hytten F, Chamberlain G (eds) Clinical physiology in obstetrics, 2nd edn. Blackwell Scientific Publications, Oxford, ch 15

Robson S, Hunter S, Boys R, Dunlop W 1989 Serial study of factors influencing changes in cardiac output during human pregnancy. American Journal of Physiology 256: 1061–1065

Rodin A, Mashiter G, Quartero R et al 1989 Thyroid function in normal pregnancy. Journal of Obstetrics and Gynaecology 10(2): 85–94

Royal College of Midwives (RCM) 1991 Successful breastfeeding, 2nd edn. Churchill Livingstone, London

Simpson K, Stakes A, Miller M 1988 Pregnancy delays paracetamol absorption and gastric emptying in patients undergoing surgery. British Journal of Anaesthesia 60: 24–27

Steer P, Alam M, Wadsworth J, Welch A 1995 Relation between maternal haemoglobin concentration and birth weight in different ethnic groups. British Medical Journal 310: 489–491

Symonds E 1992 Essential obstetrics and gynaecology, 2nd edn. Churchill Livingstone, Edinburgh

van Oppen A, Stigler R, Bruinse H 1996 Cardiac output in normal pregnancy: a critical review. Obstetrics and Gynaecology 87(2): 310–317

Wade T 1984 Skin disorders. In: Brudenell M, Wilds P (eds) Medical and surgical problems in obstetrics. John Wright, Bristol

Verralls S 1993 Anatomy and physiology applied to obstetrics, 3rd edn. Churchill Livingstone, Edinburgh

Preparing for parenthood: daily life in pregnancy

12

Lea Jamieson

This chapter considers the knowledge that is helpful when contributing to the education of pregnant women, including factors which affect learning, existing knowledge for women, exploring differing needs, and structuring sessions that answer 'real' questions for those approaching birth and parenting. It considers health in pregnancy, particularly the so-called 'minor disorders', and some of the responses which may be useful. A final focus is on situations which require immediate action.

The chapter aims to:

- explore the factors which, if considered carefully and responded to, lead to effective prenatal education

- prompt the midwife to identify the special needs of families in a particular area

- provide ideas for conducting sessions that will help to meet the needs of both men and women as they explore birth and parenting from their individual perspectives

- identify the activities of daily living that can contribute to the short- and long-term health or otherwise of the mother and baby and require a sensitive response.

Parenthood education can be interpreted in many different ways. At its broadest it describes any interaction between the midwife and the mother or parents when matters related to childbirth and parenting are discussed. This definition covers those occasions, antenatally and postnatally, when a midwife answers queries in personal conversation and builds up a mother's confidence in her ability to carry and mother a new baby. The term more obviously embraces any sessions aimed at giving information or familiarising families with the environment and experience of birth and early parenting. In order to understand parenthood education the midwife needs to understand how people learn and why they learn. This awareness exposes the rich opportunity the midwife has to enhance the couple's experience of pregnancy, childbirth and early parenting.

Economics also affect parent education. In a country where achieving safe birth is difficult, the teaching will be limited to the factors that ensure a safe outcome. In a developed country where provision for 'safe' childbirth has been achieved, teaching of parents extends to enhancing the experience and enabling the growth of skills and attitudes within parenting. A further influence occurs in a country where competition within health care is present; effective parent education can be the service which attracts the women to choose a particular unit. Units will vary in their health care philosophies and parent education may not be allocated high resources or be seen as important compared to other provision. The midwife or health professional works within a country, organisational culture and philosophy which determine the finances and influence the quality of parent education offered.

FACTORS AFFECTING LEARNING

Motivation

Motivation affects learning positively. The reader can apply this personally by examining the reasons for reading this chapter and thus identifying motivation. The student may be about to attend a first parenthood education session and would like to feel prepared or perhaps has an essay to write and feels the need for information. A midwife may have been asked to take on responsibility for more input in parent education than before. Whatever the reasons a motivated reader is in a state of readiness to learn.

Mothers are also in this state. Something very important is happening in their lives. They are hungry to satisfy their need to understand themselves and to gain the knowledge and skills required in order to cope with the coming experiences and responsibilities. Each mother will be wanting to explore her feelings and her thoughts about the amazing reality of a child growing within her. She will need to feel secure about the place of birth and after delivery she will desire to learn very quickly how to care for and nurture her offspring.

Teachers often have students with varying degrees of motivation but the mothers whom a midwife cares for will make eager demands on her which makes sharing her knowledge and expertise very rewarding. Their motivation is very high. High motivation will also cause mothers to 'shop around' and explore what different parent education opportunities might offer.

Accurate information

What governs one's choice of textbook? It may be recommended by someone whose judgement is trusted. Perhaps the reader explored parts of it and found that some information confirmed existing knowledge and gave confidence in the accuracy of the remainder. The expertise and professional standing of the editors and writers may appear to guarantee sound midwifery knowledge. Whatever the reasons for choice, the source of information must be trustworthy.

Mothers need to trust the midwife to give accurate, up-to-date information. Insufficient or biased information will not aid their growth and may jeopardise their faith in other midwives. Childbirth has many areas about which individuals need to form opinions after amassing factual, circumstantial and personal information. For example a mother needs to explore the different ways in which her pain can be soothed in labour. If, after considering and discussing the options freely, she chooses to have epidural analgesia it would be inappropriate to request a home delivery. The midwife must help the mother to understand the implications of one choice as it may rule out another. If a mother with a history of back complaints is an unsuitable candidate for epidural anaesthesia, it is unhelpful to explore this form of analgesia in depth with her. Ultrasound and home birth are other areas where the midwife must be well informed. Booklets on both these issues, prepared by the Association for Improvements in the Maternity Services (Beech & Robinson 1994, Tew 1993) and reprinted in 1996, provide helpful referenced reading that is also readily accessible to women. It may seem obvious to encourage further careful exploration but often stock answers and information are given by professionals who fail to give a more individually tailored response.

Presentation

The presentation of information affects learning. If the midwife is able to present relevant information in a way that interests the mothers and their partners, she will enhance their learning both on a one-to-one and a group basis. This may mean being ready to discuss the mother's case notes with her, explaining graphs pertaining to ultrasound or hormone assays, and deciphering and interpreting such abbreviations as *Vx*, *Vert*, *Ceph* and *NAD*. If a midwife who is preparing a session wishes it to be relevant and interesting, this will entail forward planning. She may invite other mothers to share their experiences or breast feed their babies during the discussion. She may use films and slides. The room needs to be welcoming and refreshments should be organised in advance.

Environment

Physical comfort and emotional state affect the attention one can give. If the reader is in a noisy situation, or expects to be disturbed at any moment, is cold or even feeling unhappy or worried about something, study will have less significance and concentration may be lost. The midwife should apply the same principle in parenthood education. Physical needs should usually be attended to first. Discovering the feelings of the mother and determining what she sees as a priority will enable the midwife to begin with that area which is most relevant and important to the mother. For example, if a mother coming to clinic has had her anxieties aroused by an old wives' tale she needs to be assured that it has no relevance before she can grasp information about, say, the alpha-fetoprotein blood test. Equally a woman in clinic cannot begin to listen to the midwife explaining how her baby is lying if the surroundings are noisy and her privacy is constantly threatened.

Learning by example

In every interaction with a midwife the mother learns about midwives in general. She identifies midwives' attitudes and skills from the way they communicate with her and she builds up a picture of a 'midwife'. This image will help or hinder her in childbirth and early parenting. The qualities that need to be inherent in the professional approach are gentleness, kindness, understanding and empathy. A mother touched in this way during abdominal examination will be aware of the midwife's respect for her and for her unborn baby. A mother who watches a caring professional will learn by example that it is appropriate to touch and speak to a newborn baby. Whenever a midwife is in contact with mothers, their babies and their families during her working day, she is educating by example, whether consciously or otherwise. Midwives are not alone in their teaching role. All the professionals caring for the mother in pregnancy, childbirth and early parenthood are people with expertise and knowledge. The educative role is shared with colleagues such as the general practitioner and the health visitor. Midwives should be aware of their unique contribution and be professionally secure enough to join with their colleagues in parent education. Midwives who are asked to present a specific format of parent education need to be aware that this might not fulfil the women's needs but simply satisfy an organisational outcome of having offered some information. Understanding your own or an organisational bias is essential to open communications with women and effective education.

SOURCES OF EXISTING KNOWLEDGE

Preconception care

Education is a large part of this aspect of the midwife's role which has been discussed in detail in Chapter 10. The midwife must discover how much understanding the parents have gleaned from previous interaction with professionals. The professional's insight into pregnancy is important and this can be increased by reading *Pregnancy: the Inside Story* by Joan Raphael-Leff (1993). The book explores the meaning of childbearing to the inner self and such knowledge increases the sensitivity of midwives as caregivers.

Childhood role model

Each person has positive and negative experiences within his or her childhood. It is the way in which these are handled and the internal response that affect one's behaviour later. For example, Maria, a mother who is described in Michael Deakin's *The Children on the Hill* (1973), had a very sad and restrictive upbringing owing to bereavement and an insensitive family and educational environment. Maria's response was to provide for her children the antithesis to her own experience. Alternatively, another person who has been deeply hurt in childhood may, sadly, pass this abuse on to his or her own children, a fact which is commonly known (Kempe & Kempe 1978). New parents have to be able to perceive how they reacted to the role model set by their own parents. A midwife who seeks to help them to do this must first discover the positive and negative aspects of her own experience during childhood. She must become sensitive to her internal response which may result in strong opinions or definite attitudes that need to be identified and even modified. This journey in self-awareness helps the midwife to aid parents in their own individual growth. This is discussed further later in the chapter.

Raphael-Leff (1991, 1993) clearly describes the changing relationships that accompany childbirth and the emotional experiences which occur during the three maturational phases of pregnancy. She identifies both the facilitator's and regulator's approach and the midwife is aided in her teaching by familiarity with such concepts. They link well when considering the influence of the role model and judgements hurtfully made in families.

Family life and school

Schools differ in the amount of teaching which they offer in health care, life skills and related subjects. A survey by Prout (1986) suggests that teenagers gain quite an extensive understanding of antenatal care and that the strategies to enhance knowledge and encourage clinic attendance should take this awareness into account. A midwife is often invited to describe her role to a group of secondary school children or highlight the needs of the unborn baby to primary school children. Professional input which builds on their present knowledge will be valuable and relevant to the children. The relationship with the professional must be open and caring with an atmosphere of mutual trust and respect. This may mean that school groups covering areas such as preconception care, antenatal care and childbirth need to be small and intimate to be effective. This early contact with a midwife will contribute to the children's idea of what a midwife is like.

In parenthood education sessions, awareness of the couple's existing knowledge is vital if the midwife is to build from that point.

EDUCATION DURING PREGNANCY

Much has been written about the time and place for parenthood education. This chapter began by identifying every interaction with a midwife as an opportunity to teach by example. If a midwife chooses, she can make her communication specific and valuable to the individual mother.

Hospital

The booking visit (see Ch. 13) is an excellent opportunity for the midwife to describe the aims of antenatal care and to give the mother an overall concept of what to expect. She can help the mother to become aware of how valuable constant care of herself will be to her unborn baby. If the mother experiences respect she will enjoy her contribution to the growth of a healthy baby. A clinic visit which leaves a mother feeling undervalued as a woman, frustrated and anxious about her pregnancy means that each professional involved has failed to maximise the opportunity to build up the mother and enhance her experience of pregnancy. In the words of Oakley (1980):

> Reproduction is not just a handicap and a cause of second-class status; it is an achievement, the authentic achievement of women.

Midwives aware of these two attitudes within society will be able to actively present the positive view to the mother.

Different stages of pregnancy offer different opportunities for information giving and discussion. For example, nausea and vomiting may be bothersome early in pregnancy and heartburn later. The mother's need for specific advice requires a response from the midwife. Ideally the pace is determined by the mother. The midwife, cognisant that anxieties, embarrassment and lack of trust inhibit communication, will allow time for feelings to be shared and will provide an environment free from interruption. This will enable the mother to go from the clinic emotionally and intellectually satisfied, with her questions answered.

Sometimes major difficulties occur in pregnancy, such as unemployment of a husband, eviction from the home or bereavement. If the midwife has created a caring, listening environment the mother will feel free to seek help. The midwife may need to mobilise other members of the health care team to resolve some of the problems. The clinic should be a point of contact and help.

A clinic visit may provide an opportunity to work through a birth plan in which a mother's personal preferences are noted. This discussion can acknowledge her desires and expectations, inform her of what to expect and help her to adapt her plans in the face of changing circumstances. Ideally the mother should relate to a small number of midwives throughout her pregnancy so that they are all aware of her hopes and aspirations for the birth and able to discuss them sensitively during her visits.

Home

The home provides privacy and an opportunity to meet other important members of the family, such as the husband or a toddler. When a midwife visits at home, delicate topics can be discussed. These may include anxieties about sibling jealousy or the changing relationship within a marriage. In the comfort of a sitting room the midwife acquires an identity which is separate from 'the clinic' and she is more easily seen as a trusted friend. In this setting the mother may feel free to discuss such intimate matters as lovemaking and the relationship with her in-laws. In turn, the midwife gains first-hand knowledge of the mother's home setting and can share her experience gained from other women to inform and guide the situation.

The community or team midwife has the best opportunity for continuity of care and can slowly build up trust. She can evaluate the degree of the mother's understanding and introduce a little more information at each meeting or research to provide specific information requested by a mother.

A midwife can use home visits to provide education on labour and mothering for the single girl or teenager who is too shy or reluctant to attend sessions elsewhere. Sensitivity to needs and future wishes may lead the midwife to visit in everyday clothes rather than in a uniform.

Parenthood education sessions

Effective parenthood education sessions ideally would follow the principles already outlined in this chapter. The midwife explores how she can meet the needs of the mothers in her care. Midwives in different parts of the country will be presented with different problems in terms of the mix of social classes and ethnic groups.

Specialised needs

In considering the special needs of families in a particular area it might be helpful to address the questions listed in Box 12.1. The possible questions are endless but each district has a population with specific needs and the midwife who explores the demographic picture will at least begin to identify which problems she is likely to face. There will be recognition of any dissonance between her own

---

Box 12.1 Questions designed to explore the special needs of families in a particular area

- What types of social deprivation may be encountered?
- Is drug or alcohol abuse a possibility?
- Is there a large number of single mothers?
- Is the area one where young families are constantly moving so that little stability is afforded by neighbours and friends?
- Is the area frequented by gypsies or wandering folk who may be difficult to reach and care for?
- Is the area high in unemployment, making daytime sessions for both husbands and wives a viable proposition?
- Does the area contain immigrant families or other groups whose perception of birth and child care differs from that of the potential educators?
- Does the area include Forces families with support but the uncertainty of frequent home changes?

culture, values and race, increasing the need for sensitivity to differing beliefs and past experiences.

Timing

Sessions should be timed in such a way as to meet the needs of the parents as nearly as possible. Some areas may offer preconception sessions which include advice concerning the actual pregnancy. More frequently, the first parenthood education sessions will consist of one or two early meetings in order to discuss topics such as diet, alcohol consumption, smoking, work hazards, fatigue and minor disorders of pregnancy. Meeting other women in this way helps to reduce the feeling of isolation which pregnant women experience.

A longer series of sessions is usually planned for the third trimester when many women have given up work or will shortly be doing so. In the last weeks preparation for labour is the main interest. Multigravid women become more concerned about the baby during the last month and it may be helpful to arrange special sessions for them during this period. If toddlers are brought, they can be included in aspects such as the tour of the hospital and see tiny babies in the postnatal ward, possibly being breast fed. Saving this visit until the later weeks of pregnancy helps to ensure that toddlers will retain the memory until their own brother or sister is born.

If a woman wishes to attend with her partner or has chosen to continue working until late in the pregnancy, evening or weekend sessions will usually be needed. Other sessions should be arranged at times which will suit the clients.

The length of each session depends on accommodation and the needs of the midwife and the mother. Women will not be able to concentrate if they have to get away to collect children from school or playgroup. The attention span is at most 20 minutes before a change of activity is needed. During pregnancy a woman finds it even more difficult to concentrate for long, and sessions should allow for frequent breaks and opportunities for discussion and sharing.

Recruitment

The best advertisement for sessions is the satisfied mother in the community. If the sessions are interesting and valuable, mothers will spread the news to one another. The programme, especially new sessions such as toddler tours, couples sessions and single or 'solo' sessions need to be advertised. In society today we are accustomed to professional advertising. In the same way, posters about parenthood sessions need to capture interest, give clear information and be professionally executed. Health education departments will often have suitable material. If a midwife has to produce a poster herself, the use of transfer lettering or a stencil can give a professional look. A personal invitation sent to every mother with her booking letter produces good results and makes use of postage already accounted for. A personal word from the midwife at a clinic visit reinforces the information and makes the mother feel welcome. It is vital that there is a thorough knowledge of parent education available, for example clinic midwives need to know of any new ventures such as breast feeding workshops or postnatal support groups. Colleagues can both enthuse and encourage women if they have sufficient information. Equally, knowing about local active birth classes, aquarobics, baby swims, National Childbirth Trust or PIPPIN (Parents in Partnership–Parent Infant Network) provision shows an awareness of differing needs and an acceptance of alternatives for the women. Women have an awareness of the Baby Friendly Initiative and the continuity, choice and control promulgated by *Changing Childbirth* (DH 1993). The midwife who is teaching or giving care ideally appreciates the local Baby Friendly status or the progress towards it and the application of Changing Childbirth action points within the Unit. The latter is specific to England but the Baby Friendly Hospital Initiative is worldwide.

Minority groups

Addressing the questions listed in Box 12.1 may have brought to light the needs of single mothers, immigrant families, young families with minimal support, gypsies and families suffering from poor housing, unemployment or eviction. Such situations need specific help and support. Where there is bereavement or chronic illness it might be helpful to put a mother in touch with a self-help group or voluntary organisation.

Pregnancy itself produces minority groups such as:

- the mother having twins or triplets
- the mother who is to have a planned caesarean section
- the mother who has had in vitro fertilisation
- the mother with a drug-induced pregnancy
- the mother who has previously experienced the tragedy of a perinatal death or sudden infant death.

Parents planning to adopt are a minority group often missed by midwife educators. Sessions which teach practical skills and help to develop an awareness of the emotions which *all* new parents experience are helpful to them.

All these groups can benefit from sharing with other mothers and couples who have similar experiences to their own. The initial involvement often leads to very long-standing friendships. People who share their feelings share themselves and trust results.

Format of groups

In order to allow exchange within a group and opportunity for every member to participate and learn according to her or his needs, the group should consist of no more than 15 members (Abercrombie 1974). Hospitals and communities which cater for large numbers of deliveries, 2000–5000 per year, need to coordinate their services so that there are sufficient groups to keep the numbers small and so that the facilities are fully utilised. A central booking system enables the mothers to attend sessions near their own homes when possible and yet equalises the numbers. This approach has been successfully adopted in some health districts (Zander & Chamberlain 1984). The mothers who book late and the ones who, though invited, choose not to make their arrangements until late in pregnancy are the ones who may not be able to attend the sessions of their choice but can still be accommodated by this method. Figure 12.1 shows a booklet which advertises parent education sessions.

Grouping people with similar needs eases the work of the educator. Mothers having second or third children can meet together to brush up their knowledge and to reflect on their last labours and plan the integration of each new baby into the family. Whereas a second-time mother may be useful in a group of first-time mothers, her needs are different from theirs. It is wisest to invite her specifically to share her experiences and to offer her alternative sessions which meet her differing needs.

The actual schedule of classes offered in any health district must be planned with the location of centres in mind as well as the groups who need to attend. It is valuable if sessions offered by health visitors can be coordinated with those run by midwives and this may be the responsibility of a parent education coordinator for the district. Varying lengths of courses may be needed. Couples or primigravid mothers attending on their own may need between four and eight sessions, while mothers expecting a second or third baby probably need no more than two or three. 'Solos' often appreciate an open group where attendance is welcome throughout pregnancy and a 'special focus' group for women expecting twins or a caesarean birth may only need a single meeting. Many of the groups which do not cater for the partner as a rule may be able to arrange an evening when the 'dads' can come along.

Content of sessions

The content must match the needs of the mothers. The midwife's own plan should be flexible. She should respond to needs which are stated at the beginning of the sessions and adapt during a session if anxieties and fears become apparent. If the midwife conducting a session discovers, for instance, that a recent television programme on postnatal depression has disturbed the mothers, she should respond by discussing the subject to their satisfaction before continuing. During the introductory session the midwife must offer the mothers an idea of her aims and ask for their suggestions for possible content. The mothers and their partners should be invited to say which areas they hope will be covered in order to satisfy their needs and also to state which additional subjects would interest them. Lists made by parents vary and give the midwife an excellent insight into the perceived needs of the group. Couples might state that both partners would like to see the environment for

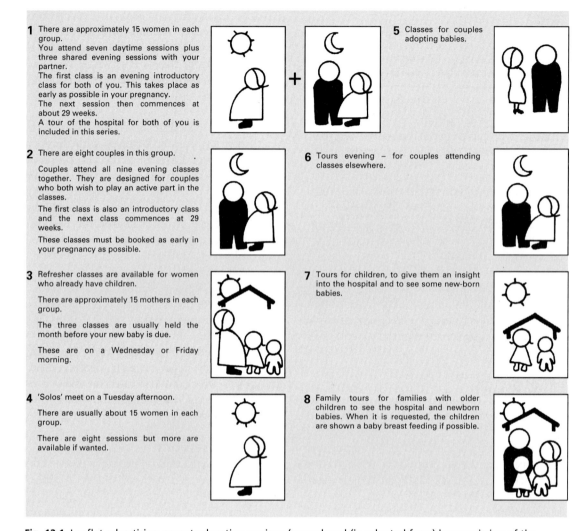

1 There are approximately 15 women in each group.
You attend seven daytime sessions plus three shared evening sessions with your partner.
The first class is an evening introductory class for both of you. This takes place as early as possible in your pregnancy.
The next session then commences at about 29 weeks.
A tour of the hospital for both of you is included in this series.

2 There are eight couples in this group.

Couples attend all nine evening classes together. They are designed for couples who both wish to play an active part in the classes.

The first class is also an introductory class and the next class commences at 29 weeks.

These classes must be booked as early in your pregnancy as possible.

3 Refresher classes are available for women who already have children.

There are approximately 15 mothers in each group.

The three classes are usually held the month before your new baby is due.

These are on a Wednesday or Friday morning.

4 'Solos' meet on a Tuesday afternoon.

There are usually about 15 women in each group.

There are eight sessions but more are available if wanted.

5 Classes for couples adopting babies.

6 Tours evening – for couples attending classes elsewhere.

7 Tours for children, to give them an insight into the hospital and to see some new-born babies.

8 Family tours for families with older children to see the hospital and newborn babies. When it is requested, the children are shown a baby breast feeding if possible.

Fig. 12.1 Leaflet advertising parent education sessions (reproduced (in adapted form) by permission of the Norwich Health Authority).

delivery and to discuss how they might support one another emotionally during labour. The group might ask to learn the practical skill of baby massage. Questions may be asked which seek to evaluate the progressiveness of the unit in which the baby is to be born. Such groups need a confident, competent midwife who can understand their approach and satisfy their particular requests. Another group may be less demanding and almost unable to be clear about what they want but with encouragement will become enthusiastic and enjoy suggesting items for inclusion in their sessions.

It is unwise to prescribe what the content of any programme should be. The outline in Box 12.2 suggests a number of questions to which mothers may require to find answers.

A midwife who wishes to build up trust in the group and to help the individuals to grow and change must always accept the other person's perception without being judgemental.

Approaching sessions from the perspective of the mother and her partner enables the midwife to be effective as an educator. A midwife who decides to offer parenthood education needs to develop

---

Box 12.2 Questions it is helpful to explore in a parent education programme

Questions for parents to ask themselves

Besides needing factual answers to their questions, mothers and their partners may be helped to explore their feelings and attitudes to pregnancy and parenthood. The midwife may be able to enhance the mother's perception of herself and build up her self-esteem. She can respond to worries about an unfavourable outcome and broach the subject of emergency intervention and help to prepare for changes in the plans. She can use other people's experiences to help the new parents to imagine how they will deal with their own and to consider ways of coping.

Questions for expectant mothers
- What does antenatal care consist of?
- Why is it done?
- How will I know that all is well?
- What influences the choice of where to have the baby?
- How has and might pregnancy affect me (psychologically/physically)?
- What do I like about being pregnant?
- What do I not like about being pregnant?
- What is my attitude towards birth? Can I trace where this comes from?
- What do I need to know about the process of labour, physically, emotionally and practically?
- What awareness do I have of my own body's ability to give birth?
- Do I trust my body?
- Who and what may help me at this time?
- What makes labours so different?
- What are the possible outcomes which I need to understand and anticipate?

- What are my attitudes and feelings towards the whole experience?
- What will give me confidence at this time in myself, in my partner, my family, my midwife and my attendants?
- What skills can I master which will help me to feed and nurture my baby?

Questions for a second or subsequent pregnancy
- Has the care changed since last time?
- Will my labour be different?
- Will I feel the same afterwards?
- Can I avoid jealousy between my present child and the new baby?
- How can I ease or help their relationship?
- Will I be able to love the baby as much as the first child?

Questions for unsupported women
- What will I need if I decide to keep the baby?
- How can I budget?
- How will I cope with loneliness?
- How do other people feel in my position?
- How do they cope?
- How can I increase my support network?

Questions for partners
- What is my attitude towards birth?
- What is my experience of birth so far?
- How does my life experience contribute?
- Do I trust my wife's body to give birth?
- What confidence do I have in myself as a supporter?
- Who will support me?
- What strengths do I have?
- What will my feelings be towards the baby?

---

an awareness of some of her own attitudes, biases and prejudices. She needs to explore the ways in which she can enhance learning and must face her own limitations in order to make appropriate use of others who can help her to cover areas in which she feels insecure. An example is inviting a health visitor to discuss how other children can be helped to accept a new brother or sister or to explain about immunisation. Books which enlarge knowledge of the psychological processes of childbirth include those by Gross (1989), Michaels & Goldberg (1988), Niven (1992) and Raphael-Leff (1991, 1993). Parr (1998) of PIPPIN would add insight.

The most successful childbirth educator will be someone with sufficient knowledge of childbirth and parenting, an openness to the validity of others'

thoughts and ideas, an enthusiasm in planning and conducting the sessions and an honesty and acceptance of the recipients' evaluation. The latter point ensures a response to mothers' changing needs within society in keeping with *The Patient's Charter* (DH 1992). A chapter on evaluation is included in *Health Promotion in Midwifery* (Crafter 1997) and this enables the midwife to consider all aspects which could enhance a future approach. *Changing Childbirth* (DH 1993) is also a source of identifying what women say they want from the maternity services and guides the midwife in her practice. In placing the woman at the centre of the service provision, it focuses on her choice and control rather than the need of the professional to control the care.

Session structure

Traditionally, parent education sessions have been approximately 2 hours weekly over a specified period. Workshops covering a day or a half-day can be held. One example is breast-feeding workshops (Jamieson 1990, Jamieson & Long 1997). These workshops which target knowledge, skills and attitudes are very effective in enabling mothers to breast feed successfully. The prolonged time increases the depth of relationship both with professionals and with other mothers. Other subject areas that suit this approach are 'Help yourself to antenatal care – benefits and options', 'Preparing for the birth experience', 'Understanding mothering' and 'Knowledge and skills needed for bottle feeding'. Workshops may be a valid approach for teams to ensure an individualised approach with continuity of prenatal care and teaching. Sometimes there can be a loss of the socialising benefits of the consecutive sessions but the skilled facilitator can maximise the opportunities for the women. Part of the sessions can be used for relaxation and focusing on skills which are needed in labour. An obstetric physiotherapist may lead this part. If the midwife educator is alone, she is able to integrate the exercises with the rest of the session and make links with attitudes and strengths of the individuals. No one approach or skill needs emphasis but a range giving the mother a choice for different experiences of labour. Opportunities for socialising are vital, as friendships formed can give great support in the early months and even years of parenting. Clulow (1982) supports such a view in his book *To Have and To Hold*:

Preparation for parenthood involves more than alerting couples to the likely effects of children upon their marriage. There is a limit to the usefulness of information to parents, although imparting information provides a reason for couples and services to meet. Preparation for the emotional impact of parenthood means establishing relationships which can be called upon later as an aid to integrating experience once that experience has been lived through. The partnership between parents is not alone in requiring preparation. Partnerships between families and the services available to them need to be established before they are required. In addition, the partnerships within the relevant helping agencies will affect the ability of those directly in touch with families to provide an integrated service. In all three contexts, the containing relationship can serve as midwife to the emerging family unit, enabling those involved both to have and to hold the new life generated by birth. Developing such relationships is a proper objective for preparative and preventive services.

Equally a quotation from a mother's letter to her teacher (Close 1980) helps to show how attitudes are important:

You managed to communicate to me your conviction that it is possible to participate willingly and constructively in the experience of childbirth, through knowledge.

The whole conception of assistance rather than resistance was completely revolutionary to me, apparently my environment had encouraged me to have an irresponsible attitude physically, I simply refused to examine and understand the workings and functions of my body.

The realisation that I could assist the course of my labour, give birth rather than unwillingly allow a child to be dragged from me, created a confidence I had always felt lacking in myself. I do believe that it is a pervasive feeling of inferiority in women that helps to make childbirth the nightmare it undoubtedly is for so many. It was your insistence that we could help ourselves if we wanted to that gave me the courage to attempt it. You really revealed a way of thinking to me, one which I have found myself applying in many other situations besides labour.

Another mother gives insight into structuring the session (Perkins 1980):

I think rather than talk blindly on, they ought to let people ask. You go in, and they give a talk, very helpful really, but they might put you on a subject, or a small item, that will trigger something off and you sit and think 'shall I ask, because I've got that'. At the end they say 'any questions' and they sit looking at one another, and I think that instead of them sitting talking they ought to let you all talk, because it is then that you spill your fears.

Time should be allowed within the session for current anxieties to be broached. Sometimes this will mean shortening the intended input and being prepared to use different methods if time is curtailed by the group.

The midwife as facilitator of the group must be aware of her own attitudes and ideas in the knowledge that example is a powerful teacher. Variety will help each person to come expecting to enjoy the session and to be distracted from the physical discomfort of pregnancy. The midwife may share her own feelings about a recent birth in a way which will help the couples to identify with her as a person and as a midwife. There should always be a break for social exchange and refreshment.

If the session has covered the more disturbing aspects such as forceps delivery and caesarean section or if members of the group have led the discussion into puerperal depression or stillbirth, the session should close on a lighter note. This is possible by looking forward to the next week or by inviting the couples to think about their ex-pected babies. A group should never leave on a sad or anxious note.

Box 12.3 gives a basic framework for couples' sessions. It is not to be copied, simply to be used as an example of content. Each teacher and each group needs to sort out the areas to be covered within the constraints of their own time and facili-ties. The contents need to be reviewed and altered as the participants experience pregnancy and as the educator grows in skill and perception.

HEALTH IN PREGNANCY

In her contact with pregnant women, whether in a group or singly, the midwife has ample oppor-tunities to discuss a healthy lifestyle for pregnancy in terms of diet, exercise and personal habits. Sometimes the mother will ask for the midwife's guidance. It is often helpful to link advice to a specific problem which the woman is experiencing, such as a minor disorder of pregnancy, because at such times the woman will be more receptive to health information. Chapter 10 discusses health related to preconception care and most of the information also applies during pregnancy itself.

Box 12.3 Suggested plan for couples' sessions

Session 1
Introduction
Meeting the babies, listening to their heartbeats
Your expectations and requests
Video showing birth with a focus on responsive relationships

Session 2
Introduction to labour
Visit to delivery suite

Session 3
Labour (continued); skills that help pain relief
Caesarean delivery
Forceps delivery
Relaxation and breathing techniques
Positions for labour

Session 4
Parents sharing their own experience of childbirth and early parenting
Special care nursery
Visit to postnatal ward

Session 5
Video showing baby's attributes and communication skills
Communication with a baby
Bathing a baby
Relaxation exercises

Session 6
Breast feeding knowledge, skills and attitudes
Relaxation/distraction techniques

Session 7
Support networks
Postnatal realities
Parenting: planning a postnatal reunion

Daytime (optional)
Baby massage
Limbering up for labour: exercises for women
Active birth exercises
Aquanatal classes

Diet in pregnancy

Diet is important on three counts: the health of the woman herself, her developing fetus and the alleviation of minor disorders of pregnancy. Some women will not be conversant with the main foods in terms of protein, fat and carbohydrates, fibre, vitamins and minerals, but can readily understand food groups (see Ch. 10). In addition, the midwife may explain that a regular intake of food ensures a regular supply for the unborn baby and should encourage the mother to avoid rushing meals or missing them.

Of particular importance is the intake of protein for the growth of new tissue. Meat, fish and cheese are prime sources, but cheaper sources may be advised such as peas, beans and lentils, milk and eggs. Two minerals are vital in pregnancy: calcium and iron. Milk, cheese and eggs supply the former; soft cheeses such as Brie are best avoided because they have sometimes been found to carry listeria, and eggs must be cooked thoroughly in order to destroy any salmonella that may be present. Iron is found in red meat and offal but pregnant women are advised to avoid liver and liver products since liver may contain excessive vitamin A. Pâté may also be contaminated with listeria. Dark green vegetables and red fruits also contain some iron.

Vitamin C helps the absorption of iron, and mothers should be encouraged to eat good quantities of fresh fruit and vegetables – at least half a kilogram per day. These will also contribute to the fibre content of the diet which helps to prevent constipation. Other high-fibre foods include wholemeal bread, cereals and pulses. A certain amount of carbohydrate is required to provide energy but mothers should be encouraged to avoid a high sugar intake and to choose instead starches, which are absorbed more slowly.

Some mothers may need specialised advice. Those on low incomes or who are unsupported may need help with budgeting and with making sensible choices. It may have to be pointed out that a filled wholemeal roll is more nourishing and costs less than a fizzy drink and a packet of crisps. New vegetarians may need advice from the dietitian to ensure that the range of foods they eat is adequate to supply all their nutritional requirements.

Alcohol

The inadvisability of drinking alcohol whilst pregnant has received much press coverage. Mothers may want to discuss with the midwife the fact that because they did not suspect pregnancy, they have taken alcohol up to the time of missing the first period. Moderate to high levels of alcohol have been found to give rise to fetal problems so a mother who only drinks occasionally may be reassured. No safe level of alcohol consumption has been established, therefore it is wise to stop drinking alcohol prior to conception (see Ch. 10).

Smoking

There is already plenty of literature which discourages the pregnant woman from smoking but the midwife needs to be aware of the social pressures and advertising that give a contrary message. Smoking can be a response to stress and it is inappropriate to add to the woman's stress by being over-directive and insensitive to her needs. If she can stop, the outlook for herself and the fetus is improved; if this proves very difficult, she should try to cut down. Smoking is linked with intrauterine growth retardation, preterm labour and an increase in the perinatal mortality rate. The mother herself is at increased risk of chest infections and thromboembolic disorders.

As smoking becomes less acceptable socially it is to be hoped that fewer women will present in pregnancy as smokers; those who do are likely to be those who find it most difficult to give up. Understanding that smoking reduces the baby's oxygen and food supply may motivate a mother to stop but this is not always so. It is helpful if the midwife finds out what triggers the smoking and suggests ways of cutting down (see Box 12.4). A smoky environment will not be good for the baby in the future and it is important to discuss this aspect. At all times the midwife must be sensitive to the particular circumstances of the woman, taking care not to lay a burden upon her that she is powerless to respond to.

Box 12.4 Tips for giving up or cutting down smoking

- Leave a longer stub.
- Use filter tips.
- Keep hands busy.
- Only smoke when sitting down.
- Do not inhale.
- Cut out the first cigarette of the day and the last one at night.
- Try chewing gum or sucking peppermints.

Sexual intercourse

Sometimes couples fear that sexual intercourse in pregnancy may harm the baby. It is absolutely safe and normal unless special conditions pertain. If the woman is nauseated in early pregnancy she may feel disinclined to have intercourse but the couple can be encouraged to find other ways of being loving. Libido varies throughout pregnancy and the middle trimester is usually the time of most vitality. Towards the end of pregnancy when the abdomen is large, couples sometimes have to adopt different positions.

There are certain situations when caution is advised. If a mother has a history of miscarriages she should avoid intercourse in the early months, especially at the times when her period would usually have started. If any bleeding is seen at any stage the couple should abstain and seek advice.

Some women experience contractions following intercourse due to the prostaglandins in seminal fluid and oxytocin release at orgasm. These will usually pass off with rest. After an episode of pre-term labour which has been successfully averted, abstention should be advised for the same reason.

Exercise and sport

If a mother is used to taking regular exercise such as walking, swimming, riding or cycling, there is no reason why she should not continue for as long as she feels comfortable. Pregnancy is not a time to try out strenuous new sports and the more energetic sports such as squash and wind-surfing will probably need to be discontinued fairly early. A woman could continue to swim quite safely until term and can even do her pregnancy exercises in the water. The mother's own comfort and desire can be used as a guideline. (Exercise is discussed more fully in Chapter 45.)

Travel

Travel is sometimes unavoidable in pregnancy, for example, in Forces families. Airlines ask for a doctor's certificate stating that a pregnant woman is fit to travel and they prefer not to take women beyond the 32nd week. Mothers can and do fly safely after this time, however. Prior to 32 weeks' gestation a holiday abroad can be very refreshing and of benefit to a couple sharing the experience of looking towards parenting. An important consideration is whether any immunisations are needed because it is not wise to be immunised in pregnancy. The woman should be fastidious about washing fruit and sterilising unsafe drinking water. Sunbathing is often not enjoyed because the mother is already feeling over-warm owing to an increase in her basal metabolic rate.

Long, unbroken journeys by whatever transport should be avoided. If travel is essential, taking extra fluids and making definite breaks can ease any discomfort. It is important for the woman to carry up-to-date details of her pregnancy or her own notes or records, so that should something unforeseen occur the information needed is readily at hand.

Clothing

This reflects the mother's taste and financial position but loose cool clothing will be the most comfortable. Pinafore dresses and dresses made of ready-gathered material can accommodate the changing shape for longer. Unfortunately, pregnant women often get bored with their maternity dresses, however pretty, because they cannot afford enough to ring the changes. Fashions with loose and flowing lines make it easier for the mother's clothes to accommodate pregnancy in the early months.

Jeans can be made with elastic insets either at the side or at the front to accommodate a growing baby. The feet sometimes spread and shoes need to be comfortable. They should not tip the mother forward. Breasts usually increase in later pregnancy by at least two bra sizes. If the mother intends to breast feed, she should buy a suitable bra which opens at the front rather than simply a larger ordinary one. The National Childbirth Trust and main stores often offer a fitting service and advise on size and comfort for the individual mother.

MINOR DISORDERS OF PREGNANCY

Minor disorders are only minor inasmuch as they are not life-threatening. As soon as a midwife becomes pregnant and experiences the fatigue of early pregnancy coupled with nausea and vomiting she realises the inaccuracy of the description. A minor disorder may escalate and become a serious complication of pregnancy. Where sickness develops into hyperemesis gravidarum, a condition which began as a minor disorder has become a life-threatening abnormality. The role of the midwife is to be always alert to any developing complications and refer appropriately. She must, as always, educate; when the changes of pregnancy are understood they are easier to tolerate and unnecessary anxiety is alleviated. She should also provide practical advice to ease the situation as far as is possible and listen attentively to the reality of the experience for the mother.

Causes of minor disorders can be divided into hormonal changes, accommodation changes, metabolic changes and postural changes. Every system of the body adjusts and is affected by pregnancy. In order to make reference easy, the disorders will be dealt with by systems. The mother will only need advice pertinent to some. The skill of the midwife is in anticipating the need for knowledge in the mother in order to equip her to cope with the experience of pregnancy. She also meets the mother's need for specific knowledge when she presents with a discomforting or worrying symptom.

Digestive system

Nausea and vomiting.   This presents between 4 and 16 weeks' gestation. Hormonal influences are cited as the most likely cause. Human chorionic gonadotrophin is found in large amounts until the placenta takes over from the corpus luteum at around 12 weeks. Oestrogen and progesterone are also contributors; the transient nausea which may occur when a woman takes the contraceptive pill corroborates this. The sickness is not confined to 'early morning' but can occur at any time in the day. The smell of food cooking will often cause the mother to retch. The midwife can explain the probable reasons and encourage the mother to look positively towards a resolution of the sickness which should occur between 12 and 16 weeks; understanding the cause provides comfort. Mothers often find salads tempting and light snacks more tolerable than full meals. Carbohydrate snacks at

bedtime and before rising can prevent hypoglycaemia which is often implicated as a cause of nausea and vomiting. It is always important to remember that other conditions such as appendicitis, unrelated to pregnancy, can present with vomiting so the midwife must be vigilant in her history taking. If vomiting becomes severe, the mother may lose weight and become dehydrated and ketotic. This condition is called hyperemesis gravidarum and warrants specialised care and appropriate referral.

Heartburn.   This is a burning sensation in the mediastinal region. Progesterone relaxes the cardiac sphincter of the stomach and allows reflux of gastric contents into the oesophagus. Heartburn is most troublesome at about 30–40 weeks' gestation because at this stage the stomach is under pressure from the growing uterus.

The advice varies according to the severity of the condition. If the heartburn is occasional, the reflux can be prevented by avoiding bending over whilst housekeeping and kneeling to clean the bath or to make the beds. Small meals take up less room in the reduced stomach space and are digested more easily. Sleeping with more pillows than usual and lying on the right side semi-reclining can sometimes help. For persistent heartburn the doctor may prescribe antacids.

Excessive salivation (ptyalism).   This occurs from 8 weeks' gestation and is thought to be caused by the hormones of pregnancy. It may accompany heartburn. Explanation and attentive listening are helpful.

Pica.   This is the term used when a mother craves certain foods or unnatural substances such as coal. The cause is unknown but hormones and changes in metabolism are blamed. The midwife needs to be aware that this condition can occur and to seek medical advice if the substance craved is potentially harmful to the unborn baby.

Constipation.   Progesterone causes relaxation and decreased peristalsis of the gut, which is also displaced by the growing uterus. It is helpful to increase the intake of water, fresh fruit, vegetables and wholemeal foods in the diet. A glass of warm water in the morning, before tea or breakfast, may activate the gut and help regular bowel movements. Exercise is helpful, especially walking. Aperients are considered only as a last resort: a bulk-increasing agent would be the first choice. Constipation is sometimes associated with the taking of oral iron. The condition can aggravate haemorrhoids and early common-sense advice may avoid much discomfort for the mother. A midwife should be alert to the possibility of constipation if a mother complains of abdominal discomfort and be aware that a full rectum is a cause of non-engagement of the fetal head at term.

Musculoskeletal system

Backache. This is fully discussed in Chapter 45 with advice regarding sitting and posture. The midwife's role is to educate the mother to understand her changing centre of gravity as the fetus grows and which postures to adopt. The hormones sometimes soften the ligaments to such a degree that some support is needed. When the woman appreciates this, she is reassured that once birth has occurred the ligaments will return to their pre-pregnant strength. Backache must never be dismissed lightly as it is associated with urinary tract infection and with the onset of labour especially when the fetal occiput is posterior.

Cramp. The cause of leg cramp in pregnancy is unknown. It may be due to ischaemia or result from changes in pH or electrolyte status. The mother may be advised to dorsiflex the foot (see Ch. 45) and to raise the foot of the bed about 25 cm. It may be helpful to make gentle leg movements whilst in a warm bath prior to settling for the night. This enhances circulation and removes waste products from muscle. Other remedies used are vitamin B complex and calcium.

Genitourinary system

Frequency of micturition. This occurs in the early weeks of pregnancy when the growing uterus is still situated within the pelvis and competes for space required by the bladder. In the latter weeks the fetal head usually enters the pelvis and reduces the space available. The midwife may reassure the

mother, having excluded other causes of bladder irritability such as infection. She may also explain that the problem is resolved when the uterus rises into the abdomen after the 12th week.

Leucorrhoea. This is the term used for the increased white, non-irritant vaginal discharge in pregnancy. If the mother finds the discharge disturbing, it is helpful to offer simple advice concerning personal hygiene. She should wear cotton underwear and avoid tights. Washing with plain water twice a day should be adequate and a mild cream is preferable to talcum powder. The midwife should exclude the possibility of infections such as thrush and trichomonas. Both are dealt with in Chapter 18.

Circulatory system

Fainting. In early pregnancy fainting may be due to the vasodilatation occurring under the influence of progesterone before there has been a compensatory increase in blood volume. Avoiding long periods of standing is helpful, as is being quick to sit or lie down if she feels slightly faint.

Later in pregnancy a mother may feel faint while lying flat on her back. The weight of the uterine contents presses on the inferior vena cava and slows the return of blood to the heart. Turning the mother quickly onto her side will bring about a rapid recovery. The midwife has to explain to the mother that this occurs in about 10% of pregnant women and that she would be wise not to lie on her back except during abdominal examination. Explanation will give the mother confidence to know what to do if she feels faint and will help to ensure her safety.

Varicosities. Progesterone relaxes the smooth muscles of the veins and results in sluggish circulation. The valves of the dilated veins become inefficient and varicosities result. Varicose veins may occur in the legs, anus (haemorrhoids) and vulva. The situation is compounded by pelvic congestion. The midwife must be aware of mothers at risk, for example, those with a family history of varicose veins and those doing work which demands long periods of standing or sitting. Exercising the calf muscles by rising onto the toes or making circling movements with the ankles will help the venous return. In the early days of pregnancy, resting with the legs vertical against the wall for a short time will drain the veins. Support tights increase comfort and should be put on before rising or after resting with the legs elevated.

The avoidance of constipation by fibre in the diet and adequate fluids will reduce exacerbation of haemorrhoids. If appropriate, topical applications should be recommended and medical advice sought.

Vulval varicosities are rare and very painful. A panty-girdle or sanitary pad may give support. The midwife should listen and offer appropriate advice. She should also be aware of the risk of haemorrhage from a ruptured vein during delivery.

Skin

The mother observes her skin changes closely and will often comment upon the linea nigra and the areola of the breasts. If chloasma occurs, which is a butterfly-shaped area of pigmentation over the face, the mother may be reassured that this will diminish as soon as the baby is born. Sometimes there is generalised itching which often starts over the abdomen. This is thought to have some connection with the liver's response to the hormones in pregnancy and with raised bilirubin levels. It clears as soon as the baby is born and comfort can be gained from local applications. An antihistamine such as Piriton (chlorpheniramine) is often prescribed. If a mother complains of vulval irritation, infection, such as thrush, and glycosuria as a result of diabetes must be excluded before advising on cotton underwear and perhaps washing with unscented soap.

Nervous system

Carpal tunnel syndrome. The mother complains of numbness and 'pins and needles' in her fingers and hands. This usually happens in the morning but it can occur at any time of the day. It is caused by fluid retention which creates oedema and pressure on the median nerve. Wearing a splint at night with the hand resting high on two or three pillows sometimes brings relief. Carpal tunnel syndrome usually resolves spontaneously following

delivery. The doctor may prescribe diuretics but the conservative approach is favoured.

Insomnia

This must never be dismissed lightly. There are physical reasons for sleep disturbance such as nocturnal frequency and difficulty in getting comfortable in bed because of the growing fetus. The increased blood supply to the uterus on lying down sometimes causes the baby to move a lot, just as the mother wishes to sleep. This may be overcome by going to bed earlier in the hope that the baby will have an active time earlier and allow the mother to sleep when she wants to.

Remembering the increased anxieties which pregnancy may bring, the midwife may ask the mother what dreams or thoughts she has as she falls asleep. Talking through some of the very common fears of pregnancy may help a mother to come to terms with her own anxieties. It is common to dream of delivering 'monsters' or animals and also to dream that the baby is born dead. Sensitive listening and expressing that the mind is presenting fears through dreams can be helpful. Knowing that it is very common is reassuring.

Later in pregnancy it is wise to recommend that the mother has a lie-in in the morning or has a rest in the afternoon when sleep often comes easily. This may help to prevent the tiredness and some of the depression that can occur in the last trimester of pregnancy. Sharing her feelings can result in a sense of normality and lightness for the mother and can greatly enhance her perception of care and experience of pregnancy.

It is thought that the hormonal changes towards the end of pregnancy also contribute to periods of depression for some women. Self-confidence in pregnancy is also labile and knowing that this is normal can make the experience easier to cope with. It can be frustrating for a woman to feel bouncy and excited one week and the next to feel so insecure that she cannot go into a shop. Explaining such responses helps both the mother and her partner. If a midwife is concerned that the mother's moods are not simply those of normal pregnancy, medical aid should be sought. The minor disorders can provide the midwife with opportunities to advise the mother and help her to achieve the most comfortable and safe pregnancy possible. She will be alert to any need for referral.

Disorders which require immediate action

Most minor disorders can escalate into a more serious complication of pregnancy. Mothers should be encouraged to seek advice if at any time they feel unwell or the signs exceed what they have been led to expect. In addition there are certain incidents which should always be reported to the midwife or doctor. These are:

- vaginal bleeding
- reduced fetal movements
- frontal or recurring headaches
- sudden swelling
- rupture of the membranes
- premature onset of contractions
- sudden nausea or sickness
- epigastric pain
- maternal anxiety for whatever reason.

The mother can be reassured that her pregnancy is likely to proceed smoothly and without complication. It adds to her security if she knows clearly when she should seek the help of a professional.

READER ACTIVITIES

1. Talk to several newly delivered women. Find out what they wished they had learned in their parent education classes.

Repeat the exercise with a similar number of women whose babies are about 28 days old.

Next ask the same question of a number of women during a subsequent pregnancy.

Compare the findings. How do women's perceived needs change with time and experience?

2. Devise a scheme for evaluating a series of parent education classes. If you have an opportunity, carry out such an evaluation. Reflect on your findings and identify the things that you would change as a result.

ACKNOWLEDGEMENTS

I should like to record my thanks to the late Miss Gillian Barnard and all the mothers and fathers who generously shared their experiences with me.

REFERENCES

Abercrombie M L J 1974 Aims and techniques of group teaching. Society for Research in Higher Education, London
Beech B, Robinson J 1994 Ultrasound? Unsound. Association for Improvements in the Maternity Services, London
Close A 1980 Birth report. NFER Publishing, Windsor
Clulow C F 1982 To have and to hold. University Press, Aberdeen
Crafter H (ed) 1997 Health promotion in midwifery. Arnold, London
Deakin M 1973 The children on the hill. Quartet, London, ch 2
Department of Health (DoH) 1992 The patient's charter. HMSO, London
Department of Health (DoH) 1993 Changing childbirth. Report of the expert maternity group. HMSO, London
Gross J 1989 Psychology and parenthood. Open University Press, Milton Keynes
Jamieson L 1990 Breast feeding knowledge and skills shared in a midwife–mother partnership. In: A midwife's love, skill and knowledge. International Congress of Midwives

Proceedings, Japan, pp 196–197
Jamieson L, Long L 1997 Promoting breastfeeding. In: Crafter H (ed) Health promotion in midwifery. Arnold, London, ch 14
Kempe R S, Kempe C H 1978 Child abuse. Fontana/Open Books, London, ch 2
Michaels G Y, Goldberg W A (eds) 1988 The transition to parenthood. Current theory and research. Cambridge University Press, Cambridge
Niven C 1992 Psychological care for families before, during and after birth. Butterworth-Heinemann, Oxford
Oakley A 1980 Women confined. Martin Robertson, Oxford
Parr M 1998 A new approach to parent education. British Journal of Midwifery 6(3): 160–165
Perkins E R 1980 Education for childbirth and parenthood. Croom Helm, London
Prout A 1986 Teenage girls' knowledge of antenatal care and its implications for school-based preventive strategies. Health Education Journal 44: 193–197

Raphael-Leff J 1991 Psychological processes of childbearing. Chapman & Hall, London

Raphael-Leff J 1993 Pregnancy: the inside story. Sheldon Press, London

Tew M 1993 Safety in childbirth. Association for Improvements in the Maternity Services, London

Zander L, Chamberlain G 1984 Pregnancy care for the 1980s. Royal Society of Medicine and Macmillan Press, London, section V, ch 22

FURTHER READING

Beech B, Robinson J 1994 Ultrasound? Unsound. Association for Improvements in the Maternity Services, London

Cobb J 1980 Babyshock. Hutchinson, London

Henderson C, Jones K 1997 Essential midwifery. Mosby, London

Kitzinger S 1977 Education and counselling for childbirth. Baillière Tindall, London

Nichols F, Humenick S 1988 Childbirth education: practice, research and theory. W B Saunders, London

Priest J, Schott J 1991 Leading antenatal classes: a practical guide. Butterworth-Heinemann, Oxford

Scott Peck M 1978 The road less traveled. Simon and Schuster, New York

Sherr L 1995 The psychology of pregnancy and childbirth. Blackwell Science, Oxford

Tew M 1993 Safety in childbirth. Association for Improvements in the Maternity Services, London

Antenatal care

Sarah Das

Antenatal care refers to the care that is given to an expectant mother from the time that conception is confirmed until the beginning of labour. In addition to monitoring the progress of the pregnancy, it aims to provide appropriate support for the woman and her family whatever the outcome of the pregnancy and information which will allow them to make sensible and informed choices.

The chapter aims to:

- discuss the initial assessment visit, defining its objectives and considering the significance of the different components of the history taken by the midwife

- describe the physical examination of the woman at the initial assessment and during subsequent visits

- detail the methods used during abdominal examination to check the growth of the fetus, its position and heart rate

- emphasise the contribution of skilled communication to sensitive and effective antenatal care.

Until very recently the large majority of pregnant women in the UK received a pattern of antenatal care that had seen little change since 1929 (MoH 1929). This traditional pattern of care consisted of visits at monthly intervals to 28 weeks of gestation, then fortnightly until 36 weeks and finally weekly visits until the birth of the baby. Many people have questioned the benefits of such a routine system of care and there has been much recent research to explore a more flexible approach to both the timing of visits and place of consultation. This has been in an attempt to achieve improved maternal and perinatal morbidity and increase consumer satisfaction.

Following on from the work of Marion Hall and colleagues (Hall et al 1980) and the recommendation for organisational change to be made to antenatal care from the 'Changing Childbirth' report (DH 1993), Sikorski et al (1996) conducted a randomised controlled trial on low-risk pregnant women, to compare the acceptability and effectiveness of a reduced antenatal visit schedule of six to seven routine visits with the traditional 13 routine visits. The results showed no differences in clinical outcome between the two groups but twice as many women in the reduced-visit group were dissatisfied with the frequency of attendance when compared to women who received the full range of visits. A substantial number of women in both groups felt that the gaps in their care were too long, with women in the reduced-visit group feeling less remembered from one visit to the next. The need to provide a more individualised, flexible approach to care with increased psychosocial support for those pregnant women who needed it was one of the main conclusions of this study.

An example of how antenatal care could be tailored to meet the needs of particular women was explored by Oakley et al (1990). Oakley conducted a randomised controlled trial to look at the effect of providing social support to women who had previously had one or more babies with a birthweight less than 2500 g. A group of women who had an increased likelihood of being socially disadvantaged in pregnancy were identified and additional support was given to the 'intervention' group of women by a research midwife. The midwife visited this group of women a minimum of three times during their pregnancy. She could be contacted by phone 24 hours a day, gave practical advice and information when asked, made referrals to other health care professionals as necessary but did not give any clinical care.

The results demonstrated that both women and babies in the intervention group experienced improved outcomes in several ways compared with the control group. There were fewer admissions to hospital during pregnancy and fewer very low birthweight babies, with babies generally needing less neonatal intensive care and mothers also reporting that their babies appeared healthier in the first few weeks of life.

When questioned a year later, women felt less anxious about their babies and more positive about motherhood. In 1996 Oakley et al looked at the same group of women, and the psychological and health benefits in the intervention group had continued compared with women in the control group.

Aims of antenatal care

- To support and encourage a family's healthy psychological adjustment to childbearing.
- To promote an awareness of the sociological aspects of childbearing and the influences that these may have on the family.
- To build up a trusting relationship between the family and their caregivers which will encourage them to participate in and make informed choices about the care they receive.
- To monitor the progress of pregnancy in order to ensure maternal health and normal fetal development.
- To recognise deviation from the normal and provide management or treatment as required.
- To ensure that the woman reaches the end of her pregnancy physically and emotionally prepared for the birth of her baby.
- To help and support the mother in her choice of infant feeding; to promote breast feeding in a sensitive manner and give advice about preparation for lactation when appropriate.
- To offer the family advice on parenthood either in a planned programme or on an individual basis.

These aims can only be achieved if the service provided is acceptable to women and their families. This has become more apparent in recent years. Women now have more control over their fertility. They are more likely to have planned the pregnancy and, if not, will have had the opportunity to discontinue it. Many factors have led to a decrease in maternal and perinatal mortality. Women expect a healthy outcome for themselves and their babies and have therefore become less worried about complications and more concerned with the emotional aspects of the experience. Both these factors will influence the type of care that women expect to receive. Education through schools, magazines, television and lay childbirth organisations all emphasise the normality of pregnancy and childbirth. Families are encouraged to participate fully in decision-making and to expect emotional satisfaction from the childbearing experience.

In order to respect these views, professionals must be approachable and flexible and inspire trust and confidence. They must give adequate and unbiased information in order to help families make sensible informed choices.

For its part, the family needs to have realistic expectations of the future and unrealistic demands must be discussed sensitively in the antenatal period. Counselling and discussion must be used to negotiate an acceptable compromise. If this is not attempted, there may be confrontation and breakdown in communication when the expectation is not met. This is even more likely when the family is under stress such as during an emergency when the required action is in conflict with the expressed wishes of the woman and her family. The whole concept of consenting to medical intervention becomes a nonsense if women receive inadequate information with which to make decisions about their care. Ultimately, the woman has the right to refuse treatment for herself and infringement of this could be considered as assault, but the law is less specific when intervention is deemed necessary to protect the fetus.

The midwife requires good communication skills in order to explore a woman's perception of the care she will receive. Together they may use this knowledge to formulate a care or birth plan as a progressive record of the individual needs and wishes of the woman. The woman must be made to feel that she is participating in the birth process. The current trend for women to hold their own maternity records is heightening this sense of participation in their care.

THE INITIAL ASSESSMENT (BOOKING VISIT)

This assessment should take place as soon as possible after pregnancy has been confirmed. Advice should be given early because the fetal organs are almost completely formed by the 12th week of pregnancy. Maternal nutrition, infection, smoking or drug-taking may all have a profound effect on the fetus during this time.

The early few weeks may leave the mother feeling exhausted, nauseous and bewildered about the changes occurring in her body. Unless referral is early she may be denied the midwife's support at this important time. It has been suggested that midwives should be more involved with the confirmation of pregnancy so that an earlier contact would be made. A midwife could then be available for support and counselling should the pregnancy fail. Unfortunately, the risk of early fetal loss often means that the initial assessment is postponed until the pregnancy is more established. Inefficient administration also leads to slow referral.

There are many schemes available, each with different options for place of antenatal care, birth and length of stay in hospital. Most entail one consultation with the hospital obstetric team to determine the suitability of the option.

This is probably the woman's first introduction to the team that is to care for her during pregnancy. First impressions are often lasting and the reception she receives at this visit is likely to colour the rest of her experience. For this reason the midwife must be friendly and adopt a woman-centred approach. Much of the visit is concerned with exchange of information (see Box 13.1). Ideally,

---

Box 13.1 Objectives for the initial assessment

- To assess levels of health by taking a detailed history and to employ screening tests as appropriate.
- To ascertain baseline recordings of weight, height, blood pressure and haemoglobin level in order to assess normality. These values are used for comparison as the pregnancy progresses.
- To identify risk factors by taking accurate details of past and present obstetric and medical history.
- To provide an opportunity for the woman and her family to express any concerns they might have regarding this pregnancy or previous obstetric experiences.
- To give advice on general health matters and those pertaining to pregnancy in order to maintain the health of the mother and the healthy development of the fetus.
- To begin building a trusting relationship in which realistic plans of care are discussed.

most of it should be conducted in the woman's home, away from the bustle of the busy clinic. This allows the midwife to get to know her in her own environment. The midwife may meet other members of the family and in this way gain a more holistic view of the woman's needs.

If the initial assessment must be done in the hospital, it is possible to humanise the process. It is helpful to write to the woman in advance and to advise her of the probable length of the interview, explaining what will happen and who she will see. This will allow her to make preparation for the visit. She may wish to bring a friend or her partner for support. Hospitals can be daunting to those who are not used to them. Two heads are better than one when trying to find the antenatal clinic amongst the many different departments. Children should be welcomed. Involving a toddler in the excitement of early pregnancy paves the way for future trust and lessens the fear of the mother going away should she require hospital admission. Crèche facilities are a great advantage, but if not available, a well-stocked toy cupboard will provide some distraction and allow the woman and midwife to talk. Making the assessment room as informal as possible helps to put the woman at ease.

The midwife requires many skills to achieve the aims of this visit and not least of these is her ability to communicate. More than 10 years ago the World Health Organization recommended that 'The training of health care professionals should include communication techniques in order to promote sensitive exchange of information between members of the health team and the pregnant woman and her family' (WHO 1985). The whole thrust of the 'Changing Childbirth' initiative 8 years later still emphasised these basic principles of care as a means of achieving increased satisfaction for women in pregnancy and childbirth (DH 1993). Listening skills involve showing real interest in the woman as a person, using verbal and nonverbal responses to encourage her to talk freely. The midwife must also be able to analyse the information and elicit further details in order to complete the picture. Communication skills also encompass writing accurate, comprehensive yet concise records of information. This is vital when using a team approach to care and especially so where women will have responsibility for their own records in pregnancy. Repeated questioning on the same topic not only undermines a woman's confidence in the service but also wastes time that could be used for more important purposes.

The midwife also requires clinical skills in order to carry out the physical examination of the woman which can include screening tests such as cervical smear, high vaginal swab and venepuncture.

First impressions

A midwife can gain much from observing a woman right at the start of their first meeting. Does she respond to a smile? She may appear nervous or shy. A long wait or the prospect of an assessment that she has undergone in other pregnancies may have made her irritable. Perhaps she is distressed at the failure of contraception; unresolved anger may lead to unresponsive behaviour. The most likely response is that of nervous but happy anticipation, as this visit is a further confirmation of a wanted pregnancy. Whatever the response it is essential to acknowledge it, clarify the situation and use the information gained to establish a rapport with the woman and then conduct the assessment with sensitivity. It may be that she will need to talk about previous experiences or unresolved problems before she can clear her mind and attend to the business in hand. This should be encouraged. If she is ambivalent about the pregnancy, she may value counselling from an abortion agency in order to become aware of her choices before finally accepting the pregnancy; adoption may be an acceptable alternative. Even a woman who has planned and welcomed her pregnancy needs time to discuss her fears and anxieties.

Observation of physical characteristics is also important. Posture and gait can indicate back problems or previous trauma to the pelvis. She may be lethargic, which suggests extreme tiredness, malnutrition or depression.

Midwifery history

Although it is very helpful to use a prepared list to ascertain salient information, it is important to resist the temptation to read out a list of questions. It is much more effective to couch questions in conversation leading from one topic to another.

Social history

It is important to assess the response of the whole family to the pregnancy. An additional child may mean overcrowding in the home or even the threat of eviction. A woman may doubt her ability to care for other children during the pregnancy, birth or afterwards; teenage children particularly may be unhappy about their mother being pregnant. The client may herself be a teenager or even younger, still under her parents' care and they may not wish to support her during the pregnancy. Special groups have been formed in some areas to give support to teenagers facing childbirth and motherhood and the midwife should offer to introduce the client to such a group. Financial problems arise in any family, with unemployment being common in some districts. It is not the midwife's responsibility to solve family problems but she must be sympathetic, have a thorough understanding of the financial benefits that are available and be able to refer a family to other professionals as appropriate. The Maternity Alliance is one such organisation. Chapter 46 explains the financial benefits.

Environmental factors must be considered when assessing needs during the pregnancy. Studies show that perinatal mortality and morbidity rates are higher in families in social classes IV and V who are more likely to live in poor conditions. Poor housing, lack of hot water, inadequate heating and insufficient money to take a healthy diet or buy items for the baby are all issues that must be addressed. The social worker should be informed if the family wishes, but in deprived inner-city areas the situation is unlikely to improve quickly. The midwife should be aware that women in deprived areas have greater health care needs and should offer realistic advice in order to help them to use all the resources available.

General health

General health should be discussed and good habits reinforced, giving further advice when required.

Exercise is important. Most activities may be continued during pregnancy. The woman's own body is a good indicator of when she should slow down or stop.

The importance of restricting alcohol and nicotine intake is stressed. It may be unrealistic to expect a woman to stop smoking altogether during pregnancy. Exhortations about the effect of smoking on the fetus may exacerbate her fears about the pregnancy so much that she actually increases her intake. Some women even see a bonus in the fact that smoking causes the baby to be smaller. The midwife must give practical advice to help the woman to cut down and give details of organisations such as QUIT who will provide useful ideas and support for reducing smoking in pregnancy. One of the key messages from the Foundation for the Study of Infant Deaths was that cigarette smoking in pregnancy increases the risk of babies dying from the sudden infant death syndrome (Blair et al 1996) (see Ch. 12).

Alcohol abuse is less common but can affect the baby (see Ch. 43 for fetal alcohol syndrome). In order to be sure of safety, no alcohol at all should be taken during pregnancy. Up to one glass of wine per day or the equivalent is probably acceptable.

Education for parenthood is provided in most areas (see Ch. 12). Sessions should be planned with individual needs in mind, providing for such diverse groups as experienced mothers, first-time mothers, gay couples, teenage mothers, single parents or couples. There may be some women who do not easily fit into a particular group and it might be possible to meet their needs during antenatal visits. It may be beneficial for a community midwife to visit them at home.

Menstrual history

Determining expected date of delivery (EDD). It is necessary to ascertain the approximate date on which the baby was conceived in order to predict a date of giving birth and calculate gestational age at any point in pregnancy. In this way actual fetal size can be compared with expected size.

The EDD is calculated by adding 9 calendar months and 7 days to the date of the first day of the woman's last menstrual period. This method assumes that:

- conception occurred 14 days after the first day of the last period: this is only true if the woman has a regular 28-day cycle
- the last period of bleeding was true menstruation: implantation of the ovum may cause slight bleeding.

The midwife must enquire about the normal cycle and amount of bleeding in order to assess the reliability of the calculation. If necessary, the midwife should explain to the woman how to calculate when her last menstrual period was and help her to do this.

If the woman has taken oral contraceptives within the previous 3 months, this may also confuse estimation of dates because breakthrough bleeding and anovular cycles lead to inaccuracies.

The EDD which is calculated by dates is sometimes confirmed by assessing uterine size vaginally or more commonly by early ultrasound scan. Bimanual examination carries a risk of abortion and should be avoided, particularly for women who have a previous history of spontaneous abortion.

Some women become pregnant with an intra-uterine contraceptive device (IUCD) still in place. Although the pregnancy is likely to continue normally, the position of the IUCD should be determined using ultrasound techniques. If it is not evident during delivery the uterus should be explored after labour in order to retrieve it.

Fetal movements are first felt by a multigravid woman at about 16 weeks, and by 20 weeks by a primigravid woman.

Obstetric history

Past childbearing experiences have an important part to play in predicting the likely outcome of the present pregnancy. The way in which a woman will respond to pregnancy, labour and the puerperium cannot be known until she has had at least one child. For this reason the woman who has not been pregnant before, a primigravida, needs closer observation to ensure that all remains normal. Women who have already had one healthy pregnancy are less likely to develop pregnancy-induced hypertension, unless this is the first pregnancy with a new partner. Adequate pelvic capacity can also be assumed if the fetus is of a similar size to previous babies delivered vaginally. Uterine efficiency is better after the first labour (see Ch. 21). If a woman has had more than five previous births she is considered at high risk particularly of postpartum haemorrhage.

Previous termination of pregnancy is usually discussed although it may cause the woman embarrassment or distress. A sympathetic non-judgemental approach is required in order to elicit information and encourage the woman to talk freely about her feelings. Sometimes feelings of guilt or shame are not expressed or resolved at the time of the abortion. This may lead to their suppression, which could interfere with emotional adjustment to the present pregnancy. In rare cases techniques employed in termination may affect the viability of subsequent pregnancies. Dilatation and curettage could contribute to incompetence of the cervix and cases of later uterine rupture have also been cited (see Ch. 29). Any form of abortion occurring in a Rhesus negative woman requires prophylactic administration of anti-D immuno-globulin. If applicable, the woman should be asked if this was administered.

It should be discussed with the woman whether she would prefer any confidential information to be recorded in a clinic-held summary of her pregnancy and not in the record that she will take home with her.

Repeated spontaneous abortion may indicate such conditions as genetic abnormality, hormonal imbalance or incompetent cervix. Diagnosis of the cause often depends on the time at which the abortion occurred. Screening or treatment may be necessary in the present pregnancy. The woman will also be more anxious about the pregnancy and will be relieved when it progresses past the date of previous abortions. She may be overanxious, requiring extra time and support. Minor disturbances in pregnancy may cause her undue worry, and preoccupation with the pregnancy may lead to difficulties in her home life. She will feel reassured if she hears the fetal heart or sees the image of an ultrasound scan and this may also help her partner. He can assist her to assess the normality of her symptoms and encourage confidence.

In order to give a summary of a woman's child-bearing history, the descriptive terms *gravida* and *para* are used.

Gravid means pregnant. Gravida means a pregnant woman; a subsequent number indicates the number of times she has been pregnant regardless of outcome.

Para means having given birth. A woman's parity refers to the number of times that she has given birth to a child, live or still, excluding abortions.

A *grande multigravida* is a woman who has been pregnant five times or more: this tells nothing of outcome.

A *grande multipara* is a woman who has given birth five times or more.

For completeness of the history, reference to old case notes should be made. The woman may not remember everything about past experiences and obstetric or medical detail is sometimes of least importance to her. It should be remembered that this is a very good reason always to involve the woman in the process of her care and wherever possible avoid the use of medical jargon both in conversation with the woman and when recording information in her records. The fact that labour was augmented with Syntocinon or that the woman required two injections after the birth of the baby may not be of significance to her but to the midwife such facts will indicate that there may have been inefficient uterine action or a post-partum haemorrhage.

Complications in previous childbearing may be relevant to the present pregnancy. High-risk factors listed in Box 13.2 will determine the frequency of antenatal visits and alert staff to appropriate screening techniques. The place of antenatal care will be determined by the availability of support services, senior obstetric staff and experienced midwives. Place of birth will also be influenced by these criteria but in all cases the ultimate decision is taken by the mother who must be involved in making the decision.

Medical history

Medical conditions also influence pregnancy. These range from the severe cardiac conditions to the more common but important urinary tract infection (UTI). During pregnancy both the mother and the fetus may be affected.

• Urinary stasis and reflux occur during pregnancy. A urinary tract infection (UTI) can easily develop into pyelonephritis which may lead to premature labour.

• Pregnancy predisposes to deep vein thrombosis and pulmonary embolism.

• Essential hypertension predisposes to pregnancy-induced hypertension (PIH) which results in reduced placental function, fetal intrauterine growth retardation, fetal compromise, possible antepartum haemorrhage.

• Asthma, epilepsy, infections, psychiatric disorders and so on require drug treatment which may affect early fetal development.

Major medical complications such as diabetes and cardiac conditions require the involvement and support of a medical specialist (see Ch. 16).

Family history

Certain conditions are genetic in origin, others are familial or have racial characteristics and some occur because of the social environment in which the family lives.

Genetic disease in the baby is much more likely to occur if his biological parents are close relatives such as first cousins.

It is known that diabetes, although not genetically inherited, leads to a predisposition in other family members, particularly if they become pregnant or obese. Hypertension also has a familial component. Multiple pregnancy has a higher incidence in certain families and races.

Examples of conditions which are common in particular races are spina bifida, sickle cell anaemia and thalassaemia.

It was suggested as long ago as 1965 that there may have been a possible link between fetal malformation and insufficient intake of folic acid (Hibbard & Smithells 1965). It is now known that supplementation of folic acid reduces the incidence of fetal neural tube defects by up to 70%. For this reason the Department of Health recommends that women increase their folate supplement before conception and in the first trimester of pregnancy (McLeod et al 1996).

Box 13.2 Factors that require additional antenatal surveillance or advice

Box 13.2 Factors that require additional antenatal surveillance or advice

Initial assessment
Age less than 18 years or over 35 years
Grande multiparity (more than four previous births)
Vaginal bleeding at any time during pregnancy
Unknown or uncertain EDD

Past obstetric history
Stillbirth or neonatal death
Baby small or large for gestational age
Congenital abnormality
Rhesus isoimmunisation
Pregnancy-induced hypertension
Two or more terminations of pregnancy
Two or more spontaneous abortions
Previous preterm labour
Cervical cerclage in past or present pregnancy
Previous caesarean section or uterine surgery
Ante- or postpartum haemorrhage
Precipitate labour

Maternal health
Previous history of deep vein thrombosis or pulmonary embolism
Chronic illness
Hypertension
History of infertility
Uterine anomaly including fibroids
Smoking
Family history of diabetes

Examination at the initial assessment
Blood pressure 140/90 or above
Maternal weight over 85 kg or less than 45 kg (the latter may depend on racial origin)
Maternal height less than 5 feet (150 cm or less)
Cardiac murmur detected
Other pelvic mass detected
Rhesus negative blood group
Blood disorders

Tuberculosis is more common in living conditions which are poor and cramped, where it spreads easily.

PHYSICAL EXAMINATION

Screening procedures play an important part in ascertaining normality. Clinical observation such as height, weight and abdominal examination can be enhanced by sophisticated biochemical assessments and ultrasound investigations.

Height of over 160 cm is indication of a normal-sized pelvis. Some authorities believe shoe size to be significant whilst others identify stature as of greater importance (Frame et al 1985, Mahmood et al 1988). Factors which may be thought to affect the fetal size include the genetic contribution of the father but this only has a modest influence; the mother tends to grow a fetus to suit her pelvis.

A woman who is short in stature may come from a small-sized race or family or she may be stunted because of poor nutrition in utero or in childhood.

At about 36 weeks' gestation when the fetus is almost fully grown the pelvic size is reassessed. The fetal head is an excellent pelvimeter and if it will engage in the pelvic brim there is little cause for concern about cephalopelvic disproportion.

Weight. Obesity is associated with an increased risk of gestational diabetes and PIH.

To be accurate, weight should always be measured using the same scales and the woman asked to wear similar clothing each time she is weighed. Women may record their own weight at home, without clothes, in order to overcome these problems.

Blood pressure is taken in order to ascertain normality and provide a baseline reading for comparison throughout pregnancy. It may be falsely elevated if a woman is nervous or anxious; long waiting times can cause additional stress. If this is the case it is good practice to recheck the blood pressure when the woman is more relaxed, remembering that she should always be in the same position to ensure a comparable reading. Brachial artery pressure is highest when she is sitting and lower when she is in the recumbent position. An adequate blood pressure is required to maintain placental perfusion but systolic blood pressure of 140 mmHg or diastolic pressure of 90 mmHg at booking is indicative of hypertension and could cause damage to the placenta.

It has, until recently, been the convention to record the Korotkoff 4 (K4) sound (muffled, fading sound) for the diastolic pressure in pregnant women in the belief that the K5 (absence of sound) is not always present (Herbert & Alison 1996). However, in a recent study involving 85 pregnant women to compare the accuracy of recording K4 compared with K5, K4 was heard in fewer than half of measurements compared with K5, which was identified in all measurements. Listening for Korotkoff 5 in pregnancy was therefore recommended except in rare cases when it is absent (Shennan et al 1996). Steps that can be taken to increase accuracy of blood pressure measurement and recording are listed in Box 13.3.

Urinalysis is performed to exclude abnormality. At the first visit a midstream specimen is sent to the laboratory for culture to exclude asymptomatic bacilluria. This condition exists when a culture is grown of a specific bacterium that exceeds 10^6 organisms per ml urine. As it is symptomless the woman is unaware of disease. Pyelonephritis can readily develop because of the changes in the renal tract during pregnancy.

Other possible findings during subsequent routine urinalysis include:

- ketones due to increased maternal metabolism caused by fetal need or because of vomiting
- glucose caused by higher circulating blood levels, reduced renal threshold or disease
- protein due to contamination by vaginal leucorrhoea, or disease such as UTI or PIH.

See Chapters 16 and 17 for further information.

Blood tests taken at the initial assessment determine *ABO blood group* and *Rhesus (Rh) factor*. Antibody screening is performed followed by titration if present. Normal follow-up of a woman whose blood group is Rh negative will include further blood samples at 28, 32, 36 and 40 weeks, to ensure that the pregnancy is not stimulating antibody activity. Rhesus negative women who have threatened miscarriage, amniocentesis or any other uterine trauma should have anti-D gammaglobulin within a few days of the event. If the titration demonstrates a rising antibody response, more frequent assessment will be made in order to plan management by a specialist in Rhesus disease (see Ch. 42).

Haemoglobin (Hb) estimations are performed (see Ch. 11 for normal values), and in some areas ferritin levels are also taken in order to assess the adequacy of iron stores. Haemoglobin estimation is repeated at 28 weeks when the physiological effects of haemodilution are becoming more apparent and at 36 weeks to ensure that any anaemia is treated prior to birth. Iron supplementation is not considered necessary in women who are taking adequate dietary iron and who have a normal Hb at initial assessment. If necessary, the decision to use supplements should be made on an individual basis and not as a policy decision. Gastrointestinal upsets are common as a result of oral iron and many women find tablets unpleasant. If the woman is vegetarian, fasting for cultural reasons or has an aversion to foods that contain iron, the iron content of the diet should be determined. Frequent conceptions and breast feeding may deplete iron stores and necessitate replacement.

Iron tablets should be taken with meals to reduce gastrointestinal symptoms. If more than one tablet is necessary, they should be taken separately, one in the morning and one in the evening. Maximum absorption will be achieved by divided dosage and adequate intake of vitamin C. The intestinal mucosa have a limited ability to absorb iron and when this is exceeded extra iron is excreted in the stools.

Venereal Disease Research Laboratory (VDRL) test for syphilis is still performed despite this being a rare disease these days. Not all positive results indicate active syphilis. Early testing will allow a woman to be treated in order to prevent infection of the fetus (see Ch. 18).

Human immunodeficiency virus (HIV) antibodies. Routine screening to detect HIV infection is still controversial. There are many views as to the ethical issues involved in screening (see Ch. 18). It is important to gain informed consent for any blood tests undertaken and offer appropriate counselling before the screening is carried out.

Rubella immune status is determined by measuring the rubella antibody titre. Women who are not immune must be advised to avoid contact with anyone suffering from the disease and may be offered termination of pregnancy if they have been exposed. Vaccination is offered during the puerperium and subsequent pregnancy must be avoided for at least 3 months.

Other blood disorders may be sought in members of certain ethnic groups. In some areas testing may be done to screen for sickle cell disease or thalassaemia. If a woman either has or is a carrier of one of these diseases her partner's blood should also be tested. The couple will be given genetic counselling and management during pregnancy will be explained (see Ch. 16).

Routine screening for hepatitis is becoming more common and it may soon be recommended that all pregnant women be screened routinely for the disease. Screening tests for cytomegalovirus and toxoplasmosis are not routinely done in pregnancy. In view of the low prevalence of toxoplasmosis, a health education programme may be more effective in further reducing the incidence (Wang & Smaill 1989).

Screening for fetal abnormality. Details of this programme are given in Chapter 20.

Midwife's examination

Most of the midwife's examination is performed by exchange of information between the woman and herself rather than physical examination. Communication will be more effective if for most of the time the woman is sitting in a comfortable position, feeling that she has the attention of the midwife.

At the *initial assessment* visit certain aspects of the examination will be more relevant than others but the midwife will explain to the woman what she will be looking for at different stages in the pregnancy.

The midwife's general examination of the woman should follow an orderly direction; for example she may start by looking at the woman's face and then progress downwards to finish with an inspection of her legs and feet. The order should be planned so that after the initial discussion, the woman moves from chair to couch for examination. She should then be invited to return to her chair and asked if she has any final questions.

General appearance. The usual social contact gives the midwife opportunity to look at the woman's face and assess her health. Her general manner will indicate vigour and vitality. Women who are anaemic, depressed, tired or ill appear lethargic, are not interested in their appearance and are likely to be unenthusiastic about the assessment.

Lack of energy may be a temporary state. Early pregnancy is particularly tiring as the fetus is growing at its fastest. A woman often feels exhausted and morning or evening sickness may leave her debilitated. Her sleeping pattern should be discussed and advice given as necessary. If she has other young children, they require constant attention and energy and the midwife should help the mother to find ways of sharing the child care responsibility. Perhaps she could involve a relative or a neighbour or join a playgroup scheme to allow her to rest during the day. Working women are unlikely to be able to rest during the day and many need to sleep as soon as they return home. Most men are now ready to take a greater share in household tasks. The midwife should encourage the mother to accept support from her partner.

Minor disorders of pregnancy may be a nuisance; Chapter 12 discusses these and suggests remedies.

If at any time the midwife notices any sign of ill health she should pass this information on to her obstetric colleagues.

Breast examination may be linked to the discussion of infant feeding which will take place at this visit. Breast feeding should be promoted in a sensitive manner and information given about the benefits to both mother and baby (see Ch. 36). Whether or not a woman wishes to breast feed, the midwife should ask permission to examine the breasts. A woman may feel embarrassed at the prospect and the midwife must be aware of her feelings and gain her cooperation. The breast should be gently palpated with the flat of the hand to feel for any lumps. The nipple should be drawn forward to see if it is protractile; the woman may prefer to do this herself. This may be an appropriate opportunity to demonstrate to the woman how to carry out breast examination herself and it is a good lifelong skill for her to acquire. The midwife will observe the changes due to pregnancy and note the evidence of hormonal activity.

The woman will appreciate information about the changes taking place in her body. Some are distressed by the increase in breast size, others by the obvious large blue veins that are appearing or the increase in areola size. Increasing abdominal size may be an acceptable body change but breast changes may not have been anticipated. For some women breast size and appearance are an important part of their body image (see Ch. 2). Partners may also regret the changes. Unless psychological adjustment is made, the woman may feel that she is no longer attractive, which could lead to strain in the relationship. The midwife has a responsibility to counsel the woman who had not realised the extent to which pregnancy would change her body. It may be that she only imagines her partner to be unattracted. Honest discussion between the woman and her partner and reassurance that these changes will reverse in the puerperium may help to resolve anxieties. A good relationship in which the couple feel able to share anxieties and fears will minimise the difficulties in making the transition to motherhood.

Elimination should be discussed at every visit. During the initial assessment the midwife should ask the woman about her normal bowel habit. Dietary advice may be necessary at this visit or later in the pregnancy when hormonal changes may alter normal function. Oral iron supplementation during pregnancy may cause changes in bowel movement.

Routine urinalysis is carried out at every visit. Frequency of micturition is common in early pregnancy and recurs during late pregnancy. The midwife should enquire about the presence of any dysuria that the woman may be experiencing and alert her obstetric colleagues to it.

Vaginal discharge increases in pregnancy. The woman should be asked during the initial assessment if she has noticed any increase or changes. Once the woman has identified what is normal she will then be able to report any changes to the midwife during subsequent visits. If the discharge is itchy, causes soreness, is any colour other than creamy-white or has an offensive odour, infection must be suspected and investigated.

Later in pregnancy the woman may report a change from leucorrhoea to a discharge which has the colour and consistency of egg white. It may be tinged with blood. Mucoid loss is evidence of cervical changes and if it occurs before the 37th week of pregnancy should be reported to the obstetrician.

Vaginal bleeding at any time during the pregnancy should be reported to the obstetrician who will investigate its origin. In early pregnancy spotting may occur at the time when menstruation would have been due. Women who have suffered miscarriage in the past will be particularly worried. Early bleeding is not uncommon; the midwife should advise the woman to rest at this time and avoid sexual intercourse until the pregnancy is more stable.

Abdominal examination should be performed at each physical examination. At the initial assessment the midwife will observe for signs of pregnancy. It is unlikely that the uterus will be palpable abdominally before the 12th week of gestation. If previously it has been retroverted it may not be palpable until the 16th week. See below for a description of the method of examination and an explanation of findings.

Oedema is not likely to be in evidence during the initial assessment but occurs as the pregnancy progresses. A degree of oedema is normal and correlates with a healthy outcome to the pregnancy. The midwife must ensure that the observed oedema is physiological and not excessive. This could be associated with pregnancy-induced hypertension. Physiological oedema occurs after rising in the morning and worsens during the day; it is often associated with daily activities or hot weather. At visits later in pregnancy the midwife should ask the woman if she has noticed any swelling.

Often the woman has noticed that her rings feel tighter and her ankles are swollen. The midwife should test for pitting oedema in the lower limbs by applying fingertip pressure for 10 seconds over the tibial bone. If pitting oedema is present a depression will remain when she removes her finger. Pitting oedema that reaches the knee should be reported to the obstetrician.

Varicosities are more likely to occur during pregnancy and are a predisposing cause of deep vein thrombosis. The legs should be examined at every visit and any abnormality discovered must be reported to the doctor. The woman should be asked to remove her trousers, thick tights and footwear to allow the midwife to make a thorough examination of her legs. It is often easier if the woman stands up for this examination because both the back and front of the legs can be visualised. The midwife should inspect the legs for varicosities and record their position and condition. This will enable comparison to be made at future visits. Advice about support stockings is given as appropriate. The midwife also observes for reddened areas of the calf which may be caused by phlebitis. Areas that appear white as if deprived of blood could be caused by deep vein thrombosis. The midwife, using the whole of her cupped hand, feels gently along the length of the calf to assess normal warmth of the leg and to exclude irregularity in the shape of the calf. The woman should be asked to report any tenderness that she feels either during the examination or at any time during the pregnancy.

Medical examination

Many doctors still perform this examination as they see it as an opportunity to ascertain health, using screening tests.

Heart and lungs are examined to exclude disease. A soft systolic murmur is heard in 50% of pregnant women but all other abnormality would be referred for the physician's opinion.

A vaginal examination is sometimes performed. A Papanicolaou smear may be taken for cervical cytology, any cervical erosion would be noted and the examination would also exclude abnormality of the genital tract and pelvic masses.

Some practitioners order ultrasound scans to confirm the gestational age of the fetus.

ABDOMINAL EXAMINATION

Aims of abdominal examination

Women do not always appreciate the importance of attending for regular examination but the skilful midwife will be able to explain that the chief aim is to establish and affirm the normal, especially as the pregnancy progresses. The specific aims are:

- to observe signs of pregnancy
- to assess fetal size and growth
- to assess fetal health
- to diagnose the location of fetal parts
- to detect any deviation from normal.

Preparation

The general examination will have been conducted with the mother sitting or standing but during the abdominal examination she must lie on the couch. It is difficult to ask questions while lying in this position and the midwife must explain her findings fully when the woman is sitting up again. The midwife should ensure that the woman has emptied her bladder within 30 minutes before abdominal palpation. Not only will this aid comfort but measurement of fundal height will be more accurate. It is unnecessary for the woman to undress completely as long as her clothes are loose enough to allow access to the abdomen. Modesty is an important aspect of Islam and women of this faith will wish to keep their arms and legs covered. All women appreciate privacy and respect of their feelings by minimising exposure. The woman should be lying comfortably with her arms by her sides.

Method

Inspection

The size of the uterus is assessed roughly by eye. A distended colon or obesity may give a false impression. Multiple pregnancy or polyhydramnios will enlarge both the length and breadth of the uterus whereas a large baby increases only the length.

The shape of the uterus is longer than it is broad when the lie of the fetus is longitudinal as occurs in 99.5% of cases. If the lie of the fetus is transverse, the uterus is low and broad.

The multiparous uterus lacks the snug ovoid shape of the primigravid uterus.

Occasionally it is possible to see the shape of the fetal back or limbs. In posterior positions of the occiput a saucer-like depression is seen at or below the umbilicus.

Fetal movement is evidence of fetal life and aids in the diagnosis of position.

Contour of the abdominal wall.   A full bladder may be visible and is more obvious in the later weeks of pregnancy. The umbilicus becomes less dimpled as pregnancy advances and may protrude slightly in later weeks.

When the woman is erect, lightening may be evident (see Ch. 11).

Lax abdominal muscles in the multiparous woman may allow the uterus to sag forwards: this is known as *pendulous abdomen* or anterior obliquity of the uterus. In the primigravida it is a serious sign as it may be due to pelvic contraction.

Skin changes.   The condition of the skin is noted. Any stretch marks are observed. A linea nigra may be seen. This is a dark line of pigmentation running longitudinally in the centre of the abdomen below and sometimes above the umbilicus. Explanation may be needed if the woman is concerned. A line of hair in the same position should alert the midwife to the possibility of an android pelvis.

Scars may indicate previous obstetric or abdominal surgery.

Palpation

The hands should be clean and warm: cold hands do not have the necessary acute sense of touch; they tend to induce contraction of the abdominal and uterine muscles and the mother resents the discomfort of them. Arms and hands should be relaxed and the pads, not the tips, of the fingers used with delicate precision. The hands are moved smoothly over the abdomen in a stroking motion in order to avoid causing contractions.

Estimating the period of gestation.   The following method of assessing the period of gestation does not always produce an accurate result because the size and number of fetuses and the amount of amniotic fluid vary. Variations in maternal size and parity may also affect the estimation.

In order to determine the height of the fundus the midwife places her hand just below the xiphisternum. Pressing gently, she moves her hand down the abdomen until she feels the curved upper border of the fundus. She notes the number of finger breadths which can be comfortably accommodated between the two (see Fig. 13.1). An alternative and increasingly popular method is to measure the distance of the fundus from the symphysis pubis using a tape measure. This is plotted on a chart which gives average findings for gestational age – a symphysis–fundal height chart. The height of the fundus correlates well with gestational age, especially during the earlier weeks of pregnancy (see below).

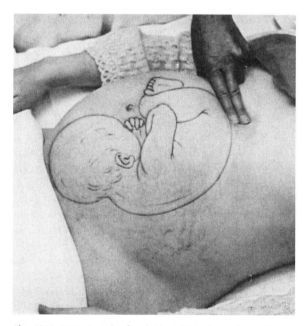

Fig. 13.1 Assessing the fundal height in finger breadths below the xiphisternum.

The overall size of the uterus must be considered along with the height of the fundus. If the uterus is unduly big, the fetus may be large but multiple pregnancy or polyhydramnios may be suspected. When the uterus is smaller than expected, the most likely explanation is that the woman is mistaken in the date of her last menstrual period but retarded intrauterine growth may be suspected. The experienced midwife will be able to estimate the size of the fetus itself, judging by the size of the head and fetal parts.

Fundal palpation is carried out in order to determine whether it contains the breech or the head. This information will help to diagnose the lie and presentation of the fetus.

Watching the woman's reaction to the procedure, the midwife lays both hands on the sides of the fundus, fingers held close together and curving round the upper border of the uterus. Gentle yet deliberate pressure is applied using the palmar surfaces of the fingers to determine the soft consistency and indefinite outline that denotes the breech. Sometimes the buttocks feel rather firm but they are not as hard, smooth or well defined as the head. With a gliding movement the fingertips are separated slightly in order to grasp the fetal mass, which may be in the centre or deflected to one side, and to assess its size and mobility. The breech cannot be moved independently of the body as can the head (see Fig. 13.2).

The head is much more distinctive in outline, being hard and round; it can be ballotted between the fingertips of the two hands because of the free movement of the neck.

Lateral palpation is used to locate the fetal back in order to determine position. The hands are placed on either side of the uterus at about umbilical level (see Fig. 13.3). Gentle pressure is applied with alternate hands in order to detect which side of the uterus offers the greater resistance. More detailed information is obtained by feeling along the length of each side with the fingers. This can be done by sliding the hands down the abdomen while feeling the sides of the uterus alternately. Some midwives prefer to steady the uterus with one hand and, using a rotary movement of the

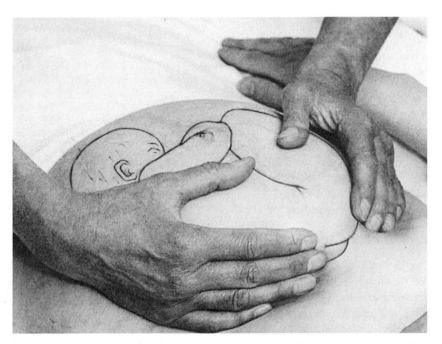

Fig. 13.2 Fundal palpation. Palms of hands on either side of the fundus, fingers held close together palpate the upper pole of the uterus.

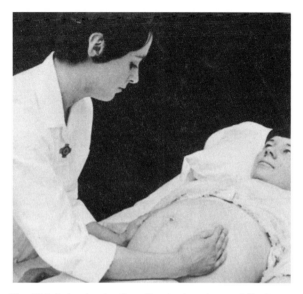

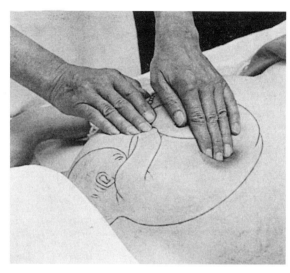

Fig. 13.4 'Walking' the fingertips across the abdomen to locate the position of the fetal back.

Fig. 13.3 Lateral palpation. Hands placed at umbilical level on either side of the uterus. Pressure is applied alternately with each hand.

opposite hand, to map out the back as a continuous smooth resistant mass from the breech down to the neck; on the other side the same movement reveals the limbs as small parts that slip about under the examining fingers.

'Walking' the fingertips of both hands over the abdomen from one side to the other is an excellent method of locating the back (see Fig. 13.4). The fingers should be dipped into the abdominal wall fairly deeply. The firm back can be distinguished from the fluctuating amniotic fluid and the receding knobbly small parts. To make the back more prominent, fundal pressure can be applied with one hand and the other used to 'walk' over the abdomen.

The anterior shoulder can be located by palpating from the neck upwards and inwards. Its height will vary with the station of the head.

Pelvic palpation.   Palpation of the lower pole of the uterus just above the pelvis should not cause discomfort to the woman.

The midwife should ask the woman to bend her knees slightly in order to relax the abdominal muscles and suggest that she breathes steadily through an open mouth. Relaxation may be helped

if she sighs out slowly. The sides of the uterus just below umbilical level are grasped snugly between the palms of the hands with the fingers, held close together, pointing downwards and inwards (see Fig. 13.5).

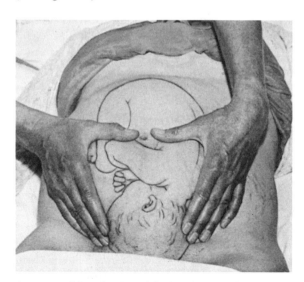

Fig. 13.5 Pelvic palpation. If the hands are in the correct position, the outstretched thumbs will meet at about umbilical level. The fingers are directed inwards and downwards.

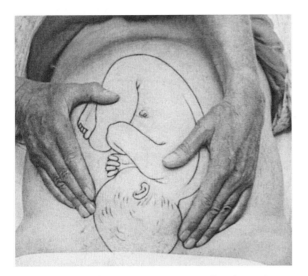

Fig. 13.6 Method of pelvic palpation used to determine position in a vertex presentation. The higher cephalic prominence (the sinciput) will be on the side opposite to the back.

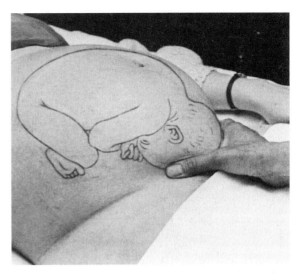

Fig. 13.7 Pawlik's manoeuvre. The lower pole of the uterus is grasped with the right hand, the midwife facing the woman's head.

If the head is presenting, a hard mass with a distinctive round, smooth surface will be felt. In order to determine if the vertex is presenting, the occipital and sincipital prominences are located (see Fig. 13.6). If the head is well flexed the sinciput will be felt on the opposite side from the back and higher than the occiput. If the head is deflexed the prominences are on the same level. If the head is extended as in a face presentation the bulk of the head is felt on the same side as the back. The midwife will also estimate how much of the fetal head is palpable above the pelvic brim.

The two-handed grip is favoured because it is the most comfortable for the woman and gives the most information. *Pawlik's manoeuvre* is sometimes used to judge the size, flexion and mobility of the head but the midwife must be careful not to apply undue pressure. The midwife grasps the lower pole of the uterus between her fingers and thumb which should be spread wide enough apart to accommodate the fetal head (see Fig. 13.7).

Auscultation

Auscultation usually forms part of each abdominal examination and follows any procedure in order to assess fetal well-being. The sound may be simulated by tapping the fingers together very close to one's ear. Like all heart beats it is a double sound but more rapid than the adult heart. Pinard's fetal stethoscope is commonly used to hear the fetal heart. It is placed on the mother's abdomen and at right angles to it (see Fig. 13.8). The ear must be in close, firm contact with the stethoscope but the hand should not touch it while listening because extraneous sounds are produced. The stethoscope should be moved about until the point of maximum intensity is located where the fetal heart is heard most clearly. Increasingly, ultrasound equipment is used for this purpose so that the woman may also hear the fetal heartbeat.

Findings

No single piece of information should ever be considered in isolation from other findings. The

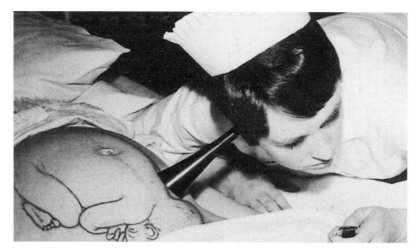

Fig. 13.8 Auscultation of the fetal heart. Vertex left occipitoanterior.

midwife, in making her diagnosis, assesses all the information which she has gathered from inspection, palpation and auscultation and draws the one conclusion which accounts for all of the factors. If one fact does not fit in with the rest she must think again.

Gestational age

During pregnancy the uterus is expected to grow at a predicted rate and in early pregnancy uterine size will usually equate with the gestation estimated by dates (see Fig. 13.9). Later in pregnancy, increasing uterine size gives evidence of continuing fetal growth but is less reliable as an indicator of gestational age.

Multiple pregnancy increases the overall uterine size and should be diagnosed by 24 weeks' gestation. In a singleton pregnancy the fundus reaches the umbilicus at 22–24 weeks and the xiphisternum at 36 weeks. In the last month of pregnancy lightening occurs and the fetus sinks down into the lower pole of the uterus. The uterus becomes broader and the fundus lower. In the primigravida strong abdominal muscles encourage the fetal head to enter the brim of the pelvis.

Lie

The lie of the fetus is the relationship between the long axis of the fetus and the long axis of the

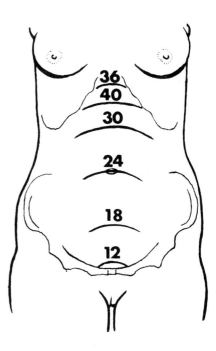

Fig. 13.9 Growth of the uterus, showing the fundal heights at various weeks of pregnancy.

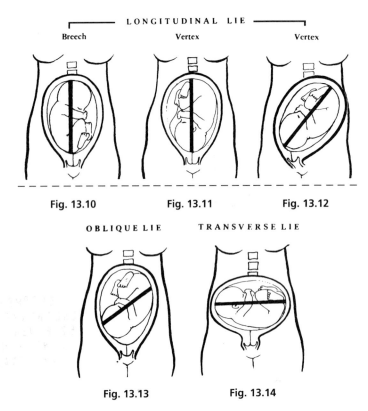

LONGITUDINAL LIE

Breech   Vertex   Vertex

Fig. 13.10   Fig. 13.11   Fig. 13.12

OBLIQUE LIE   TRANSVERSE LIE

Fig. 13.13   Fig. 13.14

Figs 13.10–13.14 The fetal lie.
Figures 13.10, 13.11 and 13.12 depict the longitudinal lie. Confusion sometimes exists regarding Figure 13.12 which gives the impression of an oblique lie, but the fetus is longitudinal in relation to the uterus and merely moving the uterus abdominally rectifies the presumed obliquity.
Figure 13.13 shows an oblique lie because the long axis of the fetus is oblique in relation to the uterus.
Figure 13.14 shows the true transverse lie with shoulder presentation.

uterus (see Figs 13.10–13.14). In 99.5% of cases the lie is longitudinal owing to the ovoid shape of the uterus; the remainder are oblique or transverse. Oblique lie, when the fetus lies diagonally across the long axis of the uterus, must be distinguished from obliquity of the uterus, when the whole uterus is tilted to one side (usually the right) and the fetus lies longitudinally within it. When the lie is transverse the fetus lies at right angles across the long axis of the uterus. This is often visible on inspection of the abdomen.

Attitude

Attitude is the relationship of the fetal head and limbs to its trunk. The attitude should be one of flexion. The fetus is curled up with chin on chest and arms and legs flexed, forming a snug, compact mass which accommodates itself to the uterine cavity. Flexion of the fetal head enables the smallest diameters to present to the pelvis and results in an easier labour.

Presentation

Presentation refers to the part of the fetus which lies at the pelvic brim or in the lower pole of the uterus. There are five presentations (see Figs 13.15–13.20). The approximate incidence of each presentation is given below:

- vertex 96.8%
- breech 2.5%

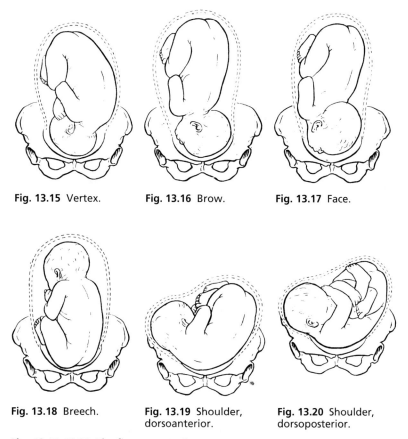

Fig. 13.15 Vertex.   **Fig. 13.16** Brow.   **Fig. 13.17** Face.

Fig. 13.18 Breech.   **Fig. 13.19** Shoulder, dorsoanterior.   **Fig. 13.20** Shoulder, dorsoposterior.

Figs 13.15–13.20 The five presentations.

- shoulder 0.4% (1 in 250)
- face 0.2% (1 in 500)
- brow 0.1% (1 in 1000).

Vertex, face and brow are all head or cephalic presentations. When the head is flexed the vertex presents; when it is fully extended the face presents and when partially extended the brow presents (see Figs 13.21–13.24). It is more common for the head to present because the bulky breech finds more space in the fundus which is the widest diameter of the uterus and the head lies in the narrower lower pole. The muscle tone of the fetus also plays a part in maintaining its flexion and consequently its vertex presentation.

Denominator

Denominate means to give a name to; the denominator is the name of the part of the presentation which is used when referring to fetal position. Each presentation has a different denominator and these are as follows:

- in the vertex presentation it is the occiput
- in the breech presentation it is the sacrum
- in the face presentation it is the mentum.

Although the shoulder presentation is said to have the acromion process as its denominator, in practice the dorsum is used to describe the position. In the brow presentation no denominator is used.

Position

Position is the relationship between the denominator of the presentation and six points on the pelvic brim (see Fig. 13.25). In addition, the denominator may be found in the midline either anteriorly

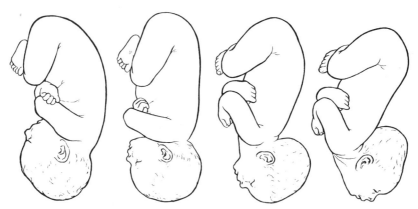

Fig. 13.21 Vertex (well-flexed head). **Fig. 13.22** Vertex (deflexed head). **Fig. 13.23** Brow. **Fig. 13.24** Face.

Figs 13.21–13.24 Varieties of cephalic or head presentation.

or posteriorly, especially late in labour. This position is often transient and is described as direct anterior or direct posterior.

Anterior positions are more favourable than posterior positions because when the fetal back is in front it conforms to the concavity of the mother's abdominal wall and can therefore flex better. When the back is flexed, the head also tends to flex and a smaller diameter presents to the pelvic brim. There is also more room in the anterior part of the pelvic brim for the broad biparietal diameter of the head.

Positions in a vertex presentation are summarised in Box 13.4.

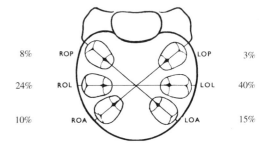

Fig. 13.25 Diagrammatic representation of the six vertex positions and their relative frequency: LOA = left occipitoanterior; LOL = left occipitolateral; LOP = left occipitoposterior; ROA = right occipitoanterior; ROL = right occipitolateral; ROP = right occipitoposterior.

Box 13.4 Positions in a vertex presentation

Left occipitoanterior (LOA). The occiput points to the left iliopectineal eminence; the sagittal suture is in the right oblique diameter of the pelvis (Fig. 13.26).

Right occipitoanterior (ROA). The occiput points to the right iliopectineal eminence; the sagittal suture is in the left oblique diameter of the pelvis (Fig. 13.27).

Left occipitolateral (LOL). The occiput points to the left iliopectineal line midway between the iliopectineal eminence and the sacroiliac joint; the sagittal suture is in the transverse diameter of the pelvis (Fig. 13.28).

Right occipitolateral (ROL). The occiput points to the right iliopectineal line midway between the iliopectineal eminence and the sacroiliac joint; the sagittal suture is in the transverse diameter of the pelvis (Fig. 13.29).

Left occipitoposterior (LOP). The occiput points to the left sacroiliac joint; the sagittal suture is in the left oblique diameter of the pelvis (Fig. 13.30).

Right occipitoposterior (ROP). The occiput points to the right sacroiliac joint; the sagittal suture is in the right oblique diameter of the pelvis (Fig. 13.31).

Direct occipitoanterior (DOA). The occiput points to the symphysis pubis; the sagittal suture is in the anteroposterior diameter of the pelvis.

Direct occipitoposterior (DOP). The occiput points to the sacrum; the sagittal suture is in the anteroposterior diameter of the pelvis.

In breech and face presentations the positions are described in a similar way using the appropriate denominator.

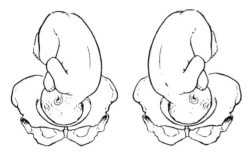

Fig. 13.26 Left occipitoanterior.

Fig. 13.27 Right occipitoanterior.

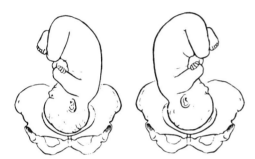

Fig. 13.28 Left occipitolateral.

Fig. 13.29 Right occipitolateral.

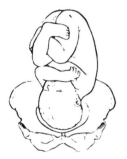
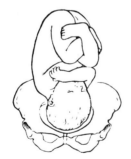

Fig. 13.30 Left occipitoposterior.

Fig. 13.31 Right occipitoposterior.

Figs 13.26–13.31 Six positions in vertex presentation.

Engagement

Engagement is said to have occurred when the widest presenting transverse diameter has passed through the brim of the pelvis. In head presentations this is the biparietal diameter and in breech presentations the bitrochanteric diameter. Engagement is an important sign that the maternal pelvis is likely to be adequate for the size of the particular fetus and that a vaginal delivery may be expected.

In a primigravid woman the head normally engages between about the 36th and 38th week of pregnancy but in a multipara this may not occur until after the onset of labour. When the vertex presents and the head is engaged the following will be evident on clinical examination:

- less than half of the fetal head is palpable above the pelvic brim (see Fig. 13.32)
- the head is not mobile
- the sinciput is felt less than 5 cm above the brim
- the anterior shoulder is little more than 5 cm above the brim.

On rare occasions the head is not palpable abdominally because it has descended deeply into the pelvis.

If the head is not engaged, the findings are as follows:

- more than half of the head is palpable above the brim
- the head may be high and freely movable but it can also be partly settled in the pelvic brim and consequently *immobile*
- the sinciput may be 7.5 cm above the brim.

If the head remains unengaged in a primigravid woman at 38 weeks, the possibility of cephalo-pelvic disproportion should be borne in mind. The midwife will refer the woman to the obstetrician who may assess the pelvis clinically, taking the size of the fetal head into account.

Assessment of pelvic capacity

The size of the obstetric conjugate can be estimated by measuring the diagonal conjugate per vaginam.

The diagonal conjugate is measured from the lower border of the symphysis pubis to the centre of the promontory of the sacrum. This is usually 12–13 cm, approximately 2 cm longer than the measurement of the obstetric conjugate. The examination is usually carried out after the 36th week of pregnancy when the vagina and pelvic floor are softer and maximum pelvic joint relaxation has occurred, making the procedure less uncomfortable.

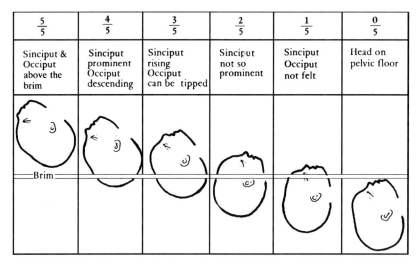

$\frac{5}{5}$	$\frac{4}{5}$	$\frac{3}{5}$	$\frac{2}{5}$	$\frac{1}{5}$	$\frac{0}{5}$
Sinciput & Occiput above the brim	Sinciput prominent Occiput descending	Sinciput rising Occiput can be tipped	Sinciput not so prominent	Sinciput Occiput not felt	Head on pelvic floor

Fig. 13.32 Descent of the fetal head estimated in fifths palpable above the pelvic brim.

Method. The woman should be given the opportunity to empty her bladder. She then lies in the dorsal position with her knees drawn up. Cleanliness is maintained and modesty observed. The first two fingers of the gloved hand are lubricated with obstetric cream and inserted into the vagina. An effort is made to reach the sacral promontory although only the long-fingered will be able to contact it. If bone is encountered, the fingers should be directed further upwards. No bone is felt above the promontory because the fifth lumbar vertebra recedes.

The point where the examining hand is in contact with the lower border of the symphysis pubis is marked by the forefinger of the other hand and after withdrawal the distance between that point and the tip of the middle finger is measured with a ruler. On subtracting 2 cm, the measurement of the obstetrical conjugate is obtained.

The cavity and outlet can also be assessed. The ischial spines are palpated to see if they are prominent, which would indicate a reduced bispinous diameter. Two fingers are placed in the greater sciatic notch; this will determine whether it is adequate. The curve of the sacrum is noted. Before removing the fingers, the pubic arch is examined to see whether the angle is about 90°. Two fingers can normally be accommodated in the apex of the arch. Finally the distance between the two tuberosities can be gauged by asking the woman to lie on her side and inserting a closed fist between the tuberosities. This is a very rough guide to the anatomical outlet. The amount of maternal tissue and fat will vary as will the size of the individual's fist but one might ascertain whether the outlet is small, average or large.

In the multigravid woman engagement often does not occur until labour has commenced. If, during palpation, it is thought that the present fetus is much larger than previous vaginally delivered babies, further investigations are required.

It is usual to avoid diagnosing cephalopelvic disproportion until either X-ray evidence is unequivocal or until after the onset of labour. The reason for this is that the force of labour contractions encourages flexion and moulding of the fetal head and the relaxed ligaments of the pelvis allow the joints to give. This may be sufficient to allow engagement and descent. Other causes of a non-engaged head at term include:

- occipitoposterior position
- full bladder
- wrongly calculated gestational age
- polyhydramnios
- placenta praevia or other space-occupying lesion

- multiple pregnancy
- pelvic brim inclination of more than 80° as occurs in a high assimilation pelvis.

Presenting part

The presenting part of the fetus is the part which lies over the cervical os during labour and on which the caput succedaneum forms. It should not be confused with presentation.

ONGOING ANTENATAL CARE

It has been stressed that all the information gathered will enable a decision to be made about the subsequent care offered to the pregnant woman and her family.

A woman who has a high number of risk factors identified during the initial assessment visit or who develops complications during pregnancy (see Box 13.5) will be invited to attend for antenatal care at the hospital unless a scheme exists where consultant obstetricians visit community clinics.

The timing and number of visits will depend on the individual (see introduction to this chapter).

New schemes of antenatal care encourage referral to the midwife much earlier in pregnancy. This would help to make the midwife's support and advice far more effective. The frequency of visits could be decided upon between the woman and her attendant with the option of self-referral if necessary between agreed visits. Should any risk factors develop during pregnancy, the woman will be invited to attend more frequently and the planned place of birth will be reviewed.

Options for women with few or no risk factors

- Shared care between midwife and GP with key visits to hospital clinic: birth mostly takes place in hospital.
- Midwife-led care in hospital or community: birth sometimes takes place at home but mostly in hospital.
- Shared care between midwife and GP: birth sometimes takes place at home, in a GP unit attached to the hospital or in the main hospital.
- Shared care between a hospital midwife and senior obstetrician: birth in hospital.
- Care by an independent midwife. The woman's GP will have been informed and have agreed to be involved as necessary. The birth will often be at home.

Purpose of continuing antenatal care

- To continue to observe for maternal health and freedom from infection.
- To assess fetal well-being.
- To ascertain that the fetus has adopted a lie and presentation that will allow vaginal delivery.
- To offer an opportunity to express any fears or worries about pregnancy or labour.
- To ensure that the mother and family are confident to decide when labour has commenced and that they have telephone numbers to use if they wish to seek advice.
- To discuss any views about the conduct of labour and formulate a birth plan if required.

At each visit the midwife will examine the woman, employing the same systematic approach discussed earlier. Some women offer information readily but others will require sensitive questioning.

In order to evaluate the effectiveness of advice or treatment given during a previous visit, good record-keeping is essential. The importance of legible, signed entries in records giving relevant instructions for ongoing care cannot be over-emphasised. This is even more important when the care is being shared between practitioners.

Box 13.5 Risk factors arising during pregnancy

- Fetal movement pattern changed
- Hb lower than 10 g/dl
- Poor weight gain, weight loss
- Proteinuria, glycosuria, bacilluria
- BP systolic of or above 140 mmHg, diastolic of or above 90 mmHg
- Uterus large or small for dates
- Excess or decreased liquor
- Malpresentation
- Head not engaged in primigravid woman by 38 weeks
- Any vaginal bleeding
- Premature labour
- Vaginal infection

In many areas women carry their own pregnancy records, in others the records are used only in the hospital with the woman carrying a short summary of her care. The first indicator of success in the 'Changing Childbirth' report (DH 1993) recommends that all women should be entitled to carry their own notes.

Indicators of fetal well-being

- Increasing maternal weight in association with increasing uterine size compatible with the gestational age of the fetus.
- Fetal movements which follow a regular pattern throughout pregnancy.
- Fetal heart rate which should be between 110 and 150 beats per minute during auscultation.

Eliciting information about recent fetal movement will reassure the mother. Patterns of fetal movements are a reliable sign of fetal well-being. Evidence of at least 10 movements a day is considered acceptable. The midwife would, however, expect that these movements had occurred within a 12-hour period. The period of observation usually starts at 9 a.m. but fetal activity is often greatest during the late evening. If this is normal for a particular fetus, then a period of observation should be identified which includes the time during which the fetus is most active. The same time period should be used each day to allow for comparison. If the fetus is taking progressively longer each day to achieve 10 movements, this indicates that the fetus is becoming compromised in utero. It is imperative that the woman is asked to inform the labour ward if the fetus has not moved 10 times in the 12-hour period or if its pattern of activity changes greatly. She should not wait for the next antenatal appointment or even the next day but ring immediately no matter how late at night. The midwife explains that cardiotocographic monitoring will then be performed to ascertain fetal condition.

Many women believe that it is normal for the fetus to become less active before labour. The midwife can point out that although the type of movement changes because of reduced space, fetal activity should continue throughout pregnancy and labour.

Preparation for labour

During the latter weeks of pregnancy, labour should be discussed. Most hospitals provide a list to remind women what they are likely to need while in hospital. A woman who has decided to give birth at home is visited by her midwife to make final arrangements for the birth (see Ch. 3). In both cases it is important to ensure that women know whom to contact if they are worried or have begun labour.

During pregnancy a birth plan may have been formulated; there should be an opportunity for revision as parents' wishes or original plans may have changed. The midwife should allow time for discussion about the birth plan. She should explain the likely course of labour and the policies adopted by the maternity unit, or any other matters relating to the birth which she feels need clarification. Most parents are agreeable to change when necessary and are often ready to consider alternatives if the need arises. This is all the more likely if they feel that their needs have been fully considered and that they have been well informed and are involved in decision-making. Parents' wishes should be recorded in the case notes so that they are readily available for labour. Finally the midwife should reinforce how to recognise the onset of labour, emphasising the normal pattern of events, with clear instructions about who to contact both in normal labour and if events deviate from the normal.

READER ACTIVITIES

1. During an initial assessment visit, plan an individualised schedule of antenatal care with a woman. Discuss the acceptability of the plan with an experienced midwife.

2. A week after an initial assessment visit, arrange to meet the woman and assess her level of understanding of everything which took place during the assessment. (Often women are

confused by medical jargon and the volume of information given to them at this first visit.)

3. Assessment of fetal size is a skill which requires practice. In order to maximise your practice, try to estimate the weight of the fetus when palpating women near the end of their pregnancies. Check your estimation by visiting the mother and baby after delivery.

It is also very helpful to visit the Special Care Baby Unit in order to visualise the size of babies at earlier gestational ages, but remember that not all preterm babies are the birthweight expected for their gestation.

4. Compose a letter inviting a woman to attend the antenatal clinic or GP surgery for her initial assessment. Assume that she is primigravid and knows nothing about the procedure. Explain in the letter what will happen at this visit and what she should expect. Evaluate the letter by showing it to a woman who has recently attended the booking clinic and ask her how it might be improved upon.

5. Consider a room in your hospital where the initial assessment takes place. List five ways in which it could be made less clinical for the duration of the interview.

6. A woman who is 34 weeks' pregnant requests to give birth to her baby at home. List the reasons why you think this may or may not be possible and then discuss these reasons with an experienced midwife.

USEFUL ADDRESSES

Confidential Enquiry into Stillbirths & Deaths in Infancy (CESDI)
Chiltern Court
188 Baker Street
London NW1 5SD

The Foundation for the Study of Infant Deaths (FSID)
14 Halkin Street
London SW1X 7DP
Tel: 0171 235 0965

The Maternity Alliance
(Educational & Research Trust Registered Charity No. 285804)
45 Beech Street
London EC2P 2LP
Tel: 0171 588 8582

QUIT
Victory House
Tottenham Court Road
London W1P 0HA
Tel: 0171 388 5775
Helpline: 0800 002200 (Quitline)

REFERENCES

Bisson D L, Golding I, MacGillivray P et al 1990 Blood pressure lability. Contemporary Reviews in Obstetrics and Gynaecology 2: 11–15

Blair P, Bensley D, Smith I, Bacon C, Taylor E 1996 Smoking and the sudden infant death syndrome: results from 1993–5 case-control study for confidential enquiry into stillbirths and deaths in infancy. British Medical Journal 313: 195–198

Department of Health 1993 Changing childbirth: report of the expert maternity group. HMSO, London

Frame S, Moore J, Peters A et al 1985 Maternal height as a predictor of pelvic disproportion: an assessment. British Journal of Obstetrics and Gynaecology 92: 1239–1245

Hall M H, Chng P K, MacGillivray I 1980 Is routine antenatal care worth while? Lancet 1: 78–80

Herbert R A, Alison J A 1996 Cardiovascular function. In: Hinchliff S M, Montague S E, Watson R (eds) Physiology for nursing practice, 2nd edn. Baillière Tindall, London

Hibbard E D, Smithells R W 1965 Folic acid metabolism and human embryopathy. Lancet i: 1254–1256

McLeod S, Gillies A, Carter Y, Wilson S 1996 Folic acid: an essential ingredient for making babies? British Journal of Midwifery 4(8): 404–406

Mahmood T A, Campbell D M, Wilson A W 1988 Maternal height, shoe size and outcome of labour in white primigravidas: a prospective study. British Medical Journal 297: 515–517

Ministry of Health 1929 Maternal mortality in childbirth. Antenatal clinics: their conduct and scope. HMSO, London

Oakley A, Rajan L, Grant A 1990 Social support and pregnancy outcome. British Journal of Obstetrics and Gynaecology 97: 155–162

Oakley A, Hickey D, Rajan L 1996 Social support in pregnancy: does it have long term effects? Journal of Reproductive and Infant Psychology 14: 7–22

Shennan A, Gupta M, Halligan A, Taylor D J, de Swiet M 1996 Lack of reproducibility in pregnancy of Korotkoff phase IV as measured by mercury sphygmanometry. Lancet 347: 139–142

Sikorski J, Wilson J, Clement S, Das S, Smeeton N 1996 A randomised controlled trial comparing two schedules of antenatal visits: the antenatal care project. British Medical Journal 312: 546–553

Wang E, Smaill F 1989 Infection in pregnancy. In: Chalmers I, Enkin M, Keirse M (eds) Effective care in pregnancy and childbirth, Oxford University Press, Oxford, vol 1, ch 34, pp 534–564

World Health Organization 1985 Appropriate technology for birth. Lancet 2: 436–437

FURTHER READING

Department of Health 1993 Changing childbirth: report of the expert maternity group. HMSO, London

Methven R 1989 Recording an obstetric history or relating to a pregnant woman? A study of the antenatal booking interview. In: Robinson S, Thomson A (eds) Midwives, research and childbirth. Chapman & Hall, London. Vol 1, ch 3, pp 42–71

QUIT 1996 Helping smokers to quit: a handbook for the practice and community nurse, health visitor and midwife, 2nd edn. Department of Health, London, Tel: 0171 388 5775

14

Abnormalities of early pregnancy

Christine V. Shiers

This chapter deals with conditions that occur within the first 20 weeks of pregnancy. Many of these are potentially life-threatening for the mother, so recognition and prompt treatment is vital for her well-being.

The chapter aims to:

- consider the three main categories of loss in early pregnancy – spontaneous abortion, induced abortion and ectopic pregnancy

- describe hydatidiform mole, which occurs much less frequently but still accounts for the loss of a pregnancy

- emphasise the need for midwives to be able to offer support and care for mothers early in pregnancy

- discuss conditions such as hyperemesis and fibroids, which affect a smaller number of women but can each cause considerable discomfort during pregnancy.

Mothers are encouraged by midwives to seek their professional advice as early as possible in pregnancy. Increased knowledge and understanding of the abnormalities that can occur in early pregnancy will help to improve the quality of midwifery care offered to the mothers at this time.

BLEEDING IN PREGNANCY

Vaginal bleeding during pregnancy is abnormal. It is a cause of concern to mothers, particularly to those who have a previous experience resulting in fetal loss. Any reports of bleeding should be viewed seriously by the midwife. If the woman presents with a history of bleeding in the current pregnancy it is important to establish when it occurred. How much blood was lost, the colour of the loss and whether it was associated with any pain should be noted. If the symptoms have subsided it is important to advise the mother to report any recurrence.

Assessment of the fetal condition will depend on gestation. Ultrasound scanning can confirm viability of the pregnancy before heart sounds are audible or movements felt. In the second trimester use of ultrasound equipment can elicit the heart sounds, and note of fetal movements may also be made.

Implantation bleeding

As the trophoblast erodes the endometrial epithelium and the blastocyst implants, a small vaginal blood loss may be apparent to the mother. It occurs around the time of expected menstruation, and may be mistaken for a period, although lighter. It is of significance if the estimated date of delivery is to be calculated from menstrual history.

Cervical eversion

This condition is commonly and erroneously known as a cervical erosion. The cervix is lined with two distinct cell types. Columnar epithelium lines the cervical canal, reaching the external os. The structure changes abruptly and stratified squamous epithelial cells cover the vaginal aspect of the cervix, and continue along the vagina itself (Fig. 14.1).

High levels of oestrogen encourage the proliferation of columnar epithelial cells, found in the cervical canal. These then occupy a wider area, including the vaginal aspect of the cervix, encroaching on the squamous epithelial cells (metaplasia). The junction between them is everted into the vagina. This eversion, or ectropion as it is more correctly described, is a physiological response to the hormonal changes in pregnancy. Hyperactivity of the endocervical cells increases the quantity of vaginal discharge. As the cells are vascular it may also cause intermittent bloodstained loss, or

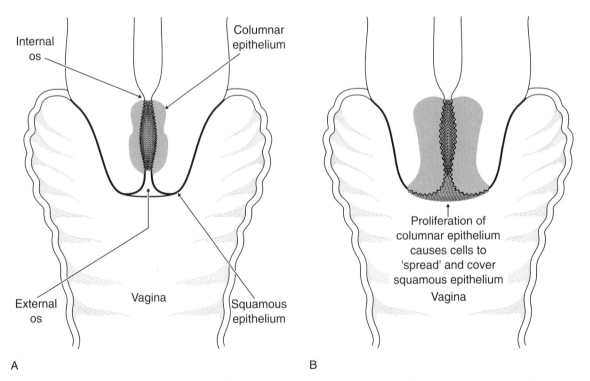

A   B

Fig. 14.1 Cervical eversion: (A) columnar epithelium becomes profuse in pregnancy; (B) cervical eversion caused by growth of columnar epithelial cells, the cervix appears reddened.

spontaneous bleeding. Bleeding following sexual intercourse is common with eversion. The eversion will usually disappear during the puerperium. Normally, eversion requires no treatment in pregnancy.

Cervical polyps

Small, vascular pedunculated growths attached to the cervix may bleed during pregnancy. They can be visualised on speculum examination and no treatment is required during pregnancy, unless bleeding is profuse or a cervical smear suggests malignancy.

Carcinoma of the cervix

Carcinoma of the cervix is the most frequently diagnosed cancer in pregnancy. It is a treatable condition if detected early and 80% of cases detected in pregnancy are diagnosed in the first or second trimester. The incidence in pregnancy is in a range of 1 in 2000–5000 women (Peel 1995). It is the commonest carcinoma in women worldwide, and a major contributor to mortality in women in developing countries.

Cervical intraepithelial neoplasia (CIN) is the precursor to invasive cancer of the cervix. If the condition is detected at this stage, treatment can be given and the cytology reverts to normal. The principal screening test used is the Papanicolaou smear.

Clinical signs

Bleeding is the most common symptom, with vaginal discharge being the next most common. As symptoms may be mistakenly diagnosed as symptoms of pregnancy there may be delay in diagnosis.

A Papanicolaou smear test (Box 14.1) will detect atypical cells on the surface of the cervix, or within the endocervix. When changes are detected a repeat smear test followed by colposcopy is indicated. Colposcopy allows the cervix to be visualised with a powerful light source and examined microscopically to reveal the extent of the lesion. Abnormality or CIN can be detected as visible changes on the cervix. Biopsies can be taken to reveal the extent of the lesion.

Box 14.1 Papanicolaou smear test

- The test allows identification and treatment of pre-malignant changes to cervical cells and detection of cervical cancer.
- Early diagnosis of cervical cancer increases the long-term survival rates.
- The Pap smear is a painless investigation in which the cervix is visualised using a speculum. Shaped spatulas are used to remove a layer of cells from the cervix and the area of the vagina surrounding the cervix. The area includes the squamocolumnar junction.
- National guidelines in the UK recommend that all personnel carrying out smear tests be properly trained. All results should be available within 6 weeks of the smear being taken and 80% of women should have results within 4 weeks.
- Lack of information, embarrassment, fear of pain during the test and fear of the results have been cited as reasons for women failing to attend appointments for the screening test.

As with any investigation, the mother and her partner should be fully informed about any tests and treatments that are offered. She should be aware of when and from whom results will be available. Adequate time should be made to ensure that the results are discussed in a non-hurried manner. A positive test result following a smear test will cause anxiety to the mother and her family and it is important that accurate information is available along with supportive counselling.

Treatment

Treatment depends on the stage of the disease and gestation. Laser treatment or cryotherapy following colposcopy can be carried out on an outpatient basis and will result in the destruction of the abnormal area of cells.

Cone biopsy under general anaesthesia involves excision of cervical tissue and is both a diagnostic tool and a treatment but may increase the risk to the mother. The cervix is highly vascular in pregnancy and the risk of haemorrhage is high, as is the possibility of causing the mother to miscarry. Delaying treatment until the end of pregnancy is an option for women who are found to have early changes in cervical cytology.

If the changes to the cervix are advanced and diagnosis is made in the first or second trimester, the mother may have to make a choice as to whether to terminate the pregnancy in order to undergo treatment. If diagnosis is made later in pregnancy, a decision to deliver the fetus may be taken to allow the mother to commence treatment.

Midwives have a role in explaining the value of regular smear tests to mothers. National guidelines in the UK recommend that every woman between the ages of 20 and 64 has a cervical smear test every 5 years. Where there is no evidence of a recent smear having been carried out, it may be appropriate for a smear to be taken during pregnancy. Simple explanations about the procedure can help overcome anxieties about the smear test.

Cervical screening is an important element of the 6 week postnatal examination (see Ch. 31). Women should be encouraged to continue to attend for regular cervical smear tests on completion of their pregnancy.

Spontaneous abortion

Spontaneous abortion is defined as the involuntary loss of the products of conception prior to 24 weeks' gestation. The fetus is said to be viable or capable of sustaining life outside of the uterus from 24 weeks' gestation in the UK. Bleeding after 24 weeks is classed as an antepartum haemorrhage.

Terminology
The terms miscarriage and spontaneous abortion are synonymous, the former being more acceptable to women who have experienced such a loss (Moulder 1995).

Incidence
15% of all confirmed pregnancies are said to result in a miscarriage, some 80% of which happen in the first trimester.

Aetiology
The causes of miscarriage in most instances remain unknown.

Fetal causes. Where a cause is determined, 50% of miscarriages are due to chromosomal abnormalities of the conceptus. Genetic and structural abnormalities are also said to cause pregnancy loss.

Maternal causes. Spontaneous early pregnancy loss has been attributed to the following maternal influences:

- Structural abnormalities of the genital tract such as retroversion of uterus, bicornuate uterus and fibroids.
- Infections such as rubella, listeria and chlamydia.
- Maternal diseases. Management and control of medical conditions such as diabetes, renal disease and thyroid dysfunction have reduced the risk of miscarriage in affected women. Where these conditions are not well controlled the risk of miscarriage remains (Edmonds 1992).
- Environmental factors. Excessive consumption of alcohol and cigarette smoking, including passive exposure to cigarette smoke, have been found to increase the risk of miscarriage.

Regan et al (1989) found that previous obstetric history was an important predictor of spontaneous abortion. Multigravidae are significantly more at risk than primigravidae, with miscarriage in the previous pregnancy being a prime indicator of risk.

There are several types of spontaneous abortion (Fig. 14.2):

- threatened
- inevitable
- complete
- incomplete
- missed
- septic.

In first trimester miscarriage, the embryo or fetus succumbs prior to the abortion. Later losses may involve a fetus who is still alive.

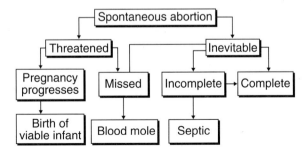

Fig. 14.2 Classification of spontaneous abortion/ miscarriage.

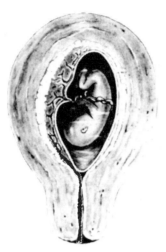

Fig. 14.3 Threatened abortion: slight vaginal bleeding; cervical os closed.

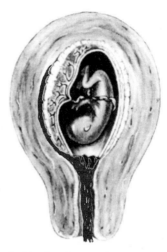

Fig. 14.4 Inevitable abortion: moderate to heavy vaginal bleeding; cervical dilatation; and fetal membranes ruptured.

Threatened abortion (Fig. 14.3)

As any vaginal bleeding in pregnancy is abnormal, so any vaginal blood loss in early pregnancy should be thought of as a threatened miscarriage until shown otherwise. In a threatened miscarriage, blood loss may be scanty, with or without low backache and cramp-like pains. The pain may resemble dysmenorrhoea or period pains (Moulder 1995). The cervix remains closed and the uterus soft, with no tenderness when palpated. The symptoms may continue over a period of time.

Traditionally mothers have been advised to rest, but there is a lack of research evidence to suggest this as effective in preventing miscarriage. 70–80% of all mothers, diagnosed as having a threatened miscarriage in the first trimester, continue with their pregnancies to term. If the bleeding settles and the pregnancy continues, subsequent management should take account of the possibility of intrauterine growth retardation, due to poor placental function. There is also an increased risk of a preterm labour.

If the loss persists, the pain may become rhythmical and the uterus contracts to expel its contents as the miscarriage becomes inevitable.

Inevitable abortion (Fig. 14.4)

Vaginal bleeding is heavy, with clots or products of conception. Blood loss may be heavy and the mother in a shocked state. The uterus, if palpable, may be smaller than expected. The membranes can rupture at this time, and amniotic fluid will be seen. The cervix dilates and, on examination, products may be seen in the vagina, or protruding through the os. Blood loss may be excessive and, if needing to be controlled, Syntocinon 20 units intravenously or ergometrine 0.5 mg intravenously, or intramuscularly, can be given.

Some cases of spontaneous loss present with the mother in a state of shock that is out of proportion to the revealed blood loss. This is caused by products of conception becoming trapped in the cervix and will resolve with their removal.

The pain experienced by the mother at this time may be as intense as that felt during labour. Adequate analgesia should be available and the mother's privacy and dignity protected. Care should be provided on a ward where staff are practised in caring for mothers having a miscarriage (Kohner 1995). The woman and her partner need to be kept informed of what is happening. Depending on gestation, an identifiable body or complete embryo may be lost. In some cases nothing is identifiable. The couple need to be prepared for these eventualities (Moulder 1995).

Incomplete abortion (Fig. 14.5)

Remnants of placenta remain within the uterine

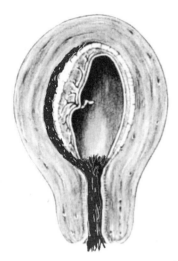

Fig. 14.5 Incomplete abortion: heavy and profuse vaginal bleeding; cervical os dilated.

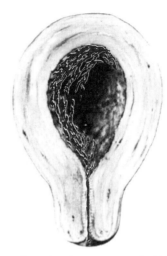

Fig. 14.6 Complete abortion: scanty vaginal bleeding; cervical os closed; fetus, placenta and membranes expelled.

cavity, contributing to the degree of bleeding which may be heavy and profuse. Intravenous or intramuscular ergometrine 0.5 mg may be given to control the loss. Evacuation to remove any retained tissue should be done under general anaesthetic, once the mother is in a stable condition. Treatment of hypovolaemia may be required prior to anaesthesia.

Incomplete miscarriage contributes to the mortality and morbidity of women worldwide.

Complete abortion (Fig. 14.6)

The conceptus, placenta and membranes are expelled completely from the uterus. The pain stops, and signs of pregnancy will regress. The uterus, on palpation, is firmly contracted and an empty cavity is seen on ultrasound examination. No further medical intervention is required, although support through the aftermath of pregnancy loss should be available. Mothers should be advised to seek advice if bleeding recurs or a temperature develops.

Missed abortion

This term is applied when the embryo dies, despite the presence of a viable placenta, and the sac is retained. Embryo death usually occurs before 8 weeks' gestation but the mother's body does not

recognise its demise. A brown loss originating from the degeneration of placental tissue may present, and threatened miscarriage is suspected. Women report a reduction and then cessation of the symptoms of pregnancy. Uterine growth stops and diagnosis can be confirmed by ultrasound scan.

Treatment of a missed abortion is evacuation of the uterus by dilatation and curettage under general anaesthetic. During the operation, the cervical canal is gently dilated to allow a small curette to be introduced into the uterine cavity. The curette is used to remove any retained products. Prostaglandins, inserted vaginally, make the cervix favourable prior to dilatation and curettage. This avoids trauma to the cervix, caused by forcible dilatation, and reduces the risk of cervical incompetence in subsequent pregnancies. There is a risk of hypofibrinogenaemia when the fetus has been retained for some weeks (see Ch. 15).

This condition is sometimes referred to as blighted ovum.

Septic abortion

This condition is most commonly a complication of induced or incomplete abortion, and is due to ascending infection. In addition to the signs of miscarriage, the mother complains of feeling unwell and may have a headache, nausea, and be pyrexial. It may present as either a localised infection in the uterine tubes and the uterine cavity, or as generalised septicaemia with peritonitis.

Blood culture and vaginal swabs should be taken to identify the cause of the infection. Intravenous antibiotics should be given, commencing with both a broad spectrum antibiotic and one effective against anaerobic infection.

Sequelae to early pregnancy loss

Midwives need to support the mother and her family at a time of uncertainty and anxiety. The effect of the loss of a baby at this time is under-estimated by professionals, who often see it as a routine clinical situation (Cecil & Slade 1996). Language used should be appropriate, in recognition that the mother will be grieving for her lost baby (Moulder 1995). Feelings of failure and inadequacies may be expressed by the mother, as she blames herself, or some action, for the loss of her child. She may also be afraid that she is incapable of bearing children (Iles 1989).

Interpreters who are trained in bereavement support should be available where staff have problems communicating to parents in their own language. Facilities should also be accessible for visually or hearing impaired parents to have information communicated effectively to them (Kohner 1995).

Regardless of gestation the parents may want to see and hold the baby. Some parents may want to see the loss when there is no body. Parents also need information on how the remains will be disposed. Under 24 weeks' gestation the baby is not registrable in the UK, therefore is not legally required to be buried or cremated. All hospitals and maternity units should have guidance for parents, and staff knowledgeable in the local procedures. Written information should be available, explaining the choices available.

Follow-up after miscarriage is needed, with parents able to receive further information about their loss and be offered advice regarding future pregnancies.

Induced abortion

Termination of pregnancy before 24 weeks' gestation is legal in the UK within the terms of current legislation. Amendments to The Abortion Act 1967 came into force in 1991 which made the termination of pregnancy legal in certain circumstances after 24 weeks.

Midwives will primarily be caring for mothers for whom termination of pregnancy is an option they are considering as a result of the antenatal screening or diagnostic tests offered. The aim of these investigations is to detect specific fetal abnormalities. The family need to be given accurate, factual information about the investigations and the possible anomaly as well as the options available in their local area to enable an informed choice to be made about termination (see Ch. 20).

All women who are opting to terminate a pregnancy need adequate support and counselling, both before and after the procedure. Social, medical and psychological factors all contribute to the decision.

There are five identified areas that allow grounds for ending a pregnancy before 24 weeks' gestation. Two medical practitioners are required to certify that one or more of the following apply:

1. Continuation of the pregnancy would involve risk greater than if the pregnancy were terminated, of injury to the physical or mental health of the pregnant woman or any existing children of her family.
2. Termination is necessary to prevent grave permanent injury to the physical or mental health of the woman.
3. The continuance of the pregnancy would involve risk to the life of the pregnant woman, greater than if the pregnancy were terminated.
4. There is substantial risk that if the child were born it would suffer such physical or mental abnormalities as to be seriously handicapped. (Abortion Act 1967, as amended by Human Fertilisation and Embryology Act 1990)

Furthermore, termination of pregnancy is permitted under the Acts, after 24 weeks, where the woman's life is at risk or where, as in Clause 4 of the Act, there is a substantial risk of the child being born seriously physically or mentally disabled.

Methods

Abortion can be carried out in the first trimester, using vacuum aspiration, dilatation and evacuation under general anaesthetic. Medical methods using mifepristone and prostaglandin are licensed for use up to the 63rd day from the first day of a woman's last menstrual period (UK Multicentre Trial 1990). Mifepristone is an antiprogesterone compound that blocks the action of progesterone, a hormone essential for the maintenance of the pregnancy. It is taken orally, on licensed premises, in the presence of a doctor or nurse. By blocking progesterone with mifepristone the sensitivity of the uterus to prostaglandin rises. A low-dose vaginal prostaglandin pessary is inserted to effect the termination (Norman 1991).

In the second trimester medical methods are used. Extrauterine prostaglandin, accompanied by large doses of oxytocin, produces uterine contractions. The mother experiences labour pains and the process may be protracted.

The mother needs to be cared for in a single room, privacy being protected at all times. She should be offered information about the process so she is aware of what is happening. Adequate analgesia should be available and supportive staff identified to care for the mother and her family throughout the procedure (Kohner 1995). It may be appropriate for the named midwife to care for the mother during her termination.

Amendments to the Abortion Act 1967 in 1991 allowed for the reduction of multiple pregnancies where one or more of the fetuses, but not all, may be terminated (Paintain 1994).

International perspective

Induced abortion contributes to the worldwide maternal mortality statistics. In the developing world unsafe abortion is one of the five main causes of direct maternal death (Kwast 1991).

Infection is a possible consequence of any abortion but is more common following an induced abortion. Septic abortion remains a major complication of an illegal abortion or one carried out in non-sterile conditions.

Maternal mortality

Early pregnancy mortality figures for the triennium 1991–1993 include three deaths following spontaneous miscarriage, and five following induced abortion. Deaths have reduced in the UK since abortion has been legalised. Sepsis and rupture of the uterus remain factors in these deaths (DH et al 1996).

Ethical issues

Within the terms of the Abortion Act 1967, if an individual has a conscientious objection, he or she is not required to assist with abortion. Midwifery practice may involve assisting with blood tests or amniocentesis, the results of which could lead to a termination. The duty of care and exercise of professional accountability means that mothers should be given the necessary information and advice.

Professional guidelines require the midwife to care for clients in a non-judgemental manner. This applies when caring for a mother terminating a current pregnancy and to mothers who have undergone termination in a previous pregnancy.

Recurrent miscarriage

Recurrent miscarriage is defined as the loss of three or more consecutive pregnancies (Stirrat 1990a). This is a problem that affects 1% of all women, and the risk of further abortion increases with each pregnancy lost.

The incidence of recurrent miscarriage suggests that there are significant underlying causes and the loss of the pregnancy is not chance. Factors associated with recurrent miscarriage include:

1. *Genetic causes.* Abnormal parental karyotype, of which the most common is translocation.

2. *Immunological factors.* Women with a history of recurrent pregnancy loss have been found to lack an immunoglobulin G (IgG) blocking agent. In a normal pregnancy the IgG coats the fetal antigens and prevents rejection of the fetus.

3. *Hypersecretion of luteinising hormone.* This may act on the oocyte, causing it to age, or on the endometrium, resulting in errors in implantation. Mothers with polycystic ovaries have reduced fertility, and an increased risk of early pregnancy loss (Clifford & Regan 1994).

4. *Infection.* The role of infection in recurrent early pregnancy failure is unclear. Alteration of

the normal vaginal flora may contribute to recurrent miscarriage when loss or reduced levels of lactobacilli occur with the condition bacterial vaginosis. Presence of this in the first trimester has been found to increase the risk of second trimester miscarriage and preterm labour (Hay et al 1994, Kurki et al 1992). *Toxoplasma gondii*, listeria and cytomegalovirus are infective agents associated with pregnancy loss, but their action in recurrent loss remains uncertain (Clifford & Regan 1994, Stirrat 1990b).

5. *Structural anomalies.* Both uterine abnormalities and cervical incompetence have been attributed as causes of recurrent loss, although it is thought that too much emphasis has been given to their contribution (Rai et al 1996, Stirrat 1990b)

In many cases no causative factor is identified. Mothers should be referred to specialist clinics, where a screening service is available, thus enabling a probable cause to be identified (Rai et al 1996).

Cervical incompetence

Cervical incompetence is said to occur when painless dilatation of the cervix occurs as pregnancy progresses, allowing the membranes to bulge through the cervical os into the vagina. As the intrauterine pressure increases, the membranes may rupture, resulting in miscarriage within the second trimester, or preterm birth.

Causes of incompetence are uncertain. Trauma to the cervix such as might be caused during dilatation and curettage or induced abortion appear to contribute to the risk. Cone biopsy of the cervix may also be a possible cause. The incompetence may be due to a congenital weakness.

Treatment for subsequent pregnancies is by cervical cerclage. At 14 weeks' gestation a non-absorbable suture is inserted at the level of the cervical os. This remains in situ until 38 weeks or the onset of labour, when it is removed.

ECTOPIC PREGNANCY

An ectopic pregnancy is one where implantation occurs at a site other than the uterine cavity. Sites can be in the uterine tube, ovary, cervix and the abdomen (Fig. 14.7).

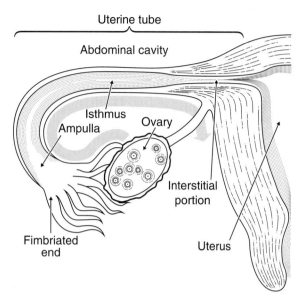

Fig. 14.7 Sites of implantation in ectopic pregnancy.

The incidence of ectopic pregnancies has been rising – currently 1% of all pregnancies are ectopic. The maternal mortality rate in the UK associated with ectopic pregnancy is falling, accounting for 4.2% of the direct and indirect deaths in the triennium 1991–1993 (DH et al 1996).

The life-threatening outcome of this condition means that prompt and appropriate treatment is needed by the mother. Midwives need to be aware of the possibility of ectopic pregnancy being responsible for abdominal pain and bleeding in early pregnancy.

Tubal pregnancy

In tubal pregnancy, implantation can occur at any point along the tube, although the ampulla is the most common site. The isthmus is next in frequency, and the interstitial portion least common.

Causes of ectopic pregnancy

Any alteration of the normal function of the uterine tube in transporting the gametes contributes to the risk of ectopic pregnancy.

• Congenital abnormalities of the tube.
• Previous infection. This may alter the ciliated lining, or the peristaltic action of the tube. Infection can also leave adhesions both inside

and surrounding the tube, restricting normal function.

• Surgery on the uterine tube.
• Use of intrauterine contraceptive devices.
• Assisted reproductive techniques.

Physiology of tubal pregnancy

In uterine pregnancy the blastocyst embeds in the decidua and the trophoblast erodes the maternal tissue anchoring the developing embryo. In tubal cyesis, the blastocyst rapidly erodes the epithelium and becomes attached to the muscle layer. It grows and expands within the wall, distending the tube. Maternal vessels are exposed and the pressure caused by the resultant blood flow can destroy the embryo.

The uterus increases in size, and changes associated with early pregnancy occur in the body. Degrees of change take place within the endometrium, under the influence of hormones. Vaginal bleeding associated with ectopic pregnancy is derived from degeneration of the decidua, which is passed in fragments, or as a decidual cast.

Outcomes of tubal pregnancy (Fig. 14.8)

1. Tubal abortion. The developing conceptus separates and is expelled through the fimbriated end of the uterine tube. This outcome is more common with ampullary implantation.
2. Tubal mole. Bleeding around the embryo results in its death. The blood clots around the conceptus, enclosing it. Products are retained in the tube, and may need to be removed.
3. Tubal rupture. The wall is distended by the pregnancy and penetrated by the trophoblast to such an extent that it ruptures. This can be gradual or occur as an acute episode.
4. Abdominal pregnancy.

Clinical presentation

It is rare for a tubal pregnancy to remain asymptomatic beyond 8 weeks. It can be difficult to diagnose, but delay may endanger the life of the mother. Where the midwife suspects that ectopic pregnancy may be the cause of symptoms, she must refer the mother promptly to hospital.

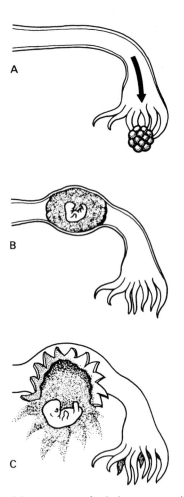

Fig. 14.8 Possible outcomes of tubal pregnancy: (A) tubal abortion; (B) tubal mole; (C) tubal rupture.

The mother may present with a history of amenorrhoea, followed by some vaginal spotting. This precedes the onset of abdominal pain, often localised in nature, described also as sharp and stabbing. The mother complains of dizziness and nausea and she can have shoulder pain, indicative of bleeding into the peritoneal cavity. Acute symptoms are the result of tubal rupture, and relate to the degree of haemorrhage there has been.

Ultrasound enables an accurate diagnosis of tubal pregnancy, making management more proactive. Vaginal ultrasound combined with the use of sensitive tests, which detect the presence of human chorionic gonadotrophin, has meant that diagnosis is made earlier and reduces risk of rupture (Cacciatore et al 1990, Stabile & Grudinskas 1994).

Treatment focuses on the removal of trophoblast and efforts are directed to preserving, where possible, the affected tube. If the tube ruptures, shock may ensue; therefore resuscitation followed by laparotomy is needed. Management of ectopic pregnancy is moving towards more conservative approaches, with less invasive treatments being assessed (Bhatt & Taylor 1995).

The mother should be offered follow-up support and information regarding subsequent pregnancies. As with any loss during pregnancy, the midwife should be sensitive to her client's need to grieve.

Abdominal pregnancy

Abdominal pregnancy is rare. Fetal development may take place in the abdominal cavity and follows early rupture or abortion of a tubal pregnancy. The placenta remains attached to the uterine tube, but expands and attaches to neighbouring organs. The fetus develops within the peritoneal cavity but the majority of these pregnancies do not survive. If this happens in early pregnancy the fetus may be reabsorbed or calcification occurs. In some cases infection can develop, resulting in an abscess with the potential to rupture and cause peritonitis and septicaemia.

In very rare cases abdominal pregnancy proceeds to term. On palpation the lie may be persistently abnormal and fetal parts readily felt. Reports describe the uterus as being enlarged, due to hormonal activity, and felt separate from the fetus. Delivery is by laparotomy, with individual surgeons assessing the dangers involved with the separation and delivery of the placenta. Separation may be followed by major haemorrhage that is uncontrollable. Leaving the placenta in situ may result in infection but is considered to be the safer option.

The baby may be found to have compression deformities due to oligohydramnios.

Ectopic pregnancy and maternal mortality

In the Confidential Enquiry into Maternal Deaths for the triennium 1991–1993 there were eight reports of direct maternal deaths due to ectopic pregnancy. Comparisons with previous reports are difficult, owing to changes in data collection. The findings state that all the deaths were associated with substandard care (DH et al 1996).

The need for early diagnosis is essential, and facilities to make an accurate diagnosis should be widely available. Midwives need to be aware of the facilities for early pregnancy screening in their area. Midwives encourage mothers to seek their advice as early as possible in pregnancy and the midwife may be the professional called on in the first instance. Accurate, comprehensive booking information may highlight those women for whom ectopic pregnancy is a risk.

GESTATIONAL TROPHOBLASTIC DISEASE

Gestational trophoblastic disease is a general term covering both the benign hydatidiform mole and choriocarcinoma, which is malignant. A third condition, placental site trophoblastic tumour, exists but is outside the remit of this chapter.

Hydatidiform mole

Hydatidiform mole is the term applied to a gross malformation of the trophoblast in which the chorionic villi proliferate and become avascular. They are found in the cavity of the uterus and, very rarely, within the uterine tube.

The incidence of hydatidiform mole in the western world is between 0.5–2.5 in 1000 pregnancies (Bracken 1987). The risk rises to 1 in 50 where the mother has previously had a molar pregnancy. Risk is also increased for women under 20 and over 40 years of age, and for women of Asian origin (Bagshawe et al 1986). As this condition can lead to the development of cancer, accurate diagnosis, treatment and follow-up is essential.

For the midwife caring for a mother who is diagnosed as having a molar pregnancy it is important to recognise the psychological as well as physical needs of the mother, who will grieve for the loss of her pregnancy, and baby. Although the condition is curable, stress will inevitably affect the mother and her family as she comes to terms with a potentially life-threatening condition. She will require advice and counselling on subsequent pregnancies.

Two forms of mole have been identified, one of which carries an increased risk of the mother subsequently developing choriocarcinoma (Lawler et al 1991).

Complete hydatidiform mole

This type of mole contains no evidence of embryo, cord or membranes. Death occurs prior to the development of the placental circulation (Szulman 1988). The chorionic villi alter to form clear, hydropic vesicles, which hang in clusters from small pedicles, giving the appearance of a bunch of grapes. The size of vesicles varies, from being barely visible, to a few centimetres in diameter. Hyperplasia affects the syncytiotrophoblast and the cytotrophoblast layers. The mass occupies the uterine cavity and can be large enough to mimic an advanced gestation.

In a normal pregnancy the trophoblast erodes the decidua to anchor the conceptus, and this ability means that the developing mole is more than capable of penetrating beyond the site of implantation. The myometrium can be involved and, more rarely, the veins. Rupture of the uterus with massive haemorrhage is a possible outcome.

Complete moles usually have 46 chromosomes of paternal origin only. A haploid sperm fertilises a so-called empty egg, the maternal chromosomes being lost (Lawler et al 1991). The paternal chromosomes alone duplicate. Choriocarcinoma can develop from this type (Bagshawe et al 1986).

Partial mole

Evidence of an embryo, fetus or amniotic sac may be found, as death occurs around the eighth or ninth week. Hyperplasia of the trophoblast is confined to the single syncytiotrophoblast layer and is less widespread than in complete moles. Chromosome analysis will usually show this to be triploid, with 69 chromosomes, i.e. three sets of chromosomes, one maternal and two paternal. It can be difficult to differentiate between a partial mole and a missed abortion on histology. This has a clinical significance because although the risk to the mother of developing choriocarcinoma from a partial mole is slight, follow-up is still essential (Szulman 1988, Yedema et al 1993).

Clinical features

Symptoms vary, according to the type of mole developing. Exaggerated signs of pregnancy, appearing by 6–8 weeks, are characteristic of complete hydatidiform mole. For partial mole the signs may be less obvious.

Bleeding or a bloodstained vaginal discharge after a period of amenorrhoea is the commonest symptom which may present as the first sign of abnormality. Rupture of a vesicle may result in a light pink or brown vaginal discharge. The vesicles can detach and be passed vaginally allowing diagnosis, if not already suspected, to be made.

Anaemia, as a result of the gradual loss of blood, can be a problem in some cases. Medical intervention may be needed where excessive nausea and vomiting, due to high levels of human chorionic gonadotrophin, result in the mother requiring treatment for hyperemesis gravidarum. Hyperthyroidism has been detected in cases of molar pregnancy and requires to be treated prior to evacuation of the mole (Goldstein & Berkowitz 1994). Pre-eclampsia developing early in pregnancy is suggestive of the presence of a hydatidiform mole.

On examination, the uterine size exceeds that expected for gestation. On palpation, the uterus feels 'doughy' or elastic, and it does not contract. Mothers with a partial mole may not show signs of increased growth. No fetal parts or movements are felt and the fetal heart is not heard, although this may be in keeping with expected findings, depending on gestation. Diagnosis is confirmed by ultrasound scan and serum human chorionic gonadotrophin levels.

Treatment

The aim of treatment is to remove all trophoblast tissue. In some cases the hydatidiform mole aborts spontaneously. Where this does not occur, vacuum aspiration or dilatation and curettage is necessary. Spontaneous expulsion of the mole carries less risk of malignant change.

All women who have been treated for hydatidiform mole in the UK are recorded on a central register. In the majority of cases removal of the mole results in resolution of the condition. In about 10% of cases the trophoblast tissue does not die off completely. For this reason and the possibility of developing a malignancy, women confirmed as having a complete mole require follow-up over a 2-year period. Following treatment, surveillance of urinary levels of human chorionic gonadotrophin should demonstrate a reduction of level, with a return to normal after 6–8 weeks: rising levels are suggestive of recurrence (Bagshawe et al 1986).

Pregnancy should be avoided during the follow-up period. Intrauterine contraceptive devices are contraindicated because of risks of perforation and infection and hormonal methods of contraception are not prescribed until levels of human chorionic gonadotrophin have returned to normal (Sapire 1990).

The midwife can provide support and explanations of the importance of this protracted period of screening. An understanding of the condition should help the midwife to plan care in subsequent pregnancies.

Choriocarcinoma

Choriocarcinoma is a malignant neoplasm, which can develop as a consequence of a molar pregnancy. The growth actively invades the myometrium, putting the mother at risk of severe haemorrhage in the first instance. The mother is also at risk of developing lung, hepatic and cerebral metastases if the neoplasm goes undetected.

Choriocarcinoma can also occur after a normal term gestation, or a termination of pregnancy.

Administration of anti-D immunoglobulin in early pregnancy

Anti-D immunoglobulin was introduced to reduce the risk of iso-immunisation in Rhesus negative women (see Ch. 42). It has been demonstrated that significant fetomaternal haemorrhage can occur following early pregnancy loss. Anti-D 250 IU is the normal dose given before 20 weeks' gestation.

Women who have an ectopic pregnancy should have their blood group identified, and it is recommended that anti-D is given if found to be Rhesus negative. Retrospective analysis has shown that women in this group are particularly at risk of sensitisation.

Women who are Rhesus negative and have had evacuation of a hydatidiform mole should also have anti-D administered (NBTSIWP 1991).

RETROVERSION OF THE UTERUS

When the long axis of the uterus is directed backwards during pregnancy, the uterus is said to be retroverted.

In the first trimester, retroversion of the uterus is said to occur in 11% of all pregnancies (Weekes et al 1976). It is associated with a slightly increased risk of early pregnancy bleeding and abortion. This is due to compression of the uterine vessels decreasing blood flow to the decidua (Gibbons & Paley 1969). As pregnancy progresses most cases correct spontaneously, the uterus rising out of the pelvis into the abdomen, causing no further problems.

Incarceration of the retroverted gravid uterus

If the retroverted uterus fails to rise out of the pelvic cavity by the 14th week, it is said to be incarcerated. This situation occurs in 1 in 3000 pregnancies. Causes include congenital anomalies of the pelvis and uterus. A history of conditions such as pelvic adhesions, endometriosis, fibroids or ovarian tumours may contribute to the condition.

The growing uterus is confined within the pelvis, beneath the sacral promontory. Pressure causes abdominal discomfort, and a feeling of pelvic fullness, low abdominal or back pain. Frequency of micturition, dysuria and paradoxical incontinence are the result of the urethra being elongated as the cervix increasingly is displaced. Compression of the bladder neck leads to urinary retention. Urinary stasis can result in infections developing, including pyelonephritis (Myers & Scotti 1995). The mother may also complain of rectal pressure and constipation with impaction of faeces.

On examination, the bladder will be palpable abdominally. The fetal heart may be difficult to auscultate if the bowel is full. The midwife, recognising a deviation from normal, will send for medical aid while assessing the mother's condition (UKCC 1994). Catheterisation to relieve the retention of urine is needed. An indwelling catheter is used to keep the bladder empty, enabling the uterus to rise out of the pelvis.

Anterior wall sacculation occurs in extreme cases when the uterus remains entrapped. In this situation the lower portion of the uterus continues to expand and extend, forming a pouch to accommodate the fetus. Uterine rupture can result, and bladder rupture due to overextension, or from necrosis of the bladder wall during manual correction, has been reported.

FIBROIDS (LEIOMYOMAS)

These are firm, benign tumours of muscular and fibrous tissue, ranging in size from the very small to very large. The incidence of detectable fibroids in pregnancy is 1%, the lowest risk being in Caucasian women but risk increases in Afro-Caribbean women and women over 35 years old.

Types of fibroid

Intramural. These are embedded within the wall of the uterus, separated from the myometrium by a capsule of connective tissue. They are most common, and are often the cause for enlargement of the non-pregnant uterus.

Subserosal. These lie below the perimetrium, and may be irregular in shape. Subserosal fibroids can become pedunculated.

Submucosal. These are found within the endometrium, or decidua. They can be difficult to detect on abdominal examination. They can cause bleeding, and become both infected and necrotic.

Fibroids can be found in both upper and lower segments of the uterus; they can be singular, but most are multiple. Fibroids are found most often in the body of the uterus.

Effect of pregnancy on fibroids

Ultrasound monitoring of fibroids has demonstrated that they do not significantly increase in size during pregnancy (Aharoni et al 1988, Davis et al 1990). The same factors that influence uterine growth were thought to affect the fibroid, the walls of the fibroid containing hormone receptors. The fibroid does, however, become more vascular and oedematous, making it softer and more difficult to detect on palpation.

Effect of fibroids on pregnancy

Early pregnancy loss is associated with submucosal fibroids, where implantation occurs over the fibroid. Mild abdominal pain may occur that resolves without treatment (Aharoni et al 1988).

Lower segment or cervical fibroids may be felt on vaginal examination. Outcome of pregnancy is dependent on the position of the fibroid, and in some situations obstruction may occur. Fibroids located in the lower segment or on the cervix can prevent descent of the fetal head, causing malpresentation and obstructed labour. Caesarean section is more likely where the fibroid is situated in the lower segment (Vergani et al 1994).

Red degeneration of fibroids

During pregnancy, rapid growth can cause degeneration of a fibroid as it exceeds the available blood supply. The central core necroses, and bleeding occurs into the middle. The tumour takes on a reddish appearance. The mother experiences severe abdominal pain that is acute in nature (Katz et al 1989), the affected area is tender on palpation, and she may also have a low-grade pyrexia. Other causes of pain need to be excluded – typically, appendicitis or placental abruption need to be considered.

Referral for ultrasound scan aids differential diagnosis of the pain, as the relationship between the placental site and the focus of pain can be established. The degeneration can be seen clearly on ultrasound (Chudleigh & Pearce 1992). The pain is normally relieved by rest and analgesia; no other treatment is required (Rice et al 1989).

HYPEREMESIS GRAVIDARUM

Vomiting that starts before the 20th week of pregnancy and requires intervention is known as hyperemesis gravidarum. Nausea and vomiting are common symptoms in pregnancy, occurring in 50% of all pregnancies and normally self-limiting. Severe nausea and vomiting leads to dehydration, electrolyte imbalance and weight loss. It is a condition affecting approximately 1 in 1000 pregnant women.

The aetiology of hyperemesis is uncertain, endocrine and psychological factors being proposed. Rising levels of oestrogen and human chorionic gonadotrophin appear to be significant. Hyperemesis occurs more often where mothers have a multiple pregnancy, or a hydatidiform mole, both of which are associated with increased hormone levels. Simultaneous occurrence of hyperthyroidism and hyperemesis has been reported (Crump & Aten 1992), suggesting transient thyroid dysfunction as a possible cause.

In addition to multiple pregnancy and molar pregnancy, hyperemesis is known to be associated with first pregnancies and with a history of unsuccessful pregnancies (Fairweather 1968). In a proportion of cases, psychological factors associated with rejection or ambivalence may be implicated (Deuchar 1995). Women with a previous history of hyperemesis are likely to experience it in subsequent pregnancies (Fairweather 1968). However, women with vomiting in early pregnancy had improved pregnancy outcomes, compared to those who did not suffer from vomiting (Klebanoff et al 1985, Weigel & Weigel 1989).

Historically, hyperemesis was a contributory factor to maternal mortality statistics, until understanding and management of dehydration and electrolyte imbalance ensured that some treatment was available (Hod et al 1994).

The midwife should enquire of all women attending for early antenatal care whether they are experiencing nausea or vomiting. Causes of vomit-ing not due to pregnancy, such as urinary tract infection or gastroenteritis, need to be excluded.

Diagnosis is made where there is a history of persistent, severe nausea and vomiting in early pregnancy. A mother suspected of suffering from hyperemesis presents as being unable to retain food or fluids. She may have lost weight, and be distressed by her symptoms. The woman requires admission to hospital for assessment, and management of symptoms.

A history of the frequency and severity of the bouts of vomiting is taken. The mother's appearance is noted, including any dryness or inelasticity of the skin. In severe cases jaundice may be apparent. This indicates hepatic involvement, a late sign, and one associated with the condition being neglected.

Additional signs of dehydration such as rapid pulse, low blood pressure and dry furred tongue may be seen. The mother's breath may smell of acetone, a sign of ketosis. Ptyalism may occur, contributing to the dehydration, but may not be a cause of complaint as the mother is retching and vomiting (Abell & Riely 1992).

Elevated haematocrit, alterations in electrolyte levels and ketonuria are associated with dehydration. Hypovolaemia and electrolyte imbalance are corrected by intravenous infusion. Vitamin supplements can be given parenterally, particularly where hyperemesis has been prolonged. Initially nothing is given by mouth, to allow time for the vomiting to be controlled. Gradual introduction of fluids and diet as her condition improves is closely monitored.

The mother should be encouraged to rest and may be cared for in a single room. The distress caused by repeated vomiting can be marked. Some women may be prescribed a mild sedative if they appear agitated. Supportive psychotherapy or counselling has been used to treat some cases of hyperemesis (Deuchar 1995). Small palatable meals on a regular basis help to encourage the mother to regain her appetite.

The use of antiemetics in pregnancy received widespread publicity when links were found between thalidomide and severe malformations of children born to mothers who had taken the drug for morning sickness. Currently antihistamines are the recommended pharmacological treatment for nausea and vomiting, no antiemetic being approved for treatment.

If hyperemesis is left untreated the mother's condition worsens. Wernicke's encephalopathy is a complication associated with a lack of vitamin B_1 (thiamine). Hepatic and renal involvement lead to coma and death. Termination of pregnancy may reverse the condition and has a place in preventing maternal mortality.

READER ACTIVITIES

1. Identify a booking interview you have been involved in, where the mother presented with a history of previous early pregnancy loss.

Write down how you explored the issue of her previous loss.

How do you feel about the interview, having reflected on it? What might you do differently, when in a similar situation again?

2. A 24-year-old mother you are caring for tells you she has never had a cervical smear. How will you respond?

Visit your local health promotion department and local clinics and review the information available for women on cervical screening.

How can you in your role as a midwife increase health awareness amongst women?

USEFUL ADDRESSES

Miscarriage Association
Clayton Hospital
Northgate
Wakefield
West Yorkshire
WF1 3JS

SAFTA (Support around Termination for Abnormality)
73 Charlotte Street
London W1P 1LB

SANDS (Stillbirth and Neonatal Death Society)
28 Portland Place
London W1N 4DE

REFERENCES

Abell T L, Riely C A 1992 Hyperemesis gravidarum. Gastroenterology Clinics of North America 21(4): 835–847

Abortion Act 1967. HMSO, London

Aharoni A, Reiter A, Golan D, Paltiely Y, Sharf M 1988 Patterns of growth of uterine leiomyomas during pregnancy. A prospective longitudinal study. British Journal of Obstetrics and Gynaecology 95: 510–513

Bagshawe K D, Dent J, Webb J 1986 Hydatidiform mole in England and Wales 1973–83. Lancet ii: 673–675

Bhatt A N, Taylor D J 1995 Advances in the treatment of ectopic pregnancy. In: Bonnar J (ed) Recent advances in obstetrics and gynaecology. Churchill Livingstone, Edinburgh, vol 19, ch 1, pp 1–14

Bracken M B 1987 Incidence and aetiology of hydatidiform mole: an epidemiological review. British Journal of Obstetrics and Gynaecology 94: 1123–1135

Cacciatore B, Stenman U-H, Ylostalo P 1990 Diagnosis of ectopic pregnancy by vaginal ultrasonography in combination with a discriminatory serum hCG of 1000 IU/l (IRP).

British Journal of Obstetrics and Gynaecology 97: 904–908

Cecil R, Slade P 1996 Miscarriage. In: Niven C, Walker A (eds) Conception, pregnancy and birth. Butterworth Heinemann, Oxford, vol 2, ch 7, p 89

Chudleigh P, Pearce J M 1992 Obstetric ultrasound, 2nd edn. Churchill Livingstone, Edinburgh, ch 2, p 24

Clifford K A, Regan L 1994 Recurrent pregnancy loss. In: Studd J (ed) Progress in obstetrics and gynaecology. Churchill Livingstone, Edinburgh, vol 11, ch 6, pp 97–110

Crump W J, Aten L A 1992 Hyperemesis, hyperthyroidism or both? Journal of Family Practice 35(4): 450–456

Davis J L, Ray-Mazumder S, Hobel C J, Baley K, Sassoon D 1990 Uterine leiomyomas in pregnancy: a prospective study. Obstetrics and Gynaecology 75(1): 41–44

Deuchar N 1995 Nausea and vomiting in pregnancy: a review of the problem with particular regard to psychological and social aspects. British Journal of Obstetrics and Gynaecology 102: 6–8

Department of Health, Welsh Office, Scottish Home and

Health Department, Department of Health and Social Services, Northern Ireland 1996 Report on confidential enquiries into maternal deaths in the United Kingdom 1991–1993. HMSO, London

Edmonds D K 1992 Spontaneous and recurrent abortion. In: Shaw R W, Soutter W P, Stanton S L (eds) Gynaecology. Churchill Livingstone, Edinburgh, ch 15, pp 205–218

Fairweather D I 1968 Nausea and vomiting in pregnancy. American Journal of Obstetrics and Gynecology 102(1): 135–173

Gibbons J M, Paley W B 1969 The incarcerated gravid uterus. Obstetrics and Gynecology 33: 842–845

Goldstein D P, Berkowitz R S 1994 Current management of complete and partial molar pregnancy. Journal of Reproductive Medicine 39(3): 139–146

Hay P E, Lamont R F, Taylor-Robinson D, Morgan D J, Ison C, Pearson J 1994 Abnormal bacterial colonisation of the genital tract and subsequent pre-term delivery and late miscarriage. British Medical Journal 308: 295–298

Hod M, Orvieto R, Kaplan B, Friedman S, Ovadia J 1994 Hyperemesis gravidarum: a review. Journal of Reproductive Medicine 39: 605–612

Human Fertilisation and Embryology Act 1990 HMSO, London

Iles S 1989 The loss of early pregnancy. Clinical Obstetrics and Gynaecology 3(4): 769–791

Katz V L, Dotters D J, Droegemueller W 1989 Complications of uterine leiomyomas in pregnancy. Obstetrics and Gynecology 73(4): 593–596

Klebanoff M A, Koslowe P A, Kaslow R, Rhoads G G 1985 Epidemiology of vomiting in early pregnancy. Obstetrics and Gynecology 66: 612–616

Kohner N 1995 Pregnancy loss and the death of a baby. Guidelines for professionals. SANDS, London

Kurki T, Sivonen A, Renkonen O-V, Savia E, Ylikorkala O 1992 Bacterial vaginosis in early pregnancy and pregnancy outcome. Obstetrics and Gynecology 80(2): 173–177

Kwast B E 1991 Maternal mortality: the magnitude and the causes. Midwifery 7: 4–7

Lawler S D, Fisher R A, Dent J 1991 A prospective genetic study of complete and partial hydatidiform moles. American Journal of Obstetrics and Gynecology 164(5): 1270–1277

Moulder C 1995 Miscarriage. Women's experiences and needs. Pandora, London

Myers D L, Scotti R J 1995 Acute urinary retention and the incarcerated, retroverted, gravid uterus. A case report. Journal of Reproductive Medicine 40: 487–490

National Blood Transfusion Service Immunoglobulin Working Party (NBTSIWP) 1991 Recommendations for the use of anti-D immunoglobulin. Prescribers Journal 31: 137–145

Norman J 1991 Antiprogesterones. British Journal of Hospital Medicine 45: 372–375

Paintain D 1994 Induced abortion. In: Clements R V (ed) Safe practice in obstetrics and gynaecology. A medico-legal handbook. Churchill Livingstone, Edinburgh, ch 28, p 355

Peel K R 1995 Premalignant and malignant disease of the cervix. In: Whitfield C R (ed) Dewhurst's textbook of obstetrics and gynaecology for postgraduates, 5th edn. Blackwell Science, Oxford, ch 46, pp 717–737

Rai R, Clifford K, Regan L 1996 The modern preventative treatment of recurrent miscarriage. British Journal of Obstetrics and Gynaecology 103: 106–110

Regan L, Braude P R, Trembath P L 1989 Influence of past reproductive performance on risk of spontaneous abortion. British Medical Journal 229: 541–545

Rice J P, Kay H H, Mahoney B S 1989 The clinical significance of uterine leiomyomas in pregnancy. American Journal of Obstetrics and Gynecology 160(5): 1212–1216

Sapire K E 1990 Contraception and sexuality in health and disease, UK edn. McGraw-Hill, Maidenhead, pp 114–115

Stabile I, Grudinskas J G 1994 Ectopic pregnancy – what's new? In: Studd J (ed) Progress in obstetrics and gynaecology. Churchill Livingstone, Edinburgh, vol 11, ch 17, pp 281–309

Stirrat G M 1990a Recurrent miscarriage I: definition and epidemiology. Lancet 336: 673–675

Stirrat G M 1990b Recurrent miscarriage II: clinical associations, causes and management. Lancet 336: 728–733

Szulman A E 1988 The biology of trophoblastic disease: complete and partial hydatidiform moles. In: Beard R W, Sharp F (eds) Early pregnancy loss, mechanisms and treatment. Springer-Verlag, London, pp 309–316

UK Multicentre Trial 1990 The efficacy and tolerance of mifepristone and prostaglandin in first trimester termination of pregnancy. British Journal of Obstetrics and Gynaecology 97: 480–486

United Kingdom Central Council for Nursing, Midwifery and Health Visiting (UKCC) 1994 The midwife's code of practice. UKCC, London, p 5

Vergani P, Ghidini A, Strobelt N, Roncaglia N, Locatelli A, Lapinski R, Mangioni C 1994 Do uterine leiomyomas influence pregnancy outcome? American Journal of Perinatology 11(5): 356–358

Weekes A R L, Atlay R D, Brown V A, Jordan E C, Murray S M 1976 The retroverted gravid uterus and its effect on the outcome of pregnancy. British Medical Journal 1: 622–624

Weigel M, Weigel R M 1989 Nausea and vomiting of early pregnancy and pregnancy outcome. An epidemiological study. British Journal of Obstetrics and Gynaecology 96: 1304–1311

Yedema K A, Verheijen R H, Kenemans P, Schijf C P, Borm G F, Segers M F, Thomas C M 1993 Identification of patients with persistent trophoblastic disease by means of a normal human chorionic gonadotrophin regression curve. American Journal of Obstetrics and Gynecology 168(3): 787–792

FURTHER READING

Dimond B 1994 Legal aspects of midwifery. Books for Midwives, Hale, ch 25, pp 239–246

Hord C E, Delano G E 1996 Reducing maternal mortality from abortion: the midwife's role in abortion care. In: Murray S F (ed) Midwives and safer motherhood. Mosby, London, ch 5, pp 63–78

McDonald M 1996 Loss in midwifery. Guidelines for midwives. Baillière Tindall, London

United Kingdom Central Council for Nursing, Midwifery and Health Visiting (UKCC) 1996 Guidelines for professional practice. UKCC, London

Problems of pregnancy

Helen Crafter

15

Problems of pregnancy range from the mildly irritating to life-threatening conditions. Fortunately the life-threatening ones are rare because of improvements to the general health of the population, improved social circumstances and lower parity. However, as women delay childbearing (an increasing phenomenon in the developed world) they become more at risk of medical disorders associated with increasing age, such as malignancy, placenta praevia and problems associated with obesity. Regular antenatal checks beginning early in pregnancy are valuable in both preventing complications and their ensuing problems, and contributing to timely diagnosis and treatment.

The chapter aims to:

- provide an overview of the medical problems of pregnancy

- describe the role of the midwife in relation to the identification, assessment and management of different disorders

- consider the needs of both parents for continuing support and reassurance when a disorder has been diagnosed.

The midwife's role

The midwife's role in relation to the medical problems associated with pregnancy is clear. At initial and subsequent encounters with the pregnant woman it is essential that an accurate health history is obtained. General and specific physical examinations must be carried out and the results meticulously recorded. The examination and recordings give direction towards future referral and management. Whilst the elements of antenatal care are routine for the midwife they will be very individual for the mother in her care.

Where the midwife detects in the health of the

mother or fetus a deviation from the norm, she must refer that woman to a registered medical practitioner (UKCC 1993).

The midwife will continue to offer the woman care and support throughout her pregnancy and beyond. The woman who develops problems during her pregnancy is no less in need of the midwife's skilled attention and, indeed, her condition and psychological state may be considerably improved by the midwife's continued presence and support.

ABDOMINAL PAIN IN PREGNANCY

Abdominal pain is a common complaint in pregnancy. It is probably suffered by all women at some stage, and therefore presents a problem for the midwife in distinguishing the physiologically normal (for instance mild indigestion or muscle stretching) and the pathological but not dangerous (for instance degeneration of a fibroid) from the dangerously pathological requiring immediate referral to the appropriate medical practitioner for urgent treatment (for instance ectopic pregnancy or appendicitis).

The midwife should take a detailed history and perform a physical examination in order to reach a decision as to whether to refer the woman. Treatment will depend on the cause (Box 15.1), and the maternal and fetal conditions.

Many of the pregnancy-specific causes of abdominal pain in pregnancy listed in Box 15.1 are dealt with in this and other chapters. For many of these conditions abdominal pain is one of many, and not necessarily an overriding, symptom. However, an observant midwife may be crucial to a safe pregnancy outcome for a woman presenting with abdominal pain.

Uterine fibroid degeneration

The problems experienced in early pregnancy, as outlined in Chapter 14, may continue throughout the pregnancy as the muscle fibres continue to hypertrophy and the fibroid (myoma) enlarges. Approximately 10% of women with uterine fibroids will experience acute pain, as fibroids situated

---

Box 15.1 Causes of abdominal pain in pregnancy (Clewell 1994)

Pregnancy-specific causes
- Physiological
  - Round ligament pain
  - Braxton Hicks contractions
  - Miscellaneous discomfort in late pregnancy
  - Severe uterine torsion
- Pathological
  - Ectopic pregnancy
  - Miscarriage
  - Uterine fibroids
  - Urinary tract infection
  - Placental abruption
  - Preterm labour
  - Severe pre-eclampsia
  - Uterine rupture

Incidental causes
- Physiological
  - Heartburn, excessive vomiting, constipation
- Common pathology
  - Appendicitis
  - Bowel obstruction
  - Cholecystitis
  - Renal disease
  - Inflammatory bowel disease
  - Acute pancreatitis
  - Peptic ulcer
  - Torsion of the ovary
- Rare pathology
  - Rectus haematoma
  - Sickle crisis
  - Malignant disease
  - Porphyria
  - Arterial haemorrhage

---

within the myometrium may receive a diminished blood supply and, as the pregnancy progresses, there may be central core necrosis.

If the fibroid or fibroids were not diagnosed prior to pregnancy or in its early stages, diagnosis can be made at any stage by ultrasound, especially if a fibroid is seen where the pain is located. Often fibroids are easily palpable. The pain usually subsides within 4–7 days with adequate explanation to the woman, rest and analgesia. The pregnancy will usually progress to term. However, the pain is often recurrent, especially if more than one fibroid is present.

Occasionally, enlargement of the fibroid may impede the progress of labour. Rupture of the uterus at the affected site is a possibility which should always be considered when caring for the woman in labour.

Severe uterine torsion

As it grows during pregnancy, the uterus usually rotates to the right by no more than 40 degrees. On rare occasions, the uterus rotates by more than 90 degrees and this may cause abdominal pain in the latter half of pregnancy. There is almost always a predisposing factor in such cases of acute torsion, the most common being fibroid, congenital malformation of the uterus, adnexal mass or a history of pelvic surgery (Clewell 1994).

The condition is usually managed conservatively by bedrest, altering the maternal position to correct the torsion spontaneously. Analgesia may be required and the well-being of the mother and fetus should be monitored, as in the rare severe cases the mother can become shocked and the fetus deprived of oxygen. In such cases a laparotomy will be performed as it is said to be difficult to make a clear diagnosis without surgical evidence. Delivery by caesarean section may be performed, either preceded or followed by manipulation of the uterus.

PELVIC ARTHROPATHY

Pelvic arthropathy is characterised by abnormal relaxation of the ligaments supporting the pubic joint. This is brought about by high levels of pregnancy hormones, particularly relaxin. The result of the relaxation is increased mobility of the joint; the pubic bones move up and down alternately as the woman walks. Strain on the sacroiliac joints may also occur, particularly in grande multiparae.

The woman will complain of pain in the pubic region, and also of backache, at any time from the 28th week of pregnancy. Pain may be experienced in the abdominal muscles owing to an attempt to stabilise the bones by muscular action. On examination, the mother will complain of tenderness over the symphysis pubis.

The midwife should note whether there is any history of pelvic fractures which may be aggravated by the pregnancy. Otherwise the midwife should explain to the mother the cause of this condition and advise her that as much rest as possible will be beneficial, especially as the pregnancy advances and abdominal distension increases. A supportive panty girdle and comfortable shoes may also help when the woman is up and about.

The midwife should notify the doctor of this condition and of the advice which she has given. Advice and treatment from an obstetric physiotherapist will be of great help to the woman. In severe cases, bedrest may be necessary. A fracture board will be required.

The ligaments should slowly return to normal following delivery. Postnatal physiotherapy will aid the strengthening and stabilisation of the joint.

ANTEPARTUM HAEMORRHAGE (APH)

Bleeding from the genital tract in late pregnancy, after the 24th week of gestation and before the onset of labour, is referred to as an antepartum haemorrhage. This may place the life of the mother and unborn child at risk.

Effect on the fetus

Fetal mortality and morbidity are increased as a result of severe vaginal bleeding in pregnancy. Stillbirth or neonatal death may occur. Premature placental separation and consequent hypoxia may result in the birth of a child who is mentally and physically impaired.

Effect on the mother

If bleeding is severe, it may be accompanied by shock and disseminated intravascular coagulation. The mother may die or be left with permanent ill health.

These events are infrequently seen by practitioners in the UK.

Types of antepartum haemorrhage

If bleeding from local lesions of the genital tract (*incidental causes*) is excluded, vaginal bleeding in late pregnancy is confined to placental separation due to *placenta praevia* or *placental abruption* (Table 15.1).

Table 15.1 Causes of bleeding in late pregnancy (Konje & Wally 1994)

Cause	Incidence (%)
Placenta praevia	31
Abruption	22
'Other bleeding'	47
Marginal	(60.0)
'Show'	(20.0)
Cervicitis	(8.0)
Trauma	(5.0)
Vulvovaginal varicosities	(2.0)
Genital tumours	(0.5)
Genital infections	(0.5)
Haematuria	(0.5)
Vasa praevia	(0.5)
Other	(0.5)

Note: Konje & Wally do not explain the lost 2.5% of 'Other bleeding'.

Initial appraisal of a woman with antepartum haemorrhage

When a woman first loses blood per vaginam during pregnancy, she has little idea of the cause and will find the episode frightening and disturbing. She may call the midwife or present herself at hospital. Her first need is for a feeling that someone capable is in control of the situation. She will fear that she is losing her baby; her partner may fear for the life of both mother and child. The midwife's role at this stage is to be supportive and ascertain as much detail as possible of the history and the circumstances surrounding the blood loss. This will assist both in assessing the woman's condition and in making a diagnosis. However, the midwife will also be aware that antepartum haemorrhage is unpredictable and the woman's condition can deteriorate rapidly at any time; she must therefore make a rapid decision as to the urgency of need of a medical and/or paramedic presence, often at the same time as observing and talking to the woman and her partner.

Sometimes, bleeding which the woman had presumed to be from the vagina will in fact be from haemorrhoids. The midwife should consider this differential diagnosis and confirm or exclude this as soon as possible by careful questioning and examination.

Assessment of physical condition

Maternal condition. The first priority is the well-being of the mother. The midwife will look for any pallor or breathlessness which may indicate shock. She will weigh up the woman's emotional state as she greets her and begins to ask for a history of events. She must generate the trust of both partners and remain calm.

Observation of pulse rate, respiratory rate, blood pressure and temperature will be made and recorded. The midwife must assess the amount of blood lost in order to ensure adequate fluid replacement. She will discuss with the couple how much has been lost earlier and should ask to see all soiled articles, retaining them for the doctor's inspection.

A gentle abdominal examination is made, observing for signs that the woman is going into labour. *On no account must any vaginal or rectal examination be made nor may an enema or suppository be given to a woman suffering from an antepartum haemorrhage, as these procedures could exacerbate the bleeding.*

Fetal condition. The mother should be asked if the baby has been moving as much as normal. The midwife must attempt to auscultate the fetal heart and may use ultrasound apparatus to obtain the information.

Factors to aid differential diagnosis

The location of the placenta is perhaps the most critical piece of information which will be needed in order to make a correct diagnosis; initially the midwife will not usually have this fact at her disposal. If she is able to elicit the following information from her observations and talking to the woman and her partner, it will help her to arrive at a provisional diagnosis:

Pain. Did the pain precede bleeding and is it continuous or intermittent?

Onset of bleeding. Was this associated with any event such as coitus?

Amount of visible blood loss. Is there any reason to suspect that some blood has been retained in utero?

Colour of the blood. Is it bright red or darker in colour?

Degree of shock. Is this commensurate with the amount of blood visible or more severe?

Consistency of the abdomen. Is it soft or tense and board-like?

Tenderness of the abdomen. Does the mother resent abdominal palpation?

Lie, presentation and engagement. Are any of these abnormal when taking account of parity and gestation?

Audibility of the fetal heart. Is the fetal heart heard?

Ultrasound scan. Does a scan suggest that the placenta is in the lower uterine segment?

The relevance of the findings from these observations is further discussed in the context of the various causes of antepartum haemorrhage.

Supportive treatment

After emotional reassurance the first need is for restoration of physical condition. This will necessitate fluid replacement with a plasma expander and later with whole blood. If the mother is in severe pain she must have strong analgesia to help counteract shock. If the midwife is in attendance at home she must summon the emergency obstetric unit where this exists, or alternatively the ambulance service. If she carries intravenous equipment she should site an infusion. The obstetric registrar or paramedic will carry and infuse a plasma expander before transfer of the woman to hospital.

Subsequent management depends on the definite diagnosis.

Placenta praevia

The placenta is partially or wholly implanted in the lower uterine segment on either the anterior or posterior wall. The anterior location is less serious than the posterior.

The lower uterine segment grows and stretches progressively after the 12th week of pregnancy.

In later weeks this may cause the placenta to separate and severe bleeding can occur. Bleeding is caused by shearing stress between the placental trophoblast and maternal venous blood sinuses. In some instances bleeding may be precipitated by coitus. Placenta praevia places the mother and fetus at high risk and it constitutes an obstetric emergency. Medical assistance is vital if the lives of the mother and fetus are to be saved. Women with suspected placenta praevia should be transferred to a consultant obstetric unit either at the request of the general practitioner or via the obstetric emergency service.

Degrees of placenta praevia

Type 1 placenta praevia. The majority of the placenta is in the upper uterine segment (Figs 15.1 and 15.5). Vaginal delivery is possible. Blood loss is usually mild and the mother and fetus remain in good condition.

Type 2 placenta praevia. The placenta is partially located in the lower segment near the internal cervical os (marginal placenta praevia) (Figs 15.2 and 15.6). Vaginal delivery is possible, particularly if the placenta is anterior. Blood loss is usually moderate, although the conditions of the mother and fetus can vary. Fetal hypoxia is more likely to be present than maternal shock.

Type 3 placenta praevia. The placenta is located over the internal cervical os but not centrally (Figs 15.3 and 15.7). Bleeding is likely to be severe, particularly when the lower segment stretches and the cervix begins to efface and dilate in late pregnancy. Vaginal delivery is inappropriate because the placenta precedes the fetus.

Type 4 placenta praevia. The placenta is located centrally over the internal cervical os (Figs 15.4 and 15.8) and torrential haemorrhage is very likely. Vaginal delivery should not be considered. Caesarean section is essential in order to save the lives of the mother and fetus.

Indications of placenta praevia

Bleeding per vaginam is the only sign and it is painless. The uterus is not tender or tense. The

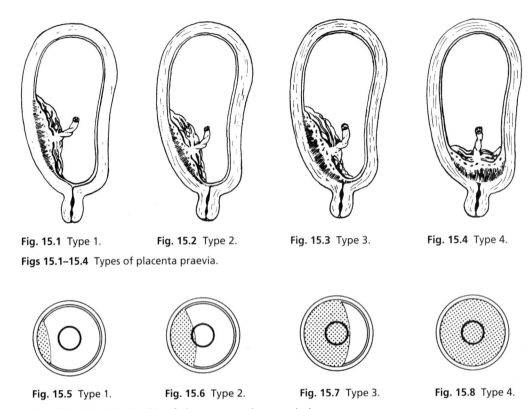

Fig. 15.1 Type 1.   **Fig. 15.2** Type 2.   **Fig. 15.3** Type 3.   **Fig. 15.4** Type 4.

Figs 15.1–15.4 Types of placenta praevia.

Fig. 15.5 Type 1.   **Fig. 15.6** Type 2.   **Fig. 15.7** Type 3.   **Fig. 15.8** Type 4.

Figs 15.5–15.8 Relationship of placenta praevia to cervical os.

presence of placenta praevia should be considered when:

- the fetal head remains unengaged in a primigravida
- there is a malpresentation, especially breech
- the lie is oblique or transverse
- the lie is unstable, usually in a multigravida.

Localisation of the placenta using ultrasonic scanning will confirm the existence of placenta praevia and establish its degree.

Assessing the mother's condition

The amount of vaginal bleeding is variable. Some mothers may have a history of a small repeated blood loss at intervals throughout pregnancy. Others may have a sudden single episode of vaginal bleeding after the 20th week but severe haemorrhage occurs most frequently after the 34th week of pregnancy.

The haemorrhage may be mild, moderate or severe, is often not associated with any particular type of activity and may occur at rest. The colour of the blood is bright red, denoting fresh bleeding. The low placental location allows all of the lost blood to escape unimpeded and a retroplacental clot is not formed. For this reason pain is not a feature of placenta praevia.

General examination. If the haemorrhage is slight the woman's blood pressure, respiratory rate and pulse rate may be normal. In severe haemorrhage, however, the blood pressure will be low and the pulse rate raised due to shock. The degree of shock correlates with the amount of blood lost per vaginam. Respirations are also rapid and the mother may have air hunger due to a reduction in the number of red blood cells in the circulation available for the uptake of oxygen. The mother's colour will be pale and her skin cold and moist.

Abdominal examination. The midwife may find that the lie of the fetus is oblique or transverse and the fetal head may be high in a primigravida near term. The uterine consistency is normal and pain is not experienced by the mother when her abdomen is palpated.

The midwife should not attempt to do a vaginal examination as this could precipitate a torrential haemorrhage and worsen the situation.

An attempt should be made to quantify the amount of blood lost and all blood-soaked material used by the mother should be saved. Although this will not provide an accurate estimation of the quantity, it may be a helpful clue in assessing fluid replacement.

Assessing the fetal condition

The mother should be asked whether fetal activity has been normal. She may be aware of diminution or cessation of fetal movements which may occur if fetal hypoxia is severe. In some instances she may report that her fetal movements have been excessive which is another indication of severe fetal hypoxia.

The midwife should assess the fetal condition using an ultrasound fetal monitor such as a cardiotocograph or hand-held device. A Pinard fetal stethoscope may be used if these are not available. Fetal oxygenation depends upon the proportion of the placenta remaining attached. Fetal hypoxia is an emergency and medical assistance should be called urgently.

Management of placenta praevia

The management of placenta praevia depends on:

- the amount of bleeding
- the conditions of mother and fetus
- the location of the placenta
- the stage of the pregnancy.

Conservative management is appropriate if bleeding is slight and the mother and fetus are well. The woman will be kept in hospital at rest until bleeding has stopped. A speculum examination will have ruled out incidental causes. Further bleeding is almost inevitable if the placenta encroaches into the lower segment and therefore it is usual to require the woman to remain in hospital for the rest of the pregnancy. Placental function is monitored by means of fetal kick charts and antenatal cardiotocography. Ultrasound scans are repeated at intervals in order to observe the position of the placenta in relation to the cervical os as the lower segment grows. Fetal growth is also monitored as placental perfusion across the lower segment is less efficient than that in a fundally situated placenta, and intrauterine growth retardation may result.

A woman who is asked to stay in hospital for many weeks will have particular psychological and social needs. If she has other children, she will be anxious to know that good arrangements have been made for their care and they must be allowed to visit her frequently. She should be offered parent education and sometimes it may be possible to continue with the group she has been attending. Occupational therapy may help to alleviate the boredom often felt during long-stay hospital admission. A visit to the Special Care Baby Unit, perhaps with her family, and answering any questions she has may also help to prepare her for the possibility of preterm delivery.

A decision will be made as to how and when the woman will be delivered. If the woman does not have further severe bleeding she will be delivered when the fetus reaches maturity, vaginally if the placental location allows. Vaginal ultrasound allows for a more accurate estimation of placental site, on which the decision about mode of delivery will be based.

Vaginal delivery is usual with Type 1 placenta praevia and possible with Type 2 unless the placenta is situated immediately above the sacral promontory where it is vulnerable to pressure from an advancing fetal head and may impede descent. The degrees of placenta praevia which are amenable to vaginal delivery may be termed minor. Labour is likely to be induced from 37 weeks' gestation.

The midwife should be aware that even if vaginal delivery is achieved, there remains a danger of postpartum haemorrhage because the placenta has been situated in the lower segment where there is paucity of oblique muscle fibres and therefore the living ligature action will be poor.

Active management. Severe vaginal bleeding

will necessitate immediate delivery by caesarean section regardless of the location of the placenta. This should take place in a unit with facilities for special care of the newborn especially if the baby will be preterm.

Blood will be taken for a full blood count, cross-matching and clotting studies. An intravenous infusion will be in progress and several units of blood may need to be transfused quickly. In an emergency it may be necessary to give group O blood, if possible of the same Rhesus group as the mother.

An anaesthetist will be involved in the woman's care in assessing her fluid requirements and output and helping her to make a decision about regional or general anaesthesia (if she is able).

During the assessment and preparation for theatre the mother will be extremely anxious and the midwife must comfort and encourage her, giving her as much information as possible. The partner will also need to be supported, especially if he has to wait outside the theatre during the operation.

If the placenta is situated anteriorly in the uterus, this may complicate the surgical approach as it underlies the site of the normal incision.

In major degrees of placenta praevia (Types 3 and 4) caesarean section is required even if the fetus has died in utero. This will prevent torrential haemorrhage and possible maternal death.

Incidence

Placenta praevia occurs in 0.5% of all pregnancies. It is more common in multigravidae, with an incidence of 1 in 90 deliveries. (Placenta praevia rates rise in women with increasing age and increasing parity.) In primigravidae the incidence is 1 in 250 deliveries. Its aetiology is unknown but raised incidence is also seen in women who smoke and those who have had a previous caesarean section. The recurrence rate for women who have had a previous placenta praevia is in the order of 4–8%.

Complications include:

- maternal shock, resulting from blood loss and hypovolaemia
- anaesthetic and surgical complications, which are more common in women with major

degrees of placenta praevia, and in those for whom preparation for surgery has been suboptimal (DH et al 1996)
- placenta accreta in up to 15% of women with placenta praevia
- air embolism, an occasional occurrence when the sinuses in the placental bed have been broken
- postpartum haemorrhage: occasionally uncontrolled haemorrhage will continue, despite the administration of oxytocic drugs at delivery – even following the best efforts to control it, a caesarean hysterectomy may be required to save the woman's life
- maternal death, a very rare outcome of this condition (DH et al 1996)
- fetal hypoxia and its sequelae due to placental separation
- fetal death, depending on gestation and amount of blood loss.

Placental abruption

Premature separation of a normally situated placenta occurring after the 22nd week of pregnancy is referred to as placental abruption. The aetiology of this type of haemorrhage is not always clear but it is often associated with pregnancy-induced hypertension or with a sudden reduction in uterine size. Rarely, direct trauma to the abdomen may partially dislodge the placenta.

Unlike inevitable haemorrhage which is due to placenta praevia, placental abruption is an accidental occurrence of haemorrhage in 2% of all pregnancies. Accidental in this context does not denote trauma.

Partial separation of the placenta causes bleeding from the maternal venous sinuses in the placental bed. Further bleeding continues to separate the placenta to a greater or lesser degree. If blood escapes from the placental site it separates the membranes from the uterine wall and drains through the vagina. Blood which is retained behind the placenta may be forced into the myometrium and it infiltrates between the muscle fibres of the uterus. This extravasation can cause marked damage and if observed at operation the uterus will appear bruised and oedematous. This is termed Couvelaire uterus or uterine apoplexy. There is no vaginal bleeding, but the mother will have all the signs and symptoms of hypovolaemic shock, caused by concealed bleeding into the muscle of the uterus. The concealed haemorrhage causes uterine enlargement and extreme pain.

A combination of these two situations where some of the blood drains via the vagina and some is retained behind the placenta is known as a mixed haemorrhage.

Types of placental abruption

The blood loss from a placental abruption may be defined as revealed, concealed or mixed haemorrhage as described above. An alternative classification, based on the degree of separation and therefore related to the condition of the mother and baby, is of mild, moderate and severe haemorrhage. The midwife cannot rely on visible blood loss as a guide to the severity of the haemorrhage; on the contrary the most severe haemorrhage is that which is totally concealed.

Assessing the mother's condition

There may be a history of pregnancy-induced hypertension. A recent history of headaches, nausea, vomiting, epigastric pain and visual disturbances may be a feature. Road traffic accidents are probably the most likely cause of trauma to the abdomen. External cephalic version injudiciously performed may result in placental separation. The midwife should be aware of the possibility of placental separation after the birth of a first twin or loss of copious amounts of amniotic fluid.

The mildest degrees of placental abruption are relatively pain-free, although the mother may experience a slight localised pain. The blood loss is revealed. More severe degrees are associated with abdominal pain and the midwife should enquire as to the time of onset and whether the bleeding (if any) began simultaneously or later.

General examination. The woman is likely to be anxious, experiencing abdominal pain and her skin will be pale and moist if she is shocked. On clinical examination the mother may have obvious oedema of the face, fingers and pretibial area of the lower limbs due to pre-eclampsia.

The blood pressure and pulse should be taken immediately. A low blood pressure and raised pulse rate are signs of shock; if the mother has pregnancy-induced hypertension the blood pressure may be within normal limits, having been raised prior to the haemorrhage. The respirations may be normal or rapid and reduced oxygenation may lead to air hunger. The temperature will usually be normal but, as placental abruption may be caused by severe infection, it should be taken.

The amount of any visible blood loss should be estimated and its colour noted. Freshly lost blood is bright red; blood that has been retained in utero for any length of time changes to a brown colour.

Abdominal examination. Concealed haemorrhage may lead to uterine enlargement in excess of gestation. The uterus has a hard consistency and there is guarding on palpation of the abdomen. Palpation may be difficult and should not be attempted if the uterus is rigid and excessively painful. Fetal parts may not be palpable. In less severe cases palpation should be kept to a minimum in order to avoid further damage. The nature and location of the pain should be established.

The fetal heart is unlikely to be heard with a fetal stethoscope if there has been any concealed haemorrhage; an ultrasound scanner, cardiotocograph or hand-held device should be used. If the haemorrhage is severe, fetal death is a common outcome.

Assessing the fetal condition

The woman may be aware of a cessation of fetal movements. It is said that excessive fetal movements may also occur as a result of profound hypoxia. A cardiotocograph recording will give more complete information about fetal condition, as will an ultrasound scan of the heart chambers. Failure to elicit heart sounds with a Pinard stethoscope is not confirmation of fetal death.

The midwife should take care how she conveys information about the fetus to the mother. If the heart is inaudible on first examination, she should explain that a fetal monitor is needed to establish the condition of her baby. If fetal heart sounds can be detected with ultrasonic apparatus, this will be of great comfort to the mother. It is rarely, if ever, appropriate to attempt to conceal fetal death from the mother.

Management

Any woman with a history suggestive of placental abruption needs urgent medical attention. She should be transferred speedily to a consultant obstetric unit, preferably by the emergency obstetric service. The general practitioner may be called to the home in the first instance.

On arrival at the hospital the woman is admitted to the delivery suite and the registrar or consultant obstetrician is informed. The midwife should offer the woman comfort and encouragement by attending to her physical and emotional needs, including her need for information.

Pain exacerbates shock and must be alleviated. As it may be extreme, a suitable analgesic would be morphine 15 mg or pethidine 100–150 mg. If the woman has had a narcotic drug prior to admission, the midwife must alert those in attendance to the fact that analgesia has been given.

The acute pain of concealed haemorrhage from placental abruption is due to the extravasation of blood between the muscle fibres of the uterus. This must be differentiated from the pain of uterine contraction due to the onset of labour and from subcapsular liver haemorrhage as a result of pre-eclampsia. The nature of the pain should be discussed because labour may supervene following placental abruption.

Shock may be due to hypovolaemia, to extravasation and consequent pain or to consumptive coagulopathy. The latter is due to tissue damage and the liberation of thromboplastins into the circulation with resulting disseminated intravascular coagulation. This is discussed later in this chapter.

If blood is not available for immediate transfusion, hypovolaemia may be reduced by administering a suitable plasma expander. Letsky (1995) favours the use of Haemaccel which does not interfere with platelet function or subsequent blood grouping and cross-matching of blood. It also helps to improve renal function. However, this is only a temporary palliative and blood transfusion must follow as quickly as possible.

The woman should rest on her side in order to prevent vena caval occlusion and aortic compression by the gravid uterus. If shock becomes severe and medical assistance cannot be immediately obtained, or intravenous access secured, placing the woman flat or in a semi-recumbent position with the legs only raised will help to sustain the circulation to her upper body for a short period. However, under no circumstances should the foot of the bed be elevated as this will cause pooling of blood in the vagina and is unlikely to reduce shock.

Observations

As the maternal and fetal conditions become apparent following admission to the delivery suite, decisions will be made about management. If resuscitation of the woman is required her condition should be stabilised before surgery is undertaken. Likewise, if the woman and fetus are not in imminent danger (or the fetus has died) some time will elapse before surgery is considered, and at this time it is crucial that the midwife maintains continual and accurate observations.

The mother's blood pressure and pulse rate should be taken at frequent intervals, which will depend on the severity of her condition. If a pyrexia is present the temperature may be recorded every 1–2 hours; if the woman is not feverish, a 4-hourly recording is adequate. A central venous line is usually inserted in order to monitor the central venous pressure 2-hourly or more frequently as necessary (see Ch. 25). If the haemorrhage is not severe enough to warrant intravenous infusion, a cannula will be sited in case the haemorrhage suddenly worsens.

Urinary output is accurately assessed by the insertion of an indwelling catheter. Oliguria or anuria indicates suppression of renal function which may persist until a postpartum diuresis occurs. The urine should be tested for the presence of protein, which may also be linked to pre-eclampsia. Fluid intake must also be recorded accurately and fluid balance assessed with the aid of the central venous pressure recordings.

Fundal height and abdominal girth are measured hourly. An increase indicates continued bleeding behind the placenta. If the fetus is alive, the fetal heart rate should be monitored continuously with the aid of a cardiotocograph.

Any deterioration in the maternal or fetal conditions must be immediately reported to the obstetrician.

Investigations

As soon as practicable following admission a full blood count, cross-match and clotting studies will be obtained. Blood samples may be needed at intervals in order to monitor the progress of the condition. If pre-eclampsia is suspected blood urea and electrolytes will also be measured.

Management of different degrees of placental abruption

Mild separation of the placenta. In this case the placental separation and the haemorrhage are slight. Mother and fetus are in a stable condition. There is no indication of maternal shock and the fetus is alive with normal heart sounds. The consistency of the uterus is normal and there is no tenderness on abdominal palpation. It may be difficult to differentiate this condition from placenta praevia and from an incidental cause of vaginal bleeding.

An ultrasound scan can determine the placental location and identify any degree of concealed bleeding. Fetal condition should be continually assessed while bleeding persists by frequent, if not continuous, monitoring of the fetal heart rate. Subsequently cardiotocography should be carried out once or twice daily because any degree of abruption by definition involves partial separation of the placenta.

If the woman is not in labour and the gestation is less than 37 weeks she may be cared for in an antenatal ward for a few days. She may then go home if there is no further bleeding and the placenta has been found to be in the upper uterine segment. Women who have passed the 37th week of pregnancy will have labour induced, often by amniotomy. Further bleeding or evidence of fetal distress may indicate that a caesarean section is necessary.

Moderate separation of the placenta. This describes placental separation of about one-quarter. Up to 1000 ml of blood may be lost, some of which will escape per vaginam and some be retained behind the placenta as retroplacental clot or extravasation into the uterine muscle. The mother will be shocked, with a raised pulse rate and a lowered blood pressure. There will be a degree of uterine tenderness and abdominal guarding. The fetus may be alive although hypoxic; intrauterine death is a possibility.

The immediate aims of care are to reduce shock and to replace blood loss. Fluid replacement should be monitored with the aid of a central venous pressure line (see above). The fetal condition should be assessed with continuous cardiotocography if the fetus is alive, in which case immediate caesarean section may be indicated once the woman's condition is stabilised.

If the fetus is in good condition or has already died, vaginal birth may be contemplated. Such a delivery is advantageous because it enables the uterus to contract and control the bleeding. The spontaneous onset of labour frequently accompanies moderately severe placental abruption but if it does not, amniotomy is usually sufficient to induce labour. Oxytocin may be used with great care if necessary. Delivery is often quite sudden after a short labour. The use of drugs to attempt to stop labour is usually inappropriate.

Moderate separation of the placenta may on occasion deteriorate into a more serious degree of separation.

Severe separation of the placenta. This is an acute obstetric emergency; at least two-thirds of the placenta has become detached and 2000 ml of blood or more are lost from the circulation. Most or all of the blood will be concealed behind the placenta. The woman will be severely shocked to a degree far beyond what might be expected from the amount of visible blood loss. The blood pressure will be lowered; the reading may lie within the normal range owing to a preceding hypertension. The fetus will almost certainly be dead. The woman will have very severe abdominal pain with excruciating tenderness; the uterus has a board-like consistency.

Features associated with severe haemorrhage are coagulation defects, renal failure and pituitary failure.

Treatment is the same as for moderate haemorrhage. Whole blood should be transfused rapidly and subsequent amounts calculated in accordance with the woman's central venous pressure. Labour may begin spontaneously in advance of amniotomy and the midwife should be alert for signs of uterine contraction causing periodic intensifying of the abdominal pain. However, if bleeding continues or a compromised fetal heart rate is present, caesarean section may be required as soon as the woman's condition has been adequately stabilised. The woman requires constant explanation and psychological support, despite the fact that because of her shocked condition she may not be fully conscious. Pain relief must also be considered. The woman's partner will also be very concerned, and should not be forgotten in the rush to stabilise the woman's condition.

Care of the baby

Preparation should be made for an asphyxiated baby. The paediatrician must be present at the birth to resuscitate the infant. The baby may require neonatal intensive care following delivery and the staff of the neonatal unit will have been alerted. In addition to the insult of the haemorrhage the baby may suffer from the effects of preterm delivery and her or his stay in the neonatal unit may be prolonged.

A baby who is born in good condition will of course require minimal resuscitation and may be transferred to the postnatal ward with her or his mother.

Psychological care

When a woman has a placental abruption she and her partner must be kept fully informed of what is happening at all times. The doctor should have a full and frank discussion with them about the events and the prognosis. The midwife should ensure that the partner is offered support and adequate explanation if the woman requires emergency surgery or if her condition deteriorates suddenly. Whenever possible he should continue to be present and he may need another member of the family to share the burden.

If the fetus is alive, a midwife from the neonatal unit should visit the couple in order to introduce herself and explain where the baby will be cared for after delivery. The partner should be encouraged to visit the unit.

When the baby is born, if it is at all possible, the parents should be given a chance to see and handle their child before she or he is transferred to the neonatal unit. It is most helpful to have a photograph taken which the mother can keep beside her, and the father should visit the baby at the earliest opportunity. Later the mother will be taken to see the baby, if necessary in her bed or in a wheelchair. As soon as she is able, she will be encouraged to participate in caring for her baby.

At a suitable time following her recovery, the mother must be invited to discuss the events and the prognosis for her baby. She may ask about the possibility of haemorrhage occurring in future pregnancies and can usually be reassured.

Complications

- Disseminated intravascular coagulation is a complication of moderate to severe placental abruption.
- Postpartum haemorrhage may occur as a result of the Couvelaire uterus and disseminated intravascular coagulation or both. Intravenous ergometrine 0.5 mg is given at delivery as a prophylactic measure.
- Renal failure may occur as a result of hypovolaemia and consequent poor perfusion of the kidneys.
- Pituitary necrosis is another possible consequence of prolonged and severe hypotension.

BLOOD COAGULATION FAILURE

Normal blood coagulation

Haemostasis refers to the arrest of bleeding. Its function is to prevent loss of blood from the blood vessels. It depends on the mechanism of coagulation. This is counterbalanced by fibrinolysis which ensures that the blood vessels are reopened in order to maintain the patency of the circulation.

Blood clotting occurs in three main stages:

• When tissues are damaged and platelets break down, *thromboplastin* is released.

• In the presence of *calcium* ions thromboplastin leads to the conversion of *prothrombin* into *thrombin*.
• Thrombin is a proteolytic (protein-splitting) enzyme which converts *fibrinogen* into *fibrin*.

Fibrin forms a network of long, sticky strands which entrap blood cells to establish a clot. The coagulated material contracts and exudes serum which is plasma depleted of its clotting factors.

This is the final part of a complex cascade of coagulation involving a large number of different clotting factors. These factors have been assigned numbers in order of their discovery and a summary of the process is shown in Figure 15.9.

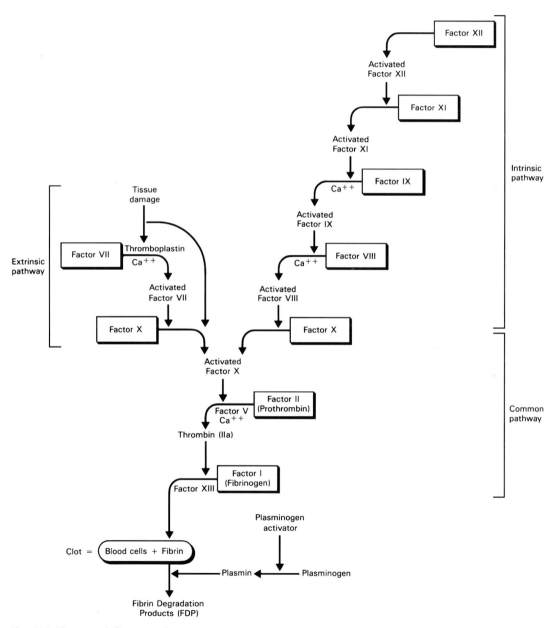

Fig. 15.9 The coagulation cascade.

It is equally important for a healthy person to maintain the blood as a fluid in order that it can circulate freely. The coagulation mechanism is normally held at bay by the presence of heparin which is produced in the liver.

Fibrinolysis is the breakdown of fibrin and occurs as response to the presence of clotted blood. Unless fibrinolysis takes place, coagulation will continue. It is achieved by the activation of a series of enzymes culminating in the proteolytic enzyme plasmin. This breaks down the fibrin in the clots and produces fibrin degradation products (FDPs).

Disseminated intravascular coagulation (DIC)

This is a situation of inappropriate coagulation within the blood vessels which leads to the consumption of clotting factors. As a result clotting fails to occur at the bleeding site.

Aetiology

DIC is never a primary disease – it always occurs as a response to another disease process. Such an event triggers widespread clotting with the formation of microthrombi throughout the circulation. Clotting factors are used up. The DIC triggers fibrinolysis and the production of FDPs. FDPs reduce the efficiency of normal clotting. A paradoxical feedback system is therefore set up, clotting being the primary problem, but haemorrhage being the predominant clinical finding.

When DIC occurs during or after delivery, the reduced level of clotting factors and the presence of FDPs prevent normal haemostasis at the placental site. FDPs inhibit myometrial action and prevent the uterine muscle from constricting the blood vessels in the normal way. Torrential haemorrhage may be the outcome. Visible blood loss may be observed to remain uncoagulated for several minutes and even when clotting does occur, the clot is unstable.

Microthrombi may cause circulatory obstruction in the small blood vessels. The effects of this vary from cyanosis of fingers and toes to cerebrovascular accidents and failure of organs such as the liver and kidneys.

Events which trigger DIC

There are a number of obstetric events which may precipitate DIC:

- placental abruption
- intrauterine fetal death including missed abortion
- amniotic fluid embolism
- intrauterine infection including septic abortion
- pre-eclampsia and eclampsia.

Each of the conditions is dealt with in the appropriate chapter and only those aspects relating to DIC are discussed here.

Placental abruption. Owing to the damage of tissue at the placental site large quantities of thromboplastin are released into the circulation and may cause DIC. If the placenta is delivered as soon as possible after the abruption the risk of DIC is reduced.

Intrauterine fetal death. If a dead fetus is retained in utero for more than 3 or 4 weeks thromboplastins are released from the dead fetal tissues. These enter the maternal circulation and deplete clotting factors. If labour does not follow fetal death spontaneously, it should be induced. If fetal death is known to have occurred some time previously, clotting studies should be performed prior to induction of labour and if DIC is diagnosed the appropriate medical action should be taken.

Amniotic fluid embolism. If death does not occur from maternal collapse, DIC may develop. Thromboplastin in the amniotic fluid is responsible for setting off the cascade of clotting.

Intrauterine infection. The causes of this include septic abortion, hydatidiform mole, placenta accreta and endometrial infection before or after delivery. DIC is caused by endotoxins entering the circulation and damaging the blood vessels. Therefore as well as treating the DIC, the infection itself must be aggressively treated with antibiotics. It should be noted that if the woman develops haemolytic septicaemia any blood administered may be destroyed by the bacteria in the bloodstream. The baby may need treatment following delivery if the infection was antepartum. In post-partum infection any retained products must be evacuated from the uterus.

Pre-eclampsia and eclampsia. The exact aetiology of pregnancy-induced hypertension is unknown and the factors which precipitate DIC as a complication of this condition are unclear. FDPs are increased in the serum and urine which indicates that fibrinolysis is taking place.

Although some authors argue that the haemolysis, elevated liver enzymes and low platelets (HELLP) syndrome is a variant form of DIC, there is not universal agreement on this (Blake et al 1993).

Management

The midwife should be aware of the conditions which may cause DIC. She should be alert for signs that clotting is abnormal and the assessment of the nature of the clot should be part of her routine observation during the third stage of labour. Oozing from a venepuncture site or bleeding from the mucous membrane of the mother's mouth and nose must be noted and reported.

As well as a full blood count and blood grouping, the doctor will carry out clotting studies and also measure the levels of platelets, fibrinogen and FDPs.

Treatment involves the replacement of blood cells and clotting factors in order to restore equilibrium. This is usually done by the administration of fresh frozen plasma and platelet concentrates. Banked red cells will be transfused subsequently. The use of fresh whole blood is not now common, partly because the screening processes undertaken in the modern transfusion service can take up to 24 hours and the components are best given separately. In situations where the transfusion service is not so sophisticated, whole blood will be used.

Care by the midwife

DIC causes a frightening situation which demands speed of recognition and of action. The midwife has to maintain her own calmness and clarity of thinking as well as helping the couple to deal with the situation in which they find themselves. Frequent and accurate observations must be maintained in order to monitor the woman's condition.

Blood pressure, pulse rate and temperature are recorded. The general condition is noted. Fluid balance is monitored with vigilance for any sign of renal failure.

The father in particular is likely to be baffled by a sudden turn in events when previously all seemed to be under control. The midwife must make sure that someone is giving him appropriate attention and he will need to be kept informed of what is happening and be excluded as little as possible. The carers need to be aware that he may find it impossible to absorb all that he is told and he may require repeated explanations. He may be the best person to help the woman to understand. The death of the mother is a real possibility and this may be one of the rare situations when the midwife finds herself needing to minister to a grieving partner.

HEPATIC DISORDERS AND JAUNDICE IN PREGNANCY

The metabolic changes in pregnancy influence hepatic function. These changes are brought about by the increased hormone levels. Some liver disorders are specific to pregnant women, and some pre-existing or coexisting disorders may complicate the pregnancy (Box 15.2).

Intrahepatic cholestasis of pregnancy (ICP)

This is an idiopathic condition which begins in pregnancy, usually in the third trimester but occasionally as early as the first trimester. It resolves spontaneously following delivery but has a

---

Box 15.2 Hepatic disorders of pregnancy

Specific to pregnancy
- Intrahepatic cholestasis of pregnancy (ICP)
- Acute fatty liver in pregnancy
- Pre-eclampsia and eclampsia (see Ch. 17)
- Severe hyperemesis gravidarum (see Ch. 14)
- Intrahepatic cholestasis of pregnancy (ICP)

Pre- or coexisting in pregnancy
- Gall bladder disease
- Hepatitis

40–60% recurrence rate in subsequent pregnancies (Walters 1994). It has a prevalence of 1–2 cases per 1000 pregnancies and its cause is unknown although genetic, geographical and environmental factors would appear to be at play. It is not a life-threatening condition for the mother but she is at increased risk of preterm labour, fetal distress and meconium staining and her stillbirth risk is increased by 15% without active management of her pregnancy. These problems are thought to be due to disturbances in fetal steroid metabolism.

Affected women will firstly start to notice pruritus at night, and may complain of fatigue and insomnia because of this. Two weeks later, 50% of women affected will develop mild jaundice which will persist until the birth. Fever, abdominal discomfort and nausea and vomiting are not uncommon symptoms. Women may notice that their urine is darker and stools paler than usual.

If this condition is suspected, blood will be tested for an increase in bile acids, serum alkaline phosphatase, bilirubin and transaminases. Hepatic viral studies and an ultrasound scan of the hepatobiliary tract, and an autoantibody screen (for primary biliary cirrhosis) are also indicated as of value in excluding differential diagnoses. The woman will be prescribed local antipruritic measures, for instance antihistamines, and advised to keep any sores, caused by scratching, clean. Because of concern about the implications of this condition for the fetus, the resultant jaundice and the severity of the itching, this woman will require sensitive psychological care. She will be prescribed a vitamin K supplement as her absorption will be poor (and the resulting hypoprothrombinaemia will predispose her to obstetric haemorrhage). Fetal wellbeing should be monitored and elective delivery considered when the fetus is mature (usually at 35–38 weeks of gestation) or earlier if the fetal condition appears to be compromised by the intrauterine environment.

The woman can be advised that her pruritus will resolve within 3–14 days following birth. She should be carefully monitored if she uses oral contraception in the future. The pruritus is often so severe and distressing that many women who have suffered from this condition will avoid future pregnancy.

Acute fatty liver of pregnancy (AFLP)

This is a rare condition of unknown aetiology which affects 1:10 000–1 000 000 pregnancies. It is frequently fatal for the mother and baby unless there is a speedy diagnosis and the correct treatment is given.

Typically, an obese woman will present with vomiting and a headache in her third trimester. She will quickly complain of malaise and severe abdominal pain, followed by jaundice and drowsiness. Fagan (1995) comments that over 50% of these women have symptoms of pre-eclampsia (hypertension and proteinuria), and so there is an inherent danger that the pre-eclampsia will mask the presentation of AFLP.

The condition is diagnosed by the clinical picture. The woman's liver is tender but not enlarged, and an ultrasound or computerised tomography (CT) scan of the liver demonstrates fatty infiltration. Liver biopsy is contraindicated owing to the risk of coagulopathy. The liver enzymes are moderately raised and the woman will also quickly show signs of renal failure and will become hypoglycaemic.

Management will firstly involve correcting any coagulopathy by measures such as infusing fresh frozen plasma. The woman must be delivered immediately. Caesarean section is said to have many advantages for the baby but it is safest for the mother to deliver vaginally if this is possible. Epidural analgesia is contraindicated in all but the mildest cases owing to the coagulopathy problems, unless these have been corrected first.

Convalescence is prolonged but usually complete. In the few cases where further pregnancy has been undertaken and recorded in the medical literature, recurrence has been low.

Gall bladder disease

Pregnancy appears to increase the likelihood of gallstone formation but not the risk of developing acute cholecystitis. Diagnosis of gall bladder disease is made by listening to the woman's previous history and/or an ultrasound scan of the hepatobiliary tract. She will require symptomatic treatment of the biliary colic by analgesia, hydration, nasogastric suction and antibiotics. Surgery should be avoided if at all possible.

Viral hepatitis (B)

Viral hepatitis is the most common cause of jaundice in pregnancy (Fagan 1995). It affects approximately 1:1000 pregnancies and has an incubation period of 1–6 months. Symptoms include nausea, vomiting, anorexia, pain over the liver, mild diarrhoea, jaundice lasting several weeks and malaise. Fever is rare and for many the disease is asymptomatic, or mimics mild influenza. Its main spread is by blood, blood products and sexual activity but it can also be transmitted across the placenta. It is more common in tropical and developing countries, especially where nutrition is poor and the use of barrier contraceptives is limited but it is also a particular problem among injecting drug users who share needles in the western world.

In the healthy adult 90% of cases resolve completely within 6 months. In the remaining 10% hepatitis B surface antigen (HBsAg) remains in the serum and the woman is considered to be a chronic carrier. Some of these will clear the antigen in the next 6 months and the rest will develop chronic active hepatitis, and the symptoms described above will also continue. A few will develop hepatic failure which can result in death unless liver transplantation is available (see Box 15.3). If hepatitis B is transmitted from mother to fetus and immunisation does not prevent infection in the baby, the child will be at increased risk of liver cancer in later life (Pastorek 1994). In pregnancy the risk is considered to be greater to the fetus than the mother through transplacental passage of the virus and particularly through blood and body fluids at birth.

Diagnosis is made from the woman's history of her symptoms and lifestyle. Serological studies will be performed but it can be difficult to distinguish from other forms of viral hepatitis during the acute presentation, before antibodies have formed. Treatment is of the symptoms as they arise. Infection control measures should be instituted where the woman is considered to be infectious, and information not only about the disease, but also nutrition and sexual advice should be

---

Box 15.3 Pregnancy and liver transplantation

There have now been a small number of pregnancies in women who have undergone liver transplantation before or during their pregnancy, many with successful outcomes. Although not desirable, liver transplantation in women of childbearing age is becoming increasingly common and such women now have the opportunity to consider having a family. However, the risks to pregnancy are great and these women require expert medical and midwifery care at a specialised centre equipped to deal with all of the complications, both of a physical and psychological nature, that such women may face.

---

offered. Liver function will be monitored and fetal condition assessed. Household contacts should be offered immunisation once their HBsAg seronegativity is established. Sexual partners should be traced and offered testing and vaccination. Postnatally the mother will be encouraged to accept vaccination for the baby. Advice about breast feeding remains controversial.

SKIN DISORDERS

Many skin changes are noticed by pregnant women, most so common as to be described as physiological.

Treatment of pre-existing skin disorders, such as eczema or psoriasis, should continue as required, bearing in mind that some topical agents should be used with caution in pregnancy.

Many women suffer from physiological pruritus in pregnancy, especially over the abdomen. Often reassurance, and the application of calamine lotion over the affected area, will suffice. However, for some women, pruritus with or without a rash will be a symptom of a more serious condition. Generalised pruritus should always be referred to a medical practitioner, as it may be a symptom of conditions such as intrahepatic cholestasis, liver or thyroid disease, lymphoma or scabies.

Herpes gestationis (pemphigoid gestationis)

This is a disease specific to pregnancy which usually occurs in the mid-trimester and persists into the postnatal period, although sometimes it starts after the birth. It affects 1 : 60 000 pregnancies and its aetiology is unknown although it is thought that the condition is initiated by a maternal response to paternal antigens and persists under the influence of pregnancy hormones. Despite its name this skin condition is not related to the herpes virus – the misnomer came about in the 19th century when 'herpes' referred to skin blisters, rather than the virus.

The woman will complain of generalised itching and a burning sensation, and an erythematous rash will appear. This is initially over the abdomen and it spreads to involve the remainder of the trunk and limbs. Blisters develop which may become infected and purulent, especially if the woman scratches.

The midwife should refer the woman to a medical practitioner and be supportive to her throughout her care. The lesions should be kept clean and may be covered to prevent the woman scratching. A diet high in vitamins should be encouraged. The woman will usually have her labour induced at about the 37th week of pregnancy as there is controversial evidence that there is a greater incidence of intrauterine growth retardation and raised infant mortality with the condition, suggestive of a link with placental insufficiency. The fetus may have a rash when born and will need paediatric examination for any skin lesions, although these are usually clinically mild.

Without excessive scratching or secondary infection, the woman's lesions will heal without scarring. The condition may recur in subsequent pregnancies, especially with the same consort.

DISORDERS OF THE AMNIOTIC FLUID

Normal amniotic fluid increases in amount throughout pregnancy from a few millilitres until 38 weeks when there is about a litre. After this it diminishes to approximately 800 ml at term. Amniotic fluid is not static; the water of which it is largely composed is changed every hour and the solutes are changed about every 3 hours.

There are two chief abnormalities of amniotic fluid: polyhydramnios (or hydramnios) and oligohydramnios.

Polyhydramnios

Polyhydramnios has been defined as being a quantity of amniotic fluid which exceeds 1500 ml, although definition by amount is now being superseded by definition by ultrasound measurement of pools of liquor around the fetus. It occurs in 0.9% of pregnancies (Hill et al 1987).

Causes

- Oesophageal atresia
- Open neural tube defect
- Multiple pregnancy, especially in the case of monozygotic twins
- Maternal diabetes mellitus
- Rarely, Rhesus iso-immunisation is associated with polyhydramnios
- Chorioangioma, a rare tumour of the placenta
- In many cases, the cause is unknown.

Types

Chronic polyhydramnios is gradual in onset, usually from about the 30th week of pregnancy. It is the most common type.

Acute polyhydramnios is very rare. It occurs at about 20 weeks and comes on very suddenly. The uterus reaches the xiphisternum in about 3 or 4 days. It is frequently associated with monozygotic twins or severe fetal abnormality.

Recognition

The mother may complain of breathlessness and discomfort. If the polyhydramnios is acute in onset, she may have severe abdominal pain. The condition may cause exacerbation of symptoms associated with pregnancy such as indigestion, heartburn and constipation. Oedema and varicosities of the vulva and lower limbs may be present.

Abdominal examination. On inspection the uterus is larger than expected for the period of gestation and is globular in shape. The abdominal skin appears stretched and shiny with marked striae gravidarum and obvious superficial blood vessels.

On palpation the uterus feels tense and it is difficult to feel the fetal parts but the fetus may

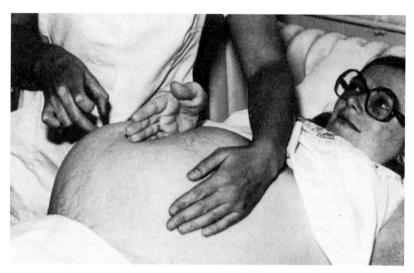

Fig. 15.10 Eliciting a fluid thrill in polyhydramnios.

be ballotted between the two hands. A fluid thrill may be elicited by placing a hand on one side of the abdomen and tapping the other side with the fingers (Fig. 15.10). A wave of fluid will move across from the side which is tapped and is felt by the opposite examining hand. It may be helpful to measure the abdominal girth (Fig. 15.11), particularly in cases of acute polyhydramnios, in order to observe the rate of increase.

Auscultation of the fetal heart is difficult because

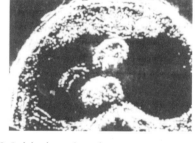

Fig. 15.12 Polyhydramnios: ultrasonogram.

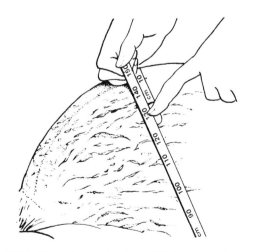

Fig. 15.11 Measuring abdominal girth in a case of polyhydramnios.

the quantity of fluid allows the fetus to move away from the stethoscope.

Ultrasonic scanning may be used to confirm the diagnosis of polyhydramnios (Fig. 15.12). The liquor volume is estimated by measuring 'pools' of liquor around the fetus in each of the four quadrants, and an amniotic fluid index (AFI) allocated. Scanning may reveal a multiple pregnancy or fetal abnormality. X-ray examination is not often performed and the images are usually hazy if there is a large quantity of amniotic fluid.

Complications

- Maternal ureteric obstruction
- Increased fetal mobility leading to unstable lie and malpresentation

- Cord presentation and prolapse
- Premature rupture of the membranes
- Placental abruption when the membranes rupture
- Premature labour
- Increased incidence of caesarean section
- Postpartum haemorrhage
- Raised perinatal mortality rate.

Management

The cause of the condition should be determined if possible. The woman may be admitted to a consultant obstetric unit. Subsequent care will depend on the condition of the woman and fetus, the cause and degree of the polyhydramnios and the stage of pregnancy. Diabetes mellitus will be managed as an entity; the polyhydramnios is managed much as in other cases. The presence of fetal abnormality will be taken into consideration in choosing the mode and timing of delivery. If gross abnormality is present, labour may be induced; if the fetus is suffering from an operable condition such as oesophageal atresia, it may be appropriate to arrange transfer to a neonatal surgical unit.

Mild asymptomatic polyhydramnios is managed expectantly. The woman is not necessarily admitted to hospital, but should be advised that if she suspects that her membranes have ruptured immediate admission is recommended. She should be encouraged to get adequate rest, and if she is working it may be helpful to discuss commencing maternity leave, although the physical nature of her job and the stress which may be engendered by stopping work should be assessed with the woman before making recommendations. She will require detailed explanation of the condition and support from her health professionals as she is likely to become deeply fearful for the well-being of her child. Regular ultrasound scans will reveal if the polyhydramnios is progressive or not.

For a woman with symptomatic polyhydramnios, an upright position will help to relieve any dyspnoea and she may be given antacids to relieve heartburn and nausea. If the discomfort from the swollen abdomen is severe therapeutic amniocentesis, or amnioreduction, may be considered. However, this is not without risk, as infection may be introduced or the onset of labour provoked.

No more than 500 ml should be withdrawn at any one time. It is at best a temporary relief as the fluid will rapidly accumulate again and the procedure may need to be repeated.

The drug indomethacin reduces fetal urine production and consequently amniotic fluid, but its administration is still in its experimental phase until the risks have been more fully ascertained.

Acute polyhydramnios managed by amnioreduction has a poor prognosis for the baby. The usual course of events is that the fluid continues to increase at an alarming rate, the membranes rupture spontaneously and the fetus or fetuses are born, grossly premature, in a river of amniotic fluid.

The woman may need to have labour induced in late pregnancy if the symptoms become worse. The lie must be corrected if it is not longitudinal and the membranes will be ruptured cautiously, allowing the amniotic fluid to drain out slowly in order to avoid altering the lie and to prevent cord prolapse. Placental abruption is also a hazard if the uterus suddenly diminishes in size.

Labour is usually normal but the midwife should be prepared for the possibility of postpartum haemorrhage. The baby should be carefully examined for abnormalities and the patency of the oesophagus ascertained by passing a nasogastric tube.

Oligohydramnios

Oligohydramnios is an abnormally small amount of amniotic fluid. At term it may be 300–500 ml but amounts vary and it can be even less. When diagnosed in the first half of pregnancy it is often found to be associated with renal agenesis (absence of kidneys) or Potter's syndrome in which the baby also has pulmonary hypoplasia; when diagnosed at any time in pregnancy before 37 weeks it may be due to fetal abnormality or to preterm premature rupture of the membranes where the amniotic fluid fails to reaccumulate. The lack of amniotic fluid reduces the intrauterine space and over time will cause compression deformities. The baby has a squashed-looking face, flattening of the nose, micrognathia and talipes. The skin is dry and leathery in appearance.

Oligohydramnios also occurs in the postmature

pregnancy and is believed to be linked with the development of placental insufficiency. As placental function reduces, so too does perfusion to the fetal organ systems including the kidneys. The decrease in fetal urine formation leads to oligohydramnios, as the major component of amniotic fluid is fetal urine.

Recognition

On inspection, the uterus appears smaller than expected for the period of gestation. The mother who has had a previous normal pregnancy may have noticed a reduction in fetal movements. When the abdomen is palpated the uterus is small and compact and fetal parts are easily felt. Breech presentation is possible. Auscultation is normal.

Ultrasonic scanning will enable differentiation from intrauterine growth retardation (although both may occur together where there is placental insufficiency). Renal abnormality may be visible on the scan.

Management

The woman may be admitted to hospital. If the ultrasound scan demonstrates renal agenesis the baby will not survive. Liquor volume will also be estimated from the ultrasound scan, and if renal agenesis is not present further investigations will include checking with the woman the possibility of preterm rupture of the membranes by careful questioning. Placental function tests will also be performed.

Where fetal anomaly is considered not to be lethal, or the cause of the oligohydramnios is not known, amnioinfusion with normal saline, Ringer's lactate or 5% glucose may be performed in order to prevent compression deformities and hypoplastic lung disease, and prolong the pregnancy. However, the procedure is still at an experimental stage as its benefits and possible harm are not yet adequately understood.

In cases of normal but prolonged pregnancy, where a woman does not wish to have her pregnancy induced, Arulkumaran (1994) suggests that it may be useful to measure the AFI twice weekly, as fluid can reduce remarkably quickly and is highly suggestive of reduced placental function. However, in 1995 Montan & Malcus demon-

strated that the normal reduction in amniotic fluid in prolonged pregnancy (which they defined as 42 completed weeks of gestation) had no correlation with adverse fetal and neonatal outcome. Furthermore, Larsen et al (1995) studied certain aspects of the morphology of a small number of both mature and postmature placentae and discovered no significant physiological changes, although acknowledging that further studies of postmature placental structure are required. Oligohydramnios in prolonged pregnancy is a poorly understood phenomenon, and its management therefore remains highly controversial.

Preterm prelabour rupture of the membranes is dealt with separately below.

In the case of a woman with oligohydramnios, labour may intervene or may be induced because of the possibility of placental insufficiency. Epidural analgesia may be indicated because uterine contractions are often unusually painful with this condition. Impairment of placental circulation or cord compression may result in fetal hypoxia and therefore continuous fetal heart rate monitoring is desirable. Constriction rings are a possibility owing to the small amount of amniotic fluid. In rare cases the membranes may adhere to the fetus. Also, if meconium is passed in utero it will be more concentrated and represent a greater danger to an asphyxiated baby as she or he is born.

PRETERM PRELABOUR RUPTURE OF THE MEMBRANES (PPROM)

This condition occurs before 37 completed weeks of gestation where rupture of the fetal membranes occurs without the onset of spontaneous uterine activity resulting in cervical dilatation. (Term prelabour rupture of the membranes is discussed in Ch. 21.)

PPROM affects 2% of pregnancies. Placental abruption is evident in 4–7% of women who present with PPROM. The condition has a 21–32% recurrence rate in subsequent pregnancies of affected women (Svigos et al 1994). It may be associated with cervical incompetence (although it is likely that uterine contractions accompany the rupture of membranes with this condition). It is now believed that there is a strong association between PPROM and maternal vaginal colonisation with potentially pathogenic microorganisms and a long-term multicentre trial started in the UK in 1993 (Medical Research Council Antibiotic Uncertainty Trial – ORACLE) to study the role of antibiotics in both PPROM and preterm labour. To date the evidence suggests that if antibiotics are taken in PPROM, pregnancy is prolonged, but the effect on infant morbidity is unknown (Mercer et al 1997). The ORACLE trial continues.

Risks of PPROM

These include:

- labour which may intervene at any time, resulting in a preterm birth
- chorioamnionitis, which may be followed by fetal and maternal systemic infection if not treated promptly
- oligohydramnios if prolonged PPROM occurs, with associated fetal problems including pulmonary hypoplasia
- psychosocial problems resulting from uncertain fetal and neonatal outcome and long-term hospitalisation
- cord prolapse
- malpresentation associated with prematurity
- primary antepartum haemorrhage.

Management

Because the pathophysiology of PPROM is poorly understood the management is controversial.

Psychological consideration of the woman's and couple's circumstances must always be considered with PPROM as it is known to be an extremely disturbing condition for parents, not least because causes and predictions of the outcome cannot be given. If PPROM is suspected, the woman will be admitted to the delivery suite where a careful history is taken and rupture of the membranes confirmed by a sterile speculum examination of any pooling of liquor in the posterior fornix of the vagina. Very wet sanitary towels over a 6-hour period will also offer a reasonably conclusive diagnosis if urine leakage has been excluded, but a positive nitrazine test should not be considered conclusive when it is the only sign (Svigos et al

1994) because infection can produce a vaginal discharge with an alkaline pH. Digital vaginal examination should be avoided to reduce the risk of introducing infection. Observations must also be made of the fetal condition from the fetal heart rate (an infected fetus may have a tachycardia) and maternal infection screen, temperature and pulse, uterine tenderness and any purulent or offensively smelling vaginal discharge. A decision on future management will then be made.

If the woman has a gestation of less than 32 weeks, the fetus appears to be uncompromised and APH and labour have been excluded, she will be managed expectantly. She is likely to be hospitalised and offered frequent ultrasound scans to check the growth of the fetus and the extent and complications of any oligohydramnios. She should be given corticosteroids as soon as PPROM is confirmed in case delivery occurs, and if labour intervenes, tocolytic drugs will be considered to prolong the pregnancy. Known vaginal infection will be treated with antibiotics and prophylactic antibiotics may be offered to women without symptoms of infection. Sometimes the leak will reseal (especially if it is a hindwater leak) and the pregnancy may proceed with no further complications (Svigos et al 1994). However, if the membranes rupture before 24 weeks of gestation the outlook is not good; the fetus is likely to succumb either to the problems caused by oligohydramnios or those caused by preterm birth.

If the woman is more than 32 weeks pregnant, the fetus appears to be compromised, and APH or intervening labour is suspected or confirmed, active management will ensue. Method of delivery will be decided and induction of labour or caesarean section performed.

MALIGNANT DISEASE IN PREGNANCY

It is estimated that 1:1000 pregnancies are complicated by cancer (Slocumb & Pastorek 1994). The most common malignancies associated with pregnancy are, in descending frequency: cervix, breast, melanoma, ovary, thyroid, leukaemia, lymphoma and colorectum (Allen & Nisker 1986, quoted in Slocumb & Pastorek 1994). The incidence of cancer occurring alongside pregnancy increases as women delay childbearing. Further details on cervical carcinoma can be found in Chapter 14, particularly in relation to cervical smears.

Pregnancy may adversely affect the course of the disease, and cancer in the mother can metastasise to the placenta and fetus, melanoma being the most likely to do so.

If cancer is discovered before pregnancy is embarked upon, it should be treated and followed up before pregnancy is attempted. Once successfully treated and as long as the reproductive organs are not damaged, pregnancy is rarely contraindicated for medical reasons.

However, cancer discovered during pregnancy leads to a whole host of management dilemmas. The options involve balancing the effects of the treatment, the disease and delivery on both the mother and her fetus.

If the woman is in early pregnancy her first dilemma may be whether or not to continue with the pregnancy. If she continues, the next dilemma will be whether to treat the disease during the pregnancy or wait until delivery, as both chemotherapy and radiation therapy may have toxic effects, particularly on the fetus. Surgery is the treatment least likely to affect the pregnancy adversely, particularly if it takes place in later pregnancy but it may not be the treatment of first choice for the particular condition.

Elective preterm delivery is often favoured by medical practitioners involved in the woman's care and the woman herself, after which her condition can be assessed and more appropriate treatment of the disease administered.

Needless to say, the support of the midwife throughout pregnancy is likely to be crucial to this woman's psychological well-being.

OBESITY OR FAILURE TO GAIN WEIGHT IN PREGNANCY

The value of regular, routine weighing of women whilst pregnant is debatable. Surprisingly little is known about the effectiveness of weighing as a screening procedure to predict obstetric outcome or even the clinical implications for pregnancy.

However, it is becoming increasingly clear that women who have a poor diet and their fetuses are at greater risk than well-nourished women (Dallison & Lobstein 1995).

Weight is no more than a very crude indicator of a woman's health status in pregnancy. The midwife's observation of a very obese woman, or a very thin one, should alert her to some of the risks such women may face during pregnancy and the longer-term risks to both women and their children.

Quetelet's index (weight in kg/height in m^2) is commonly used to assess women's prepregnancy weight, with a view to classifying them as thin (less than 20); normal (20–25); mildly obese (25–30) and obese (30 or more). Further details on the Quetelet index can be found in Chapter 10.

A woman who starts pregnancy while obese, or puts on an excessive amount of weight during pregnancy, is at greater risk of hypertensive disturbances, including pregnancy-induced hypertension. She is also at greater risk of gestational diabetes and both of these conditions make her more likely to be delivered by caesarean section. She is also at increased risk of urinary tract infection, uncertain fetal position, postpartum haemorrhage and thrombophlebitis. She is more likely to give birth to a large for gestational age infant, although if her pregnancy has been otherwise uncomplicated she is not statistically at greater risk of cephalopelvic disproportion or shoulder dystocia (Wildschut 1994). She is also more prone to wound infection following operative delivery. Obesity may also be associated with malnourishment from essential nutrient deficiency.

As well as excessive weight increase during pregnancy being a greater risk factor for the onset of hypertensive disorders, its sudden onset may signal occult oedema. If such weight gain is noted by the woman or the midwife it is prudent to take the woman's blood pressure and test her urine for protein.

Once oedema has been excluded, the midwife should make tactful attempts to discuss the woman's diet with her, when it becomes apparent that her weight may raise her risk of complications. It is debatable at what point the midwife should intervene with such a discussion. Ideally all women should be given the opportunity to discuss diet, as well as other general lifestyle factors, from as early on in their pregnancy as possible, or even before, and at regular intervals thereafter. Overweight women will often themselves express concerns to a friendly and generally supportive midwife and the midwife should be able to take such opportunities to discuss diet, nutrition, exercise and the reasons why excessive weight gain in pregnancy is undesirable. Referral to a dietician may be helpful, as strict dieting in pregnancy is dangerous. Blood pressure measurements should always be taken accurately with a correctly sized cuff, and gestational diabetes and urinary tract infection screened for. Routine weighing is rarely of any practical benefit, and may only reduce a woman's self-esteem and make her dread her antenatal appointments. The midwife should also bear in mind that obesity can be a symptom of another disease, such as hypothyroidism, polycystic ovarian syndrome or Cushing's disease, and in such cases diet will have minimal effect on weight.

Conversely, the midwife may observe that a woman appears to be thin during her pregnancy and not laying down healthy fat stores. Detailed discussion should attempt to elicit the quality and quantity of the woman's diet and her weight pattern over previous years. Some women are naturally very slim and remain so because of genetic factors and a high metabolic rate, going on to produce a healthily sized infant. Of the rest, a medical disorder such as a malabsorption condition may be present, or starvation, if the woman has been living until recently in a country struck by famine.

The midwife needs to be aware that pregnant women can be afflicted by anorexia nervosa and/or bulimia, often chronic conditions that may have been previously undetected, despite their obsessive nature, or labelled 'dieting'.

Where a woman is suffering from nutritional deprivation she is at greater risk of anaemia, preterm birth and intrauterine growth retardation and its sequelae including birth asphyxia and perinatal death. Bulimia may be wrongly diagnosed as hyperemesis gravidarum.

The midwife's role in the care of such women will depend on the cause. She should always involve the medical practitioner because of the risk of intrauterine growth retardation, and in cases with a medical cause. Where an eating disorder such as anorexia nervosa or bulimia is suspected or admitted to, the involvement of a clinical psychologist or psychiatrist may be of value but, of course, the woman must be amenable to this. (It should also be said that if a midwife cares for a woman who has resolved a former eating disorder it would be most inappropriate to suggest that the woman requires psychiatric support in her pregnancy because of her history.) Dietary discussion and advice, including the use of supplements such as multivitamins and referral to a dietician, should be discussed with the woman. Quality of nutrition is as important, if not more so, than quantity. Where a woman is known to be suffering from an eating disorder, the importance of non-judgemental support of all of her carers cannot be overestimated in maintaining her well-being. As with the obese woman, some of the problem may lie with lowered self-esteem.

PROBLEMS ASSOCIATED WITH PREGNANCY FOLLOWING ASSISTED CONCEPTION

The rate of assisted conceptions has risen dramatically in the last few years, not least because of increasing understanding of the human reproductive cycle, its failings and technological advances that can correct childlessness from a variety of causes.

Couples who achieve pregnancy following assisted conception may be at greater risk of complications during the pregnancy than those who conceive naturally, for a number of reasons.

The cause of the fertility problem may be a medical problem in itself, which will be aggravated by pregnancy, such as some forms of malignancy and their treatments. It is also known that with some forms of assisted conception there is an increased rate of multiple pregnancy which will in turn increase the risk of pre-eclampsia, preterm labour and so on. Women who undergo assisted conception are by definition of an older age group, either having previously tried for some time to conceive a child naturally or having fertility problems because of their increased age. Increased maternal age has slight associations with multiple pregnancy and pre-eclampsia and the older a woman is, the more lifetime she has lived to develop a medical problem such as essential hypertension or diabetes mellitus or a gynaecological problem such as fibroids.

The desire for a child by many couples will override potential risk to the woman and a couple may present a compelling case to the fertility clinic whose help they seek.

Also, women who achieve pregnancy with medical assistance are more likely to be closely monitored, particularly with ultrasound scans and perhaps closer follow-up of otherwise mild symptoms. The couple themselves may feel greatly reassured to have their pregnancy the subject of such close medical scrutiny. However, the combination of the increased use of technology and the stress, engendered by searching for problems (which in today's open environment means explaining what each problem may entail) in a so-called 'precious pregnancy', can themselves invoke a perception of a more complicated pregnancy than may actually be the case.

Specific problems

- Increased risk of ectopic pregnancy following assisted conception, especially ovulation induction and in vitro fertilisation and its derivatives, e.g. gamete intrafallopian transfer (GIFT) (Edwards & Brody 1995).
- Multiple pregnancy and its sequelae.
- Higher miscarriage rate, particularly if the woman has a condition such as incompetent cervix or septate uterus which predisposes her to miscarriage. However, although early miscarriage rates appear to be higher in women with assisted conception, this is almost certainly because of a higher detection rate due to intensive monitoring of hormone levels and ultrasound scans from very early pregnancy, and heavy bleeding at the time the menstrual period was expected – normally a woman would not have been aware that she was pregnant.
- More vaginal bleeding requiring hospital admission. Edwards & Brody (1995) also found that women with an assisted conception had a 3% placenta praevia rate as opposed to 1.4% seen in controls.

Interestingly, there does not appear to be a greater incidence of chromosomal abnormality following assisted conception.

READER ACTIVITIES

1. Formulate a list of questions you would ask a pregnant woman with acute abdominal pain of unknown cause. What information would each of your questions give you, in making an accurate provisional report to medical personnel?

2. Return to the list of factors to aid differential diagnosis of antepartum haemorrhage. Using the information given in the chapter, how will the answers to these questions help the midwife to decide whether the placenta is likely to be in a normal situation or to be a placenta praevia? How will the answers affect her actions?

3. How may the midwife recognise:

   a. polyhydramnios
   b. oligohydramnios?

4. Consider how the midwife may best offer emotional support to a woman who experiences otherwise uncomplicated preterm prelabour rupture of the membranes in the mid-trimester.

5. What are the advantages and disadvantages of weighing women in pregnancy?

6. Ask a woman who has had a complication of pregnancy the best and worst aspects of the midwifery care that she has experienced.

ACKNOWLEDGEMENTS

I would like to thank Sara Kenyon for her help with the section on preterm prelabour rupture of the membranes, and Sheila Culloty for her comments regarding clinical midwifery care.

REFERENCES

Arulkumaran S 1994 Prolonged pregnancy. In: James D K, Steer P J, Weiner C P, Gonik B (eds) High risk pregnancy management options. W B Saunders, London, ch 16, pp 217–228

Blake P G, Martin J N, Perry K G 1993 Disseminated intravascular coagulation, autoimmune thrombocytopenic purpura, and haemoglobinopathies. In: Knuppel R A, Drukker J E (eds) High risk pregnancy a team approach. W B Saunders, Philadelphia, ch 28, pp 561–596

Clewell W H 1994 Abdominal pain. In: James D K, Steer P J, Weiner C P, Gonik B (eds) High risk pregnancy management options. W B Saunders, London, ch 34, pp 605–622

Dallison J, Lobstein T 1995 Poor expectations. NCH Action For Children, London

Department of Health, Welsh Office, Scottish Office Home and Health Department, Department of Health and Social Services, Northern Ireland 1996 Report on confidential enquiries into maternal deaths in the United Kingdom 1991–1993. HMSO, London

Edwards R G, Brody S A 1995 Principles and practice of assisted human reproduction. W B Saunders, Philadelphia

Fagan E A 1995 Disorders of the liver, biliary system and pancreas. In: de Swiet M (ed) Medical disorders in obstetric practice. Blackwell Science, Oxford, ch 9, pp 321–378

Hill L M, Breckle R, Thomas M L, Fries J K 1987 Polyhydramnios: ultrasonically detected prevalence and neonatal outcome. Obstetrics and Gynecology 69: 21–25

Konje J C, Wally R J 1994 Bleeding in late pregnancy. In: James D K, Steer P J, Weiner C P, Gonik B (eds) High risk pregnancy management options. W B Saunders, London, ch 9, pp 119–136

Larsen L G, Clausen H V, Andersen B, Graem N 1995 A stereologic study of postmature placentas fixed by dual perfusion. American Journal of Obstetrics and Gynecology 172(2) (part 1): 500–507

Letsky E A 1995 Coagulation defects. In: de Swiet M (ed) Medical disorders in obstetric practice. Blackwell Science, Oxford, ch 3, pp 71–115

Mercer B M, Miodovnik M, Thurnau G R et al 1997 Antibiotic therapy for reduction of infant morbidity after preterm premature rupture of the membranes: a randomized controlled trial. JAMA 278(12): 989–995

Montan S, Malcus P 1995 Amniotic fluid index in prolonged pregnancy: a cohort study. Journal of Maternal–Fetal Investigation 5(1): 4–7

Pastorek J G 1994 Viral diseases. In: James D K, Steer P J, Weiner C P, Gonik B (eds) High risk pregnancy management options. W B Saunders, London, ch 29, pp 481–508

Slocumb C O, Pastorek J G 1994 Malignant disease. In: James D K, Steer P J, Weiner C P, Gonik B (eds) High risk pregnancy management options. W B Saunders, London, ch 32, pp 567–595

Svigos J M, Robinson J S, Vigneswaran R 1994 Premature rupture of the membranes. In: James D K, Steer P J, Weiner C P, Gonik B (eds) High risk pregnancy management options. W B Saunders, London, ch 12, pp 163–172

United Kingdom Central Council for Nursing, Midwifery and Health Visiting 1993 Midwives Rules. UKCC, London

Walters B N J 1994 Hepatic and gastrointestinal disease. In: James D K, Steer P J, Weiner C P, Gonik B (eds) High risk pregnancy management options. W B Saunders, London, ch 25, pp 385–397

Wildschut H I J 1994 Maternal weight and weight gain. In: James D K, Steer P J, Weiner C P, Gonik B (eds) High risk pregnancy management options. W B Saunders, London, ch 6, pp 67–74

16

Common medical disorders associated with pregnancy

Carmel Lloyd   Victoria Margaret Lewis

Pregnancy may be complicated by a variety of disorders and conditions that can profoundly affect the woman and her fetus. This chapter describes the most common cardiac, respiratory, renal, haematological, metabolic, infectious, neurological and autoimmune conditions which may complicate pregnancy. The pathophysiology of these disorders may adversely affect the pregnancy. Similarly, the physiological changes occurring in pregnancy may modify the clinical course of these disorders and their management.

The chapter aims to:

- outline the common medical disorders

- describe the effects of the different disorders on the woman and her fetus or neonate

- identify the treatment required and implications for midwifery care

- consider the midwifery care and support required by the client and her family during pregnancy, labour and the postnatal period.

Medical disorders which predate pregnancy are important because of the way that pregnancy affects them, and because of the way in which the disorder, or the treatment, affects the pregnancy; they are also important for their social and psychological consequences. For example, a woman with anaemia not only has a medical problem but may become tired and depressed, she may find herself unable to cope with existing children and she may have to take time off from her employment. Her ideals about the place of confinement and the conduct of her labour may be compromised and the added anxiety of her medical condition may increase her need for pain-relieving drugs; anxiety has even been shown to decrease uterine efficiency in some species (Naaktegeboren 1989). Postnatally, the woman's lactation may suffer and her ability to enjoy her baby may be inhibited, which may predispose her to postnatal psychological problems. It can be seen that the woman's physical, social and psychological conditions are inseparable.

When the midwife is assessing the needs of the woman and her family and planning their care, this interplay of social, psychological and physical factors is important. If the medical problem is one that is likely to continue into the next pregnancy, the midwife can use the postnatal period to begin preconception care and advice. If the midwife can make the experience of this pregnancy a positive one, the woman will be encouraged to seek contact with the maternity services early in subsequent pregnancies or even before.

CARDIAC DISEASE

Trends in cardiac disease

The overall incidence of cardiac disease in pregnancy is falling in Europe and North America, largely owing to the lower incidence of rheumatic heart disease (less than 1% in the UK). However, the number of women with congenital cardiac defects who survive to childbearing age is increasing as medical and surgical care improves (de Swiet 1995). Coronary artery disease is also increasing. In the developing world rheumatic heart disease is still the most common cardiac problem. In parts of Africa, cardiomyopathy is often seen during pregnancy or the puerperium although it is rare in the UK. To manage pregnancy effectively in a patient with heart disease the normal compensatory changes in the cardiovascular system that occur during pregnancy must be understood. These normal responses are only detrimental to the mother and fetus if heart disease is present (Nolan 1990).

Changes in cardiovascular dynamics during pregnancy

In normal pregnancy the cardiovascular dynamics alter in order to meet the increased demands of the fetoplacental unit. This increases the workload of the heart quite significantly.

The major cardiac changes to occur are:

- an increase in cardiac output by 40%
- an increase in blood volume by 35%

- a decrease in total peripheral resistance (Nolan 1990).

These changes commence in early pregnancy and gradually reach a maximum at the 30th week, where they are maintained until term. Oestrogens and prostaglandins are thought to be the mediators of the alterations in haemodynamics during pregnancy (de Swiet 1995). These changes are associated with several clinical signs:

- The increased cardiac output may produce a physiological systolic flow in one-third of pregnant women.
- The heart dilates and a third heart sound is common.
- As the uterus enlarges, the heart may be displaced upwards by the growing uterus.
- During the third stage of labour 300–400 ml of blood is added to the circulating volume by the contracting uterus (Nolan 1990).

Classification

The New York Heart Association classification based on exercise tolerance is useful for describing the extent of the immediate problem but has little predictive value:

I. No symptoms during ordinary physical activity
II. Symptoms during ordinary physical activity
III. Symptoms during mild physical activity
IV. Symptoms at rest (Benson 1983).

It used to be said that women would deteriorate by one grade in pregnancy, but it is now thought more useful to consider the prognosis for each specific problem. For example, valvular incompetence may improve during pregnancy as peripheral resistance drops and more blood flows in the right direction, whereas the woman with mitral stenosis may deteriorate three grades in a matter of hours.

Rheumatic heart disease

Valvular lesions predominate in rheumatic heart disease which constitutes approximately 50% of all heart disease seen in pregnancy (Nolan 1990).

Mitral and aortic valve incompetence. Pregnancy can be helpful in this case as it lowers the pressure in the arterial system, encouraging blood to flow the right way through the valves. There is, however, a risk of endocarditis (Landon & Samuels 1996).

Mitral stenosis. A non-pregnant woman with this condition already requires an increase in left atrial pressure in order to push blood through the mitral valve. As the demand for cardiac output rises in pregnancy, pressure in the left atrium rises still further. This may lead to back pressure in the pulmonary system and pulmonary oedema. The left atrium, unable to cope with the demands made upon it, begins to fibrillate and heart failure may occur (de Swiet 1995).

Congenital heart disease

The most common congenital defects which may remain uncorrected during the childbearing years are:

- atrial septal defect
- patent ductus arteriosus
- ventricular septal defect.

All of these are openings which allow communication between the right and left sides of the heart or, in the case of patent ductus arteriosus, between the pulmonary artery and the aorta (McAnulty et al 1988). Problems arise when pulmonary vascular resistance rises, as it does in pre-eclampsia, and blood flows from the right side to the left instead of passing through the lungs, leading to cyanosis. This may also happen in the third stage of labour when there is a sudden return of blood to the heart (Landon & Samuels 1996).

Risk to mother and fetus

Any structural defect, whether congenital or acquired, predisposes the woman to bacterial endocarditis and thromboemboli. The most recent confidential enquiry reported an increase in deaths due to cardiac disease, the majority being attributed to deaths of women with acquired heart disease (DH et al 1996). This emphasises the need for expert attention from obstetricians, cardiologists and anaesthetists for this group of patients (Celermajer & Deanfield 1991).

In rheumatic heart disease (RHD) the maternal mortality is low and pregnancy does not affect long-term survival. The fetal outcome in RHD is usually good and little different from that in patients who do not have heart disease (de Swiet 1995). Maternal mortality is most likely in those conditions where pulmonary blood flow cannot be increased as, for example, in Eisenmenger's syndrome (DH et al 1996).

During pregnancy, fetuses of women with heart disease are generally growth retarded and fetal loss may be high. However, there is no increase in the perinatal mortality rate (PMR) although there is an increased incidence of congenital heart disease (CHD) in children born to mothers who have CHD themselves (Nolan 1990).

Women with artificial heart valves run a risk of developing thromboemboli unless anticoagulants are given. There is debate about the choice of drug. The oral anticoagulant warfarin crosses the placenta and is known to be teratogenic in the first 13 weeks of pregnancy (Landon & Samuels 1996); it also predisposes the fetus and neonate to haemorrhage. Heparin is not passed to the fetus but it is thought by some doctors to be less effective in reducing thromboemboli. Some doctors prescribe subcutaneous heparin throughout pregnancy; others prescribe heparin in early pregnancy then warfarin until 36 weeks, reverting to subcutaneous heparin which is given until the day of delivery. Heparin and warfarin are given again after delivery. Warfarin appears in breast milk but there is no evidence that it harms the baby although some doctors prefer not to prescribe it. Whilst the mother is taking warfarin the prothrombin time is monitored.

Preconception care and advice

A woman who knows that she has cardiac disease would be wise to seek advice from both a cardiologist and an obstetrician before becoming pregnant so that the risks of her condition can be discussed. In some cases, preconception surgery such as mitral valvotomy may be advised (Shabetai 1988). The woman should be helped to control obesity, cut down smoking and choose a diet which will prevent anaemia in order to minimise risk. It is advisable that family size should be limited, as the risks increase with each pregnancy. Contraceptive advice is therefore an important aspect of management.

Antenatal care

Diagnosis of cardiac disease in some women may only be made during antenatal visits. The midwife may detect a problem when taking the woman's history. Breathlessness, fatigue, swollen ankles and palpitations may all be attributable to the normal changes associated with pregnancy but if they were present before the pregnancy began they may indicate something more sinister and the woman must be referred to a cardiologist. Diagnosis will be made with the aid of the clinical picture, radiography, electrocardiography (ECG) and echocardiography (de Swiet 1995).

Assessment of the problem and its prognosis can be made at a combined cardiac and obstetric clinic where the couple can discuss the options open to them. Where there is no evidence of a cardiac lesion, no further follow-up will be required. Some women may have a mild lesion with no haemodynamic effect, in which case pregnancy may not be affected, although prophylactic antibiotic cover in labour is recommended (de Swiet 1995). For those with a significant lesion with real or potential haemodynamic implications, the future of the pregnancy needs to be considered and careful counselling given. If termination of pregnancy is decided upon, it is preferable that this should be done in the first trimester, as termination after 16 weeks' gestation is no safer than later delivery (James 1989).

Management. All pregnant women with heart disease should be managed in a combined obstetric–cardiac clinic by an obstetrician and a cardiologist (de Swiet 1995). In this way most pregnancies in women with heart disease will be successful. The aim of management is to maintain or improve the physical and psychological well-being of mother and fetus. This involves keeping a steady haemodynamic state and preventing complications. The major maternal complications are:

• bacterial endocarditis

• thromboemboli
• cyanosis
• heart failure.

The risk factors for heart failure include:

• infections, particularly urinary tract infection (UTI)
• hypertension
• anaemia
• multiple pregnancy
• obesity
• smoking (de Swiet 1995).

Physical care. Depending on the woman's condition, antenatal clinic visits may be more frequent than usual. Women with cardiac disease will require the same health and dietary advice as other pregnant women, although each mother must be considered individually. An important aspect of care is that of dental treatment and antibiotic cover to eliminate sources of sepsis and reduce the risk of endocarditis (Shabetai 1988). In late pregnancy it may be advisable to restrict activity or admit the woman to hospital for rest and close monitoring. Obstetric management in pregnancy includes early ultrasound examination of the fetus to confirm gestational age and detect congenital abnormality. Thereafter, those women who do not have haemodynamically significant heart disease require no special obstetric management (de Swiet 1995). However, in those women who do, the fetus should be monitored for the following:

• assessment of fetal growth and amniotic fluid volume both clinically and by ultrasound
• monitoring the fetal heart rate by cardiotocography
• measurement of fetal and maternal placental blood flow indices by Doppler ultrasonography (de Swiet 1995).

Social care. With more frequent antenatal visits the midwife may need to give advice about assistance with fares or transport to the hospital. If the mother is required to reduce her physical activity and leave work earlier than she had planned, the midwife may need to give advice regarding the Employment Protection Act and any DSS benefit to which she may be entitled (see Ch. 46). If the problem is complex, referral to a social worker will be appropriate. A woman who finds it necessary to restrict her activities in the home could be put in contact with the home help service.

Psychological care. Psychological support by the midwife is important during pregnancy, particularly at times when there are intercurrent problems which may require admission to hospital. Consideration must particularly be given to the emotional stress caused by a woman being separated from her other children.

Intrapartum care

The first stage of labour

The least stressful labour for a woman with cardiac disease will be spontaneous in onset and result in a vaginal delivery. The midwife should inform the anaesthetist and cardiologist that the woman has been admitted. Blood may be cross-matched in case of need. Oxygen and resuscitation equipment should be available and functioning. Observations of pulse and respiratory rate should be made every 15 minutes. The heart may be monitored by ECG. Deviations from the normal, such as breathlessness and tachycardia, should be reported immediately. Blood pressure and fetal condition should be carefully monitored and recorded. As these women are at an increased risk from endocarditis it would seem prudent to administer antibiotic prophylaxis in labour and for 48 hours after delivery (de Swiet 1995).

Positioning. The mother will need encouragement to adopt a position in which she is comfortable. It is important to remember that women with heart disease are particularly sensitive to aortocaval compression by the gravid uterus in the supine position. This results in marked hypotension and maternal and fetal distress (de Swiet 1995). Positions such as the lithotomy position in which the feet are higher than the trunk are best avoided because of the risk of acute heart failure resulting from the sudden increase of venous return to the heart.

Fluid balance. Women with significant heart disease require care concerning fluid balance in labour. Indiscriminate use of intravenous crystalloid fluids will lead to an increase in circulating blood volume, which women with heart disease will find difficult to cope with and they may easily develop pulmonary oedema (de Swiet 1995).

Pain relief. Women with heart disease usually have quite rapid, uncomplicated labours. The midwife should help the woman to use the techniques that she has learned for coping with stress, as she and her labour companion are likely to be very anxious. In the majority, an epidural would be the analgesia of choice, inserted by a skilled anaesthetist. It is effective analgesia which decreases cardiac output and heart rate. It causes peripheral vasodilatation and decreases venous return which alleviates pulmonary congestion. Nitrous oxide and oxygen (Entonox) and pethidine are usually considered safe but it is wise to consult a doctor before administering any form of pain-relieving drug to a woman with this condition.

Preterm labour. If the woman should labour prematurely beta-sympathomimetic drugs such as salbutamol, widely used for the treatment of premature labours, are not recommended. The vasodilatory side-effects cause tachycardia and an increase in circulatory blood volume which may lead to the development of pulmonary oedema and heart failure. In addition, these drugs have metabolic effects which may further impair myocardial function (de Swiet 1995).

Induction is only considered safe if the benefits outweigh the disadvantages. A failed induction leads to caesarean section and a risk of sepsis which is especially dangerous for a damaged heart. Labour is not usually induced for uncomplicated heart disease. If it is necessary to induce labour, the use of prostaglandins is advocated but with caution as they are potent vasodilators and cause a marked rise in cardiac output (Willis et al 1987). Interaction of any drugs the woman may be taking with the prostaglandin must be considered prior to administration in case of adverse side-effects (de Swiet 1995). Oxytocin by intravenous infusion causes a degree of fluid retention and it is important for the midwife to keep a careful record of fluid balance if this is used.

The second stage of labour

This should be short and without undue exertion on the part of the mother. Prolonged pushing with held breath such as the Valsalva manoeuvre, which is undesirable for healthy women, may be dangerous for a woman with heart disease. It raises the intrathoracic pressure, pushes blood out of the thorax and impedes venous return, with the result that cardiac output falls. Midwives may need to suggest to the woman that she avoids holding her breath and follows her natural desire to push, giving several short pushes during each contraction. In this way she will also avoid facial petechiae and subconjunctival haemorrhages. Some doctors perform a forceps delivery electively (de Swiet 1995), while others see no reason for this if the woman is expected to deliver quickly and easily. Some midwives and doctors advocate delivery in the left lateral position (Shabetai 1988).

The third stage of labour

No ergot-containing preparations should be used for the third stage of labour (James 1989) as it causes a tonic contraction which returns 300–500 ml of blood to the venous system (de Swiet 1995). Syntocinon may be used in order to prevent haemorrhage as it has less effect on blood vessels than ergometrine. If the woman is in heart failure, oxytocics should be avoided. In the case of actual haemorrhage, Syntocinon can be given by infusion accompanied by intravenous frusemide to prevent pulmonary oedema (de Swiet 1995).

Postnatal care

During the first 48 hours following delivery the heart must cope with the extra blood from the uterine circulation and it is important to monitor the woman's condition closely during this time. A 4-hourly record of her temperature will help in the early detection of infection.

The baby is examined very carefully for any sign of hereditary heart disease. Breast feeding is not contraindicated unless the woman is in heart failure. Her drugs may be transmitted through breast milk and she may need advice on any possible effect on the baby. Antibiotic cover may continue for up to 2 weeks after the birth.

When the woman has discussed the implications of future pregnancies on her condition with the cardiologist and obstetrician, she may need help to choose a suitable method of family spacing. The intrauterine contraceptive device has been associated with an increased risk of infection which may lead to endocarditis. The combined pill increases the risk of thromboembolism and hypertension but the progesterone-only pill and barrier methods with spermicides are suitable alternatives. Sterilisation, if chosen, is usually delayed for 2–3 months after delivery.

On her return home the woman may benefit from extra help in the house. Friends and relatives often fulfil this need but the home help service could be approached.

RESPIRATORY DISORDERS

Asthma

Asthma is the most common respiratory disease encountered during pregnancy, affecting 3% of women in their childbearing years (Littlejohns et al 1989). Effective treatment of this condition is readily available and consists of prevention of attacks rather than relief from them. Unfortunately there are many health professionals and members of the public who remain misinformed regarding the management of asthma. They therefore need to be educated in order to reduce the continuing morbidity and mortality associated with this disease which is largely preventable (Moore-Gillon 1994).

The effects of pregnancy on asthma are variable and dependent upon the many factors which may trigger an attack, for example allergens, chest infections and emotional state. Added to this is the problem of a woman reducing or discontinuing her medication for fear of harming her baby (Moore-Gillon 1994). To date all medications commonly used in the management of asthma such as the beta-agonists (salbutamol, terbutaline), methylxanthines (aminophylline), cromoglycate (Intal), oral steroids and inhaled beclomethasone (Becotide) have not demonstrated any evidence of teratogenic effect (Moore-Gillon 1994). It is difficult to predict how pregnancy will be affected by asthma as studies are inconclusive, demonstrating that some women experience no change in symptoms during pregnancy whilst others have a distinct worsening of the disease (Awadh & Fleetham 1995).

Management

Any woman identified at booking with diagnosed or suspected asthma should be referred to a chest physician for assessment of her condition. Wherever possible, joint consultancy with an obstetrician is ideal in order that consistency in the management of care is communicated to all health professionals involved. This is a good opportunity to ensure that any medication prescribed to the woman is taken correctly whilst giving her an opportunity to discuss any fears that she may have regarding the treatment and the pregnancy. Continual monitoring of peak flow should be included as part of the management of this condition.

If during the pregnancy there are any difficulties in controlling the asthma, the woman should be admitted to hospital (de Swiet 1995). Labour, however, is not usually complicated by asthma attacks (Landon & Samuels 1996). This is thought to be due to an increase in cortisone and adrenaline from the adrenal glands during labour thus preventing asthma (de Swiet 1995). If an asthma attack does occur, it should be treated with the same rapidity and medication as an attack outside of pregnancy (Moore-Gillon 1994). There are certain drugs which should be avoided in pregnancy and labour because of their bronchospasm action; these are intravenous, intra-amniotic and transcervical prostaglandins (Schatz 1992). Any woman who has received corticosteroids in pregnancy should have increased doses for the stress of labour and delivery, normally hydrocortisone 100 mg intramuscularly 6-hourly and for 24 hours after delivery (de Swiet 1995, Landon & Samuels 1996).

Breast feeding should be encouraged, particularly as it may protect infants from developing certain allergic conditions (Kelnar & Harvey 1995). None of the drugs used in the treatment of asthma, except tetracycline and iodides, is likely to be secreted in breast milk in sufficient quantities to harm the neonate (de Swiet 1995).

In conclusion, asthma is a common condition affecting many women in pregnancy. Although generally pregnancy is successful, good control of the woman's asthma will further improve the quality for the mother and inevitably the fetus. It is imperative therefore that women and health professionals are aware of maintaining treatment of asthma throughout pregnancy in order to prevent a potentially life-threatening exacerbation of the condition.

Cystic fibrosis

Cystic fibrosis (CF) is a genetic disorder found in Caucasians which has an incidence of 1:2000 live births (Nakielna 1995). It is an autosomal recessive disease of the exocrine glands which causes production of excess secretions with abnormal electrolyte concentrations resulting in the obstruction of the ducts and glands (Kent & Farquharson 1993). This affects the pancreas, sweat glands, respiratory, digestive and reproductive tracts. Consequently fertility in females is reduced, possibly because of the abnormally low water content of the cervical mucus (Kopito et al 1973). However, owing to improved diagnosis and treatment of this condition, more women are surviving to become pregnant (de Swiet 1995). Treatment includes prophylactic antibiotics with regular physiotherapy and postural drainage. In addition, careful attention to nutritional support is necessary, particularly when pregnancy is planned (Nakielna 1995). When planning a pregnancy, a woman with CF and her partner should discuss with their specialist the potential effects that pregnancy will have on her condition and the risks to the fetus. For example, the risk of the infant having the disease is 1:40 if the father is of unknown genetic make-up (Nakielna 1995); the incidence rises to 1:2 if the father is a genetic carrier. All infants will be carriers of the CF gene (Hilman et al 1996).

Management

A multidisciplinary team should be responsible for the woman with CF during her pregnancy. This would include the CF physician, obstetrician, nutritionist or dietitian, physiotherapist and midwife (Nakielna 1995). Pregnancy is well tolerated by women with CF if their lung function and nutritional status are good. An essential part of obstetric care is therefore early recognition and prompt treatment of acute exacerbations of CF or infections (Hilman et al 1996).

During labour, particular attention should be given to fluid and electrolyte balance as women with CF may easily become hypovolaemic due to the loss of large quantities of sodium in sweat. They are also intolerant of overhydration (de Swiet 1995). At delivery, pulse oximetry monitoring of the mother is recommended as well as giving supplementary oxygen (Hilman et al 1996). If the second stage of labour becomes prolonged, instrumental delivery is recommended (de Swiet 1995). Caution should be exercised with inhalational anaesthesia and therefore, if a caesarean section is required, epidural anaesthesia is recommended (de Swiet 1995).

Breast feeding is not contraindicated in well-nourished women who maintain an adequate calorie intake (Nakielna 1995). Studies have highlighted that the condition of women with CF is at an increased risk of deterioration following pregnancy (Hilman et al 1996). In addition, their infants are at risk of low birthweight or preterm delivery and the sequelae associated with these conditions (Hilman et al 1996).

In summary, women with mild pulmonary disease and good nutritional status are expected to do well. In contrast, women with severe complications associated with their CF are likely to have a poor outcome and therefore should be advised against becoming pregnant (Nakielna 1995).

Pulmonary tuberculosis

The prevalence of pulmonary tuberculosis in the UK is between 0.5 and 1%. The incidence of tuberculosis increased by 12% in the poorest 30% of the population in England and Wales between 1988 and 1992 (Bhatti et al 1995).

Effects on the woman

The onset of primary tuberculosis is often insidious, producing night sweats, weight loss, anorexia, coughing, purulent sputum, haemoptysis (as the blood vessels in the lung are eroded), low-grade fever and general malaise (Ebrahim 1993). The overall effect this has is to debilitate the woman,

making her less able to cope with pregnancy and her existing family. Although pregnancy makes extra demands on her respiratory system, dyspnoea may not be the principal problem. Transplacental infection of the fetus is rare but possible and there is a suggestion that the risks of abortion may be increased (Benson 1983).

Management

The woman will be under the care of an obstetrician and a chest physician during her pregnancy. If there are clinical signs of tuberculosis or the woman is known to have been in contact with tuberculosis, a chest X-ray is performed during the third month, at term and 6 months after delivery. A full-size plate is used as this involves a lower dose of radiation (Landon & Samuels 1996). The fetus is protected by a lead apron. Sputum specimens are taken and any pleural effusions may be aspirated to help identify the organism (de Swiet 1995). Most treatment is given on an outpatient basis, although the woman may be admitted to an isolation unit if her sputum test is positive because the disease is communicated by droplet infection. The rest of her household will also be referred for investigation.

The treatment for tuberculosis includes rest (physical and emotional), hospitalisation if the disease is moderate or advanced, and chemotherapy (Benson 1983). None of the drugs available for treating tuberculosis is ideal. Table 16.1 gives those used, their doses and reported side-effects. Treatment is usually with isoniazid and ethambutol during the first trimester; rifampicin may be used after that (de Swiet 1995). If treatment is begun soon enough the sputum test will be negative by the time the baby is born, although drug therapy is likely to continue for 9 months.

Some women are admitted for rest during the last 2 weeks of pregnancy. Part of the midwife's role is to consider the woman's social and domestic situation. If she has financial difficulties or poor housing the help of a social worker will be needed. She may welcome information about other people or organisations who could care for existing children during the day while she rests. An examination of her eating habits and subsequent dietary counselling may help to improve her nutritional status.

Table 16.1 Drugs used in the treatment of tuberculosis

Drug	Dose	Reported side-effects
Isoniazid	5 mg/kg/day	Abnormalities seen in animals. Interferes with pyridoxine metabolism. Supplements are needed. Found in significant amounts in breast milk
Ethambutol hydrochloride	15–20 mg/kg/day	No effects on fetus apparent
Rifampicin	6–12 mg/kg/day	Increased incidence of neural tube defects: not usually given in first trimester
Streptomycin sulphate	1 g/day i.m.	Fetal auditory and vestibular nerve damage

Intrapartum care

If the mother is infectious, she should be allocated a single room during her stay in hospital. Problems in labour stem from fatigue and reduced lung function and the midwife should seek advice before offering the woman nitrous oxide and oxygen. Episiotomy and forceps delivery may be advocated to reduce the strain of the second stage. Unnecessary blood loss can be avoided by careful management of the third stage. The interaction between her regular medication and the drugs given in labour may be important; for example, streptomycin potentiates the effect of muscle-relaxing drugs (BMA and RPS 1996).

Postnatal care

Separation of the baby from his family is not always necessary. The baby can be vaccinated with an isoniazid-resistant BCG (bacille Calmette–Guérin) whilst being protected from the disease by the prophylactic use of isoniazid syrup 25 mg/kg/day. The vaccine becomes effective in 3–6 weeks as shown by a positive Mantoux test. Without vaccination the child has a 50% chance of catching the disease (Landon & Samuels 1996). If any of the baby's family is infected with an isoniazid-resistant organism, separation will be advised until the baby is Mantoux positive.

Breast feeding is contraindicated if the woman has an active infection. Mothers taking antituberculous therapy should be encouraged to breast feed since the infant will receive a maximum of 20% of the normal infant dose by this route (Snider 1984). Women who breast feed whilst still undergoing treatment may need their medication altered.

Caring for a child at home makes great demands on the woman. If it is possible for her to have extra help in the home, this could be arranged in advance of her return. Friends, relatives or the home help service could be contacted. Midwives should explain that poor nutrition, stress and overtiredness will encourage a recurrence of active disease.

Family planning advice is an integral part of postnatal and preconception care as it is advisable for the woman to avoid further pregnancies until the disease has been quiescent for at least 2 years. When choosing her method of family planning, the woman needs to be aware that rifampicin reduces the effectiveness of oral contraception (BMA and RPS 1996). Long-term medical and social follow-up is necessary in order to monitor the disease and its treatment and to provide help for the socially and economically disadvantaged.

RENAL PROBLEMS

A knowledge of the effects of pregnancy on the urinary tract and on renal function will assist the midwife to understand the impact of pregnancy on existing urinary tract disease and the predisposition pregnant women have to develop urinary tract infection (see Ch. 11).

Tests of renal function

Creatinine is a product of muscle breakdown and is excreted by the kidney at a regular rate; for this reason it is a useful indicator of renal function. The glomerular filtration rate rises by 50% during pregnancy, leading to a greater clearance of creatinine; the plasma creatinine level falls but rises again during the third trimester.

Plasma urea levels follow a similar pattern.

Asymptomatic bacteriuria (ASB)

A diagnosis of ASB is defined as bacteriuria with more than 100 000 organisms per millilitre of urine from a clean voided specimen (Duff 1984). ASB occurs in 2–10% of pregnant women owing to the physiological changes in the urinary tract during pregnancy. If ASB is not identified and treated, 25% of these women will develop symptomatic urinary tract infection (Barnick & Cardoza 1991).

Routine analysis of a midstream specimen of urine in pregnancy is controversial because of the high costs involved (Davison 1995). It is important therefore that a good history is obtained by the midwife when booking a woman antenatally to identify those women at significant risk of this condition. A woman with a history of a previous urinary tract infection with bacteriuria gives the most positive prediction (Davison 1995) and subsequently warrants specific screening.

The consequences of this condition in pregnancy represent a significant risk to both mother and fetus. Symptomatic infections may be implicated in delivery of low birthweight infants, whilst acute pyelonephritis is associated with preterm labour (Davison 1995, Eschenbach 1988).

The penicillins and cephalosporins appear to be the drugs of choice for initial treatment and are administered for between 7 and 14 days (Barnick & Cardoza 1991). A urine sample should be obtained for culture 1 week after therapy is discontinued and thereafter at regular intervals throughout the pregnancy to ensure that reinfection has not occurred (Davison 1995).

Pyelonephritis

Pyelonephritis occurs in 1–2% of all pregnancies (Barnick & Cardoza 1991). The causative organism is often *Escherichia coli* (*E. coli*). Bacteriuria in early pregnancy is a predisposing factor. Intrauterine growth retardation and preterm labour are associated with pyelonephritis and there is a suggestion that there may be an increase in congenital abnormality (Samuels 1996a). The mother feels extremely unwell and usually has a marked pyrexia which may reach 40°C. Rigors may occur. Maternal and fetal heart rates are accelerated. The mother may be nauseated and vomit to the point of dehydration. Pain and tenderness over the loins may be accompanied by muscle guarding. The pain follows the path of the ureters and radiates down to the suprapubic region. The mother may complain of scalding on micturition and a desire to pass urine even when her bladder is empty. Examination of the urine shows it to be cloudy. If the infecting organism is *E. coli*, the urine will usually be acid, but with other organisms may be acid or alkaline.

Management of acute pyelonephritis

If the mother exhibits any of the above symptoms, the midwife must refer to a doctor immediately as it may be a life-threatening condition (Barnick & Cardoza 1991). Admission to hospital is usual and the midwife should help the mother to arrange for care of any other children. A midstream specimen of urine (MSU) should be sent to the laboratory for culture and sensitivity testing.

An appropriate antibiotic will be prescribed; this will be given intravenously at first and orally as the condition improves (Davison 1987). In some centres antibiotics may be continued for as long as 6 weeks and nitrofurantoin given until 2 weeks after delivery (Samuels 1996a). A further MSU may be required 48 hours after commencement of treatment and this should be repeated at intervals after resolution of the infection in order to ensure that there is no recurrence.

Intravenous fluids may also be required to correct dehydration and an accurate record of fluid balance must be kept. During the early stages of the illness, the woman will be confined to bed and the midwife should take steps to prevent complications of immobility such as deep vein thrombosis and constipation. The midwife must monitor uterine activity as there is a risk of labour commencing when the temperature rises. It may be necessary to reduce the temperature by the use of tepid sponging and antipyretics prescribed by the doctor

(Davison 1987). The temperature and pulse should be recorded at least 4-hourly.

The mother may be in considerable pain which may be eased by a heat pad applied to her back. Buscopan 20 mg may be used to relieve pain and antiemetics given to counteract nausea. Follow-up excretion urography is often carried out 3 months postnatally as persistent or recurrent infection, with or without symptoms, may be associated with an abnormality of the renal tract (Barnick & Cardoza 1991).

Chronic renal disease

The chances of a woman becoming pregnant decrease with declining renal function; pregnancy is rare if the kidneys are functioning at less than 50% efficiency. A pregnant woman with pre-existing renal disease is considered to be at high risk of pre-eclampsia; intrauterine growth retardation, preterm birth and perinatal mortality are increased. The woman's own condition is likely to deteriorate. Hospital delivery is essential. Disagreement exists over whether it is pregnancy or pregnancy complications which cause deterioration in renal condition. It is argued that the physiological increase in glomerular filtration can shorten the life of a damaged kidney (Brenner et al 1982).

During pregnancy proteinuria tends to increase (Samuels 1996a). A loss of more than 30% of protein in 24 hours leads to oedema. Damage to the kidney tubules causes an activation of the renin–angiotensin system, leading to salt and water retention and a consequent rise in blood pressure. Production of erythropoietin may be reduced, leading to anaemia. The presence of chronic infection predisposes the mother to superimposed acute infection. The outcome of pregnancy depends on the degree of renal dysfunction, the blood pressure and episodes of infection. Termination of pregnancy or early induction of labour may be offered if the renal condition deteriorates severely.

Examples of pre-existing renal disease are:

- polycystic kidney disease
- glomerular nephritis
- chronic pyelonephritis
- renal calculi
- nephrotic syndrome.

The implications for mother and baby and the management vary according to the condition.

Management

Apart from routine monitoring of the pregnancy (see Ch. 13), the aim of management is to prevent deterioration in renal function. This will necessitate more frequent attendance for antenatal care and the midwife may need to help the mother make the necessary arrangements. Renal function tests are performed at intervals throughout the pregnancy. The emergence and severity of hypertension and pre-eclampsia are monitored by recording blood pressure and estimating urea, creatinine clearance and total protein excretion levels. Admission to hospital is advised if there is evidence of fetal compromise, if renal function deteriorates and proteinuria increases or if the blood pressure rises (Samuels 1996a). In severe cases it may be necessary to transfer the woman to a renal unit for dialysis. If pregnancy remains uncomplicated, some doctors suggest induction of labour at 38 weeks while others hope for spontaneous labour and delivery at term.

Renal transplant

The fertility of women who have had successful transplants is greater than that of women on haemodialysis. There is an increase in ectopic pregnancy as a result of pelvic adhesions but pregnancy does not affect the acceptance of the graft or the survival of the recipient.

Women are advised to wait 2 years after the transplant before attempting to become pregnant as this allows time for the success of the graft to be evaluated (Davison 1987). Preconception advice is particularly important as the woman must be in optimal health before embarking on a pregnancy. The choice of contraceptive must be made with care because the combined pill may raise the woman's blood pressure and the intrauterine contraceptive device may predispose her to infection.

Davison (1987) suggests the following indicators for successful pregnancy and delivery:

- good health for 2 years following transplant

- stature compatible with good obstetric outcome
- no proteinuria
- no significant hypertension
- no evidence of graft rejection
- no evidence of distension of the renal pelvis and calyces on a recent excretory urogram
- plasma creatinine of 180 μmol/l or less
- limited drug therapy, for example prednisolone 15 mg/day or less and azothioprine 2 mg/kg/day or less.

Management

Immunosuppressive therapy is continued during pregnancy, which makes the woman more vulnerable to infections such as cytomegalovirus. Hypertension, proteinuria, urinary tract infection, anaemia, intrauterine growth retardation and premature delivery are all more common. The midwife must be aware of these possible deviations.

During pregnancy the woman should be seen by both the obstetrician and a nephrologist. Clinic visits will be more frequent. Fetal well-being, renal function, blood pressure, haemoglobin and the status of the graft will all be assessed.

During labour steroid therapy may be increased and antibiotics may be prescribed. Special care should be taken to prevent infection and monitor fluid balance.

The baby will be more prone to infection as the mother's immunosuppressive therapy reduces the number of antibodies crossing the placental barrier. The midwife should discuss with the parents ways in which the risk of infection can be minimised. The baby's adrenal function may also be depressed (Samuels 1996a). Long-term follow-up of mother and baby is usually undertaken.

THE ANAEMIAS

Anaemia is a reduction in the oxygen-carrying capacity of the blood which may be due to:

- a reduced number of red blood cells
- a low concentration of haemoglobin, or
- a combination of both.

Physiological anaemia of pregnancy

During pregnancy, maternal plasma volume gradually expands by 50%, an increase of approximately 1200 ml by term. Most of the rise takes place before 32–34 weeks' gestation and thereafter there is relatively little change (Letsky 1987). The total increase in red blood cells is 25%, approximately 300 ml, which occurs later in pregnancy. This relative haemodilution produces a fall in haemoglobin concentration, thus presenting a picture of iron deficiency anaemia. However, it has been found that these changes are not pathological but represent a physiological alteration of pregnancy necessary for the development of the fetus. Normal changes occurring in the blood during pregnancy are summarised in Box 16.1.

Iron requirements in pregnancy

During pregnancy approximately 1500 mg iron is needed for:

- the increase in maternal haemoglobin (400–500 mg)
- the fetus and placenta (300–400 mg)
- replacement of daily loss through stools, urine and skin (250 mg)
- replacement of blood lost at delivery (200 mg)
- lactation (1 mg/day).

Routine screening for anaemia

The criteria used for diagnosing true anaemia in

Box 16.1 Normal blood changes in pregnancy

- Red blood count (RBC). The concentration of red blood cells falls from $4.2 \times 10^{12}/l$ to $3.8 \times 10^{12}/l$.
- Mean cell volume (MCV). The average volume of a red cell fluctuates within the non-pregnant range 77–93 femtolitres (one-thousand-million-millionth of a litre).
- Mean cell haemoglobin (MCH). The average amount of haemoglobin (Hb) in a red cell falls within the non-pregnant range of 26–32 picograms.
- Mean cell haemoglobin concentration (MCHC) indicates how well filled with Hb the cells are. This remains within the non-pregnant range of 32–36 g/dl.
- Packed cell volume (PCV) or haematocrit (Hct) may fall from 0.45–0.33 l/l (45–33%).

pregnancy vary. In 1972 the World Health Organization definition was an Hb level of less than 11 g/dl but many doctors only begin to investigate and treat anaemia when the Hb falls below 10.5 g/dl. Studies in the developing world have demonstrated that many women show no ill effects with an Hb of 10 g/dl. Murphy et al (1986) suggest that the optimal booking haemoglobin is between 10.4 and 13.2 g/dl.

Attempts to detect iron deficiency in pregnancy, however, are not confined to measuring haemoglobin concentration. This is because the normal indices used in laboratory investigations are unreliable in pregnancy. Enkin et al (1995) state that mean cell volume may be the most useful as it is not closely related to haemoglobin concentration and declines quite rapidly in the presence of iron deficiency. It is suggested that parameters which do not rely on relationships to the plasma volume are more useful guides to iron deficiency, for example the total body iron stores (Romslo et al 1983). These can be estimated by measuring serum ferritin which is the body's major iron store protein. Serum ferritin concentration falls in proportion to the decrease in iron stores. Non-pregnant serum ferritin levels are 30 µg/l in women with the following variations found in pregnancy: 90 µg/l in the first trimester, 30 µg/l in the second trimester falling to 15 µg/l in the third trimester (Torrance 1992). Pregnant women are usually screened at their first antenatal visit and thereafter at monthly intervals from the 28th week.

Some doctors prescribe iron supplements for all pregnant women although there is little evidence to support this practice; some give it to those at risk of anaemia while some only use iron to treat anaemia if it occurs. Many doctors avoid giving iron during the first trimester of pregnancy owing to the gastrointestinal side-effects. It may be more appropriate to administer prophylactic iron therapy in the third trimester of pregnancy. During this time the maternal iron stores become depleted due to the increasing fetal demand. Indications for prophylactic iron therapy include:

- previous anaemia
- dietary conditions
- chronic blood loss

- low haemoglobin on booking
- close family spacing.

Oral iron preparations given prophylactically consist of one of the iron salts, either alone or in combination with folic acid. Pregaday contains ferrous fumarate 304 mg (this has 100 mg iron) and folic acid 350 µg. Iron may also be combined with ascorbic acid or other vitamins.

Iron deficiency anaemia

Iron deficiency in women is usually due to blood loss resulting from excessive menses, postpartum haemorrhage or iron deprivation from previous pregnancies. About 95% of pregnant women with anaemia have the iron deficiency type (Benson 1983).

Anaemia in the developing world

In developed countries it is estimated that approximately 2% of women are anaemic; in the developing world this figure may be as high as 50% and this contributes to the high rate of maternal mortality. Iron, folic acid and vitamin B_{12} deficiencies are more common; the unavailability of correct food, food taboos and eating and cooking customs all play a part. In order to help prevent anaemia, midwives must not only understand the medical problem but also any social circumstances that give rise to it. Other contributory causes to the high incidence of anaemia include infections such as amoebic dysentery, malaria (particularly *Plasmodium falciparum*) and *Clostridium welchii*, which cause increased haemolysis. Hookworm (*Ancylostoma duodenale*), which is a parasite found in the tropics, lives in the duodenum and gains its nutrition from the host's blood, causing anaemia. The ova of the worm may be found in the woman's stools. The haemoglobinopathies are discussed later.

Causes

- Reduced intake or absorption of iron. This includes dietary deficiency and gastrointestinal disturbance such as morning sickness.
- Excess demand such as multiple pregnancy, frequent or numerous pregnancies, chronic inflammation, particularly of the urinary tract.

• Blood loss, for example from menorrhagia before conception, bleeding haemorrhoids, antepartum or postpartum haemorrhage, hookworm.

Signs and symptoms

• Pallor of mucous membranes
• Fatigue
• Fainting
• Tachycardia and palpitations
• Dyspnoea.

The associated risks of anaemia (Hb <10.4 g/dl)

Mother (Horn 1988):

• Reduced enjoyment of pregnancy and motherhood owing to fatigue
• Reduced resistance to infection caused by impaired cell-mediated immunity
• Reduced ability to withstand postpartum haemorrhage
• Potential threat to life.

Fetus/baby (Horn 1988, Murphy et al 1986):

• Increased risk of intrauterine hypoxia and growth retardation
• Preterm birth (< 37 completed weeks)
• Low birthweight (< 2500 g)
• Increased risk of perinatal morbidity and mortality.

Prevention

The midwife can help to identify the woman at risk of anaemia by taking an accurate medical, obstetric and social history. This may reveal a pre-existing problem or a woman whose racial origin or lifestyle puts her at risk of anaemia. It may also suggest that the woman is suffering from the effects of anaemia.

Advice and explanations which are appropriate to the particular woman can be given, taking into account health and religious and cultural preferences. Women need to be taught about the sources of iron and ways in which absorption can be increased. Iron intake is closely linked with calorie intake; 2000 kcal per day will contain approxi-

mately 12–14 mg of iron, sufficient to cover the recommended daily amount of 13 mg for pregnant women (Torrance 1992). However, absorption of iron is complex and is influenced by the bioavailability of the iron as well as dietary factors or habits.

Iron is most easily absorbed in the form found in red meat. It is also found in whole-grain products such as wholemeal bread. Egg yolks contain iron but it is less well absorbed. Where the diet is mainly vegetarian, iron is of low bioavailability. Absorption of iron is inhibited by tea and coffee but enhanced by ascorbic acid which is present in orange juice and fresh fruit (Torrance 1992). Generally speaking, those taking a well-balanced diet would not be expected to develop iron deficiency although Cook (1976) found that 20% of menstruating women were deficient in iron.

Investigation

A low Hb concentration only indicates that the woman is anaemic; it does not reveal the cause. Iron deficiency is microcytic, that is, it produces small red cells; the MCV falls first, followed by the MCH, Hct and Hb. By the time the Hb falls, the iron stores will already be depleted. Lack of iron is demonstrated by measuring the serum iron level which will be reduced (normal range 11–30 µmol/l) and the serum iron-binding capacity which will be raised (normal range 54–75 µmol/l). Serum ferritin levels show changes before the Hb falls and correspond well with iron stores but the test is expensive. A midstream specimen of urine should be taken to exclude urinary tract infection which will affect erythropoiesis.

Management

The midwife's role lies in helping the woman to understand the condition, its cause and treatment. The dietary advice already discussed will help her to increase her iron intake. Fatigue may be lessened if other family members can share the workload. It is sometimes appropriate to arrange day care for other children.

Oral iron. The daily dose of iron for treating anaemia is between 120 and 180 mg in divided doses. Two examples are:

- ferrous sulphate: 200 mg tablets contain 60 mg iron
- ferrous gluconate: 300 mg tablets contain 35 mg iron.

Side-effects of oral iron.
The woman should be warned that her stools may turn black but that this does not mean that iron is not being absorbed. Other side-effects are dose related and include nausea and epigastric pain and diarrhoea or constipation. These discomforts may be reduced by taking iron after meals. Some women find one form of iron salts more tolerable than another.

Parenteral iron.
If iron is given intramuscularly or intravenously it bypasses the gastrointestinal tract. This is not a common method of treatment owing to its unpleasant side-effects, although it is an advantage for women who are unable to take, tolerate or absorb oral iron. Bypassing the gastrointestinal tract does not affect the rate of haemoglobin increase. Women receiving parenteral iron do not require any further iron therapy during pregnancy. Parenteral iron is contraindicated for women who have liver or renal disorders.

Intramuscular iron is given in the form of iron sorbitol 50 mg/ml. The dose is 1.5 mg iron/kg bodyweight daily or weekly. Injections should not be given in conjunction with oral iron as this enhances toxic effects such as headache, dizziness, nausea and vomiting. The injection should be given deep into the muscle to prevent staining of the skin, formation of abscesses and fat necrosis.

Total dose iron infusion is given as iron dextran 50 mg/ml in a slow intravenous infusion of normal saline. The dosage is calculated by taking account of bodyweight and the Hb concentration deficit. Side-effects include allergic reaction which may take the form of severe anaphylactic shock; joint pain, occurring within 24 hours of the infusion, is not uncommon. A test dose must be given and the woman's condition monitored strictly during and immediately following the infusion according to local procedure. Women who are prone to allergies should not receive this form of iron.

Blood transfusion is used rarely to treat severe iron deficiency anaemia. It may be used to raise the Hb level quickly if delivery is imminent.

Folic acid deficiency anaemia

Folic acid is needed for the increased cell growth of both mother and fetus but there is a physiological decrease in serum folate levels in pregnancy. Anaemia is more likely to be found towards the end of pregnancy when the fetus is growing rapidly. It is also more common during winter when folic acid is more difficult to obtain and in areas of social, economic and nutritional deprivation. Complications which arise in pregnancy as a result of folate deficiency include abortion, antepartum haemorrhage and preterm labour (Letsky 1987). More recently (1991) the Medical Research Council (MRC) Vitamin Study Research Group found a positive correlation between folate deficiency and neural tube defects.

Causes

- Reduced dietary intake.
- Reduced absorption.
- Interference with utilisation; drugs such as anticonvulsants, sulphonamides and alcohol are folate antagonists.
- Excessive demand and loss. In haemolytic anaemia there is an increased demand for production of new red cells and consequently for folic acid. Multiple pregnancy also results in an increased demand.

Prevention

The risk of folic acid deficiency can be reduced by advising pregnant women on correct selection and preparation of foods which are high in folic acid. Folic acid is found in leafy green vegetables such as Brussels sprouts, broccoli and spinach but is destroyed easily by prolonged boiling or steaming. Other sources include peanuts, chick peas, bananas and citrus fruits. It is also found in avocado pears, asparagus and mushrooms but these are expensive sources. Following the MRC trial in 1991, the Department of Health Expert Advisory Group recommended that all women of childbearing age should eat more folate-rich foods, eat food fortified with folic acid such as bread and cereals and take a folic acid supplement of 0.4 mg per day (DH 1992). It is important for the following conditions in pregnancy that folic acid is prescribed at the correct dose, usually 5 mg per day (Letsky 1987):

- folate deficiency
- malabsorption syndrome
- haemoglobinopathy
- epilepsy requiring anticonvulsant treatment
- multiparity
- multiple pregnancy
- adolescence.

Investigation

The signs and symptoms are varied and may be mistaken as 'minor disorders of pregnancy' such as pallor, lassitude, weight loss, depression, nausea and vomiting, glossitis, gingivitis and diarrhoea. Examination of the red cell indices will reveal that the red cells are reduced in number but enlarged in size. The condition is termed macrocytic or megaloblastic anaemia. The MCV rises; the MCH may remain the same but as there are fewer cells the Hb level falls.

Management

Treatment, once megaloblastic anaemia has been diagnosed, requires folic acid therapy. Folic acid is available in oral and intramuscular forms, the usual daily dose being between 5 and 15 mg in divided doses. This is usually well tolerated with no side-effects.

Vitamin B$_{12}$ deficiency anaemia

Deficiency of vitamin B$_{12}$ also produces a megaloblastic anaemia. Vitamin B$_{12}$ levels fall during pregnancy but anaemia is rare because the body draws on its stores. Deficiency is most likely in vegans, who eat no animal products at all, and therefore vitamin B$_{12}$ supplements should be taken during pregnancy. Folic acid should not be given in cases of vitamin B$_{12}$ deficiency as it can hasten subacute degeneration of the spinal cord (Letsky 1987).

Haemoglobinopathies

This term describes inherited conditions where the haemoglobin is abnormal. Haemoglobin consists of a group of four molecules, each of which has a haem unit which is made up of an iron porphyrin complex and a protein chain. The position of the amino acids in the protein chain determines the type of haemoglobin produced. Adult Hb (HbA) has two alpha and two beta chains while fetal Hb (HbF) has two alpha and two gamma chains. By 6 months of age 96% of a baby's Hb is HbA.

The type of protein chain is genetically determined. Defective genes lead to the formation of abnormal haemoglobin; this may be as a result of impaired globin synthesis (thalassaemia syndromes) or from structural abnormality of globin (haemoglobin variants such as sickle cell anaemia). These conditions prevail in certain geographical areas as the heterozygous (trait) form of thalassaemia and sickle cell offers some protection against malaria. It is found mainly in people whose families come from Africa, the West Indies, the Middle East, the Eastern Mediterranean and Asia (Anionwu & Jibril 1986).

As these conditions are inherited and in the homozygous form can be fatal, screening of the population at risk should be carried out. Blood is examined by electrophoresis which detects the different types of haemoglobin. Prospective parents who are known to have (or carry genes for) abnormal haemoglobin need genetic counselling in order to help them make an informed decision before embarking on a pregnancy (Anionwu 1983, West 1988). All women in the at-risk population are screened in early pregnancy and where possible their partners. If both parents are carriers there is a 1:4 chance that the fetus will be homozygous (Fig. 16.1). This raises considerable ethical and moral issues concerning screening of the fetus and possible termination of the pregnancy (Adams 1994).

Thalassaemia

This condition is most commonly found in people of Mediterranean, African, Middle and Far Eastern origin. The basic defect is a reduced rate of globin chain synthesis in adult haemoglobin. This leads to ineffective erythropoiesis and increased haemolysis with a resultant inadequate haemoglobin content. The red cell indices show a low Hb and MCHC

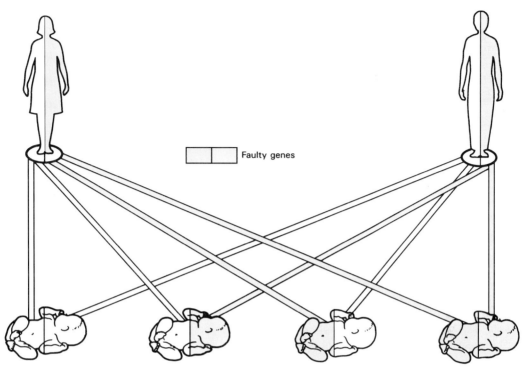

Faulty genes

Fig. 16.1 The inheritance of thalassaemia when both parents are heterozygous.

level but raised serum iron level. Definitive diagnosis is obtained by electrophoresis. The severity of the condition depends on whether the abnormal genes are inherited from one parent or from both. Figure 16.1 shows the possible offspring from a couple who each carry one faulty gene. There are also different types of thalassaemia depending on whether the alpha or beta globin chain synthesis is affected. Box 16.2 shows the number of abnormal genes in each type of thalassaemia.

Box 16.2 Types of thalassaemia and their inheritance

Alpha chains are formed by 2 genes from each parent.
Beta chains are formed by 1 gene from each parent.

Therefore:

Alpha thalassaemia major	= 4 defective alpha genes
Alpha thalassaemia intermedia	= 3 defective alpha genes
Alpha thalassaemia minor	= 2 or 1 defective alpha genes
Beta thalassaemia major	= 2 defective beta genes
Beta thalassaemia minor	= 1 defective beta gene

Alpha thalassaemia major. This condition is more commonly found in Southeast Asia. The child inherits abnormal genes from both parents. Rapid red cell breakdown produces a severe anaemia which is incompatible with extrauterine life (Letsky 1987).

Beta thalassaemia major. The defective genes present result in severe haemoglobin deficiency which may result in cardiac failure and death in early childhood. The use of frequent blood transfusion increases the possibility of survival to childbearing age. However, the constant breakdown of red cells from donated blood results in an accumulation of iron in the body which must be removed by an iron-chelating agent in order to prevent toxicity. Pregnancy in transfusion-dependent thalassaemia is rare and should be monitored closely by the obstetrician and haematologist. It may be preferable for the woman to be referred to a specialist centre where members of staff giving care are experienced in managing this condition. The woman is likely to suffer from severe anaemia and congestive heart failure. Folic acid supplementation is essential and repeated blood transfusions will be required. Iron supplements should only be given if the serum iron levels are low (Samuels 1996b). The midwife has a role to play in supporting the woman and in maintaining links with other departments such as haematology, social work and voluntary bodies, for example UK Thalassaemia Society (107 Nightingale Lane, London N8 7QY).

Alpha and beta thalassaemia minor. The heterozygous condition is the more common form of thalassaemia and produces an anaemia which is similar to iron deficiency in that the Hb, the MCV and the MCH are all lowered. A deficiency in iron is not, however, usually a problem because red cells are broken down more rapidly than normal and the iron is stored for future use. In pregnancy, oral iron and folate supplements are necessary in order to maintain the iron stores. Parenteral iron should never be given. Blood transfusions may be required if the haemoglobin is thought to be inadequate for the stress of labour and blood loss at delivery (Letsky 1987).

Sickle cell disorders

Sickle cell disorders are found most commonly in people of African or West Indian origin. In this condition defective genes produce abnormal haemoglobin beta chains; the resulting Hb is called HbS. In sickle cell anaemia (HbSS) abnormal genes have been inherited from both parents while in sickle cell trait (HbAS) only one abnormal gene has been inherited.

Sickle cell anaemia (HbSS). Sickle cells have an increased fragility and shortened life span of 17 days resulting in chronic haemolytic anaemia and causing episodes of ischaemia and pain; these are known as sickle cell crises. Women with sickle cell anaemia may be subfertile but those who do become pregnant may already have organ damage. This occurs as a result of the sickling crises which may occur whenever oxygen concentration is low. Precipitating factors include psychological stress, cold climate and extreme temperature changes, smoking-induced hypoxia, strenuous physical exer-

tion and fatigue, respiratory disease, infection and pregnancy (Anionwu & Jibril 1986). When subjected to low oxygen tension, HbS contracts, damaging the cell and causing it to assume a sickle shape. Damaged cells block capillaries and the resulting infarction leads to pain, affecting particularly the bones, joints and abdominal organs. Emboli may be thrown off into the circulation, which may threaten life.

Antenatal care. All women in groups at risk are screened. Haematological investigations show a reduced haemoglobin level and electrophoresis demonstrates abnormal haemoglobin patterns in both the heterozygous and homozygous forms (Chamberlain et al 1988). Those who are diagnosed as having sickle cell anaemia should be referred to a specialist sickle cell centre with trained haemoglobinopathy counsellors. Monitoring of pregnancy is performed at regular intervals under the joint supervision of obstetricians and haematologists with back-up from the haematology laboratory.

Regular monitoring of the haemoglobin concentration is required throughout pregnancy and folate supplements should be given. A blood transfusion every 6 weeks may be necessary to maintain an adequate haemoglobin level. During pregnancy it is important that women with sickle cell anaemia avoid situations which may precipitate a crisis. Should these occur, admission to hospital is required and treatment involves rest, rehydration, treatment of infection, pain relief, oxygen therapy and blood transfusion.

Pregnancy is considered hazardous to women who have sickle cell anaemia and complications which may occur include urinary tract infection, spontaneous abortion, pre-eclampsia, preterm labour and intrauterine growth retardation. Both fetal and maternal mortality rates are increased (Tuck & White 1981). The midwife's role is to identify preventive measures as well as to provide social and psychological support.

Intrapartum care. During labour the midwife must ensure that the woman is kept well hydrated with intravenous fluids, and given prophylactic antibiotics, effective analgesia, preferably epidural, and oxygen therapy if needed. The fetus should be monitored closely for signs of distress.

Postnatal care. Prevention of puerperal sepsis is paramount; therefore antibiotic cover is continued throughout the postnatal period. Neonatal testing of all babies at risk must be undertaken by obtaining a cord blood sample at delivery. The sickle cell test does not yield positive results until the age of 3–4 months as fetal haemoglobin (HbF) recedes. A positive test does not distinguish between sickle cell trait and sickle cell anaemia; therefore all children showing positive results should be investigated and followed up by the haematologist. In order to prevent the high incidence of infant mortality from sickle cell anaemia, early diagnosis combined with prophylaxis against infection, parental education and adequate follow-up are recommended (Streetly et al 1993).

Sickle cell trait (HbAS). This is usually asymptomatic. The blood appears normal, although the sickle screening test is positive. There is no anaemia even under the additional stress of pregnancy.

Combinations of abnormal haemoglobins

Sickle cell haemoglobin C anaemia (HbSC) is a mild variant of HbSS more commonly found in Ghanaians. It presents with normal or near-normal levels of Hb. Owing to its mildness, neither the woman nor the obstetrician is aware of its presence or its complications. Women with HbSC may have mild sickling episodes; therefore close supervision is required to avoid any stimulus to a crisis such as hypoxia, dehydration or trauma. This particularly applies immediately after delivery. These women should be managed during labour in the same way as those with HbSS.

Sickle cell disease may be combined with beta thalassaemia.

Other rare inherited disorders

Glucose-6-phosphate dehydrogenase (G6PD) deficiency is found in Africa, Asia and Mediterranean countries. It is inherited through an X-linked gene and is therefore seen predominantly in males. G6PD is an enzyme necessary for the survival of the red cell. When it is deficient, red blood cells are destroyed in the presence of certain substances. These include fava beans, sulphonamides, vitamin K analogues, salicylates and camphor (found in products such as Vicks VapoRub). Clinically G6PD deficiency takes two forms:

- Jaundice in the neonatal period, usually occurring on the second or third day of life, reaching a maximum by the sixth day and subsiding by the end of the first week.
- Acute self-limiting haemolysis precipitated by contact with the substances listed above. This may be indirect contact via the placenta or breast milk. Death from haemolysis is rare.

Spherocytosis is found in Northern Europe. In this condition the red cells are spherical instead of biconcave and are easily destroyed. In this disease the abnormal gene is dominant. It may cause a haemolytic jaundice in the neonate.

DIABETES MELLITUS

Carbohydrate metabolism in pregnancy

The fetus obtains glucose from its mother via the placenta by a process of facilitated diffusion (Smith 1995). From the 10th week of pregnancy there is a progressive fall in the maternal fasting glucose level from 4 mmol/l in early pregnancy to 3.6 mmol/l at term. During the third trimester the mother begins to utilise fat stores which were laid down during the first two trimesters. This results in a rise in free fatty acids and glycerol in the bloodstream and the woman will become ketotic more easily (de Swiet 1995).

The fetoplacental unit alters the mother's carbohydrate metabolism in order to make glucose more readily available. The placenta manufactures human placental lactogen (HPL) which produces a resistance to insulin in the maternal tissues (Johnson & Everitt 1995). This results in blood glucose levels which are higher after meals and remain raised for longer than in the non-pregnant state. Oestrogen and progesterone contribute to these changes and at the end of pregnancy cortisol levels rise, which also leads to a rise in blood glucose.

More insulin is produced, sometimes two or three times as much as in the non-pregnant state

(Oates & Beischer 1987). The extra demands on the pancreatic beta cells can precipitate glucose intolerance or overt diabetes in women whose capacity for producing insulin was only just adequate prior to pregnancy. If a mother was already diabetic before pregnancy, her insulin needs will be increased (Landon 1996).

Glycosuria in pregnancy

Glucose is more liable to appear in the urine of a pregnant woman for the following reasons:

- In a non-diabetic the blood glucose remains within normal limits but the glomerular filtration rate rises. Glucose passes through the proximal convoluted tubule faster than it can be reabsorbed.
- In the diabetic, the rise in blood glucose leads to more glucose in the glomerular filtrate because of the lowering of the renal threshold for glucose.
- Renal tubular damage interferes with glucose reabsorption and may be revealed for the first time during pregnancy.

Glycosuria in pregnancy is not diagnostic of diabetes nor can it be used as a monitor of diabetes in the pregnant woman. Two episodes, however, are regarded as an indication for a glucose tolerance test (Jowett & Nichol 1986).

Gestational diabetes

Certain women are at special risk of developing diabetes during pregnancy and may be identified when the history reveals one or more of the following (Carpenter 1995):

- diabetes in a first-degree relative
- recurrent abortion
- unexplained stillbirth
- congenital abnormality
- a baby whose birthweight was greater than the 97th centile for gestational age, for example a baby weighing more than 4360 g at 40 weeks
- previous gestational diabetes or impaired glucose tolerance
- persistent glycosuria.

In addition the woman may exceed the normal weight range by more than 20% (Landon 1996). The progressive increase in insulin demand during

pregnancy can make latent diabetes appear. This may resolve after the pregnancy. Some women show a slightly impaired glucose tolerance during pregnancy which returns to normal after delivery.

Detection of diabetes in pregnancy

Women considered to be at risk of gestational diabetes undergo a glucose tolerance test. This will indicate whether they have normal or impaired glucose tolerance or have developed diabetes. The criteria for carrying out this test vary but have relied historically upon the presence of the risk factors listed above and also heavy or repeated glycosuria (Landon 1996). Before proceeding to a full glucose tolerance test, a fasting blood sample may be examined for glucose.

Glucose tolerance tests vary slightly but the aim is always to assess the body's response to a glucose load. The woman is asked to fast for a period of time. The fasting blood glucose level is estimated and the woman is given a measured amount of glucose in the form of a drink such as Lucozade 353 ml which provides 75 g glucose. Blood samples are obtained at intervals for glucose estimation and the results compared with a normal range. The blood glucose level will rise initially but should return to normal within a given length of time. This time will vary with the amount of glucose administered. It would be considered abnormal if, between 28 and 34 weeks of pregnancy, glucose levels in two out of four venous samples exceeded the following (WHO 1980):

- Fasting   8.0 mmol/l
- 1 hour after ingestion of 75 g glucose   11.0 mmol/l
- 2 hours after ingestion of 75 g glucose   9.0 mmol/l
- 3 hours after ingestion of 75 g glucose   7.0 mmol/l.

The effect of pregnancy on diabetes

In the early stages of pregnancy diabetic control may be complicated by nausea and vomiting. As the fetus grows the mother needs more carbohydrate and ketosis is induced more easily, particularly in the later stages of pregnancy. The diabetic who is controlled by diet may become dependent on insulin. Blood sugar must be kept within narrow limits in order to avoid exacerbating the effects of the diabetes. Women who have had diabetes since childhood and already have nephropathy or retinopathy must be monitored carefully for signs of any deterioration of their condition (de Swiet 1995).

The effect of diabetes on pregnancy

When diabetes is well controlled its effect on pregnancy may be minimal. If the control is inadequate there may be complications. Maternal haemoglobin (Hb) can become irreversibly bound to glucose; this is termed glycosylated Hb and it normally constitutes 4–8% of the woman's total Hb, increasing during hyperglycaemia (Saunders et al 1980). Fertility is reduced and should conception occur there is an increased risk of spontaneous abortion, stillbirth and fetal abnormality. The perinatal mortality rate among infants of diabetic mothers is markedly increased compared with that of non-diabetic mothers (Bradley 1990). Diabetic women are more prone to urinary tract infection and they have a greater susceptibility to *Candida albicans*. The incidence of pre-eclampsia and of polyhydramnios is also increased (Benson 1983).

Effects on the fetus

The effect of uncontrolled diabetes on the fetus is partially due to disturbed maternal metabolism. Severe maternal ketosis can cause intrauterine death and sometimes maternal death and therefore warrants immediate admission to hospital if suspected (de Swiet 1995). Fetal blood glucose is similar to that of the mother and it is thought that congenital abnormality is caused by fetal hyperglycaemia during the first trimester of pregnancy. No particular congenital abnormality is typical but the rare combination of sacral agenesis and neurological defects is most often seen in babies of diabetic mothers. Neural tube defects are twice as common amongst babies of diabetic mothers and defects in the kidney and heart are also seen (Hollingsworth & Resnik 1988).

Glycosylated Hb releases oxygen poorly to the fetus and this may lead to intrauterine growth retardation. A compensatory fetal polycythaemia develops and will result in neonatal jaundice when the excess red cells are broken down (Roberton 1992). This is exacerbated by relative immaturity of liver enzymes in these babies. Babies of mothers with poorly controlled diabetes may be large (macrosomic) rather than small. The fetus responds to the extra glucose by producing more insulin which can increase its body fat and muscle mass (Roberton 1992). Birthweight and body length are both greater and the kidneys and adrenal cortex are larger. The head circumference and brain size are normal, however.

Prepregnancy care of the known diabetic

As pregnancy complications are reduced if diabetes is well controlled, a diabetic woman should consult her physician for preconception care and advice. Pregnancy may lead to a deterioration of the diabetes; for this reason she must be carefully examined for the presence of renal, cardiovascular or retinal changes before becoming pregnant. The woman will need to continue using some form of contraception while improving control of her diabetes. She may be advised to use the progesterone-only pill, which reduces the risk of arterial changes associated with the combined oral contraceptive pill, or barrier methods which reduce the possibility of intrauterine infection caused by an intrauterine contraceptive device. The midwife will offer advice on weight control and giving up smoking. She will also remind women of the importance of early antenatal care because of the effects of pregnancy on insulin requirements. All women with diabetes should be told by those who care for them how essential it is to ensure that their diabetes is well controlled before considering a pregnancy (de Swiet 1995).

Antenatal care

A woman with diabetes should be advised to book to have her baby in a hospital with a neonatal intensive care unit. She should be seen at a combined antenatal and diabetic clinic. The woman is seen as often as is required in order to maintain good diabetic control; this may entail fortnightly visits until 28 weeks' gestation and then weekly until term. The midwife should remember the woman's predisposition to urinary and vaginal infections and alert her to signs and symptoms so that she will seek treatment as soon as possible. It is important to pay particular attention to the maintenance of hygiene.

It is necessary to assess the progress of the pregnancy in the normal way and to detect any complications. Alpha-fetoprotein screening results must be interpreted in the light of the fact that open neural tube defects have been found at lower levels in diabetic mothers. Fetal growth and detailed anomaly scans must be observed carefully because of the risk of either growth retardation, macrosomia or fetal abnormality. Examination of maternal weight and of her abdomen will help the midwife to detect polyhydramnios. In addition, the woman must be examined for any sign of diabetic complications. In severe cases such complications may provide sufficient grounds for termination of the pregnancy.

Control of diabetes in pregnancy

The aims of diabetic control in pregnancy are to avoid hypoglycaemia, to maintain the preprandial blood glucose between 4.0 and 5.5 mmol/l and to ensure that the postprandial peak does not exceed 7.2 mmol/l (Bradley 1990, James 1989). The dietitian should be consulted and will advise the woman on her nutritional requirements. Special attention will be paid to such problems as nausea and vomiting and the woman might need advice on the importance of maintaining an adequate calorie intake. A diet which is high in fibre produces a more constant blood glucose because the carbohydrate is released for absorption more slowly (Luke & Murtagh 1995). The need for carbohydrate increases as the fetus grows and the diet must be reviewed frequently. 24-hour urine samples can be taken to estimate glucose loss.

Subcutaneous insulin provides the best method of control for most women. A combination of a short- and an intermediate-acting insulin is usually given twice daily before breakfast and the evening meal (Bradley 1990). The dose must be adjusted during pregnancy as insulin requirements increase

(de Swiet 1995). In the case of a newly diagnosed diabetic, the midwife's role will include teaching the woman how to measure her blood glucose and give herself injections. Insulin is absorbed most quickly from the upper arm, then from the abdomen and more slowly from the thigh (Landon & Gabbe 1995). The same area should be used at the same time each day so that the rate of absorption is predictable. The midwife will also ensure that the woman understands her dietary requirements and is able to complete any records accurately. The woman is usually given a kit containing glucagon which can be administered subcutaneously in the event of severe hypoglycaemia. The woman and members of her family should be taught how and when to use it. Some women are able to alter their insulin dose once they are familiar with the variations in their own glucose pattern. Some centres have a doctor on call 24 hours a day to advise women on any concerns they may have. Diabetic women may be admitted to hospital because of poor diabetic control, a destabilising illness or obstetric complications.

Monitoring diabetic control. As far as possible the woman monitors her own diabetes at home. The purpose of these home blood glucose measurements is:

- to detect hyperglycaemia and hypoglycaemia
- to measure changes of blood glucose during a 24-hour period
- to assess blood glucose control in times of special need so that insulin dosage can be readjusted accordingly
- to obtain a full blood glucose profile; samples should be taken at the following times:
  - before the morning injection
  - 1–2 hours after breakfast
  - before lunch
  - 1–2 hours after lunch
  - before the evening injection
  - 1–2 hours after the evening meal
  - before bedtime
  - at some point during the night (Landon 1996).

The woman should try to do two home profiles before visiting the diabetic clinic; this will give a clearer picture of what is happening (Knopfler

1989). She may need to be taught how to take capillary blood samples and test them using a reflectance meter. Some women also test their urine but a reliable estimation cannot be obtained during pregnancy (see Glycosuria in pregnancy).

At the clinic random blood glucose estimations may be carried out in order to check the woman's self-monitoring. Blood samples for estimation of glycosylated haemoglobin (HbA$_1$) are often taken throughout pregnancy in order to gain a retrospective picture of the blood glucose levels over a 6-week period. The HbA$_1$ levels reflect overall control and correlate with the blood glucose profiles. In a non-diabetic person the HbA$_1$ level averages 6 mmol/l throughout pregnancy. In a diabetic pregnancy, levels of 5–8.5 mmol/l should be aimed for. A rise in HbA$_1$ in a woman with pre-existing diabetes during the first trimester is associated with an increase in fetal abnormality (Oates & Beischer 1987).

Management of labour and delivery

If diabetes has been well controlled, the risk of stillbirth is small. The former practice of routine delivery between 35 and 37 weeks of pregnancy is unnecessary. Fetal lungs mature more slowly when the mother is diabetic and it is important to take this into account if induction of labour is being considered (Bourbon & Farrell 1985). Ideally, labour should be allowed to commence spontaneously at term but poor diabetic control or a deterioration in maternal or fetal condition may necessitate earlier, planned delivery (Bradley 1990).

If labour begins prematurely, beta-sympathomimetics such as ritodrine hydrochloride or salbutamol may be used to relax the uterus in order to allow the fetal lungs more time to mature. These drugs increase insulin requirements and blood glucose must be monitored frequently while they are being administered. Steroids such as dexamethasone which may be used to aid lung maturation also increase insulin requirements (de Swiet 1995). Some doctors prefer not to attempt inhibition of preterm labour in diabetic women because of this.

Control of diabetes in labour

Although regimens for diabetic control vary, the aim is to maintain blood glucose between 4 and 5 mmol/l. Maternal hyperglycaemia leads to an increase in fetal insulin production which will cause neonatal hypoglycaemia. See Figure 16.2 for an example of a regimen for diabetic control in labour. If labour is induced, some women will be allowed a light breakfast while others will receive nil orally and the insulin dose will be adjusted accordingly.

The midwife should monitor fetal condition continually throughout labour using electronic fetal monitoring. A paediatrician should be present during delivery, especially if labour has been induced, as a baby with immature lungs may require resuscitation. Polyhydramnios increases the risk of malpresentation, cord prolapse and uterine inertia during labour. Birth asphyxia is more common in both the macrosomic and the growth-retarded baby. The large baby is prone to birth injuries. Shoulder dystocia is a possible hazard to which the midwife must be alert during delivery. Caesarean section is not indicated for diabetes alone and should be reserved for obstetric indications (Bradley 1990).

Postnatal care

Mother
Carbohydrate metabolism returns to normal very quickly after delivery of the placenta and insulin requirements will fall rapidly. The woman can resume her prepregnancy regimen. Owing to increased nutritional demands, a diabetic mother who is breast feeding should be encouraged to increase her carbohydrate intake by 50 g a day (de Swiet 1995) and may need to adjust her insulin requirements according to a preprandial blood glucose estimation. Poor diabetic control will interfere with lactation. Although small amounts of insulin may enter breast milk these are destroyed in the baby's stomach. The diabetic woman is more prone to infection and delayed healing. The midwife may need to advise her to change her pads frequently in order to keep any wound clean and dry.

Gestational diabetes. A woman with gestational diabetes requiring insulin will stop this immediately after delivery. A postpartum glucose tolerance test should be performed approximately 3

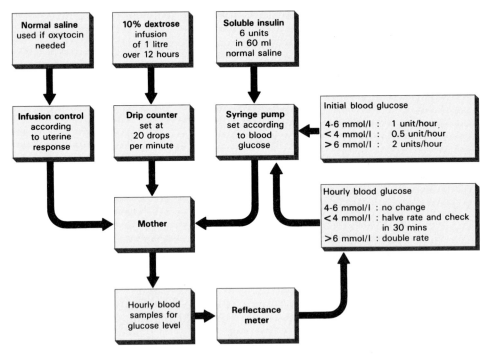

Fig. 16.2 The management of diabetes during labour.

months after delivery. If this is normal, the woman should be warned that the condition may recur in a subsequent pregnancy (de Swiet 1995). All women who have had gestational diabetes, particularly those who are overweight, are encouraged to keep to their diet for the rest of their lives, regardless of whether their glucose tolerance test is normal (Knopfler 1989).

Baby

Asphyxia is common in both macrosomic and growth-retarded babies. The former are also prone to birth injuries because of their size. The baby must be examined carefully at birth as there is an increased risk of congenital abnormality. After birth, the baby continues to produce more insulin than he needs. As he is no longer receiving high levels of glucose from his mother, hypoglycaemia may occur. To prevent this complication the baby should be fed soon after delivery. Monitoring of neonatal blood glucose is often undertaken on the postnatal ward. If the baby's blood glucose is unstable he may be admitted to a neonatal unit for

monitoring. Fetal hyperinsulinism results in polycythaemia. The destruction of many red cells and the relative immaturity of the liver in the newborn predispose the baby to jaundice (Roberton 1992).

INFECTION

Pregnancy produces a degree of altered immunoresponsiveness which helps to prevent fetal rejection but predisposes the woman to infection. The physiological events of childbearing also predispose her to urinary and vaginal infections (Duff 1996) and if she is already the mother of small children the likelihood of exposure to the viral diseases of childhood is increased. Midwives taking a detailed medical history from the pregnant woman should note any infections that she has had while pregnant and during the previous 3 months. An infection in pregnancy may cause discomfort only, whilst others result in potentially serious maternal disease or adverse pregnancy outcome such as abortion or premature labour (Eschenbach 1988).

Transmission of infection to the fetus can occur as follows:

- via the transplacental route, for example the human immunodeficiency virus (HIV) and rubella
- by ascending via the vagina after rupture of the membranes, for example faecal bacteria
- as the baby passes through the birth canal, for example herpes simplex and hepatitis B.

(Infection of the neonate is dealt with in Ch. 42.)

Viral infections are commonly transmitted via the placenta; some bacteria such as *Treponema pallidum* of syphilis and *Listeria monocytogenes*, and protozoa such as *Toxoplasma gondii* are also transferred. The effect on the fetus is variable and includes abortion, fetal death and stillbirth and major or minor morphological abnormality (Hurley 1995). The earlier the fetus is infected the more severe the problem and some conditions may not always be apparent at birth, for example deafness. Most of these infections gain access to the fetus via the placenta. The degree to which the fetus is affected is generally dependent on:

- the virulence of the infecting organism
- the mother's resistance to disease
- the stage of fetal development.

Immunisation. If the woman is planning to go abroad during or shortly after pregnancy she may wish to discuss vaccination. Immunisation in pregnancy with a killed vaccine is generally considered safe. Some vaccines, however, such as cholera and typhoid, are contraindicated because they can produce pyrexia which may cause spontaneous abortion or preterm delivery. Live vaccines such as rubella can damage the fetus and therefore must not be used during pregnancy (Eschenbach 1988). Polio vaccine is only advocated if the woman is travelling to a country where the disease is endemic and then a killed vaccine is used in preference to the live oral type.

Care of the woman with an infection

If the woman contracts an infection she should be cared for in isolation from other pregnant women.

Investigations of the cause of infection include careful history taking, blood culture and culture of a high vaginal swab, a throat swab and a urine sample as appropriate. Blood samples for blood count, antibody titres and immunoglobulin M (IgM) determination may also be required (Hurley 1995).

Treatment
Antimicrobial therapy is undertaken with care. Overuse of broad-spectrum antibiotics has produced resistant organisms and some antibiotics are contraindicated in pregnancy because of their effect on the fetus. Sulphonamides, when given close to the time of delivery, can produce neonatal jaundice (Priest 1990). Co-trimoxazole, which is prescribed for urinary tract infection, is a folate antagonist and is therefore avoided in the first trimester of pregnancy (Davison 1995). Later it can be given in conjunction with folic acid supplements and the midwife can discuss with the woman ways of increasing her dietary intake of folic acid. The aminoglycosides such as streptomycin cause fetal auditory nerve damage, while tetracycline stains the child's deciduous teeth (Priest 1990).

Viral infections

According to Best & Banatvala (1990) the list of viruses that may cause congenital infections is growing. These include rubella virus, cytomegalovirus, varicella zoster virus, the human immunodeficiency viruses (HIV I and HIV II) and human parvovirus B19.

Congenital rubella
This is usually the result of a primary maternal infection. A secondary attack which produces clinical illness in the mother is not thought to put the fetus at risk. If the mother contracts rubella during the first 10 weeks of pregnancy there is a 90% risk that the fetus will be affected. Between 12 and 16 weeks the fetal infection rate is about 50% and the risk of defects is 25%. Although infection may occur after 16 weeks, defects do not necessarily follow. Defects not identified at birth may become evident later. Up to 20% of apparently normal newborn infants develop defects

later on. Careful follow-up of potentially infected babies is therefore necessary (Benson 1983).

All women have their rubella antibody titre assessed during the antenatal period. If they are shown to be susceptible to the disease they are advised to avoid contact with anyone who may be infectious. They will be offered the vaccination during the postnatal period and advised to take precautions to avoid becoming pregnant for 3 months. Should a non-immune woman contract rubella during a critical period of fetal development she may be offered a termination of pregnancy (Kelnar & Harvey 1995). The rubella vaccination programme has substantially reduced the susceptibility among women of childbearing age and the introduction of the measles, mumps and rubella vaccine in October 1988 for children aged 1–2 years should reduce the circulation of the virus in the community (Logan & Peckham 1991).

Varicella zoster virus (chickenpox)

This presents a risk both in early pregnancy and at term. Morgan-Capner (1991, p. 155) states that 'there have been a number of reports of infants with characteristic abnormalities, such as microcephaly and skin scarring, after maternal varicella in the first 20 weeks of pregnancy'. Equally the risk to the neonate is substantial if maternal infection occurs near or soon after delivery. Because of these risks, hyperimmune varicella zoster immune globulin (VZIG) can be offered to susceptible mothers in contact with chickenpox or shingles. In addition, Sills et al (1987) recommended the use of prophylactic acyclovir for those babies at risk. Best & Banatvala (1990, p. 1152) recommend the use of ultrasonography to monitor women who have acquired varicella in the first 20 weeks of pregnancy, 'as it is the only method for detecting defects induced by varicella such as severe scarring and limb deformities'.

Bacterial infections

With the advent and increasing use of convenience foods, pregnant women are becoming more susceptible to food-borne organisms and to developing subsequent infections such as listeriosis. This may be responsible for abortion, fetal disease or death depending upon the severity of the infection and the duration of pregnancy (DH 1991).

Listeriosis

The bacterium which is the cause of listeriosis, *Listeria monocytogenes*, is widespread in the environment. It can be found in soil, dust, mud, vegetation, silage, sewage and most of the animals that have been tested. Thus access to the human food chain is easily gained. Foods implicated in the outbreaks of listeriosis are raw vegetables, coleslaw, milk, soft cheeses and meat pâté. Cook-chill catering is also a hazard as the organism has the unusual characteristic of being able to grow, albeit slowly, at temperatures as low as 2°C (Levy 1989).

Infection in pregnancy may vary from a mild 'flu-like' to a severe illness. This may precipitate premature birth or abortion and cause meningitis in neonates or adults whose immunity to infection is impaired (Scott 1993). When intrauterine infection is present, amniotic fluid may be heavily contaminated and, at birth, attendant staff's hands, clothing and equipment will also become contaminated.

The diagnosis is made by culturing the organism from blood and/or cerebrospinal fluid. In the event of infection, the mother and child are treated with large doses of penicillin or erythromycin (Benson 1983). It is important that the midwife and other health professionals who come into contact with the mother give simple, but comprehensive, education on personal, environmental and food hygiene. This is in order to reduce the risk of fetal morbidity and mortality (Levy 1989).

Protozoal infections

Toxoplasmosis

This is a multisystem disease caused by the protozoan *Toxoplasma gondii* and results in spontaneous abortion, preterm labour, stillbirth and congenital malformations (Benson 1983). The parasite is endemic in Europe and less common in the UK. It is capable of infecting all mammals but is most commonly found in cats. These domestic pets hunt rodents harbouring the parasite and subsequently excrete infective oocytes in the faeces. Human infection follows hand-to-mouth contact after disposal of cat litter or ingestion of undercooked meat from cattle or sheep grazed in contaminated fields (Ibarra 1992).

Parasitaemia can result in fetal infection acquired transplacentally; the fetal bloodstream is invaded by parasites. If the primary infection of the mother occurs in the first or second trimester, the damage to the fetus is high. The principal locus of the infection is the central nervous system leading to developmental and neurological damage; 10–15% of babies born with congenital toxoplasmosis will die (Griffiths 1990). The disease can only occur in the fetus when there is acute maternal infection, hence those mothers who have antibodies before conception are safe. Those mothers who have no antibodies must be advised to eat only well-cooked meat during their pregnancy and to avoid handling cat litter.

In today's society pregnant women have become more likely to travel abroad and may be exposed to certain endemic diseases such as malaria and tuberculosis. Equally, the rising immigrant population within the UK may be more at risk of carrying these diseases.

Malaria

This is a parasitic infection which is carried by mosquitoes, the most common causative organism being *Plasmodium falciparum*. It may cause infertility and complicates pregnancy. Parasitisation of the placental site, especially in primigravid women, may result in spontaneous abortion, intrauterine growth retardation, preterm delivery, stillbirth and neonatal death (Prien-Larsen & St Jeanquist 1993).

Exacerbation or relapse of malaria, which occurs in infections with some malaria species (*P. vivax* and *P. ovale*), is also common during pregnancy and the resultant high fever may precipitate abortion or the onset of preterm labour (Molyneux 1997). Diagnosis in pregnancy is often difficult because of the non-specific symptoms resembling viral or bacterial infections (Prien-Larsen & St Jeanquist 1993). However, it is imperative that a detailed history is taken from any pregnant woman who has recently travelled to an area of endemic disease, particularly if she presents with a pyrexia.

The midwife should also be vigilant for any signs of mosquito marks if a woman has recently returned from a high-risk country (R Coppen, personal communication, 1996). If there are any suspicions that malaria could be a possible cause, the doctor should be notified as well as the Department of Health as it is a communicable disease.

Severe complications of malaria include cerebral malaria, massive haemolysis and acute renal failure; this is more commonly found with *Plasmodium malariae* infection. It is essential that antimalarial drugs are administered intravenously and started as soon as possible as delay may prove fatal (Nathwani et al 1992). The prevention and treatment of malaria during pregnancy is complicated by the increasing resistance of *Plasmodium falciparum* to chloroquine. In zones with chloroquine-resistant malaria, quinine is the treatment of choice (Molyneux 1997). Pregnant women planning to travel in hot countries should be advised to avoid geographical areas where chloroquine-resistant malaria is endemic. In addition, no antimalarial drug is completely safe for use during pregnancy (Nathwani et al 1992). If a pregnant woman must be treated for malaria, it is recommended that advice be sought from experts such as the National Hospital for Tropical Diseases, London.

Approximately 10% of infants born of women with plasmodial infection will have plasmodia in cord blood samples (Benson 1983). Although relatively protected during early infancy by maternal antibodies and fetal haemoglobin, infants will become susceptible to infection with malaria. Neonatal antimalarial therapy is recommended in these cases (de Swiet 1995). The parasite is not thought to be transmitted in milk, but breast feeding should be discouraged in women with clinical evidence of malaria (Benson 1983). Women receiving any antimalarial agent who are breast feeding should be told that their infants are not protected against malaria.

EPILEPSY

The prevalence of epilepsy in the general population is 1:200 and it affects 0.3–0.5% of pregnant women (Donaldson 1995). Between 1985 and

1996, nine women died as a result of status epilepticus during pregnancy (DH et al 1996). It is important that midwives are aware of the complications which may occur and closely monitor women with epilepsy in order to reduce the risk of maternal death and fetal loss.

Antenatal care

In general, women whose epilepsy is well controlled have few problems from their condition in pregnancy. Most of the complications to pregnancy are increased when the epilepsy is poorly controlled (Saunders 1989). Preconception advice is therefore important as it allows time for changes in medication and stabilising the condition prior to pregnancy. Care should be shared between the neurologist, the obstetrician and the midwife, preferably at a combined clinic as this maximises professional surveillance of the woman's condition without the added stress of multiple hospital appointments (Lindsay 1990).

The physiological changes of pregnancy produce a haemodilution and an increased metabolism of anticonvulsant drugs which lead to a fall in the plasma concentration. This results in difficulties with controlling seizures as pregnancy progresses. It is important to monitor the plasma concentration of anticonvulsant therapy on a monthly basis so that a therapeutic range is maintained (Donaldson 1995). The dosage may need to be altered again in the postnatal period.

Complications of anticonvulsant therapy

Women on anticonvulsant therapy become folic acid deficient and may develop macrocytic anaemia. Folic acid deficiency has also been associated with neural tube defects and other congenital malformations such as orofacial clefts and congenital heart defects (Saunders 1989). Abnormalities are more common if anticonvulsant drugs are prescribed in high concentration and particularly if more than one is used. In spite of these potential problems most babies are unaffected and 90% are born normal. Folic acid supplementation (4 mg/day) should be commenced before or early in pregnancy and continued throughout pregnancy to prevent congenital malformations and the development of anaemia in the woman (Rutherford & Rubin 1996). Carbamazepine is not a folate antagonist and appears to be relatively safe in terms of teratogenicity; it is considered to be the drug of choice in pregnancy. Antenatal care should include a detailed anomaly scan, which will detect any fetal abnormalities and allow the option of terminating the pregnancy. Long-term phenytoin treatment produces vitamin D deficiency and therefore women affected should receive supplementary vitamin D throughout pregnancy.

Intrapartum and postnatal care

Care during labour and delivery is not likely to be any different from that of other mothers. Seizures are more likely to occur in conditions such as sleep deprivation, hypoglycaemia, anaemia, stress or hyperventilation. Anticonvulsant therapy should therefore be maintained throughout labour and careful observation by the midwife is required during labour and the early postnatal period (RCM 1997a,b). Safety precautions in the home are important and should be discussed with the woman and her partner (RCM 1997a,b). In addition, women should be advised not to bathe on their own as there appears to be an increased susceptibility to seizures while taking baths in the postnatal period (DH et al 1996). Advice is also given about how to minimise risks when feeding, bathing and transporting the baby. All methods of contraception are available to women with epilepsy. Oral contraceptives are less effective with most anticonvulsants as they induce hepatic enzymes which metabolise oestrogen faster. These women will require oral contraceptives with higher dosage of oestrogens.

Effect on fetus and neonate

According to Donaldson (1995), when status epilepticus occurs, one-third of mothers and half of the fetuses do not survive. A single seizure may cause fetal morbidity from hypoxia or placental abruption. Anticonvulsants cross the placenta freely and decrease production of vitamin K leading to the risk of haemorrhagic disease. This can be prevented by routine administration of vitamin K to the mother from 36 weeks' gestation and to the baby shortly after birth (Brodie 1990). The rate of clearance of anticonvulsant drugs varies according to the drug. Newborn infants may therefore suffer harmful effects from the anticonvulsant level and, as a group, tend to be less efficient at feeding and gain weight more slowly. A minority will suffer withdrawal symptoms such as tremor, excitability and convulsions. Anticonvulsants pass into the breast milk in relatively small quantities. Breast feeding is not contraindicated unless sedative drugs are used such as phenobarbitone, primidone or benzodiazepines. In this case bottle feeding is recommended (Rutherford & Rubin 1996).

AUTOIMMUNE DISEASE AND PREGNANCY

Autoimmune diseases are multifactorial with genetic, environmental, hormonal and viral influences (Nicholas 1988). They are more prevalent in women and often have their onset in the childbearing years. They broadly fall into two groups:

1. multisystem disease such as systemic lupus erythematosus (SLE)
2. tissue- or organ-specific disorders such as idiopathic thrombocytopenic purpura (ITP) and autoimmune thyroid disease.

They are characterised by the production of autoantibodies which are antibodies synthesised by an individual against a component of her own body. The management of these diseases in pregnancy dictates specific care taking into consideration the possible effects of drug therapy on the fetus (Jones 1994).

The aim of this section is to give the reader a brief overview of these conditions. Owing to the complexities of autoimmune disease it is suggested that further reading is undertaken to increase the depth of knowledge (see list of further reading at the end of the chapter).

Systemic lupus erythematosus

Systemic lupus erythematosus (SLE) is an autoimmune disease which upsets the normal immunity of a person (Hughes 1994). It is a multisystem disease which affects women in their reproductive years (Hawkins & Lim 1988). Its peak onset is between the ages of 15 and 40 years and the female:male ratio can be as high as 9:1. It also appears to be commoner in the Afro-Caribbean population (Cervera et al 1990).

SLE is characterised by exacerbations (flares) and remissions but has no typical disease pattern, which often makes diagnosis difficult (Sala 1993). It may manifest as polyarthritis, myalgia, skin rash, alopecia, pleurisy, dyspnoea, pericarditis, proteinuria or anaemia (Hawkins & Lim 1988).

Fertility rates are normal; therefore pregnancy becomes a common management problem in this group of women (Buchanan et al 1993). The effects of SLE are variable, some studies suggest that 'flares' are more common in the second trimester of pregnancy (Buchanan et al 1993) whilst others suggest these occur in the first trimester and within 6 weeks following delivery (Sala 1993). Most studies agree that providing the disease is in remission the outcome of pregnancy is good (Hawkins & Lim 1988). Preconception counselling is therefore important to educate prospective parents about avoiding pregnancy until the disease is quiescent. It is also important to inform women that successive pregnancies do not necessarily affect an individual in the same way (de Swiet 1995).

Effects of SLE on pregnancy

During pregnancy SLE most commonly affects the renal system, the central nervous system and the placenta (Sala 1993). This may have adverse effects on the fetus as there is an increased incidence of low birthweight, prematurity and congenital heart block in the pregnancies of those women with active disease (Buchanan et al 1993). Diagnosis of pre-eclampsia is also difficult in women with SLE as hypertension, proteinuria and oedema occur in both. Despite this, the maternal mortality and long-term prognosis of SLE are not affected by pregnancy (Hawkins & Lim 1988).

Management of pregnancy

A team approach to the management of the pregnancy is necessary. The woman should be referred as soon as possible to a specialist centre; an early antenatal assessment and ultrasound scan is recommended. The frequency of the visits is dependent on the severity of the disease but should include full haematological and immunological investigations. Renal function tests, full blood count and measurements of erythrocyte sedimentation rate and complement levels should be undertaken at each visit in addition to routine antenatal screening (Nicholas 1988). Cardiotocography (CTG) is recommended from 24 weeks' gestation. It is imperative that the midwife ensures that the physical and psychological needs of the woman are met and that the pregnancy is treated as normal as far as possible.

Control and treatment of SLE is mainly dependent on drugs, commencing with simple analgesics such as paracetamol and progressing to corticosteroids, immunosuppressives, cytotoxic agents and antimalarials in the most severe cases (de Swiet 1995). Drug therapy is individualised and dependent upon the disease activity and organs involved. It is important that the woman is aware of the risks both to herself and her baby if SLE is left untreated as often women are reluctant to take drugs in pregnancy (Greener 1991).

Intrapartum care

The timing of delivery in women with this condition depends upon the severity of the disease and whether there are any other complications present such as pre-eclampsia or renal involvement (de Swiet 1995). Delivery should otherwise be at term. A woman in labour with SLE should have an evaluation of her heart and lung sounds and the physician whose care she has been under should be informed of her admission. It is important that all health professionals involved in the woman's care are aware of the risk that infection has on someone with SLE as it is one of the leading causes of death amongst these patients (Sala 1993). The midwife should ensure that careful hand washing and strict aseptic technique are adhered to, as well as limiting the number of vaginal examinations to reduce the risk of infection. Observations of vital signs need to be frequent along with measurement of fluid intake and output and assessment of urinary protein. Continuous electronic fetal monitoring is recommended in conjunction with fetal blood gas estimation because of the potential for placental involvement (Sala 1993). Vaginal delivery is aimed for where possible (Nicholas 1988). However, as a consequence of the associated problems many fetuses are delivered by planned caesarean section (de Swiet 1995). Women on long-term corticosteroid therapy should have parenteral steroid cover in labour and for 24 hours postnatally (de Swiet 1995).

Postnatal care

Following delivery of the baby, the midwife needs to encourage the woman to rest as much as possible in order to prevent an exacerbation of her SLE which is known to occur during stressful times (Sala 1993). Close monitoring of vital signs should continue for 24–48 hours after delivery. Breast feeding is generally thought to be safe if the mother is receiving non-steroid anti-inflammatory drugs or low-dose steroids. Salicylates, antimalarial and immunosuppressive agents need to be avoided (de Swiet 1995). The infant should have a careful clinical examination and undergo appropriate serological evaluation by a paediatrician in the postnatal period. The choice of contraceptives for a woman with SLE is limited as the intrauterine device is thought to increase the risk of infection (Sala 1993) whilst oral contraceptives induce exacerbation of the disease (Nicholas 1988). Barrier methods therefore represent the safest option and the midwife can help educate the woman and her partner in their proper use (Sala 1993).

Idiopathic (autoimmune) thrombocytopenia (ITP)

ITP is the most common autoimmune disease in women of childbearing age and may be recognised in 2–4% of pregnant women (Sullivan & Martin 1995). In simple terms, this condition causes increased platelet destruction by immune processes which may arise following viral infection or an allergic response to drugs (Allison 1989). If the platelet count falls below $50 \times 10^9/l$ the condition may become manifest as bleeding from mucous surfaces and episodes such as epistaxis, multiple small bruises, petechiae in the skin, postpartum uterine haemorrhage or bleeding from abdominal or perineal incisions (Allison 1989, Sullivan & Martin 1995).

Diagnosis

Diagnosis may be made following a routine full blood count with a platelet count of $<100 \times 10^9/l$, or when a pregnant women presents with repeated bleeding episodes in pregnancy (Browning & James 1990). Other causes of thrombocytopenia, such as gestational thrombocytopenia, SLE and pre-eclampsia, should be excluded before a conclusive diagnosis is made (Sullivan & Martin 1995). Samuels et al (1990) identify the difficulty in making a differential diagnosis although this is crucial in terms of maternal and neonatal complications.

Effect of ITP on pregnancy and the fetus

Maternal mortality and morbidity in ITP are now rare (Jones 1994), postpartum haemorrhage being the major risk which is directly related to the maternal platelet count at that time (Browning & James 1990). The perinatal mortality rate can be as high as 15% in extreme cases, the risk stemming from the transplacental passage of IgG antibodies to the fetus (Jones 1994). Complications to the fetus include gastrointestinal bleeding, haemopericardium, intraventricular haemorrhage and severe cutaneous manifestations of bleeding. Profound thrombocytopenia (platelet count below $50 \times 10^9/l$) may develop in infants born to women with ITP, although this is considered to be a transient neonatal condition lasting between 1 week and 4 months of life (Samuels et al 1990).

Antenatal care

Management of this condition in pregnancy is supervised by a haematologist and involves monitoring and maintaining the maternal platelet count at an acceptable level for that woman (Browning & James 1990). Corticosteroid therapy is the initial treatment of choice which will increase the maternal platelet count. If this fails, a high dose of immunoglobulin can be given intravenously (Sullivan & Martin 1995).

Intrapartum care

Decisions regarding the delivery should be on an individual basis. Induction of labour is not indicated if maternal platelets are stable (Browning & James 1990). There is no strong evidence that elective caesarean section affects the perinatal outcome (Jones 1994) and it may cause serious maternal complications (Sullivan & Martin 1995). The objective is to plan for a vaginal delivery avoiding an episiotomy and ensuring good control of the third stage of labour; intravenous ergometrine may be used prophylactically (Hawkins & Lim 1988). If an epidural is the chosen analgesia, there is the theoretical risk of the formation of an extradural haematoma when inserting the epidural cannula. This is unlikely to occur if the platelet count is $> 50 \times 10^9/l$ and the clotting studies are normal (Browning & James 1990). A paediatrician should be present at delivery and an immediate cord platelet count taken (Letsky 1995). Treatment may be required if the platelet count is $< 50 \times 10^9/l$.

Postnatal care

Once the woman has delivered, the midwife should inspect the genital tract to identify and control any bleeding sites. Strict attention to aseptic technique and careful repair of any tissue trauma is important (Sullivan & Martin 1995). Breast feeding is encouraged unless there are adverse complications (Browning & James 1990). Further investigations of this condition may be necessary in the postpartum period. Discussion with the woman and her partner regarding the risks of future pregnancies is important, and they should be advised that platelet levels need to be within normal limits prior to future conceptions (Browning & James 1990).

THYROID DISEASE

Thyroid disease is common in women of reproductive age (Becks & Burrow 1991). The incidence of thyroid disease associated with pregnancy is varied. Hyperthyroidism is reported as occurring in 2 per 1000 pregnancies and hypothyroidism complicates 9 per 1000 (Girling 1996). Thyroid disease in pregnancy can have potential adverse effects on the fetus; the fetal morbidity and mortality rates in untreated women can be as high as 50% (Sugrue & Drury 1980).

Diagnosis

The physiological changes in metabolism make this condition difficult to diagnose, because the hormonal changes and metabolic demands during pregnancy result in complex alterations in the biochemical parameters of thyroid function (Bishnoi & Sachmechi 1996).

Hyperthyroidism

The disease should be suspected in any woman who fails to gain weight satisfactorily despite a good appetite. Other symptoms include exophthalmos, eyelid lag and persistent tachycardia (Ramsay 1995). Clinical diagnosis is difficult as the physiological signs and symptoms pregnant women normally exhibit such as heat intolerance, palpitations and mood lability may mask this condition. Hyperthyroidism when poorly controlled is associated with an increase in preterm delivery, low birthweight and fetal death (Mestman 1980). The condition known as transient hyperthyroid syndrome should be considered in any woman who manifests with hyperemesis gravidarum in early pregnancy and presents with weight loss, tachycardia and vomiting with evidence of biochemical hyperthyroidism (Mestman et al 1995). This condition usually resolves spontaneously by 18–20 weeks' gestation (Bishnoi & Sachmechi 1996).

Treatment

The main form of treatment for hyperthyroidism is by means of antithyroid drugs. The most commonly used are methimazole which crosses the placenta and is secreted in the breast milk (Bishnoi & Sachmechi 1996) and the drug propylthiouracil which does this to a lesser degree. Methimazole has been linked to a scalp defect – aplasia cutis; however, van Dijke et al (1987) have not supported this. The aim of management is to use the lowest dose possible as these agents may cause goitre and hypothyroidism in the fetus (Ramsay 1995).

Antenatal care

The woman should be seen monthly by the endocrinologist during pregnancy for clinical evaluation and estimation of her thyroid levels, and medication should be adjusted accordingly (Ramsay 1995). The midwife has an important role in discussing the woman's diet with her to ensure that the demands of pregnancy and the needs of the fetus are met (Smith 1990). Diarrhoea can be a problem for women with this condition, requiring monitoring of her fluid loss and education regarding signs of dehydration and how to prevent it (Smith 1990).

Breast feeding

In women who wish to breast feed, propylthiouracil is the drug of choice as it crosses into breast milk to a lesser extent (Bishnoi & Sachmechi 1996). The dosage should not exceed 150 mg per day administered in divided doses after each feed (Mestman et al 1995). Some studies suggest that the thyroid function of an infant who is breast feeding whilst his mother is taking antithyroid drugs should be monitored (Becks & Burrows 1991). It is important to determine thyroid hormone levels before the woman leaves hospital as the disease may flare up in the postpartum period.

Hypothyroidism

Historically, hypothyroidism has been associated with infertility but more recent studies suggest that this is not as common as previously thought (Emerson 1991). It is important to diagnose the condition because of the increased rate of fetal loss and reduced IQ in these children (Girling 1996). Symptoms manifest as excessive weight gain despite poor appetite, cold intolerance and a roughening of the skin.

Diagnosis

Again diagnosis may be extremely difficult. Thyroid function measurement is taken and if low the woman is commenced on thyroxine which is titrated to normalise thyroid function (Bishnoi & Sachmechi 1996). This assessment is done on a monthly basis.

Antenatal care

Women with pre-existing hypothyroidism will require monitoring of their thyroid function during pregnancy and their medication adjusted as necessary (Bishnoi & Sachmechi 1996). Hypothyroid pregnant women tend to gain weight easily and the midwife therefore needs to observe this closely for any deviations from the expected weight gain (Smith 1990). Constipation may also prove to be a problem because it is exacerbated by both hypothyroidism and pregnancy. Dietary advice such as increasing fibre content and fluid intake may help alleviate the problem.

Postnatal care

After delivery, the neonate's thyroid status should be checked to identify whether there is any neonatal hypothyroidism present. There is no contraindication to breast feeding but the dose of thyroxine may need adjustment postpartum because of the maternal weight loss following delivery.

Postpartum thyroiditis

This is a transient thyroid dysfunction that occurs during the first year after parturition (Bishnoi & Sachmechi 1996). The condition is characterised initially by symptoms of mild hyperthyroidism followed by a transient episode of hypothyroidism and may mimic postpartum psychosis (Walfish & Chan 1985). Recovery is usually spontaneous in most women but the disorder tends to recur with subsequent pregnancies (Bishnoi & Sachmechi 1996).

READER ACTIVITIES

1. Bearing in mind the risk of food-borne infections to the pregnant woman and fetus, outline the dietary advice which you would give to a pregnant woman on her first and subsequent visits to the antenatal clinic.

2. Highlight the specific problems associated with caring for a woman with cardiac disease during labour. As a midwife, how can you ensure that this labour will have a satisfactory outcome for mother and baby?

3. Arrange a visit to the haematology laboratory and ask to be shown microscope slides showing different forms of anaemia.

4. Explore the literature on the use of iron therapy during pregnancy and clarify for yourself the advice that midwives should give concerning this controversial issue.

5. Discuss the value and cost-effectiveness of routinely carrying out urinalysis, weighing and blood pressure measurement during pregnancy.

6. Devise a care plan covering the first 24 hours after delivery for a woman who has epilepsy. Refer to the RCM booklets, *Guidelines for Midwives on the Care of Women with Epilepsy* and *Guidelines for Women with Epilepsy* (RCM 1997a,b) to assist you in this.

7. Read *Pregnancy Complicated by Thyroid Disease* by J. E. Smith (1990) (Journal of Nurse-Midwifery 35(3): 142–149) in order to gain an understanding of the physiology and role of the thyroid gland in pregnancy.

8. Design a care plan to reflect the specific midwifery care required for a woman with one of the conditions outlined in this chapter.

REFERENCES

Adams S 1994 Sickle cell disease: a case to answer? British Journal of Midwifery 2(10): 275–478

Allison J V 1989 Blood. In: Bray J J, Cragg P A, Macknight A D C et al (eds) Lecture notes on human physiology, 2nd edn. Blackwell Scientific Publications, Oxford

Anionwu E N 1983 Sickle cell disease: screening and counselling in the antenatal and the neonatal period, part 1. Midwife, Health Visitor and Community Nurse 19(3): 402–406

Anionwu E N, Jibril H B 1986 Sickle cell disease: a guide for families. Collins, London

Awadh N, Fleetham J A 1995 Asthma in pregnancy. Journal of the Society of Obstetricians and Gynaecologists of Canada 17(6): 27, 29–31

Barnick C G W, Cardoza L 1991 The lower urinary tract in pregnancy, labour and the puerperium. In: Studd J (ed) Progress in obstetrics and gynaecology. Churchill Livingstone, Edinburgh, vol 9

Becks G P, Burrows G N 1991 Thyroid disease and pregnancy. Medical Clinics of North America 75(1): 121–150

Benson B 1983 Handbook of obstetrics and gynaecology. Lange Medical Publications, California

Best R, Banatvala J E 1990 Congenital virus infections. British Medical Journal 300(5 May): 1151–1152

Bhatti N, Law M R, Morris J K, Halliday R, Moore-Gillon J 1995 Increasing incidence of tuberculosis in England and Wales: a study of the likely causes. British Medical Journal 310(6985): 967–969

Bishnoi A, Sachmechi I 1996 Thyroid disease during pregnancy. American Family Physician 53(1): 215–220

Bourbon J R, Farrell P M 1985 Fetal lung development in the diabetic pregnancy. Paediatric Research 19: 253–267

Bradley R 1990 Diabetic pregnancy. British Journal of Hospital Medicine 44(6): 386–390

Brenner B M et al 1982 Dietary protein intake and the progressive nature of kidney disease. The role of hemodynamically mediated glomerula-injury in the pathogenesis of progressive glomerular sclerosis in ageing, renal ablation and intrinsic renal disease. New England Journal of Medicine 307: 652–659

British Medical Association and Royal Pharmaceutical Society of Great Britain 1996 British national formulary. BMA, London

Brodie M J 1990 Management of epilepsy during pregnancy and lactation. Lancet 336(8712): 426–427

Browning J, James D 1990 Immune thrombocytopenia in pregnancy. Fetal Medicine Review 2: 143–157

Buchanan N M M, Khamashta M A, Kerslake S et al 1993 Practical management of pregnancy in systemic lupus erythematosus. Fetal and Maternal Medicine Review 5: 223–230

Carpenter M W 1995 Testing for gestational diabetes. In: Reece E A, Coustan D R (eds) Diabetes mellitus in pregnancy, 2nd edn. Churchill Livingstone, New York

Celermajer D S, Deanfield J E 1991 Adults with congenital heart disease. British Medical Journal 303(7 December): 1413–1414

Cervera R, Khamashta M A, Hughes G R U 1990 Lupus. Maternal and Child Health 15(8): 243–247

Chamberlain G, Gibbings C, Dewhurst J 1988 Obstetrics illustrated textbook. Lippincott/Gower, Philadelphia/London

Cook J D 1976 Evaluation of the iron status of a population. Blood 48: 449–455

Davison J M 1987 Pregnancy in renal allograft recipients: prognosis and management. Clinical Obstetrics and Gynaecology 1(4): 1027–1045

Davison J 1995 Renal disease. In: de Swiet M (ed) Medical disorders in obstetric practice, 3rd edn. Blackwell Scientific Publications, Oxford

Department of Health 1991 While you are pregnant. HMSO, London

Department of Health Expert Advisory Group 1992 Folic acid and the prevention of neural tube defects. HMSO, London

Department of Health, Welsh Office, Scottish Home and Health Department, Department of Health and Social Services, Northern Ireland 1996 Report on confidential enquiries into maternal deaths in the United Kingdom 1991–1993. HMSO, London

de Swiet M (ed) 1995 Medical disorders in obstetric practice, 3rd edn. Blackwell Scientific Publications, Oxford

Donaldson J 1995 Neurological disorders. In: de Swiet M (ed) Medical disorders in obstetric practice, 3rd edn. Blackwell Scientific Publications, Oxford

Duff P 1984 Pyelonephritis in pregnancy. Clinics in Obstetrics and Gynaecology 27: 17–20

Duff P 1996 Maternal and perinatal infection. In: Gabbe S G, Niebyl J R, Simpson J L (eds) Obstetrics: normal and problem pregnancies, 3rd edn. Churchill Livingstone, New York

Ebrahim G 1993 Paediatric practice in developing countries, 2nd edn. Macmillan Press, London

Emerson C H 1991 Thyroid disease during and after pregnancy. In: Braverman L E, Utiger R D (eds) Werner and Ingbar's The thyroid, 6th edn. Lippincott, Philadelphia

Enkin M, Keirse M J N C, Renfrew M, Neilson J 1995 A guide to effective care in pregnancy and childbirth, 2nd edn. Oxford University Press, Oxford

Eschenbach D A 1988 Infections and sexually transmitted diseases. In: Hollingsworth D R, Resnik R (eds) Medical counseling before pregnancy. Churchill Livingstone, New York

Girling J 1996 Thyroid disease in pregnancy. Maternal and Child Health 21(9): 202–205

Greener M 1991 SLE. A clinical challenge. Professional Nurse 6(10): 589–592

Griffiths G 1990 *Toxoplasma gondii* and toxoplasmosis. Nursing Standard 4(28): 28–30

Hawkins D F, Lim K B 1988 Medical disorders in pregnancy. In: Elder M G (ed) Reproduction in obstetrics and gynaecology. Heinemann Professional Publishing, London

Hilman B C, Aitken M L, Constantinescu M 1996 Pregnancy in patients with cystic fibrosis. Clinical Obstetrics and Gynaecology 39(1): 70–86

Hollingsworth D R, Resnik R (eds) 1988 Medical counseling before pregnancy. Churchill Livingstone, New York

Horn E 1988 Iron and folate supplements during pregnancy: supplementing everyone treats those at risk and is cost effective. British Medical Journal 297(6659): 1325, 1327

Hughes G 1994 Lupus: a guide for patients. Lupus Clinic, Rheumatology Department, St Thomas's Hospital, London

Hurley R 1995 Fever and infectious diseases. In: de Swiet M (ed) Medical disorders in obstetric practice, 3rd edn. Blackwell Scientific Publications, Oxford

Ibarra J 1992 Cats, dogs and young families: do they mix? Professional Care of Mother and Child 2(4): 101–103

James D 1989 High-risk pregnancies. In: Studd J (ed) Progress in obstetrics and gynaecology. Churchill Livingstone, Edinburgh, vol 7

Johnson M, Everitt B 1995 Essential reproduction, 4th edn. Blackwell Scientific Publications, Oxford

Jones W R 1994 Autoimmune disease and pregnancy. Australian and New Zealand Journal of Obstetrics and Gynaecology 34(3): 251

Jowett N I, Nichol S G 1986 Gestational diabetes – are the right women being screened? Midwifery 2(2): 98–100

Kelnar C, Harvey D 1995 The sick newborn baby, 3rd edn. Baillière Tindall, London

Kent N E, Farquharson D F 1993 Cystic fibrosis in pregnancy.

Canadian Medical Association Journal 149: 512–516

Knopfler A 1989 Diabetes in pregnancy. Positive Health Guide. Macdonald, London

Kopito L E, Kosaksy H J, Schwachman H 1973 Water and electrolytes in cervical mucus from patients with cystic fibrosis. Fertility and Sterility 24: 512–516

Landon M B 1996 Diabetes mellitus and other endocrine diseases. In: Gabbe S G, Niebyl J R, Simpson L (eds) Obstetrics: normal and problem pregnancies, 3rd edn. Churchill Livingstone, New York

Landon M B, Gabbe S G 1995 Insulin treatment. In : Reece E A, Coustan D R (eds) Diabetes mellitus in pregnancy, 2nd edn. Churchill Livingstone, New York

Landon M B, Samuels P 1996 Cardiac and pulmonary disease. In: Gabbe S G, Niebyl J R, Simpson J L (eds) Obstetrics: normal and problem pregnancies, 3rd edn. Churchill Livingstone, New York

Letsky E A 1987 Anaemia in obstetrics. In: Studd J (ed) Progress in obstetrics and gynaecology. Churchill Livingstone, Edinburgh, vol 6

Letsky E A 1995 Coagulation defects. In: de Swiet M (ed) Medical disorders in obstetric practice, 3rd edn. Blackwell Scientific Publications, Oxford

Levy J 1989 Listeria and food poisoning – a growing concern. Maternal and Child Health 14(12): 380–383

Lindsay P 1990 Epilepsy in pregnancy. Nursing Times 86(24): 36–38

Littlejohns P, Abrahim S, Anderson R 1989 Prevalence and diagnosis of chronic respiratory symptoms in adults. British Medical Journal 289: 1556–1560

Logan G S, Peckham C 1991 Congenital infections. Hospital Update 17(7): 586–591

Luke B, Murtagh M A 1995 Dietary management. In: Reece E A, Coustan D R (eds) Diabetes mellitus in pregnancy, 2nd edn. Churchill Livingstone, New York

McAnulty J H, Metcalfe J, Ueland K 1988 Cardiovascular disease. In: Burrow G N, Ferris T F (eds) Medical complications during pregnancy, 3rd edn. W B Saunders, Philadelphia

Mestman J H 1980 Management of thyroid disease in pregnancy. Clinical Perinatology 7: 371–377

Mestman J H, Goodwin T M, Montoro M M 1995 Thyroid disorders of pregnancy. Endocrinology and Metabolism Clinics of North America 24: 41–71

Molyneux M 1997 Malaria in non-endemic areas. Medicine (Protozoal Tropical Infections) 25(1): 28–31

Moore-Gillon J 1994 Asthma in pregnancy. British Journal of Obstetrics and Gynaecology 101(8): 658–660

Morgan-Capner P 1991 Viral infections in pregnancy. British Journal of Hospital Medicine 45(March): 150–157

MRC Vitamin Study Research Group 1991 Prevention of neural tube defects: results of the MRC vitamin study. Lancet 338: 132–137

Murphy J F, Newcombe R G, O'Riordan J, Coles E C, Pearson J F 1986 Relation of haemoglobin levels in first and second trimesters to outcome of pregnancy. Lancet 1(May 3): 992–995

Naaktegeboren C 1989 The biology of childbirth. In: Chalmers I, Enkin M, Keirse M J N C (eds) Effective care in pregnancy and childbirth. Oxford University Press, Oxford, vol II

Nakielna B E M 1995 Cystic fibrosis and pregnancy. Journal of the Society of Obstetricians and Gynaecologists of Canada 17(5): 453–461

Nathwani D, Currie P F, Douglas J G, Green S T, Smith N C 1992 Plasmodium falciparum malaria in pregnancy: a review. British Journal of Obstetrics and Gynaecology 99(2): 118–121

Nicholas N 1988 Rheumatic diseases in pregnancy. British Journal of Hospital Medicine 39(1): 50–53

Nolan J 1990 Heart disease in pregnancy. Maternal and Child Health 15(3): 94–96

Oates J N, Beischer N A 1987 Gestational diabetes. In: Studd J (ed) Progress in obstetrics and gynaecology. Churchill Livingstone, Edinburgh, vol 6

Prien-Larsen J C, St Jeanquist M 1993 Malaria in pregnancy – a master of masquerade. MIDIRS Midwifery Digest 3(4): 412–413

Priest J 1990 Drugs in pregnancy and childbirth. Pandora Press, London

Ramsay I D 1995 Thyroid disease. In: de Swiet M (ed) Medical disorders in obstetric practice, 3rd edn. Blackwell Scientific Publications, Oxford

Roberton N R C 1992 A manual of normal neonatal care. Edward Arnold, London

Romslo I, Haram K, Sagen et al 1983 Iron requirement in normal pregnancy as assessed by serum ferritin, serum transferrin saturation and erythrocyte protoporphyrin determinations. British Journal of Obstetrics and Gynaecology 90: 101–107

Royal College of Midwives 1997a Guidelines for midwives on the care of women with epilepsy. RCM, London

Royal College of Midwives 1997b Guidelines for women with epilepsy. RCM, London

Rutherford J M, Rubin P C 1996 Management of epilepsy in pregnancy: therapeutic aspects. British Journal of Hospital Medicine 55(10): 620–622

Sala D J 1993 Effects of SLE on pregnancy and the neonate. Journal of Perinatal and Neonatal Nursing 7(3): 39–48

Samuels P 1996a Renal disease. In: Gabbe S G, Niebyl J R, Simpson J L (eds) Obstetrics: normal and problem pregnancies, 3rd edn. Churchill Livingstone, New York

Samuels P 1996b Haematologic complications of pregnancy. In: Gabbe S G, Niebyl J R, Simpson J L (eds) Obstetrics: normal and problem pregnancies, 3rd edn. Churchill Livingstone, New York

Samuels P, Bussel J B, Braitman L E 1990 Estimation of the risk of thrombocytopenia in the offspring of pregnant women with presumed immune thrombocytopenic purpura. New England Journal of Medicine 323(4): 229–235

Saunders J, Baron M D, Shenouda F S 1980 Measuring glycosylated haemoglobin concentrations in a diabetic clinic. British Medical Journal 281: 1394–1395

Saunders M 1989 Epilepsy in women of childbearing age. British Medical Journal 299: 581

Schatz M 1992 Asthma during pregnancy: interrelationships and management. Annals of Allergy 68(1): 123–133

Scott J 1993 Reducing the client's risk of listeriosis. Modern Midwife 3(6): 22–23

Shabetai R 1988 Congenital or acquired heart disease. In: Hollingsworth D, Resnik R (eds) Medical counseling before pregnancy. Churchill Livingstone, New York

Sills J A, Gallaway A, Amegarie C, Marzouk O, Hein P, Allen K D 1987 Acyclovir prophylaxis and perinatal varicella. Lancet i: 161

Smith J E 1990 Pregnancy complicated by thyroid disease. Journal of Nurse-Midwifery 35(3): 142–149

Smith S L 1995 Hypoglycaemia in the neonate. In: Alexander

J, Levy V, Roch S (eds) Aspects of midwifery practice – a research-based approach. Macmillan, London

Snider D E 1984 Should women taking antituberculous drugs breastfeed? Archives of Internal Medicine 144: 589–590

Streetly A, Dick M, Layton M 1993 Sickle cell disease: the case for coordinated information. British Medical Journal 306(5 June): 1491–1492

Sugrue D, Drury M I 1980 Hyperthyroidism complicating pregnancy: results of treatment by antithyroid drugs in 77 pregnancies. British Journal of Obstetrics and Gynaecology 87: 970–975

Sullivan C A, Martin N J 1995 Management of the obstetric patient with thrombocytopenia. Clinical Obstetrics and Gynaecology 38(3): 521–534

Torrance C 1992 Absorption and function of iron. Nursing Standard 6(19): 25–28

Tuck S M, White J M 1981 Sickle cell disease. In: Studd J (ed) Progress in obstetrics and gynaecology. Churchill Livingstone, Edinburgh, vol 3

van Dijke C P, Heydendael R J, De Kleine M J 1987 Methimazole, carbimazole and congenital skin defects. Annals of Internal Medicine 106: 60–61

Walfish P G, Chan J Y C 1985 Postpartum hyperthyroidism. Clinics in Endocrinological Metabolism 14: 417–420

West R 1988 Ethical aspects of genetic disease and genetic counselling. Journal of Medical Ethics 14(4): 194–197

World Health Organization (WHO) 1972 Nutritional anaemias. WHO Technical Report Series No 503:29. WHO, Geneva

World Health Organization (WHO) 1980 World Health Organization Expert Committee: diabetes mellitus technical report issues. WHO, Geneva

Willis D C, Catond Levelle J P, Banner T 1987 Cardiac output response to prostaglandin E_2 induced abortion in the second trimester. American Journal of Obstetrics and Gynecology 156: 170–173

FURTHER READING

Cook M 1995 Systemic lupus erythematosus: a multifaceted problem in the child-bearing years. Hunter Valley Midwives Association Journal 13(1): 6–8

Garmel S H, D'Alton M E 1995 The management of immune thrombocytopenic purpura in pregnancy. Current Opinion in Obstetrics and Gynaecology 7(3): 229–232

Legun L A 1990 Systemic lupus erythematosus during pregnancy. Journal of Obstetric, Gynaecologic and Neonatal Nursing 19(4): 304–310

Rodin A 1989 Thyroid disease in pregnancy. British Journal of Hospital Medicine 41(3): 234–242

Smith J E 1990 Pregnancy complicated by thyroid disease. Journal of Nurse-Midwifery 35(3): 142–149

Hypertensive disorders of pregnancy

Carmel Lloyd   Victoria Margaret Lewis

Cardiovascular alterations which occur as a consequence of pregnancy may induce hypertension in women who have been normotensive prior to pregnancy or aggravate existing hypertensive conditions. Hypertensive disorders include a variety of vascular disturbances such as gestational hypertension, pre-eclampsia, HELPP syndrome, eclampsia and chronic hypertension.

This chapter aims to:

- list the classifications for hypertensive disorders in pregnancy including the main differentiating characteristics

- describe the signs, symptoms and potential sequelae of the hypertensive disorders

- provide an overview of the medical and alternative therapeutic regimens which may be utilised in the treatment of hypertensive disorders

- identify the midwifery care and support required by a woman with a hypertensive disorder.

The triennial report of maternal deaths in the UK 1991–1993 (DH et al 1996) identified that hypertensive disorders of pregnancy were the second most common cause of maternal death with 5.3 deaths per million maternities from pre-eclampsia and 3.4 deaths per million maternities from eclampsia.

PRE-ECLAMPSIA

Incidence

Between 5 and 8% of all pregnancies are complicated by hypertension and of these pre-eclampsia accounts for 80% (Llewellyn-Jones 1990). It occurs more frequently in young primigravidae, first pregnancies from a new partner and in mothers over 35 years of age. In the latter, pre-eclampsia may be superimposed upon an already existing hypertension. It is known to be associated with hydatidiform mole, multiple pregnancy and maternal diabetes and this is believed to be related to the greater mass of placental tissue. Careful observation of this condition worldwide has identified that the incidence varies with geographical location and race.

Aetiology

Although the exact nature of the primary event causing pregnancy-induced hypertension is not known, evidence accumulated over the past few years indicates that abnormal placentation may be one of the initial events in the disease process. In normal pregnancy placentation involves invasion of the decidua by the syncytiotrophoblast. During early pregnancy, the muscular walls and endothelium of the spiral arteries are eroded and replaced by trophoblast to ensure an optimum environment for the developing blastocyst. A second phase of this invasive process occurs between 16 and 20 weeks' gestation when the trophoblast erodes the myometrium of the spiral arteries. The loss of this musculoelastic tissue results in dilated vessels which are incapable of vasoconstriction; hence a low-pressure, high-blood-flow system into the placenta is produced with maximal placental perfusion (Sheppard & Bonnar 1989). In pre-eclampsia trophoblastic invasion of the spiral arteries is thought to be inhibited by some immunological mechanism (Roberts & Redman 1993). The resultant high-pressure, low-blood-flow system reduces placental perfusion.

Friedman et al (1991) and Lyall & Greer (1994) suggest that a poorly perfused trophoblast in early pregnancy releases one or more factors which damage the endothelial cells, producing vasoconstrictor substances and activating procoagulants. These effects become manifest throughout the body, producing multisystem disorder.

Pathological changes

Normotensive human pregnancy is associated with pronounced cardiovascular changes including an increase in heart rate, blood volume and cardiac output and a decrease in arterial pressure and responsiveness to angiotensin II – a potent vasoconstrictor (Gant et al 1973). Endothelial cell damage alters the vasodilator:vasoconstrictor ratio resulting in sustained hypertension.

Hypertension together with endothelial cell damage affects capillary permeability. Plasma leaks from the damaged blood vessels producing oedema within the tissues. The reduced intravascular compartment causes hypovolaemia and haemoconcentration and this is reflected in an elevated haematocrit. In severe cases the lungs become congested with fluid and pulmonary oedema develops, oxygenation is impaired and cyanosis occurs.

With vasoconstriction and disruption of the vascular endothelium the coagulation cascade is activated. Increased platelet consumption produces thrombocytopenia and may be responsible for disseminated intravascular coagulation (DIC). As the process progresses fibrin and platelet deposits occur which will occlude blood flow to many organs, particularly the kidneys, liver, brain and placenta.

In the kidney, vasospasm of the afferent arterioles results in a decreased renal blood flow which produces hypoxia and oedema of the endothelial cells of the glomerular capillaries. Glomeruloendotheliosis (glomerular endothelial damage) allows plasma proteins to filter into the urine, producing proteinuria. Renal damage is reflected by reduced creatinine clearance and increased serum creatinine and uric acid levels.

The liver is affected in severe cases where intracapsular haemorrhages and necrosis occur. Ultrasonography may show a subcapsular hepatic haematoma. Oedema of the liver cells produces epigastric pain and impaired liver function.

The brain becomes oedematous and this, in conjunction with hypertension and DIC, can produce thrombosis and necrosis of the blood vessel walls resulting in headaches, visual disturbances and a cerebrovascular accident. Other signs of central nervous system involvement include irritability, hyperreflexia and clonus.

In the uterus, vasoconstriction reduces the uterine blood flow and vascular lesions occur in the placental bed. Placental abruption can be the result. Reduction in blood flow to the choriodecidual spaces diminishes the oxygen which diffuses through the cells of the syncytiotrophoblast and cytotrophoblast into the fetal circulation within the placenta. The result is that the placental tissue becomes ischaemic, the capillaries in the chorionic villi thrombose and infarctions occur, leading to intrauterine growth retardation. Hormonal output is impaired with reduced placental function and this has serious implications for the survival of the fetus.

Classification

Several classification schemes have been proposed to aid clinical recognition of pre-eclampsia. It is important to recognise the distinction between a woman whose hypertension antedates pregnancy (chronic hypertension) and one who develops an increased blood pressure during pregnancy (pregnancy-induced hypertension). There are three major categories of hypertension during pregnancy (see Box 17.1).

Transient (gestational) hypertension is diagnosed when, after resting, the woman's diastolic blood pressure rises 25 mmHg above the basal blood pressure recorded in early pregnancy or when the blood pressure rises above 140/90 mmHg, on at least two occasions, 4 hours or more apart after the 20th week of pregnancy in a woman known to be normotensive. Oedema of the feet, ankles and pretibial region may be present.

Moderate pre-eclampsia is usually diagnosed when there is a marked rise in the systolic and dias-

tolic pressure, when proteinuria (2+ on dipstick or > 3 g/24 hours) is present in the absence of urinary tract infection and when there is evidence of generalised oedema.

Severe pre-eclampsia is diagnosed when the blood pressure exceeds 170/110 mmHg, when there is an increase in the proteinuria and where oedema is marked. The woman may complain of frontal headaches, visual disturbance and upper abdominal pain with or without vomiting. HELLP (haemolysis, elevated liver enzymes, low platelet count – see below) may be evident.

Diagnosis of pre-eclampsia

The two essential features of pre-eclampsia are hypertension and proteinuria. Oedema and excessive weight gain used to be included in the diagnostic criteria but both are variable findings and have no prognostic significance. Diagnosis is usually based on the rise in blood pressure and presence of proteinuria after 20 weeks' gestation. Symptoms are rarely experienced by the mother until the disease has arrived at an advanced state.

Blood pressure. A rise of 25 mmHg above the mother's normal diastolic pressure or an increase above 90 mmHg on two occasions elicited at least 4 hours apart when the mother has been at rest signifies that cardiovascular changes have taken place. In order to detect an incipient increase, the midwife should take the mother's blood pressure early in pregnancy and compare this with all subsequent recordings, taking into account the normal pattern in pregnancy.

Proteinuria in the absence of urinary tract infection is indicative of renal damage. Urine collections should be instigated for measurement of creatinine and protein. The amount of protein in the urine is frequently taken as an index of the severity of pre-eclampsia. Proteinuria is considered to be the most serious manifestation and a significant increase in proteinuria coupled with diminished urinary output indicates renal impairment.

Oedema of the ankles in late pregnancy is a common occurrence and may be found in 40% of pregnant mothers. It is of a dependent nature,

---

Box 17.1 Classification of hypertensive disorders of pregnancy (adapted from Roberts 1994, p. 72)

1. Pregnancy-induced hypertension: develops during pregnancy and regresses postpartum
   a. Transient (gestational) hypertension: increased blood pressure only, no proteinuria
   b. Pre-eclampsia
      (i) mild/moderate
      (ii) severe
   c. Eclampsia
2. Chronic hypertension: known hypertension before pregnancy or a rise in blood pressure >140/90 mmHg before 20 weeks
3. Chronic hypertension with superimposed pregnancy-induced hypertension

usually disappears overnight and is not significant in the absence of raised blood pressure and proteinuria. Oedema affects approximately 80% of women with pre-eclampsia. It may appear rather suddenly and be associated with a rapid weight gain (Wallenburg 1989). Generalised oedema is significant and may be classified as occult or clinical. Occult oedema may be suspected if there is a marked increase in weight but this may be due to causes other than fluid retention. Clinical oedema may be mild or severe in nature and the severity is related to the worsening of the pre-eclampsia. The oedema pits on pressure and may be found in the following anatomical areas: the face, hands, lower abdomen, vulva, sacral area, pretibial region, ankles and feet. Excessive tissue fluid responds to gravitational pull and the midwife should examine the most appropriate anatomical site in order to identify the presence of oedema.

Effects on the mother

- The condition may worsen and eclampsia may occur.
- Placental abruption may occur with all the complications stated in Chapter 15.
- Haematological disturbance can occur and the kidneys, lungs, liver and brain may be seriously damaged.
- The capillaries within the fundus of the eye may be irreparably damaged and blindness can occur.

Effects on the fetus

- Reduced placental function can result in low birthweight.
- There is an increased incidence of hypoxia in both the antenatal and intrapartum periods.
- Placental abruption, if minor, will contribute to fetal hypoxia; if major, intrauterine death will occur.
- Early delivery if the disease worsens, or if abruption occurs, will produce a preterm baby requiring resuscitation.

The midwife's role in detection

As pregnancy-induced hypertension is unlikely to be prevented, early detection and appropriate management can minimise the severity of the condition. A high standard of antenatal care will contribute to the maintenance of optimum health. The midwife is in a unique position to identify those women with a predisposition to pre-eclampsia. A comprehensive history taking at their first meeting will identify:

- adverse social circumstances or poverty which could prevent the woman from attending for regular antenatal care
- a familial tendency towards hypertension
- the mother's age and parity
- any history of renal disease
- a new partnership
- a past history of pre-eclampsia.

On subsequent visits the midwife must take note of any further predisposing factors such as a multiple pregnancy. Urinalysis and blood pressure measurement are undertaken at regular intervals throughout pregnancy. If the midwife identifies any abnormality, the woman should be referred to a registered medical practitioner so that appropriate care can be commenced. The woman may be admitted directly to the maternity unit for care and treatment. A woman with severe pre-eclampsia will require immediate admission to a maternity unit. The midwife should be sensitive to the needs of the family if the mother is admitted to hospital, especially if she is feeling well enough to be at home. Visiting may be limited to her immediate family; if the woman's condition permits, her own children should be encouraged to visit. She is likely to be anxious about the well-being of her children and their visits will allay her fears. The woman and her partner will be concerned for the current pregnancy; sensitive support and encouragement will be required of the midwife.

Management of pregnancy-induced hypertension and mild or moderate pre-eclampsia

The aims of care

The aims of care are to provide rest and a tranquil environment, to monitor the condition and to prevent it worsening by giving appropriate care and treatment. Pregnancy-induced hypertension will require close monitoring but should pre-eclampsia develop more therapeutic interventions may be required. The ultimate aim is to prolong the pregnancy until the fetus is sufficiently mature to survive, while safeguarding the mother's life. Numerous psychosocial implications are involved in caring for a woman who develops pre-eclampsia. The maternal and fetal condition together with the plan of care need to be discussed with the woman and her partner and family. Helping the woman and her partner to interpret the situation, in particular the prognosis for the pregnancy and the potential for perinatal loss, is an important consideration. The midwife is best suited for the psychological support these women require and good communication with those involved with the care of the woman and her baby is essential.

Rest. Women are advised to rest as much as possible and may be admitted to hospital to facilitate this; however, this has not been found to be cost-effective and can be disruptive to family life. In addition Tuffnell et al (1992) found that inpatient care does not improve outcomes or prevent the development of proteinuria. They recommend attendance at a day assessment unit as a means of reducing the need for antenatal admissions and the number of medical interventions. It is preferable for the woman to rest at home and to have regular visits by the midwife or general practitioner and in some instances this can be highly effective where there is the availability of distance monitoring. When proteinuria develops in addition to hypertension the risks to the mother and fetus are considerably increased. Admission to hospital is requisite to monitor and evaluate the maternal and fetal condition.

Diet. There is little evidence to support dietary intervention for preventing or restricting the advance of pre-eclampsia. As for any pregnant woman a diet rich in protein, fibre and vitamins may be recommended. There is some evidence to suggest that prophylactic fish oil in pregnancy may act as an antiplatelet agent, thereby preventing hypertension and proteinuric pre-eclampsia (Redman & Roberts 1993). Calcium supplementation is also

being investigated as it is thought that supplements maintain serum calcium levels, low values being associated with hypertension (Belizan et al 1991).

Weight gain. The efficacy of routine weighing during antenatal visits has been questioned and in many areas has now been abandoned as a form of antenatal screening for pre-eclampsia (Dawes et al 1992). However, weight gain may be useful in monitoring the progression of pre-eclampsia in conjunction with other parameters (Surratt 1993). The initial body mass index (weight in kilograms/(height in metres)^2) is considered a more useful predictor of hypertension in pregnancy, since women developing hypertension have higher body mass indices (Masse et al 1993).

Blood pressure is monitored regularly. It is important to consider several factors in assessing blood pressure.

Blood pressure should not be taken immediately after a woman has experienced anxiety, pain, a period of exercise or has smoked. A 10-minute rest period is recommended before measuring the blood pressure in these circumstances.

The position of the person in whom the blood pressure is measured is important in pregnancy. The supine and right lateral positions are not recommended in view of the effect of the gravid uterus on venous return resulting in postural hypotension. Sitting or lying in the left lateral position with the sphygmomanometer cuff approximately level with the heart is recommended (Shennan & Halligan 1996).

Blood pressure can be overestimated as a result of using a sphygmomanometer cuff of inadequate size relative to the arm circumference. Two cuffs should be available with inflation bladders of 35 cm for normal use and 42 cm for large arms. The length of the bladder should be at least 80% of the arm circumference (Petrie et al 1986).

The question of whether to use Korotkoff (K) IV (muffling sound) or V (disappearance of sound) as a measure of the diastolic blood pressure remains controversial. Rubin (1996) found that K V is easier to obtain, more reproducible and closer to intra-arterial pressure. Shennan & Shennan (1996) recommend the use of K V unless the sound is near zero when K IV should be taken.

The rounding off of the blood pressure measurements should be avoided and an attempt made to record the blood pressure as accurately as possible to the nearest 2 mmHg (Petrie et al 1986).

Urine should be tested for protein daily. If the woman or midwife identifies protein in a midstream specimen of urine, laboratory investigation is essential. Dipstick testing is an unreliable measure (Kuo et al 1992) and therefore a 24-hour urine collection is instigated in order to determine renal function. The level of protein indicates the degree of vascular damage. Reduced kidney perfusion is indicated by proteinuria, reduced creatinine clearance and increased serum creatinine and uric acid.

Abdominal examination is carried out daily. Any discomfort or tenderness should be recorded and reported immediately to the doctor as this may be indicative of placental abruption. Upper abdominal pain is highly significant and indicative of the HELLP syndrome associated with fulminating (rapid onset) pre-eclampsia (Barry et al 1994).

Fetal assessment. It is advisable to undertake a biophysical profile in order to determine fetal health and well-being. This is done by the use of the following: kick charts, cardiotocograph monitoring, serial ultrasound scans to check for fetal growth, liquor volume and fetal breathing movements and/or Doppler flow studies to determine placental blood flow (see Ch. 20).

Antihypertensive therapy. The use of antihypertensive treatment is controversial. In order to be of value 'hypotensive agents should be able to lower maternal blood pressure, reduce hospital admissions and ideally prevent the onset of proteinuria. They must also have no adverse effects on the fetal outcome and should be advantageous in reducing neonatal morbidity' (Pickles et al 1989, p. 38). In general, they have been shown to prevent increases in blood pressure and the development of severe hypertension. There is no evidence of any effect on the development of proteinuria or the prevention of fetal growth retardation or fetal death (Collins & Wallenburg 1989). Their use may be advocated as short-term therapy in order to control hypertension and thereby reduce the risk to the mother of cerebral haemorrhage as well as prolong the pregnancy until the fetus is viable. When pre-eclampsia develops late in gestation, steroids may be given to reduce the risk of neonatal respiratory distress syndrome and delivery in a unit with a neonatal intensive care facility is preferable to antihypertensive therapy.

Methyldopa is the most widely used drug in women with mild to moderate pregnancy-induced hypertension. Beta blockers such as atenolol and labetalol are becoming more popular although their use over the long term is not recommended. Butters et al (1990) reported significant growth retardation in the fetus after long-term use of beta-blockers in pregnant women with chronic hypertension. Calcium channel blockers such as nifedipine are also used to a lesser extent.

Antithrombic agents. Early activation of the clotting system may contribute to the later pathology of pre-eclampsia and as a result the use of anticoagulants or antiplatelet agents has been considered for the prevention of pre-eclampsia and intrauterine growth retardation. Aspirin is thought to inhibit the production of the platelet aggregating agent thromboxane A_2. The CLASP trial concluded that low-dose aspirin might be beneficial for those women at high risk of early-onset pre-eclampsia (CLASP Collaborative Group 1994). A large randomised trial undertaken by the ECPPA Collaborative Group (1996) found that aspirin may prevent a few preterm deliveries per 100 high-risk women treated but there were no other benefits identified. The conclusion from both trials is that the *routine* use of aspirin does not prevent pre-eclampsia or other hypertensive complications in pregnancy.

Management of labour

First stage. The midwife should remain with the mother throughout the course of labour. Pre-eclampsia can suddenly worsen at any time and it is essential to document the presence of oedema, the blood pressure, urinalysis and urinary output. Fluid balance should be monitored carefully and use of a central venous pressure line is recommended (DH et al 1996). Marked deviations should be noted and medical assistance sought. The mother should be made as comfortable as possible, which will necessitate attention to general nursing care.

Vital signs. Blood pressure is measured half-hourly. Because of the haemodynamic changes in pre-eclampsia, a number of authors recommend the measurement of the mean arterial pressure (MAP); this can be calculated by the use of an automatic blood pressure recorder such as the 'Dynamap'. The MAP is defined as systolic blood pressure plus twice the diastolic pressure divided by three. MAP reflects systemic perfusion pressure and therefore the degree of hypovolaemia, whilst measurement of diastolic pressure alone is a better indicator of the degree of hypertension (Wallenburg 1989). Observation of the respiratory rate (>16/min) should be complemented with pulse oximetry. This is a non-invasive measure of the saturation of haemoglobin with oxygen giving an indication of the degree of maternal hypoxia. The level of consciousness may be assessed hourly using a modified Glasgow coma scale (Macdonald 1994). Examination of the optic fundi can give an indication of cerebral oedema. Cerebral irritability can be assessed by the degree of hyperreflexia or the presence of clonus.

Fluid balance. The reduced intravascular compartment in pre-eclampsia together with poorly controlled fluid balance will result in circulatory overload, pulmonary oedema, adult respiratory distress syndrome and ultimately death (DH et al 1996). A central venous pressure line should therefore be utilised in order to monitor the fluid status effectively. This is inserted and supervised by an anaesthetist and measurements are taken hourly. Intravenous fluids are administered using infusion pumps and the recommended infusion rate is 85 ml/h. Syntocinon should be administered with caution as it has an antidiuretic effect. A urinary catheter is also inserted and urine output is measured hourly: > 30 ml/h reflects adequate renal function. Urinalysis to detect the presence of protein, ketones and glucose is undertaken 4-hourly.

Plasma volume expansion. Although women with pre-eclampsia have oedema they are hypovolaemic. The blood volume is low as shown by a high haemoglobin concentration and a high haematocrit. This results in movement of fluid into the extravascular compartment causing oedema. The oedema initially occurs in dependent tissues but as the disease progresses oedema occurs in the liver and brain, giving rise to the symptomatology described previously. Expansion of the blood volume may be required to improve the maternal systemic and uteroplacental circulation, thereby preventing hypoxia and reducing the effect of haemorrhage. Clear fluids will leak out and aggravate pre-existing oedema, therefore colloid solutions such as Haemaccel and Gelofusine are recommended (Macdonald 1994). These solutions increase the colloid osmotic pressure and pull fluid back into the circulation, thereby reducing the oedema and increasing the blood volume.

Pain relief. Epidural analgesia may procure the best pain relief, reduce the blood pressure and facilitate rapid caesarean section should the need arise. It is important to ensure a normal clotting screen and a platelet count > 100×10^9/l prior to insertion of the epidural.

Fetal condition. The fetal heart rate should be monitored continuously and deviations from the normal reported and acted on.

Second stage. When the second stage commences, the obstetrician and paediatrician should be notified. The midwife will continue her care of the mother and will usually deliver the baby. A short second stage may be prescribed depending on the maternal and fetal conditions and in this instance a Ventouse extraction or forceps delivery will be performed by the obstetrician.

Third stage. Ergometrine and Syntometrine will cause peripheral vasoconstriction and increase hypertension and therefore 'should not normally be used in the presence of any degree of pre-eclampsia unless there is severe haemorrhage' (DH et al 1996, p. 31). Syntocinon is the preferred agent for the management of the third stage of labour.

Care following delivery. The maternal condition

should continue to be monitored at least every 4 hours for the next 24 hours as there is still the potential danger of the mother developing eclampsia.

Signs of impending eclampsia
The following signs and symptoms will alert the midwife to the onset of eclampsia:

- a sharp rise in blood pressure
- diminished urinary output which is due to acute vasospasm
- increase in proteinuria
- headache which is usually severe, persistent and frontal in location
- drowsiness or confusion due to cerebral oedema
- visual disturbances such as blurring of vision or flashing lights due to retinal oedema
- epigastric pain which denotes liver oedema and impairment of liver function
- nausea and vomiting.

The midwife should be alert to any of these signs and summon medical assistance immediately. The aims of care at this time are to control hypertension, prevent convulsions and coma and to prevent death of the mother and fetus. Treatment is intensified to this end and delivery will be expedited by caesarean section.

HELLP SYNDROME

The syndrome of haemolysis (H), elevated liver enzymes (EL) and low platelet count (LP) was first described by Weinstein in 1982 and is generally thought to represent a variant of the pre-eclampsia–eclampsia syndrome. Pregnancies complicated by this syndrome have been associated with both poor maternal and poor neonatal outcome. Serious maternal morbidity includes: disseminated intravascular coagulation, acute renal failure, pulmonary oedema, subcapsular liver haematoma and retinal detachment (Sibai et al 1993). Infants whose mothers have HELLP syndrome are often small for gestational age and are at risk of perinatal asphyxia. The affected very low birthweight infants have relatively high incidences of leucopenia, neutropenia and thrombocytopenia (Harms et al

1995). Patients manifesting this syndrome are usually seen before term (less than 36 weeks' gestation) complaining of malaise, epigastric or right upper quadrant pain and nausea and vomiting, and some will have non-specific viral-syndrome-like symptoms. Hypertension and proteinuria may be absent or slightly abnormal (Sibai 1990).

Diagnosis
The variety of signs and symptoms makes diagnosis difficult. As women with pre-eclampsia complicated by HELLP may be normotensive and aproteinuric at presentation, blood pressure measurement and urinalysis cannot be relied on to exclude the diagnosis of pre-eclampsia. Barry et al (1994) identify upper abdominal pain as a common manifestation of the disorder, which should be investigated. Occasionally the presence of this syndrome is associated with hypoglycaemia leading to coma, severe hyponatraemia and cortical blindness. Sibai (1990) recommends that all pregnant women presenting with the above symptoms should have a full blood count and platelet and liver determinations irrespective of maternal blood pressure (Box 17.2).

Complications
Subcapsular haematoma of the liver is a rare but potentially fatal complication of the HELLP syndrome. The condition usually presents with severe epigastric pain that may persist for several hours and in addition the woman may complain of neck and shoulder pain. Barton & Sibai (1996) recommend imaging of the liver in these circumstances.

Box 17.2 Diagnosis of HELLP syndrome

Haemolysis
- Abnormal blood picture
- Increased bilirubin > 20 µmol/l
- Increased lactic dehydrogenase (LDH) > 600 IU/l

Elevated liver enzymes
- Increased serum glutamic-oxaloacetic transaminase (SGOT)/aspartame aminotransferase (AST) > 72 IU/l
- Increased LDH > 600 IU/l

Low platelets
- Platelet count $< 100 \times 10^9$/l

Treatment

Women with the HELLP syndrome should be admitted to a consultant care unit with intensive care cots available. In pregnancies less than 34 weeks' gestation conservative treatment is recommended using plasma volume expanders and pharmacological vasodilators (Visser & Wallenburg 1995). Stabilisation and significant improvement in the laboratory and clinical parameters of the HELLP syndrome may be seen in women who also receive high-dose antenatal corticosteroids (Megann et al 1994). In term pregnancies or where there is a deteriorating maternal or fetal condition, immediate delivery is recommended.

ECLAMPSIA

Eclampsia is rarely seen in developed countries today especially if there are good facilities for antenatal care. Usually pregnancy-induced hypertension is diagnosed and treatment instituted to prevent eclampsia. Occasionally pre-eclampsia is so rapid in onset and progress that eclampsia ensues before any action can be taken. In this situation pre-eclampsia is termed fulminating. In Europe and other developed countries, eclampsia is estimated to complicate around 1 in 2000 deliveries. In developing countries, the estimates vary from 1 in 100 to 1 in 1700 deliveries (Duley 1994).

Eclampsia is defined as the occurrence of one or more convulsions in association with the syndrome of pre-eclampsia. A major problem for preventing and treating eclampsia is that the cause of the condition is unknown, although there is a link between the hypertension, which may not be extreme, and cerebral disease. Redman (1988) identifies the clinical similarities between eclampsia and hypertensive encephalopathy. Whilst the condition is recognised by the advent of a grand mal convulsion it differs from other types of seizure in that the prodromal disorder is not always present before the convulsions begin. Therefore, detecting and managing imminent eclampsia is made more difficult (Redman 1988). In fulminating pre-eclampsia or eclampsia, delivery of the mother should take place as soon as possible once the condition has been stabilised by the following measures.

Care of a mother with eclampsia

The aims of immediate care are to:

- summon medical aid
- clear and maintain the mother's airway – this may be achieved by placing the mother in a semi-prone position in order to facilitate the drainage of saliva and vomit
- administer oxygen and prevent severe hypoxia
- prevent the mother from being injured.

The midwife must remain with the mother constantly and assistance with medical treatment will be required. In the first instance all effort is devoted to the preservation of the mother's life and the well-being of the baby is secondary. This may seem arbitrary but if the mother dies fetal death is inevitable. Treatment may be given as follows.

Anticonvulsant therapy

Discussion about the care of women with eclampsia has focused largely on the control of convulsions with various opinions as to the most appropriate anticonvulsant to use. Magnesium sulphate, diazepam and phenytoin are the most widely used anticonvulsants for the management of eclampsia. The rationale for their use is principally historical rather than scientific. Diazepam is widely used for control of other types of seizures and has a sedative effect. Phenytoin is also effective in controlling convulsions but has been advocated for eclampsia as there is no sedative effect.

Magnesium sulphate is thought to aid vasodilatation thereby reducing cerebral ischaemia (Belfort & Moise 1992). Results of the Collaborative Eclampsia Trial provide evidence of the superiority of magnesium sulphate over diazepam and phenytoin in terms of preventing further seizures and possibly reducing the incidence of pneumonia, artificial ventilation and admission to intensive care (ETCG 1995). Magnesium sulphate is now the recommended drug of choice for routine anticonvulsant management of women with eclampsia rather than diazepam or phenytoin (DH et al 1996, ETCG 1995). Robson (1996) and Duley (1996) suggest a loading dose of 4 g given over 15 minutes intravenously with a maintenance dose of 5 g/500 ml normal saline given as an intravenous infusion at a rate of 1 g/h until 24 hours following delivery. High levels of magnesium sulphate can be toxic and therefore the patellar reflex and respiratory rate or oxygen saturation levels should be measured hourly. In women with oliguria regular monitoring of serum magnesium levels is recommended. Calcium gluconate is the antidote for magnesium toxicity and should be readily available.

Treatment of hypertension

Intravenous hydralazine is the most useful agent to gain control of the blood pressure quickly. 10 mg should be administered slowly and the blood pressure estimated at 5-minute intervals until the diastolic pressure reaches 90 mmHg. The diastolic blood pressure is maintained at this level by titrating an intravenous infusion of hydralazine against the blood pressure.

Intravenous infusions

Care must be taken not to overload the maternal system with intravenous fluid as discussed in the management of pre-eclampsia.

The role of the midwife

The mother will require intensive care as she may remain comatose for a time or may be heavily sedated. Recordings should be carried out as previously mentioned for severe pre-eclampsia. The midwife must observe for periodic restlessness associated with uterine contraction, which indicates that labour has commenced.

The mother's partner should be informed as soon as possible. The midwife will need to give emotional support through this unexpected and anxious time. It is usual to expedite delivery of the baby as soon as possible when eclampsia occurs. In this instance caesarean section is the usual mode of delivery. Anaesthesia should be performed by an experienced anaesthetist as marked facial and laryngeal oedema may make intubation difficult or impossible (Macdonald 1994). The next of kin is usually required to give consent for surgery.

As soon as the baby is delivered, the partner should be encouraged to hold him and accompany him to the neonatal intensive care unit where he will be cared for. It is important that the partner has early interaction with the baby so that an account can be given of the baby's progress from the time of birth. Likewise, the midwife should liaise with the neonatal unit staff and explain the treatment given to the baby and the likely prognosis. A photograph is taken of the baby so that the mother can see it as soon as she recovers from the anaesthetic.

30% of eclamptic fits occur following delivery; therefore intensive surveillance of the woman should be continued for 4 days. Parameters to monitor are: a return to normal blood pressure, an increase in urine output, a reduction in oedema and a return to normal laboratory indices. Thromboelastic stockings should be worn to prevent deep vein thrombosis (Macdonald 1994). All the usual postpartum care is given and as soon as the mother's condition permits she should be taken in her bed or a chair to see her baby. Alternatively, if the baby's condition is good, he may be returned to his mother.

Complications of eclampsia

- Cardiovascular
  - vasospasm
  - pulmonary oedema
- Renal
  - ischaemia
  - oliguria
  - renal failure
- Haematological
  - hypovolaemia
  - haemoconcentration
  - thrombocytopenia
  - disseminated intravascular coagulation
  - haemorrhage
- Neurological
  - cerebral oedema
  - cerebral haemorrhage
- Hepatic
  - hepatocellular damage
  - subcapsular haematoma
  - hepatic rupture
- Fetal
  - placental abruption
  - intrauterine growth retardation

– fetal distress
– intrauterine death.

Future management

There is no indication that pregnancy-induced hypertension causes later hypertensive disease but it can bring to the fore an inherent disposition towards hypertension. Women with a history of severe pre-eclampsia before 32 weeks' gestation have a 5% risk of recurrence by this gestational age and a 15% risk of recurrence overall. There is also evidence that the risk of recurrence may be higher if the pregnancy is with a new partner (Robillard et al 1994)

Usually the blood pressure returns to normal within several weeks but the proteinuria may persist for a longer period. Six months after delivery, the mother is examined by the obstetrician and if all is well she will be discharged and advised to seek advice as soon as a subsequent pregnancy occurs. Referral to voluntary organisations such as Action on Pre-eclampsia (APEC, 31–33 College Road, Harrow, Middlesex HA1 1EJ) may provide additional information, advice and support following a pregnancy complicated by hypertensive disorders.

The mother may have very little recollection of the birth and the events surrounding it if she was unconscious or heavily sedated at the time. It is essential that the midwife enquire further if a mother gives no clear history of a previous delivery or if she says that she was ill. It is advisable to obtain the previous case notes where possible. In this way good care can be provided and prophylactic management established where indicated.

CHRONIC HYPERTENSION

Chronic hypertension has two possible causes:

• It may be a long-term problem, present before the beginning of the pregnancy, for example essential hypertension which accounts for 5% of the cases of hypertension in pregnancy.
• It may be secondary to existing medical problems such as:
    – renal disease

– systemic lupus erythematosus
– coarctation of the aorta
– Cushing's syndrome
– phaeochromocytoma, which is a rare but dangerous tumour of the adrenal medulla.

Diagnosis

Consistent blood pressure recordings of 140/90 mmHg or more, on two occasions more than 24 hours apart during the first 20 weeks of pregnancy suggest that the hypertension is a chronic problem and unrelated to the pregnancy. The diagnosis may be difficult to make because of the changes seen with blood pressure in pregnancy. This is a particular problem in women who present late in their pregnancy with no baseline blood pressure measurement. In addition, Sibai (1996) found that women with chronic hypertension showed greater decreases in their blood pressure during pregnancy than do normotensive women. Hence the chronic hypertension may be missed unless the woman is seen prior to or in early pregnancy.

Investigation

When taking a history the midwife may identify potential or existing problems which may include a known medical condition. Women with chronic hypertension tend to be older, parous and have a family or personal history of hypertension.

Accurate measurement of blood pressure is important and the midwife needs to consider the guidelines mentioned earlier. Serial blood pressure recordings should be made in order to determine the true pattern as even normotensive women show occasional peaks.

The doctor's physical examination of the woman may reveal the long-term effects of hypertension such as retinopathy, ischaemic heart disease and renal damage. Renal function tests may be performed; however, it is important to realise the extent to which the alterations in the physiological norms may affect clinical interpretation in pregnancy. Blood urate levels may help to differentiate between chronic hypertension and pre-eclampsia; they do not rise in the former as they do in the latter.

Admission to hospital or day assessment unit for

initial assessment may be necessary. The midwife can enquire about the woman's social background and investigate her physiological needs, offering her support as necessary.

Complications

The perinatal outcome in mild chronic hypertension is good. However, the perinatal morbidity and mortality is increased in those women who develop severe chronic hypertension or superimposed pre-eclampsia. Other complications are independent of pregnancy and include renal failure and cerebral haemorrhage. In 1–2% of cases hypertensive encephalopathy may develop if the blood pressure suddenly rises above 250/150 mmHg (Sibai 1996). Maternal mortality is high if phaeochromocytoma is left untreated.

Management

Mild chronic hypertension

This is defined as a systolic blood pressure of < 160 mmHg and a diastolic blood pressure of < 110 mmHg. The woman is unlikely to need antenatal admission to hospital and may be cared for in the community by the midwife and the general practitioner. The woman's condition should be carefully monitored in order to identify any preeclampsia which develops.

Severe chronic hypertension

The systolic blood pressure is > 160 mmHg and the diastolic blood pressure is > 110 mmHg. Ideally the woman will be cared for by the obstetric team in conjunction with the physician. Frequent antenatal visits are recommended in order to monitor the maternal condition. This includes blood pressure monitoring, urinalysis to detect proteinuria and blood tests to measure the haematocrit and renal function.

Antihypertensive drug therapy is used in order to prevent maternal complications but has no proven benefit for the fetus nor to the prognosis of the pre-eclamptic process. The most commonly used agent is methyldopa 1–4 g/day in divided doses. It has a sedative effect lasting 2–3 days and is generally considered safe for mother and fetus. Other drugs in common usage include labetalol, nifedipine and oral hydralazine. Sedative drugs may be given to reduce anxiety and help the woman to rest. The midwife may do much to settle anxiety by the use of counselling skills and by mobilising resources to meet social needs if required. In the rare event of a phaeochromocytoma being present the blood pressure will be treated with appropriate antihypertensive drugs during the pregnancy and the tumour resected postnatally.

Monitoring of fetal well-being and of placental function will be carried out assiduously because of the risk of fetal compromise. This would include using serial growth scans and placental blood flow studies by Doppler ultrasound (see Ch. 20). If maternal or fetal condition causes concern, the woman will be admitted to hospital. The timing of the delivery is planned according to the needs of mother and fetus. If early delivery is deemed necessary, induction of labour is preferred to caesarean section.

Renal function should be reassessed postnatally and the woman is seen by the physician with a view to long-term management of persistent hypertension. Antihypertensive therapy may be required. These drugs are excreted in breast milk but Sibai (1996) suggests there are no short-term adverse effects on the infant exposed to methyldopa, hydralazine or beta-blockers. The midwife who is advising the woman on family planning should be aware of the hypertensive effect of the combined oral contraceptive pill.

READER ACTIVITIES

1. Contact the APEC organisation and identify the information, advice and support that this organisation provides to women, their families and health professionals.

2. Research into the hypertensive disorders of pregnancy is ongoing. In order to keep up to date attend one of the national study days on pre-eclampsia organised by APEC.

REFERENCES

Barry C, Fox R, Stirrat G 1994 Upper abdominal pain in pregnancy may indicate pre-eclampsia. Student British Medical Journal 308(2): 1562–1563

Barton J R, Sibai B M 1996 Hepatic imaging in HELLP syndrome (haemolysis, elevated liver enzymes, and low platelet count). American Journal of Obstetrics and Gynecology 174(6): 1820–1827

Belizan J M, Villar J, Gonzalez L 1991 Calcium supplementation to prevent hypertensive disorders of pregnancy. New England Journal of Medicine 325: 1399–1405

Belfort M A, Moise K J 1992 Effect of magnesium sulfate on brain blood flow in preeclampsia: a randomised placebo-controlled study. American Journal of Obstetrics and Gynecology 167: 661–666

Butters L, Kennedy S, Rubin P C 1990 Atenolol in essential hypertension during pregnancy. British Medical Journal 301: 587–589

CLASP (Collaborative Low-dose Aspirin Study in Pregnancy) Collaborative Group 1994 CLASP: a randomised trial of low-dose aspirin for the prevention and treatment of pre-eclampsia among 9364 pregnant women. Lancet 343: 619–629

Collins R, Wallenburg C S 1989 Pharmacological prevention and treatment of hypertensive disorders in pregnancy. In: Chalmers I, Enkin M, Keirse M J N C (eds) Effective care in pregnancy and childbirth. Oxford University Press, Oxford, vol 1

Dawes M G, Green J, Ashurst H 1992 Routine weighing in pregnancy. British Medical Journal 304: 487–489

Department of Health, Welsh Office, Scottish Home and Health Department, Department of Health and Social Services, Northern Ireland 1996 Report on confidential enquiries into maternal deaths in the United Kingdom 1991–1993. HMSO, London

Duley L 1994 Maternal mortality and eclampsia: the eclampsia trial. MIDIRS Midwifery Digest 4(2): 176–178

Duley L 1996 Magnesium sulphate regimens for women with eclampsia: messages from the Collaborative Eclampsia Trial. British Journal of Obstetrics and Gynaecology 103(February): 103–105

Eclampsia Trial Collaborative Group (ETCG) 1995 Which anticonvulsant for women with eclampsia? Evidence from the Collaborative Eclampsia Trial. Lancet 345(June 10): 1455–1463

ECPPA (Estudo Colaborativo para Prevencao da Pre-eclampsia com Aspirina) Collaborative Group 1996 ECPPA: randomised trial of low-dose aspirin for the prevention of maternal and fetal complications in high-risk pregnant women. British Journal of Obstetrics and Gynaecology 103: 39–47

Friedman S A, Taylor R N, Roberts J M 1991 Pathophysiology of pre-eclampsia. Clinics in Perinatology 18: 661–682

Gant N F, Daley G L, Chand S 1973 A study of angiotensin II pressor response throughout pregnancy. Journal of Clinical Investigation 52: 2682–2689

Harms K, Rath W, Herting E 1995 Maternal haemolysis, elevated liver enzymes, low platelet count, and neonatal outcome. American Journal of Perinatology 12(1): 1–6

Kuo V S, Koumantakis G, Gallery E D M 1992 Proteinuria and its assessment in normal and hypertensive pregnancy. American Journal of Obstetrics and Gynecology 167(3): 723–728

Llewellyn-Jones D 1990 Fundamentals of obstetrics and gynaecology. Vol 1. Obstetrics. Faber & Faber, London

Lyall F, Greer I A 1994 Pre-eclampsia: a multifaceted vascular disorder of pregnancy. Journal of Hypertension 12: 1339–1345

Macdonald R 1994 The obstetric anaesthetist and the sick obstetric patient with special reference to fulminating pre-eclamptic toxaemia. Midwives Chronicle and Nursing Notes 107(1273): 44–48

Masse J, Forest J-C, Moutquin J-M, Marcoux S, Brideau N-A, Belanger M A 1993 A prospective study of several biological markers for early prediction of the development of pre-eclampsia. American Journal of Obstetrics and Gynecology 169: 501–508

Megann E F, Bass D, Chauhan S P 1994 Antepartum corticosteroids: disease stabilization in patients with the syndrome of haemolysis, elevated liver enzymes, and low platelets (HELLP). American Journal of Obstetrics and Gynecology 171(4): 1148–1153

Petrie J C, O'Brien E T, Littler W A, de Swiet M 1986 Recommendations on blood pressure measurement. British Medical Journal 293: 611–615

Pickles C J, Symonds E M, Broughton Pipkin F 1989 The fetal outcome in a randomized double-blind controlled trial of labetalol versus placebo in pregnancy-induced hypertension. British Journal of Obstetrics and Gynaecology 96: 38–43

Redman C W G 1988 Eclampsia still kills. British Medical Journal 296(6631): 1209–1210

Redman C W G, Roberts J M 1993 Management of pre-eclampsia. Lancet 341(June 5): 1451–1454

Roberts J 1994 Current perspectives on preeclampsia. Journal of Nurse Midwifery 39(2): 70–90

Roberts J M, Redman C W G 1993 Pre-eclampsia: more than pregnancy-induced hypertension. Lancet 341(June 5): 1447–1451

Robillard P-Y, Hulsey T C, Perianin J, Janky E, Miri E H, Papiernik E 1994 Association of pregnancy-induced hypertension with duration of sexual cohabitation before conception. Lancet 344: 973–975

Robson S C 1996 Magnesium sulphate: the time of reckoning. British Journal of Obstetrics and Gynaecology 103(February): 99–102

Rubin P 1996 Measuring diastolic blood pressure in pregnancy. British Medical Journal 313: 4–5

Shennan A, Halligan A 1996 Blood pressure measurement in pregnancy: room for improvement. Maternal and Child Health 21(3): 55–59

Shennan C, Shennan A 1996 Blood pressure in pregnancy: the need for accurate measurement. British Journal of Midwifery 4(2): 102–108

Sheppard B L, Bonnar J 1989 The maternal blood supply to the placenta. In: Studd J (ed) Progress in obstetrics and gynaecology. Churchill Livingstone, Edinburgh, vol 7

Sibai B M 1990 The HELLP syndrome (haemolysis, elevated liver enzymes, and low platelets): much ado about nothing? American Journal of Obstetrics and Gynecology 162(2): 311–316

Sibai B M 1996 Hypertension in pregnancy. In: Gabbe S G, Niebyl J R, Simpson J L (eds) Obstetrics: normal and problem pregnancies, 3rd edn. Churchill Livingstone, New York

Sibai B M, Ramadan M K, Usta I 1993 Maternal morbidity and mortality in 442 pregnancies with haemolysis, elevated liver enzymes, and low platelets (HELLP syndrome). American Journal of Obstetrics and Gynecology 169(4): 1000–1006

Surratt N 1993 Severe preeclampsia: implications for critical-care obstetric nursing. Journal of Obstetric, Gynecologic and Neonatal Nursing 22(6): 500–507

Tufnell D J, Lilford R J, Buchan PC 1992 Randomised controlled trial of day care for hypertension in pregnancy. Lancet 339(8787): 224–227

Visser W, Wallenburg H C S 1995 Temporising management of severe pre-eclampsia with and without the HELLP syndrome. British Journal of Obstetrics and Gynaecology 102(2): 111–117

Wallenburg H C S 1989 Detecting hypertensive disorders in pregnancy. In: Chalmers I, Enkin M, Keirse M J N C (eds) Effective care in pregnancy and childbirth. Oxford University Press, Oxford, vol I

Weinstein L 1982 Syndrome of haemolysis, elevated liver enzymes and low platelet count: a severe consequence of hypertension in pregnancy. American Journal of Obstetrics and Gynecology 142: 159–167

FURTHER READING

Broughton Pipkin F, Crowther C, de Swiet M, Duley L, Judd A, Lilford R J, Onwude J, Prentice C, Redman C W G, Roberts J, Thornton J, Walker J 1996 Report of a workshop: where next for prophylaxis against pre-eclampsia? British Journal of Obstetrics and Gynaecology 103(July): 603–607

Cheston T M 1996 Pre-eclampsia. In: Alexander J, Levy V, Roch S (eds) Midwifery practice: core topics 1. Macmillan, London

Redman C, Walker I 1990 Pre-eclampsia: the facts. Oxford University Press, Oxford

18

Sexually transmissible and reproductive tract infections in pregnancy

Carolyn Roth

This chapter reviews issues relating to a number of sexually transmissible and reproductive tract infections that are important in relation to pregnancy. Whilst its focus is on pregnancy, other sources of information should be consulted for consideration of the broader issues involved in the presentation, diagnosis and treatment of sexually transmissible and reproductive tract infection such as that offered by Adler (1995).

The chapter aims to:

- consider the general significance to midwives of this group of infections in pregnancy

- describe those infections that give rise to local symptoms in the vagina and vulva

- discuss other infections, some of which have a more generalised impact on the pregnant woman and newborn baby, including infection with human immunodeficiency virus (HIV).

Referral of a woman to a clinic of genitourinary medicine (GUM) which specialises in the diagnosis and treatment of many of the infections discussed here will often be most appropriate. Clinics have at their disposal a range of diagnostic facilities as well as personnel who are familiar with relevant social, psychological and physical issues and can offer counselling and facilitate contact tracing when required. Midwives should familiarise themselves with local provision so that liaison and referral between the two services are facilitated.

The range of sexually transmissible infections

A variety of organisms are capable of being transmitted sexually; in the case of some, for example group B streptococcus (GBS) and *Candida albicans*, sexual transmission is an incidental feature, whereas in others, such as *Neisseria gonorrhoeae* and *Treponema pallidum*, sexual contact is the primary mode of transmission. There are other organisms, such as HIV and hepatitis B virus (HBV), whose presence in blood and other body fluids, including semen and cervical secretions, facilitates their spread by sexual contact.

THE RELEVANCE OF SEXUALLY TRANSMISSIBLE iNFECTION FOR WOMEN OF CHILDBEARING AGE

* A number of sexually transmitted organisms (e.g. *N. gonorrhoeae* and *Chlamydia trachomatis*) cause salpingitis which may lead to chronic pelvic inflammation and permanent damage to the uterine tubes, resulting in reduced fertility and ectopic pregnancy.
* The factors which enable the sexual spread of infection – the presence of an organism within or around the genitalia or its presence in the blood and sexual secretions – also facilitate vertical (perinatal) transmission of infection, from mother to her fetus or newborn baby.
* Some perinatally acquired infections have serious and prolonged consequences for the fetus or neonate (see Ch. 42).
* Pregnancy may have an impact on the presentation and course of infection, giving rise to difficulties in diagnosis or management. Some infections, such as *human papillomaviruses* (HPV), become more virulent; some, such as GBS, are asymptomatic in the woman but may produce serious neonatal disease.
* Some infections, such as HIV and HBV, are incurable and have serious, lifelong implications for the health and infectivity status of those infected.
* The diagnosis of a sexually transmitted infection may have stressful or destructive consequences for the relationship between the woman and her partner, which may be particularly difficult to respond to during pregnancy.
* Women may experience high levels of anxiety and guilt about the implications for their babies of a perinatally transmissible infection.

Educational issues

The advent of the HIV epidemic in the 1980s stimulated educational efforts to heighten awareness about sexually transmitted infection and the necessity for people to avoid this serious, lifelong infection by changing their sexual behaviour and practising 'safer sex'. However, it is clear that women face constraints in relation to their social and sexual lives that will influence the extent to which they are able to practise sex more safely (Thomson & Holland 1994).

Suggestions on how to reduce the risk of contracting a sexually transmitted infection can be easily listed. These include using an effective barrier, such as a condom, during sexual intercourse, avoidance of multiple sexual partners and partners with other sexual partners, avoidance of sexual contact with a partner experiencing symptoms of infection or genital lesions and avoidance of genital contact with oral 'cold sores'. Anyone who places themselves at risk should have regular check-ups (Adler 1995). However, translation of these 'principles' into accessible and usable information both for pregnant women as a group and for individual women is a challenge for midwives. Barriers of language and social attitudes are two issues that need to be addressed in meeting the challenge successfully.

Social issues

For many women the balance of power in sexual relationships is such that their capacity to insist on safer sexual practices may be limited. In addition, the condom, which is the most effective barrier method to protect from sexually transmitted infection, is a method under the control of the man and, in this respect, a woman's power to control her situation is constrained (Stein 1990). Female condoms are now available and research supports their efficacy in prevention of pregnancy and sexually transmitted infection when used consistently and correctly (Farr et al 1994, Soper et al 1993). Elias & Coggins (1996) review current developments in infection prevention technology within women's personal control, but choices remain limited for the present.

Pregnancy, customarily, is a time during which use of barrier contraceptives has not been considered necessary, yet a woman's exposure to a sexually transmitted infection is as liable to occur during pregnancy as at other times of unprotected intercourse. Anatomical and immunological changes of pregnancy may increase susceptibility to some infections (Brunham et al 1990) and the consequences of sexually transmissible infection are liable to be greater during pregnancy than at other times: for example, infection of the membranes and amniotic fluid is associated with preterm delivery and there is risk of fetal exposure and puerperal maternal illness.

Midwives should seek to maximise the opportunity for women to ask questions and express concerns about their sexual health. Women need access during pregnancy, as well as postnatally, to information and supplies of condoms and spermicides.

A legacy of stigma, misinformation and guilt surrounding the issue of sexually transmitted infection has consequences for women seeking and receiving care in relation to this problem. A woman may be reluctant to report symptoms or exposure to infection because she fears judgemental attitudes from her caregivers or is worried about the risk of the confidence being disclosed to others. Many women find a speculum examination of the vagina, especially when conducted by a man, a disturbing experience; midwives and doctors should be sensitive to this distress and provide care which is acceptable to the woman, including the conduct of examinations by a midwife who has received appropriate instruction.

When infection is diagnosed during pregnancy, midwives should use the opportunity to offer information and counselling which may enable the woman to avoid future infection. It is also important that women receive a constructive response to their expression of feelings of guilt or fear. Midwives may need to spend some time considering their own attitudes around issues of sexuality, in addition to their knowledge of sexually transmissible infection. Provision of appropriate information will also require understanding and sensitivity to the particular circumstances of a woman's life, her sense of self-esteem and her attitudes about her sexuality.

Confidentiality

Ensuring the security of information which women share with their caregivers and the results of investigations carried out is essential to creating an environment in which clients feel safe to seek advice about symptoms and to discuss their concerns, and this may be particularly true in the sensitive area of sexually transmissible infection.

It is important for midwives to address the general issue of how, where and whether sensitive information is to be documented in notes. It is inappropriate to document certain information in the notes that women carry, although there may be a need to share information with other caregivers, the GP for example. Women should be consulted about how information should be documented and should, where possible, be enabled to be responsible for relaying relevant information to other professionals involved in their care.

Protection of confidentiality and establishment of a sound relationship of trust between the pregnant woman and her caregiver is best facilitated by a system of continuity of care and carer. In such a scheme, information about a woman's health status is contained amongst the small numbers of people who are actually engaged in giving her care, thus reducing the likelihood of an inadvertent breach of trust.

> As a registered ... midwife ... you are personally accountable for your practice and, in the exercise of your professional accountability, must: ... protect all confidential information concerning patients and clients obtained in the course of professional practice and make disclosures only with consent ... (UKCC 1992)

Screening

Syphilis is the only sexually transmissible infection for which there is presently a policy of routine screening during pregnancy.

Other infections do not lend themselves as easily to routine screening, since many require culture and analysis of the infecting organism rather than serological diagnosis and the tests are therefore more labour intensive and costly to perform.

It may be that the simplicity of serological testing for syphilis and the rarity of a positive diagnosis have contributed to a fairly cavalier approach to the conduct of the test. The blood specimen is usually taken as one of several during the booking visit, often without adequate explanation of the test to be performed. The result, if negative, may be recorded without further discussion with the woman (personal observation). Clearly, these practices breach the principle of informed consent and are a poor basis for establishing an effective exchange of information between a woman and her attendants. Equally, an opportunity is lost of raising the awareness and knowledge of women about the risks and prevention of sexually transmitted infections.

Where screening is carried out, it is essential that midwives have sufficient knowledge of the condition, its significance for the woman and her baby, the treatment available should the diagnosis be positive, the time it will take for a diagnostic result to be reported and other relevant details.

In addition, there must be sufficient time for discussion with the woman and to answer any questions which she might want to pose. An offer of screening should always be used to better inform women about their sexual health as well as to diagnose particular infection. (See below for discussion of HIV testing in pregnancy.)

LOCAL INFECTION OF THE VAGINA AND VULVA

The vagina, far from constituting a sterile environment, is host to a rich variety of microorganisms. These are subject to dynamic alteration in quantity and composition, reflecting at any given time a woman's current physiological state, her immunological defence mechanisms and her past exposure. Transfer and sharing of microorganisms between partners occurs during sexual intercourse, and may include the exchange of infective organisms.

There is, however, a difference between presence of an infective agent in the vagina and the existence of infection. Clinical disease may occur because of the introduction of organisms which are new to the woman or because of a redistribution of existing microbiological flora due, for example, to the physiological changes of pregnancy or the action of antibiotics. Changes may occur in a woman's susceptibility to, or the pathogenicity of, previously encountered organisms.

Fungal infections

The most common of these is *Candida albicans* (thrush), which accounts for the vast majority of fungal vulvovaginal infections, with a minority caused by organisms such as *Torulopsis glabrata* and *Candida tropicalis* (Lossick 1986).

Candida is a common inhabitant of the mouth, large intestine and vagina in 25–50% of healthy individuals and isolation of the organism does not correlate strongly with the presence of clinical disease. Colonisation of the vagina and vulva may originate from contamination of the perianal region; many women are colonised by the same organism and phenotype in different sites.

The particular environmental and biological factors which give rise to clinical infection by *C. albicans* are not understood, but some women may be more susceptible; predisposition to infection is associated with diabetes, pregnancy and the administration of antibiotics, particularly those, like penicillin, which are effective against vaginal lactobacilli.

Resistance to fungal infection depends on cell-mediated immunity and therefore compromise of this by disease such as HIV infection or immuno-suppressive therapy increases infection risk. Some individuals develop candida-specific reduced cell immunity.

The role of sexual transmission in Candida infection is not clear; although the organism is often shared by sexual partners, it is unlikely that just the deposition of the organism gives rise to infection (Lossick 1986). Tight clothes and mild skin abrasions may contribute to clinical presentation of infection.

Presentation and diagnosis

A woman may complain of vulval pruritus (itchiness) and on examination there may be evidence of vulvovaginitis and/or vulval, vaginal and cervical erythema. Dyspareunia (pain during intercourse) is a common complaint.

A vaginal discharge is common but not universal and may be scant or thick and white with a curd-like consistency. In less than 20% of cases white thrush patches may be present on the vulva or walls of the vagina (Lossick 1986).

Half of the babies born to infected women will be infected by Candida (Lossick 1986), generally involving oral or gastrointestinal infection. Such infection is usually mild, but treatment of the mother prior to delivery is clearly desirable.

Diagnosis of *C. albicans* is by detection of spores and mycelia by microscopy from a swab sent for culture (see Table 18.1).

Treatment

Vaginal infection is treated by the insertion of vaginal pessaries at night to maximise the time for local action, with cream provided for application to the vulval and perianal area.

A number of antifungal treatments are available, including:

1. Clotrimazole pessaries	100 mg for 6 nights *or* 200 mg for 3 nights *with*
Clotrimazole cream (1%)	for application to the vulva two to three times daily
2. Miconazole pessaries	150 mg for 3 nights
3. Nystatin pessaries × 2	100 000 i.u. for 14 nights *with*
Nystatin gel	100 000 i.u./g for external use.

Signs of clinical infection in a man, usually small red spots or plaques on the glans penis, should be treated with cream applied to the infected area.

Generally it is advised that sexual intercourse be avoided until after treatment is complete, perhaps to avoid local irritation which might provoke reinfection. Useful suggestions to women include daily bathing to maintain cleanliness of the perianal area but avoidance of harsh soaps or other irritants, the importance of wiping away from the vagina after defaecation, the advantages of cotton underwear, and avoidance of tights and clothing which is tight or constricting in the crotch.

Protozoal infection

The protozoan, *Trichomonas vaginalis*, is an anaerobic organism which is highly pathogenic to the epithelium in the vagina. Its prevalence varies considerably in different populations, but it is estimated on the basis of serological screening that

Table 18.1 Transport media for swabs prior to culture

Infection suspected	Type of medium	Comments
Candidiasis or gonorrhoea	Stuart's	a. White and opalescent – as oxygen content rises it becomes bluish and unsuitable for use b. Stored refrigerated. It must be at room temperature when the swab is inserted and not refrigerated again if the organism is to survive Gonococcus should be cultured within 6 hours
Group B streptococcus	Stuart's	See above
Trichomoniasis	Special medium containing a broad-spectrum antibiotic (this prevents swamping of the organism by fungal or bacterial growth)	As point (b) above. Stuart's may be used if the special medium is not available
Herpes simplex or cytomegalovirus	Viral transport medium (contains antibiotics as above)	Stored frozen; liquefied prior to insertion of swab Refrigerated if there is a delay in transport
Chlamydia trachomatis	Special medium containing antibiotics and sucrose to protect the organism	As for herpes simplex but should ideally reach the laboratory within 1 hour

about one-third of American women have been exposed to it (Lossick 1986).

The major mode of transmission is sexual intercourse. 80% of women whose partners are infected with *T. vaginalis* become infected, although the rate of female-to-male transmission is lower than this (Lossick 1986).

T. vaginalis is significant because of the severe vaginitis experienced by some infected women and also because of its common association with other sexually transmitted infections, particularly *N. gonorrhoeae* and *C. trachomatis*. Infection of the neonate seems to be uncommon.

Presentation and diagnosis

About half to two-thirds of infected women will complain of symptoms. In addition to the pruritus and burning of vaginitis, these include an increase in vaginal discharge, which may range from normal to copious, greyish in colour and somewhat bubbly in character. The green, frothy discharge and friable erythematous cervix, which are the 'classic' presenting features of infection, are rarely seen (Lossick 1986). Urethritis may also be a feature.

Asymptomatic infection may sometimes be detected on the Papanicolaou smear.

A wet swab examined immediately under a microscope will demonstrate the presence of the pear-shaped protozoan, with three to five flagellae and an undulating membrane.

Alternatively, a swab may be sent for culture in special medium (see Table 18.1).

Because of the high coincidence of trichomonal with other infections, swabs should be taken to exclude the presence of gonococcal and chlamydial infection.

Treatment

A single oral dose of metronidazole 2 g or a 5-day course of 400 mg twice daily is the treatment of choice. Although there is no evidence of a teratogenic effect in human pregnancy, metronidazole has generally been avoided in the first trimester of pregnancy because it has been found to be carcinogenic to rodents after long-term use and mutagenic for some bacteria. Burtin et al (1995) conducted

a meta-analysis of its safety in pregnancy over a 30-year period which confirmed the absence of a teratogenic risk. The authors suggest that women in need of the drug should be encouraged to use it and those exposed in early pregnancy should be reassured about its safety. Clotrimazole (see above) may also be used as local treatment for trichomonal infection in early pregnancy. A woman's partner should also be prescribed treatment with metronidazole.

Metronidazole potentiates the action of alcohol, and consumption of alcohol should be avoided while taking it. It may also potentiate the action of anticonvulsants and warfarin. Because of its excretion in breast milk, it is contraindicated for breast-feeding mothers (Erikson et al 1981).

Conventional advice suggests the avoidance of intercourse until treatment is complete.

BACTERIAL INFECTION

Bacterial vaginosis

Bacterial vaginosis is a term applied to vaginal discharge associated with a variety of anaerobic organisms including *Gardnerella vaginalis* and *Bacteroides spp*. It has been associated with postpartum pyrexia, amniotic fluid infection, preterm labour and pelvic inflammatory disease (Lossick 1986).

Presentation, diagnosis and treatment

The infection presents with a grey or white, fishy smelling discharge, which may be adherent or of normal consistency and may be more profuse than normal.

Diagnostic clues are the distinctive fishy odour of the discharge and a vaginal pH of greater than or equal to 4.5.

Treatment is with metronidazole 400 mg twice daily for 5 days.

Chlamydial infection

Chlamydia trachomatis is one of a group of intracellular parasites, closely related to Gram-negative bacteria. The organism is responsible for a number of human disorders including trachoma, inclusion conjunctivitis, nongonococcal urethritis, salpingitis, cervicitis and neonatal pneumonitis. Its prevalence in pregnant women varies widely with estimates ranging from 2–37%, with higher rates among young women, unmarried women, and women from lower socioeconomic groups and those attending inner-city antenatal clinics (Wang & Smaill 1989).

C. trachomatis is the major cause of salpingitis and pelvic inflammatory disease (PID) with their sequelae of ectopic pregnancy and infertility, and postpartum and postabortal infection. Chlamydial infection has been associated with increased risk of low birthweight, preterm rupture of membranes (Alger et al 1988) and a shorter gestation (Brunham et al 1990). It is currently the most common cause of neonatal conjunctivitis and it is estimated that from 3–18% of infants born to infected mothers will develop chlamydial pneumonia (Abel & von Unwerth 1988).

Presentation and diagnosis

The condition is often asymptomatic in the woman, although a mucopurulent cervicitis may be detected clinically, or she may present with salpingitis or the urethral syndrome (Wang & Smaill 1989).

Screening for chlamydia. In the light of its association with maternal and neonatal morbidity, detection of chlamydial infection during pregnancy could offer significant benefits, but until recently isolation of *C. trachomatis* involved extremely labour-intensive and expensive techniques. Antigen detection systems may now allow for cost-effective screening to be undertaken; Schachter & Grossman (1981) suggest that if the prevalence of maternal infection in the antenatal population exceeds 6%, it will be cost-effective to use the new techniques to identify and treat chlamydial infection in all pregnant women.

On the basis of epidemiological data, the Centers for Disease Control (CDC) in the US recommend that at least one prenatal culture for *C. trachomatis* be undertaken for pregnant women who fall into one of the following categories: age less than 20 years; unmarried; history of other sexually transmitted disease; multiple sexual partners; and a partner with multiple partners (Bell & Grayson 1986).

Where such a screening strategy is adopted, it is essential for midwives to consider how to discuss this with women and offer screening in a non-judgemental, non-discriminatory and sensitive way.

Treatment

Erythromycin, 400 mg four times a day for 7 days, is the antibiotic of choice during pregnancy.

Group B streptococcus

Group B streptococcus (GBS, *Streptococcus agalactiae*) is part of the vaginal flora of 5–25% of women. One-third or more pregnant women may be vaginal carriers of GBS during pregnancy, with intermittent and recurring colonisation.

This asymptomatic maternal infection is significant in pregnancy as the most frequent cause of overwhelming sepsis in neonates, estimated to occur from 0.6–3.7 cases per 1000 live births (Wang & Smaill 1989). The mortality rate of neonatal GBS in the US is 50% (Brunham et al 1990).

In addition, GBS has been associated with early spontaneous rupture of membranes, and with a threefold increase in preterm delivery at < 32 weeks' gestation (Brunham et al 1990).

Of the neonates of women with GBS colonisation, 65–75% will be colonised with the organism, although only 1–2% of exposed neonates will develop invasive disease (Brunham et al 1990).

Management and treatment of GBS colonisation in pregnancy

The efficacy of routine antenatal screening and treatment of GBS is limited because of the intermittent nature of maternal infection and the tendency for recurrence after treatment.

The use of a rapid screening test which can identify heavy vaginal GBS colonisation within 5 hours in women with preterm rupture of membranes would facilitate a strategy of antibiotic treatment for GBS in infected women (Wang & Smaill 1989).

The recommended treatment is intravenous administration of ampicillin (or erythromycin if the woman is allergic to penicillin), which should be continued if the result is positive or unavailable (Wang & Smaill 1989).

Gonococcal infection

Gonorrhoea is caused by *Neisseria gonorrhoeae*, a Gram-negative diplococcus, which has an affinity for columnar epithelial tissue. In women, infection occurs in the urethra or cervix. The vagina of women of childbearing age, composed of transitional and stratified squamous epithelium, is protected from being a site of infection, although resistance may be lowered in prepubertal and postmenopausal women. Colonisation of pharyngeal tissue can also occur as a result of oral sexual contact with an infected partner, as does infection of the rectum through anogenital contact.

Incidence of maternal infection varies greatly between populations, ranging from 1–5% (Wang & Smaill 1989). The rate of asymptomatic infection is high, and as many as 50% of women diagnosed in GUM clinics are asymptomatic (Adler 1985).

Effect of gonococcal infection in pregnancy

Gonorrhoea may give rise to local or systemic infection and pregnancy appears to increase the likelihood of infection presenting as arthritis or systemic disease. This apparent increase may be attributable to better follow-up during this period (Wang & Smaill 1989) or may be associated with the higher rate of pharyngeal infection in pregnancy which has been noted in some US studies and the greater risk of dissemination associated with pharyngeal colonisation (Brunham et al 1990).

Among non-pregnant women with endocervical infection, about 10–20% have clinical evidence of pelvic inflammatory disease (PID) and up to 50% of those with recent infection developed PID. Acute PID is rare in pregnancy, although positive *N. gonorrhoeae* cultures are sometimes associated with fever and pain.

The signs and symptoms which may characterise local gonococcal infection in pregnant women are:

- dysuria–sterile pyuria syndrome (urethral infection)

- cervicitis (endocervical infection)
- proctitis (rectal infection)
- conjunctivitis (ophthalmic infection).

Less common manifestations noted include acute inflammation of the Bartholin's glands (bartholinitis), endometritis and salpingitis (Wang & Smaill 1989).

Arthritis is the most common manifestation of disseminated infection. Infection usually presents with fever and rigors and there may be a characteristic purpuric-petechial rash (Wang & Smaill 1989).

Impact of gonococcal infection on pregnancy

Pregnancy complicated by endocervical gonococcal infection is associated with premature rupture of membranes, chorioamnionitis, early rupture of membranes and preterm delivery. The effect of gonococcal infection on early pregnancy is not well studied but early infection is associated with septic abortion and chorioamnionitis (Brunham et al 1990, Wang & Smaill 1989).

Intrapartum infection is associated with postpartum endometritis and upper genital tract infection (Brunham et al 1990).

Infection in the neonate

Neonatal infection most commonly presents as conjunctivitis, but infection at other body sites can occur and may be associated with a higher risk of disseminated infection (Brunham et al 1990). For further discussion see Chapter 42.

Diagnosis

Because of the presence of other Gram-negative diplococci in the female genital tract, Gram staining is not adequate for diagnosis of gonococcal infection in women and culture of the organism is required.

Swabs should be taken from the cervix and the urethral meatus. If culture is being conducted because of known contact with an infected partner, other sites of exposure such as the throat and anus should be swabbed.

Screening

Screening all women for gonococcal infection in pregnancy has been advocated by a number of authors, on the grounds of its serious effects on pregnancy and the risks of neonatal and puerperal infection (Brunham et al 1990, Wang & Smaill 1989) and the fact that a high proportion of infection in women is asymptomatic. Repeat cultures in the last trimester are suggested for women with a previous history of gonorrhoea or other sexually transmitted infection.

Treatment

Penicillin is the drug of choice, intramuscularly with probenecid 1 g orally, or ampicillin may be prescribed in a single dose orally with probenecid 1 g orally (Adler 1995). In cases of disseminated disease treatment should be administered either as penicillin intravenously or intramuscularly, with an initial dose of 10 MU per day and continued at a reduced dose for 10–14 days. If arthritis is a feature of infection, a longer therapy is indicated (Wang & Smaill 1989).

Repeat swabs should be cultured because of the rising incidence of penicillin-resistant strains of gonococcus.

Conclusions

Prevention of complications of pregnancy and neonatal disease associated with *N. gonorrhoeae* depends on early detection and treatment of infection which, it has been argued (Wang & Smaill 1989), would be best accomplished by screening of all pregnant women.

If routine screening is introduced or when testing is undertaken on an individual basis, it should be accompanied by information about how gonorrhoea is transmitted, the need for the woman's sexual partner also to be diagnosed and treated, and the use of barrier protection during sexual intercourse to reduce transmission of gonorrhoea and other infections.

Syphilis

Syphilis is an infection caused by *Treponema pallidum*, one of a family of three spirochaetes associated with human disease. In pregnancy its particular significance is the devastating effect it has on fetal well-being.

The natural course of adult infection is divided into stages (Adler 1995):

Early infectious:

- Primary: 9–60 days after exposure
- Secondary: 6 weeks to 6 months after exposure (4–6 weeks after primary infection)
- Early latent: 2 years after exposure.

Late non-infectious:

- Late latent: more than 2 years after exposure
- Neurosyphilis, cardiovascular syphilis or gummatous syphilis.

Most pregnant women diagnosed will be in the primary or secondary stages and untreated infection will affect almost all fetuses. About 20% of infants will deliver preterm, 20% will result in miscarriage or perinatal death, 20% of surviving infants will present with subclinical infection and 40% with congenital syphilis with resulting disability (Wang & Smaill 1989). Untreated early latent syphilis results in a 40% rate of prematurity or perinatal death, while about 10% of infants of mothers with untreated late syphilis will show signs of congenital syphilis with a 10 times increased perinatal death rate (Brunham et al 1990). Whereas sexual transmission of untreated infection does not usually occur after 2 years, women may remain infectious for their fetuses for much longer (Brunham et al 1990).

Prenatal diagnosis and treatment through routine serological testing in early pregnancy has been the key to the prevention of congenital syphilis in the UK. It has also contributed to the general decline in the incidence of syphilis insofar as it functions as an indirect population screening programme, facilitating referral of women to GUM clinics where contact tracing and treatment of infected partners can be initiated (Clay 1989).

In spite of the rarity of syphilis amongst women of childbearing age in England and Wales, there is evidence that there may be pockets of increase (Horner et al 1989) and calculations have demonstrated a benefit-to-cost ratio of 30 to 1 in favour of continuing screening (Williams 1985). O'Mahoney & Holland (1989) have argued in favour of performing a second screening test in late pregnancy or the introduction universally of the more sensitive *Treponema pallidum* haemagglutination test (TPHA) in addition to the Venereal Diseases Research Laboratory (VDRL) test for detection of infection. They report experience of a number of infants presenting with congenital syphilis although their mothers had had negative serology in early pregnancy.

Treatment

Penicillin is the drug of choice and the dosage depends on the stage of the woman's infection. If it is 2 years or less since the time of infection, she should receive aqueous procaine penicillin 600 000 units intramuscularly daily for 10 days. In late latent infection (more than 2 years since infection) the dosage is 900 000 units/day for 21 days.

If the woman is allergic to penicillin, erythromycin 500 mg 6-hourly for 15 days in early infection or 30 days in latent infection will be required. The baby should then be treated with penicillin at birth, because of less efficient placental transfer of erythromycin.

Ideally, case identification and treatment should be initiated in early pregnancy. Problems of third trimester diagnosis include treatment failure due to inadequate dosage of penicillin. In addition, treatment may give rise to a Jarisch–Herxheimer reaction, which may provoke uterine contractions and fetal distress (Horner et al 1989). The Jarisch–Herxheimer reaction, common in the treatment of primary and secondary syphilis, is characterised by fever and flu-like symptoms which may occur 3–12 hours after the first injection of penicillin (Adler 1995).

The baby should be examined and have serological tests done to exclude infection, even if the mother has been treated early with penicillin. Passively transmitted maternal antibodies may persist for up to 6 weeks, and therefore serological tests should be done at 6 weeks and 3 months of age.

Treatment of a woman in subsequent pregnancies is advocated by some, because of the possibility of persistent treponemes after treatment.

Adler (1995) suggests that if the woman has already been followed up for two years and discharged as cured, an alternative to retreating the mother is to carry out serology on the infant at 3 months of age to exclude infection. It is important that the woman is informed of this necessity so that she can arrange for follow-up of the baby.

Congenital syphilis

This occurs at the rate of 2 per 10 000 live births.

The infection may be diagnosed by serology in the case of a baby born to a mother known to have *T. pallidum*. Blood tests, however, can be misleading, with some babies positive with specific IgM present whilst in others all serology is negative. A 3-month follow-up is required to exclude the presence of infection. Physical characteristics of the placenta are not a useful guide to diagnosis.

Early signs may be present at birth or develop within the first 2 years but primary syphilis is not found, as the treponemes have been blood borne rather than transmitted by contact with skin or mucous membrane. Highly contagious vesicles ('syphilitic pemphigus') on the palms, soles and possibly other areas burst and leave their dull, red, raised bases exposed. Aborted or stillborn babies may have similar lesions. Ulcers can occur on the lips and mouth and, if on the larynx, the baby's cry may be thin or soundless. Ulcers of the nasal periosteum cause a purulent, bloodstained or watery nasal discharge, teeming with treponemes. Poor feeding and weight loss may be features of infection.

Periostitis produces swelling of the long bones and the resulting pain may cause the baby to behave as if he or she has a fracture. The baby may also present with patchy alopecia, hepatosplenomegaly and mild jaundice.

With treatment the prognosis is excellent if the early hazards are survived.

Late signs may develop at any time from the 2nd to the 30th year of life even if none of the early signs was exhibited. Corneal scarring can cause impaired vision or blindness; meningitis can result in convulsions, blindness and mental disability. Gummata in the nasal septum can leave deformity and there may be eighth nerve deafness. Rarely, neurosyphilis may develop. The prognosis depends on the damage which has occurred prior to treatment.

Scars and deformities resulting from syphilitic infection are known as *stigmata* and, although characteristic, are not always present. There may be a 'saddleback' depression of the nasal bridge or linear scars, known as *rhagades*, resulting from ulcers around the mouth, nares and anus. The permanent incisors may be widely spaced and have sides which converge to resemble the end of a screwdriver, the cutting edge being notched, so-called *Hutchinson's teeth*.

Management. The baby may be very ill. Intramuscular procaine penicillin 50 000 i.u. per kg bodyweight is given in divided doses over 10 days. In the presence of contagious lesions the baby must be barrier nursed until antibiotics have been given for 48 hours.

Some advocate routine lumbar puncture to look for treponemes. Follow-up is prolonged and parents will need investigation for persistent infection.

VIRAL INFECTIONS

Herpes simplex virus

Herpes simplex is one of a family of herpes viruses, which includes varicella-zoster, cytomegalovirus (CMV) and Epstein–Barr virus. All within this family share the ability to establish lifelong, persistent infection in their host and to undergo periodic reactivation. Reactivated infection may have characteristics different from the primary episode.

Infections of the mouth and lips caused by herpes simplex virus were recognised by the ancient Greeks; genital infections were described by an 18th century French physician, Astruc. Neonatal herpes infections were first documented 50 years ago (Stagno & Whitley 1990).

It was only in the mid-1960s that two herpes simplex viruses (HSV), type 1 associated with infections of the lip and oropharynx, and type 2 associated with genital infection, were demonstrated. The recognition that neonatal infection was most often associated with HSV type 2 and

that maternal viral excretion could be present at the time of delivery, suggested transmission by exposure to genital secretions at delivery. However, postnatal infection of the newborn baby with HSV type 1 from maternal or non-maternal sources, such as staff and visitors, has also been documented.

For transmission to occur the HSV virus must come into contact with mucosal surfaces or abraded skin. Viral replication occurs at the site of infection and then the virus or particles of it are transported along neurons to the ganglia where they remain dormant until there is an alteration in the host environment that gives rise to recurrence of active infection.

Presentation of infection with HSV

Primary infection of HSV type 1 in young children is usually asymptomatic, though it may present with gingivostomatitis. In young adults, primary infection is associated with pharyngitis and mononucleosis-like illness.

Primary infection with HSV type 2 usually presents with painful genital ulcers after an incubation period of less than 7 days. Skin lesions begin with erythema, progress to vesicles and then ulcers and finish with crusting. Local lesions with viral shedding may last about 12 days, with complete healing taking another week (Adler 1995). Both the vulva and cervix are involved in most primary attacks in women, but single sites may be affected.

Recurrent infection involves reactivation of the virus at the same site, rather than reinfection. Patients may experience prodromal symptoms of local tingling or numbness at the site of the lesions about 24–48 hours prior to onset of lesions. There may be fewer lesions, milder symptoms and a shorter duration in recurrent attacks.

Both primary and recurrent infection may be asymptomatic; this presents a particular problem in the case of primary infection in pregnancy, which is the situation in which the fetus is at greatest risk.

Effect of HSV infection in pregnancy

The main concerns about HSV during pregnancy are the association of primary infection with an increased risk of spontaneous abortion, prematurity and the acquisition of serious infection by the neonate (Nahmias et al 1971). Transmission of virus to the fetus or neonate is thought to occur at delivery and only rarely transplacentally (Brunham 1990). In primary maternal infection the rate of transmission has been estimated to be as high as 50% (Nahmias et al 1971); in recurrent maternal infection, however, the rate is low, with estimations of between 3 and 8% (Prober et al 1987). The difference in infection rate between the two groups of babies is attributed to the presence of a high titre of passively acquired maternal antibodies to HSV in the babies of mothers with recurrent infection (Prober et al 1987, Anon 1988).

Management of HSV in pregnancy

Recommendations for the management of late pregnancy and delivery of women with a history of genital HSV have evolved in the light of the accumulating evidence about perinatal transmission, although there have been no randomised trials to evaluate clinical policy and the evidence for recommended policy remains weak (Wang & Smaill 1989). Guidelines for the management of herpes infection in pregnancy, based on best available evidence, are offered by Smith et al (1998) and these are reflected in the discussion below.

Because most genital herpes infection is unrecognised, it is important that a careful vulval inspection is undertaken at the time of the onset of labour of all women, not just those with a history of genital herpes, in order to detect clinical signs of infection.

First episode of genital herpes in pregnancy. When this occurs in the first or second trimester of pregnancy the use of oral or intravenous acyclovir should be considered. In non-pregnant women this antiviral drug is known to shorten the duration and reduce the severity of symptoms as well as reduce the duration of viral shedding (Corey et al 1983, Mindel et al 1988). However, as acyclovir is not licensed for use in pregnancy the responsibility for prescribing rests with the physician. There is no evidence of teratogenicity (Burroughs Wellcome 1989). A detailed discussion of the risks and benefits of treatment should take place with the woman and her partner and its use should

be registered prospectively with the Acyclovir in Pregnancy Register.

When a first episode occurs in the third trimester there is an increased risk of premature labour. If labour becomes established, there is a strong rationale for treatment with intravenous acyclovir and delivery by caesarean section, on the grounds of reducing maternal viraemia and reducing exposure of the fetus to virus.

In the case of the woman who has recovered from her first episode without going into labour, because of the high risk of continued viral shedding, an elective caesarean section at 38 weeks may be prudent, especially if symptoms began within 6 weeks of the expected date of delivery.

If, following a first episode of infection in the third trimester, a vaginal delivery is unavoidable or if the membranes have been ruptured for more than 4 hours prior to caesarean section, it is suggested that mother and baby be treated with intravenous acyclovir to reduce the risk of neonatal infection. The use of fetal scalp electrodes and fetal blood sampling should be avoided to reduce the exposure of the fetus to virus.

Recurrent episodes of genital herpes. Some women may become pregnant while being treated with oral acyclovir for recurrent herpes. This is not an indication for a termination of pregnancy.

The use of continuous prophylactic oral acyclovir, which is associated with a reduction of recurrences in non-pregnant individuals (Mindel et al 1982) has not been evaluated for safety and efficacy during pregnancy. Occasional attacks of mild genital herpes may be treated with saline bathing and analgesia.

Smith et al (1998) review the considerations for the management of recurrent herpes during pregnancy and suggest the following:

• There is no indication for using sequential cultures during late gestation to predict viral shedding at term.
• The benefits of obtaining specimens for culture at delivery to detect asymptomatic viral shedding are unproven.
• Caesarean section to prevent neonatal herpes is not indicated in women who do not have genital lesions at delivery.

• Symptomatic recurrences during the third trimester will be brief and vaginal delivery is appropriate if no lesions are present at delivery.

Current practice in the UK is for women with genital lesions at the onset of labour to be delivered by caesarean section; however, there is evidence that the risks of infection of the neonate are small and the maternal risks of caesarean section must be set against these. Delivery by caesarean section in the presence of recurrent lesions was abandoned in the Netherlands in 1987, achieving a substantial reduction in caesarean sections for this indication without any apparent increase in the incidence of neonatal disease (van Everdingen et al 1993).

Women who experience recurrent HSV infection during pregnancy should be reassured that the transmission rate is very low and that antiviral therapy is available if infection of the baby occurs (see Ch. 42).

Cytomegalovirus (CMV)

This is another of the herpes group of viruses which can be found in saliva, urine, breast milk, semen and cervical secretions. Between 60 and 90% of adults carry antibodies in their blood (Mandal et al 1996). Transmission between adults usually occurs by direct contact, for example by kissing, and may be sexual. Primary infection may occasionally present similarly to glandular fever or influenza, with headache, sore throat and anorexia. There may be hepatitis with prolonged pyrexia. Subsequently the virus may remain dormant but be subject to reactivation and be excreted for many years.

Diagnosis is confirmed on culture of specimens of urine, blood or saliva, or of a swab taken from the cervix (see Table 18.1). Serology is performed for antibody levels.

Infection in pregnancy

There is increasing evidence that at any stage of pregnancy both primary and reactivated CMV infection can result in transplacental transmission to the fetus, although the results are probably most serious in primary infection. Abortion, still-birth, growth retardation and premature labour

may result. The incidence is estimated to be about 4 per 1000 live births. 2% of these develop serious problems (for example, micro- or hydrocephaly, spastic quadriplegia, psychomotor retardation and deafness). 8% have minor problems (e.g. hepato-splenomegaly and thrombocytopenia). 90% of infected infants are symptom free at birth but some will not attain their expected intellectual potential and/or will become deaf in later childhood.

If *transplacental infection* is suspected, cord blood should be examined for specific IgM and a urine sample and nasopharyngeal swab sent for culture. Treatment is supportive only and great care should be taken to avoid infection of other babies and members of staff, particularly pregnant staff. The virus may continue to be shed by the infected infant for a prolonged period.

Babies may also be infected by breast milk, but this does not cause serious disease. Transfusion of infected blood may give rise to pneumonitis, especially in preterm babies and, in some centres, only blood free of CMV antibodies is given.

Whilst it is estimated that 50% of women of childbearing age have been infected by CMV, only about 1% of their infants will be infected.

Routine screening in pregnancy does not seem to be useful; it is difficult to know what advice could be given to parents and, as attacks are often subclinical, repeated screening would be necessary.

CMV is an increasing problem and work to develop a vaccine has been slow. It is estimated that where rubella vaccination levels are high, CMV is now a more important cause of congenital abnormality.

Hepatitis B infection

Hepatitis B virus (HBV) is a major cause of chronic liver disease and carcinoma of the liver world-wide and perinatal transmission from an infected mother to her newborn is the major mode of transmission. It can also be transmitted sexually and by means of infected blood products or unsterilised equipment contaminated by infected blood, such as may occur in injecting drug use, tattooing, or as a consequence of needlestick injury in the health care setting.

Early in acute infection, hepatitis B surface

antigen (HBsAg) and hepatitis Be antigen (HBeAg), part of the core antigen, can be detected in the serum. Antibodies to HBV core antigen (which is itself not detectable in a blood test) – anti-HBc followed by anti-HBe – develop during acute illness but neither of these provides immunity. Anti-HBs appears after the disappearance of HBsAg, although there may be a gap before it can be detected.

Chronic carriage of HBV is indicated by the persistence of HBsAg more than 6 months after acute infection. The presence of HBe antigen (HBeAg) indicates continued viral activity and high infectivity, although antibody to this (anti-HBe) indicates a lower level of infectivity in chronic carriers (Mandal et al 1996).

Screening women in early pregnancy allows detection of those who carry HBV so that vaccination of the baby can be initiated within 24 hours of birth. Selective screening of women in groups with increased risk of exposure to HBV infection will fail to identify some carriers and for this reason antenatal screening of all women for HBV infection has been implemented in some maternity units.

The babies of mothers who are chronic carriers or who have been infected with HBV during pregnancy should receive hepatitis B vaccine within 24 hours of birth which will be repeated at 1 and 6 months of age. In addition, the babies of mothers who are infectious – those who have had acute hepatitis B during pregnancy and those who do not have anti-HBe antibodies – should also receive hepatitis B immunoglobulin (HBIg), administered in a different site from the vaccine, not later than 48 hours after birth, to confer immediate passive immunity. Arrangements for the supply of HBIg should be made well in advance (Salisbury & Begg 1996).

Genital warts

Genital warts are caused by the human papillomavirus (HPV) and are nearly always transmitted by sexual contact, although, rarely, a baby may acquire a laryngeal papilloma as a result of exposure at the time of delivery.

The special significance of warts in pregnancy is that they occasionally increase very dramatically in size, which may be extremely distressing for the woman and may infrequently jeopardise the possibility of a vaginal delivery.

The preferred first line of treatment for genital warts is 10–25% podophyllin, but as this is contraindicated during pregnancy because of its toxicity, the recommendation is not to treat warts at this time. Other treatments that may be attempted in pregnancy are trichloroacetic acid, cryotherapy or electrocautery (Adler 1995).

It is suggested that women presenting with genital warts should have full investigations to exclude other sexually transmitted infections. In addition, the cervix should be examined by colposcopy to exclude flat warts on the cervix, which may be associated with malignant changes. Because of the possible association between HPV and cervical intracellular neoplasia (CIN), cytological screening is recommended for women with vulval or vaginal warts or those whose partners have penile warts (Adler 1995).

Human immunodeficiency virus (HIV)

HIV is a retrovirus which may be transmitted in three ways:

- in blood
- via semen and cervical secretions during sexual intercourse
- from mother to fetus in utero, at delivery or via breast feeding.

It is recognised that there are at least two varieties of HIV, designated as HIV-1 and HIV-2. So far, in the UK, HIV-1 is the predominant form and the following discussion relates to HIV-1 unless otherwise stated.

For a full discussion of the pathophysiology of HIV and HIV-associated illness see Pratt (1995).

HIV infection in pregnancy

The distinct effect of pregnancy on the expression of maternal HIV infection has been difficult to evaluate in the absence of appropriately controlled observations (Minkoff & DeHovitz 1990, Vermund et al 1992), although pregnancy has not been confirmed to have an adverse effect on the clinical progression of HIV disease (Hankins & Handley

1992). A review of the literature suggested that adverse clinical outcomes are common among HIV-infected women, but studies had not disentangled the many confounding factors. HIV-related complications were common in pregnancy only in association with immunosuppression, in women with CD4 counts of less than 300 cells/mm³ (Vermund et al 1992).

Perinatal transmission of HIV

In Europe, the rate of maternal-to-child transmission is estimated to be between 15 and 20% (Thorne et al 1995). Higher rates are recorded elsewhere, with that in Africa estimated to be twice that of Europe (Dabis et al 1993) and, while this difference is not yet explained, it may be related to concomitant maternal infections, geographic variation in viral virulence and increased frequency of breast feeding (Scarlatti 1996).

Diagnosis of HIV infection

The diagnosis of asymptomatic adult HIV infection is made on the basis of the presence in serum of antibodies to the virus. Most individuals will produce antibodies (seroconvert) within 3 months of infection with the virus. If an HIV antibody test is carried out less than 3 months after the most recent possible exposure, during the so-called 'window of infectivity', a negative result will require a repeat test in order to take account of the possibility of late seroconversion.

Diagnostic HIV antibody testing in the UK employs two tests. The ELISA (enzyme-linked immunosorbent assay) test is highly sensitive to the presence of antibodies. Its sensitivity increases the possibility of false positive results and thus a Western blot test, which has a greater specificity for HIV, is used to confirm the presence of the antibodies. A second specimen of blood may be tested to confirm the result.

The notion of risk in relation to HIV

The prevalence of HIV in different communities and under different circumstances varies enormously. Infection with HIV, however, is linked not to who or what a person is but rather to what they do which might expose them to infection.

The activities that put individuals at risk are:

• Unprotected sexual intercourse with an infected partner. Because it is not possible to distinguish with certainty an infected from an uninfected sexual partner, unprotected intercourse with someone who has had unprotected intercourse with anyone else or has shared injecting equipment may be an infection risk.
• Using needles and syringes for injecting drug use which have been used by someone else.
• Being transfused with blood or other blood products which have not been screened for HIV infection.

If the health education and availability of testing is to serve the interests of clients, it is essential that women are offered information which will enable them to protect themselves more effectively against HIV in future, whether they decide to be tested or not.

Issues of infection control

Because it is impossible to know the HIV status of all individuals or indeed to exclude the presence of other blood-borne infections which might constitute a transmission risk, the principle of 'universal precautions' has been advocated as a basis for infection control policy (Centers for Disease Control 1988). This recommends the application, in the care of *all* clients, of measures which protect staff and others from accidental exposure to potentially infectious body fluids (see Box 18.1). In the midwifery context such fluids include blood,

---

Box 18.1 Principles of universal precautions

• When exposure to body fluids is anticipated, protective clothing should be worn.
• Spillage of fluids should be disinfected and mopped up using a hypochlorite solution 1:100 or 1:10.
• Skin accidentally exposed should be washed thoroughly with soap and water.
• Great care should be exercised in handling sharps to avoid accidental injury.
• Should injury occur, the wound should be encouraged to bleed, washed thoroughly, the accident reported to the occupational health physician and agreed local policy for follow-up implemented.

liquor, cervical secretions and cerebrospinal fluid. Chester et al (1997) propose a useful, systematic approach to infection control measures within a maternity service, based on the procedures being conducted instead of the client being cared for.

HIV antibody testing in pregnancy

The prevalence of HIV infection in childbearing women in England and Wales is rising (Unlinked Anonymous Surveys Steering Group 1995, 1996).

Department of Health (1994) guidelines encourage offering HIV testing antenatally to all women in areas where prevalence of infection is high, and the availability of requested antenatal HIV testing in other centres.

In spite of this policy, however, the proportion of infected women whose status is determined during pregnancy is disappointingly low. Thus, for example, only 22 of 322 women in London with undiagnosed infection were identified by antenatal testing in 1993 and 1994 (MacDonagh et al 1996b).

Knowing her HIV status during pregnancy can offer a woman a number of benefits. These are related to decision-making about the continuation of pregnancy, interventions aimed at reducing transmission of infection to her baby (Peckham & Gibb 1995), early detection and treatment of ill health and prophylaxis against *Pneumocystis carinii* pneumonia for her and her baby.

It is important, however, to appreciate the adverse impact on a woman of a diagnosis of HIV, perhaps especially during pregnancy, including psychological and social stress, the experience of stigma, social isolation and fear about her health, that of her baby and about breaches of confidentiality. The diagnosis may have serious consequences for a woman's personal relationships and, although knowing her status may enable her to protect an uninfected sexual partner from infection, some women choose not to confide their diagnosis.

Successful implementation of a policy encouraging antenatal testing for HIV requires that midwives and other caregivers provide the time, information and support needed for a woman to make a choice about HIV testing in an informed and knowledgeable way (Royal College of Mid-

wives 1996). Caregivers must also be able to facilitate access to whatever medical and supportive resources a woman may require in the event of a positive test result.

The pattern of provision of HIV testing varies enormously, even in those areas in which, because of their high prevalence, testing should be available for all women (MacDonagh et al 1996a). It is important that all women are offered access to early diagnosis and support which may improve the care available for them and their babies, and the obstacles to achieving this need to be identified and acted upon (MacDonagh et al 1996b).

Special considerations for care of women in relation to HIV

In the following section some of the issues that are likely to arise in relation to the care of the HIV-positive pregnant woman are highlighted. Throughout the discussion reference is made to 'the woman', although where appropriate this should be taken to include her partner or other support persons. The circumstances of women are so variable that it is difficult to find a phrase that applies equally well to all women.

Breaking the news

Receiving a diagnosis of HIV infection gives rise to shock and extreme emotion, and this is likely to be intensified in pregnancy. A woman should be told, at the time the blood specimen is taken, when to expect the result to be available and from whom she will receive it. She should be encouraged to involve her partner or a reliable close friend who might accompany her, but because of the stigma and prejudice which mark reactions to HIV infection she may need to guard against disclosure which may be detrimental to her.

Midwives must be prepared to offer the woman immediate access to a support network and formal counselling should she want it and it is important that local facilities and telephone numbers are available to midwives in advance of HIV testing.

A further appointment with the doctor and midwife should be offered in the next few days to further discuss her care and answer the questions which she will have and she should be given a phone number she can ring to make contact before that.

Termination of pregnancy?

Counselling should be offered to enable the woman to consider her plans for this pregnancy in the light of her diagnosis. The counsellor should be able to discuss the most recent available information about the impact of HIV on the mother's and baby's health in order to facilitate an informed decision.

The stage of the pregnancy, the woman's immune status, her desire for a child and her attitude about termination will all be important factors in the discussion of this issue.

Perinatal transmission and interventions for its reduction

As data accumulate, greater clarity will emerge about factors associated with transmission from mother to child (Bryson 1996, European Collaborative Study 1992). Improved understanding of the mechanisms of perinatal transmission will enable better informed decisions about continuation of and management of pregnancy, as well as strategies which may be adopted to minimise the risks of neonatal infection.

Current evidence suggests that transmission occurs transplacentally but is more common in late pregnancy and during labour (Rouzioux et al 1995). There is also some evidence suggesting that delivery by caesarean section might reduce perinatal transmission (European Collaborative Study 1994b); this is currently under investigation by means of a prospective, multicentre, randomised controlled trial.

The risk of maternal–child transmission of HIV infection is increased by breast feeding and, where safe alternatives are available, HIV-infected women should avoid breast feeding (Dunn et al 1992). However, where there are high rates of infant mortality associated with malnutrition and infectious disease, breast feeding should continue to be encouraged, regardless of HIV infection status, as the risks to the baby of artificial feeding outweigh those of vertical transmission of HIV (Global Programme on AIDS 1992).

A joint American and French multicentred study (Connor et al 1994) achieved a marked reduction of maternal–infant transmission of HIV with the administration of zidovudine to asymptomatic HIV-infected pregnant women and their newborn babies, with a reduction of the expected rate of neonatal infection from 24 to 8%. The criterion for inclusion in the study was a CD4 count of over 200 cells/mm^3 (a standardised measure of immune function) and none of the women were receiving antiretroviral therapy for their HIV infection. They had not previously been exposed to zidovudine and were between 14 and 34 weeks of pregnancy when therapy commenced. They received zidovudine orally during the pregnancy and intravenously during labour; the babies were given the drug orally for 6 weeks after birth. There were no serious side-effects associated with the regimen; some babies suffered short-term anaemia, which resolved.

A number of questions remain to be explored in order to refine the practice implications of this important study, including continued follow-up of the children for long-term side-effects, surveillance for the possibility of zidovudine-resistant HIV infection in the woman or baby, and further investigation to determine the optimal timing and length of treatment, which was variable within the study group. In addition, this strategy requires exposing all babies of infected mothers to zidovudine, although only a small proportion of them will have acquired the infection without such treatment.

The Royal College of Obstetricians and Gynaecologists (1997) recommends that women be informed of the results of the study and offered zidovudine prophylaxis, but acknowledge that modifications to the treatment regimen are to be expected and that close liaison between obstetricians and specialist physicians and virologists is essential.

Continuity of care

The midwife has an essential contribution to make in coordinating appropriate care and providing an accessible source of information and support throughout the pregnancy.

Early and regular surveillance of the woman's

general health and immune status should be organised with the appropriate specialist physician. Coordination of care with other agencies, such as the Drug Dependency Unit (DDU) should be ensured.

Early reporting, investigation and treatment of signs of HIV-related and other infections should be encouraged, with particular attention to non-specific signs such as weight loss, oral thrush and diarrhoea. The woman may experience recurrence of HSV lesions; evidence of this should be sought and investigations initiated if delivery is imminent. Because of the increased risk of CIN in the HIV-infected woman (Minkoff & DeHovitz 1990), colposcopy or cytology may be indicated.

Opportunity should be provided for the woman to meet the paediatrician who will care for the baby, and to discuss the pattern of follow-up and treatment that may be undertaken if the baby is infected.

The midwife should encourage the woman to talk about her plans for feeding and discuss the additional risk of breast feeding. If she had hoped to breast feed it is important to help her to consider how to achieve the physical closeness of breast feeding even if she decides to use formula milk. The decision not to breast feed may be an additional source of disappointment which she may want to talk about.

Discussion should also be initiated about self-care, the onset of labour, how she should manage spilled liquor, and what to expect with regard to care in labour.

Care in labour

Care by a midwife already known to the woman is desirable. This ensures that confidentiality will continue to be protected and allows care to be given within an established, supportive relationship. Suggestions for minimising risks to staff are given in Box 18.2.

Postnatal care

The midwife should discuss with the woman whether she has preference for a single room; if not, a separate room and toilet or bath facilities are not necessary. There should be adequate facil-

---

Box 18.2 Care in labour: suggestions for minimising risks to staff

- Wear waterproof protective gowns and gloves when exposure to body fluids is expected.
- Leave membranes intact to avoid unnecessary contamination with liquor.
- Avoid the use of fetal scalp electrodes and fetal blood sampling to minimise unnecessary exposure of the baby.
- Protect against splashes to the eye by wearing British Standard approved safety glasses if directly involved in care where a splash might occur, e.g. at delivery, cutting the cord.
- Masks should also be available.
- Use mechanically operated suction in preference to a mouth-operated device, if suction of the baby is required.
- Bath the baby as soon as possible after delivery, in water at 37.5°C, provided he or she is well and has a body temperature of 36.5°C or above. Rubber gloves and plastic apron should be worn; gloves should be worn when handling the baby until the bath is done.

---

ities for the safe disposal of sanitary towels and the woman should be aware of the need for immediate attention to the disinfection and cleaning of any spilled blood.

The stress and adjustment of the postnatal period is likely to be intensified for the woman who is HIV positive, complicated by anxiety about her baby's health and her own, uncertainty about the future and the long-term well-being and care of her baby. She may also lack confidence in her skills as a new mother and experience the sense of inadequacy that accompanies this. Continued care by a known midwife, familiar with the woman and her circumstances and confident to respond to her questions and doubts, is especially important at this time. The midwife should be alert to the woman's sense of isolation, loneliness and guilt and should offer support or referral to a counsellor, social worker, or contact with a self-help group as appropriate.

The midwife's daily examination should specifically elicit signs or symptoms suggestive of physical illness and emotional distress. Gloves need only be worn if exposure to blood is anticipated, for instance when examining the perineum, lochia or caesarean wound.

The mother should be encouraged to manage the baby's care herself with the support of the midwife. Gloves need only be worn by the midwife if she is carrying out cord care or nappy changing in the presence of bleeding. Gloves should be worn for invasive procedures, such as the collection of a capillary sample of blood, as for the Guthrie test, when contamination of the operator's hands is difficult to avoid.

Plans for follow-up care of the mother and baby should be reviewed prior to discharge, and the woman should be encouraged to consider the roles that might be played by the Community Midwife, GP and Health Visitor in her ongoing care. The decision to inform these caregivers of her HIV status should rest with the woman herself and arrangements for informing them should be discussed with the woman.

Discussion of contraception should be offered before her transfer home and she should be advised to use condoms as well as another method for birth control. Even if both partners are HIV positive, condoms are advisable to prevent possible exposure to other sexually transmitted infections. Evidence for a preferable additional method of contraception is lacking. An intrauterine contraceptive device (IUCD) may not be ideal because of increased risk of pelvic inflammatory disease; oral contraceptives may alter the metabolism of other drugs used in the treatment of HIV-infected women (Minkoff & DeHovitz 1990).

Some women will not have confided their HIV status to their partners, and this discussion of contraception might offer an opportunity to explore this difficult problem. Further formal counselling may assist a woman to find a way of discussing her infection with her partner.

Appointments should be arranged for follow-up cervical smear or colposcopy as well as for general assessment by the physician. She should be given appointments for the baby's follow-up assessments and should be given a contact number should any problems arise about which she needs advice.

Care and follow-up of the baby

All babies who are born to HIV-positive women will have passively acquired maternal antibodies to HIV and these may persist for as long as 18 months. Therefore, diagnosis of HIV cannot be achieved with antibody testing and confirmation of the infant's infection status may not occur for an extended period of time. The uncertainty and doubt which parents may experience at this time is an additional stress.

Data from the European Collaborative Study (1991, 1994a) have allowed a picture of the natural history of infection to be described. Progression of HIV disease is not as fast as anticipated on the basis of early findings. 23% of infected children developed AIDS before 1 year of age, and nearly 40% by age 4. 10% of the infected children died before 1 year of age, 28% before age 5. However, 2 years after an AIDS diagnosis, 48% of those children were still alive and, although immunologic abnormality became more common after 1 year of age, the proportion of infected children with significant HIV-related signs and symptoms declined (European Collaborative Study 1994a).

Treatment

It is beyond the scope of this chapter to discuss the complex issue of the treatment of women and babies with HIV disease and the opportunist infections associated with it. Current literature should be consulted for ongoing trials and case reports.

Conclusion

The woman whose pregnancy is complicated by HIV infection will face a multitude of complex physical, social and emotional challenges during her pregnancy and after. It is essential that the care she is offered acknowledges those complex needs and attempts to respond to them.

This will be best achieved by continuity of care provided by a midwife who is sensitive to the woman's needs, who is well informed about HIV infection and who can contribute to and coordinate the appropriate medical and supportive services.

READER ACTIVITIES

1. With a colleague, role play a conversation between a woman and midwife, in which the woman wants to confide her worries about having been exposed to or having symptoms of a sexually transmitted disease.

Imagine the discussion is being conducted in your familiar antenatal clinic. Spend about 10 minutes on this. If you are able to tape-record the conversation, do so. You will hear a lot in the playback that you were probably not aware of at the time.

Debrief each other after the 'consultation'.

In your discussion after this exercise you might address the following:

a. Which aspects of the conversation were difficult and which worked well for the 'midwife'?
b. Which were difficult and which worked well for the 'client'?
c. Were the (imagined) circumstances in which you carried out the conversation conducive to meeting the client's needs?
d. Did the midwife feel comfortable and confident of her knowledge and the advice she offered?

Try to explore with each other:

- why the midwife responded the way she did
- why she asked the questions she did
- why she offered the information in the way she did
- whether the client found interventions useful.

Each of you might choose to conduct the role play with another colleague or with each other taking on the opposite role.

2. Talking with women about sex and enabling them to express their concerns about sexual issues can be difficult, especially during pregnancy.

With a colleague or friend with whom you feel comfortable, try brainstorming about what it is that makes such discussion difficult – this might range from problems of language, assumptions about women and their sexual concerns, to the environment of the clinic.

Attempt to translate the results or insights of your brainstorming into a leaflet for women which might be a way of opening the possibility of discussion for them. The focus might be on 'safe sex' or another theme that you think is relevant for pregnant women.

REFERENCES

Abel E, von Unwerth L 1988 Asymptomatic chlamydia during pregnancy. Research in Nursing and Health 11(6): 359–365

Adler M 1985 Sexually transmitted diseases. In: Holland W W, Detels R, Knox G (eds) Oxford textbook of public health. Oxford University Press, Oxford, vol 3

Adler M W 1995 The ABC of sexually transmitted diseases, 5th edn. British Medical Journal, London

Alger L S, Lovchik J C, Hebel J R et al 1988 The association of Chlamydia trachomatis, Neisseria gonorrhoeae, and group B streptococci with preterm rupture of the membrane and pregnancy outcome. American Journal of Obstetrics and Gynecology 159(2): 397–404

Anonymous 1988 Virological screening for herpes simplex virus during pregnancy. Lancet (24 September): 722–723

Bell T A, Grayson J T 1986 Centers for Disease Control: guidelines for prevention and control of Chlamydia trachomatis infections. Annals of Internal Medicine 104: 524–526

Brunham R C, Holmes K K, Embree J E 1990 Sexually transmitted diseases in pregnancy. In: Holmes K K, Mardh P A, Sparling P F et al Sexually transmitted diseases, 2nd edn. McGraw Hill, New York

Bryson Y J 1996 Perinatal HIV-1 transmission: recent advances and therapeutic interventions. AIDS 10(suppl 3): S33–S42

Burroughs Wellcome 1989 Acyclovir in pregnancy registry. International interim report. June 1 1984 through June 30 1989

Burtin P, Taddio A, Ariburnu O, Einarson T R, Koren G 1995 Safety of metronidazole in pregnancy: a meta-analysis. American Journal of Obstetrics and Gynecology 172(2): 525–529

Centers for Disease Control 1988 Universal precautions for prevention of transmission of human immunodeficiency virus, hepatitis B virus and other blood borne pathogens in health care settings. Morbidity and Mortality Weekly Report 37: 377–388

Chester T, Jervis R, O'Connell T 1997 The traffic light model for universal precautions: an approach to HIV infection in maternity services. Midwives 110(1315): 194–195

Clay J C 1989 Antenatal screening for syphilis must continue. British Medical Journal 299: 409–410

Connor E M, Sperling R S, Gelber R et al 1994 Reduction of

maternal–infant transmission of human immunodeficiency virus type 1 with zidovudine treatment. Pediatric AIDS Clinical Trial, Group Protocol 076 Study Group. New England Journal of Medicine 331: 1173–1180

Corey L, Benedetti J, Critchlow C, Mertz G, Douglas J, Fife K, Fahnlander A, Remington M L, Winter C, Dragavon J 1983 Treatment of primary first-episode genital herpes simplex virus infection with acyclovir: results of topical, intravenous and oral therapy. Journal of Antimicrobial Chemotherapy 12: 79–88

Dabis F, Msellati P, Dunn D et al 1993 Estimating the rate of mother-to-child transmission of HIV: report of a workshop on methodological issues, Ghent (Belgium). AIDS 7: 1139–1148

Department of Health 1994 Guidelines for offering named HIV anti-body testing to women receiving ante-natal care. Department of Health, London

Dunn D T, Newell M L, Ades, A E, Peckham C S 1992 Risk of human immunodeficiency virus type 1 transmission through breastfeeding. Lancet 340: 585–588

Elias C J, Coggins C 1996 Female-controlled methods to prevent sexual transmission of HIV. AIDS 10(suppl 3): S43–S51

Erikson S H, Oppenheim G L, Smith G H 1981 Metronidazole in breast milk. Obstetrics and Gynecology 57: 48–50

European Collaborative Study 1991 Children born to women with HIV-1 infection: natural history and risk of transmission. Lancet 337: 253–260

European Collaborative Study 1992 Risk factors for mother-to-child transmission of HIV-1. Lancet 339: 1007–1012

European Collaborative Study 1994a Natural history of vertically acquired human immunodeficiency virus-1 infection. Pediatrics 94(6): 815–819

European Collaborative Study 1994b Caesarean section and risk of vertical transmission of HIV-1 infection. Lancet 343: 1464–1467

Farr G, Gabelnick H, Sturgen K, Dorflinger L 1994 Contraceptive efficacy and acceptability of the female condom. American Journal of Public Health 84(12): 1960–1964

Global Programme on AIDS 1992 Consensus statement from the WHO/UNICEF constitution on HIV infection and breast-feeding. Weekly Epidemiological Record 67: 177–184

Hankins C A, Handley M A 1992 HIV disease and AIDS in women: current knowledge and a research agenda. Journal of Acquired Immune Deficiency Syndrome 5(10): 957–971

Horner P J, Goldmeier D, Byrne M, Hay P E 1989 Antenatal screening for syphilis (letter). British Medical Journal 299(6704): 919

Lossick J G 1986 Sexually transmitted vaginitis. Seminars in Adolescent Medicine 2(2): 131–142

MacDonagh S E, Masters J, Helps B A, Tookey P A, Ades A E, Gibb D M 1996a Antenatal HIV testing in London: policy, uptake and detection. British Medical Journal 313: 532–533

MacDonagh S E, Masters J, Helps B A, Tookey P A, Gibb D M 1996b Why are antenatal HIV testing policies in London failing? British Journal of Midwifery 4(9): 466–470

Mandal B K, Wilkins E G L, Dunbar E M, Mayon-White R T 1996 Lecture notes on infectious diseases, 5th edn. Blackwell Science, Oxford

Mindel A, Adler M W, Sutherland S, Fiddian A P 1982

Intravenous acyclovir treatment for primary genital herpes. Lancet i: 697–700

Mindel A, Faherty A, Carney O, Patou G, Freris M, Williams P 1988 Dosage and safety of long-term suppressive acyclovir therapy for recurrent genital herpes. Lancet i: 926–928

Minkoff H L, DeHovitz J A 1990 Care of women infected with the human immunodeficiency virus. Journal of the American Medical Association 266(16): 2253–2258

Minkoff H L, Willoughby A, Mendez H et al 1990 Serious infections during pregnancy among women with advanced immunodeficiency virus infection. American Journal of Obstetrics and Gynecology 162(1): 30–34

Nahmias A J et al 1971 Perinatal risk associated with maternal genital herpes simplex virus infection. American Journal of Obstetrics and Gynecology 100: 825–833

O'Mahoney C, Holland N 1989 Antenatal screening for syphilis (letter). British Medical Journal 299: 859

Peckham C, Gibb D 1995 Mother to child transmission of the human immunodeficiency virus. New England Journal of Medicine 333(5): 298–302

Pratt R J 1995 HIV and AIDS: a strategy for nursing care, 4th edn. Edward Arnold, London

Prober C G et al 1987 Low risk of herpes simplex virus infections in neonates exposed to the virus at the time of vaginal delivery to mothers with recurrent genital herpes infections. New England Journal of Medicine 316: 240–244

Rouzioux C, Costagliola D, Burgard M, Blanche S, Mayaux M J, Griscelli C, Valleron A J 1995 Estimated timing of mother-to-child human immunodeficiency virus type 1 (HIV-1) transmission by use of a Markov model. The HIV Infection in Newborns French Collaborative Study Group. American Journal of Epidemiology 142(12): 1330–1337

Royal College of Midwives 1996 HIV & AIDS: Position Paper, Number 16, November 1996. RCM, London

Royal College of Obstetricians and Gynaecologists 1997 HIV infection in maternity care and gynaecology: working party report. RCOG, London

Salisbury D M, Begg N T (eds) 1996 Immunisation against infectious disease. HMSO, London

Scarlatti G 1996 Paediatric HIV infection. Lancet 348: 863–868

Schachter J, Grossman M 1981 Chlamydial infections. Annual Review of Medicine 3: 45–61

Smith J R, Cowan F M, Munday P E 1998 The management of herpes simplex virus infection in pregnancy. British Journal of Obstetrics and Gynaecology 105: 255–260

Soper D E, Shoupe D, Shangold G A, Shangold M M, Gutmann J, Mercer L 1993 Prevention of vaginal trichomoniasis by compliant use of the female condom. Sexually Transmitted Diseases 20(3): 137–139

Stagno S, Whitley R J 1990 Herpesvirus infection in the neonate and children. In: Holmes K K, Mardh P A, Sparling P F et al (eds) Sexually transmitted diseases, 2nd edn. McGraw Hill, New York

Stein Z A 1990 HIV prevention: the need for methods women can use. American Journal of Public Health 80(4): 460–462

Thomson R, Holland J 1994 Young women and safer (hetero)sex: context, constraints and strategies. In: Wilkenson S, Kitzinger C (eds) Women and health: feminist perspectives. Taylor and Francis, London

Thorne C, Newell M L, Dunn D, Peckham C 1995 The European Collaborative Study: clinical and immunological characteristics of HIV 1-infected pregnant women. British Journal of Obstetrics and Gynaecology 102: 869–875

United Kingdom Central Council for Nursing, Midwifery and Health Visiting (UKCC) 1992 Code of professional conduct. UKCC, London

Unlinked Anonymous Surveys Steering Group 1995 Report of the unlinked anonymous HIV prevalence monitoring programme: England and Wales. Department of Health, London

Unlinked Anonymous Surveys Steering Group 1996 Report of the unlinked anonymous HIV prevalence monitoring programme: England and Wales. Department of Health, London

van Everdingen J J E, Peeters M F, ten Have P 1993 Neonatal herpes policy in the Netherlands: five years after a consensus conference. Journal of Perinatal Medicine 21: 371–375

Vermund S H, Galbraith M A, Ebner S C, Sheon A R and Kaslow R A 1992 Human immunodeficiency virus/acquired immunodeficiency syndrome in pregnant women. Annals of Epidemiology 2(6): 773–803

Wang E, Smaill F 1989 Infection in pregnancy. In: Chalmers I, Enkin M, Keirse M (eds) Effective care in pregnancy and childbirth. Oxford University Press, Oxford

Williams K 1985 Screening for syphilis in pregnancy: an assessment of costs and benefits. Community Medicine 7: 37–42

FURTHER READING

Berer M, Ray S 1993 Women and HIV/AIDS: an international resource book. Pluto Press, London

Berer M, Ravindran T K S (eds) 1995 Pregnancy, birth control, STDs and AIDS: promoting safer sex. Reproductive Health Matters 5 May

Gordon P, Mitchell L 1988 Safer sex: a new look at sexual pleasure. Faber, London

19

Multiple pregnancy

Margie Davies

The term 'multiple pregnancy' is used to describe the development of more than one fetus in utero at the same time.

Families expecting a multiple birth have different health needs, requiring extra practical support and understanding throughout pregnancy, the postnatal period and the early years. Information and support from well-informed health care professionals from the time that the multiple pregnancy is diagnosed will help to prepare the parents and potential problems may be avoided.

The chapter aims to:

- describe how types of multiple pregnancy may be distinguished

- consider the diagnosis and management of twin pregnancy and labour and the care of the mother and babies after birth

- give an overview of the problems particularly associated with twins and higher order births and the fetal anomalies unique to the twinning process

- explain the special needs of the parents and identify the sources of help available.

Incidence

The incidence of multiple births in the UK continues to rise; in 1995 there were 9565 sets of twins born, that is 1 in 76 maternities. In the 1940s and 1950s the incidence was similar at 1 in 80 but then fell to 1 in 105 in the 1970s (see Fig. 19.1). The full explanation for the fall is unknown though smaller families and the earlier completion of families were contributing factors. The current rise is almost entirely due to the increased use of various kinds of treatments for infertility involving ovulation induction.

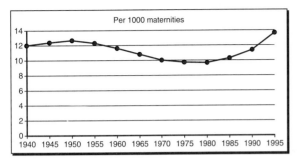

Fig. 19.1 Twinning rates England and Wales 1940–1995 (data supplied by Office of National Statistics).

The number of triplets has more than trebled in the last 12 years (Botting et al 1990); this is due to the rise in infertility treatments such as in vitro fertilisation (IVF) and ovulatory stimulating drugs, like clomiphene citrate and gonadotrophins. In 1995 there were 311 sets of triplets and 8 sets of quadruplets born in the UK.

In other parts of the world the incidences are different: in West Africa they are much higher and in Japan much lower. Triplets in the UK occur in about 1 in 3000 pregnancies and quadruplets once in every 700 000.

Naturally occurring quadruplets and more are rare, but when IVF treatments were first introduced with no limit on the number of embryos that could be replaced the incidence of quintuplets, sextuplets and septuplets increased. Survival rates in such pregnancies, however, were poor.

The Human Fertilisation and Embryology Authority (HFEA) Act 1990 requires all centres providing IVF to be licensed by the HFEA. They are now only allowed to replace a maximum of three embryos.

TWIN PREGNANCY

Types of twin pregnancy

Twins will be either monozygotic or dizygotic. Monozygotic or uniovular twins are also referred to as identical twins. They develop from one ovum and one spermatozoon which after fertilisation split into two. These twins will be of the same sex and have the same genes, blood groups and physical features such as eye and hair colour, ear shapes and palm creases. However, they may be of different sizes and sometimes have different personalities.

Dizygotic or binovular twins develop from two separate ova that are fertilised by two different spermatozoa, and are often referred to as non-identical twins. They are no more alike than any brother or sister and can be of the same or different sex. Because in any pregnancy there is a 50:50 chance of a girl or boy, half dizygotic twins will be boy and girl pairs. A quarter of dizygotic twins will be both boys and a quarter both girls. Of all twins born in the UK, two-thirds will be dizygotic and one-third monozygotic. Therefore approximately one-third of twins are girls, one-third boys, and one-third girl–boy pairs.

Determination of zygosity and chorionicity

Midwives should understand the differences between the two (Table 19.1) and why it is important.

Determination of zygosity means determining whether or not the twins are identical. In about a third of all twins born it will be obvious as the children will be of a different sex. Of the remaining same-sex twins their zygosity will usually be apparent from physical features by the time they are 2 years old, though parents are not usually prepared to wait this long. At birth, identical twins tend to have a greater weight variation than non-identical ones. In approximately two-thirds of identical twins a monochorionic placenta will confirm monozygosity. If the babies have a single

Table 19.1 Relationship between zygosity and chorionicity	
Dichorionic	Monochorionic
Two placentae (may be fused) Two chorions Two amnions	One placenta One chorion Two amnions (one amnion in monoamniotic twins is very rare)
These twins can be either dizygotic or monozygotic	These twins can only be monozygotic

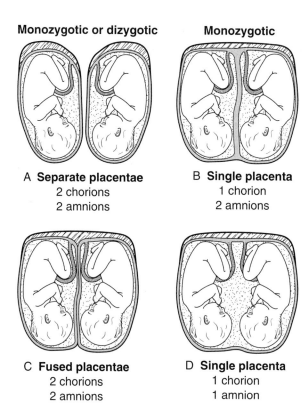

Monozygotic or dizygotic	Monozygotic
A **Separate placentae** 2 chorions 2 amnions	B **Single placenta** 1 chorion 2 amnions
C **Fused placentae** 2 chorions 2 amnions	D **Single placenta** 1 chorion 1 amnion

Fig. 19.2 Placentation of twins (after Bryan 1984).

outer membrane, the chorion, they must be monozygotic (Fig. 19.2). One-third of identical twins will have two chorions and two amnions, and either a fused placenta or two separate placentae, which is indistinguishable from the situation in nonidentical twins. This occurs when the fertilised ovum splits within the first 3 or 4 days after fertilisation and while it is still in the uterine tube. When these are seen on an early scan they appear as two separate placentae and are dichorionic diamniotic, exactly the same as non-identical twins.

Chorionicity: why is it important to know?

Monochorionic twin pregnancies have a three to five times higher risk of perinatal mortality and morbidity than dichorionic twin pregnancies (Fisk & Bennett 1995).

Prenatally the chorionicity is determined by ultrasound examination. Preferably this should be performed during the first trimester as the differences between the two types of placentation are more pronounced. The chorions forming the septum between the amniotic sacs can be seen more clearly in the first trimester of pregnancy. If the septum has a mean thickness of 2.4 mm or more then it is usually a dichorionic twin pregnancy; if it is a thin septum with a mean thickness of 1.4 mm then it is more likely to be a monochorionic pregnancy (Winn et al 1989).

Another method of determining chorionicity is by studying the septum at its base adjacent to the placenta. A tongue of placental tissue is seen ultrasonically between the two chorions and this is termed the 'twin peak' (Finberg 1992) or lambda sign (Kurtz et al 1992).

Zygosity

This can be determined in same-sexed dichorionic twins by multiple blood grouping or DNA microprobe technique. The easiest way to obtain blood is from the umbilical cords at delivery but unfortunately only a few specialist laboratories offer testing on blood groups. Provided enough blood groups are tested a reliable assessment of zygosity can be made. If any single blood group is different, the twins are definitely dizygotic (DZ). If all the blood groups tested are the same, then there is a high probability that they are monozygotic (MZ), up to 99%. The most accurate method of zygosity determination is by DNA microprobe technique but unfortunately this method is very expensive.

Zygosity determination should be routinely offered to all same-sexed twins because:

- Most parents will want to know whether or not their twins are identical.
- If parents are considering further pregnancies they will want to know their risk of having twins again. DZ twins tend to run in families and the increased risk is approximately fivefold, usually on the female side though not in all cases. MZ twins do not run in families and the risk does not change (except in rare families who carry a dominant gene for monozygotic twinning). The chance of any fertile woman having MZ twins is 1 in 300.
- It will help the twins in establishing their sense of identity; it will influence their life and family relationships.
- The information is important for genetic

reasons, not just with monogenic disorders but with any serious illness later in life.

Twins are frequently asked to be involved in research where knowledge of zygosity is essential.

Diagnosis of twin pregnancy

This is usually through ultrasound examination and the diagnosis can be made as early as 6 weeks into the pregnancy or later at the routine detailed structural scan between the 18th and 20th weeks. When booking a woman in the antenatal clinic a family history of twins should alert the midwife to the possibility of a multiple pregnancy. If the pregnancy is diagnosed at 6 weeks the woman should have the 'vanishing twin syndrome' explained to her (Landy & Nies 1995). It has been suggested that in up to 50% of twin pregnancies diagnosed at 6 weeks one fetus is lost (Bryan 1992). However, later research has questioned this high number. Occasionally one fetus may die in the second trimester and become a fetus papyraceous (Fig. 19.3) which becomes embedded in the surface of the placenta and expelled with the placenta at delivery. This is very rare and probably occurs in 1 in 12 000 live births.

The news that a woman is expecting a multiple birth should be broken to the parents in a sensitive manner (Spillman 1985). As soon as a multiple pregnancy has been diagnosed the mother should be given relevant information about multiple pregnancy, the telephone numbers of her local twins club and of national twin organisations, as well as any details of special antenatal classes that may be available. Many parents can spend weeks of unnecessary anxiety through ignorance of the help available (Spillman 1987).

Since the advent of routine ultrasound scanning it is very rare for a woman to get to delivery with undiagnosed twins but this will not apply in areas where this technology is unavailable.

Abdominal examination

Inspection. On inspection, the size of the uterus may be larger than expected for the period of gestation, particularly after the 20th week. The uterus may look broad or round and fetal movements may be seen over a wide area, although the findings are not diagnostic of twins. Fresh striae gravidarum may be apparent. Up to twice the amount of amniotic fluid is normal in a twin pregnancy but polyhydramnios is not an uncommon complication of a twin pregnancy, particularly with monochorionic twins.

Palpation. On palpation the fundal height may be greater than expected for the period of gestation. The presence of two fetal poles (head or breech) in the fundus of the uterus may be revealed on palpation and multiple fetal limbs may also be palpable. The head may be small in relation to the size of the uterus and may suggest that the fetus is also small and that there may therefore be more than one present. Lateral palpation may reveal two fetal backs or limbs on both sides. Pelvic palpation may give findings similar to those on fundal palpation although one fetus may lie behind the other and make detection difficult. Location of three poles in total is diagnostic of at least two fetuses.

Auscultation. Hearing two fetal hearts is not diagnostic as one can often be heard over a wide area in a singleton pregnancy. If simultaneous comparison of the heart rates reveals a difference of at least 10 beats per minute, it may be assumed that two hearts are being heard.

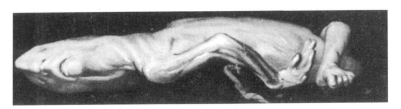

Fig. 19.3 Fetus papyraceous.

The pregnancy

A multiple pregnancy tends to be shorter than a single pregnancy. The average gestation for twins is 37 weeks, triplets 34 weeks, and quadruplets 33 weeks.

Effects of pregnancy

Exacerbation of minor disorders. The presence of more than one fetus in utero and the higher levels of circulating hormones often exacerbate the minor disorders of pregnancy. Morning sickness, nausea and heartburn may be more persistent and more troublesome than in a singleton pregnancy.

Anaemia. Iron deficiency and folic acid deficiency anaemias are common in twin pregnancies. Early growth and development of the uterus and its contents make greater demands on the maternal iron stores and in later pregnancy (after 28th week) fetal demands may lead to anaemia and cause the midwife to suspect iron or folic acid deficiency or both.

Blood tests. Haemoglobin should be tested routinely as for singletons but a special eye kept on the results as women expecting multiples are more likely to become anaemic.

Polyhydramnios. This is also common and is particularly associated with monochorionic twins and with fetal abnormalities. Polyhydramnios will add to any discomfort which the woman is already experiencing. If acute polyhydramnios occurs it can lead to miscarriage or premature labour.

Pressure symptoms. The increased weight and size of the uterus and its contents may be troublesome. Impaired venous return from the lower limbs increases the tendency to varicose veins and oedema of the legs. Backache is common and the increased uterine size may also lead to marked dyspnoea and to indigestion.

Antenatal screening

- Nuchal translucency for Down syndrome is only accurate if done before 11 weeks.
- Chorionic villus sampling (CVS) is not usually recommended in multiple pregnancy as loss rates are high.
- Amniocentesis can be performed in twin pregnancies. Most obstetricians prefer to do a dual needle insertion so there is no chance of contamination between the two sacs.
- Chorionicity should be determined in the first trimester.
- All monozygotic twins should have echocardiography performed at approximately 20 weeks' gestation, as there is a much higher risk of cardiac anomalies in these babies. In the UK at present the incidence is 32 per 1000.

Ultrasound examination

- Monochorionic twin pregnancies should be scanned every 2 weeks from diagnosis to check for discordant fetal growth, and signs of fetofetal transfusion syndrome.
- Dichorionic twin pregnancies should be scanned at 20 weeks for anomalies as with a singleton and then 4-weekly.

Antenatal preparation

Early diagnosis of a twin pregnancy and of chorionicity is extremely important in order to prepare the parents by giving them the specialist support and advice they will need.

Parent education

When a multiple pregnancy is diagnosed written information on twins or more should be made immediately available to the mother. This should include contact phone numbers of local support organisations. As soon as the multiple pregnancy is diagnosed the midwife who organises parent education should be informed. The news that they are expecting twins or more may have come as a considerable shock to the parents and the midwife should give them the opportunity to discuss any worries or problems they may have. Two babies will add a considerable financial burden to any family's income, so the midwife should check whether they would like to be referred to a social worker.

Routine parent education classes should start

earlier for twin mothers than for singleton mothers, ideally at 24–26 weeks' gestation or even earlier if a mother's work commitments allow. A specialist class for multiples should be offered at 28–30 weeks; usually one session is enough. In most hospitals these classes are held monthly, but a course of two or three held every 2 or 3 months may be preferred (Davies 1995). When planning these classes, contact with the local twins club can provide a valuable source of practical information. Mothers from the twins club are usually delighted to participate in the classes and talk on the more practical issues such as coping with two or more babies, equipment and even breast feeding. All of these will be very helpful to prospective parents (Denton & Bryan 1995). Suggestions for class topics are listed in Box 19.1.

Preparation for breast feeding

Mothers will inevitably give a lot of thought to how they are going to feed their babies, not only from the nutritional point of view but also from the practical, because it will take up a large amount of their time during the first 6 months. Mothers should be encouraged right from the beginning that it is not only possible to breast feed two, and in some cases three babies, but that it is the best way for her to feed her babies nutritionally and it can be a very rewarding experience for her as well. Many sets of twins have been entirely breast fed, some beyond their first birthdays. Very few sets of triplets are totally breast fed (Fiducia 1995) but many manage to combine breast and bottle feeding very successfully.

Early in the antenatal period the mother should be given as much information and advice as possible about both breast and bottle feeding, so she can make an informed choice on how she wants to feed her babies. Both parents should have the opportunity to talk through any worries they have regarding feeding and should be encouraged to meet with another mother who is successfully breast feeding her babies. This will give encouragement as well as a chance to talk over any practical concerns they may have (Box 19.2). Introductions can usually be made through the local twins group.

LABOUR AND DELIVERY

Onset. The higher the number of fetuses the mother is carrying, the earlier labour is likely to start. Term for twins is usually considered to be 37 weeks rather than 40, and approximately 30% of twins are born preterm, that is before 37 weeks' gestation. In addition to being preterm the babies may be light for dates and therefore prone to the associated complications of both conditions. If spontaneous labour begins very early, the chances of survival outside the uterus are small and the mother may be given drugs to inhibit uterine activity. Intravenous salbutamol and sulindac tablets are the drugs most commonly used. Known causes of preterm labour must, if at all possible, be diagnosed and treated quickly, for example urinary tract infection should be treated with antibiotics.

It is very unusual for a twin pregnancy to last more than 40 weeks; many obstetricians advise induction of labour at 38 weeks.

If the first twin is in a cephalic presentation, labour is usually allowed to continue normally to a vaginal delivery, but if the first twin is presenting in any other way (Fig. 19.4), an elective caesarean section is usually recommended.

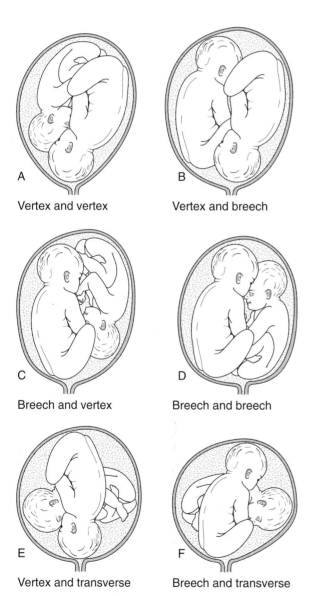

A — Vertex and vertex

B — Vertex and breech

C — Breech and vertex

D — Breech and breech

E — Vertex and transverse

F — Breech and transverse

Fig. 19.4 Presentation of twins before delivery (after Bryan 1984).

Management of labour

During the antenatal classes the mother must be warned that a multiple birth is bound to create a lot of interest and so there may be a number of people who would like to observe the birth. If the mother has any objection to this, her wishes must be respected and a record made in her notes that she only wants those concerned with her medical care to be present.

Induction of labour usually occurs around 38 weeks' gestation. The presence of complications such as pregnancy-induced hypertension, intra-uterine growth retardation or fetofetal transfusion syndrome may be reasons for earlier induction.

The majority of women expecting twins will go into labour spontaneously. Theoretically the duration of the first stage of labour should be no different from that of a single pregnancy. However, there is an increased incidence of dysfunctional labour in twin pregnancies, possibly because of overdistension of the uterus.

Labour in the mother of twins must be recognised as high risk and continuous fetal heart monitoring of both babies is essential. This can be achieved either with two external transducers or, once the membranes are ruptured, a scalp electrode on the presenting twin and external transducer on the second. If a 'twin monitor' is available both heart beats can be monitored simultaneously to give a more reliable reading. Uterine activity will also need to be monitored.

If cardiotocography is not available, use of the Doptone or Sonicaid may give more accurate recordings of the fetal heart rates than a fetal stethoscope. If the latter has to be used, two people must auscultate simultaneously so that fetal heart rates are counted over the same minute.

Whilst in labour the woman should be encouraged to adopt whichever position she finds most comfortable. A foam rubber wedge under the side of the mattress will help to prevent supine hypotensive syndrome by giving a lateral tilt. It may be preferable for her to adopt a semiprone position, well supported by pillows or a bean bag. A birthing chair or a reclining chair, if available, may be more comfortable than a delivery bed.

Regional epidural blockade is usually the pain

relief of choice in twin labours (Crawford 1978). It provides excellent analgesia and, if necessary, allows easier instrumental deliveries and also manipulation of the second twin.

The use of Entonox analgesia may be helpful, either before the epidural is in situ or during the second stage if the epidural is wearing off.

The woman should be encouraged to use whatever form of relaxation she finds helpful. If she chooses to use drugs only after other methods have failed, her wishes should be respected. The midwife should explain that if complications arise, intervention and the use of drugs may be necessary. This should be discussed long before the onset of labour.

If fetal distress occurs during labour, delivery will need to be expedited, usually by caesarean section. Action may also need to be taken if the mother's condition gives cause for concern.

If uterine activity is poor, the use of intravenous Syntocinon may be required once the membranes have been ruptured. Artificial rupture of the membranes may be sufficient in itself to stimulate good uterine activity but may need to be used in conjunction with intravenous Syntocinon. The cardiotocograph will give a good indication of the pattern of uterine activity, whether the labour is induced or spontaneous. The response of the fetal hearts to uterine contractions can be observed on the graph paper.

If the babies are expected to be premature, of low birthweight or known to have any other problems, the neonatal unit must be informed that the woman is in labour so that they can make the necessary preparations to receive the babies. When the delivery is imminent, the paediatric team should be summoned so that they may be present when the infants are born.

Throughout labour the emotional as well as the general physical condition of the mother must be considered. She requires support from the midwife and may be apprehensive about the delivery. The presence of her partner or companion will be helpful to her, and the midwife should encourage her to ask questions and express her feelings.

Management of delivery

The onset of the second stage of labour should be confirmed by a vaginal examination. The obstetrician, paediatric team and anaesthetist should be present for the delivery because of the risk of complications.

If epidural analgesia has been used it may be 'topped up' prior to delivery, either by the anaesthetist or by the midwife if qualified to do this. The possibility of emergency caesarean section is ever present and the operating theatre should be in a state of readiness to receive the mother at short notice. Monitoring of both fetal hearts should continue until delivery. Provided that the first twin is presenting by the vertex, the delivery can be expected to proceed normally, as with a singleton pregnancy. When the first twin is born, the time of delivery and the sex are noted. This baby must be labelled as 'twin one' immediately. The identity bracelets should be completed and the midwife must check them with the mother or father before they are applied to the infant's wrist and ankle. The mother may wish to hold her baby and if he is in good condition this should be encouraged. He may be put to the breast because suckling stimulates uterine contractions. If he requires active resuscitation, the paediatric team will take over his care once on the resuscitaire.

After the delivery of the first twin, abdominal palpation is made to ascertain the lie, presentation and position of the second twin and to auscultate the fetal heart. If the lie is not longitudinal, an attempt may be made to correct it by external cephalic version. If it is longitudinal, a vaginal examination is made to confirm the presentation. If the presenting part is not engaged it should be pushed into the pelvis by fundal pressure before the second sac of membranes is ruptured. The fetal heart should be auscultated again and a scalp electrode may be applied once the membranes are ruptured. If uterine activity does not recommence, intravenous Syntocinon may be used to stimulate it.

When the presenting part becomes visible, the mother should be encouraged to push with contractions to deliver the second twin. The midwife should be aware that, owing to the reduced size of the placental site following the birth of the first twin, the second fetus may be somewhat deprived of oxygen. Delivery will proceed as normal if the presentation is vertex but if the fetus presents by the breech the midwife may need to hand over the delivery to the doctor.

Delivery of the second twin should be completed within 45 minutes of the first twin as long as there are no signs of fetal distress in the second twin; if there are, the delivery must be expedited and the second twin is usually delivered by caesarean section.

An oxytocic drug is usually given intramuscularly or intravenously, depending on local policy, after the delivery of the anterior shoulder as with a singleton pregnancy.

This baby is labelled as 'twin two'. A note of the time of delivery and the sex of the child is made. The risk of asphyxia is greater for the second twin and the paediatric team may need to actively resuscitate this infant. He may need to be transferred to the neonatal unit immediately after delivery. He should, however, be shown to his mother prior to transfer and if at all possible she may cuddle him. Some units make a policy of keeping twins together which may mean that the healthy twin goes to the neonatal unit as well.

After both babies have been delivered, the midwife prepares to deliver the placenta(e). Once the oxytocic drug has taken effect, controlled cord traction is applied to both cords simultaneously and the placentae should be delivered without delay. Emptying the uterus enables bleeding to be controlled and postpartum haemorrhage prevented.

Samples of cord blood should be taken for determination of zygosity if it is the hospital's policy. The placenta(e) should be examined and the number of amniotic sacs, chorions and placentae noted (see Fig. 19.2).

If the babies are of different sexes they are dizygotic. If the placenta is monochorionic they must be monozygotic but if they are of the same sex and the placenta is dichorionic further tests will be needed (see above). Pathological examination of placenta and membranes may be needed to confirm chorionicity.

The umbilical cords should be examined and the number of cord vessels and the presence of any abnormalities noted.

Complications associated with multiple pregnancy

The high perinatal mortality associated with twinning is largely due to complications of pregnancy, such as the premature onset of labour, intrauterine growth retardation and complications of delivery. The management of multiple pregnancy is concerned with the prevention, early detection and treatment of these complications.

Polyhydramnios

Acute polyhydramnios may occur as early as 18–20 weeks. It may be associated with fetal abnormality but it is more likely to be due to the fetofetal transfusion syndrome (FFTS) also known as twin-to-twin transfusion syndrome (TTTS).

Fetofetal transfusion syndrome. This can be acute or chronic. The acute form usually occurs during labour and is the result of a blood transfusion from one fetus (donor) to the other (recipient) through vascular anastomosis in a monochorionic placenta. Both fetuses may die of cardiac failure if not treated immediately.

Chronic fetofetal transfusion syndrome can occur in up to 35% of monochorionic twin pregnancies (Fisk 1995). Most of the recent data on FFTS suggest that the placentae in these cases are charac-terised by one or more deep unidirectional arteriovenous anastomoses. This results in anaemia and growth retardation in the donor twin (the term 'stuck twin' may be used) and polycythaemia with circulatory overload in the recipient twin (hydrops). The fetal and neonatal mortality is high but some infants may be saved by early diagnosis and prenatal treatment with either amnioreduction or laser coagulation of communicating placental vessels. Selective fetocide is sometimes considered.

The midwife should always be on the lookout for the mother who complains of a rapid increase in her abdominal girth in the second trimester, as well as a uterus that feels hard and uncomfortable continuously. This is due to polyhydramnios and if not treated as an urgent obstetric problem will cause premature labour. Amnioreduction may have to be repeated on a number of occasions, as reaccumulation of fluid can occur rapidly.

Fetal abnormality

This is particularly associated with monozygotic twins.

Conjoined twins. This extremely rare malformation of monozygotic twinning results from the incomplete division of the fertilised ovum. Delivery has to be by caesarean section. Separation of the babies is sometimes possible and will depend on how they are joined and which internal organs are involved. Antenatal investigations will usually have given some indication of whether surgery will be feasible.

Acardiac malformation. This occurs in about 1 in 30 000 deliveries. In acardia, one twin presents without a well-defined cardiac structure and is kept alive through placental anastomoses to the circulatory system of the viable fetus (Moore et al 1990).

Fetus-in-fetu. In fetus-in-fetu parts of a fetus may be lodged within another fetus; this can only happen in MZ twins (Eng et al 1989).

Malpresentations

Although the uterus is large and distended, the fetuses are less mobile than may be supposed. They can restrict each other's movements, which may result in malpresentations, particularly of the second twin. After delivery of the first twin, the presentation of the second twin may change.

Premature rupture of the membranes

Malpresentations due to polyhydramnios may predispose to premature rupture of the membranes.

Prolapse of the cord

This, too, is associated with malpresentations and polyhydramnios and is more likely if there is a poorly fitting presenting part. The second twin is particularly at risk of cord prolapse.

Prolonged labour

Malpresentations are a poor stimulus to good uterine action and a distended uterus is likely to lead to poor uterine activity and consequently prolonged labour.

Monoamniotic twins

Approximately 1% of twins share the same sac. Monoamniotic twins risk cord entanglement with occlusion of the blood supply to one or both fetuses.

Locked twins

This is a rare but serious complication of twin pregnancy. There are two types. One occurs when the first twin presents by the breech and the second by the vertex, the other when both are vertex presentations. In both instances the head of the second twin prevents the continued descent of the first (Fig. 19.5).

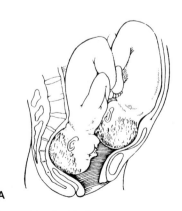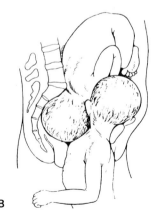

A   B

Fig. 19.5 Locked twins.

Delay in the birth of the second twin

After delivery of the first twin, uterine activity should recommence within 5 minutes. Delivery of the second twin is usually completed within 45 minutes of the first birth. In the past the delivery interval was limited to 30 minutes in an attempt to minimise complications such as cord prolapse, placental abruption and fetal distress. With the introduction of fetal heart rate monitoring the interval time between babies is not so crucial as long as the fetal condition is monitored. Poor uterine action as a result of malpresentation may be the cause of delay. The risks of such delay are intrauterine hypoxia, birth asphyxia following premature separation of the placenta and sepsis as a result of ascending infection from the first umbilical cord which lies outside the vulva. After delivery of the first twin the lower uterine segment begins to re-form and the cervical canal may have to fully dilate again.

The midwife may need to 'rub up' a contraction and to put the first twin to the breast to stimulate uterine activity. If there appears to be an obstruction, medical aid is summoned and a caesarean section may be necessary. If there is no obstruction, Syntocinon infusion may be commenced or forceps delivery considered.

Premature expulsion of the placenta

The placenta may be expelled before delivery of the second twin. In dichorionic twins with separate placentae, one placenta may be delivered separately; in monochorionic twins the shared placenta may be expelled. The risks of severe asphyxia and death of the second twin are then very high. Haemorrhage is also likely if one twin is retained in utero as this prevents adequate retraction of the placental site.

Postpartum haemorrhage

Poor uterine tone as a result of overdistension or hypotonic activity is likely to lead to postpartum haemorrhage.

Undiagnosed twins

The possibility of an unexpected undiagnosed second baby (though this is unlikely with ultra-sound scanning) should be considered if the uterus appears larger than expected after delivery of the first baby or if the baby is surprisingly smaller than expected. If an oxytocic drug has been given after delivery of the anterior shoulder of the first baby, the second baby is in great danger and delivery should be expedited. He will require active resuscitation because of severe asphyxia. The midwife must break the news of undiagnosed twins gently to the parents. These parents will require special support and guidance during the postnatal period.

Deferred delivery of the second twin

There have been several reported cases where the first twin has been born, often quite prematurely, and then there has been a long gap before labour recommences; up to 30 days or more have been reported before the second twin is delivered. This opportunity can be used to give betamethasone to the mother in cases of immaturity of the lungs. Careful observations of the mother's condition must be made during this time for signs of infection and fetal distress. The mother will need a lot of support from the midwives to cope with her anxieties for her delivered premature baby as well as still being pregnant and with her concerns for the outcome of her pregnancy.

POSTNATAL PERIOD

Care of the babies

Immediate care at delivery will involve ensuring that both babies have a clear airway. Maintenance of body temperature is vital, particularly if the infants are small and use of the overhead heater on the resuscitaire will help to prevent heat loss. The infants should not be overexposed and gentle handling is important. Identification of the infants should be clear and the parents are given the opportunity to check the identity bracelets and cuddle their babies. The infants may have to be admitted directly to the neonatal unit (NNU) from the labour ward, in which case the father should accompany them, or they will be transferred to the postnatal ward with their mother if they are in good condition.

Temperature control

Maintenance of a thermoneutral environment is essential, particularly for infants in the neonatal unit. They may need to be nursed in incubators. American studies have shown that a sick baby can benefit from sharing his incubator with his twin. In most units, wherever possible, both babies are kept together which can mean that the healthy twin goes to the neonatal unit with his brother or sister. Clothing should be light but warm and allow air to circulate. The babies' temperatures should be checked regularly and recorded. If they are below the normal range, rewarming is required.

Nutrition

Both babies may be breast fed either simultaneously or separately. The mother may choose to feed artificially but whatever her choice the midwife should support her. In the immediate postnatal days the mother may prefer to breast feed the twins separately as this gives her time with each baby. If the babies are light for dates or preterm, the paediatricians may recommend that the babies be 'topped up' after a breast feed. Expressed breast milk is the best form of nutrition for these babies. If the babies are not able to suck adequately at the breast then the mother should be encouraged to express her milk regularly for her babies. If she does not have sufficient milk for them, milk from a human milk bank can be used, which is much better for the premature babies than artificial milk (Lucas & Cole 1990) and reduces the risk of necrotising enterocolitis (NEC) (Beeby & Jeffrey 1992).

In the early postnatal days the mother may worry that her milk supply is inadequate for two babies and she should be reassured by the midwife that lactation responds to the demands made by the babies sucking at the breast. The more stimulation the breasts are given the more plentiful the milk supply. At feed times the midwife must be with the mother to offer support and advice on positioning and fixing the babies, as well as encouraging her in her ability to breast feed two babies.

As the twin babies are both more likely to be preterm or light for dates, their ability to coordinate the sucking and swallowing reflexes may be poor. If so, they may need to be fed intravenously or by nasogastric tube or cup fed (Lang 1995a,b),

depending on their size and general condition. The mother should be encouraged to participate in whatever method is used. Careful monitoring of weight gain is required. Hypoglycaemia may occur and regular capillary blood glucose estimations are essential.

Breast feeding

The advantages of breast feeding are the same as for single babies, but as twins have a higher tendency to be born prematurely and light for dates it is even more important that they should be breast fed. As well as the medical and nutritional reasons for it being better, there are the practical reasons too.

• It is cheaper: breast milk is available 24 hours a day at the correct temperature.

• There are no bottles to wash, no sterilising to organise or feeds to make up, all of which take time, something a mother of twins feels in the early days that she has very little of.

• Twins can be breast fed together or separately. If the babies are to be fed together then the feeds will only take a little longer than with a single baby.

The mother must be encouraged to get everything organised before she starts feeding. The ideal place to sit is on either a bed or a sofa so there is room to put the babies down while organising pillows, etc. In the early days a mother may need to have someone to help position the babies. It is often easier to feed them separately in the very early days as well as giving the mother a chance to get to know her babies individually. If she does feed this way to begin with, it is advisable to try to feed both together before being discharged from hospital, so that the midwife can stay with her throughout the entire feed, providing advice, support and another pair of hands.

Using pillows to support the babies, the mother is able to get herself into a comfortable sitting position (Fig. 19.6). Explain to the mother that she needs to have plenty of pillows so the weight of the babies is taken by the pillows and not by her arms as this will cause back pain.

Mothers of twins always complain that there is never enough time for cuddling, so to be able to breast feed together is a considerable advantage.

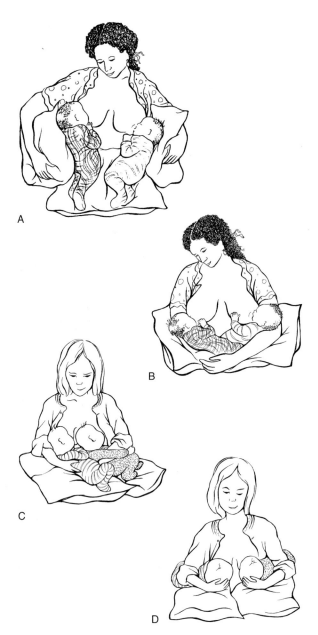

A

B

C

D

Fig. 19.6 Breast-feeding positions for twins (Illustrator: Gillian Coupland).

It is also the only way for her to hold and feed both babies at the same time. The main advantage of bottle feeding is that someone else can always help, although this can also be done by using expressed breast milk.

Prevention of infection

The principles of hygiene should be reinforced as prevention of infection is a priority. If the infants are of low birthweight they are more susceptible to infection. The mother should be encouraged to wash her hands before handling her babies and particularly after changing their nappies.

Mother–baby relationships

Mothers who have a multiple birth often find it more difficult to bond with both babies equally. This is very common and they should be reassured that they are not unusual in their feelings and in a short time will overcome these worries. If, for example, the babies are of markedly different sizes, a mother may favour one or the other, or if one baby is in the neonatal unit whilst the other is on the postnatal ward with her, she may find she bonds with the one on the ward much more quickly. In such cases the mother should be encouraged to spend as much time as practicable with the baby in the unit and to visit the NNU as soon as possible after delivery. If she has had an operative delivery she may find it difficult to care for two babies and extreme tiredness or anaemia will exacerbate the situation. She may have feelings of guilt if the delivery and immediate postnatal period have not gone as she had expected. The midwife should be alert for such circumstances and help the mother to divide her attention between both babies and to give plenty of reassurance that she is not the first mother to feel like that.

Mother–partner relationships

A mother who has had twins or more will inevitably turn to her partner for help with the care of the babies and in many families they all work well together in the care and upbringing of their children, despite the added strains and stresses a multiple birth puts on a family. But in some cases her partner may feel that she is devoting too much time to the babies and not enough to him, thus making him feel excluded, especially if when he comes home from work she is too exhausted to take any interest in him. The strain on any relationship when a new baby is born can be quite difficult for the couple to adjust to, but with a multiple birth it is even worse. The midwife should always encourage the father to be involved in the daily care of the babies, either in hospital or at home.

Care of the mother

Involution of the uterus will be slower because of its increased bulk. 'Afterpains' may be troublesome and analgesia should be offered. Some mothers may benefit from a night sedative and need adequate time to rest. A good diet is essential and if the mother is breast feeding she requires a high-protein, high-calorie diet. It is quite common for breast-feeding mothers to feel hungry between meals and they should be encouraged to keep sensible snacks to hand for such times. A dietitian may be able to offer help.

The physiotherapist or midwife should instruct the mother in her postnatal exercises and the importance of carrying these out regularly, especially to improve the muscle tone of the abdomen and pelvic floor. This will also help to improve bladder and bowel function.

The midwife must give the mother of twins extra support and help in caring for her babies as initially she may feel frightened or inadequate in what appears to her as the immensity of the task of coping with two or more babies. Her confidence will be built up by teaching her simple parenting skills and encouraging her to carry them out with increasing assurance.

The mother may feel 'in the way' if the babies are in the neonatal unit and require a lot of intensive care from the medical and nursing staff. She may also have feelings of guilt because of their prematurity and feel that it was because of something she did or did not do that they were born early. In this situation she will need time to talk her feelings through. Whilst on the neonatal unit she should always be kept up to date with the care and condition of her infants. Most units now have a named nurse caring for each baby so parents know who to talk to. If one infant is very ill or dies, the mother will experience additional psychological problems.

It is very unusual for the babies to be discharged home from the neonatal unit at different times but there are occasions when this happens. When it does happen, great demands are placed on the mother as she has to care for one baby at home and still visit the sick baby in hospital. Most units have a rooming-in policy so mothers can stay in the hospital with their babies for 2 or 3 nights before they are discharged home, to give them a chance to take over the total care of their babies and prepare them for coping at home. It is advisable for any new mother of twins or more to organise help at home for the first 2 or 3 weeks after discharge. Initially this may be in the form of her partner taking time off work. If relations or friends have offered to help, the mother should be sure to let them know what kind of help she is expecting from them before it is needed. If the parents are fortunate enough to be able to afford paid help, then they can say exactly what it is they expect to be done. There is no statutory help available for twins or triplets in England and Wales. One excellent source of help, which is free, are nursery nurse students who in their final year need practical placements in families. Local colleges of further education will be able to put midwives or mothers in contact with the nearest college which runs these courses.

The community midwife will visit daily up until the 10th postnatal day, and can visit up to the 28th day if she considers it necessary. The health visitor should also visit any time from the 11th day.

Once the mother is at home she must be encouraged to rest and catch up on her sleep during the day as much as possible and eat a well-balanced diet, in order to recover her strength and ability to cope with her family. Routine is the essence of coping with new babies and all mothers should be encouraged to establish one as soon as possible.

It may be wise to discourage visitors in the first week at home while the mother adjusts to the new circumstances. The father should be encouraged to help as much as possible.

Isolation can be a real problem for new mothers. The thought of getting two babies ready to go out can be quite fearful. In recent studies the incidence of postnatal depression has been shown to be significantly higher in twin mothers (Thorpe et al 1991). Stress, isolation and exhaustion are all significant precipitants of depression; mothers of twins are therefore bound to be more vulnerable.

Development of twins

Twins in most respects will do as well as a singleton but the one area in which they can fall behind is language. With twins the mother tends to talk to both of them together in a threesome, so there is less one-to-one communication. Inevitably she will be much busier and the temptation to leave the twins to amuse themselves is much greater. Talking to each other they act as each other's role model for language (unlike a singleton who has his mother). If one child speaks a word incorrectly his twin will copy it, reinforcing the mistake made. This is how the so-called 'secret language' of twins develops, otherwise known as cryptophasia or idioglossia. It is essential that each twin is spoken to individually as much as possible. Eye contact is vital in any relationship. If one twin is more responsive and makes eye contact more easily than the other, the mother may respond much more readily to this twin without realising it.

Identity and individuality

Parents of twins should be encouraged to think of their children as individuals. Ways to emphasise their individuality include choosing names that do not sound similar or rhyme, and avoiding the same first letter. Often parents feel a special pride in having twins and they want to preserve the twinship. This can be done by buying the same style of clothes but in different colours. Relations and friends should have this explained to them before the babies are born. They will then not be offended if the mother does not dress them in identical outfits that they have been given. The distinction can start in the postnatal ward with differently coloured blankets, or different small soft toys. As they grow up, giving them different hair styles can make children look very different. People should be encouraged to refer to the children by name, or 'the girls' or 'boys' and not 'the twins'. At birthdays or Christmas, separate cards and different presents help to retain individuality. It takes a very dedicated mother to put on two separate parties but she should ensure that each child has an individual cake and 'happy birthday' song. The twins should be given the opportunity to spend time apart. Grandparents may find it daunting to be asked to look after both children, but would really enjoy just having one child, leaving the other at home with the mother to have special time alone with her.

Siblings of multiples

An elder brother or sister of twins may find their arrival very difficult, especially if he or she has had a number of years of undivided parental attention. Parents must be alert to the feelings of their other children and include them as much as possible in all activities with the twins. A single older sibling may see her parents as a pair, the twins as a pair, and herself on her own. It can be very helpful to find a 'special friend' for her, a godparent, or teenager friend. It can be helpful if the parents arrange for the twins to have a present for the older child and also for the child to have a present to give to each of the twins. Two different small cuddly toys as the first presents the twins receive can become very special gifts.

TRIPLETS AND HIGHER ORDER BIRTHS (Fig. 19.7)

The rapidly increasing number of surviving triplets and higher order births will produce many more families needing special advice and support from health care workers. The UK Triplet Study by Botting and others (1990) revealed that the problems these families face are even greater than were previously realised.

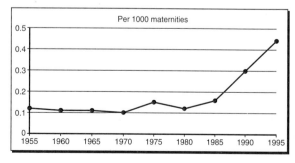

Fig. 19.7 Triplet rates England and Wales 1955–1995 (data supplied by Office of National Statistics).

A woman expecting three or more babies is at risk of all the same complications as one expecting twins, but more so. She is more likely to have a period in hospital resting before the babies are born and they will almost certainly be delivered prematurely. Perinatal mortality rates are higher for triplets than twins and the incidence of cerebral palsy is also increased (Petterson et al 1990).

The mode of delivery for triplets or more is nearly always by caesarean section. The midwives must be prepared to receive several small babies within a very short time span. It is essential the paediatric team be present as expert care will be required. The special dangers associated with these births are asphyxia, intracranial injury and perinatal death.

The main difficulties the families experience are the insufficient practical and financial help and lack of awareness by professionals of the problems.

All mothers of triplets or more must arrange for extra practical help well before the babies are born. The emotional stress and anxiety of the birth, having babies in the neonatal unit and the worries of coping with the babies when they go home will seem overwhelming if no arrangements for extra help have been made beforehand. A mother should never be expected to manage on her own. A study by the Australian Multiple Births Association (AMBA 1984) showed that it took 197.5 hours per week to care adequately for 6-month-old triplets and do the basic household tasks. Unfortunately there are only 168 hours in a week, taking no account of the mother's need to sleep!

Taking triplets out for a walk or any expedition can need major organisation, without parents having to cope with uninvited comments from passers by. Midwives can help to educate the general public who may make these comments, some of which can be insensitive and hurtful, making inferences about fertility and the parents bringing extra work on themselves.

The midwife must ensure that the mother's health visitor and, if necessary, a social worker are involved in her care. If the family are going to need extra outside help, the organisation of this must start before the babies are born. Applications to the council for rehousing may also be needed.

DISABILITY AND BEREAVEMENT

Perinatal mortality and long-term morbidity are both more common among multiple births than singletons. The perinatal mortality rate for twins is about four times that of singletons, and triplets 12 times.

Where the parents lose both or all of their babies, their tragedy will be fully acknowledged by relatives, friends and carers. However, the grief of parents following the death of one of a multiple set is often underestimated. The specific problems they face are ill understood and their needs poorly met. It often feels 'easier' to concentrate on the survivor(s), thus denying the parents essential time and space to grieve. All too often people say that they are lucky because they still have one healthy child. No one ever says that to parents who lose one of their two or three singleton children (Bryan 1986). The conflicting emotions the parents will feel and the need to grieve for the child who has died, whilst wanting to rejoice at the birth of the healthy twin, can be confusing. Birthdays and anniversaries and the constant presence of the survivor(s) are all reminders of the dead child. The parents may need help in relating to the survivor. Addresses of organisations that offer such support should be made available to the parents. Where one or more of a multiple set is disabled it is often the healthy child who needs special attention. He may feel guilt that it was something he did that caused the twin's disability and may be resentful of the attention that the other one needs or the loss of twinship. Any of these may lead to emotional and behavioural problems if not addressed early on.

EMBRYO REDUCTION

This is the reduction of an apparently healthy higher order multiple pregnancy down to two or even one embryo so the chances of survival are much higher.

This may be offered to parents who have conceived triplets or more, whether spontaneously or as a result of infertility treatments from the doctors who care for them.

The procedure is usually carried out between the 10th and 12th week of the pregnancy. Various techniques may be used, either inserting a needle under ultrasound guidance via the vagina or, more commonly, through the abdominal wall into the fetal thorax. Potassium chloride is usually used although some doctors prefer saline. Whichever technique is used, all embryos remain in the uterus until delivery. Usually the pregnancy is reduced to two embryos, but in some cases to three or even one (Bollen et al 1993). Any parents who have been offered this treatment must be given counselling, which should include:

- the advantages and disadvantages of reducing the pregnancy
- the risks of continuing with a higher multiple pregnancy
- the risks of embryo reduction
- the effects on the surviving children
- how the parents may feel afterwards
- help for the parents to reach the right decision for them
- organisations who can help them
- the offer of long-term support if and when required.

SELECTIVE FETOCIDE

This may be offered to parents with a multiple pregnancy, where one of the babies has a serious abnormality. The affected fetus is injected as described in embryo reduction, so allowing the healthy fetus to grow and develop normally. Counselling must again be offered to the parents on the lines shown above. The full impact of either of these procedures and their bereavement will often not be felt until the birth of their remaining baby(ies) many weeks later. Moreover, unlike the termination of a single pregnancy, the parents will be more aware of what could have been as they watch the surviving baby grow up. The midwife must always be aware of women who have undergone these procedures at other hospitals, as there may be very little documented in their own hospital's notes. When it comes to delivery she must be ready to offer the appropriate care and understanding in the parents' bereavement. The

bereavement should be clearly indicated in the notes so it is not forgotten when the mother comes back for her postnatal check and for future pregnancies.

SOURCES OF HELP

In the UK there is so far no statutory obligation to provide any extra help for families with twins, triplets or more. In some countries, such as Belgium, parents with triplets are automatically offered a full-time nanny for 3 years. In Britain the support provided by social services varies greatly so it is always advisable for families with triplets to apply. Health care workers should be prepared to write letters supporting any applications these families have made. In the UK a child allowance is paid to all children born. The firstborn child receives at present £2.15 more than subsequent children. In multiple pregnancies it is only the firstborn child that receives the higher allowance.

Parents should be advised to contact organisations such as Home Start, or the local colleges with nursery training courses, both of which are able to offer assistance in some cases.

TAMBA (Twins and Multiple Births Association)

This is the umbrella organisation for the 250 or so local twins clubs throughout the country. The clubs are run by parents of twins and are the best source of practical advice and support for parents expecting twins.

They also run specialist groups: Supertwins (triplets or more); Single parent group; Bereavement group; Special needs group; Health and education group; Infertility group; Adoptive parents group; and TAMBA Twinline which is a national, confidential listening and information telephone service for all parents of twins, triplets and more. It is open in the evenings and at weekends.

The Multiple Births Foundation (MBF)

The Foundation offers help and support to families as soon as their multiple pregnancy is diagnosed, as well as to couples considering treatment for infertility. It advises couples and professionals through antenatal meetings and specialist evening talks on many aspects of the development of twins, triplets and more. General twins clinics are regularly held in London, Birmingham and York; there are also special clinics held 3-monthly for supertwins (triplets or more), growth and bereavement. A telephone consultation service has been recently and very successfully established. The MBF also provides information and support to professionals through its education programme (study days, courses, lectures and publications (see below)) as well as its library and resource centre.

Preparing for Multiples. This is an educational pack containing videos, a book on multiples by Dr Elizabeth Bryan, and various booklets, leaflets and posters for use by midwives and health visitors in parenthood education, midwifery and health visitor training, and in-service staff training. It has been fully endorsed by the RCM.

Guidelines for Professionals. *Multiple Births and their Impact on Families* is a series of publications for professionals. It currently comprises three books (there are five more titles to follow):

• *Facts about Multiple Births*, by Elizabeth Bryan, Jane Denton and Faith Hallett, provides essential background and statistics with suggestions for further reading.
• *Multiple Pregnancy*, by Elizabeth Bryan, Jane Denton and Faith Hallett, has sections on infertility and pretreatment counselling, monitoring the pregnancy, antenatal care, preparation for parenting, feeding, labour and delivery, postnatal care, older siblings and higher order pregnancy. It is intended for use by infertility teams, obstetricians, neonatal nurses, ultrasonographers, family doctors, midwives, health visitors and social workers.
• *Bereavement*, by Elizabeth Bryan and Faith Hallett, focuses on the particular issues raised by the loss of a twin, triplet or higher multiple birth at any stage of infancy or childhood.

Other booklets available:

• *Multiple pregnancy and multiple birth* – information for couples considering treatment for infertility
• *Are they identical?* – zygosity determination for twins, triplets and more
• *Monochorionic twins* – when twins share a placenta
• *Preparing for twins and triplets*
• *Higher multiple pregnancies – fetal reduction*
• *Multiple pregnancy – selective fetocide*
• *Feeding twins or more*
• *When a twin or triplet dies*
• *How to get twins (or more) to sleep*
• *Individuality in twins.*

READER ACTIVITIES

1. Find out your local branch of TAMBA. If possible visit the group and talk to the parents on practical issues.
2. Think about what needs to be included in a parent education session specifically for multiple birth parents in your area.

USEFUL ADDRESSES

Multiple Births Foundation MBF
Queen Charlottes and Chelsea Hospital
Goldhawk Rd
London W6 0XG
Tel: 0181 383 8519
Fax: 0181 383 3041
E-mail: mbf@rpms.ac.uk

Home Start
2 Salisbury Rd
Leicester LE1 7GR
Tel: 01162 339955

Twins and Multiple Births Association TAMBA
PO Box 30
Little Sutton
The Wirral
L66 1TH
Tel: 0151 3480020
TAMBA Twinline: 01732 868000
Weekdays: 7 p.m. – 11 p.m.
Weekends: 10 a.m. – 11 p.m.

REFERENCES

Australian Multiple Births Association (AMBA) 1984 Proposal submitted to the Federal Government concerning 'Act of Grace' payments for triplets and quad families. Coogee, Australia

Beeby P J, Jeffrey H 1992 Risk factors for necrotising enterocolitis: the influence of gestational age. Archives of Disease in Childhood 67: 432–435

Bollen N, Campus M, Tournaye H 1993 Embryo reduction in triplet pregnancy after assisted procreation. A comparative study. Fertility and Sterility 60: 504–509

Botting B, Macfarlane A J, Price F V 1990 Three four and more: a study of triplets and higher order births. HMSO, London

Bryan 1984 Twins in the family (a parents' guide). Constable, London

Bryan E M 1986 The death of a newborn twin. How can support for parents be improved? Acta Geneticae Medicae et Gemellologiae 5: 166–170

Bryan E M 1992 Multiple pregnancy. In: Bryan E M Twins and higher multiple births, a guide to their nature and nurture. Edward Arnold, London, ch 3, pp 31–34

Bryan E M 1995 Parents of multiples clubs and clinics: the UK experience. In: Keith L, Papiernik E, Keith D, Luke B (eds) Multiple pregnancy epidemiology, gestation and perinatal outcome. Parthenon, New York, ch 52, pp 663–665

Crawford J S 1978 Principles and practice of obstetric anaesthesia, 4th edn. Blackwell, Oxford, p 218

Crawford J S 1987 A prospective study of 200 consecutive twin deliveries. Anaesthetic 42: 33

Davies M E 1995 Managing multiple births, supporting parents. Modern Midwife 5(11): 10–14

Denton J, Bryan E M 1995 Prenatal preparation for parenting twins, triplets or more: the social aspect. In: Whittle M, Ward R H (eds) Multiple pregnancy. RCOG Press, London, ch 12, p 119

Eng H L, Chuang J H, Lee T Y 1989 Fetus-in-fetu, a case report and review of the literature. Journal of Pediatric Surgery 24: 296–299

Fiducia A 1995 Breast feeding three babies at once. Twins, Triplets and More Magazine 6(3): 10–11

Finberg H J 1992 The 'twin peak' sign: reliable evidence of dichorionic twinning. Journal of Ultrasound in Medicine 11: 571–577

Fisk N 1995 The scientific basis of fetofetal transfusion syndrome and its treatment. In: Whittle M, Ward R H (eds) Multiple pregnancy. RCOG Press, London, ch 24, p 235

Fisk N, Bennett P 1995 Prenatal determination of chorionicity and zygosity. In: Whittle M, Ward R H (eds) Multiple pregnancy. RCOG Press, London, ch 6, p 56

Human Fertilisation and Embryology Authority (HFEA) Act 1990 HMSO, London

Kurtz A B, Wapne R J, Mata J et al 1992 Twin pregnancies: accuracy of first trimester abdominal ultrasound in predicting chorionicity and amnionicity. Radiology 185: 759–762

Landy H J, Nies B M 1995 The vanishing twin. In: Keith L, Papiernik E, Keith D, Luke B (eds) Multiple pregnancy, epidemiology, gestation and perinatal outcome. Parthenon, New York, ch 6, p 59

Lang S 1995a Cup feeding an alternative method of infant feeding. Archives of Disease in Childhood 71: 365–369

Lang S 1995b Cup feeding alternate method. Midwives Chronicle 107: 171–176

Lucas A, Cole T J 1990 Breast milk and neonatal necrotising enterocolitis. Lancet 336: 1519–1523

Moore T R, Gale S, Benirschke K 1990 Perinatal outcome of forty nine pregnancies complicated by acardiac twinning. American Journal of Obstetrics and Gynecology 163: 907–912

Petterson B, Stanley F, Henderson D 1990 Cerebral palsy in multiple births in Western Australia. American Journal of Medical Genetics 37: 346–351

Spillman J R 1985 'You have a little bonus my dear'. The effect on mothers of the diagnosis of multiple pregnancy. British Medical Ultrasound Society Bulletin 39: 6–9

Spillman J R 1987 The emotional impact of multiple pregnancy: the midwives' role in supporting the family. Midwives Chronicle (March): 58–62

Thorpe K, Golding J, Magillivray I, Greenwood R 1991 Comparisons of prevalence of depression in mothers of twins and mothers of singletons. British Medical Journal 302: 875–8

Winn H N, Gabrielli S, Reece E A et al 1989 Ultrasonographic criteria for the prenatal diagnosis of placental chorionicity in twin gestations. American Journal of Obstetrics and Gynecology 161: 1540–1542

FURTHER READING

Botting B, Macfarlane A J, Price F V 1990 Three four and more: a study of triplets and higher order births. HMSO, London

Bryan E M 1992 Twins and higher multiple births: a guide to their nature and nurture. Edward Arnold, London

Bryan E M 1996 Twins, triplets and more: their nature, development and care, 2nd edn. Multiple Births Foundation, London

Ward R H, Whittle M (eds) Multiple pregnancy. RCOG Press, London

20

Specialised antenatal investigations

Jean Proud

The provision of good antenatal care has always been a priority for the midwife. Working on the premise that a healthy mother produces a healthy baby, midwives for generations have been involved in educating mothers on pursuing a healthy lifestyle, not only during a pregnancy but also prior to having a family. Early consultation during the pregnancy with an appropriate health professional of the mother's choice, which may be the midwife, enables the pregnancy to be monitored so that any deviation from the normal can be detected.

Rapid advances in technology in the past few decades have meant that prenatal diagnosis of fetal anomaly has become a major part of monitoring. It has also meant that pregnancy, instead of being a time of delight, expectation and joy, can become fraught with dilemmas, anxiety and heartache, because the parents are immediately confronted with the choice of the many screening procedures that have become available.

The chapter aims to:

- distinguish between screening and diagnostic tests

- explore some of the technologies used to screen and diagnose anomalies of the fetus

- discuss the implications to the parents from a psychological as well as an ethical standpoint.

DIAGNOSIS VS SCREENING

Much confusion occurs between tests that diagnose a particular condition and those that act as a screening test for it (Proud 1995).

Diagnostic tests tell those concerned whether or not the person being tested is suffering from the disease being tested for. Because some of these tests are prohibitive because of cost, their invasive nature, or the risks involved in partaking in the test, it is sometimes preferable to identify a subgroup of the population, who are deemed more likely to have the condition. The population concerned is therefore screened to identify this subgroup of individuals who are then offered the diagnostic test.

Pregnant women are offered screening to identify the subgroups who are likely to be carrying fetuses with certain anomalies. The results of such screening give the mother and the professionals looking after her a risk factor, expressed as a ratio, as to how likely the fetus is to have a certain condition. According to the risk of the condition and the risk to the fetus of having a further test, the parents make a decision as to whether or not to proceed to have the diagnostic test or tests.

It must be remembered that the majority of women do have perfectly normal babies. Only 2% of all full-term births produce babies suffering from some form of congenital anomaly (Green & Statham 1993). Many screening tests performed on the mother are for conditions that can be corrected or cured, for example haemoglobin estimation for anaemia, whereas tests for fetal anomaly are usually performed for conditions that cannot be corrected or cured. Termination of the pregnancy is often the only option available, if the condition is found to be present, other than continuation of the pregnancy.

Women approach screening in one of two ways. They are usually quite ambivalent about screening if they have no history, family history, or suspicion of any congenital anomaly and accept all the tests that are offered to them, not for one moment thinking that they will have a fetus suffering from the conditions for which they are being screened. They are therefore devastated if the results are screen positive and are even more devastated if the eventual diagnosis proves positive. Women on the other hand who have a family history or have had a previous baby with a certain condition seek reassurance from screening, to make sure that their fetus is not suffering from that condition and their anxiety levels are much higher. They often do not allow themselves to think too much about the pregnancy or become attached to their baby until

that reassurance has been given. If the results are positive, they are devastated but almost expect it; their relief is tremendous when results prove negative. It must also be remembered that women very often accept screening for very different reasons from those for which it is offered, one obvious example being ultrasound scanning, which is usually accepted because it gives the woman a preview of her baby, not for what it might reveal.

SCREENING FOR CONGENITAL ABNORMALITIES

Maternal serum screening

Biochemical tests of the maternal serum between 15 and 20 weeks (most accurate when they are done between 16 and 18 weeks) have become widely available and are routinely offered to many women for fetal anomaly screening.

Alpha-fetoprotein

This fetal protein is present in small amounts in the maternal serum during pregnancy. It is also present in the amniotic fluid. The level rises as the pregnancy advances, normal levels becoming very variable the more advanced the pregnancy becomes.

Levels increase by about 19% per week in the second trimester of pregnancy so accuracy depends on knowledge of the gestational age of the fetus (Wald & Cuckle 1984). Levels higher than normal are found in cases of open defects of the fetus, since there is a leakage of the protein into the amniotic fluid and hence into the maternal circulation. Measurements of alpha-fetoprotein can therefore be undertaken to screen for the fetus at risk of this type of abnormality, and have been undertaken in the UK since the 1970s. High levels of alpha-fetoprotein are present in other conditions, for example intrauterine bleeding and multiple pregnancy (with the exception of monozygotic twins, because the placental area is not increased). All these conditions, however, can also be diagnosed by ultrasound scan. Not only can these conditions be diagnosed, but the size of the fetus can be measured to give an assessment of gestational age. This increases the accuracy of the test by reducing the number of false-positive results. This also helps to reduce parental anxiety for those who would otherwise needlessly undergo further tests (Wald et al 1992). If the size of the fetus is not accurately assessed, the results cannot be interpreted properly. The results are expressed in multiples of the median (MoM); for example, if the alpha-fetoprotein level at a certain gestation is known, a level twice the normal amount would be expressed as 2 MoM.

Measuring the maternal serum for open defects of the fetus has, however, largely been superseded by ultrasound, not only because ultrasound can identify and diagnose the condition by direct visualisation of the lesion, but because of the wide range of 'normal' levels which have been found to vary with race (Cuckle et al 1987, Johnson et al 1990a), maternal age and maternal weight (Johnson et al 1990b) and diabetic status. The levels have also been found to be higher in boys (Calvas et al 1990) and are also inclined to vary from day to day (Carter et al 1988). It can be seen, therefore, that only a minority of women found to be screen positive will actually have a fetus suffering from an open defect. The incidence of open defects of the fetus, particularly neural tube defects, has decreased in recent years, which may in part be due to the increased intake of folic acid in the mother's diet; therefore the predictive power of the test has waned for these abnormalities. However, there is some suggestion that high levels can be an indication that other problems may arise later in the pregnancy (Robinson et al 1989).

Because of the accuracy of ultrasound diagnosis of open defects of the fetus, samples of maternal serum are not usually collected to detect this type of anomaly alone. It is more usual to offer this type of screening to detect the fetus at risk of suffering from Down syndrome, which is suggested if the levels are low.

Maternal serum screening for Down syndrome

It has long been known that the probability of having a child with Down syndrome rises with maternal age, which is why until a few years ago screening for this condition was offered to women over a certain age. That age depended on the health district offering the programme but was usually either 35 or 37 years. At these ages, the risk of having a child with the condition equals or outweighs the risk of having a miscarriage as a result of either amniocentesis or chorionic villus sampling. These investigations enable the karyotype of fetal cells to be determined. Performed in isolation, they detected 35% of cases, which involved 7–8% of women in that age group.

Maternal serum screening, or the triple test, or Bart's test as it is sometimes known, measures a combination of biochemicals in the maternal serum and has been offered to women in many health districts for some considerable time. This test has demonstrated that 67% of cases can be detected, with a false-positive rate of 4% (Kennard et al 1995).

The level of alpha-fetoprotein in the serum is reduced by approximately 25% at 16 weeks' gestation in the fetus suffering from Down syndrome (Kennard et al 1995). Similarly, unconjugated oestriol is reduced. A more accurate estimation of this risk can be obtained by combining the two measurements with the maternal age. In this way, 45% of affected pregnancies can be identified (Wald et al 1988a). By adding to this the concentration of human chorionic gonadotrophin in the maternal serum, which is abnormally high in affected pregnancies, 60% of such pregnancies can be identified (Wald et al 1988b). Measurement of separate subunits of human chorionic gonadotrophin (free a-hCG and b-hCG) can further enhance the efficiency of the test to 65%, but the facilities for this are not widely available at present (Wald et al 1994). Maternal age still forms an important component of the test, so women over the age of 30 years are more likely to have a screen-positive result. The use of ultrasound to confirm the gestational age of the fetus again increases the efficiency of the test by a further 5% and reduces the number of false-negative and false-positive results.

It is important to emphasise to parents that measurement of these biochemicals in the maternal serum, plus maternal age in the case of Down syndrome, gives a risk factor only and does not diagnose or detect a condition of the fetus. Further tests are indicated if the risk factor is above a certain level. This level is decided by the centre undertaking and monitoring the tests, but is usually 1: 200–250, again because the risk of miscarriage by proceeding to further tests (usually amniocentesis or cordocentesis) is a similar figure.

Although antenatal serum screening for Down syndrome has become fairly universal between 15 and 22 weeks of pregnancy, earlier detection would be desirable. Various potential serum markers have been identified in the first trimester but as yet insufficient studies have been done to assess their effectiveness. Wald and colleagues have reported on the value of using a combination of several markers and have identified two that seem to have potential in successfully identifying pregnancies at risk between 8 and 14 weeks of pregnancy (Wald et al 1996). According to Wald, serum screening for Down syndrome at 10 weeks is now a possibility.

In the future, actual examination of fetal DNA in maternal serum, which might become possible, will mean that diagnosis of chromosomal anomalies by examining the maternal serum could be made.

ULTRASOUND

Most women are offered a scan at some stage during their pregnancies, usually as a routine screening procedure either in the first or the second trimester or sometimes both.

Routine vs selective scanning

The reasoning behind routine screening in the first trimester is usually associated with a maternal serum screening programme as previously described. Scanning in the second trimester, usually between 18 and 22 weeks, takes the form of fetal anomaly screening as well as confirming gestational age, a singleton pregnancy, location of the placenta and viability of the fetus.

Routine ultrasound, although widely carried out, is a controversial issue. Hall (1991) and Robinson & Beech (1993) are just some of the authors who have claimed that because its use has never been properly evaluated, that is, its use during pregnancy has never been compared with a group where ultrasound has been totally withheld, it should only be used when there are good clinical reasons. This is

also the recommended policy of the World Health Organization (WHO) and the National Institute of Health in Bethesda, USA (Wells 1987).

Several studies have compared the routine use of ultrasound with its selective use, that is, for clinical reasons only. Early studies in this category (Bakketeig et al 1984, Bennett et al 1982, Waldenstrom et al 1988, Warsof et al 1983) produced inconclusive evidence as to its usefulness as a routine screening tool. This was either because of inconclusive statistical evidence due to small numbers, or because their work was compromised in some way, but they still recommended its routine use and much of present-day practice is based on these recommendations. They claimed, despite their inability to produce significant results to that effect, that fetal and maternal outcomes were improved.

More recently, much larger studies (Bucher & Schmidt 1993, Ewigman et al 1993, Neilson 1995) have found that the use of routine ultrasound screening does not improve fetal outcome in terms of mortality or morbidity. One large study conducted in Helsinki (Saari-Kemppainen et al 1990) appeared to dispute this, but as Neilson (1995) pointed out in his meta-analysis, the conditions under which this was conducted were unrealistic in comparison with those of the normal district hospital, where routine ultrasound is normally carried out.

However, some district authorities who have tried to change a policy of routine scanning to selective use in the light of recent research, have found it almost impossible because of public demand (Proud 1995).

One of the arguments against the use of routine ultrasound, apart from the fact that its benefits are unproven, is the possibility of exposing the fetus to some potential hazard, as a result of its use. Despite extensive research, no conclusive evidence has been produced to suggest that such a hazard exists but just because none has so far come to light it does not mean that ultrasound can be considered to be completely safe. Some concern has grown since the use of Doppler ultrasound, which increases the ultrasound energy output into the tissues, has been incorporated into the routine examination (Robinson & Beech 1993).

The hypothesis that the intensive use of ultrasound imaging, plus the use of Doppler flow studies, which monitor blood flow to and from the fetus in either fetal or uterine arteries, would improve fetal outcome was the subject of a randomised controlled trial (Newham et al 1993). The results suggested that there was no improvement in terms of fetal outcome, but the researchers did observe that there was a significantly greater number of babies of low birth weight in the intensive arm of the trial, as opposed to the group having one scan only. Salveson and colleagues (1993) followed up children who had been scanned in utero and found that although no impairment was found in the neurological development of any of the children, there was a slight increase in the number of children who were left handed.

There have also been several suggestions that prenatal ultrasound causes dyslexia, delayed speech, and some delay in development in young children. This was first mooted after a joint working party between the Royal College of Radiologists and the Royal College of Obstetricians and Gynaecologists had examined the research into the safety of using ultrasound in pregnancy (Wells 1987), when they reported on a study by Stark and colleagues (1984), who had brought to light a possible link between prenatal ultrasound and dyslexia. Further studies, however, seemed to disprove this (Lyons 1985). However, Campbell and colleagues (1993), in a small study of young children, found that delayed speech seemed to be a factor among children who had experienced ultrasound in utero. Anecdotal accounts in the media suggested that other young children experienced delay in reaching certain developmental milestones (BBC broadcast, September 1996).

Further studies are needed to replicate these findings. It would also be advantageous for randomised trials to be performed, using probes which have recently come into frequent use and are placed much nearer the part to be scanned (e.g. the vaginal probe).

How does ultrasound work?

Sound emitted at a high pitch travels in a more or less straight line. At a low pitch it spreads out.

Sound that is produced at a very high pitch (ultrasound) is therefore transmitted in a narrow beam, which is produced by a type of electric gong. This gong, known as the probe or transducer, is a thin disc to which a wire is attached. The transducer transforms electrical energy to sound and back again. When the transducer is placed on the body a sound wave passes into the body and encounters a structure; a fraction of that sound is reflected back. The echo is detected electronically and transmitted onto the screen as a dot.

The amount of sound from each organ varies according to the type of tissue encountered:

• strong echoes give bright white dots, for example bone
• weaker echoes give various shades of grey according to their strength
• fluid-filled areas cause no reflection and give rise to a black image.

The real-time scanner is so called because it produces a moving picture on the screen as opposed to scanners that only give a static picture. The static picture is built up as a single crystal transducer is moved backwards and forwards across the area scanned. This type of scanner is not often seen or used nowadays.

The real-time scanner can have several types of transducer attached to it, which are interchangeable and are used according to the type of image needed and the part of the anatomy to be examined. Types of transducers in common use include: the linear array; the curved linear array; the sector; and the vaginal probe. Instead of a single crystal, all these types of transducer have many crystals that fire off electrical energy and collect the echoes very rapidly, thus producing the moving picture.

The uses of ultrasound in obstetrics

Ultrasound scanning has for some time been widely used for accurate assessment of gestational age. Women who definitely know the date of their last menstrual period, have a regular menstrual cycle and especially those who know the date of conception do not need an ultrasound scan to confirm gestational age, although many would argue that it is desirable (Giersson 1991). The case for ultrasound scanning prior to a maternal serum screening programme as advocated by Wald and colleagues (1988a) has already been discussed. It must be remembered that there is a small percentage of women in whom it is unjustifiable to date the pregnancy by ultrasound despite the fact that the measurements of the fetus may not fall within the average parameters for that age. Approximately 5% of normal fetuses lie above or below the two standard deviations from the mean of the normal measurements. However, abnormally small fetuses for gestational age could be suffering from some kind of anomaly, which could be chromosomal in origin or be due to some infection. Other factors such as maternal smoking, or drug or alcohol addiction, should also be considered and further screening might therefore be appropriate.

Measurements in common use

Ideally a series of measurements should be taken and combined to come to a conclusive result.

Linear measurements

Crown–rump length (CRL).   This is the length of the embryo from the top of the head to the rump or base of the sacrum. This measurement is only useful in the first trimester, before the spine becomes too curved, which is at approximately 10–11 weeks of the pregnancy. Accuracy is therefore limited owing to the attitude the fetus adopts while the examination is taking place. This will inevitably have some reflection on the measurement and thus the interpretation. Crown–rump length is the only conceivable measurement, however, for the very early embryo, when the parameters for norms for a certain gestation are small. Accuracy can be improved by using the vaginal probe, which enables smaller embryos to be seen and viability confirmed.

Biparietal diameter (BPD).   This is the measurement between the two parietal eminences of the fetal skull. It is useful in assessing the gestational age of the fetus during the second trimester of pregnancy and is considered by some to be the most accurate method to use for this purpose at this time, because of its stability (Warsof et al 1983). However, because the pregnancy is more advanced the parameters are wider according to gestational age. As the pregnancy advances it becomes less accurate and gestational age assessment becomes impossible because the parameters become wider still and because the shape of the head can change.

Limb lengths.   All limbs can be measured. The most usual bone to be measured in the assessment of gestational age is the femur. A short femur is thought to be associated with Down syndrome (Lockwood et al 1987). It is therefore essential that this measurement correlates with other measurements of the fetus when used for the purpose of assessing gestational age. Fetal anomalies associated with abnormal limb lengths can also be detected, for example achondroplasia.

Non-linear measurements

Head circumference (HC).   Measurements of the circumference of the head, although useful during the second trimester, are preferable in the third trimester when moulding may render the BPD less reliable. Because fetal growth is slower in the third trimester of pregnancy, it is difficult to make precise measurements of fetal age. However, when the gestational age of the fetus is known, HC is useful in helping to detect abnormal growth patterns of the fetus.

Abdominal circumference (AC).   This is measured at the bifurcation of the main portal vein. The correct cross-section of the trunk is obtained by bringing the bifurcation of the portal vein, the fetal stomach and the cross-section of the fetal spine into view on the same plane. The circumference is measured at this point. This is a useful measurement in monitoring growth patterns of the fetus but is not so useful in assessing gestational age.

HC : AC ratio.   This ratio is very useful in monitoring the growth of the fetus. The abdominal circumference is compromised before the head circumference in most instances. When both are affected simultaneously, anomalies should be suspected.

Nomograms are available for many other parts

of fetal anatomy, many of which are used in the diagnosis of fetal anomalies.

Screening for fetal anomalies

One of the principal uses of ultrasound is the detection of fetal anomalies. In this respect ultrasound can be used both as a diagnostic and as a screening tool, sometimes both at the same examination, but sometimes specifically as a diagnostic test, for example following a screen-positive high maternal serum alpha-fetoprotein result. Some anomalies are discovered during routine scanning in the first trimester and include those of missed abortion or anembryonic pregnancy (blighted ovum). Anencephaly and some of the major structural abnormalities can also be detected, so it is important that women are made aware of this ability of ultrasound, even if the first trimester scan is only requested to confirm or establish gestational age of the fetus. Nicolaides and colleagues (1992, 1994) advocated that the fetus be screened at 12 weeks' gestation to identify those at risk of having Down syndrome. This is done by measuring the area at the back of the fetal neck (the nuchal fold) while measuring the BPD. If this forms part of the routine scan at this stage, then women need to be informed.

For the majority of women, fetal anomaly screening by ultrasound is offered at 18–22 weeks' gestation. If a first trimester scan has not been performed, then the gestational age of the fetus is confirmed at this stage together with a singleton pregnancy, and the placental site is established.

By this time the fetus has moved out of the pelvis into the abdomen, so that it is easily accessible and therefore easily seen. It is also large enough for the anatomy to be examined in detail to exclude any major structural defects. Examples of these include:

- Skeletal abnormalities such as neural tube defects, absent or abnormal limbs.
- Defects of the gastrointestinal system such as gastroschisis.
- Kidney abnormalities, for example renal agenesis.
- Heart defects. Although most cardiac defects require specialist attention, major abnormalities can be detected by close examination of the four chambers. Any suspicion of abnormality then requires referral to a specialist centre.

Most of these abnormalities, when visualised, can be closely examined and a diagnosis made. Some may need referral to a regional centre for a definitive opinion. Following discussions with the parents and the relevant consultants, for example paediatricians, the prognosis of the condition is assessed and outcomes considered. These could be termination of the pregnancy, referral to a hospital containing a neonatal surgery unit specialising in a particular condition, transfer to another hospital for delivery to be in such a vicinity or, more rarely, intrauterine surgery for the abnormality to be corrected before birth or simply continuing the pregnancy.

Some anomalies can be visualised but diagnosis and prognosis prove difficult, producing many a dilemma for the professionals and subsequently for the parents. Many of these anomalies can be markers of chromosomal disease, for example extra or absent digits, talipes and cysts in the choroid plexus of the brain. In themselves they may mean nothing more than a minor problem which can be corrected at or very soon after birth. Some, as in the case of choroid plexus cysts, may disappear as the pregnancy advances but if they do not they can indicate chromosomal disorders. Combinations may be significant; for example, an infection such as toxoplasmosis may be responsible for hydrocephalus together with a fetus small for gestational age while a chromosomal anomaly like Down syndrome may be spotted through the detection of talipes together with a short femur. The detection of even one anomaly such as an extra digit places the health professionals in the dilemma of how to advise the mother. The problem of diagnosis creates anxiety for all concerned, especially the parents, and has led some consultants to question the place of routine scanning for fetal anomalies. Twining (1994, p. 34) suggests that it is 'more trouble than it is worth'.

Several studies have examined the effectiveness of routine ultrasound scanning to detect abnormalities of the fetus. Chitty and colleagues (1991) found that it can detect many abnormalities successfully, but also reported problems in counselling women. Luck (1992) found that perinatal mortality and morbidity were reduced, but again stressed the need for a well-organised counselling service for women undergoing ultrasound screening. A regional survey in Yorkshire (Brand et al 1994) examined the efficiency of ultrasound diagnosis in utero by correlating the ultrasound findings with cytogenetics, postmortem findings and paediatric examinations following delivery. Although they found that termination of pregnancy was performed for a correct prognosis in 99.5% of cases, they admitted over- and underdiagnosis of major anomalies in 2.4% of cases. Two fetuses were terminated for abnormalities which were found to be less severe than predicted by ultrasound. Other studies have produced similar results including that of Chitty and colleagues (1991).

Ultrasound in the third trimester can also bring to light anomalies that were perhaps not detected at previous scans, or have developed as the pregnancy advances. One such anomaly is diaphragmatic hernia. Scanning at any stage of the pregnancy can therefore reveal anomalies of the fetus, a fact of which the parents should be made aware.

Scanning in the third trimester of pregnancy

Estimation of the gestational age is not possible in the third trimester owing to the wide parameters equivalent to gestational age, but it is useful to measure the various parameters to monitor growth patterns both of the macrosomic fetus as well as the small for gestational age fetus, when the clinical situation indicates it.

It is just as important to recognise the large fetus as it is the small. The large fetus can cause problems at delivery, due to cephalopelvic disproportion and/or shoulder dystocia. Very often there is no cause, but sometimes it is associated with maternal diabetes mellitus. Some obstetricians therefore like these fetuses to be serially scanned in order to monitor their growth, which will sometimes indicate the optimal mode of delivery.

Small babies can be divided into two groups:

1. symmetrically small babies
2. asymmetrically small babies.

Symmetrically small babies. Here both parameters (HC and AC) are reduced. The condition usually becomes apparent early in the pregnancy. Very often they are perfectly normal, but miniature, babies at the lower end or below the normal range of measurements. They are, however, genetically determined to be small and are not abnormal. Some, however, are small because of infection such as toxoplasmosis, chromosomal anomalies or drug or alcohol addiction. Some may be small as a result of maternal malnutrition.

Asymmetrically small babies. This type of growth retardation usually becomes apparent later in the pregnancy and is said to be due to 'placental insufficiency'. The placenta fails in its ability to supply the fetus initially with nutrients and then, if the condition goes unnoticed, its ability to supply oxygen. Detection of the condition is therefore an early warning sign that oxygen supply to the fetus will decline in the near future. The abdominal circumference becomes reduced as the liver stores of glycogen are diminished. The head circumference continues to grow at the normal rate.

Monitoring fetal growth by ultrasound

To monitor the growth of the fetus, it is essential to establish its size prior to 24 weeks' gestation, including the HC and AC measurements. In conditions where monitoring the growth is desirable because of a poor obstetric history, or maternal or fetal conditions, serial scanning every 4 weeks is ideal. The measurements are charted so that the growth curve can be easily observed. Intrauterine growth retardation (IUGR) is the term applied to the fetus whose growth curve is less than was expected. This does not necessarily mean that the baby will be small for dates. For example, a fetus might start on the upper limits of normal for gestational age and yet be born near the lower limits of normal. It might retain a HC at the upper level but the AC curve would be seen to flatten off. This baby would be suffering from IUGR but the birthweight might be well within normal limits, whereas a fetus commencing life on the lower limits of normal but remaining at that level would not. However, both might be called small for dates.

Scanning for placental location

This is useful following antepartum haemorrhage or detection of a low-lying placenta earlier in the pregnancy. Approximately 20–30% of women will be found to have a low-lying placenta at the second trimester scan, but only 5% will be found to have placenta praevia at term (Chudleigh & Pearce 1983). The apparent movement of the placenta occurs because of the growth of the uterus and the formation of the lower segment. The diagnosis of a low-lying placenta during the second trimester should therefore be followed by a repeat scan after 36 weeks' gestation to note the relationship between the lower edge of the placenta and the internal os. If it remains low, a diagnosis of placenta praevia is made. Scans before 36 weeks are unnecessary as the true picture cannot be obtained before this.

Fetal weight estimation

Obstetricians often ask for this to be calculated when trying to decide on the mode of delivery, for example in cases of preterm labour. Both sonographers and clinicians should be aware that there is a margin of error of up to 160 g/kg of fetal weight in this estimation. Formulae are available for sonographers to calculate fetal weight, having obtained several combinations of fetal measurements.

Routine scanning in the third trimester is not usual as studies examining its usefulness in this respect have found no advantage in terms of fetal outcome (Neilson et al 1984).

Observational studies of fetal behaviour have been found to be useful as an indication for fetal well-being (Manning et al 1980) but have in the main been superseded by studies of fetal or maternal blood flow, which give more information as to the fetal condition. However, measurements of liquor volume and sometimes the appearance of the placenta have been found to be useful, especially if there is thought to be inadequate placental function (Proud & Grant 1987).

Doppler ultrasound

Ultrasound transmitted into the body in a narrow beam is transferred back at the same frequency when the object is still. When moving there is a change in the frequency. This is known as the Doppler shift. The frequency increases or decreases according to whether the movement is towards or away from the source of energy.

Blood flow can be measured using this method, providing the diameter of the vessel through which it is flowing is known. Uterine and fetal blood flow can be assessed in this fashion. In some units this has become a routine part of the scan at 18–20 weeks. It was hypothesised that the fetus at risk of compromise could be identified. However, in a study on a low-risk population the benefits of this procedure were found to be negligible (Tyrell et al 1993). When the clinical situation demands, it is a useful measurement.

Psychological and ethical considerations

The rapid advances in screening techniques both by maternal serum screening and by ultrasound have outstripped considerations regarding the psychological effects they have on women, a subject which Marteau (1989, 1990, 1993) has constantly drawn to public attention.

Alongside the psychological effects of such testing are the ethical dilemmas which constantly face health care professionals and the parents, not only when ambiguous results are encountered, as previously discussed, but in the decisions that have to be made as a result of them. In the first instance, decisions need to be made concerning the existence of the tests, whether to partake in them or not. Decisions then have to be made as how to proceed following a screen-positive result to obtain a definite diagnosis of a fetal abnormality and, following a positive result from this, as to how to proceed to procure a satisfactory outcome. This usually involves decisions as to whether or not to terminate the pregnancy. Everyone involved with prenatal screening is unique in their reaction to it, which will depend on a variety of differing values, resulting from cultural, religious and environmental beliefs and differing circumstances. No two people will feel the same. This is important for midwives to remember when discussing these issues with the parents either before entering a screening programme or following it when discussing the results. The parents will not have the same views as the midwife, because they come from different standpoints and sometimes the parents will not agree, for the same reason. Section 33(i) of the Midwives Rules (UKCC 1993) makes the midwife's position very clear when it states that the midwife shall achieve the following outcome: 'have an appreciation of the influence of social, political and cultural factors, in relation to health care and advising on the promotion of health'.

The offer of screening

Just offering screening to women raises anxiety levels as thoughts of abnormality are brought to the parents' minds (Shickle & Chadwick 1994). Marteau (1990) points out that this anxiety will remain raised in some mothers until the baby is born even if results are negative, but these levels can be reduced by adequate counselling, preferably by discussing the procedure with the parents, backed up by a written explanation.

In a further study, Smith & Marteau (1995) discovered that although maternal serum screening is often fairly adequately discussed with women and usually presented as optional, ultrasound is not discussed in the same way and is very rarely presented as optional, despite the fact that it reveals similar information. In fact ultrasound reveals more definitive information in many respects. This was probably because ultrasound was seldom viewed as a screening test, a situation Proud (1995) also discovered, when questioning midwives about the amount of information they gave women before they attended their first scan.

She found that midwives seemed to assume that women want scans and therefore fail to give much information, feeling it to be a waste of valuable time. This does mean, however, that many women are undergoing the procedure without giving informed consent. MIDIRS have sought to rectify this by campaigning for women's choice and publishing supporting literature both to give to women and for midwives to use when imparting information. Women do enjoy scans but there are a number who, when informed about their potential to detect anomalies, decline (Green 1990).

Proud (1995) discovered a lack of knowledge among midwives about the tests on offer and found them to be guilty of manipulating and withholding information to influence women's choice. Either they used these tactics as an excuse or deliberately practised them, in order that parents would comply with obstetricians' wishes and hospital policies, when confronted with screening programmes. This practice means that parents are coerced into accepting tests they may regret when confronted with screen-positive and/or ambiguous results.

Particular problems relating to scanning

For the majority of women, the scan is the highlight of the pregnancy; many remark that seeing the fetus on the screen makes them realise for the first time that they are pregnant. It is therefore a time of great joy. In most hospitals, partners and children are welcome, although for some sonographers this causes problems of concentration and, as this examination is primarily an investigative test, this should be respected and the sonographer's wishes adhered to. Sometimes difficulties can arise if anomalies are discovered or suspected during the examination and the visitors who happen to be present are not the next of kin. Confidential disclosures can inadvertently be given to them. If it is the practice to discuss diagnosis and prognosis during the scan, then this scenario can be very difficult. Policies within each department should take these situations into consideration and women must be made aware of the possibility of disclosure.

The sonographer. Most ultrasound scanning takes place within the imaging department, where the operator is usually a radiographer with at least a diploma in medical ultrasound. Occasionally, a midwife or member of another discipline with a similar qualification will perform the scan. Untrained personnel should be discouraged from scanning. It is unsafe practice, because wrong techniques are potentially dangerous and it is unfair to the mother, who has a right to expect trained personnel to care for her in every aspect of her pregnancy.

Seeing the baby. Most mothers regard the scan as the occasion when they will see their baby for the first time but a great deal depends on the communication skills of the operator (Roberts 1986). It is a time when relationships between the fetus and the family can become established and several studies have examined this effect (Reading & Cox 1982, Reading & Platt 1985, Reading et al 1988).

Difficulties can arise when something abnormal is revealed on the screen, especially in cases when the scan operator is not at liberty to reveal the results of the scan. The mother very quickly becomes aware that something is wrong. Despite any effort to proceed as normal, it is difficult for the sonographer to disguise the concern and increased concentration when this occurs.

When developing a routine scanning programme, arrangements should be made to deal with this eventuality. The results of the scan should be discussed with the parents either during or immediately following the scan. It is inhuman to ask the woman to return at a future date for such discussions.

THE MIDWIFE'S RESPONSIBILITY REGARDING PRENATAL SCREENING

The extent to which midwives are involved in prenatal screening varies widely. Some are never involved, but as midwives take on caseloads caring for women from the time they become pregnant until their care is taken over by the health visitor, then all midwives will, to some extent, need to involve themselves in preparing and counselling women through the process.

Section 5.3 of 'The Midwife's Code of Practice' states that the midwife shall 'prescribe or advise on the examinations necessary for the earliest possible diagnosis of pregnancies at risk' (UKCC 1994).

When giving information to women about the screening tests available it is important to include the following information:

- why the test is offered
- why the test is available
- what the test involves
- when and how the results will be given.

Screening should never be offered to women 'to make sure the baby is all right'. Not all anomalies can be detected by any one test, neither is there a test for all anomalies and some may develop after the test has taken place. Making sure the baby is all right implies that if it is not all right the condition can be rectified, which of course in most instances it cannot (Green et al 1991).

In order to advise women regarding the tests that are available, the midwife needs to keep up to date with current technological advances. This means, in the light of the post-registration education and practice recommendations, identifying areas within his or her practice that need updating and correcting them by undertaking any periods of study that may be necessary (UKCC 1990).

Information given to women should also include how the woman needs to prepare herself, for example by attending with a full bladder for a scan.

The midwife also needs to be available for women when ambiguous or screen-positive results plunge them and their partners into a period of anxiety as they try to make decisions regarding further tests and/or termination of the pregnancy.

INVASIVE PROCEDURES UNDERTAKEN DURING PREGNANCY

A mother who is to undergo an invasive investigative procedure will usually fall into that category of women who know they are at considerable risk of having a baby with some congenital abnormality. Possible exceptions to this are the women over 35 years of age whose fetus is being screened for Down syndrome in areas where maternal serum screening is not available. There is also a small percentage of women who request amniocentesis instead of maternal serum screening.

Amniocentesis

Most women are very anxious as they approach amniocentesis, having arrived at this point following screening tests that revealed them to be at high risk of having a baby with some abnormality, or having a family history of, or a previous baby with, a congenital defect. Joan Raphael-Leff (1993, p. 144) described this time as a 'watershed, – not a medical procedure, but a life event'. The results could mean termination of the pregnancy, the prospect of bringing up a handicapped child, the prospect of having a fetus or child needing surgery to correct some major defect or, hopefully, the intense relief that the fetus has not got the suspected condition. Sometimes, however, this relief is not apparent until the baby is born and sometimes not for a long time after. Unfortunately there is often a long wait for the results, a fact that Green (1990) has discussed in her book *Calming or Harming* where she reviews studies that have examined women's reactions to prenatal screening. This long wait was the worst factor that women found about this test. The reason for the long wait is that the procedure itself involves the removal of fetal epithelial cells from the amniotic fluid, which then have to be cultured before karyotyping can be done. During this time, the parents often feel 'in limbo', often denying their pregnancy, refusing to become too attached to the fetus.

The normal time for the procedure to take place is between 16 and 18 weeks' gestation, when approximately 20 ml of amniotic fluid is removed and sent for analysis.

For the group of women opting for amniocentesis instead of maternal serum screening, or where the latter is not available, early amniocentesis is desirable. Early amniocentesis can also be offered to women when measurement of the nuchal fold by ultrasound scan suggests a fetus having Down syndrome (Salveson & Groble 1995). Early amniocentesis has been made possible by improved techniques of filtration. Fetal cells can be extracted from very small amounts of fluid and used to determine the karyotype. The obvious advantage of early amniocentesis is that if a fetal abnormality is detected and the mother wishes to terminate the pregnancy, it can be undertaken at an earlier stage, when the procedure is easier to accomplish and before fetal movements are felt by the mother. Although some authorities consider that this procedure should be regarded as experimental (Wilson 1995) and the results sometimes take longer and the success rate is not quite up to that of amniocentesis performed later in the pregnancy, it can be a real advantage for many women (Vega et al 1996). The fluid can also be examined for alpha-fetoprotein levels, obviating the necessity for maternal serum screening or ultra-sound for this purpose at a later date (Crandall & Chua 1995).

Other reasons for amniocentesis. These include:

- Rhesus iso-immunisation of the mother
- maternal illness which may affect the fetus
- parents being carriers of genetic disease, for example cystic fibrosis
- suspected infection of the fetus, for example toxoplasmosis
- assessment of fetal maturity to estimate the lecithin–sphingomyelin ratio.

Other investigations have largely replaced amniocentesis in many instances.

Technique of amniocentesis

An ultrasound examination is performed and the placenta localised and a pool of liquor found. The woman's bladder should be empty and strict asepsis observed throughout the procedure. The skin is cleaned and dried and the doctor inserts a needle and stilette through the abdominal wall into the uterus under direct ultrasound guidance. This means that a suitable pool of liquor is identified by ultrasound avoiding placental tissue and the needle is inserted under direct ultrasound visualisation, so that the tip is seen to be in the centre of the pool. This reduces the number of bloody taps and abortive attempts at the procedure. The needles most commonly used are 20- or 22-gauge spinal needles or a Medicut cannula. Local anaesthetic may be used but is not always considered necessary. 10–20 ml of amniotic fluid are withdrawn for analysis, or a smaller amount if the amniocentesis is performed in the first trimester. If a stilette is not used the first 2 ml may be contaminated and should be discarded.

If the woman has a Rhesus negative blood group, a Kleihauer test for fetal red cells should be performed and anti-D immunoglobulin administered to the mother to prevent Rhesus iso-immunisation.

Following the procedure, the fetal heart must be auscultated, if necessary with a Sonicaid, or demonstrated on scan. The woman must be given clear information about when to expect the results of the test and the obstetrician may wish to advise her about her activities in the next few days.

Risks of amniocentesis

Maternal:

- Infection
- Haematoma
- Antepartum haemorrhage
- Rhesus iso-immunisation
- Fetal loss.

Fetal:

- Death
- Haemorrhage
- Abortion
- Preterm labour
- Amniotic fluid leakage
- Respiratory problems
- Orthopaedic abnormalities.

The risk factor is said to be 0.5–1% (MRC European Trial of Chorionic Villus sampling 1991, Tabor et al 1986).

Chorionic villus biopsy

This procedure is usually undertaken during the first trimester of pregnancy, although in theory it can be undertaken at any stage. Other methods are, however, more effective and efficient in the second and third trimesters.

Anaesthesia is said not to be required. Under ultrasound guidance the technique is exactly the same as that of amniocentesis if the abdominal route is used, except the placenta is located and chorionic villi are extracted instead of amniotic fluid. If the cervical route is preferred a spectrum is introduced vaginally and a sample of the chorionic villi is aspirated via a syringe or suction pump. Examination of the villi may yield information about congenital abnormality. Because of the nature of the sample a fetal karyotype is much quicker to obtain.

Nowadays, chorionic villus sampling (CVS) is usually carried out via the abdominal route, which is believed to be safer. When comparing the results of this procedure with second trimester amniocentesis (MRC European Trial of Chorionic Villus sampling 1991) it was found that miscarriage following CVS was greater. These results were corroborated by Halliday and colleagues (1992) but the loss rate depended very much on the competence of the operator and the gestation at which the sampling was carried out. It was less if the procedure was carried out after 10 weeks' gestation. The risk of miscarriage is quoted as being between 2% and 4% (Saura et al 1994). Other disadvantages of this procedure are the higher risk of results failure and ambiguous results from mosaicism, which may mean that the woman will have to undergo amniocentesis at a later date.

A study in Oxford (Firth et al 1991) reported a possible association between CVS and limb deformities. This led to further studies (Firth et al 1994, Kuliev et al 1992) which concluded that, although the reasons for this phenomenon were still open to discussion, it was associated with CVS before 10 weeks' gestation. For this reason the procedure is rarely performed before that time.

Cordocentesis (fetal blood sampling)

This technique is used to take a sample of fetal blood during pregnancy in order to screen for chromosomal abnormalities, haemoglobinopathies and other disorders affecting the blood or cells. Under ultrasound guidance, as before, the needle is directed to the base of the umbilical cord. These blood samples are then sent for fetal karyotyping, which takes approximately 2–5 days. The risk of miscarriage following this procedure is said to be 1% but greatly depends on the condition of the fetus prior to the procedure (Weiner 1988). Sometimes this technique is performed on a fetus that is already greatly compromised.

This same procedure can be used to sample any type of tissue including muscle and skin.

Fetoscopy

This is a technique whereby direct visualisation of the fetus is undertaken via an endoscope. The fetal loss rate is said to be 5% (Hobbins & Mahony 1974) and, although it was used in the 1970s and early 1980s to examine the fetus and take samples of skin and muscle for biopsy, it is rarely performed these days as it has been superseded by other tests.

Embryoscopy

Endoscopic visualisation of the developing embryo is now possible by passing the endoscope through the cervix. This enables access to the fetal circulation in the first trimester.

Selective termination/reduction

This can be performed transabdominally or transcervically in a multiple pregnancy. The chorionic sacs are identified and the needle tip is placed at the site of the fetal heart of the selected fetus. An injection of 1–2 ml of potassium chloride is given until the fetal heart stops.

Fetal therapy

There are certain conditions that are amenable to fetal surgery. These include shunting to overcome renal obstruction, fetal ascites and repair of diaphragmatic hernia. Success rates are variable and the procedures are somewhat controversial, but no doubt as techniques improve these procedures will become more acceptable and available for affected fetuses.

The decision to terminate the abnormal fetus

The decision to terminate a pregnancy can have devastating results. The mother takes a positive decision to 'kill' her baby, so, whatever the stage of the pregnancy, the parents should be given time to come to a decision following positive diagnoses of fetal anomalies and should not be hassled to make up their minds, even if the pregnancy is fairly advanced. These couples need extensive counselling regarding all the options available to them, not just about the decision to terminate the pregnancy. Some abnormalities can be corrected in utero or neonatally, although these procedures very often carry great risks and very often the prognosis following such procedures is poor. The parents do need to be informed and also to be assured of support from the professionals throughout this time of decision-making and through whatever outcome they decide to take.

If they do decide on termination, they can be put in touch with Support Around Termination for Fetal Abnormality (SATFA), which is a support association for those who decide to abort an abnormal fetus.

THE USES OF RADIOLOGY IN OBSTETRICS

Radiology in obstetrics is used mainly to supplement and confirm findings which have been made on clinical examination during pregnancy. It is used rarely since ultrasound scanning has come into its own.

Radiation hazards

The risks involved in the use of radiology must be balanced against the advantages to mother and fetus.

An increased mutation rate in the germ cells in the mother and child may affect future generations by causing congenital disease and abnormalities.

Attempts to prevent these dangers are being made by the use of modern radiological techniques, namely shielding the maternal and fetal gonads and shorter wave lengths. During childbearing years, X-ray examinations of abdomen, pelvis and hips should only be made during the 10 days following a menstrual period to avoid the possibility of irradiation during early pregnancy.

Because of adverse publicity, many mothers are worried about the hazards of radiography during pregnancy. They need a great deal of reassurance and careful explanation as to why the investigation is thought to be necessary.

Lateral pelvimetry

Radiography to determine pelvic size and shape might be indicated in the following circumstances:

- history of injury or disease of the pelvis and spine
- previous difficult delivery
- cases of maternal limp or deformity
- suspected cephalopelvic disproportion

Infertility

In cases of infertility, radio-opaque substances may be injected into the uterus and uterine tubes (hysterosalpingogram) to demonstrate the patency or non-patency of the tubes.

READER ACTIVITY

Design a suitable prenatal screening programme and accompanying protocol for a maternity unit. This should include any counselling service considered appropriate to accompany such a programme.

REFERENCES

Bakketeig L, Eik-Nes S H, Jacobsen G, Ulsten M K, Brodkorb C J, Balstad P, Eriksen B C, Jorgenson N P 1984 Randomised controlled trial of ultrasonographic screening in pregnancy. Lancet ii: 207–211

Bennett M J, Little G, Dewhurst C J, Chamberlain G 1982 Predictive value of ultrasound measurements in early pregnancy: a randomised controlled trial. British Journal of Obstetrics and Gynaecology 22: 161–168

Brand I R, Kaminopetros P, Cave M, Irving H, Lilford R 1994 Specificity of antenatal ultrasound in the Yorkshire Region: a prospective study of 2261 ultrasound detected anomalies. British Journal of Obstetrics and Gynaecology 101: 392–397

Bucher N, Schmidt J G 1993 Does routine ultrasound scanning improve outcome in pregnancy? Meta analysis of various outcome measures. British Medical Journal 307: 13–17

Calvas P, Bourrouillou G, Smilovici W 1990 Maternal serum alpha-fetoprotein and fetal sex. Prenatal Diagnosis 10: 134–135

Campbell J D, Elford R W, Brant R F 1993 Case-control study of prenatal ultrasonography exposure in children with delayed speech. Canadian Medical Ultrasound Journal 149(10): 1435–1439

Carter P, Howell R J S, Kitau M J 1988 Day to day variation in the levels of alpha-fetoprotein in maternal serum. Journal of Obstetrics and Gynaecology 9: 32–36

Chitty L S, Hunt G H, Moore J, Lobb M 1991 Effectiveness of routine ultrasonography in detecting fetal structural abnormalities in a low risk population. British Medical Journal 303: 1165–1169

Chudleigh P, Pearce M J 1983 Obstetric ultrasound. Churchill Livingstone, Edinburgh, pp 186–188

Crandall B F, Chua C 1995 Detecting neural tube defects by amniocentesis between 15–20 weeks gestation. Prenatal Diagnosis 15(4): 339–343

Cuckle H S, Nanchahal N J, Wald N J 1987 Maternal serum alpha-fetoprotein and ethnic origin. British Journal of Obstetrics and Gynaecology 94: 1111–1112

Ewigman B, Crane J, Frigoletto F, LeFevre M, Bain R, McNellis D and the RADIUS Study Group 1993 Effect of prenatal ultrasound screening on perinatal outcome. New England Journal of Medicine 329(12): 821–827

Firth H V, Boyd P A, Chamberlain P F, Mackenzie I Z, Lindenbaum R H, Huson S M 1991 Severe limb abnormalities after chorionic villus sampling at 56–66 days gestation. Lancet 337: 1091

Firth H V, Boyd P A, Chamberlain P F, Mackenzie I Z, Morris-Kay G M, Huson S M 1994 Analysis of limb reduction defects in babies exposed to chorionic villus sampling. Lancet 343: 1069–1071

Giersson R T 1991 Ultrasound instead of last menstrual period as the basis of gestational age assignment. Ultrasound in Obstetrics and Gynaecology 1: 212–219

Green J M 1990 Calming or harming? Galton Institute, London, pp 19–25

Green J, Statham H 1993 Testing for fetal abnormality in routine antenatal care. Midwifery 9: 124–135

Green J M, Statham H, Snowden C 1991 Screening for fetal abnormalities: attitudes and experiences. In: Chard T, Richards M P M (eds) Benefits and hazards of the new obstetrics for the 1990s. Mackeith Press, London, pp 65–89

Hall M H 1991 Health of pregnant women. British Medical Journal 303: 460–462

Halliday J L, Lumley J, Sheffield L J, Robinson H P, Renou P, Carlin J B 1992 Importance of complete follow-up of spontaneous fetal loss after amniocentesis and chorionic villus sampling. Lancet 340: 886–890

Hobbins J, Mahony M 1974 In utero diagnosis of haemoglobinopathies: techniques for obtaining fetal blood. New England Journal of Medicine 290: 1065

Johnson A M, Palomaki G E, Haddow J E 1990a Maternal serum alpha-fetoprotein levels in pregnancies among black and white women with open spina bifida: a United States collaborative study. American Journal of Obstetrics and Gynecology 162(2): 328–331

Johnson A M, Palomaki G E, Haddow J E 1990b The effect of adjusting maternal serum alpha fetoprotein levels for maternal weight in pregnancies with fetal open spina bifida. American Journal of Obstetrics and Gynecology 163(1): 9–11

Kennard A, Goodburn S, Golightly S, Piggott M 1995 Serum screening for Down's syndrome. Midwives 108(1290): 207–210

Kuliev A M, Modell B, Jackson L 1992 Limb abnormalities and chorionic villus sampling. Lancet 340: 668

Lockwood M D, Benacerraf M D, Krinsky A, Blakemore K 1987 A sonographic screening method for Down's syndrome. American Journal of Obstetrics and Gynecology 157: 803–808

Luck C A 1992 Value of routine ultrasound scanning at 19 weeks: a four year study of 8849 deliveries. British Medical Journal 304: 1474–1478

Lyons E A 1985 Long term follow-up study of children exposed to ultrasound in utero. In: Kossof G, Barnett S (eds) Proceedings of the first symposium on the safety of ultrasound in obstetrics and gynaecology. Sydney, p 23

Manning F A, Platt L D, Sipos L 1980 Antepartum fetal evaluation: development of biophysical profile. American Journal of Obstetrics and Gynecology 136: 787–795

Marteau T 1989 Psychological costs of screening. British Medical Journal 299: 527

Marteau T 1990 Reducing the psychological costs. British Medical Journal 301: 2126–2127

Marteau T 1993 Psychological consequences of screening for Down's syndrome, still being given too little attention. British Medical Journal 307: 146–147

MRC European Trial of Chorionic Villus Sampling 1991 MRC working party on the evaluation of chorionic villus sampling. Lancet 337: 1491–1499

Neilson J P 1995 Routine early pregnancy ultrasound. Cochrane Database of Systematic Reviews, Issue 2. Update Software, Oxford

Neilson J P, Munjanja S P, Whitfield C R 1984 Screening for small for dates fetuses. A controlled trial. British Medical Journal 289: 1179–1182

Newham J P, Evans S F, Michael C A, Stanley F J, Landau L I 1993 Effects of frequent ultrasound during pregnancy: randomised controlled trial. Lancet 342: 887–890

Nicolaides K H, Azar G, Byrne D, Mansur C, Marks K 1992 Fetal nuchal translucency: ultrasound screening for chromosomal defects in first trimester of pregnancy. British Medical Journal 304: 867–869

Nicolaides K H, Brizot M, Snijders R J 1994 Fetal nuchal translucency: ultrasound screening for fetal trisomy in the first trimester of pregnancy. British Journal of Obstetrics and Gynaecology 101: 782–786

Proud J 1995 Information given to women prior to undergoing ultrasound examination in pregnancy. Unpublished Dissertation for MSc, University of Surrey

Proud J, Grant A 1987 Third trimester grading by placental ultrasonography as a test of fetal wellbeing. British Medical Journal 294: 1641–1644

Raphael-Leff J 1993 Psychological processes of childbearing. Chapman & Hall, London

Reading A E, Cox D N 1982 The effects of ultrasound examination on maternal anxiety levels. Journal of Behavioural Medicine 5: 237–247

Reading A E, Platt L D 1985 Impact of fetal testing on maternal anxiety. Journal of Reproductive Medicine 30: 907–910

Reading A E, Cox D N, Campbell S 1988 A controlled prospective evaluation of the acceptability of ultrasound prenatal care. Journal of Psychometric Obstetric Gynaecology 8: 191–198

Roberts J 1986 The consumer's viewpoint on ultrasound in pregnancy. Bulletin of the British Medical Ultrasound Society (Feb/Mar): 18–19

Robinson J, Beech B 1993 Ultrasound ??? unsound. AIMS Quarterly Journal 5(1): 3, 8

Robinson L, Grau P, Crandall B F 1989 Pregnancy outcomes after increasing maternal serum alpha-fetoprotein levels. Obstetrics and Gynaecology 74: 17–20

Saari-Kemppainen A, Karjalainen O, Ylostalo P, Heinonen O P 1990 Ultrasound screening and perinatal mortality: controlled trial of systematic one-stage screening in pregnancy. Lancet 336: 387–391

Salveson K A, Vatten L J, Eik-Nes S H, Hugdahl K, Bakketeig L S 1993 Routine ultrasonography in utero and subsequent handedness and neurological development. British Medical Journal 307: 159–163

Salveson D R, Goble O 1995 Early amniocentesis and fetal nuchal translucency in women requesting karyotyping for advanced maternal age. Prenatal Diagnosis 15(10): 971–974

Saura R, Gauther B, Taine L 1994 Operator experience and fetal loss rate in transabdominal CVS. Prenatal Diagnosis 14: 70–71

Shickle D, Chadwick R 1994 The ethics of screening: is 'screenitis' an incurable disease? Journal of Medical Ethics 20: 12–18

Smith D, Marteau T 1995 Detecting fetal abnormality: serum screening and fetal anomaly scans compared. British Journal of Midwifery 3(3): 133–136

Stark C R, Orleans M, Haverkamp A, Murphy J 1984 Short and long term risks after exposure to diagnostic ultrasound in utero. Obstetrics and Gynaecology 63: 194–200

Tabor A, Philip J, Madsen M, Bang J, Obel E, Norgaad-Pederson B 1986 Randomised controlled trial of genetic amniocentesis in 4,606 low risk women. Lancet 1: 1267

Twining P 1994 Routine obstetric ultrasound is more trouble than it's worth. BMUS Bulletin 2(1): 34–35

Tyrell S, Mason G C, Lilford R J, Porter J 1993 Randomised comparison of routine versus highly selective use of Doppler ultrasound in low risk pregnancies. British Journal of Obstetrics and Gynaecology 100: 130–133

United Kingdom Central Council for Nursing, Midwifery and Health Visiting (UKCC) 1990 Post-registration education and practice project (PREP). UKCC, London

United Kingdom Central Council for Nursing, Midwifery and Health Visiting (UKCC) 1993 Midwives rules. UKCC, London

United Kingdom Central Council for Nursing, Midwifery and Health Visiting (UKCC) 1994 The midwife's code of practice. UKCC, London

Vega M D, Cueva P, Leal C 1996 Early amniocentesis at 10–12 weeks gestation. Prenatal Diagnosis 16(4): 307–312

Wald N J, Cuckle H S 1984 Open neural-tube defects. In: Wald N J (ed) Antenatal and neonatal screening. Oxford University Press, Oxford

Wald N J, Cuckle H S, Densem J W, Nanchahal K, Canick J A, Haddow J E, Knight G J, Palomaki G E 1988a Maternal serum unconjugated oestriol as an antenatal test for Down's syndrome. British Journal of Obstetrics and Gynaecology 95: 334–341

Wald N J, Cuckle H S, Densem J W, Nanchahal K, Royston P, Chard T, Haddow J E, Knight G J, Palomaki G E, Canick J A 1988b Maternal serum screening for Down's syndrome in early pregnancy. British Medical Journal 297: 883–887

Wald N J, Cuckle H S, Densem J W, Kenward A, Smith D 1992 Maternal serum screening for Down's syndrome: the effect of routine ultrasound scan determination of gestational age and adjustment for maternal weight. British Journal of Obstetrics and Gynaecology 99: 144–149

Wald N J, Densem J W, Smith D, Klee G G 1994 Four-marker serum screening for Down's syndrome. Prenatal Diagnosis 14: 707–716

Wald N J, George L, Smith D, Densem J W, Petterson K 1996 Serum screening for Down's syndrome between 8 and 14 weeks of pregnancy. British Journal of Obstetrics and Gynaecology 103: 407–412

Waldenstrom U, Nilson S, Fall O, Axelsson O, Ekland G, Lindberg S, Sjodin Y 1988 Effects of one-stage ultrasound screening in pregnancy: a randomised controlled trial. Lancet ii: 585–588

Warsof S, Pearce M, Campbell S 1983 The present place of

routine ultrasound screening. In: Campbell S (ed) Clinics in obstetrics and gynaecology. Recent advances. Sanders, London, vol 10(3): 445–457

Weiner C P 1988 The role of cordocentesis in fetal diagnosis. Clinics in Obstetrics and Gynaecology 31: 285–292

Wells P N T 1987 The safety of diagnostic ultrasound. Report of a British Institute of Radiology working group. British Journal of Radiology (suppl 20): 1–43

Wilson R D 1995 Early amniocentesis a clinical review. Prenatal Diagnosis 15(13): 1259–1273

FURTHER READING

Abramsky L, Chapple J 1994 Prenatal diagnosis. Chapman & Hall, London

Chudleigh P, Pearce M 1995 Obstetric ultrasound. How, why and when. Churchill Livingstone, Edinburgh

Green J 1992 Calming or harming? A critical review of psychological effects of fetal diagnosis on pregnant women. Galton Institute, London

Proud J 1994 Understanding obstetric ultrasound. A guide for midwives and other health professionals. Books for Midwives Press, Hale, Cheshire

Labour

The first stage of labour: physiology and early care

Patricia Cassidy

The transition from pregnancy to labour is a sequence of events that begins gradually. The first stage of labour, although difficult to diagnose, is usually recognised by the onset of regular uterine contractions and culminates in complete dilatation of the cervix.

The chapter aims to:

- describe the onset of labour, its causes and diagnosis, and how it can be recognised by the mother

- describe the changes taking place in the uterus as labour progresses and their effects on the fetus and membranes

- discuss the care of the mother, both of her comfort and well-being and in assessing the progress of labour

- look at the process and importance of record-keeping during labour.

The physiological transition from pregnancy to motherhood heralds an enormous change in each woman physically and psychologically. It is a time when every system in the body is affected and the experience represents a major *rite de passage* in the woman's life.

During pregnancy the fetomaternal unit nourishes and protects the growing fetus, the body of the uterus remaining relaxed and the cervix closed (Fig. 21.1). As parturition approaches the non-progressive Braxton Hicks contractions experienced during pregnancy alter to become the progressive form of labour. The cervix which hitherto was firm and closed becomes soft and dilatable and a life-giving force pervades the woman's body. Accompanying the physical changes are feelings of great intensity varying from excited anticipation to fearful expectancy. The midwife who is the caregiver must exercise great sensitivity at this time in order

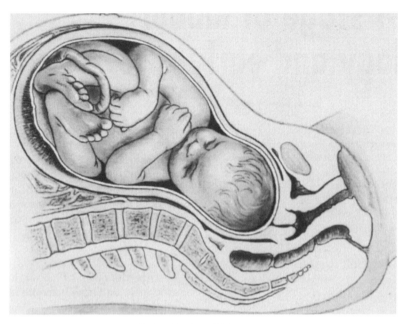

Fig. 21.1 Fetus in utero at the beginning of labour.

to meet the needs of the individual woman and her family.

Labour is described as the process by which the fetus, placenta and membranes are expelled through the birth canal.

Normal labour occurs at term and is spontaneous in onset with the fetus presenting by the vertex. The process is completed within 18 hours and no complications arise.

Three stages of labour are described:

The first stage is that of dilatation of the cervix. It begins with regular rhythmic contractions and is complete when the cervix is fully dilated.

The second stage is that of expulsion of the fetus. It begins when the cervix is fully dilated and is complete when the baby is completely born.

The third stage is that of separation and expulsion of placenta and membranes and also involves the control of bleeding. It lasts from the birth of the baby until the placenta and membranes have been expelled.

THE ONSET OF LABOUR

The onset of labour is the common pathway for all pregnancies and the recognition that the process has started is not always easy. Sound judgement at such a stressful point in a woman's life is difficult. A woman may construe herself to be labouring only to be diagnosed as being in false labour or 'niggling'. The complex physical, psychological and emotional experience of labour affects every woman differently. It is the woman herself who contributes most to the birth process and she should be encouraged to trust her own instincts and listen to her body.

Prelabour (Calder 1985, Gibb 1988) is the term given to the last few weeks of pregnancy during which time a number of changes occur.

Lightening (Figs 21.2 and 21.3). 2–3 weeks before the onset of labour the lower uterine segment expands and allows the fetal head to sink lower; it may engage. The fundus no longer crowds the lungs, breathing is easier, the heart and stomach can function more easily and the woman experi-

muscles are in good tone the uterus will be braced into an upright position which helps the fetal head to engage. In the multigravida the abdominal muscles tend to be more lax and, as a result, the abdomen becomes somewhat pendulous so that the fetal head may not engage.

Walking is more difficult because the symphysis pubis is more mobile and relaxation of the sacroiliac joints may give rise to backache.

Relief of pressure at the fundus results in an increase in pressure within the pelvis, which may be accounted for by the presence of the fetal head, venous congestion of the whole area and relaxation of the pelvic joints. Vaginal secretion also becomes more profuse at this time.

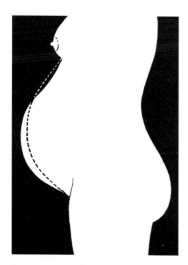

Fig. 21.2 Lightening. The dotted line shows the shape of the uterus prior to lightening.

ences a relief which is known as lightening. The symphysis pubis widens and the pelvic floor becomes more relaxed and softened, allowing the uterus to descend further into the pelvis.

In a primigravid woman when the abdominal

Frequency of micturition. Congestion in the pelvis limits the capacity of the bladder, requiring it to be emptied more often. Laxity of the pelvic floor muscles may give rise to poor sphincter control and a degree of stress incontinence.

Spurious labour. Many women experience contractions before the onset of true labour, which may be painful and may even be regular for a time,

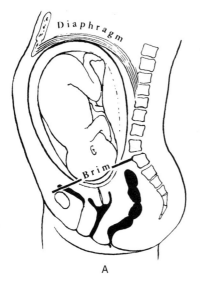
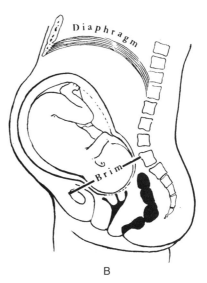

A   B

Fig. 21.3 (A) *Prior to lightening.* The fundus crowds the diaphragm. The lower uterine segment is not soft and has not stretched to accommodate the fetal head which therefore remains high. The lower segment is 'V' shaped. (B) *After lightening.* The fundus sinks below the diaphragm and breathing is easier. The lower segment is 'U' shaped; it has softened and dilated so that the head sinks down into it and may partly enter the pelvic brim.

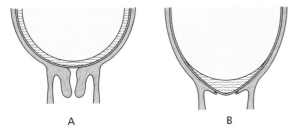

Fig. 21.4 (A) The cervix before effacement. (B) The cervix after effacement. The cervical canal is now part of the lower uterine segment.

causing a woman to think that labour has started. The two features of true labour which are absent are retraction, and dilatation of the cervix (see below). It is important to note that the discomfort the woman is conscious of is not false, the contractions she is experiencing are real but have not yet settled into the rhythmic pattern of 'true' labour.

Taking up of the cervix. The cervix is drawn up and gradually merges into the lower uterine segment (see Fig. 21.4). In the primigravida this may result in complete effacement but in the multigravida a perceptible canal remains.

During the prelabour period many women feel cumbersome, ungainly and tired. Mood swings are common and a surge of energy may be experienced. Anxiety can increase the production of adrenaline which inhibits uterine activity and may in turn prolong labour (Niven 1992, Seitchik 1987, Wuitchik et al 1989). The attitude of the midwife and the advice and guidance she gives during pregnancy influence not only the progress of labour but also the relationship of both partners to each other and to their baby after it is born (Halldorsdottir & Karlsdottir 1996, Nolan 1995).

Causes of the onset of labour

The exact cause of the onset of labour remains uncertain but it would appear to be multifactorial in origin, being a combination of hormonal and mechanical factors. Maternal oestrogen reaches optimum levels in the last weeks of pregnancy, resulting in the formation of oxytocic receptors in uterine muscle cells and opposing the quiescent action of progesterone. This, coupled with the rise in *prostaglandins* provoked by changes in the decidua

and membranes, results in uterine contractions. What is responsible for initiating these changes is unclear but it is thought that fetal factors are involved, possibly related to the high levels of *oxytocin* present in the fetal circulation during labour. Emotional and physical stresses operate on the maternal hypothalamus triggering the release of oxytocin. The mutually coordinated effects of oxytocin and prostaglandin initiate the rhythmic contractions of true labour.

Uterine activity also results from mechanical stimulation of the uterus and cervix. This may be brought about by overstretching as in the case of a multiple pregnancy or pressure from a presenting part which is well applied to the cervix (Allman et al 1996, Beazley 1995).

The onset of labour is a process, not an event; therefore it is very difficult to pinpoint exactly when the painless (sometimes painful) contractions of prelabour develop into the progressive rhythmic contractions of established labour.

Diagnosing the onset of labour is extremely important since it is on the basis of this finding that decisions are made which will affect the management of labour (Gee & Olah 1993, O'Driscoll & Meagher 1993). It is part of the remit of the midwife to ensure that women have sufficient information to assist them to recognise the onset of true labour. Contact with the midwife should be made when regular, rhythmic, uterine contractions are experienced, occurring at 10-minute intervals and perceived as uncomfortable or painful.

Contractions will usually be accompanied or preceded by a bloodstained mucoid 'show'. Occasionally the membranes will rupture, which should always be reported to the midwife.

PHYSIOLOGY OF THE FIRST STAGE OF LABOUR

Duration

The length of labour varies widely and is influenced by parity, birth interval, psychological state, presentation and position, pelvic shape and size, and the character of uterine contractions. By far the greater part of labour is taken up by the first stage and it is common to expect the active phase (see below) to be completed within 12 hours. On average the primigravida will take most of this time while the multigravida might expect to reach the second stage within 6 hours or so. In the individual case, averages can prove extremely misleading since 'The time of onset of labour is judged retrospectively and is not always easy to identify' (Whittle 1995, p. 571).

Uterine action

Fundal dominance (Fig. 21.5)
Each uterine contraction starts in the fundus near one of the cornua and spreads across and downwards. The contraction lasts longest in the fundus where it is also most intense but the peak is reached simultaneously over the whole uterus and the contraction fades from all parts together. This pattern permits the cervix to dilate and the strongly contracting fundus to expel the fetus.

Polarity
Polarity is the term used to describe the neuromuscular harmony that prevails between the two poles or segments of the uterus throughout labour. During each uterine contraction these two poles act harmoniously. The upper pole contracts strongly and retracts to expel the fetus; the lower pole contracts slightly and dilates to allow expulsion to take place. If polarity is disorganised, the progress of labour is inhibited.

Contraction and retraction
Uterine muscle has a unique property. During labour the contraction does not pass off entirely but muscle fibres retain some of the shortening of contraction instead of becoming completely relaxed (see Fig. 21.6). This is termed retraction. It assists in the progressive expulsion of the fetus; the upper segment of the uterus becomes gradually shorter and thicker and its cavity diminishes.

In the period before labour becomes established, uterine contractions occur every 15–20 minutes and may last for about 30 seconds. They are fairly weak and may even be imperceptible to the mother. They usually occur with rhythmic regularity and the intervals between them gradually lessen while the length and strength of the contractions gradually

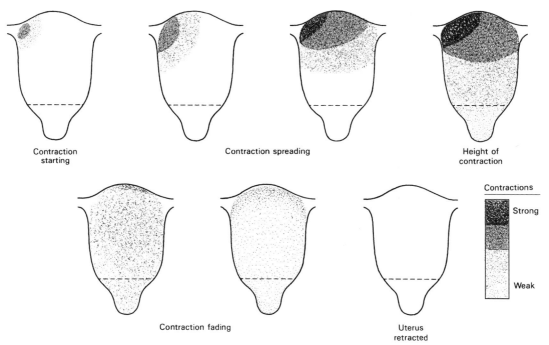

Contraction starting

Contraction spreading

Height of contraction

Contraction fading

Uterus retracted

Contractions

Strong

Weak

Fig. 21.5 Series of diagrams to show fundal dominance during uterine contractions.

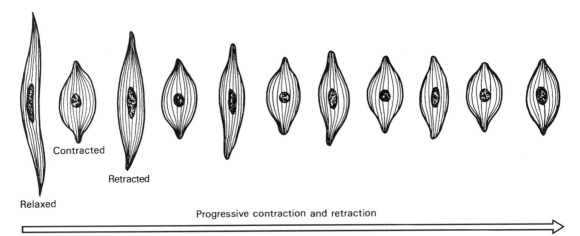

Contracted

Retracted

Relaxed

Progressive contraction and retraction

Fig. 21.6 Diagram to show how uterine muscle retains some shortening after each contraction.

increase. By the end of the first stage they occur at 2- to 3-minute intervals, last for 50–60 seconds and are very powerful.

Formation of upper and lower uterine segments

By the end of pregnancy the body of the uterus has divided into two segments which are anatomically distinct (see Fig. 21.7). The upper uterine segment is mainly concerned with contraction and is thick and muscular while the lower segment is prepared for distension and dilatation and is thinner. The lower segment has developed from the isthmus

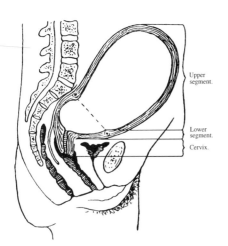

Fig. 21.7 Birth canal before labour begins.

Upper segment.

Lower segment.

Cervix.

and is about 8–10 cm in length. When labour begins, the retracted longitudinal fibres in the upper segment pull on the lower segment causing it to stretch; this is aided by the force applied by the descending head or breech.

The retraction ring

A ridge forms between the upper and lower uterine segments which is known as the retraction or Bandl's ring. It is customary to use the former term to describe the physiological retraction ring and to reserve the term Bandl's ring for an exaggerated degree of the phenomenon which becomes visible above the symphysis in obstructed labour.

The normal retraction ring gradually rises as the upper uterine segment contracts and retracts and the lower uterine segment thins out to accommodate the descending fetus. Once the cervix is fully dilated and the fetus can leave the uterus, the retraction ring rises no further (see Fig. 21.8).

Cervical effacement

Effacement refers to the inclusion of the cervical canal into the lower uterine segment. According to conventional obstetric belief this process takes place from above downward, that is the muscle fibres surrounding the internal os are drawn upwards by the retracted upper segment and the cervix merges into the lower uterine segment. The cervical canal widens at the level of the internal os

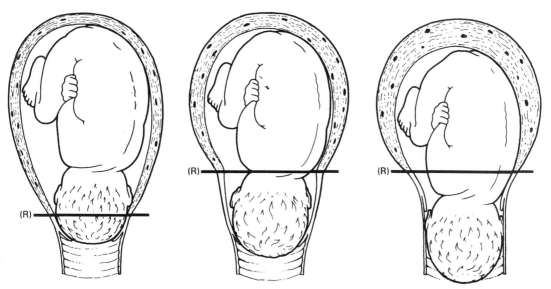

Fig. 21.8 Diagram showing the retraction ring between the upper and lower uterine segments.

while the condition of the external os remains unchanged (Cunningham et al 1989, O'Driscoll & Meagher 1993).

However, an alternative mechanism of cervical effacement has been suggested which indicates that the tissues in the region of the external os are taken up first. By an outward unrolling movement, the cervix thins from the external os upwards, leaving the internal os to be affected last (Beazley 1995, Olah et al 1993).

Effacement may occur late in pregnancy or may not take place until labour begins. In the primigravida the cervix will not dilate until effacement is complete, whereas in the multigravida effacement and dilatation may occur simultaneously.

Cervical dilatation

Dilatation of the cervix is the process of enlargement of the os uteri from a tightly closed aperture to an opening large enough to permit passage of the fetal head. Dilatation is measured in centimetres and full dilatation at term equates to about 10 cm.

Dilatation occurs as a result of uterine action and the counter-pressure applied by the bag of membranes and the presenting part. A well-flexed fetal head closely applied to the cervix favours efficient dilatation. Pressure applied evenly to the cervix causes the uterine fundus to respond by contraction (Beazley & Lobb 1983, Ferguson 1941).

Show. As a result of the dilatation of the cervix, the operculum, which formed the cervical plug during pregnancy, is lost. The woman will see a bloodstained mucoid discharge a few hours before or within a few hours after labour starts. The blood comes from ruptured capillaries in the parietal decidua where the chorion has become detached and from the dilating cervix. There should never be more than bloodstaining; frank bleeding is abnormal.

As the first stage ends, there is often a small loss of bright red blood which heralds the second stage.

Mechanical factors

Formation of the forewaters

As the lower uterine segment stretches, the chorion becomes detached from it and the increased intrauterine pressure causes this loosened part of the sac of fluid to bulge downwards into the dilating internal os, to the depth of 6–12 mm. The well-flexed head fits snugly into the cervix and cuts off the fluid in front of the head from that which surrounds the body. The former is known as the forewaters and the latter the hindwaters.

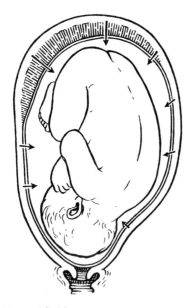

Fig. 21.9 General fluid pressure.

The effect of separation of the forewaters is to prevent the pressure applied to the hindwaters during uterine contractions from being applied to the forewaters and keeps the membranes intact during the first stage.

General fluid pressure (Fig. 21.9)
While the membranes remain intact, the pressure of the uterine contractions is exerted on the fluid and, as fluid is not compressible, the pressure is equalised throughout the uterus and over the fetal body and is known as general fluid pressure. When the membranes rupture and a quantity of fluid emerges, the placenta is compressed between the uterine wall and the fetus during contractions and the oxygen supply to the fetus is thereby diminished. Preserving the integrity of the membranes, therefore, optimises the oxygen supply to the fetus and it also helps to prevent intrauterine infection.

Rupture of the membranes (Fig. 21.10)
The physiological moment for the membranes to rupture is at the end of the first stage of labour when the cervix becomes fully dilated and no longer supports the bag of forewaters. The uterine

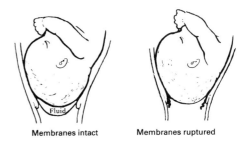

Membranes intact   Membranes ruptured

Fig. 21.10 Rupture of the membranes.

contractions are also applying increasing force at this time.

Membranes may sometimes rupture days before labour begins or during the first stage. If for any reason there is a badly fitting presenting part, the forewaters are not cut off effectively and the membranes rupture early but in some cases no reason is apparent. Occasionally the membranes do not rupture even in the second stage and appear at the vulva as a bulging sac covering the fetal head as it is born; this is known as the caul.

Routine amniotomy during the first stage of labour has no beneficial or adverse effects and should never be done without the mother's informed consent and a positive indication (Henderson 1990, Thornton & Lilford 1994).

Fetal axis pressure (Fig. 21.11)
During each contraction the uterus rears forward and the force of the fundal contraction is transmitted to the upper pole of the fetus, down the long axis of the fetus and is applied by the presenting part to the cervix. This is known as fetal axis pressure and becomes much more significant after rupture of the membranes and during the second stage of labour.

RECOGNITION OF THE FIRST STAGE OF LABOUR

Recognition by the mother
It is the woman herself who usually diagnoses the onset of labour and many women are apprehensive in case they misdiagnose the beginning of this process. Education during the prenatal period is

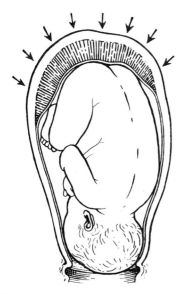

Fig. 21.11 Fetal axis pressure.

important to enable the woman to recognise the beginning of labour and thus avoid expending energy preparing for an occurrence which is not yet about to happen.

Show. It is quite common to lose a jelly-like discharge in late pregnancy but when a pink jelly-like loss is noted, labour is likely to be imminent or under way. It may be lost after a vaginal examination.

Contractions. Braxton Hicks contractions are more noticeable in late pregnancy and some women experience them as painful. They are irregular or their regularity is not maintained and they often last more than 1 minute. True labour contractions exhibit a pattern of rhythm and regularity, usually increasing in length, strength and frequency as time goes on. When the woman first feels contractions she may only be aware of backache but if she places a hand on her abdomen she may perceive simultaneous hardening of the uterus. Contractions will be short initially, lasting 30–40 seconds, and may be as much as half an hour apart. The midwife can advise the woman to continue with her normal activities until she feels unable to cope on her own.

Rupture of the membranes. The woman will have little difficulty in recognising a sudden gush of fluid as rupture of the membranes and she should be instructed to inform the midwife immediately if this happens. It is less easy to recognise a dribble of amniotic fluid and the easiest way to distinguish it from urine is by the smell. If she is certain that it is urine, she need take no action, but if she has any doubt, she should contact the midwife. The midwife may pass a speculum and test the fluid in the vagina with a nitrazine swab. The swab will change from orange to navy blue in the presence of amniotic fluid.

Confirmation by the midwife

The midwife has the opportunity to make an objective assessment of the events recounted by the woman. She will examine the abdomen to evaluate the character of the contractions and, during a vaginal examination, she can assess the state of the cervix and the uterine os. Table 21.1 will help to differentiate between true and spurious labour.

INITIAL EXAMINATION AND CARE

Welcoming the mother and her partner

When she comes to the realisation that labour has started the woman may be aware of a mixture

Table 21.1 Differential diagnosis of true and spurious labour	
True labour	Spurious labour
Uterine contractions	
Always present	Not always present
Rarely exceed 60 seconds	May last 3–4 minutes
Recur with rhythmic regularity	Are erratic
Are accompanied by abdominal tightening, discomfort or pain	May or may not be painful
Are often accompanied by backache	Not accompanied by backache
The cervix	
The cervix is shortened	The cervix does not shorten progressively
The os is dilating progressively	There is no increase in dilatation
The membranes feel tense during a contraction	The membranes do not become tense
Show is usually present	There is no show

of emotions. Most women anticipate labour with a degree of anxiety which is influenced by cultural expectations and previous childbirth experiences. Stress is an essential component of the childbirth process and although labour is an intensely personal experience each individual will have expectations of labour which may be positive or negative.

By the time labour starts a decision will have been reached about where the woman will give birth. Some women may choose to deliver the baby at home, some in hospital and some may wish to labour as long as possible at home but give birth to the baby in hospital. Whatever choice the woman makes she 'must be the focus of maternity care. She should be able to feel she is in control of what is happening to her and be able to make decisions about her care' (DH 1993).

Ideally the woman should know her own midwife and be able to contact her when labour starts. Where this is not possible, it is crucial that the first meeting between the midwife, the labouring woman and her partner establishes a rapport which sets the scene for the remainder of labour. If she is going to hospital the woman may worry about the reception she and her companion will receive and the attitude of the people attending her. In addition, an unfamiliar environment may provoke feelings of vulnerability and rob her of confidence. Comfortable surroundings, a welcoming manner and a midwife who greets the woman as an equal in a partnership will engender feelings of mutual respect, thus enabling the woman to relax and respond positively to the forces of labour (Raphael-Leff 1993).

The midwife must make an immediate assessment of whether delivery is imminent and, if so, admission procedures are curtailed and preparation is made for the birth.

Taking a history

The present labour

Taking the history of labour begins with the woman's telephone call to the midwife. If possible, the midwife should speak to the woman herself rather than to the partner. The woman's name, case number, exact location and the number of the telephone from which she is speaking should be obtained. If the membranes have ruptured or the contractions are strong and frequent, the midwife should visit the woman or advise her to make her way to the hospital. Providing that there is no complication and labour is not well advanced, the woman may remain at home as long as she feels comfortable and confident. If labour is preterm, admission to hospital is always advised (see Ch. 22).

The initial examination will include details of when labour started, whether the membranes have ruptured and the frequency and strength of the contractions. The midwife should remember that the woman will be very conscious of her body and therefore unable to pay attention or respond while experiencing a contraction. Case notes should be readily available for information concerning the pregnancy and to verify the hospital case number. Since the woman has embarked on an intensely energy-demanding process, enquiry should be made as to whether she has been deprived of sleep and also what food she has recently ingested.

Thought should be given to the social circumstances, particularly the care of other children and whether the partner is available and has been contacted.

Past history

If the woman has booked for a hospital delivery, a full history will have been taken and should be available, either in the case notes or on the co-operation card. Of particular relevance at the onset of labour are:

- parity
- character of previous labours, especially if operative delivery was necessary
- weights of previous babies
- condition of previous babies
- evidence of cephalopelvic disproportion
- age, especially if considered particularly young or old for childbearing
- maternal disease such as pre-eclampsia, anaemia, diabetes or heart disease
- Rhesus iso-immunisation.

Birth plan

Admission of a woman in labour provides the opportunity for the midwife to discuss with each individual and her partner any plans which may have already been prepared by them. An outline may be present in the case notes or the couple may bring the plan with them. Some women will not have prepared a birth plan and, if this is the case, the midwife can encourage the couple to consider any preferences which they may have. A birth plan simply means that a pregnant woman has discussed with her midwife the kind of birth she would like. Frequently the husband or partner is involved in this forward planning which should be a flexible proposal which can be reviewed and revised during labour (DH 1993). To welcome the woman who is being admitted in labour, to introduce oneself and to ascertain how she would like to be addressed should help establish a trusting relationship. Whether or not they are already identified in a birth plan the midwife should explore the following issues:

- her chosen birth companion
- her choice of clothes for labour
- games or a radio or cassette player
- ambulation
- pain relief
- episiotomy
- position for delivery
- Syntometrine
- cutting the umbilical cord
- feeding the baby after birth.

An individual plan of labour should then be drawn up, based on the woman's wishes and the midwife's observations.

General and abdominal examination of the mother

In order to assess accurately the general condition of the mother and her progress in labour, the midwife must make a thorough examination which begins at the first meeting. The mother's general demeanour will give an impression of how she is coping with contractions. If she is upright, her build, stature and gait will be evident; height and shoe size should also be noted. The woman will often be flushed with the exertions of labour: pallor or cyanosis give cause for concern.

The woman is asked to empty her bladder and a specimen of the urine is tested for protein, glucose and ketones. Her temperature is taken and should be normal. If it is elevated, a cause should be sought. If there is evidence of infection such as gastroenteritis or upper respiratory tract infection, precautions should be taken to avoid spread to other women or babies. The pulse rate is counted although not during a uterine contraction which increases the heart rate slightly. Blood pressure is recorded and the doctor is notified if it is raised. With the woman lying on an examination couch, she is examined for oedema. Slight swelling of the feet and ankles is normal, but pretibial oedema or puffiness of the fingers or face should be reported.

A detailed abdominal examination as described in Chapter 13 should be carried out and recorded. Initial observations form a baseline for those carried out throughout labour. The abdominal examination will be repeated at intervals in order to assess descent of the head. This is measured by the number of fifths palpable above the pelvic brim and recorded (see Fig. 13.32).

Vaginal examination

A vaginal examination should always be preceded by an abdominal examination and the woman's bladder must be empty. With the combination of external and internal findings, the skilled midwife will have a very detailed picture of the progress of labour.

Indications

- To make a positive diagnosis of labour
- To make a positive identification of presentation
- To determine whether the head is engaged in case of doubt
- To ascertain whether the forewaters have ruptured or to rupture them artificially
- To exclude cord prolapse after rupture of the forewaters, especially if there is an ill-fitting presenting part
- To assess progress or delay in labour
- To apply a fetal scalp electrode
- To confirm full dilatation of the cervix
- In multiple pregnancy to confirm the lie and

presentation of the second twin and in order to puncture the second amniotic sac (see Ch. 19).

The midwife should realise that a vaginal examination is not always the only way of obtaining this information and that careful, continuous observation of the labouring mother will enable her to avoid making unnecessary vaginal examinations.

Under no circumstances should a midwife make a vaginal examination if there is any frank bleeding unless the placenta is positively known to be in the upper uterine segment.

Method

A vaginal examination during labour is an aseptic procedure. If it is done carelessly there is a risk of introducing organisms into the vagina. Vaginal examination packs containing sterile swabs and bowls should be available along with sterile disposable gloves.

The midwife should first explain the procedure carefully to the woman and give her an opportunity to ask questions. In order to obtain the most information, the woman is usually asked to lie on her back but the technique can be adapted to suit other positions if necessary. During the examination the thighs should be separated and the knees bent but in order to avoid unnecessary exposure the woman can be asked to move and uncover herself when the midwife is ready to begin.

The midwife washes her hands thoroughly and puts on her gloves. The vulva is swabbed using the non-dominant hand. The first two fingers of the dominant hand are dipped into antiseptic cream and gently inserted downwards and backwards into the vagina while the labia are held apart by a thumb and finger of the other hand. The fingers are directed along the anterior vaginal wall and should not be withdrawn until the required information has been obtained. The vagina is gently explored but while turning the hand the thumb must not be brought into contact with the anus where it may be contaminated, nor the clitoris where it may cause great discomfort.

Findings

External genitalia. Before cleansing the vulva,

the midwife should observe the labia for any sign of varicosities, oedema or vulval warts or sores (see Ch. 18). She notes whether the perineum is scarred from a previous tear or episiotomy. Some cultures practise female circumcision (excision of the clitoris and possibly the labia minora) and scarring from this operation would also be evident. She should also note any discharge or bleeding from the vaginal orifice. If the membranes have ruptured the colour and odour of any amniotic fluid are noted. Offensive liquor suggests infection and green fluid indicates the presence of meconium which may be a sign of fetal distress.

Condition of the vagina. The vagina should feel warm and moist. The walls are soft and distensible. A hot, dry vagina is a sign of obstructed labour and should never be found with modern obstetric care. If the woman has a raised temperature the vagina will feel correspondingly hot but should not be dry. If the walls are firm and rigid a longer labour can be anticipated and the presence of scar tissue from a previous perineal wound may cause delay in the second stage of labour. In a multiparous woman, a cystocele may be found. A loaded rectum may be felt through the posterior vaginal wall.

The cervix (Fig. 21.12). As the examining fingers reach the end of the vagina they are turned so that their sensitive pads face upwards and come into contact with the cervix. Palpate around the fornices and sense the proximity of the presenting part of the fetus to the examining finger. A spongy feeling between the fingers and the presenting part may indicate the possibility of undiagnosed placenta praevia. The os uteri is located by gently sweeping the fingers from side to side. It will normally be situated centrally but sometimes in early labour it will be very posterior. In the rare event of a sacculated retroverted gravid uterus the cervix may be located in an extreme anterior position.

The midwife must assess the length of the cervical canal. A long, tightly closed cervix indicates that labour has not yet started. The cervical canal may be partially or completely obliterated depending on the degree of effacement (see above). In a primigravida the cervix may be completely effaced but still closed; in this case it will be closely applied

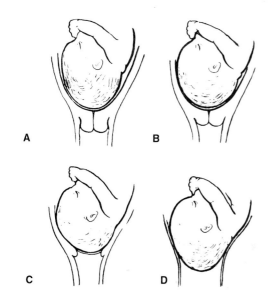

Fig. 21.12 The cervix before and during labour: (A) cervix before labour; (B) cervix partly taken up; (C) cervix dilating – membranes applied to head between contractions; (D) cervix fully dilated – membranes ruptured.

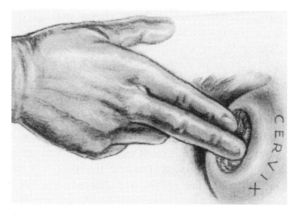

Fig. 21.13 Cervix 4 cm dilated.

to the presenting part and can easily be confused with a completely dilated cervix until the small tell-tale depression in the centre is found.

The consistency of the cervix is noted. It should be soft and elastic and applied closely to the presenting part. If it is tight, rigid or unyielding, labour may be prolonged; poor application is associated with an ill-fitting presenting part.

The uterine os. Dilatation of the cervix, that is the distance across the opening, is estimated in centimetres (Fig. 21.13). 10 cm dilatation equates to full dilatation (Fig. 21.14). In preterm labours the smaller fetal head will pass through the os at a smaller diameter. At the point where the maximum

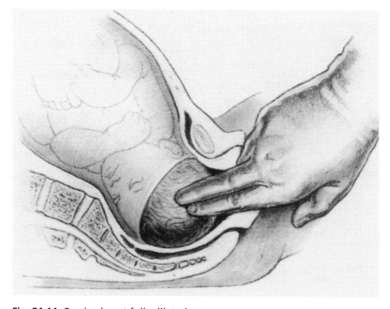

Fig. 21.14 Cervix almost fully dilated.

diameters of the fetal head have passed through the os, the cervix can no longer be felt.

The midwife should always take care to feel for the cervix in every direction as a lip of cervix frequently remains in one quarter only, usually anteriorly (see also Bishop score, Ch. 26).

The forewaters. Intact membranes can be felt through the dilating os. When felt between contractions they are slack but will become tense when the uterus contracts and the fluid behind them is then more readily appreciated. The consistency of the membranes can be likened to cling film. When the forewaters are very shallow it may be difficult to feel the membranes.

If the presenting part does not fit well, some of the fluid from the hindwaters escapes into the forewaters, causing the membranes to protrude through the cervix. This will be more exaggerated in obstructed labour. Bulging membranes are more likely to rupture early and in this case they will not be felt at all. Following rupture of the membranes the midwife needs to satisfy herself that the cord has not prolapsed.

If the forewaters are felt following a leakage of amniotic fluid it may be supposed that the hindwaters have ruptured.

Level or station of the presenting part. The presenting part is defined as the part of the fetus lying over the uterine os during labour. In order to assess the descent of the fetus in labour, the level of the presenting part is estimated in relation to the maternal ischial spines. The distance of the presenting part above or below the ischial spines is expressed in centimetres (see Fig. 21.15). As a caput succedaneum may form over the presenting part care must be taken to relate the bony part to the spines and not the oedematous swelling. Moulding of the fetal skull can also result in the presenting part becoming lower without any appreciable advance of the head as a whole. The midwife must bear in mind that the fetus follows the curve of Carus and it is impossible to judge the station precisely. The purpose of making this estimate is to assess progress and it is therefore valuable for the same person to make all the vaginal examinations on any particular mother.

Identity of the presentation. In 96% of cases

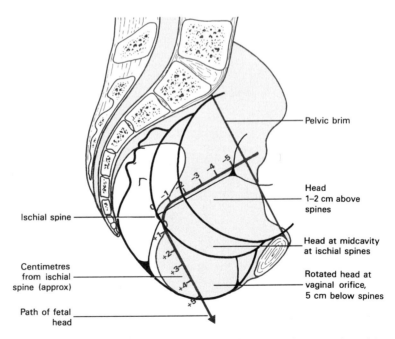

Fig. 21.15 Diagram to show stations of the fetal head in relation to the pelvic canal.

the vertex presents and is recognised by feeling the hard bones of the vault of the skull and the fontanelles and sutures. For details of the findings in face, brow, breech and shoulder presentations see Chapter 27.

Position. By feeling the features of the presenting part, the position of the presentation can be deduced. The vertex has the fewest diagnostic features but being the most common presentation is the one with which the midwife must become most familiar.

Commonly, the first feature to be felt, even in early labour, is the sagittal suture. Its slope should be noted; most frequently it will be in the right or left oblique diameter of the pelvis, or it may be transverse. Later it rotates into the anteroposterior diameter of the pelvis (see Fig. 21.16).

The sagittal suture should be followed with the finger until a fontanelle is reached. If the head is well flexed, this will be the posterior fontanelle which is recognised because it is small and triangular, with three sutures leaving it. The anterior fontanelle is diamond-shaped, covered with membrane, and four sutures leave it. The location of the fontanelle(s) in relation to the pelvis will give information as to the whereabouts of the occiput.

Moulding (see Ch. 52) can be judged by feeling the amount of overlapping of the skull bones and can also give additional information as to position. The parietal bones override the occipital bone and the anterior parietal bone overrides the posterior.

An understanding of the mechanism of labour (see Ch. 24) will help the midwife to appreciate the significance of flexion, rotation and descent as determinants of progress in labour.

Pelvic capacity. Although the capacity of the pelvis may have been assessed antenatally, the midwife should take the opportunity to assure herself of its adequacy as she completes her vaginal examination. She will feel the ischial spines which should be blunt and note the size of the subpubic angle which should be about 90° and accommodate the two examining fingers. Prominent ischial spines and a reduced subpubic angle are unfavourable features associated with the android pelvis.

Completion of the examination. As the midwife withdraws her fingers from the vagina she should note any blood or amniotic fluid and compare this with the observations made earlier. Finally the midwife should remove her gloves and

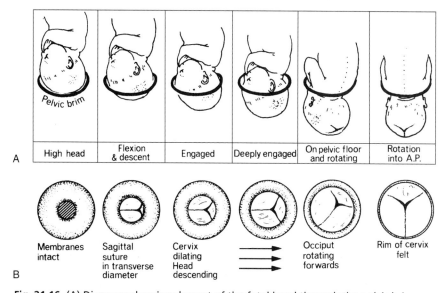

Fig. 21.16 (A) Diagrams showing descent of the fetal head through the pelvic brim. (B) Diagrams showing dilatation of the cervix and rotation of the fetal head as felt on vaginal examination.

auscultate the fetal heart prior to assisting the mother to find a comfortable position.

Keeping the woman fully informed of her progress in labour shows sensitivity to her needs and is an integral component of the support provided by the midwife. The midwife records her findings.

CLEANLINESS AND COMFORT

Bowel preparation

If there has been no bowel action for 24 hours or the rectum feels loaded on vaginal examination the woman should be consulted and asked if she would like an enema or suppositories. A small, low-volume disposable enema may be administered or two glycerine suppositories. There is no evidence to suggest a full rectum causes delay in the progress of labour (Drayton 1990).

Perineal shave

Research has shown that perineal shaving is unnecessary and does not improve infection rates. Dislike of the procedure and abrasions sustained cause discomfort for many women and detract from the positive experience of labour (Drayton 1990).

Bath or shower

Immersion in a bath inevitably allows some of the water to enter the vagina. Some see this as opening a potential gate to infection and prefer to advise women with ruptured membranes to take a shower. Others regard this risk as insignificant and consider that the comfort and relaxing effect of a warm bath outweigh the small disadvantage.

In addition to the cleansing of the whole body, soaking in a warm bath may relieve pain and the woman may choose to rest in the bath for a long time. The midwife should invite the mother who is mobile to have a bath or shower whenever she wishes during labour.

Clothing

It is entirely up to the individual woman what she wears in labour. If in hospital she may prefer to wear the loose gown offered or she may feel more comfortable wearing her own choice of clothing. As long as she is aware that the garment may become wet and bloodstained and that she may require more than one, there is no reason to restrict her choice.

RECORDS

The midwife's record of labour is a legal document and must be kept meticulously. Each event must be written down immediately after its occurrence and should be authenticated with the midwife's full signature. An accurate record of the early part of labour provides the basis for management as labour progresses.

The partogram. In recent years the partogram or partograph has been widely accepted as an effective means of recording the progress of labour. It is a chart on which the salient features of labour are entered in a graphic form and therefore provides the opportunity for early identification of deviations from normal. Figure 21.17 shows one example of a partogram which is a visual means of recording all observations and includes a pictorial record of the rate of cervical dilatation. The charts are usually designed to allow for recordings at 15-minute intervals and include:

- fetal heart rate
- maternal temperature
- pulse
- blood pressure
- details of vaginal examinations
- strength of contractions
- frequency of contractions in terms of the number in 10 minutes
- fluid balance
- urine analysis
- drugs administered.

The cervicograph is the diagrammatic representation of the dilatation of the cervix charted against the hours in labour (see Fig. 21.18). Studies have shown (Friedman & Sachtleben 1965, Pearson 1981) that the cervical dilatation time of normal labour has a characteristic sigmoid curve. This curve can be divided into two distinct parts – the latent phase and the active phase.

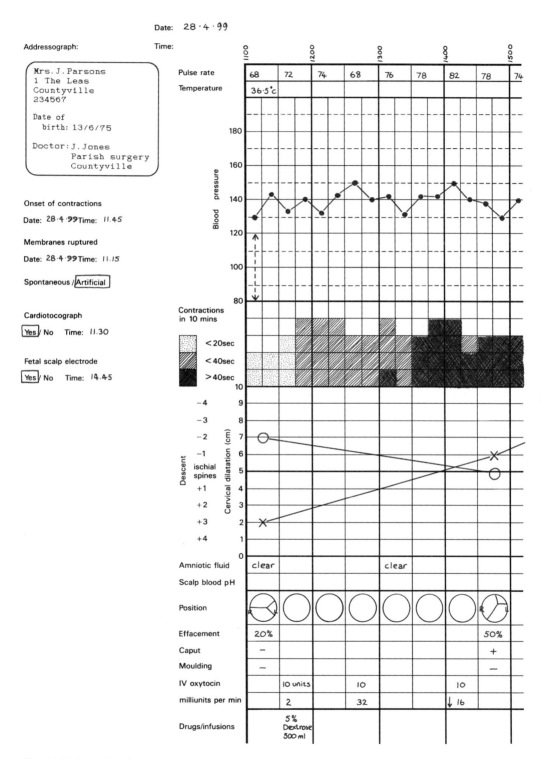

Fig. 21.17 Example of a partogram.

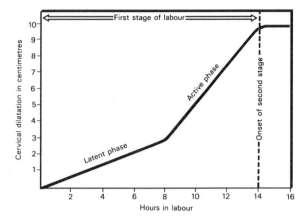

Fig. 21.18 Example of a cervicograph.

The latent phase is the period of effacement which begins with the onset of labour and ends when the cervix is 3 cm dilated. In a primigravida this phase lasts from 6–8 hours.

The active phase is the phase of acceleration and is much more rapid. It proceeds at a rate of 1–1.5 cm per hour and a rate of 1 cm an hour in the active phase is commonly accepted as the cut-off between normal and abnormal labour. The World Health Organization has produced a partograph which it recommends should be used in all labour wards worldwide. The inclusion of preset lines clearly differentiates normal from abnormal progress in labour, thus alerting staff to the possibility of prolonged labour (WHO 1988).

The disadvantage of using such prescribed parameters of normal is the temptation to make all women fit predetermined criteria for normality. The rate of progress in labour must be considered in the context of the woman's total well-being.

Midwifery record

In some cases the partogram may allow space for a certain amount of comment but usually the midwife will keep a separate written account in which she records her observations of the woman's psychological condition and any other details not included on the graph. If any changes in the birth plan become necessary, the midwife will note down how these were discussed with the woman and her partner and with what outcome. In this way the woman will feel involved in any decisions made, which encourages feelings of being in control and enhances the birth experience (Walker et al 1995).

If it becomes necessary to call a doctor, the midwife records the times and the nature of the message sent, including whether the doctor was informed, consulted or summoned to be present. Similarly she will note the doctor's response.

Medical notes

The obstetric record is shared between the midwife and the doctor. The doctor makes notes of his or her findings when he or she visits and any prescriptions made. The midwife usually enters the summary of labour and initial details about the baby.

Drug records

As well as being entered on the partogram, doses of drugs are recorded on the prescription sheet, in the summary of labour and, in the case of controlled drugs, in the Controlled Drug Register.

INFORMATION TO THE FAMILY

The day on which the baby is born is one of great excitement for the whole family. The partner should be encouraged to act as spokesman and pass on all the news to family and friends.

The person who is the birth companion should be included fully as labour is discussed with the mother and may prove invaluable in interpreting and reinforcing what the midwife wishes to convey to her, as a labouring woman does not always find it easy to concentrate on what she is being told. If the companion is not the partner, the midwife should enquire how he will be kept informed. At all times, priority is given to the closest relatives and the midwife should not divulge information over the telephone unless she is assured that the woman and her partner wish her to do so.

The midwife who communicates with the couple effectively and with sensitivity can enhance their experience and help them to feel secure and supported whatever the circumstances and environment.

READER ACTIVITIES

1. Establish a relationship with a group of women after 36 weeks of pregnancy.

   a. Ask the women to recall information gained from family and friends about the start of labour.

   b. Positively reinforce correct information verbalised.

   c. Provide information necessary to fill in knowledge gaps to ensure each individual can differentiate between Braxton Hicks and the regular contractions of true labour.

   d. Role play the onset of labour by encouraging each individual to feel her own fundus and time intervals between contractions.

2. Select a woman whom you have cared for in labour. Following the normal delivery of her baby invite a student midwife to:

   • examine the baby's head

   • identify caput succedaneum and moulding

   • identify sutures and fontanelles.

   a. Using the information obtained encourage the student to determine the position which had been adopted in utero.

   b. Explain how this knowledge was obtained on vaginal examination.

   c. Discuss the advantages of knowing the position adopted by the fetus in utero.

REFERENCES

Allman A C J, Genevier E S, Johnson M R, Steer P J 1996 Head to cervix force: an important physiological variable in labour. 1. The temporal relation between head to cervix force and intrauterine pressure during labour. British Journal of Obstetrics and Gynaecology 103: 763–768

Beazley J M 1995 Natural labour and its active management. In: Whitfield C (ed) Dewhurst's textbook of obstetrics and gynaecology for postgraduates, 5th edn. Blackwell Science, Oxford, ch 21

Beazley J M, Lobb M O 1983 Aspects of care in labour. Churchill Livingstone, New York

Calder A A 1985 Human labour – an interaction of muscle and gristle. In: The role of prostaglandins in labour. International Congress and Symposium Series Number 92. Royal Society of Medicine Services, London

Cunningham F G, MacDonald P C, Grant N F 1989 Williams obstetrics, 18th edn. Prentice-Hall International (UK), London

Department of Health 1993 Changing childbirth: report of the expert maternity group (Chairman Lady Julia Cumberlege). HMSO, London

Drayton S 1990 Midwifery care in the first stage of labour. In: Alexander J, Levy V, Roch S (eds) Intrapartum care: a research based approach. Macmillan, Houndmills

Ferguson J K 1941 A study of the motility of the intact uterus at term. Surgery, Gynecology and Obstetrics 73: 359–366

Friedman E A, Sachtleben M R 1965 Station of the fetal presenting part. American Journal of Obstetrics and Gynecology 93(4): 522–529

Gee H, Olah K S 1993 Failure to progress in labour. In: Studd J (ed) Progress in obstetrics and gynaecology. Churchill Livingstone, New York, vol 10, ch 10

Gibb D 1988 A practical guide to labour management. Blackwell Scientific, Oxford

Halldorsdottir S, Karlsdottir S I 1996 Journeying through labour and delivery: perceptions of women who have given birth. Midwifery 12: 48–61

Henderson C 1990 Artificial rupture of the membranes. In: Alexander J, Levy V, Roch S (eds) Intrapartum care: a research based approach. Macmillan, Houndmills

Nolan M 1995 Supporting women in labour: the doula's role. Modern Midwife (March): 12–15

Niven C 1992 Psychological care for families: before, during and after birth. Butterworth Heinemann, Oxford

O'Driscoll K, Meagher D 1993 Active management of labour, 3rd edn. Mosby, London

Olah K S, Brown J S, Gee H 1993 Cervical contractions: the response of the cervix to oxytocic stimulation in the latent phase of labour. British Journal of Obstetrics and Gynaecology 100: 635–640

Pearson J 1981 Partography. Nursing Mirror (July 8): xxv–xxix

Raphael-Leff J 1993 Pregnancy: the inside story. Sheldon Press, London

Seitchik J 1987 The management of functional dystocia in the first stage of labour. Clinical Obstetrics and Gynecology 30(1): 42–49

Thornton J G, Lilford R J 1994 Active management of labour: current knowledge and research issues. British Medical Journal 309: 366–369

Walker J M, Hall S M, Thomas M C 1995 The experience of labour: a perspective from those receiving care in a midwife led unit. Midwifery 11(3): 120–129

Whittle M 1995 The management and monitoring of labour. In: Chamberlain G (ed) Turnbull's obstetrics, 2nd edn. Churchill Livingstone, New York, ch 30

World Health Organization 1988 The partograph: a managerial tool for the prevention of prolonged labour.

Section I: The principle and strategy. Section II: A user's manual. WHO/MCH/88.3 and WHO/MCH/88.4. WHO, Geneva

Wuitchik M, Bakal D, Lipshitz J 1989 The clinical significance of pain and cognitive activity in latent labour. Obstetrics and Gynecology 73(1): 25–41

FURTHER READING

Albers L L, Krulewitch C J, Lydon-Rochelle M T 1995 Maternal age and labor complications in healthy primigravidas at term. Journal of Nurse-Midwifery 40(1): 4–12

Bastian H 1992 Confined, managed and delivered: the language of obstetrics. British Journal of Obstetrics and Gynaecology 99: 92–93

Belbin A 1996 Power and choice in birthgiving: a case study. British Journal of Midwifery 4(5): 264–267

Clinical Standards Advisory Group 1995 Women in normal labour: report of a CSAG committee on women in normal labour. HMSO, London

Dodds R, Goodman M, Tyler S (eds) 1996 Listen with mother (consulting users of maternity services). Books for Midwives Press, Cheshire

Middle C, Macfarlane A 1995 Labour and delivery of 'normal' primiparous women: analysis of routinely collected data. British Journal of Obstetrics and Gynaecology 102: 970–977

Nelki J, Bond L 1995 Positions in labour: a plea for flexibility.

Modern Midwife (Feb): 19–22

Philpott R H, Castle W M 1972 Cervicographs in the management of labour in primigravidae I. The alert line for detecting abnormal labour and II. The action line and treatment of abnormal labour. Journal of Obstetrics and Gynaecology of the British Commonwealth 79: 592–598 and 599–602

Robinson S, Thomson M (eds) 1994 Midwives, research and childbirth. Chapman & Hall, London, vol 3

Rothwell H 1995 Medicalisation of childbirth. British Journal of Midwifery 3(6): 318–322

Steele R 1995 Midwifery care during the first stage of labour. In: Alexander J, Levy V, Roch S (eds) Aspects of midwifery practice: a research-based approach. Macmillan, Basingstoke, ch 2

Tew M 1995 Safer childbirth?, 2nd edn. Chapman & Hall, London

Watson V 1994 Maternal position in the second stage of labour. Modern Midwife (July): 21–24

Management of the first stage of labour

22

Patricia Cassidy

It is the responsibility of the midwife to ensure the safety of the milieu within which women labour and give birth. Emotional support, physical care and clinical skills are equally important to ensure a satisfactory outcome for mother and baby.

The chapter aims to:

- stress the importance to the woman of comfort, companionship and privacy during labour

- discuss the care of the woman with particular reference to safety and emotional support

- describe the process of monitoring both the progress of labour and the condition of the mother and fetus

- consider the active management of labour and the management of preterm labour.

Labour, the culmination of pregnancy, is an event with great psychological, social and emotional meaning for the mother and her family. In addition, the woman may experience stress and physical pain, and danger may lurk around the corner. The midwife who is the caregiver should display tact and sensitivity, respect the needs of the individual and provide an environment within which each woman can labour and give birth with dignity.

ENVIRONMENT

Women may choose to give birth in their own home where they control the environment and feel comfortable in their own surroundings, or they may wish the security of a hospital birth where facilities are readily available for prompt and efficient action should an emergency arise. Soft furnishings, the use of colour and the arrangement of furniture can help to soften a hospital atmosphere with its implications of sickness and institutional rules. The attitude of the staff, however, is much more important than physical surroundings. Anxiety will affect the mother's perception and understanding (Ball 1994, Niven 1992), therefore it is essential that the labouring woman is welcomed and encouraged to feel at ease and that the midwife spends time actively listening as the woman recounts the details of the onset of labour. A trusting atmosphere between a woman and her caregivers, a feeling of being among friends and a knowledge of the skills required to cope with the stresses of labour set the scene for a positive childbirth experience (Crowe & von Baeyer 1989, Kitzinger 1985, Raphael-Leff 1993).

EMOTIONAL SUPPORT

The midwife has a traditional role to fulfil, that is being 'with woman' by monitoring the progress of labour and assessing the physical status of mother and fetus. In addition, emotional support is provided by exercising skill in imparting confidence, expressing caring and dependability and being an advocate for the childbearing woman. The midwife should display a tolerant non-judgemental attitude, ensuring that the woman is accepted whatever her reactions and behaviour may be. Women who feel in control of their own bodies, who retain control of their behaviour and who feel they have an active part in decision-making have a more satisfactory birth experience (Green et al 1990).

Companion in labour

Research has shown that continuous one-to-one support of a woman during labour creates a strong feeling of security and satisfaction (Ball 1994, Hodnett & Osborn 1989a,b) and is associated with a reduction in the length of labour, fewer perinatal complications and a reduced incidence of oxytocin augmentation (Klaus et al 1986). The woman herself is the one who cares most about her baby and therefore she is central to all the decisions made about care during labour. Her chosen companion, whether sexual partner, friend or family member, should understand this. Ideally he or she would be involved in prelabour preparation and decision-making, have participated in compiling a birth plan

and have contingency plans drawn up in the event of everything not remaining straightforward. Admission to hospital is always a traumatic experience and the company of a supportive companion can help reduce anxiety. During labour the companion can keep the woman company, walk with her if she is ambulant in early labour, support her decisions about pain relief and encourage her with breathing techniques. Providing encouragement and reassurance that labour is progressing is also important, as is helping with physical comfort such as back-rubbing or providing cool cloths or sips of water. The midwife may have to double as the companion since not all women are glad to have a husband or companion present. In some areas a midwife will be assigned to a particular woman and remain with her through her entire labour.

The companion must be encouraged to attend to his (or her) own need for rest and refreshment so that he or she has the necessary stamina to see the labour right through. The midwife should assess events and advise the companion as to the best time to take a break.

The midwife should appreciate that the companion may need direct support at times. This is particularly evident when a sudden emergency develops. If, for instance, a caesarean section becomes necessary, the midwife must delegate someone to keep the companion fully informed and ensure that he or she is not abandoned and left uncared for.

Explanation

Midwives must also provide support by giving information which encompasses ensuring that the woman understands events, feels free to ask questions and is aware of how labour is progressing. Before performing an examination, explanations should be given of what is about to be done and why. Following the procedure, the midwife should provide feedback on progress and verbal reinforcement that the woman is capable of managing her own labour, and involve both woman and companion if decisions have to be made about care (Fleissig 1993, Steele 1995).

Privacy

An unfamiliar setting, the presence of strangers and too many people entering and leaving the room increase stress for the woman, her partner and the midwife. To ensure privacy, individuals should knock before entering, be introduced to all in the room and give an explanation for their presence. Equally, the woman has a right to remain alone with her partner if she so wishes and the midwife considers it safe for both mother and fetus.

PREVENTION OF INFECTION

The very nature of the care given during labour may expose both mother and fetus to the risk of infection. The midwife has a responsibility to acquaint herself with the risks, prepare the woman physically during the antenatal period and be scrupulous in her attention to hygiene and asepsis in order to prevent infection occurring.

Mother's well-being during pregnancy

Sound general health is one of the best measures available to resist infection. Antenatal care aims to build up resistance and encourage a healthy lifestyle mainly through education. Information about diet, exercise and hygiene all contribute (see Ch. 12). Socioeconomic deprivation is one of the biggest impediments to antenatal health.

Factors affecting resistance

The blood. The haemoglobin level should be adequate and anaemia should be corrected if necessary. White blood cells are needed to fight invading organisms and usually their ability to do so correlates with general health and absence of fatigue.

Nutritional status. In developed countries nutritional status is usually fairly good, although poverty may lead to malnutrition. This may result as much from eating an unwise selection of foods as from being too hard up to buy food. Education in using economical yet nutritious foods, including how to prepare them, may be an invaluable contribution from the midwife.

The skin and membranes. An intact skin provides an excellent barrier to organisms and it is important to protect its integrity. This involves the avoidance of surgical wounds whenever possible,

including perineal lacerations and episiotomy. The fetal membranes should also be preserved intact unless there is a positive indication for their rupture which would outweigh the advantage of their protective functions (Thornton & Lilford 1994).

Hygiene. A clean body and environment will reduce the organisms which have access to the mother. This implies the need for barrier methods to be used when caring for women with any transmissible infection such as gastroenteritis, hepatitis or human immunodeficiency virus (HIV) infection.

Rest. A tired, exhausted woman will not be able to combat infection and if the mother has been deprived of sleep and rest prior to admission or during labour, the midwife may need to create an opportunity for sleeping, if necessary by offering a mild sedative drug.

The avoidance of prolonged labour is an important factor in preventing infection.

General hygiene and care of the environment

Hospitals are notorious sources of infection which can be resistant to antibiotic treatment. A modern maternity unit should be constructed so as to limit the spread of such infection. It should be sited at a distance from any source of pathogenic organisms and should be designed for easy and effective cleaning and in a way which will reduce the transfer of airborne organisms. Traffic in and out of a delivery unit should be restricted to people having direct business there and individual rooms should be treated on the same basis. Baths, sinks and toilets should be scrupulously cleaned and disinfected between users as necessary. Beds and rooms are also cleaned thoroughly after use. It is the responsibility of the midwife to ensure that high standards of cleanliness are maintained even if she does not have managerial control over domestic services.

Personal hygiene is important for both mothers and their attendants. The woman should be encouraged to bathe and wash as necessary to maintain personal freshness and the midwife must wash her hands before and after examining the mother and wear gloves when handling used sanitary pads, bloodstained linen or body fluids. The midwife will wish to pay particular attention to her own hygiene as she is in close proximity to the woman and is working in a very warm environment.

Asepsis and antisepsis

A woman's perineal area is bound to be contaminated and procedures such as vaginal examination and delivery itself can never be completely sterile. However, the midwife must always use sterile equipment and aseptic technique in order to avoid introducing foreign organisms into the genital tract.

Restriction of invasive techniques

Certain invasive techniques, such as the performance of vaginal examinations, are necessary during labour but the midwife should aim to reduce these to a minimum and ensure that she has a sound reason before embarking on a procedure. Women whose labours are prolonged are at particular risk of infection and are often subjected to a number of invasive procedures including the administration of intravenous fluids. Where progress in labour is slow and it is necessary to involve a doctor, the midwife can avoid a vaginal examination being duplicated by inviting the doctor to do it in the first instance.

POSITION AND MOBILITY

The adoption of the upright position during labour will facilitate efficient uterine contractions, shorten the latent phase and reduce the need for analgesia (Andrews & Chrzanowski 1990, Kakol 1989). Flexibility during labour allows the mother to seek and find the position most suited to her. She may walk about, rock, adopt a kneeling position or squat. The all-fours position may be comfortable if the fetus is in an occipitoposterior position as it relieves the associated backache. Midwives should accommodate the mother's wish to choose her own position remembering that, if a recumbent position is adopted, compression of the inferior vena cava may occur with consequent supine hypotension. Therefore, if the mother wishes to lie down, a lateral position is preferable and this allows the midwife to auscultate the fetal heart and monitor uterine contractions.

Other factors governing choice

Analgesia. If the mother has accepted or requested narcotic analgesia, she will be unable to walk around because she will be unsteady on her feet after receiving the narcotic. A lateral position or supported sitting is suitable.

Epidural analgesia normally demands that a woman should be in bed either sitting up or lying on her side. In some centres a combined spinal epidural block is now available which allows women to walk about during labour (Morgan & Kadim 1994) (see Ch. 23).

Monitoring. The use of a cardiotocograph may appear to limit the choice of position. A telemetric apparatus allows the woman to walk around freely, provided that she remains within a given range. A conventional cardiotocograph does not necessarily confine the woman to bed but accurate external monitoring of uterine contractions may be difficult if she is very mobile.

Fetal condition. The supine position allows the uterus to compress the inferior vena cava, resulting in maternal hypotension. This not only reduces placental blood flow and thereby fetal oxygenation but also inhibits effective uterine action. More upright positions or a lateral position are to be preferred.

Intravenous infusion. The siting of an intravenous infusion should not in itself prevent mobility as the mother may walk around with a drip stand. The midwife should, however, take account of the reason for the infusion as this may influence the choice of position.

Complications. A woman who has had an antepartum haemorrhage or who has ruptured membranes when the fetal head is still high will be confined to bed.

NUTRITION

Advice prior to admission

The woman's need in labour is for energy and it is carbohydrate that will provide it. Foods such as toast, breakfast cereal, yogurt, fruit juice, tea, plain biscuits and clear broth are easily digested. Ice cream and jelly may also be refreshing. Fluids may be taken freely although women tend to reduce their drinking as labour progresses (Roberts & Ludka 1994).

Intake in early labour

Opinions are divided and policies vary between hospitals. In many units, when there is little risk of the woman needing a general anaesthetic, she may take a low-fat, low-residue diet according to appetite, in order to give her energy and ensure that she is not hungry. However, in some centres, women receive nothing to eat after labour is established and are allowed only ice chips to suck. The latter policy stems from 'the widespread concern that eating and drinking during labour will put women at an increased and unacceptable risk of regurgitation and aspiration of gastric contents' (Johnson et al 1989, p. 827). Aspirated contents from the stomach may contain undigested food and predispose to airway obstruction; if fasting, the strongly acidic gastric juice can cause a chemical pneumonitis if inhaled (Mendelson's syndrome). The cardiac sphincter, rendered inefficient by the effects of progesterone, allows a passive leak of stomach contents into the pharynx when loss of consciousness is induced with general anaesthesia. This, combined with the oedema of the pharynx so often present in pregnancy, makes intubation by the anaesthetist a difficult procedure.

Different foods and fluids empty from the stomach at different rates and gastric emptying is prolonged following the administration of narcotic analgesia. Johnson and colleagues point out that there is, however, 'no guarantee that withholding food and drink during labour will ensure that the stomach will be empty in the event that general anaesthesia should become necessary' (p. 829). In an effort to reduce gastric volume and decrease the gastric acidity of the labouring woman, prophylactic antacids may be administered (see Ch. 28).

Glycogenic and fluid requirements

The vigorous muscle contractions of the uterus during labour demand a continuous supply of glucose. If this is not obtained from the diet, the body will start to metabolise protein and fat stores in an effort to provide glucose (gluconeogenesis) without which uterine muscle inertia will occur. This relatively inefficient method of producing glucose results in the occurrence of ketoacidosis. If no food is allowed, an intravenous infusion may be sited to correct the homeostatic imbalance by providing glucose and fluids. Care must be taken to assess the individual's needs and to avoid maternal fluid overload. High concentrations of glucose may artificially increase fetal blood glucose levels, thereby causing fetal hyperinsulinism (Lowe & Reiss 1996, Steele 1995).

Comfort

If the woman is permitted to follow her inclinations for drinks she is unlikely to become dehydrated. Simple measures such as brushing her teeth or using a mouthwash can help relieve the discomfort of a dry and uncomfortable mouth.

BLADDER CARE

The woman should be encouraged to empty her bladder every 1½–2 hours during labour. The midwife should not rely on the mother to request to use the toilet as the sensation of needing to micturate may be reduced, particularly if there is an effective epidural block in progress. If the woman is ambulant she may visit the toilet; the quantity of urine passed should be measured and a specimen obtained for testing. If the woman expresses a desire to defaecate, she may be confusing the sensation with that of imminent delivery.

A full bladder may initially prevent the fetal head from entering the pelvic brim and later impede descent of the fetal head. It will also inhibit effective uterine action. In all cases of delay in labour the midwife should ascertain whether the bladder is full and encourage the woman to empty it. If the bladder remains full, the bladder neck can become nipped between the fetal head and the symphysis pubis. This may give rise to bruising which can slough during the puerperium, leaving a vesicovaginal fistula.

Retention of urine. Urinary retention in labour may occur in association with hypotonic uterine action. A woman who is unable to visit the toilet may find it difficult to empty her bladder into a bedpan. The midwife should provide privacy and ensure maximum comfort by placing the bedpan on a stool or chair or letting the woman adopt a squatting position on the bed. The sound or feel of water can also help to trigger the micturition reflex. If the bladder is incompletely emptied or the woman is unable to void for some hours it will become necessary to pass a catheter.

Catheterisation. A plastic disposable catheter is used. If difficulty is encountered while introducing the catheter, the sterile, gloved forefinger of the non-dominant hand should be inserted into the vagina and placed along its anterior wall. The tip of the catheter can then be felt and if it is directed parallel with the finger in the vagina, the catheter will enter the bladder without injury to the urethra. If the catheter is obstructed by the fetal head, upward pressure on the head by the finger in the vagina will permit passage of the catheter.

OBSERVATIONS

Mother

Reaction to labour

As with other life events, women vary in their reactions to labour. Some may view the contractions experienced as a positive, motivating, life-giving force. Others may feel them as pain and resist them. One woman may welcome the event with excitement because soon she will see her baby, another may be glad the pregnancy is over and with it the cumbersome ungainliness she experienced. However she views labour, the preparatory phase of pregnancy is at an end and within a relatively short period a baby will be born. There may be feelings of apprehension and fear in case she does not conform to the social expectations of her culture, anxiety in case the experience is painful and concern about her ability to control pain (Niven 1992). As labour progresses she may feel less confident in her ability to cope with the relentless nature of the contractions which control her body. The midwife, with her skilful observations, can do much to encourage and help the mother whose

expectation is 'to be sustained by another human being, to have relief from pain, to have a safe outcome for self and fetus, to have attitudes and behaviour accepted and to receive bodily care' (Mackey & Lock 1989).

If the midwife concentrates her attention on the woman, she can help to absorb and deflect some of her anxieties. Accurate and easy to understand information about the progress of labour will provide encouragement and consultation about methods of pain relief will increase feelings of being in control (Ball 1994, Lovell 1996). The management of pain is discussed in Chapter 23.

Vital signs

Pulse rate. A steady pulse rate is an indication that the woman is in good condition. If the rate increases to more than 100 beats per minute it may be indicative of infection, ketosis or haemorrhage. A rising pulse rate is also a key sign of a ruptured uterus (see Ch. 29).

It is usual to record the pulse rate every 1 or 2 hours during early labour and every 15–30 minutes when labour is more advanced.

Temperature. This should remain within the normal range. Pyrexia is indicative of infection or ketosis. Temperature should be recorded every 4 hours.

Blood pressure is measured every 4 hours unless it is abnormal, when more frequent recordings are necessary. The blood pressure must be monitored very closely following the instillation of local anaesthetic into the epidural space (see Ch. 28).

The effect of labour may be to further elevate a raised blood pressure and the midwife must bear this in mind when caring for a woman who has had pre-eclampsia or essential hypertension during pregnancy. Hypotension may be caused by the supine position, shock or as a result of epidural anaesthesia.

Urinalysis

All urine passed during labour must be tested for glucose, ketones and protein. Ketones may occur as a result of starvation or maternal distress when all available energy has been utilised. Unless the mother has recently eaten a large quantity of carbohydrate, glucose is only found in the urine following intravenous administration. A trace of protein may be present following rupture of the membranes but more significant proteinuria may indicate worsening pre-eclampsia.

Fluid balance

A record should be kept of all urine passed to ensure that the bladder is being emptied (see above). If an intravenous infusion is in progress, the fluids administered must be recorded accurately. It is particularly important to note how much fluid remains if a bag is changed when only partially used.

Progress

Abdominal examination

An initial abdominal examination is carried out when the midwife first examines the mother. This should be repeated at intervals throughout labour in order to assess the length, strength and frequency of contractions and the descent of the presenting part. The method is described in Chapter 13.

Contractions.   The frequency, length and strength of the contractions should be noted. The strength of a contraction cannot be judged by the reaction of the woman but always by laying a hand on the uterus and noting the degree of hardness during a contraction and by timing its length. Some women appear to experience pain and yet the contractions may be neither long nor strong and very little is accomplished; other women appear to suffer very little, yet good progress is made.

When a uterine contraction begins, it is painless for a number of seconds and painless again at the end, so the midwife is aware of the approach of a contraction before the woman feels it and this knowledge can be utilised when giving inhalational analgesia (see Ch. 23). The uterus should always feel softer between contractions. Contractions which are unduly long or very strong and in quick succession give cause for concern as fetal hypoxia may develop.

If a cardiotocograph is in use, the contractions will be recorded electronically. This may be done by means of an external pressure transducer positioned over the uterine fundus and kept in place by an abdominal belt. For effective monitoring the belt must be relatively tight which may cause discomfort to the mother. The midwife must remember that such external monitoring cannot accurately measure the strength of uterine contractions. The size of the peak shown on the tracing is directly related to the ease with which contractions can be felt and not to the intensity of the contraction itself. The thickness of the abdominal wall will affect the reading as will movement of the mother.

If an accurate measurement of the intensity of uterine contractions is required, an internal transducer should be passed into the uterine cavity. A fluid-filled catheter is sometimes used but this has the disadvantage that it may become blocked with vernix, meconium or blood clot. A transducer-tipped catheter avoids this problem and is easier to place.

Descent of the presenting part.   During the first stage of labour, descent can be followed almost entirely by abdominal palpation. It is usual to describe the level in terms of the fifths of the head which can still be felt above the brim (see Figs 13.32 and 21.16).

In the primigravida the fetal head is usually engaged before labour begins. If this is not the case, the level of the head must be estimated frequently by abdominal palpation in order to observe whether the head will pass through the brim with the aid of good contractions.

When the head is engaged, the occipital protuberance can only be felt with difficulty from above but the sinciput may still be palpable, owing to increased flexion of the head, until the occiput reaches the pelvic floor and rotates forwards.

Vaginal examination

While it is not essential to examine the woman vaginally at frequent intervals, it may be useful to do so when progress is in doubt or another indication arises (see Ch. 21). The features which are indicative of progress are effacement and dilatation of the cervix, and descent, flexion and rotation of the fetal head.

Effacement and dilatation of the cervix. In normal labour the primigravid cervix effaces before dilating, whereas in the multigravida these two events occur simultaneously. In many centres, dilatation of the cervix up to 3 cm is discounted when calculating the length of labour because of the difficulty of deciding prospectively whether a small amount of dilatation indicates that true labour has begun. (See also latent and active phases of labour, Ch. 21.)

Progressive dilatation is monitored as labour continues and charted on either the partograph or the cervicograph. This will allow for early detection of abnormal progress and indicate when intervention is likely (Figs 21.17 and 21.18).

Descent. When assessed vaginally, the level or station of the presenting part is estimated in relation to the ischial spines which are fixed points at the outlet of the bony pelvis. During normal labour the head descends progressively (see Fig. 21.15). The midwife must be aware, while estimating whether the head is lower than previously, that marked moulding or a large caput will give a false impression of the level of the fetal head.

Flexion. In vertex presentations, progress depends on increased flexion. The spine is attached nearer to the back of the skull than the front. When the head is driven down onto the pelvic floor it encounters resistance: a lever principle causes the anterior part of the head to flex because there is less counter-pressure on it from above. The midwife assesses flexion by the position of the sutures and fontanelles. If the head is fully flexed, the posterior fontanelle becomes almost central; if the head is deflexed, both anterior and posterior fontanelles are palpable.

Rotation is assessed by noting changes in the position of the fetus between one examination and the next. The sutures and fontanelles are palpated in order to determine position. If insufficient information is gained to make a definitive diagnosis, a record is made of what *is* felt and the findings will be evaluated with the abdominal findings at the time and compared with the findings of earlier or later vaginal examinations.

The fetus

Fetal condition during labour can be assessed by obtaining information about the fetal heart rate and patterns, the pH of the fetal blood and the amniotic fluid.

The fetal heart

The fetal heart may be assessed intermittently or continuously.

Intermittent recording. This term is used when the fetal heart is auscultated at intervals using a monaural fetal stethoscope (Pinard's) or a Doppler ultrasound apparatus (Doptone or Sonicaid). The following assessments of the fetal heart can be made:

Rate. This should be counted over a complete minute in order to allow for variations. The rate should be between 120 and 160 beats per minute (bpm). The Doppler apparatus can be used throughout a contraction but listening during a contraction with a monaural stethoscope is uncomfortable for the woman and the fetal heart sounds may be inaudible. Normally the rate is maintained during a contraction and immediately after it. Episodes of fetal bradycardia may suggest hypoxia (see below).

Rhythm. The normal fetal heart has a coupled beat which should remain steady. Any noticeable irregularity in the rhythm may give cause for concern.

Continuous recording (Fig. 22.1). This depends on the use of electronic apparatus in the form of a fetal heart monitor. Continuous recording usually combines a fetal cardiograph and a maternal tocograph in a cardiotocograph apparatus (CTG). This presents a graphic record of the response of the fetal heart to uterine activity as well as information about its rate and rhythm. The CTG can be applied for periods of about 20 minutes (periodic cardiotocography) or be used for the whole of labour (continuous cardiotocography).

Method. An ultrasound transducer may be strapped to the abdomen at the point where the fetal heart is heard at maximum intensity. This

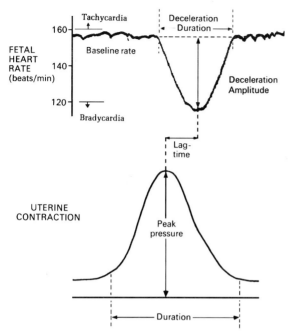

Fig. 22.1 Terms used in describing continuous fetal heart traces.

applying an electrode to the fetal scalp over a bone. In order to achieve this the membranes must be ruptured and the cervix be at least 2–3 cm dilated. The electrode is connected to the CTG by electrical wiring. A small scalp wound is inevitable but this rarely causes problems.

Internal cardiography may be used in conjunction with telemetry to monitor the fetal heart when the mother wishes to move away from the machine. A portable battery-operated transmitter is carried about by the ambulant woman. The scalp electrode transmits the fetal heart recording by radio to the cardiotocograph where it is recorded on the strip chart. It is impossible to obtain a recording of uterine activity when the mother is walking about but if she depresses a hand-held button at the onset of each contraction the strip chart will be marked accordingly.

Findings. The cardiotocograph provides information on:

- baseline fetal heart rate
- baseline variability
- response of the fetal heart to uterine contractions.

Baseline fetal heart rate. This is the fetal heart rate between uterine contractions. A rate more rapid than 160 bpm is termed *baseline tachycardia* (Fig. 22.2); a rate slower than 120 bpm is *baseline*

method is non-invasive and does not require rupture of the membranes. The quality of the fetal heart recording may be affected by the thickness of the abdominal wall, fetal position, maternal or fetal movement and uterine contractions.

A better-quality recording may be obtained by

PROLONGED ACCELERATION PATTERN

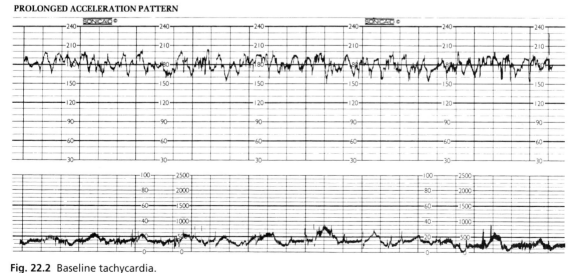

Fig. 22.2 Baseline tachycardia.
Figures 22.1–22.8 are reproduced from *Fetal heart rate patterns and their clinical interpretation* (Sonicaid Obstetrics) by kind permission of Sonicaid Limited, Chichester, West Sussex.

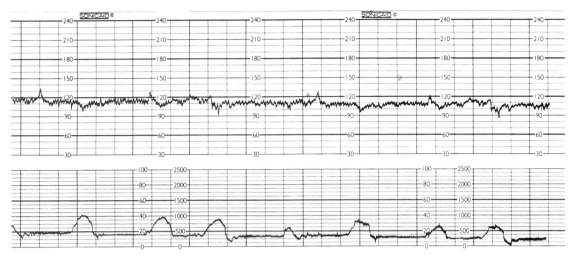

Fig. 22.3 Baseline bradycardia – normal.

bradycardia (Fig. 22.3). Either may be indicative of hypoxia but fetal tachycardia may be associated with maternal ketosis and in some fetuses the baseline rate is constant at between 110 and 120 bpm. Continuous compression of the umbilical cord, as in cord prolapse, will result in a prolonged, severe bradycardia.

Baseline variability (Figs 22.4, 22.5 and 22.6). Electrical activity in the fetal heart results in minute variations in the length of each beat. This causes the tracing to appear as a jagged, rather than a smooth, line. The baseline rate should vary by at least 5 beats over a period of 1 minute. Loss of this variability may indicate fetal hypoxia but may also be noted for a short period after the administration

of maternal pethidine which depresses the cardiac reflex centre in the fetal brain. Periods of 'fetal sleep' also cause a reduction in variability and commonly last for 20–30 minutes even in advanced labour (Gibb 1988, Lowe & Reiss 1996).

Response of the fetal heart to uterine contractions. The fetal heart rate will normally remain steady or accelerate during uterine contractions. In order to assess the significance of fetal heart rate decelerations accurately, their exact relationship to uterine contractions must be noted. An *early deceleration* begins at or after the onset of a contraction, reaches its lowest point at the peak of the contraction and returns to the baseline rate by the time the contraction has finished. On the

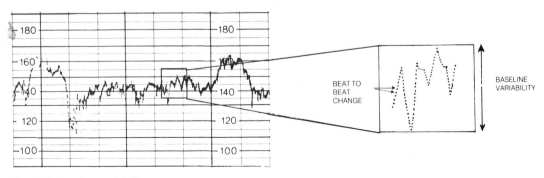

Fig. 22.4 Baseline variability.

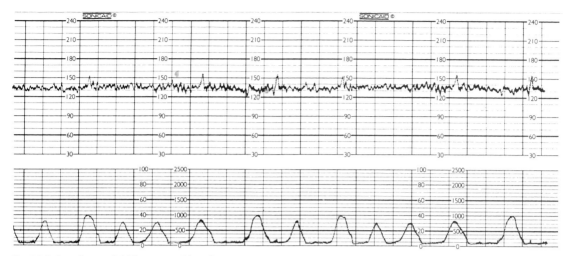

Fig. 22.5 Baseline variability: normal baseline rate.

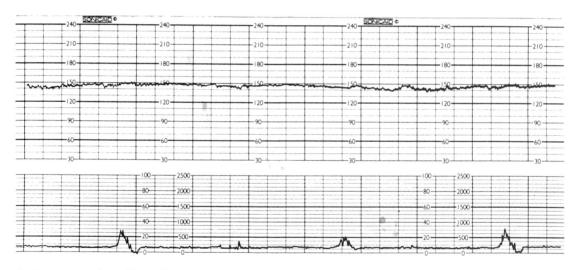

Fig. 22.6 Uncomplicated loss of baseline variability: normal rate, no decelerations.

graph it produces a mirror image of the contraction (Fig. 22.7). An early deceleration is commonly associated with compression of the fetal head, for example as it engages, but may indicate early fetal hypoxia.

A *late deceleration* begins during or after a contraction, reaches its nadir after the peak of the contraction and has not recovered by the time that the contraction has ended (Fig. 22.8). Sometimes the deceleration has barely recovered by the onset of the next contraction. The *time lag* between the peak of the contraction and the nadir of the deceleration is more significant of severity than the drop in the fetal heart rate. If this occurs the doctor must be informed as it always indicates fetal hypoxia. A vaginal examination should be performed to exclude prolapse of the cord as late decelerations are suggestive of cord compression.

Interpretation of recordings. If contact is lost, artefacts may appear on the tracing which can be confused with abnormal fetal heart patterns,

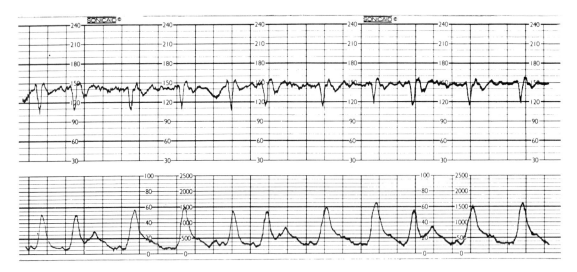

Fig. 22.7 Early decelerations.

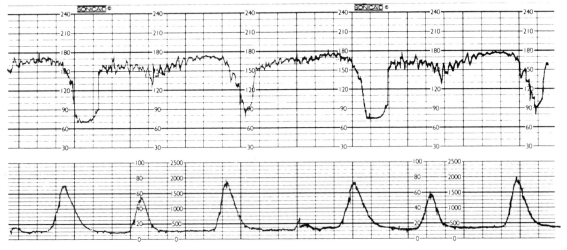

Fig. 22.8 Late decelerations.

especially decelerations. However, the midwife is cautioned against disregarding abnormalities of the tracing on the assumption that the machine is 'playing up'. An attempt should be made to improve the quality of the recording and the fetal heart rate should be checked using a monaural stethoscope or Doppler apparatus.

Some mothers will request avoidance of electronic monitoring. This request should be respected as research has not confirmed a need for continuous monitoring in normal labour (Pello et al

1988, Umstad et al 1995). The mother will not usually object to the use of hand-held Doppler apparatus to monitor the fetal heart; her concern is commonly that she wishes to be free to move around. Some units will suggest a 20-minute period of monitoring on admission with or without additional periods throughout labour.

Fetal blood sampling

The fetus who has become hypoxic will also become acidotic as the pH of its blood is lowered.

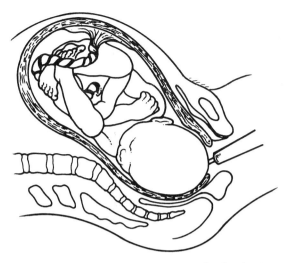

Fig. 22.9 Fetal blood sampling. Access to fetal scalp via amnioscope passed through the cervix.

The normal pH of fetal blood is 7.33 or above. If it falls below 7.25 in the first stage of labour, careful surveillance is required: in the second stage of labour a level as low as 7.15 may be acceptable provided delivery is imminent (Ritchie 1995). Cardiotocograph recording of the fetal heart may suggest hypoxia but acidosis can only be confirmed by fetal blood sampling.

An amnioscope is passed through the cervix to provide access to the fetal scalp (Fig. 22.9). A small blade is used to puncture the skin and 0.5 ml of blood is collected in a heparinised capillary tube. The specimen must be analysed immediately. While it is in transit to the blood gas analyser, care must be taken to ensure that the blood is not allowed to clot and does not come into contact with atmospheric oxygen. To prevent clotting an iron filing is added to the tube and moved backwards and forwards with a magnet to mix the heparin with the blood. The ends of the capillary tube are sealed with wax to prevent spillage and exclude air during transit.

Amniotic fluid

Following rupture of the membranes amniotic fluid escapes from the uterus continuously and may provide information about the condition of the fetus. This fluid should normally remain clear.

If the fetus becomes hypoxic, meconium may be passed as hypoxia causes relaxation of the anal sphincter. The amniotic fluid becomes green as a result of meconium staining. Amniotic fluid which is a muddy yellow colour or which is only slightly green may signify previous distress from which the fetus has recovered.

If the breech is presenting and is compacted in the pelvis, the fetus may pass meconium because of the compression of the abdomen; a fetus presenting by the breech is also prone to fetal distress and may pass meconium as a result of hypoxia.

In the rare case of a fetus who is severely affected by Rhesus iso-immunisation the amniotic fluid may be golden-yellow owing to an excess of bilirubin.

Bleeding which is of sudden onset at the time of rupture of the membranes may be the result of a ruptured vasa praevia and is an acute emergency (see Ch. 29).

Fetal distress

Fetal distress occurs when the fetus suffers oxygen deprivation and becomes hypoxic. Severe hypoxia may result in the baby being stillborn or he may be asphyxiated at birth and suffer brain damage.

Signs of fetal distress. Any or all of the following may be present:

- fetal tachycardia which is an early sign of oxygen deprivation
- fetal bradycardia or fetal heart rate decelerations related to uterine contractions
- passage of meconium-stained amniotic fluid.

Management of fetal distress. When signs of fetal distress occur the midwife must call a doctor. If Syntocinon is being administered, it must be stopped and the woman placed in a favourable position, usually on her left side. In cases of maternal oxygen lack, such as eclampsia or shock due to antepartum haemorrhage, oxygen may be given via a face mask. The doctor may wish to take a sample of fetal blood for testing and arrangements should be made for this.

If fetal distress is more than transient, delivery will be expedited. In the first stage of labour this will necessitate caesarean section. In the second stage of labour an episiotomy may be sufficient to effect delivery but failing this a forceps delivery or Ventouse extraction may be performed. In all cases of delivery following fetal distress the presence of a paediatrician is desirable.

PRETERM LABOUR

Preterm labour (for causes, see Ch. 37) is defined as labour occurring before the 37th completed week of pregnancy, and judging whether it has started or not is just as difficult regardless of the period of gestation. Of all women who present for help because of preterm uterine contractions, between 30 and 50% will have spontaneous cessation of contractions and pregnancy will continue (Pearce 1985). Increased perinatal survival attributed to increased neonatal facilities and appropriately trained personnel has altered policies towards management of the woman in preterm labour. If the labouring woman is not in an area where there is a special care unit and resident neonatal staff, she should be transferred there as quickly as possible. Betamimetic drugs to suppress uterine contractions (tocolysis) may be administered until the woman has been transferred to such a centre. Ritodrine hydrochloride (Yutopar) and salbutamol (Ventolin) are commonly used betamimetic drugs. Side-effects include maternal tachycardia, palpitations and hypotension and fetal tachycardia. The main contraindications are hypertension, haemorrhage, rupture of the membranes and drug incompatibilities.

Tocolytic drugs are administered by intravenous infusion commencing with the minimum recommended dose which is increased at 10- to 20-minute intervals. When contractions reduce to one every 15 minutes or less the dose should be stabilised and the infusion maintained for a further 24 hours before gradually tapering off the administration of the drug (Walkinshaw 1995).

Management of preterm labour

No attempt should be made to arrest labour if pregnancy has advanced to 34 weeks' gestation and the fetus is estimated to have grown to 2500 g (Pearce 1985). Generally speaking the more preterm the fetus the greater the risks from labour

and delivery. Skilled care is required for the woman and the fetus during labour. The mother is faced with an unexpected emotional crisis because of the interruption of the normal progress of pregnancy. The high perinatal mortality rate means the woman and her partner have to face the possibility of the death or disability of their baby. The fetus is at risk of hypoxia and therefore continuous electronic heart rate monitoring is advisable. To reduce the risk of intraventricular haemorrhage an episiotomy should be performed unless there is a very relaxed vaginal outlet. Caesarean section may be undertaken if there is an abnormal presentation or the infant is expected to be of very low birth weight. If the mother requires analgesia during labour, narcotics which cross the placental barrier and depress the fetal respiratory centre should be avoided. The presence of a paediatrician at delivery will ensure that skilled resuscitation is carried out promptly. For management of the baby, see Chapter 37.

ACTIVE MANAGEMENT OF LABOUR

The active management of labour movement originated in 1968 when Kieran O'Driscoll was elected Master at the National Maternity Hospital in Dublin. The term 'active management of labour' is used to describe a range of policies which purport to achieve efficient uterine action, thereby preventing prolonged labour in primigravidae. Obstetricians are involved in the supervision of normal labour with the aim 'not to expose anyone to the stress of labour for more than 12 hours' (O'Driscoll & Meagher 1993, p. 35).

The components of active management include:

Accurate diagnosis of labour. O'Driscoll and Meagher (1993) stress the importance of the accuracy of this diagnosis since it is the fundamental decision on which all subsequent management is based. Labour is judged to have started when the woman experiences regular, painful uterine contractions accompanied by either show, rupture of the membranes or complete effacement of the cervix.

Early rupture of the membranes. One hour

after labour is diagnosed an amniotomy is performed and the colour of the liquor is noted.

Monitoring of cervical dilatation. Progress during the first stage of labour is measured in terms of dilatation of the cervix and requires regular vaginal examinations. These are carried out hourly for the first 3 hours then at 2-hourly intervals, ideally by the same person. The degree of cervical dilatation is charted on a partograph. Progressive cervical dilatation at the rate of 1 cm per hour is considered acceptable. Should cervical dilatation not proceed at this predetermined rate, intravenous oxytocin is administered.

Continuous professional support for the mother. The attendance of a support person throughout labour is crucial. This is usually the midwife who will monitor fetal and maternal well-being as well as provide psychological support.

Since active management was first described by O'Driscoll, maternity units elsewhere have adopted some or all of these components in an attempt to improve the outcome of labour for both mother and baby. Now the term active management popularly refers to early rupture of membranes followed by the administration of intravenous oxytocin to ensure cervical dilatation at the rate of 1 cm per hour.

Disadvantages

Whereas some women are pleased to be guaranteed delivery within a specified time, others are more interested in achieving delivery by natural means and dislike the suggestion of intervention. Maternal preference must be taken into account when offering active management of labour.

In active management the membranes are artificially ruptured in order to shorten the labour but this is at the cost of the advantages of intact membranes. Some would also question the advantage of speed for its own sake. If the membranes are intact, hydrostatic pressure is applied evenly to the placental surface and to the fetus and the amniotic sac prevents the entry of pathogenic organisms.

It is less easy to take advantage of an upright position if active management is practised. However, the midwife may still be able to assist a mother to use positions which favour uterine action, such as the left lateral or a kneeling position, if necessary by putting a mattress on the floor.

Contractions augmented by Syntocinon may be experienced as more painful than those of spontaneous labour. This may in turn necessitate the use of pain-relieving drugs, which may disappoint the woman who had hoped to manage without them.

The midwife's role

If a policy of active management is practised, it is the midwife's responsibility to inform the mother fully of what procedures to expect and to enable her to make decisions based on accurate, unbiased information. Where possible, practice should be research-based and responsive to the needs of the individual (Clinical Standards Advisory Group 1995). Whatever the woman's wishes, the midwife should provide supportive care and endeavour to achieve a satisfactory outcome for the mother.

RECORDS

Throughout the first stage of labour the midwife must keep meticulous records of all events and of the woman's physical and psychological condition and the condition of her fetus (see Ch. 21). While observing the progress of labour she should be alert for signs of the second stage (see Ch. 24).

An individualised approach to care will attempt to follow the plan which was devised in pregnancy. If the woman changes her mind as her labour progresses, adjustments can be made. Whether or not a formal birth plan has been prepared, the midwife who is caring for the woman should communicate effectively with her, evaluate whether the labour is proceeding as expected and listen to her requests. A comprehensive record of the discussions which take place about changes in plan or about proposed measures which the midwife may suggest will ensure that the closest possible attention is paid to achieving the outcome that the parents are hoping for and also provide an excellent documented history of the labour.

READER ACTIVITIES

1. After caring for a particular woman through the whole of her labour attempt to measure the quality of care which has been provided.

Select the appropriate case notes and examine records for midwifery observations. Then review with the mother the events of her childbirth experience. Show an interest in finding out how the mother feels about her labour. Initiate dialogue by asking questions, such as:

- 'Tell me about ...'
- 'Can you tell me how you felt about ...?'

These require more than a yes or no answer and by describing a situation the woman should understand it better herself.

Allow the mother to express any feelings of anger or embarrassment or pride in her achievement. In this way emotional support is provided by the midwife as the woman talks through her feelings and compares what she expected to happen with the actual event.

2. Re-examine the case notes following the interview with the mother to identify areas where care could have been improved.

REFERENCES

Andrews C M, Chrzanowski M 1990 Maternal position, labour and comfort. Applied Nursing Research 3(1): 7–13

Ball J A 1994 Reactions to motherhood, 2nd edn. Books for Midwives Press, Cheshire

Clinical Standards Advisory Group 1995 Women in normal labour: report of a CSAG committee on women in normal labour. HMSO, London

Crowe K, von Baeyer C 1989 Predictors of a positive childbirth experience. Birth 16(2): 59–63

Fleissig A 1993 Are women given enough information by staff during labour and delivery? Midwifery 9: 70–75

Gibb D 1988 A practical guide to labour management. Blackwell Scientific Publications, Oxford

Green J M, Coupland V A, Kitzinger J V 1990 Expectations, experiences and psychological outcomes of childbirth: a prospective study of 825 women. Birth 17(1): 15–24

Hodnett E D, Osborn R W 1989a Effects of continuous intrapartum professional support on childbirth outcomes. Research in Nursing and Health 12: 289–297

Hodnett E D, Osborn R W 1989b A randomized trial of the effects of montrice support during labor: mothers' views two to four weeks postpartum. Birth 16(4): 177–183

Johnson C, Keirse M J N C, Enkin M, Chalmers I 1989 Nutrition and hydration in labour. In: Chalmers I, Enkin M, Keirse M J N C (eds) Effective care in pregnancy and childbirth. Oxford University Press, Oxford, vol 2, pp 827–832

Kakol K 1989 Position in labour – does mother know best? Professional Nurse 4(July): 481–484

Kitzinger S 1985 What do women want? In: Studd J (ed) The management of labour. Blackwell Scientific Publications, Oxford, ch 2

Klaus M H, Kennell J, Robertson S, Sosa R 1986 Effects of social support during parturition on maternal and infant morbidity. British Medical Journal 293: 585–587

Lovell A 1996 Power and choice in birthgiving: some thoughts. British Journal of Midwifery 4(5): 268–272

Lowe N K, Reiss R 1996 Parturition and fetal adaptation.

Journal of Obstetric Gynecological and Neonatal Nursing 25(4): 339–349

Mackey M C, Lock S E 1989 Women's expectations of the labor and delivery nurse. Journal of Obstetric Gynecological and Neonatal Nursing 18(November/December): 505–512

Morgan B M, Kadim M Y 1994 Mobile regional analgesia in labour. British Journal of Obstetrics and Gynaecology 101: 839–841

Niven C 1992 Psychological care for families: before, during and after birth. Butterworth-Heinemann, Oxford

O'Driscoll K, Meagher D 1993 Active management of labour, 3rd edn. Mosby, London

Pearce M J 1985 The management of preterm labour. In: Studd J (ed) The management of labour. Blackwell Scientific Publications, Oxford, ch 4

Pello L C, Dawes G S, Smith J, Redman C 1988 Screening of the fetal heart rate in early labour. British Journal of Obstetrics and Gynaecology 95: 1128–1136

Raphael-Leff J 1993 Pregnancy – the inside story. Sheldon Press, London

Ritchie J W 1995 Fetal surveillance. In: Whitfield C (ed) Dewhurst's textbook of obstetrics and gynaecology for postgraduates, 5th edn. Blackwell Science, Oxford, ch 28

Roberts C C, Ludka L M 1994 Food for thought. Childbirth Instructor Magazine (Spring): 25–29

Steele R 1995 Midwifery care during the first stage of labour. In: Alexander J, Levy V, Roch S (eds) Aspects of midwifery practice: a research-based approach. Macmillan Press, Hampshire, vol 4, ch 2

Thornton J G, Lilford R J 1994 Active management of labour: current knowledge and research issues. British Medical Journal 309: 366-369

Umstad M, Permezel M, Pepperell R 1995 Litigation and the intrapartum cardiotocograph. British Journal of Obstetrics and Gynaecology 102: 89–91

Walkinshaw S A 1995 Preterm labour and delivery of the preterm infant. In: Chamberlain G (ed) Turnbull's obstetrics, 2nd edn. Churchill Livingstone, New York, ch 33

FURTHER READING

Berg M, Lundgren I, Hermansson E, Wahlberg V 1996 Women's experience of the encounter with the midwife during childbirth. Midwifery 12: 11–15

Dover S L, Gauge S M 1995 Fetal monitoring – midwifery attitudes. Midwifery 11: 18–27

Flint C 1986 Sensitive midwifery. Heinemann, London

Henderson J 1996 Active management of labour and caesarean section rates. British Journal of Midwifery 4(3): 132–149

Jones A 1996 Psychotherapy following childbirth. British Journal of Midwifery 4(5): 239–243

Kwast B E 1994 World Health Organization partograph in the management of labour. Lancet 343: 1399–1404

Lichy R, Herzberg E 1993 The waterbirth handbook. Gateway Books, Bath

O'Reilly S, Hoyer P J P, Walsh E 1993 Low-risk mothers: oral intake and emesis in labour. Journal of Nurse-Midwifery 38(4): 228–235

Peacock J, Anderson H R, Bland J M 1995 Preterm delivery: effects of socioeconomic factors, psychological stress, smoking, alcohol and caffeine. British Medical Journal 311: 531–536

Robinson-Walsh D, Stewart J (eds) 1993 Labours of love (the stories of childbirth in parents' own words). Aurora Publishing, Bolton

Shennan A, Cooke V, de Swiet M, Lloyd-Jones F, Morgan B 1995 Blood pressure changes during labour and whilst ambulating with combined spinal epidural analgesia. British Journal of Obstetrics and Gynaecology 102: 192–197

Simkin P T 1992 Just another day in a woman's life? Part II: Nature and consistency of women's long-term memories of their first birth experiences. Birth 19(2): 64–81

Pain relief and comfort in labour

Ruth Bevis

This chapter explores the variety of ways in which midwives use their skills to achieve for each woman in labour and her partner an experience which they regard as positive.

The chapter aims to:

- give an overview of the factors affecting perception of pain and individual reactions to it

- consider the physiology of pain with particular reference to the sources of pain in labour

- discuss the importance in the management of pain of support through reassurance, encouragement, information giving and the provision of a relaxing environment

- describe those aspects of physical care that relate particularly to comfort

- describe strategies of pain relief that make use of the body's own control mechanisms

- consider pharmacological methods of relieving pain in labour other than regional anaesthesia which is discussed in Chapter 28.

Labour is one of the major events in a woman's life. If she is living in the UK it is no longer an inevitable annual occurrence, but one which is generally seen as a significant emotional and physical experience. Its memory will remain with her; negative impressions may give rise to psychological sequelae with implications for the whole family (Freely 1995). Women are therefore wanting to take control of their bodies, make informed choices and to be treated as individuals.

Melzack (1984) states that the pain of labour is rarely surpassed and frequently exceeds the woman's antepartum expectations. Rickford & Reynolds (1987) suggest that it is not that women underestimate the pain, but tend to overestimate their ability to cope with it. Women rarely appreciate fully the incessant nature and prolonged duration of pain in a first labour, as well as the debilitating effect of loss of sleep.

'Comfort' in labour is not merely an emotional or physical relieving of malaise and pain. It is a complex process in which the midwife (meaning 'with woman') or 'sage-femme' (wise woman) combines research-based knowledge and skills with warmth, empathy and sensitivity in order to provide a birth environment which is safe, caring and conducive to a satisfying birth experience (Page 1995).

PERCEPTION OF PAIN

The way in which an individual perceives and reacts to pain is affected by many different factors (Melzack & Wall 1988, Moore 1997).

Fear and anxiety will heighten the individual's response to pain (Simkin 1986). Fear of the unknown, fear of being left alone to cope with an experience such as labour and fear of failing to cope well will increase anxiety. A previous bad experience will also increase anxiety.

Personality plays a part and the woman who is naturally tense and anxious will cope less well with stress than one who is relaxed and confident.

Fatigue. The woman who is already fatigued by several hours of labour, perhaps preceded by a period when sleep was disturbed by the discomforts of late pregnancy, will be less able to tolerate pain.

Cultural and social factors also play a part. Some cultures expect stoicism while others encourage expression of feeling (Hayes 1997, Schott & Henley 1996). The perception of pain may be altered if the woman has experienced pain and hardship previously.

Expectations colour the experience. The woman who is realistic in her expectations of labour and about her likely response to it is probably the best equipped, as long as she feels confident that she will receive the help and support she needs and is assured that she will receive appropriate analgesia.

PHYSIOLOGY OF PAIN

Pain pathways

The *pain pathway* or ascending sensory tract (Fig. 23.1) originates in the sensory nerve endings at the site of trauma. The impulse travels along the sensory nerves to the dorsal root ganglion of the relevant spinal nerve and into the posterior horn of the spinal cord. This is known as the *first neuron*.

The *second neuron* arises in the posterior horn, crosses over within the spinal cord (the sensory decussation) and transmits the impulse via the medulla oblongata, pons varolii and the midbrain to the thalamus.

From here it travels along the *third neuron* to the sensory cortex.

Acute pain. Such sensations are transmitted along *A delta fibres*, which are large-diameter nerve fibres, dealing with acute pain. This type of pain is perceived as pricking pain which is readily localised by the sufferer.

Chronic pain. The pathway for chronic pain is slightly different; the nerve fibres involved are of smaller diameter and are called *C fibres*. Chronic pain is often described as burning pain, which is difficult to localise.

Neurotransmitters. Transmission of nervous stimuli is effected or inhibited by substances called neurotransmitters. These may be excitatory or inhibitory. They interact to maintain equilibrium of pain appreciation. An example of an *excitatory neurotransmitter* is acetylcholine, and one of an *inhibitory neurotransmitter* is enkephalin. Local anaesthetic solutions act by competing for the acetylcholine receptors on the neuron and blocking the action.

Inhibitory mechanisms. The thalamus, hypothalamus and parts of the cerebral cortex are known collectively as the *limbic system*. This system links the endocrine and autonomic nervous systems and regulates certain visceral functions. Some emotions arise in the limbic system and it has a part to play in inhibition of the pain response.

There is a substance in the dorsal roots of the spinal cord called *substantia gelatinosa*. If a pain

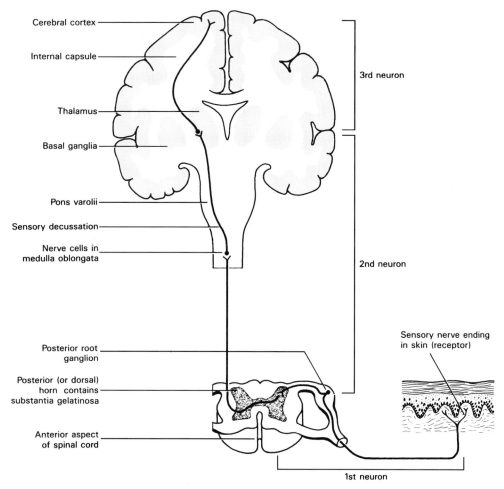

Fig. 23.1 The sensory pathway showing the structures involved in the appreciation of pain (reproduced from Bevis 1984 by courtesy of Baillière Tindall).

stimulus is not sufficiently strong, or if it is super-seded by a different stimulus, the substantia gelati-nosa may inhibit its passage. In the *gate control theory* the substantia gelatinosa is likened to a gate. Pain impulses must be sufficiently strong to open the gate in order to ascend the sensory tract any further. The gate may be closed by a competing stimulus such as local application of heat or cold.

Endogenous opioids play an important part in pain inhibition. Opioid receptors are found at various points in the central nervous system and the body produces opiate-like substances which give natural analgesia. The two main classes of endogenous opioid are the *endorphins* and the *enkephalins*. It is thought that several methods of pain relief stimulate the production of endogenous opioids and also activate the gate control system.

Pain in labour

The pain experienced by the woman in labour is caused by the uterine contractions, the dilatation of the cervix and, in the late first stage and the second stage, by the stretching of the vagina and pelvic floor to accommodate the presenting part. These painful stimuli are said to be transmitted by thoracic, lumbar and sacral nerves. A study by Bonica (1994) demonstrated that the sacral nerves do not transmit the pain of cervical dilatation.

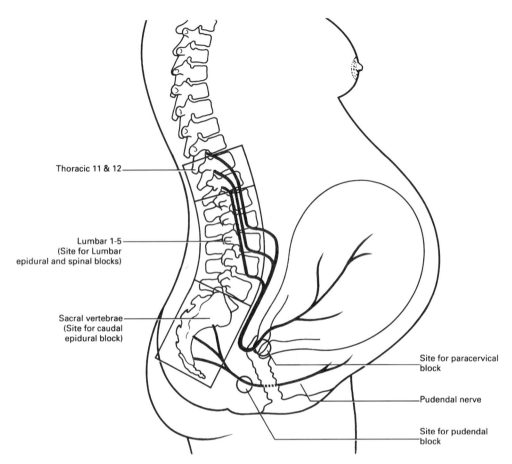

Fig. 23.2 Pain pathways in labour, showing the sites at which pain may be intercepted by local anaesthetic technique (reproduced from Bevis 1984 by courtesy of Baillière Tindall).

The nerve supply of the uterus passes to the last two thoracic nerves, T11 and T12, via the paracervical plexus (Fig. 23.2). These nerves transmit the pain caused by cervical dilatation. In the later first stage T10 and the first lumbar nerve, L1, are also involved. The pudendal nerve relays the pain impulses from the stretching of the pelvic floor to sacral nerves S2, S3 and S4. (For more detailed texts see Guyton 1987, Moore 1997, Wall & Melzack 1994.)

PSYCHOLOGICAL SUPPORT

Preparation for labour

At some stage in her pregnancy every woman will realise the inevitability of the delivery of her baby. Not every woman will experience labour but the mother who delivers by planned caesarean section will also have fears and anxieties and will wonder just how she will cope with the experience.

Giving information. Ideally, every pregnant woman should have the opportunity to form a relationship with one particular midwife (DH 1993) so that advice may be given consistently and the woman become relaxed and feel able to ask for information freely. In this way each woman is able to obtain as much information as she wishes. Some will state that they do not wish to be told too many details, while others feel reassured if they know exactly what they may expect (Priest & Schott 1991).

Discovering what level of information is required

and meeting the individual woman's needs present the midwife with a challenge. It is best done in an informal, relaxed setting and on a one-to-one basis.

It is more difficult to give information to a group of women, since some are likely to become anxious if too much information is given. The best approach when talking to a group of women is probably to attempt to meet the perceived needs of the majority and to offer an opportunity for further discussion with those who would like it.

The giving of information is supplemented by handing out leaflets and recommending books to read. Some women will wish to attend additional classes such as those run by the National Childbirth Trust (NCT).

Reassuring women that they will be given appropriate analgesia and telling them what is available are very important parts of the information given.

Allaying anxiety.   While every woman is likely to be apprehensive about some aspect of pregnancy or labour, many fears will be unfounded. Some women may be anxious at the thought of being given an episiotomy, for example, and if this is no longer routine practice in the local maternity unit a needless fear may be allayed.

Many old wives' tales are still in circulation and a discussion of these may be useful. The pregnant woman is often the recipient of such misinformation just when she is especially vulnerable. Some women seem unable to resist the temptation to recount their own horrific experiences to the innocent primigravida, although of course women who have experienced childbirth are often a great source of support and constructive advice.

Participation in planning.   Entering hospital for any reason is often seen as a dehumanising experience. The person becomes a 'patient' as he or she enters the building and assumes the sick role. Personal clothing is removed, an identity band is attached to the wrist and the person begins to feel helpless.

Women having babies have been no less prone to these experiences and during the 1980s many complained that they had no control over what was done to them. A normal physiological process had become medicalised (Martin 1987, Oakley 1984). Giving back to the woman as much control as possible reduces her feeling of helplessness and increases her ability to tolerate the sensations of labour (Choucri 1997, Lovell 1996). This may begin by encouraging her to consider her particular needs and wishes and to discuss these with the midwife.

The birth plan is commonly used (see Ch. 21). This is a document which the woman compiles together with the midwife, on which she states her preferences for care during and after labour. Completing this document provides a useful opportunity for discussion of pain relief and the exchange of information between the woman and her midwife. Choice and control are now seen as essential elements in the woman's birth experience (DH 1993).

Couples who are able to participate in planning their care in this way will feel that they matter to the professionals and are likely to be less apprehensive about the whole experience of entering hospital. The midwife should remember that for many young couples a hospital is an alien, unfamiliar environment associated with sickness and death and that they may have had no personal experience of it.

Meeting staff.   Meeting the staff of the labour ward and seeing the environment will be very helpful to many women. If the use of equipment is explained it will seem less clinical and fearsome. The team approach to care is designed to offer continuity of care and of caregiver to each woman so that she has the reassuring experience of meeting familiar people throughout her contact with the maternity service. The woman is allocated to a team of 6–12 midwives and will get to know them during her pregnancy: hopefully the midwife giving care in labour is therefore not a stranger.

Support during labour

The environment.   A relaxed, homely atmosphere will help the woman and her partner feel at ease more quickly. The attitude of the staff is very important, perhaps more so than the physical details of the environment.

The labour room must be furnished in such a way that an emergency may be dealt with swiftly and efficiently and for this reason the clinical aspect can never be removed. However, wallpaper and curtains in attractive, restful colours and the use of screens to hide equipment soften the clinical appearance of the room. Furniture now includes less formal items and rocking chairs, reclining chairs and bean bags are in widespread use.

Lighting should be versatile. Many women prefer subdued lighting or semi-darkness while they are in labour but it may be necessary to direct an efficient light onto the working area.

Piped music may be a source of irritation, but women may be encouraged to bring cassette players with tapes of their own choice and possibly personal headphones.

A television set may be a useful distraction for the woman in early labour and a pleasant sitting room with a variety of comfortable chairs is a desirable provision.

The midwife should endeavour to ensure that there are as few intrusions into the labour room as possible and should aim to maintain an unhurried, peaceful atmosphere (Flint 1986).

A supportive companion is a great source of strength to the woman in labour and provides the continuity which the staff cannot always promise (see Ch. 21) (Hodnett 1993). Some men are unwilling companions during labour and couples should be encouraged to be honest about this. Some women may feel that a female companion is more appropriate for them.

Midwife means 'with woman' and she aims to be a supportive companion, working with the woman and her partner (Halldorsdottir & Karlsdottir 1996). The ability to develop such a rapport is an essential midwifery skill.

Mobility. If the woman can be encouraged to be upright and mobile, labour is likely to progress more quickly (Melzack et al 1991) and the woman will feel more in control, especially if she is encouraged to change position from time to time in order to become as comfortable as possible.

Giving information. The couple should be kept fully informed of progress and all developments during the course of labour. Any treatment or intervention, imminent or probable, should be anticipated and explained. The prospective parents should be involved in the decision-making, and no procedure should be carried out without their informed consent (Thiroux 1986).

Relaxation techniques. If the woman has been taught relaxation techniques she should be reminded of them and supported as she puts her knowledge into practice. The midwife should be careful to discover just how the woman has been taught and should follow the same method.

If the woman has not attended classes, the midwife will aim to give her very simple instructions in breathing techniques and to encourage the use of these (see Ch. 45).

Conversation. When a woman is in labour there are times to talk and times to be silent. A companionable, sympathetic silence is infinitely preferred by most women in advanced labour. At this stage a woman is becoming tired and each contraction requires her complete concentration and all the physical and emotional reserves she can muster. She may close her eyes and become rather distant at this stage. If she is very aware of what is going on in her body, she is concentrating on the baby's progress and her own response and inconsequential conversation is inappropriate. Conversation over the woman is even more inappropriate; attention should be focused on her and her needs throughout the labour.

When silence seems appropriate, touch and facial expressions become more important.

Encouragement. The midwife should aim to encourage the woman throughout her labour. Most women will reach a stage when they feel they cannot continue any longer and will despair. Just a few quiet words of praise after each contraction or some non-verbal encouragement will often suffice. The woman who is made to feel she is coping and progressing very well will usually respond by continuing to do so. The midwife whose communication skills are well developed and who responds with warmth and enthusiasm will usually achieve this.

PHYSICAL CARE

The details of physical care are covered in Chapters 21 and 22 but the following points relate particularly to comfort.

Hygiene and comfort

The woman in labour will become very hot and will perspire profusely so that she will appreciate the opportunity to have a bath or shower if she feels able. A warm bath may be very comforting for the woman with backache and she may enjoy soaking herself in deep warm water.

If the woman is not able to get up she will appreciate frequent sponging, particularly of her face and neck, with cold water.

A clean, cool gown will be appreciated and a fan is comforting.

Her mouth will feel much fresher if she can clean her teeth or have a mouthwash. She may like to have some ice to suck.

Position

Women may need help to find a position which is comfortable. Leaning forward with the arms resting on a convenient windowsill, table or shelf during a contraction may help the woman to cope with backache. She may prefer to sit astride or kneel on a chair, leaning on the back of it. The midwife should make use of wedges, bean bags and pillows. A rocking chair provides a soothing, rhythmic distraction during contractions and the motion probably encourages release of endogenous opioids; most rocking chairs give good support to the back. A reclining chair also gives good support, but a fully recumbent position should be avoided because of the risk of aortocaval occlusion.

Birthing beds and chairs are designed specifically for women in labour and most are very versatile. Ideally they are used for delivery only and the woman is encouraged to walk about and use alternative positions (Fig. 23.3) during the first stage of labour.

An alternative position may be described as any position other than recumbent, semi-recumbent or sitting on the bed; the woman follows her natural instincts and finds a position and movements, such as pelvic rocking, which feel right for her, making use of gravity to assist descent of the presenting part. An upright or kneeling position also allows maximum 'give' of the pelvic girdle, whereas sitting causes pressure over the sacrum and coccyx. Women wishing to have an active birth will certainly want to make full use of alternative positions but any woman in normal labour may benefit from freer mobility.

In *active birth* the woman participates fully in her labour, is very aware of all that is going on within her body and aims to respond to these events naturally. She will have prepared herself during her pregnancy by exercising in order to be aware of her pelvic floor and to control these muscles. She may also practise squatting. She will not wish to have any form of medical intervention if this can be avoided. She may use any position she finds comfortable, such as squatting, kneeling on all fours or kneeling upright. Most women prefer such positions if they have the confidence to try them and they find that they can cope with the contractions better than when sitting on the bed (Balaskas 1991).

Physical contact

The woman may not wish to talk but she may find physical contact comforting. Her partner should be encouraged to hold her hand, rub her back, sponge her face or just cuddle her. Some couples may wish to practise *effleurage*, where the partner strokes the woman's abdomen and thighs, or similar techniques. Those who are wanting an active birth may wish to try nipple or clitoral stimulation to encourage the release of oxytocin from the pituitary gland and so stimulate uterine contractions in a natural way. This will also stimulate the production of endogenous opioids, giving some natural analgesia. The midwife should be sensitive to each couple's wishes and should respect them. It may be appropriate at times to leave the couple alone together, if that is what they prefer.

The woman's partner may support her in her chosen alternative position, although this becomes a physical endurance test after a time and the midwife may have to suggest practical alternatives.

Some women become very irritable as labour

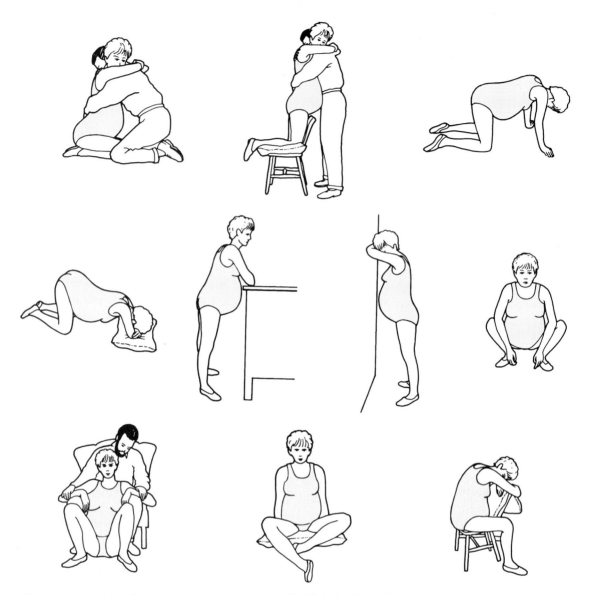

Fig. 23.3 Some of the alternative positions women may find helpful during labour.

progresses and find any touch annoying and intrusive.

The midwife should not be afraid to make sensitive use of physical contact herself but should learn to recognise when this becomes irritating and inappropriate.

Care of bladder and bowels
This is discussed more fully in Chapters 21 and 22

but care of the bladder and bowels is an important aspect of the mother's comfort.

Pain relief in labour may be considered in two categories. Some methods support the natural physiological responses to labour pain; the release of endogenous opioids and the gate mechanism. Pharmacological methods provide a chemically based adjunct to the physiological processes, which may not support but override them.

TECHNIQUES WHICH SUPPORT THE PHYSIOLOGICAL PROCESSES

Psychophysical methods of coping with pain

History

In the 1930s Grantly Dick-Read (1943) postulated that fear of the unknown led to muscular tension, thus increasing the pain of labour. He maintained that in order to break this vicious circle, it was necessary to give women more information and then to teach them specific methods of relaxing. The relaxation techniques were also intended to serve as a distraction.

Michel Odent (1984) advocates a natural approach, allowing women to feel in control of their bodies and what happens to them and encouraging them to respond instinctively to labour.

Melzack (1984) claims that painless childbirth is an unattainable ideal, based on flawed assumptions.

Certainly only a small minority of women will enjoy a painless labour. Indeed such an experience may prove very stressful if it involves a precipitate delivery at home or en route to hospital, without skilled support and assistance.

Pain, like stress, has a positive function if experienced in moderation, in an environment where the subject receives support.

Melzack discusses the issue of 'prepared childbirth training' and finds that the reported effects of such preparation are controversial and apparently contradictory. Some studies suggest that the pain itself is not reduced but that the emotional response to the pain may be. The final issue is not one of measures on a pain-rating scale, but of the woman's feelings of satisfaction with the experience and the support offered, together with her resulting sense of self-worth and achievement (Choucri 1997).

Principles

The principles in psychophysical methods of pain relief are to allay anxiety, encourage relaxation, provide distraction and to encourage a positive attitude.

Today it is well recognised that if women feel that they have choice and control, even if this is not absolute, they are likely to feel more satisfied with their birth experience, even if the experience does not match up to their hopes or expectations (Choucri 1997, Langer 1983, Lovell 1996, Morgan et al 1982). Knowing that the locus of control is at least partly within herself will tend to alleviate anxiety and enable the woman to feel positive (Raphael-Leff 1991).

Massage

The woman who is suffering from backache or pain during her labour may find appropriate massage very soothing. The midwife or partner may perform circular massage over the lumbosacral area, reducing friction with the use of talcum powder, body lotion or massage oil.

Deep massage is given by applying pressure with the heel of the hand, the knuckles or an object such as a tennis ball.

Some women may find it comforting to have abdominal massage; light circular strokes over the whole abdomen may be soothing, using both hands and passing the fingertips lightly up from the symphysis pubis, across the fundus of the uterus and down either side of the abdomen. Some may prefer a similar two-handed technique across the lower abdomen, where the pain of uterine contractions is usually felt. Women may like to do this for themselves.

If the woman finds it difficult to relax any part of herself, such as her face, she may benefit from sensitive use of massage in that area.

Transcutaneous electrical nerve stimulation (TENS)

This method of pain relief in labour has been gaining in popularity since the mid-1980s. It has been welcomed by many because it is non-pharmacological and not surgically invasive. Women like the idea of having some control and there may even be an element of distraction for the woman as she adjusts and experiments with it. It does not appear to have any residual effect on the fetus or the mother if used correctly.

It is thought to work by interrupting pain

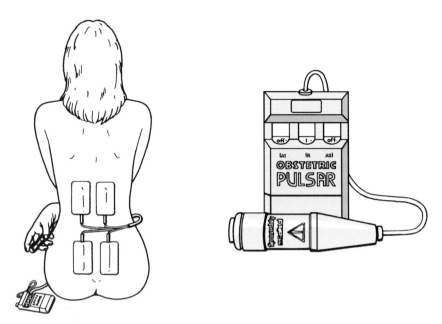

Fig. 23.4 TENS equipment in use, showing the electrodes in position on the back (reproduced by courtesy of Spembly Medical Company Ltd).

transmission along the sensory pathway and by stimulating production of endogenous opioids.

Electrodes are attached to the woman's back on the skin areas, known as *dermatomes*, overlying the nerve endings of thoracic and lumbar nerves T10 to L1, and over those of sacral nerves S2 to S4 (Fig. 23.4). Electrodes may also be placed on the woman's abdomen. It is important that these are accurately placed if the woman is to receive maximum benefit. The equipment is operated by the mother and this adds to its acceptability by women. Ideally the mother should become familiar with the equipment during pregnancy. The apparatus is activated by pressing a small button which causes a small electric current to pass through the electrodes. The electric current may be low frequency and intermittent (*pulsed*) or high frequency and continuous. Low frequency TENS stimulates the release of endogenous opioids while high frequency current closes the pain gate. As the pain of labour intensifies the woman increases the intensity of the electric current and graduates from low frequency to high frequency current. She may feel this as tingling, or as a sharper electric shock sensation. Some women will not tolerate

this and for some it will not provide adequate analgesia when used alone. It is most effective when started in early labour and so many women hire their own TENS apparatus. Because there are no residual effects the woman may receive some other form of pain relief whenever she feels the need except that she cannot use TENS in the bath or birthing pool.

Many women will be keen to persevere with its use because they do not want drugs or invasive techniques such as epidural or spinal anaesthesia.

Some anaesthetists and obstetricians are sceptical as to its efficacy but many midwives feel that if it is safe and acceptable to women, many of whom express great satisfaction, then it is a welcome adjunct to the other methods of pain relief in labour.

It is probably most useful for the multigravid woman, who may expect a shorter labour, though many primigravidae will also find it beneficial. It will be most helpful for the woman who is highly motivated to use it and who is confident that it will be effective.

In 1991 the UKCC approved TENS for use

by midwives on their own responsibility provided that:

- they have received adequate and appropriate instruction; this is to be determined by local policy
- safety standards conform to those laid down by the Department of Health Medical Devices Directorate or the equivalent body in Scotland, Wales or Northern Ireland.

The midwife must be aware of certain contraindications to the use of TENS. These are:

- any woman with a cardiac pacemaker
- any woman with epilepsy, unless she has had a thorough medical examination
- the woman should not drive while using TENS
- TENS should be stopped immediately if any skin reaction occurs at the electrode placement sites.

TENS may occasionally interfere with certain electronic fetal monitors, although Davies (1997) suggests that this is not a major problem. If this is suspected, TENS apparatus should be switched off to obtain an accurate trace from the monitor. A different fetal monitor may be satisfactory.

For more detailed information on all aspects of the use of TENS, the reader is referred to Davies (1997).

The use of water for labour and delivery

(See also Alderdice et al 1995, Balaskas & Gordon 1992, Burns & Greenish 1993, Garland 1995, Royal College of Midwives 1994.)

Soaking in a warm bath is a recognised comfort to relieve aches, pains and stress. There has been a significant increase in interest in the effectiveness of warm water for pain relief in labour.

The first beneficial effect appears to be relaxation and increased well-being. Secondary to this, and as a direct effect of the water, there is thought to be a reduction of pain perception. Tactile and thermal receptors are stimulated by warm water, and the response to this is to reduce pain stimulus at the dorsal column 'closing the gate' to pain.

The woman will feel less cumbersome and be more mobile in water and can more readily experiment with alternative positions.

It is recommended that the woman should be immersed to the level of the nipples, and should keep her abdomen under water for maximum benefit.

The water temperature is thought to be important, and the temperature should be closely monitored and kept between 36 and 38°C just before and during the second stage of labour.

Criteria commonly cited for using a birthpool are:

- the woman must be at 37 weeks' gestation or more with a singleton pregnancy
- presentation must be cephalic
- labour should have commenced spontaneously
- the cervix must be dilating – some centres specify dilatation of 4 or 5 cm
- there must be no signs of fetal distress and when the membranes rupture the liquor must be clear
- there must be no deviations from normal such as raised blood pressure or ante- or intrapartum haemorrhage.

The benefits and risks of waterbirths are not adequately researched to date (Alderdice & Marchant 1997, Garland & Jones 1997).

Many midwives feel that they have insufficient experience and skills to undertake delivery in water. If the midwife feels she is competent to offer care in labour to the woman who wishes to use water for labour, she may find that the woman is then reluctant to leave the bath when she is ready to deliver.

The midwife has a professional responsibility to ensure that she has the knowledge and skills necessary to carry out any of her professional duties competently, safely, and within local guidelines.

ALTERNATIVE METHODS OF PAIN RELIEF

(See also Moore & Holden 1997, Tiran & Mack 1995.)

Many mothers are anxious to avoid pharmacological or invasive methods of pain relief in labour and this contributes to the popularity of complementary methods of analgesia which are coming into more common use.

Acupuncture. The mode of action of this ancient practice, which originated in China and the Far East, is not fully understood. It may be related to stimulating the release of endogenous opioids as well as interruption of the transmission of pain stimuli. It is said to relate to the flow of energy within the body which occurs along specific pathways or 'meridians', and to restore balance within these where necessary.

Women may wish to employ this method of pain relief but may have difficulty in finding a practitioner who is willing to be available whenever they commence labour. The presence of the acupuncturist would need to be negotiated.

One variant of acupuncture is electro-acupuncture, where the acupuncture needle is stimulated electrically so that it vibrates slightly at the acupuncture site, so enhancing its efficacy. Another is acupressure, where the appropriate site is massaged, or pressure is applied in a particular way.

Reflexology is similar to acupressure, but is a distinct technique. Again, it has its origins in Eastern medicine.

Homeopathy. Homeopathy works on the principle that 'like cures like' in order to restore healthy balance within the body. Homeopathic remedies used in childbirth may be given to boost flagging morale and lift the mother's spirits; others include raspberry leaf tea to encourage cervical dilatation and caullophyllum to stimulate uterine contractions. Arnica has soothing and healing properties, and helps reduce bruising.

Herbalism. Herbalism is the forerunner of the modern pharmaceutical industry and uses combinations of natural plant extracts. Herbalists claim that their remedies improve general health and physiological balance, as well as improving strength and stamina.

Aromatherapy. This involves the use of aromatic oils, some of which are definitely contraindicated in pregnancy and labour. The essential oils used are concentrated extracts of plants and flowers which are thought to restore balance within the mind and body. These substances probably work mainly through the limbic system, that part of the brain where emotion and memory are effected. The essential oils are mixed with carrier oils and may then be used for massage, as a bath oil or in an oil burner. Aromatherapy oils should not be used in a birthpool, as they could have adverse effects on the baby if he comes into direct contact with them.

Yoga and meditation are claimed to have a calming effect, assist the mother in becoming attuned to her body, and give a focus for distraction from pain and tension.

Hypnosis. A few medical practitioners offer hypnosis as a pain-relieving technique. Women are usually taught self-hypnosis and in suitable subjects it may be successful.

Midwives who are interested in alternative forms of pain relief must be aware of their professional responsibilities and parameters of practice, detailed in the Standards for the Administration of Medicines (UKCC 1992), The Midwife's Code of Practice (UKCC 1994) and Guidelines for Professional Practice (UKCC 1996).

They should be prepared to make a thorough study of the remedies available, their uses and mode of action and the possible side-effects (see also Ch. 44 for a fuller discussion of complementary therapies).

PHARMACOLOGICAL METHODS OF PAIN RELIEF

Sedatives and analgesics

(See also Bevis 1997.)

Sedatives such as temazepam may be given to women in early labour, to encourage sleep and rest.

Analgesics which are used in early labour are in the mild-to-moderate analgesic range, for example paracetamol or co-dydramol.

Such drugs are usually included in the standing orders which allow a midwife to administer specified drugs in certain situations at her own discretion.

Narcotics

A narcotic is a strong analgesic drug with some sedative properties. Narcotic drugs include the opioids.

Pethidine

Pethidine (meperidine in the USA) has been used as an analgesic for women in labour since the 1940s. Although other drugs have been introduced from time to time, none shows any distinct advantage over pethidine.

Pethidine, given by intramuscular injection, appears to give satisfactory analgesia to some individuals but not to others. Some women afterwards claim that they felt unpleasantly drowsy and detached in labour but did not have adequate pain relief. They may complain of nausea or may vomit following the administration of pethidine.

An important side-effect of pethidine is that it reduces gastric motility, which is already slowed during labour. This means that gastric contents remain in the stomach, becoming more acid as labour progresses. Vomiting is an unpleasant side-effect but the risk of aspiration of acid stomach contents, if anaesthesia is required in an obstetric emergency, is the greater concern (Reynolds 1993). It is therefore common practice to give ranitidine with pethidine; this inhibits secretion of gastric hydrochloric acid. Metoclopramide will stimulate gastric emptying without stimulating gastric acid secretion, and thus has an antiemetic effect.

Pethidine may be given together with a tranquilliser such as promethazine. Although not as effective as metoclopramide, promethazine has some antiemetic action. These drugs make the woman feel relaxed and potentiate the analgesia.

Infants of mothers who received pethidine during labour may be slow to establish spontaneous respiration at birth because the respiratory centre is depressed. As alternative methods of analgesia such as epidural are available, it should not be necessary to give large total doses of pethidine. It is generally believed that the baby is less likely to be affected if pethidine is not given between 2 and 4 hours before delivery. Reynolds (1990) argues that this is not the case; Morrison et al (1973) showed that neonatal respiratory depression is likely to be greater if pethidine is given several hours before delivery, but much less marked if given within 1 hour of birth. Kuhnert et al (1985) studied the use of low doses of pethidine and found similar neonatal outcomes. Such effects are influenced by maternal metabolism of drugs, the degree and speed of transfer of drug and metabolites from maternal to fetal circulation, and the ability of the fetus to process and excrete both.

The baby whose mother received pethidine during labour is also likely to be affected in more subtle ways. Detailed neurobehavioural studies show that these babies tend to be slightly less alert, suck less frequently and demonstrate reduced peak sucking pressures when feeding (Rajan 1994). They show a slightly slower response to light and sound, a less brisk Moro reflex and tend to be less cuddly and consolable (Brazelton 1973). These very subtle effects are said to last for up to 48 hours but some authorities state that these babies are affected for much longer periods, possibly several months.

Parents have often read about these effects on the baby in the popular medical press and may be unduly anxious. They need careful advice to enable them to make an informed decision regarding pain relief in labour.

In obstetric units where active management of labour is practised an initial dose of 50 mg of pethidine may be given. This may be repeated after 30 minutes if it is not effective (O'Driscoll et al 1993).

In some units a patient-controlled analgesia (PCA) device may be used. This is designed to administer a small intravenous dose of pethidine on demand from the mother. In-built safety mechanisms include a time limit so that the dose may not be repeated too frequently. Rayburn et al (1989) found that women who used a PCA device tended to avail themselves of higher total doses than women whose analgesia was controlled by staff; this has important implications for the newborn baby.

It is easy to give a standard dose of pethidine to women in labour without considering variations in bodyweight. Thus a large lady would receive the same amount of analgesic as a small, slim woman, when it would be appropriate to give her a considerably larger amount. This may account in part for the apparent inadequacy of opioid analgesia in labour (Bevis 1997).

Other opioid drugs

Diamorphine or morphine may be used instead of pethidine. All these drugs have similar disadvantages. Some authorities feel that diamorphine offers better analgesia; it certainly gives the woman a pleasant feeling of detachment and well-being. Those who do not favour its use fear the possibility of addiction and it is more likely than pethidine to cause respiratory depression in the neonate.

Opioid antagonist. The action of the opioid drugs may be reversed by the use of the opioid antagonist naloxone (Narcan). Naloxone will reverse any respiratory depression caused by the opioid but will also reverse the analgesic effect. It acts by competing for the opioid receptors and blocking them, so that the opioid is rendered ineffective. Very occasionally the naloxone may become ineffective before the opioid has been excreted. The opioid may then become effective again.

The most common use of naloxone in obstetrics is when it is given to the baby who is born with respiratory depression due to the administration of an opioid to the mother (see Ch. 34).

Pentazocine

Pentazocine (Fortral) has not enjoyed great popularity. Its analgesic effect is said to be equivalent to that of pethidine and it does cause less nausea and vomiting. It is also less likely to cause respiratory depression in the infant but if this effect is seen, naloxone is effective in reversing it. Some women who have received pentazocine have complained of unpleasant dreams and of feeling hot and sweaty and they have disliked it for these reasons.

Meptazinol

Meptazinol (Meptid) was introduced in the mid-1980s, and may well have advantages over pethidine as the side-effects, although similar, are less marked. It is claimed to give rise to less respiratory depression in the neonate.

Inhalational analgesia

With the advent of epidural analgesia inhalational methods of analgesia have become less widely used but they still have their place.

They offer effective pain relief for the majority of women, with the advantage that all their effects are short-lived and they do not give rise to any complications in the neonate.

One approved inhalational analgesic agent is available for use by the midwife in the UK without medical supervision, provided she has been trained in its use. This agent is Entonox.

Entonox

Entonox is the trade name used to describe an equal mixture of oxygen and nitrous oxide. Nitrous oxide is used in higher concentrations as a general anaesthetic.

Physical qualities. Entonox is colourless and odourless; women may complain of a smell associated with its use but this arises from the black rubber tubing and not from the gas itself.

Equipment. In major obstetric units Entonox is usually piped to each labour room (Fig. 23.5). Alternatively a medium-sized cylinder on a wheeled

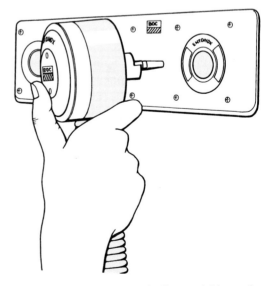

Fig. 23.5 Entonox apparatus; pipeline model (reproduced by courtesy of British Oxygen Company Ltd).

stand may be used and is easily moved from room to room (Fig. 23.6). The community midwife may obtain Entonox in a small cylinder which is fairly easy to transport; the apparatus is compact but quite heavy (Fig. 23.7).

Piped Entonox comes from a bank of large cylinders situated at a central point. These must be checked and maintained so that there is always a good supply of full cylinders.

Cylinders should always be stored on their sides rather than upright. Nitrous oxide is heavier than oxygen and the two gases may separate in extreme cold (below −7°C). If the cylinder is kept on its side the two gases may be remixed more effectively before use. The temperature of the storage site should be kept above 10°C. If the cylinders have been subjected to freezing conditions, they should be kept in a temperature of at least 10°C for 2 hours prior to use, or placed for 5 minutes in a bath of warm water (no hotter than 35°C), keeping the part of the cylinder above the neck dry. Afterwards the cylinder is inverted at least three times to mix the contents.

Entonox apparatus. This is manufactured by

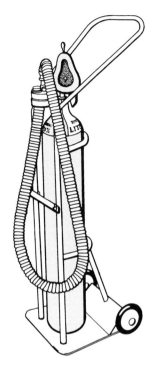

Fig. 23.6 Entonox apparatus; hospital cylinder model (reproduced by courtesy of British Oxygen Company Ltd).

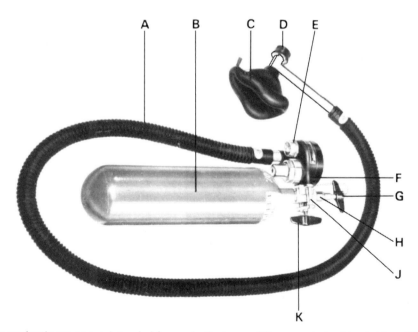

Fig. 23.7 Entonox analgesic apparatus, intended for use in the home: (A) corrugated rubber tubing; (B) 500-litre cylinder; (C) face mask; (D) expiratory valve; (E) cylinder pressure gauge; (F) demand regulator; (G) cylinder valve key; (H) pin-index valve; (J) cylinder yoke; (K) cylinder yoke key. (Reproduced by courtesy of British Oxygen Company Ltd.)

the British Oxygen Company (BOC) and is probably the most commonly used device for delivering nitrous oxide and oxygen in midwifery practice in the UK. The apparatus and the cylinder are made so that neither will fit any other equipment. They fit together by means of matching pins and holes (the pin index system). The cylinder is blue with a blue and white quartered shoulder. The apparatus has a demand valve which opens on inspiration by the user and the angle-piece attached to the mask or mouthpiece has an expiratory valve which prevents exhaled gas from being rebreathed. A cylinder pressure gauge indicates when the cylinder is becoming empty.

When Entonox is provided to the labour room from a piped supply the demand valve and non-return expiratory valve are still incorporated. In some units *scavenging equipment* to extract expired gases from the room may be fitted.

Principles involved. It is important that the mother be instructed correctly if she is to obtain maximum benefit from inhalational analgesia.

Entonox does not flow continuously from the cylinder but must be obtained by the woman's own inspiratory efforts. She must therefore be instructed to fit the mask firmly over her nose and mouth, or close her lips firmly round the mouthpiece, and take a steady breath in. Care must be taken to avoid hyperventilation; if this occurs the woman will complain of dizziness and numbness of the face and hands. She exhales into the mask or mouthpiece, which has an expiratory valve attached.

Analgesia is obtained from Entonox within about 20 seconds and the maximum effect is felt after about 45–60 seconds. The mother is instructed to start using the Entonox as soon as the contraction starts and to continue until the peak of the contraction has passed. The midwife needs to help the woman to recognise when a contraction is starting as there will be no pain at first.

The mother should be persuaded, for her own safety, to hold the mask or mouthpiece herself, since part of the principle of self-administration is that she will drop it if she takes too much of the gas.

Use with narcotics. For most primigravid women Entonox does not provide adequate analgesia alone and is often used in conjunction with pethidine. Ideally it is not used for long periods of time, although it is excreted quickly and is therefore thought not to have any residual effects.

Effects on the fetus. Because Entonox is excreted quickly from the mother via her lungs it is not thought to have any residual effect on the fetus. It will cross the placenta following the *concentration gradient*; this means that if levels are higher in the mother Entonox will pass from her to the fetus and vice versa, so that the situation is one of continual change.

The midwife's responsibilities
In the UK the United Kingdom Central Council for Nursing, Midwifery and Health Visiting (UKCC) lays down both rules and guidelines governing the midwife's practice (see Ch. 9).

Training and supervision. The midwife who is involved in the administration of inhalational analgesia is only permitted to do this if she has been trained and supervised in the use of both the agent and the apparatus concerned. Although her employer has a responsibility in this, the midwife herself is expected to seek further help and training if she does not feel confident in this area.

There are four types of apparatus approved for use by midwives on their own responsibility. These are:

* the original BOC Entonox apparatus described above
* the PneuPac apparatus
* the SOS Nitronox – midwifery model
* the Peacemaker.

Care of equipment. The equipment used must be serviced and maintained at the prescribed intervals. The community or independent midwife takes the responsibility for this herself, while in hospital practice it may be delegated to the appropriate service department or a midwifery manager. However, the individual midwife still has a responsibility to check equipment before use, and not to use it if there is any question at all as to its safety.

Selection of women. The use of inhalational analgesia is rarely contraindicated. The midwife must check the woman's medical history and if she has any reason to consider that inhalational analgesia may be an unwise choice, she should seek a medical opinion.

READER ACTIVITIES

1. Devise a study designed to find out how newly delivered women's expectations of labour differed from the reality.

Aim to elicit how they felt they could have been better prepared in the antenatal period, and also try to evaluate the support they received from their carers during labour.

Run a pilot study to test the format, but discuss the procedure with a mentor first.

2. Select some case notes of recently delivered women in your care, including some with one or more complications and investigate the management of their pain.

Discuss with a group of colleagues the care and support these women received. Attempt to evaluate their care.

Consider what kind of support you would wish to have if you were in these circumstances.

REFERENCES

Alderdice F, Marchant S 1997 Water in labour. In: Moore S (ed) Understanding pain and its relief in labour. Churchill Livingstone, Edinburgh

Alderdice F A, Renfrew M J, Marchant S et al 1995 Labour and birth in water in England and Wales: survey report. British Journal of Midwifery 3(7): 375–382

Balaskas J 1991 New active birth, revised edn. Thorsons, London

Balaskas J, Gordon Y 1992 Waterbirths. Thorsons, London

Bevis R 1997 Drugs in labour. In: Moore S (ed) Understanding pain and its relief in labour. Churchill Livingstone, Edinburgh

Bonica J J 1994 Labour pain. In: Wall P, Melzack R (eds) Textbook of pain. Churchill Livingstone, Edinburgh

Brazelton T B 1973 Neonatal behavioral assessment scale. Clinics in Developmental Medicine 50. Heinemann, London

Burns E, Greenish K 1993 Pooling information. Nursing Times 89(8): 47–49

Choucri L 1997 Care by midwives: women's experiences. In: Moore S (ed) Understanding pain and its relief in labour. Churchill Livingstone, Edinburgh

Davies R 1997 Transcutaneous nerve stimulation. In: Moore S (ed) Understanding pain and its relief in labour. Churchill Livingstone, Edinburgh

Department of Health (DH) 1993 Changing childbirth: report of the expert maternity group. HMSO, London

Dick-Read G 1943 Revelation of childbirth: the principles and practice of natural childbirth, 2nd edn. William Heinemann, London

Flint C 1986 Sensitive midwifery. Heinemann, London

Freely M 1995 Team midwifery – a personal experience. In: Page L (ed) Effective group practice in midwifery. Blackwell Science, Oxford

Garland D 1995 Waterbirth. Books for Midwives Press, Cheshire

Garland D, Jones K 1997 Waterbirth – updating the evidence. British Journal of Midwifery 5(6): 368–373

Guyton A C 1987 Basic neuroscience: anatomy and physiology. W B Saunders, Philadelphia

Halldorsdottir S, Karlsdottir S 1996 Journeying through labour and delivery: perceptions of women who have given birth. Midwifery 12(2): 48–61

Hayes L 1997 A cultural experience of pain. In: Moore S (ed) Understanding pain and its relief in labour. Churchill Livingstone, Edinburgh

Hodnett E 1993 Support from caregivers during childbirth. In: Enkin M W, Keirse M J N C (eds) Effective care in pregnancy and childbirth. Vol 2: Childbirth. Oxford University Press, Oxford

Kuhnert B R, Luin P, Kennard M J et al 1985 Effects of low doses of meperidine on neonatal behavior. Anesthesia and Analgesia 64: 335–342

Langer E J 1983 The psychology of control. Sage Books, Beverley Hills

Lovell A 1996 Power and choice in birthgiving: some thoughts. Midwifery 4(5): 268–272

Martin E 1987 The woman in the body. Open University Press, Milton Keynes

Melzack R 1984 The myth of painless childbirth. Pain 19: 321–337

Melzack R, Wall P D 1988 The challenge of pain, 2nd edn. Penguin Books, Harmondsworth

Melzack R, Belanger E, Lacroix R 1991 Labour pain: effect of maternal position on front and back pain. Journal of Pain and Symptom Management 6(8): 476–480

Moore S 1997 Physiology of pain. In: Moore S (ed) Understanding pain and its relief in labour. Churchill Livingstone, Edinburgh

Moore S, Holden M 1997 Complementary medicine for pain control in labour. In: Moore S (ed) Understanding pain and its relief in labour. Churchill Livingstone, Edinburgh

Morgan B M, Bulpitt C J, Clifton P et al 1982 Analgesia and satisfaction in childbirth (the Queen Charlottes 1000 mother survey). Lancet ii: 808–810

Morrison J C et al 1973 Metabolites of meperidine related to fetal depression. American Journal of Obstetrics and Gynecology 15: 1132–1137

Oakley A 1984 The captured womb: a history of medical care in pregnancy. Basil Blackwell, Oxford

Odent M 1984 Birth reborn. Souvenir Press, London

O'Driscoll K, Meagher D, Boylan P 1993 Active management of labour, 3rd edn. Mosby Year Books, Europe

Page L 1995 Putting principles into practice. In: Page L (ed) Effective group practice in midwifery: working with women. Blackwell Science, Oxford

Priest J, Schott J 1991 Leading antenatal classes: parenthood in prospect. Butterworth-Heinemann, Oxford

Rajan L 1994 The impact of obstetric procedures and analgesia and anaesthesia during labour and delivery on breast feeding. Midwifery 10: 87–103

Raphael-Leff J 1991 Psychological processes of childbearing. Chapman & Hall, London

Rayburn W, Leuschen M P, Earl R et al 1989 Intravenous meperidine during labour: a randomised comparison between nursing and patient-controlled administration. Obstetrics and Gynecology 74(5): 702–706

Reynolds F 1990 Pain relief in labour. British Journal of Obstetrics and Gynaecology 97: 757–759

Reynolds F 1993 Pain relief in labour. British Journal of Obstetrics and Gynaecology 100: 979–983

Rickford W J K, Reynolds F 1987 Expectations and experiences of pain relief in labour. In: Society for Obstetric Anesthesiology and Perinatology (Abstracts) 163. Halifax, Nova Scotia

Royal College of Midwives 1994 The use of water during labour: position statement. RCM, London

Schott J, Henley A 1996 Culture, religion and childbearing in a multiracial society. Butterworth-Heinemann, Oxford

Simkin P 1986 Stress, pain and catecholamines in labour. Part II – Stress associated with childbirth events. Birth 13: 234–240

Thiroux J P 1986 Ethics – theory and practice. Macmillan Publishing Company, New York

Tiran D, Mack S 1995 Complementary therapies for pregnancy and childbirth. Baillière Tindall, London

United Kingdom Central Council for Nursing, Midwifery and Health Visiting (UKCC) 1991 Registrar's Letter 8/1991 14/5/91. UKCC, London

United Kingdom Central Council for Nursing, Midwifery and Health Visiting (UKCC) 1992 Standards for the administration of medicines. UKCC, London

United Kingdom Central Council for Nursing, Midwifery and Health Visiting (UKCC) 1994 The midwife's code of practice. UKCC, London

United Kingdom Central Council for Nursing, Midwifery and Health Visiting (UKCC) 1996 Guidelines for professional practice. UKCC, London

Wall P, Melzack R 1994 Textbook of pain. Churchill Livingstone, Edinburgh

FURTHER READING

Bevis R 1984 Anaesthesia in midwifery. Baillière Tindall, London

Bogod 1992 Options for pain control in labour. Maternal and Child Health 17(7): 214–217

Bradley C, Brewin C R, Duncan S L B et al 1983 Perceptions of labour: discrepancies between midwives' and patients' ratings. British Journal of Obstetrics and Gynaecology 90: 1176–1179

Caldeyro-Barcia R 1979 The influence of maternal position on time of spontaneous rupture of the membranes, progress in labour and fetal head compression. Birth and the Family 6(1): 7–15

Chamberlain G, Wraight A, Steer P (eds) 1993 Pain and its relief in childbirth. Churchill Livingstone, Edinburgh

Dickersin K 1993 Pharmacological control of pain during labour. In: Chalmers I, Enkin M W, Keirse M J N C (eds) Effective care in pregnancy and childbirth. Vol 2: Childbirth. Oxford University Press, Oxford

Heywood A M, Ho E 1990 Pain relief in labour. In: Alexander J, Levy V, Roch S (eds) Midwifery practice – intrapartum care. Macmillan Press, London

Kitzinger S 1987 Giving birth – how it really feels. Victor Gollancz, London

McFarlane A 1977 Psychology of childbirth. Fontana, London

Mander R 1992 The control of pain in labour. Journal of Clinical Nursing 1: 219–223

Moir D D 1986 Obstetric anaesthesia and analgesia, 5th edn. Baillière Tindall, London

Niven C 1990 Coping with labour pain – the midwife's role. In: Robinson S, Thomson A M (eds) Midwives, research and childbirth 3. Chapman & Hall, London

Nursing Times 1993 Complementary therapy. Special Issue, Autumn 1993

Polden M 1985 Transcutaneous nerve stimulation in labour and post-caesarean section. Physiotherapy 71(8): 350–353

Rajan L 1993 Perceptions of pain and pain relief in labour: the gulf between experience and observation. Midwifery 9: 136–145

Simkin P 1989 Non-pharmacological methods of pain relief during labour. In: Chalmers I, Enkin M W, Keirse M J N C (eds) Effective care in pregnancy and childbirth. Vol 2: Childbirth. Oxford University Press, Oxford

Thomson A M, Hillier V F 1994 A re-evaluation of the effect of pethidine on the length of labour. Journal of Advanced Nursing 19(3): 448–456

Waldenstrom V 1988 Midwives' attitudes to pain relief during labour and delivery. Midwifery 4(2): 48–57

Physiology and management of the second stage of labour

Edith M. Hillan

The second stage of labour is a time when the whole tempo of activity changes. The mother's passive control during the long hours of the first stage is replaced by intense physical effort and exertion for a comparatively short period. Both parents require stamina, courage and confidence in the skill of the attendant midwife. Excitement and expectation mount as the birth becomes imminent. A happy outcome will depend upon a successful partnership between professionals and parents. A mother will never forget the midwife who delivered her baby.

The chapter aims to:

- consider the diagnosis of the second stage of labour

- describe the sequence of events during this stage in normal labour

- discuss the care of the mother and her partner and the observations required

- review the positions that the mother may adopt and their relative advantages and disadvantages

- describe the process of delivery

- consider the rationale for episiotomy, together with its risks and benefits, and describe the techniques of episiotomy and perineal repair.

PHYSIOLOGICAL CHANGES

The second stage of labour begins when the cervix is fully dilated and ends with the baby's birth. A knowledge of the physiological processes and of the actual mechanism of delivery forms the basis for determining midwifery care.

The physiological changes result from a continuation of the same forces which have been at work during the first stage of labour but activity is accelerated once the cervix has become fully dilated. This acceleration, however, does not occur abruptly. There may be a lull before the woman experiences the full expulsive nature of the second stage contractions.

Uterine action

Contractions become stronger and longer but may be less frequent, allowing both mother and fetus a recovery period during the resting phase. The membranes often rupture spontaneously at the onset of the second stage. The consequent drainage of liquor allows the hard, round fetal head to be directly applied to the vaginal tissues and aid distension. Fetal axis pressure increases flexion of the head which results in smaller presenting diameters, more rapid progress and less trauma to both mother and fetus.

The contractions become expulsive and as the fetus descends further into the vagina, pressure from the presenting part stimulates nerve receptors in the pelvic floor (Ferguson's reflex) and the woman experiences the need to push. This reflex may initially be controlled to a limited extent but becomes increasingly compulsive, overwhelming and involuntary during each contraction. The mother's response is to employ her secondary powers of expulsion by contracting her abdominal muscles and diaphragm.

Soft tissue displacement

As the hard fetal head descends, the soft tissues of the pelvis become displaced. Anteriorly, the bladder is pushed upwards into the abdomen where it is at less risk of injury during fetal descent. This results in the stretching and thinning of the urethra so that its lumen is reduced. Posteriorly, the rectum becomes flattened into the sacral curve and the pressure of the advancing head expels any residual faecal matter. The levator ani muscles dilate, thin out and are displaced laterally, and the perineal body is flattened, stretched and thinned. The fetal head becomes visible at the vulva, advancing with each contraction and receding during the resting phase until crowning takes place and the head is born. The shoulders and body follow with the next contraction, accompanied by a gush of amniotic fluid. The second stage culminates in the birth of the baby.

Recognition of the commencement of the second stage of labour

The transition from the first to the second stage is not always clinically apparent. Several of the signs are presumptive and not a reliable index that this stage has been reached. Nevertheless the midwife should be able to diagnose the onset of the second stage of labour. The purpose is not to impose a time limit on its duration but to conserve maternal energy and minimise the avoidable soft tissue trauma caused by premature pushing.

Presumptive signs and differential diagnoses

Expulsive uterine contractions. It is possible for a woman to feel a strong desire to push before the cervix is fully dilated, especially if the fetus is in an occipitoposterior position, the rectum is full or the woman is highly parous.

Rupture of the forewaters. This may occur at any time during labour.

Dilatation and gaping of the anus. Deep engagement of the presenting part and premature maternal effort may produce this sign during the latter part of the first stage.

Appearance of the presenting part. Excessive moulding may result in the formation of a large caput succedaneum which can protrude through the cervix prior to full dilatation. Similarly a breech presentation may be visible when the cervix is only 7–8 cm dilated.

Show. This must be distinguished from bleeding due to partial separation of the placenta or that caused by ruptured vasa praevia.

Congestion of the vulva. Enthusiastic premature pushing may also cause this.

The appearance of several presumptive signs may indicate that the second stage of labour has been reached.

Confirmatory evidence

Confirmation of the onset of second stage can only be established by performing a vaginal examination. No cervix can be felt on examination. Although the midwife should be reluctant to perform repeated vaginal examinations, she should conduct the delivery on the basis of accurate observation and assessment of progress.

THE MECHANISM OF NORMAL LABOUR

As the fetus descends, soft tissue and bony structures exert pressures which force him to negotiate the birth canal by a series of passive movements. Collectively, these movements are called the mechanism of labour. There is a mechanism for every presentation and position which can be delivered vaginally. Knowledge and recognition of the normal mechanism enables the midwife to anticipate the next step in the process of descent which in turn will dictate her conduct of the delivery. Her understanding and constant monitoring of these movements ensure that normal progress is recognised, the delivery safely completed and early assistance sought should any delay occur. During vaginal delivery the fetal presentation and position will govern the exact mechanism as the fetus responds to external pressures.

Principles common to all mechanisms are:

- descent takes place throughout
- whichever part leads and first meets the resistance of the pelvic floor will rotate forwards until it comes under the symphysis pubis
- whatever emerges from the pelvis will pivot around the pubic bone.

During the mechanism of normal labour the fetus turns slightly to take advantage of the widest available space in each plane of the pelvis. The widest diameter of the pelvic brim is the transverse: at the pelvic outlet the greatest space lies in the anteroposterior diameter.

At the onset of labour, the commonest presentation is the vertex and the most common position either left or right occipitoanterior; therefore it is this mechanism which will be described. When

these conditions are met, the way that the fetus is normally situated can be described as follows:

- the lie is longitudinal
- the presentation is cephalic
- the position is right or left occipitoanterior
- the attitude is one of good flexion
- the denominator is the occiput
- the presenting part is the posterior part of the anterior parietal bone. (See Ch. 13 for definitions of these terms.)

Main movements

Descent. Descent of the fetal head into the pelvis often begins before the onset of labour. In primigravidae it usually occurs during the latter weeks of pregnancy when engagement of the head provides confirmation that vaginal delivery is probable. In multigravidae muscle tone is lax and therefore engagement may not occur until labour actually begins. Throughout the first stage of labour the forces of contraction and retraction aid descent. Following rupture of the forewaters and full dilatation of the cervix, maternal effort speeds progress.

Flexion. This increases throughout labour. The fetal spine is attached nearer the posterior part of the skull; pressure exerted down the fetal axis will be more forcibly transmitted to the occiput than the sinciput. The effect is to increase flexion which results in smaller presenting diameters which will negotiate the pelvis more easily. At the onset of labour the suboccipitofrontal diameter, 10 cm, is presenting; with greater flexion the suboccipitobregmatic diameter, 9.5 cm, presents. The occiput becomes the *leading part*.

Internal rotation of the head. During a contraction the leading part is driven downwards onto the pelvic floor. The resistance of this muscular diaphragm brings about rotation. As the contraction fades, the pelvic floor rebounds, causing the occiput to glide forwards. Resistance is therefore an important determinant of rotation. (This explains why rotation is often delayed following epidural anaesthesia which causes relaxation of pelvic floor muscles.) The slope of the pelvic floor determines the direction of rotation. The muscles are gutter-shaped and slope down anteriorly, so whichever part of the fetus first meets the lateral half of this slope will be directed forwards and towards the centre. In a well-flexed vertex presentation the occiput leads and meets the pelvic floor first and rotates anteriorly through one-eighth of a circle. This causes a slight twist in the neck of the fetus as the head is no longer in direct alignment with the shoulders. The anteroposterior diameter of the head now lies in the widest (anteroposterior) diameter of the pelvic outlet, facilitating an easy escape (Fig. 24.1). The occiput slips beneath the sub-pubic arch and crowning occurs when the head no longer recedes between contractions and the widest transverse diameter (biparietal) is born. If flexion is maintained, the suboccipitobregmatic diameter, 9.5 cm, distends the vaginal orifice.

Extension of the head. Once crowning has occurred the fetal head can extend, pivoting on the suboccipital region around the pubic bone. This releases the sinciput, face and chin which sweep the perineum and are born by a movement of extension. The suboccipitofrontal diameter, 10 cm, distends the vaginal outlet.

Restitution. The twist in the neck of the fetus which resulted from internal rotation is now corrected by a slight untwisting movement. The occiput moves one-eighth of a circle towards the side from which it started (Fig. 24.2).

Internal rotation of the shoulders. The shoulders undergo a similar rotation to that of the head to lie in the widest diameter of the pelvic outlet, namely anteroposterior. The anterior shoulder is the first to reach the levator ani muscle and therefore rotates anteriorly to lie under the symphysis pubis. This movement can be clearly seen as the head turns at the same time (*external rotation of the head*) (Fig. 24.2). It occurs in the same direction as restitution and the occiput of the fetal head now lies laterally.

Lateral flexion. The shoulders are born sequentially, usually the anterior shoulder first. The anterior shoulder slips beneath the sub-pubic arch and the posterior shoulder passes over the perineum. This enables a smaller diameter to distend the

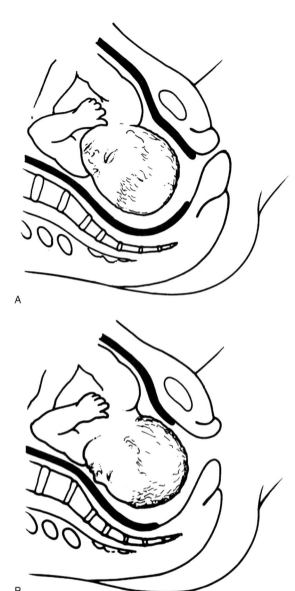

A

B

Fig. 24.1 (A) Internal rotation of the head begins. (B) Upon completion, the occiput lies under the symphysis pubis.

vaginal orifice than if both shoulders were born simultaneously. The remainder of the body is born by lateral flexion as the spine bends sideways through the curved birth canal.

Duration of the second stage

Once the onset of the second stage has been con-

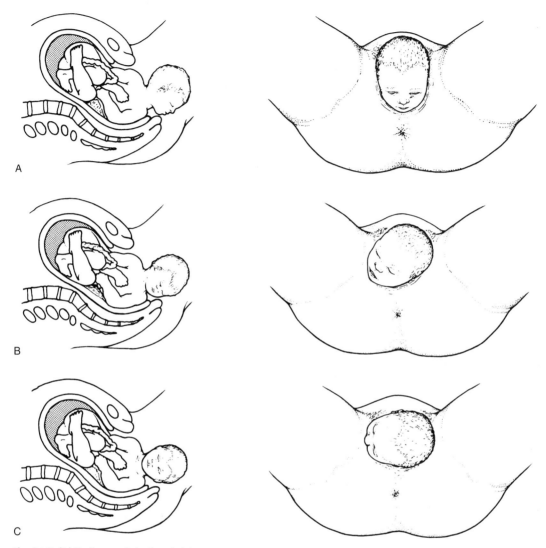

Fig. 24.2 (A) Delivery of the head. (B) Restitution. (C) External rotation.

firmed a woman should not be left without a midwife in attendance, especially if she is to be delivered at home. Accurate observation of progress is vital, for the unexpected can always happen. The duration of the second stage is difficult to predict with any degree of certainty. In multigravidae it may last as little as 5 minutes; in primigravidae the process may take 2 hours. More important than the time factor is the evidence of progressive descent and the condition of mother and fetus. There is no good evidence to suggest that the imposition of an upper time limit for

duration of second stage improves the outcome for mother or baby (Sleep et al 1989). Two phases in progress may be recognised, the latent phase during which descent and rotation occur followed by the active phase with descent and the urge to push.

The latent phase

This begins at full cervical dilatation although the presenting part may not yet have reached the pelvic outlet. The soft tissues of the vagina and pelvic floor gradually stretch and thin under the pressure of the advancing fetal head. The woman may experience little expulsive urge until the head has descended sufficiently to exert pressure on the rectum and perineal tissues. The head will then become visible.

There is scant evidence that active pushing during the latent phase achieves much, apart from exhausting and discouraging the mother. On the contrary, uterine supports and vaginal and perineal muscle may become strained and damaged as a result of the woman's efforts to push before these tissues have been able to stretch gradually (Benyon 1957). This same study showed that spontaneous delivery was not speeded by maternal effort at this stage. Passive descent of the fetus should be allowed to continue until the head is visible at the vulva.

Active phase

Once the fetal head is visible the woman will probably experience a compulsive urge to push. In the absence of this reflex, the midwife's instruction and encouragement may enable the mother to use her contractions effectively to expedite delivery but such intervention is rarely needed.

The recognition of the two phases of descent is particularly important if an effective epidural is in progress as there is little benefit in allowing the analgesia to wear off until the active phase has been reached.

The time taken to complete the second stage will vary considerably between mothers; clearly it should not be allowed to continue for many hours. However, in the presence of regular contractions, good maternal and fetal condition and progressive descent, considerable flexibility in duration should be allowed.

MIDWIFERY CARE

Care of the parents

The couple will now realise that the birth of their baby is imminent. They may feel excited and elated but at the same time anxious and frightened by the dramatic change in pace. The midwife's calm approach and information about what is happening can safeguard a cooperative partnership. This is critical at a time when a woman may feel a lack of control over events which can result in a sensation of panic. This is especially true when a supportive companion is not present. In this situation the midwife's role is even more important. The relationship of trust which she is able to build up during the earlier stages of labour will help to establish the mother's confidence in her skills. In order to achieve this, it is eminently preferable that the same midwife should look after the couple throughout labour. It may not always be possible but continuity of care is advantageous for both parents and professional. The partner's wishes about being present at the actual birth should have been fully discussed with the couple and documented prior to the start of labour.

In practice, even the most reluctant of partners may decide to change his mind and witness the birth. He is then able to offer his continued support and the couple can share the climactic moment when their baby is born. If, however, the father chooses not to be present, his wishes should be respected. In this case the mother should be given the opportunity to select another companion of her choice.

Throughout the second stage of labour the parents need explanations of events; the midwife should praise and congratulate the mother on her hard work, regardless of apparent progress, so that she is encouraged to participate actively.

Observations during the second stage of labour

Four factors determine whether the second stage may safely continue and these must be carefully monitored:

* uterine contractions
* descent of the presenting part
* fetal condition
* maternal condition.

Uterine contractions. The strength, length and frequency of contractions should be assessed continuously. They are usually stronger and longer than during the first stage of labour, lasting up to 1 minute with a longer resting phase between. The posture and position adopted by the mother may influence the contractions. The left lateral or the upright position may improve their effectiveness.

The progress of descent.   Progress is observed by noting the descent of the fetal head as it advances during contractions and recedes afterwards. This becomes apparent during the active phase. Initially, descent occurs slowly, especially in primigravidae, but it accelerates during the active phase. It may occur very rapidly in multigravidae. If descent is progressive, it should not be necessary for the midwife to make a further vaginal examination. If, however, there is a delay in progress of more than half an hour, a vaginal examination should be performed. This will confirm whether or not internal rotation of the head has taken place, the station of the presenting part and whether a caput succedaneum has formed. If the occiput has rotated anteriorly, the head is well flexed and caput succedaneum is not excessive it is likely that progress will continue.

If there is anxiety about either fetal or maternal condition, a doctor must be notified. In these circumstances vaginal assessment may be delayed until his arrival.

Fetal condition.   The liquor amnii is observed for signs of meconium staining. As the fetus descends, fetal oxygenation may be less efficient owing to either cord or head compression or to reduced perfusion at the placental site. The midwife should learn to recognise the normal changes in fetal heart rate patterns during the second stage, so that assistance may be sought at the earliest indication of fetal distress whilst avoiding the risk of unwarranted interference (see Ch. 22).

Maternal condition.   The midwife's observation includes an appraisal of the mother's ability to cope emotionally as well as an assessment of her physical well-being. Maternal pulse rate is usually recorded quarter-hourly and blood pressure hourly, provided that these are within normal limits.

Pushing

The urge to push may come before the vertex is visible. In order to conserve maternal effort and allow the vaginal tissues to stretch passively, the mother should be helped to avoid active pushing

at this stage. She should be asked to find a comfortable position and encouraged not to push. Often lying in the left lateral position relieves pressure on the rectum and improves placental blood flow. The breathing exercises learned during pregnancy may help her to control this urge (see Ch. 45).

Once the head becomes visible the woman should be encouraged to follow her own inclinations in relation to expulsive effort. Few women need formalised instruction on how to push; the desire is so overwhelming that the response becomes involuntary and compelling. Her pushing effort will be regulated in response to the varying intensity of her contractions. Most women fall into their own rhythm after the first few exertions. Attempts to override spontaneous efforts by encouraging sustained pushing accompanied by prolonged breath-holding (the Valsalva manoeuvre) may result in potentially adverse haemodynamic consequences (Nikodem 1995a). The mother is therefore the best judge of when and how to push. This concept is endorsed by Inch (1982) who advocates that mothers should be allowed 'to follow their physiological inclinations'. This results in maximum pressure being exerted at the height of a contraction, which is beneficial. Delaying active pushing in this way allows the vaginal muscles to become taut and prevents bladder supports and the transverse cervical ligaments from being pushed down in front of the baby's head. This may help to prevent prolapse and urinary incontinence in later life (Benyon 1957).

Some mothers may become frightened by the overwhelming urge and cry out. This may help a woman to cope with the contractions and she should feel free to express herself in this way. If, however, these sounds are an embarrassment to the mother or cause distress to other couples, the woman may wish to use the Entonox mask to inhale the analgesia or simply to help to muffle the sound. The midwife's gentle reassurance and praise will help to boost confidence, enabling the mother to assert her control over events. The atmosphere should be calm and the pace unhurried.

Maternal comfort and hygiene

As a result of her exertions the woman usually feels very hot and sticky and she will find it soothing to have her face and neck sponged with a cool flannel. Her mouth and lips may become very dry. Sips of iced water are refreshing and a moisturising cream can be applied to her lips. Her partner may help with these tasks as a positive contribution to ease her discomfort. Pain relief remains important but this is discussed further in Chapter 23.

Bladder care

As the fetus descends into the pelvis, the bladder is particularly vulnerable to damage from the pressure of the advancing head. The bladder base may become compressed between the pelvic brim and the fetal head. The risk of trauma is greatly increased if the bladder is distended. The woman should be encouraged to pass urine at the beginning of the second stage unless she has recently done so. Small amounts of urine may dribble during contractions.

Position

General considerations

The position the mother may choose to adopt is dictated by several factors:

• *Maternal and fetal condition*. If there is any concern about the well-being of either the woman or her baby then a need for frequent or continuous monitoring may limit the choices available to her.

• The *mother's personal preference* should always be a primary consideration.

• *The environment*. For reasons of safety and privacy it may not be possible to consider all the alternative positions.

• The *midwife's confidence* in her own skills to supervise the delivery when the mother prefers to adopt a posture with which she has little or no experience. However, a real understanding of the mechanism of labour should enable the midwife to adapt to any position that the woman wishes to adopt.

A full discussion of these issues should take place during pregnancy and the woman's preference should be ascertained and documented. The physiotherapist and midwife in partnership may advise about preparatory exercises which may be necessary to enable a particular position such

as squatting to be sustained. Practicalities such as physical support and protection of furnishings and carpets should also be discussed.

The semirecumbent or supported sitting position, with the thighs abducted, is the posture most commonly encouraged in western cultures. There is evidence to suggest that if the mother lies flat on her back, vena caval compression is increased, resulting in hypotension, and this can lead to reduced placental perfusion and diminished fetal oxygenation (Humphrey et al 1974, Kurz et al 1982). The efficiency of uterine contractions may also be reduced. Unless she is well supported, it may be difficult for a mother to direct her pushing efficiently and if she is semirecumbent, her weight is on her sacrum, which directs the coccyx forwards and reduces the pelvic outlet. Dorsal positions afford the midwife good access and a clear view of the perineum (Fig. 24.3).

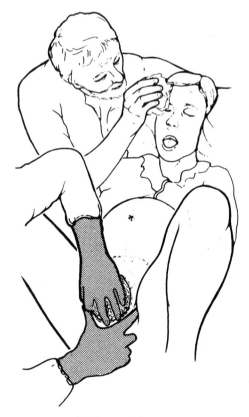

Fig. 24.3 Supported sitting position.

Squatting, kneeling or standing (Fig. 24.4). In western countries these positions have been encouraged only in recent years. In primitive cultures where women follow their own inclinations, the majority choose to adopt a variation or combination of these postures (Russell 1982). Science supports their choice. Radiological evidence demonstrates an increase of 1 cm in the transverse diameter and 2 cm in the anteroposterior diameter of the pelvic outlet when the squatting position is adopted. This produces a 28% increase in the overall area of the outlet when comparing the supine with the squatting position, resulting in obvious benefit to the progress and ease of delivery (Russell 1969).

The birthing chair is an attempt to reconcile the advantages of an upright posture with ease of access to the perineum. Women using birthing chairs are, however, at increased risk of postpartum haemorrhage (Stewart et al 1983, Turner et al 1986). This may arise as a consequence of perineal trauma exacerbated by obstructed venous return which is reflected in the excessive perineal oedema and haemorrhoids reported in women who spend long periods of time in birthing chairs (Cottrell

& Shannahan 1986). This tendency to postpartum haemorrhage is unlikely to be due to increased risk of bleeding from the placental site.

Left lateral position. This is not widely used in current practice. The perineum can be clearly viewed and uterine action is effective but an assistant may be required to support the right thigh. It provides an alternative for women who find it difficult to abduct their hips. The mother usually turns back into the dorsal position for delivery of the placenta. During this manoeuvre she should keep her knees together to prevent the uterus from filling with air; the contracted fundus should be supported by the midwife's hand.

In a review of studies examining upright versus recumbent positions during the second stage of labour, Nikodem (1995b) showed there were clear advantages for women in adopting an upright position. Women who were upright experienced less discomfort, less difficulty in bearing down, fewer abnormal deliveries and less perineal or vaginal trauma and vulval oedema when compared with women who delivered in a recumbent position. The only apparent disadvantage of upright positions is that they tend to be associated with an increased incidence of labial tears. More women who delivered in upright positions expressed a positive response about the delivery position. The perceived advantages included less pain and backache.

Whichever position the mother chooses, she is most likely to trust a midwife who allows her freedom of choice and active participation in her labour. Flexibility is the keynote. Positive and dramatic effects can be achieved by encouraging the mother to change and adapt her position in response to the way her body feels (Fig. 24.5).

Leg cramp is a common occurrence whichever posture is adopted. It can be relieved by massaging the calf muscle, extending the leg and dorsiflexing the foot.

Preparation for delivery

Once the onset of the second stage has been confirmed the midwife should make preliminary

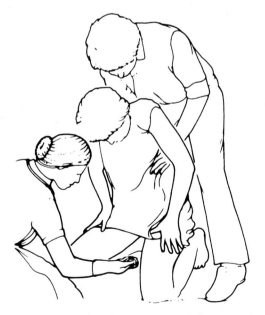

Fig. 24.4 Squatting/kneeling position with father lending support.

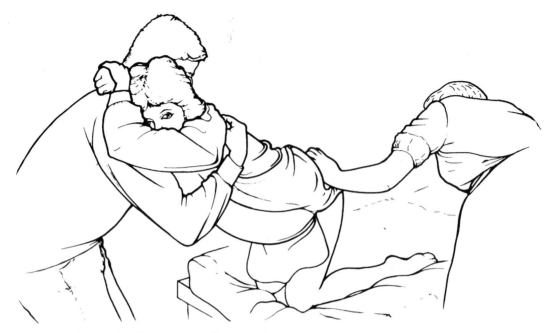

Fig. 24.5 A change of position can sometimes speed progress.

preparations for delivery. There is usually little urgency if the woman is primigravid but multigravidae may progress very rapidly.

The room in which the delivery is to take place should be warm with a spotlight available so that the perineum can be easily observed. The woman may wish other family members to witness the birth, especially if delivery is taking place at home. A clean area should be prepared to receive the baby and waterproof covers provided to protect the bed and floor. A sterile delivery pack which includes cord clamps, a midwife's gown and rubber gloves are placed to hand. An oxytocic agent (commonly Syntometrine 1 ml) is prepared in readiness for the active management of the third stage or for use during an emergency and is checked by a second person. It must be kept separate from any neonatal drugs to avoid risk of error. Some units favour the use of Syntocinon, 5 or 10 units, as the oxytocic since it avoids the side-effects of ergometrine, but if greater weight is placed on a lower blood loss, Syntometrine would be the drug of choice (McDonald et al 1997; see also Ch. 25).

A warm cot and clothes should be prepared for the baby. In hospital a heated mattress may be used; at home, a *warm* water bottle (as opposed to a hot water bottle) can be placed in the cot.

Neonatal resuscitation equipment must be thoroughly checked and readily accessible and should include portable oxygen equipment for home deliveries.

Conducting the delivery

The midwife's skill and judgement are crucial factors in minimising maternal trauma and ensuring a safe delivery for the baby. These qualities are acquired by experience but certain basic principles should be applied whatever the expertise of the accoucheuse. They are:

- observation of progress
- prevention of infection
- emotional and physical comfort of the mother
- anticipation of normal events
- recognition of abnormal developments.

Asepsis

During delivery both mother and baby are particularly vulnerable to infection. Care must be taken to observe meticulous aseptic technique when preparing sterile equipment. Sterilised surgical gloves must be worn during the delivery for the protection of both mother and midwife.

The time at which the midwife decides to scrub up will vary. If the mother is multigravid it is wise to prepare as soon as the fetal head becomes visible: in primigravidae the head usually takes a little longer to advance over the perineum. Once she has put on her gown and gloves the midwife prepares her sterile equipment. This includes the following main items:

• warm antiseptic solution
• cotton wool and pads
• cord scissors and clamps.

Delivery of the head

Throughout these preparations the midwife must not be distracted from monitoring the descent of the fetus. She must either watch the advance of the fetal head or control it with her hand or both. Quick action may be necessary if advance is rapid.

The perineum is swabbed, the delivery area draped with sterile towels and a pad used to cover the anus. There is currently no evidence to show whether or not the practice either of guarding or of massaging the perineum is effective in minimising spontaneous trauma. With each contraction the head descends. As it does so the superficial muscles of the pelvic floor can be seen to stretch, especially the transverse perineal muscles. The head recedes during the resting phase, which allows these muscles to thin gradually. The skill of the midwife in ensuring that the active phase is unhurried helps to safeguard the perineum from trauma.

The midwife places her fingers on the advancing head to monitor descent and prevent expulsive crowning which may result in perineal laceration. As the perineum distends, the decision is made as to whether an episiotomy is necessary. Light pressure on the head is maintained so that its birth is controlled. For her part, the mother can achieve control by gently blowing or 'sighing' out each breath in order to avoid pushing. The midwife will have prepared her to listen for instructions and the partner can be very supportive in relaying these. Delivery of the head in this way may take two or three contractions but delicate control will avoid unnecessary maternal trauma (Fig. 24.6).

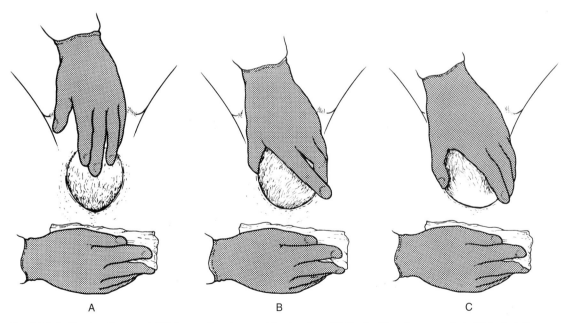

Fig. 24.6 Delivering the head. (A) Preventing too rapid extension. (B) Controlling the crowning. (C) Easing the perineum to release the face.

Once crowned, the head is born by extension as the face appears at the perineum. During the resting phase before the next contraction the midwife has time to check that the cord is not around the baby's neck. If found, it should, if possible, be slackened to form a loop through which the shoulders may pass. If tightly applied, it may still be possible to deliver the baby without cutting the cord by keeping the head near the perineum as the shoulders deliver, rather than attempting to place the baby on the mother's abdomen. If, however, the cord is very tightly wound around the neck, two artery forceps are applied 3 cm apart and the cord is severed between the two clamps. Great care must be taken that in this confined space other tissues are not clamped in error. When cutting the turgid cord it is always a wise precaution to hold a swab over the area as it is incised. This will reduce the risk of the attendants being sprayed with blood during the procedure. Once severed, the cord may be unwound from around the neck.

The mother may now be able to see and touch her baby's head and assist in delivery of the trunk.

Delivery of the shoulders

Restitution and external rotation of the head must occur in order to deliver the shoulders safely and to avoid perineal laceration. External rotation shows that the shoulders are rotating into the antero-posterior diameter of the pelvic outlet which is the largest space. The midwife proceeds to deliver one shoulder at a time to avoid overstretching the perineum. A hand is placed on each side of the baby's head, over the ears, and downward traction is applied. This allows the anterior shoulder to slip beneath the symphysis pubis while the posterior shoulder remains in the vagina. If the third stage is to be actively managed, the assistant is instructed to give intramuscular Syntometrine 1 ml or Syntocinon 5–10 units. When the axillary crease is seen, the head and trunk are guided in an upward curve to allow the posterior shoulder to escape over the perineum (Fig. 24.7). The midwife or mother may now grasp the baby around the chest to aid the birth of the trunk and lift the baby towards the mother's abdomen. This not only allows the mother immediate sighting of her baby and close skin contact with him but removes the baby from the

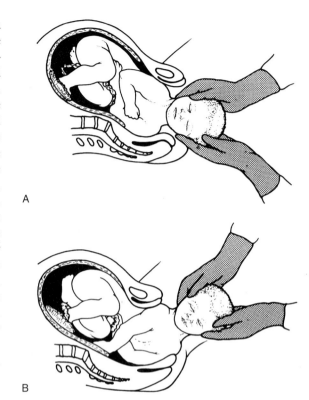

Fig. 24.7 (A) Downward traction releases anterior shoulder. (B) An upward curve allows the posterior shoulder to escape.

gush of liquor which accompanies release of the body. The time of birth is noted.

The cord is severed at whatever time is considered appropriate (see Ch. 34). The baby is dried and warmly wrapped to prevent cooling. Swabbing of the eyes and aspiration of mucus during and immediately following delivery are not considered to be necessary providing the baby's condition is satisfactory. Oral mucus extractors should not be used because of the risks of mucus which is contaminated with a virus such as the hepatitis virus or human immunodeficiency virus (HIV) entering the operator's mouth.

The moment of birth is both joyous and beautiful. The midwife is privileged to share this unique and intimate experience with the parents.

Episiotomy

This is an incision through the perineal tissues

which is designed to enlarge the vulval outlet during delivery. The UKCC sanctions its use by midwives, advocating prior infiltration of the perineum. As this is a surgical incision it is essential that the mother gives consent prior to the procedure. A detailed discussion should take place during pregnancy so that each woman is aware of the indications for and implications of the intervention. She should be assured that its use is selective and discretional. The mother's personal wishes for her own care should be clearly documented and respected.

The risks and benefits of episiotomy have been well reviewed (Banta & Thacker 1982, Hofmeyr & Sonnendecker 1987). The rationale for its use depends largely on the need to minimise the risk of severe, spontaneous, maternal trauma and to expedite the birth when there is evidence of fetal distress. During a normal delivery the indications for its use are few (Box 24.1) and the midwife should adopt a restrictive policy.

Research evidence generated by randomised, controlled trials has provided sound scientific evidence on which practice may be based. Sleep and colleagues (1984) demonstrated that the liberal (51%) use of episiotomy during normal deliveries resulted in few advantages for mothers in terms of healing and comfort, either at 10 days or at 3 months postpartum, when compared with a restrictive (10%) episiotomy policy. On the contrary, the liberal use of episiotomy is associated with higher rates of perineal trauma (Harrison et al 1984), although it does seem to protect against

anterior trauma around the labia and urethra. This, however, appears not to influence the incidences of pain on intercourse and of urinary incontinence either in the short or longer term (Sleep & Grant 1987). The midwife should use her skills to avoid this intervention if at all possible.

The timing of the incision

An episiotomy involves incision of the fourchette, the superficial muscles and skin of the perineum and the posterior vaginal wall. It can therefore successfully speed delivery only when the presenting part is directly applied to these tissues. If the episiotomy is performed too early it will fail to release the presenting part and haemorrhage from cut vessels may ensue. In addition, the levator ani muscles will not have had time to be displaced laterally and may be incised as well. If performed too late there will not be enough time to infiltrate with a local anaesthetic. There is also little reason for superimposing an episiotomy if a tear has already begun.

Types of incision

There are two main directions of incision:

Mediolateral. This begins at the midpoint of the fourchette and is directed at a 45° angle to the midline towards a point midway between the ischial tuberosity and the anus. This line avoids the danger of damage to both the anal sphincter and Bartholin's gland but it is the more difficult to repair. This is the incision largely used by midwives in the UK.

Median. This is a midline incision which follows the natural line of insertion of the perineal muscles. It is associated with reduced blood loss but a higher incidence of damage to the anal sphincter. It is the easier to repair and results in less pain and dyspareunia. This incision is favoured in the USA.

Infiltration of the perineum

The perineum should be adequately anaesthetised prior to the incision. Lignocaine is commonly used, 0.5% 10 ml or 1% 5 ml. The advantage of the more concentrated solution is that a smaller volume is needed. Lignocaine takes 3–4 minutes to take

---

Box 24.1 Indications for episiotomy

Justifiable indications
- To speed delivery if there is fetal distress.
- Prior to an assisted delivery such as forceps or Ventouse extraction.
- To minimise the risk of intracranial damage during preterm and breech delivery.

Dubious indications
- To prevent overstretching of the perineal muscles with the intention of preventing the longer-term problem of prolapse and stress incontinence.
- To reduce the risk of spontaneous 'explosive' trauma where the midwife has intuitive concern.

effect and, if possible, two or three contractions should be allowed to occur between infiltration and incision. The timing is not always easy to calculate but it is better to infiltrate and not perform an episiotomy than to incise the perineum without an effective local anaesthetic (see Ch. 28).

Method of infiltration. The perineum is cleansed with antiseptic solution. Two fingers are inserted into the vagina along the line of the proposed incision in order to protect the fetal head. The needle is inserted beneath the skin for 4–5 cm following the same line. The piston of the syringe should be withdrawn prior to injection to check whether the needle is in a blood vessel. If blood is aspirated, the needle should be repositioned and the procedure repeated until no blood is withdrawn. Lignocaine is continuously injected as the needle is slowly withdrawn. Some practitioners inject the whole amount in one operation. Anaesthesia is, however, more effective if about one-third of the amount is used at first and two further injections are made, one either side of the incision line (Fig. 24.8). The needle must be redirected just before the tip is withdrawn.

The incision. A straight-bladed, blunt-ended pair of Mayo scissors is usually used. The blades should be sharp to ensure a clean incision. (Some doctors prefer to use a scalpel for this reason.) Two fingers are inserted into the vagina as before and the open blades are positioned (see Fig. 24.8). The incision is best made during a contraction when the tissues are stretched so that there is a clear view of the area and bleeding is less likely to be severe. A single, deliberate cut 4–5 cm long is made at the correct angle. Delivery of the head should follow immediately and its advance must be immediately controlled in order to avoid extension of the episiotomy. If there is any delay before the head emerges, pressure should be applied to the episiotomy site between contractions in order to minimise bleeding. Postpartum haemorrhage can occur from an episiotomy site unless bleeding points are compressed.

Perineal repair

Midwives who have had instruction and supervised practice in suturing the perineum and are judged to be proficient may carry out the procedure. Trauma is best repaired as soon as possible after delivery in order to secure haemostasis and before oedema forms. It is also much kinder to the mother to complete this aspect of her care without undue delay and while the tissues are still anaesthetised. Prior to commencement the mother must be made as warm and comfortable as possible. The lithotomy position is usually chosen as it affords a clear view of the area. Other positions may be more appropriate in the home setting. A good, directional light is essential and the operator should be seated comfortably during the procedure.

The trolley, set with the appropriate instruments, antiseptic solution, suture materials and local anaesthetic, should be prepared before the mother's legs are placed in the stirrups. This minimises the time spent in this uncomfortable, undignified position and reduces the risks of complications such as deep vein thrombosis. The midwife scrubs and puts on sterile gown and gloves. The perineum is cleaned with warm antiseptic solution. Blood oozing from the uterus may obscure the field of vision, so a taped vaginal tampon may be inserted into the vault of the vagina. The tape is secured to the towelling drapes by a pair of forceps as a reminder that it must be removed upon completion of the procedure. Both insertion and removal should be recorded. The full extent of the trauma is assessed and explained to the mother. The procedure for repair should also be outlined so that she is aware of what is happening.

Spontaneous trauma may be of the labia anteriorly, the perineum posteriorly or both. A gentle, thorough examination must be carried out to assess the extent of the trauma accurately and to determine whether a doctor should carry out the repair, if it is extensive.

Anterior labial tears. It is debatable whether or not these should be sutured. Much depends upon the control of bleeding as the labia are very vascular. A suture may be necessary to secure haemostasis.

Posterior perineal trauma. Spontaneous tears are usually classified in degrees which are related to the anatomical structures which have been traumatised. This classification only serves as a guideline

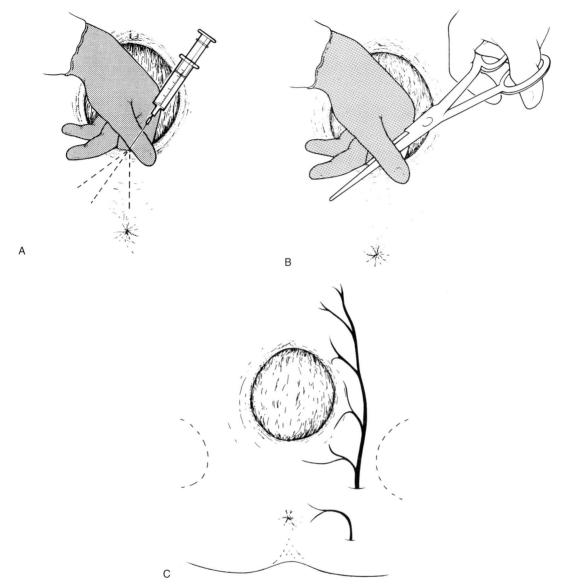

Fig. 24.8 (A) Infiltrating the perineum. (B) Performing an episiotomy. (C) Innervation of the vulval area and perineum.

because it is often difficult to identify the structures precisely.

- *1° tear* involves the fourchette only.
- *2° tear* involves the fourchette and the superficial perineal muscles, namely the bulbocavernosus and the transverse perineal muscles and in some cases the pubococcygeus.
- *3° tear.* In addition to the above structures there is damage to the anal sphincter.

- *4° tear.* This classification is sometimes used to describe trauma which extends into the rectal mucosa.

Third and fourth degree tears should be repaired by an experienced obstetrician. A general anaesthetic or effective epidural or spinal anaesthetic is necessary.

Prior to the commencement of repair, infiltration of the wound with local anaesthetic will be required. It is unlikely that any perineal infiltration carried out before delivery will be sufficient to ensure the mother's comfort during the procedure. Lignocaine 1% is used and time must be allowed for it to take effect before repair begins. If an epidural block is in progress, a 'top up' should be given.

The apex of the vaginal incision is identified and the posterior vaginal wall repaired from the apex downwards (Fig. 24.9). A continuous suture affords better haemostasis. The suture material recommended is polyglycolic acid (see below). The thread should not be pulled too tightly as oedema will develop during the first 24–48 hours. Care must be taken to identify other vaginal lacerations which should also be repaired. The deeper interrupted sutures are then inserted to repair the perineal muscles. Good approximation of tissue is important. The subsequent strength of the pelvic floor will depend largely upon adequate repair of this layer. For skin closure, a continuous subcuticular suture (see Fig. 24.9) results in fewer short-term problems than interrupted transcutaneous suturing techniques (Johanson 1995).

The best choice of method and materials for repair is debated. Grant (1986) highlights the lack of controlled trials to evaluate the different techniques and suture materials in terms of improved maternal comfort and reduced morbidity. This is likely to be of greatest significance in the choice for skin closure. In studies comparing the use of absorbable sutures (Dexon, Vicryl, chromic catgut) with non-absorbable sutures (silk, nylon), it has been shown that women sutured with absorbable sutures generally experience less pain and use less analgesia in the immediate postpartum period (Johanson 1995). Of the absorbable materials most commonly used, polyglycolic acid sutures (Dexon, Vicryl) cause less pain than chromic catgut but may cause significant irritation in a small number of women. On the basis of currently available evidence, both the deep layers and the skin should be sutured with polyglycolic acid sutures (Grant 1989).

Whatever the choice of material or type of suture, repair of the skin edges should begin at the fourchette so that the vaginal opening is properly aligned. When the wound has been closed, any

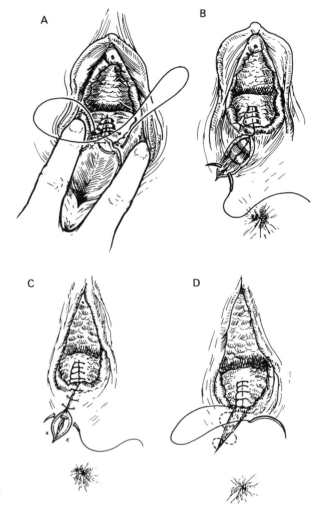

Fig. 24.9 Perineal repair. (A) A continuous suture is used to repair the vaginal wall. (B) Three or four interrupted sutures repair the fascia and muscle of the perineum. (C) Interrupted sutures to the skin. (D) Subcuticular skin suture.

further vulval lacerations should be repaired. Anterior labial tears occur more frequently when episiotomy has been avoided. This trauma does not appear to cause additional maternal discomfort 10 days after delivery (Sleep et al 1984).

The sutured areas should be inspected in order to confirm haemostasis before the vaginal pack is removed. A vaginal examination is made to ensure that the introitus has not been narrowed. Upon completion a rectal examination is made in order to ensure that no sutures have penetrated the rectal mucosa. Any such sutures must be removed to prevent fistula formation. It is essential to warn the mother before this examination is performed.

The area is cleaned and a sterile sanitary pad positioned over the vulva and perineum. The mother's legs are then gently and simultaneously removed from lithotomy support and she is made comfortable. The nature of the trauma and repair should be explained to her and information given on whether or not sutures will need to be removed.

If the midwife suspects damage to the upper vagina, cervix, anal sphincter or rectal mucosa, a senior obstetrician should be notified as this repair will be outside her province. A general anaesthetic is occasionally necessary if the trauma is extensive.

Records

It is the responsibility of the midwife conducting the delivery to complete the labour record. This should include details of any drugs administered, of the duration and progress of labour, of the reason for performing an episiotomy and of perineal repair. This information is recorded on the mother's notes and may be duplicated on her domiciliary record as well as in the birth register. Details of the baby's condition including Apgar score are also recorded.

The birth notification must be completed within 36 hours of delivery (see Ch. 48). This may be undertaken by anyone present at the birth but is usually carried out by the midwife. The notification is sent to the medical officer in the health district in which the baby was born.

The development of computerised records has minimised the need for duplication of information and has also reduced the time spent by midwives in completing several sets of documents. Computerised data are subject to the Data Protection Act 1984.

READER ACTIVITIES

1. What information is given to women who attend parentcraft classes in your area of practice in relation to perineal management at delivery and perineal care postpartum? It may prove enlightening to replicate part of Lyn Cater's study (1984). Following childbirth, women were invited to draw on a prepared diagram the direction and extent of perineal damage they believed they had sustained during delivery. The results highlighted how ill-prepared and poorly informed most women were; such findings have important implications for practice.

2. In the unit in which you work search for documents which influence or dictate any aspect of practice related to second stage management, for example the imposition of an upper limit of duration or an episiotomy policy. These documents may be guidelines for practice, defined standards of care or policy statements.

When were these documents compiled and by whom?

Are any of the recommendations supported by research evidence?

What can you do to change, improve or remove such limitations on practice?

REFERENCES

Banta D, Thacker S B 1982 The risks and benefits of episiotomy. Birth 9(1): 25–30
Benyon C 1957 The normal second stage of labour. Journal of Obstetrics and Gynaecology, British Empire 64: 6.1
Cater L 1984 A little knowledge.... Nursing Mirror 159(11): ii–viii
Cottrell B H, Shannahan M D 1986 Effect of the birth chair on duration of second stage labor and maternal outcome. Nursing Research 35: 364–367
Grant A 1986 Repair of episiotomies and perineal tears. British Journal of Obstetrics and Gynaecology 93: 176–178

Grant A 1989 Repair of perineal trauma after childbirth. In: Chalmers I, Enkin M, Keirse M J N C (eds) Effective care in pregnancy and childbirth. Oxford University Press, Oxford, pp 1170–1181
Harrison R F, Brennan M, North P M, Reed J V, Wickham E A 1984 Is routine episiotomy necessary? British Medical Journal 288: 1971–1975
Hofmeyr G J, Sonnendecker E W W 1987 Elective episiotomy in perspective. South African Medical Journal 71: 357–359
Humphrey M D, Chang A, Wood E C, Morgan S, Hounslow D 1974 A decrease in fetal pH during the second stage of

labour when conducted in the dorsal position. Journal of Obstetrics and Gynaecology, British Commonwealth 81: 600–602

Inch S 1982 The second stage. Birthrights. Hutchinson, London, pp 117–144

Johanson R B 1995 Continuous vs interrupted sutures for perineal repair. In: Keirse M J N C, Renfrew M J, Neilson J P, Crowther C (eds) Pregnancy and childbirth module of the Cochrane Database of Systematic Reviews (database on disk and CD-ROM). The Cochrane Collaboration, Issue 2. Update Software, Oxford. Available from BMJ Publishing Group, London

Kurz C S, Schneider H, Hutch R, Hutch A 1982 The influence of maternal position on the fetal transcutaneous oxygen pressure. Journal of Perinatal Medicine 10(suppl 2): 74–75

McDonald S, Prendiville W J, Elbourne D 1997 Prophylactic Syntometrine vs oxytocin in the third stage of labour. In: Neilson J P, Crowther C A, Hodnett E D, Hofmeyr G J (eds) Pregnancy and childbirth module of the Cochrane Database of Systematic Reviews (updated 1 September 1997). Available in the Cochrane Library (database on disk and CD-ROM). The Cochrane Collaboration, Issue 4, Update Software, Oxford

Nikodem V C 1995a Sustained (Valsalva) vs exhalatory bearing down in second stage of labour. In: Keirse M J N C, Renfrew M J, Neilson J P, Crowther C (eds) Pregnancy and childbirth module of the Cochrane Database of Systematic Reviews (database on disk and CD-ROM). The Cochrane

Collaboration, Issue 2. Update Software, Oxford. Available from BMJ Publishing Group, London

Nikodem V C 1995b Upright vs recumbent position during second stage of labour. In: Keirse M J N C, Renfrew M J, Neilson J P, Crowther C (eds) Pregnancy and childbirth module of the Cochrane Database of Systematic Reviews (database on disk and CD-ROM). The Cochrane Collaboration, Issue 2. Update Software, Oxford. Available from BMJ Publishing Group, London

Russell J G B 1969 Moulding of the pelvic outlet. Journal of Obstetrics and Gynaecology 76: 817–820

Russell J G B 1982 The rationale of primitive delivery positions. British Journal of Obstetrics and Gynaecology 89(September): 712–715

Sleep J, Grant A 1987 West Berkshire perineal trial: three-year follow up. British Medical Journal 295: 749–751

Sleep J, Grant A, Garcia J, Elbourne D, Spencer J, Chalmers I 1984 West Berkshire perineal management trial. British Medical Journal 289: 587–590

Sleep J, Roberts J, Chalmers I 1989 Care during the second stage of labour. In: Chalmers I, Enkin M, Keirse M J N C (eds) Effective care in pregnancy and childbirth. Oxford University Press, Oxford, pp 1129–1144

Stewart P, Hillan E, Calder A A 1983 A randomised trial to evaluate the use of a birth chair for delivery. Lancet i(June 11): 1296–1298

Turner M J, Romney M L, Webb J B, Gordon H 1986 The birthing chair: an obstetric hazard? Journal of Obstetrics and Gynaecology 6: 232–235

FURTHER READING

Johnstone F D, Aboelmagd M S, Harouni A K 1987 Maternal posture in the second stage and fetal acid base status. British Journal of Obstetrics and Gynaecology 94: 753–757

Knauth D G, Haloburdo E P 1986 Effect of pushing techniques in birthing chair on length of second stage of labour. Nursing Research 35: 49–51

Roberts J 1980 Alternative positions for child birth. Part II. Journal of Nurse-Midwifery 25(5): 13–19

Roberts J E, Goldstein S A, Gruener J S, Maggio M, Mendez-Bauer C 1987 A descriptive analysis of involuntary bearing down efforts during the expulsive phase of labour. Journal of Obstetric, Gynecologic and Neonatal Nursing 16: 48–55

Stewart K S 1984 The second stage. In: Studd J (ed) Progress in obstetrics and gynaecology. Churchill Livingstone, Edinburgh, vol 4, pp 197–216

25

Physiology and management of the third stage of labour

Sue McDonald

During the third stage of labour, the focus shifts from the mother's concentrated exertions of birth to her newborn infant. There is a sense of emotional and physical relief. Yet, for the mother, this has the potential to be the most dangerous stage of labour when the skill and expertise of the midwife will be crucial factors in facilitating a safe, healthy outcome.

The chapter aims to:

- describe the mechanism of placental separation and descent together with the normal physiological factors that ensure haemostasis

- consider the use of oxytocic drugs in third stage management and the timing of clamping of the umbilical cord

- discuss the midwife's care of the mother during and immediately after delivery of the placenta and membranes

- describe the causes and management of postpartum haemorrhage.

PHYSIOLOGICAL PROCESSES

These are a continuation of the processes and forces at work during the earlier stages of labour. It is an understanding of these changes which guides the midwife's practice. During the third stage, separation and expulsion of the placenta and membranes occur as the result of an interplay of mechanical and haemostatic factors. The time at which the placenta actually separates from the uterine wall may vary. It may shear off during the final expulsive contractions accompanying the birth of the baby or remain adherent for some considerable time. The third stage usually lasts between 5 and 15 minutes but any period up to 1 hour *may* be considered to be within normal limits.

Separation and descent of the placenta

Mechanical factors

The unique characteristic of uterine muscle lies in the power of retraction. During the second stage of labour the uterine cavity progressively empties, enabling the retraction process to accelerate. Thus by the beginning of the third stage the placental site has already begun to diminish in size. As this occurs the placenta itself becomes compressed and the blood in the intervillous spaces is forced back into the spongy layer of the decidua. Retraction of the oblique uterine muscle fibres exerts pressure on the blood vessels so that blood does not drain back into the maternal system. The vessels during this process become tense and congested. With the next contraction the distended veins burst and a small amount of blood seeps between the thin septa of the spongy layer and the placental surface, stripping it from its attachment (Fig. 25.1). As the surface area for placental attachment reduces, the relatively non-elastic placenta begins to detach from the uterine wall.

Separation usually begins centrally so that a retroplacental clot is formed (Fig. 25.2). This may further aid separation by exerting pressure at the midpoint of placental attachment so that the increased weight helps to strip the adherent lateral borders. This increased weight also helps to peel the membranes off the uterine wall so that the clot, thus formed, becomes enclosed in a membranous bag as the placenta descends, fetal surface first. This process of separation (first described by Schultze) is associated with more complete shearing of both placenta and membranes and less fluid blood loss (Fig. 25.3). Alternatively, the placenta may begin to detach unevenly at one of its lateral borders. The blood escapes so that separation is unaided by the formation of a retroplacental clot. The placenta descends, slipping sideways, maternal surface first. This process (first described by Matthews Duncan in the 19th century) takes longer and is associated with ragged, incomplete expulsion of the membranes and a higher fluid blood loss.

Once separation has occurred, the uterus contracts strongly, forcing placenta and membranes to fall into the lower uterine segment (Fig. 25.4) and finally into the vagina.

Haemostasis

The normal volume of blood flow through the placental site is 500–800 ml per minute. At placental separation this has to be arrested within seconds or serious haemorrhage will occur. The interplay of three factors within the normal physiological processes which control bleeding are critical in minimising blood loss and the serious sequelae of maternal morbidity and/or mortality which may result. They are:

1. Retraction of the oblique uterine muscle fibres in the upper uterine segment through which the tortuous blood vessels intertwine. The resultant thickening of the muscles exerts pressure on the torn vessels, acting as clamps, so securing a ligature action. This is shown in Figure 25.1. It is the absence of oblique fibres in the lower uterine segment that explains the greatly increased blood loss that usually accompanies placental separation in placenta praevia.

2. The presence of vigorous uterine contraction following separation brings the walls into apposition so that further pressure is exerted on the placental site.

3. The achievement of haemostasis. There is evidence to suggest that there is a transitory activation of the coagulation and fibrinolytic systems during, and immediately following, placental separation (Bonnar et al 1970). It is believed that this protective response is especially active at the placental site so that clot formation in the torn vessels is intensified. Following separation, the placental site is rapidly covered by a fibrin mesh utilising 5–10% of the circulating fibrinogen.

MANAGEMENT OF THE THIRD STAGE

The midwife's care of the mother should be based on an understanding of the normal physiological processes at work. Her actions can help to reduce the very real risks of haemorrhage, infection, retained placenta and shock, any of which may increase maternal morbidity and even result in death. A mother's ability to withstand these complications depends, to a large degree, upon her general condition and the avoidance of debilitating, predisposing

A

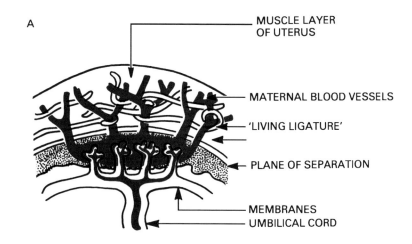

MUSCLE LAYER
OF UTERUS

MATERNAL BLOOD VESSELS

'LIVING LIGATURE'

PLANE OF SEPARATION

MEMBRANES
UMBILICAL CORD

B

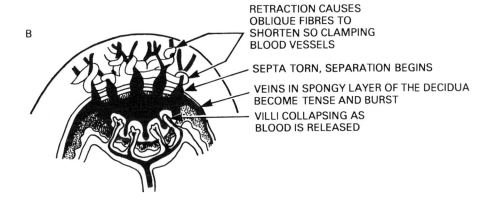

RETRACTION CAUSES
OBLIQUE FIBRES TO
SHORTEN SO CLAMPING
BLOOD VESSELS

SEPTA TORN, SEPARATION BEGINS

VEINS IN SPONGY LAYER OF THE DECIDUA
BECOME TENSE AND BURST

VILLI COLLAPSING AS
BLOOD IS RELEASED

C

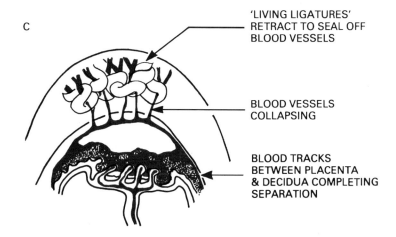

'LIVING LIGATURES'
RETRACT TO SEAL OFF
BLOOD VESSELS

BLOOD VESSELS
COLLAPSING

BLOOD TRACKS
BETWEEN PLACENTA
& DECIDUA COMPLETING
SEPARATION

Fig. 25.1 The placental site during separation: (A) uterus and placenta before separation; (B) separation begins; (C) separation almost complete.

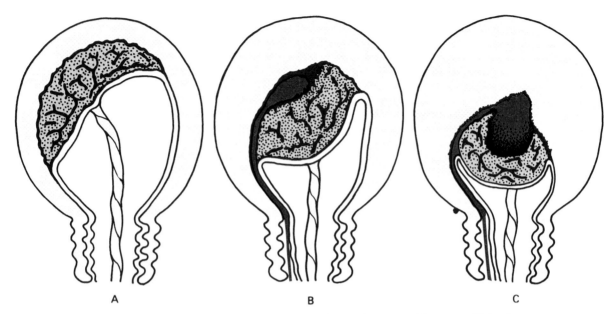

Fig. 25.2 The mechanism of placental separation: (A) uterine wall partially retracted but not sufficiently to cause placental separation; (B) further contraction and retraction thicken uterine wall, reduce placental site and aid placental separation; (C) complete separation and formation of retroplacental clot. *Note.* The thin lower segment has collapsed like a concertina following the birth of the baby.

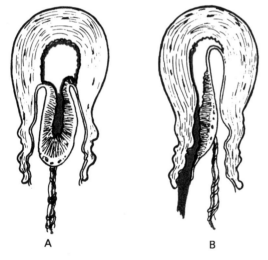

Fig. 25.3 Expulsion of the placenta: (A) Schultze method; (B) Matthews Duncan method.

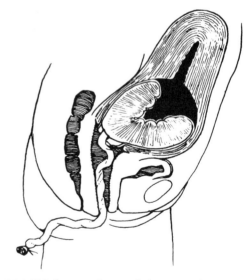

Fig. 25.4 Third stage: placenta in lower uterine segment.

problems such as anaemia, ketosis, exhaustion and prolonged hypotonic uterine action. Factors that may influence the risk of haemorrhage are discussed in more detail later in this chapter under 'Complications of the third stage of labour'.

Oxytocic agents

These are drugs that stimulate the uterus to contract. They may be administered at crowning of the baby's head, at delivery of the anterior shoulder of the baby, at the end of the second stage of labour or following the delivery of the placenta.

Ergometrine-based oxytocics such as Syntometrine are more likely to be associated with the risk of side-effects such as maternal hypertension, nausea and vomiting. During the antenatal period it is important to discuss the use of oxytocic drugs during the third stage with each mother, explaining their use in relation to the events of labour and the method of placental delivery. It is also important to understand and be able to communicate the different applications of oxytocic use.

Prophylactic use of oxytocics, is the *routine* administration of an oxytocic *at the time of birth of the baby*, given as a precautionary measure for the prevention of postpartum haemorrhage regardless of the assessed risk status of the woman. Prophylactic oxytocic administration is part of *active management*, a policy of labour management widely practised throughout the developed world. It usually comprises the administration of an oxytocic drug, clamping of the umbilical cord immediately following birth of the baby and delivery of the placenta by the use of controlled cord traction.

Therapeutic oxytocic administration implies the *subsequent use* of an oxytocic to either stop bleeding once it has occurred or to maintain the uterus in a contracted state when there are indications that excessive bleeding is likely to occur. This oxytocic administration practice is more consistent with a physiological or *expectant management* philosophy of care. In this event, routine administration of an oxytocic drug is withheld, the umbilical cord is left unclamped until cord pulsation has ceased and/or the mother requests it to be clamped and the placenta is expelled by use of gravity and maternal effort.

Emergency use usually indicates an event of uncontrolled haemorrhage.

If a woman specifically requests that oxytocic drugs be withheld from routine use in her third stage care, the midwife should clarify the circumstances in which this decision may be reversed. If an oxytocic drug is *not* to be used, the woman's preference for care must be recorded in her notes antenatally. Some would wish the record to be signed by the mother. It would be prudent for the midwife to notify her supervisor of such a request if it is contrary to local guidelines. In practice one of the following oxytocic drugs is usually used.

Intravenous ergometrine 0.25 mg

This acts within 45 seconds; therefore it is particularly useful in securing a rapid contraction where hypotonic uterine action results in haemorrhage. If a doctor is not present in such an emergency, a midwife may give the injection. Prendiville et al (1988a) in an overview of the choice of oxytocics for use in the third stage found that there was no supportive evidence for the continued routine use of intravenous ergometrine, which is associated with an increased risk of retained placenta. If an intravenous cannula is not already in situ, any difficulty encountered in locating a vein or sudden movement by the woman may result in failed venepuncture or at least a delay in administration.

Syntometrine

A 1-ml ampoule contains 5 units of Syntocinon and 0.5 mg ergometrine and is administered by intramuscular injection. The Syntocinon acts within 2 minutes, and the ergometrine within 6–7 minutes (Fig. 25.5). Their combined action results in a rapid uterine contraction enhanced by a stronger, more sustained contraction lasting several hours. It is usually administered as the anterior shoulder of the baby is delivered, thus stimulating good uterine action at the beginning of the third stage. The use of Syntometrine or any ergometrine-based drug is associated with side-effects such as elevation of the blood pressure, nausea and vomiting.

CAUTION. No more than two doses of ergometrine 0.5 mg should be given as it can cause headache, nausea and hypertension. Great caution is required where a hypertensive state already presents and its use is usually contraindicated.

Syntocinon

Syntocinon is a synthetic form of the natural oxytocin produced in the anterior pituitary, is free from side-effects and safe to use in a wider context

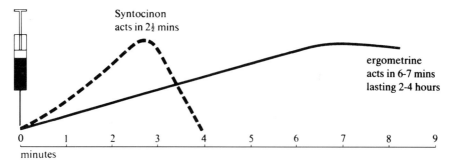

Fig. 25.5 The rapid action of Syntocinon in comparison with ergometrine.

than Syntometrine. It can be administered both as an intravenous and an intramuscular injection.

Research evidence to date suggests that this is an effective oxytocic choice where routine prophylactic management of the third stage of labour is practised (Khan et al 1995, McDonald et al 1993).

Prostaglandins

The use of prostaglandins for third stage management has up until now been more often associated with the *treatment* of postpartum haemorrhage than with *prophylaxis*. This may be partly due to it being substantially more expensive than the already discussed oxytocics. Prostaglandin agents are also associated with side-effects such as diarrhoea (Chua et al 1995) and cardiovascular complications of increased stroke volume and heart rate (Van Selm et al 1995). Prostaglandin administration is most effective when used intramurally (injected directly into the uterine wall) or by intrauterine irrigation (Peyser & Kupfermine 1990). The procedures are time consuming and invasive and the expertise required for undertaking the procedures is unlikely to always be readily available in routine labour management.

More recently, results from an observational study using a prostaglandin E_1 analogue (misoprostol), suitable for oral administration, has been reported (El-Refaey et al 1997). The authors suggest that misoprostol, which is rapidly absorbed, not prone to problems of temperature control and does not require the use of sterile syringes and needles, may be a suitable uterotonic agent for use in the prophylactic management of the third stage of labour. This is an important issue, particularly in relation to developing world settings, where approximately 90% of deaths related to postpartum haemorrhage occur.

Further appropriately designed trials are currently being undertaken in conjunction with the World Health Organization to assess the future value of this drug for management of the third stage of labour.

Clamping of the umbilical cord

This may have been carried out during delivery of the baby if the cord was tightly around the neck. However, opinions vary as to the most beneficial time for clamping the cord during the third stage of labour (Inch 1985). Early clamping is carried out in the first 1–3 minutes immediately after birth regardless of whether the cord pulsation has ceased. It has been suggested that this practice:

• may reduce the volume of blood returning to the fetus by as much as 75–125 ml, especially if clamping occurs within the first minute (Montgomery 1960). This in turn may reduce neonatal haemoglobin levels in the short term but, in the only published study to assess longer-term outcomes, by 6 weeks after birth the haemoglobin levels in these babies had been restored (Pau-Chen & Tsu-Shan 1960).

• may prematurely interrupt the respiratory function of the placenta in maintaining O_2 levels and combating acidosis in the early moments of life. This may be of particular importance in the baby who is slow to breathe.

• may result in lower neonatal bilirubin levels but the effect on the incidence of clinical jaundice is unclear (Prendiville & Elbourne 1989).

• may increase the likelihood of fetomaternal transfusion as a larger volume of blood remains in the placenta. Venous pressure is further increased as retraction continues and may be sufficiently high to rupture surface placental vessels, thus facilitating the transfer of fetal cells into the maternal system. This may be a critical factor where the mother's blood group is Rhesus negative (Ladipo 1972).

• may result in the truncated umbilical vessels containing a quantity of clotted blood, which provides an ideal medium for bacterial growth. Heavier placental weight has also been associated with early cord clamping (Newton et al 1961).

Proponents of late clamping suggest that no action be taken until cord pulsation ceases or until the placenta has been completely delivered, thus allowing the physiological processes to take place without intervention. Postulated advantages include:

1. The route to the low-resistance placental circulation remains patent which provides the newborn with a safety valve for any raised systemic blood pressure. This may be critical when the baby is preterm or asphyxiated, as raised pulmonary and central venous pressures may exacerbate the difficulties in initiating respiration and accompanying circulatory adaptation (Dunn 1985).

2. A reduction in the length of time for the cord to separate postnatally.

3. The transfusion of the full quota of placental blood to the newborn. This may constitute as much as 40% of the circulating volume depending on when the cord is clamped and at what level the baby is held prior to clamping (Yao & Lind 1974) and therefore may be important in maintaining haematocrit levels. The neonatal effects associated with increased placental transfusion include higher mean birthweight and higher neonatal haematocrit accompanied by an increase in the incidence of jaundice (Prendiville et al 1988b).

There is very little evidence concerning how much, if any, oxytocic the baby receives following birth. In five documented cases of accidental administration of an adult dose of Syntometrine to a newborn infant, no long-term adverse effects were reported (Whitfield & Salfield 1980).

Another factor, which may influence the amount of placental transfusion, is the use of an oxytocic agent prior to the completion of labour. This may precipitate a strong uterine contraction with resultant overtransfusion of the baby.

Is the timing of oxytocic administration and cord clamping clinically important in influencing the incidence of postpartum haemorrhage?

A randomised controlled trial undertaken in Western Australia during 1992/93 set out to answer that question. The data from 963 women at term, randomly allocated to receive one of four timing options during the third stage of labour, revealed that a stringent policy of immediate administration of the oxytocic and immediate cord clamping may not provide an added benefit for risk reduction of postpartum haemorrhage. It was, however, also noted that the longer the oxytocic administration was delayed, the more likely blood loss was to increase (McDonald 1996). Timing of cord clamping appeared to be less of an issue, probably owing to the normal physiological process of transfer being completed within the first 2–3 minutes of birth for the majority of term infants.

Care should be taken to apply the clamp to the cord end nearer the baby, 3–4 cm clear of the abdominal wall to avoid pinching the skin or clamping a portion of gut, which, in rare instances, may be in the cord. A greater length of cord is left when umbilical vessels are needed for transfusion, for example in preterm babies and cases of Rhesus haemolytic disease.

DELIVERY OF THE PLACENTA AND MEMBRANES

Controlled cord traction is believed to reduce blood loss, shorten the third stage of labour and therefore minimise the time during which the mother is at risk from haemorrhage. It is designed to enhance the normal physiological process. Successful results depend upon understanding the principles of placental separation described at the beginning of this chapter.

If controlled cord traction is to be used, there are several checks to be made before proceeding:

- that an oxytocic drug has been administered
- that it has been given time to act
- that the uterus is well contracted
- that counter-traction is applied
- that signs of placental separation and descent are present. (At the beginning of the third stage, a strong uterine contraction results in the fundus being palpable below the umbilicus (Fig. 25.6). It feels broad as the placenta is still in the upper segment. As the placenta separates and falls into the lower uterine segment there is a small fresh blood loss, the cord lengthens, the fundus becomes rounder, smaller and more mobile as it rises in the abdomen above the level of the placenta.)

It is important not to manipulate the uterus in any way as this may precipitate incoordinate action. No further step should be taken until a strong contraction is palpable. If tension is applied to the umbilical cord without this contraction, then uterine inversion may occur. This is an acute obstetric emergency with life-threatening implications for the mother. The action to be taken in such an event is detailed in Chapter 29.

There is debate about whether controlled cord traction (CCT) should be applied before or after the signs of placental separation have been noted. Levy & Moore (1985) observed that blood loss was reduced when CCT was delayed until lengthening of the cord and a trickle of fresh blood loss had been observed.

When controlled cord traction is the preferred method of management, the following sequence of actions is usually undertaken.

Once the uterus is found on palpation to be contracted, one hand is placed above the level of the symphysis pubis with the palm facing towards the umbilicus exerting pressure in an upwards direction. This is counter-traction. The other hand, firmly grasping the cord, applies traction in a downward and backward direction following the line of the birth canal (Fig. 25.7). Some resistance may be felt but it is important to apply steady tension by pulling the cord firmly and maintaining the pressure. Jerky movements and force should be avoided. The aim is to complete the action as one continuous, smooth, controlled movement. However, it is only possible to exert this tension for 1 or 2 minutes as it may be an uncomfortable procedure for the mother and the midwife's hand will tire.

SUMMARY OF FUNDAL HEIGHTS DURING THIRD STAGE

A, **At the beginning of third stage**	2.5 cm below	15 cm above
B, **Placenta in lower segment** (separated)	1.5 cm above	19 cm above
C, **End of third stage** (placenta expelled)	4 cm below	14 cm above
	The umbilicus	**The symphysis pubis**

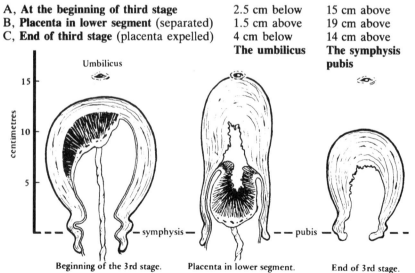

Fig. 25.6 Fundal height relative to the umbilicus and symphysis pubis.

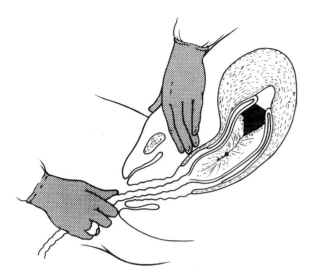

Fig. 25.7 Controlled cord traction.

Downward traction on the cord must be released *before* uterine counter-traction is relaxed. If the manoeuvre is not immediately successful there should be a pause before the uterine contraction is again checked and a further attempt is made. Should the uterus relax, tension is temporarily released until a good contraction is again palpable. Once the placenta is visible it may be cupped in the hands to ease pressure on the friable membranes. A gentle upward and downward movement or twisting action will help to coax out the membranes and increase the chances of delivering them intact. Artery forceps may be applied to gradually ease them out of the vagina. This process should not be hurried; great care should be taken to avoid tearing the membranes.

Recent evidence suggests that active management of the third stage of labour shortens it and results in less blood loss, fewer blood transfusions and a reduced need for therapeutic oxytocics (Prendiville et al 1997).

A sterile receiver should be placed against the perineum to collect blood loss and receive the placenta. If artery forceps are used to clamp the cord it is useful if they are moved and reapplied near the vulva so that they can be used to provide a handhold when applying cord traction. If a clamp is not applied, the cord is best held firmly by winding it around the hand so that tension can be applied without losing grasp of the slippery surface.

Expectant management allows the physiological changes within the uterus, which occur at the time of birth, to take their natural course with minimal intervention and normally excludes the administration of oxytocic drugs. The processes of placental separation and expulsion are quite distinct from one another and the signs of separation and descent must be evident before maternal effort can be used to expedite expulsion. If the mother is sitting or squatting at this stage, gravity will aid expulsion.

If good uterine contractions are sustained, maternal effort will usually bring about expulsion. The mother simply pushes as during the second stage of labour. Encouragement is important, as by now she may be exhausted and the contractions will feel weaker and less expulsive than those during the second stage of labour. Providing that fresh blood loss is not excessive and the mother's condition remains good and her pulse rate normal, there need be no anxiety. This spontaneous process can take from 20 minutes to an hour to complete. It is important that the midwife monitors uterine action by placing a hand lightly on the fundus. She can thus palpate the contraction whilst checking that relaxation does not result in the uterus filling with blood. Vigilance is crucial as it should be remembered that the longer the placenta remains undelivered the greater the risk of bleeding because the uterus cannot contract down fully whilst the bulk of the placenta is in situ. Dombrowski et al (1995) found that the frequency of haemorrhage increased between 10 and 40 minutes after the birth of the baby. Patience and confidence are required on the part of the midwife to secure a successful conclusion. An oxytocic agent is usually not administered unless uterine tone is poor.

Encouraging the mother to suckle the baby may enhance these physiological changes. This will result in the reflex release of oxytocin from the posterior lobe of the pituitary gland, which helps to secure good uterine action.

There is an increasing amount of appropriate, rigorously conducted research evidence available which strongly suggests that the prophylactic administration of an oxytocic significantly reduces the risk of postpartum haemorrhage. It has also been highlighted by the wide range of 'risk status' of women included in several studies that it is in fact very difficult to define a group of women who are not at risk for postpartum haemorrhage (Begley 1990, Khan et al 1997, McDonald et al 1993, Prendiville et al 1988b).

Position of the mother

The effect of the position adopted by the mother at the time of placental delivery is still largely unclear. It may vary according to the mother's personal preference, the normality of progress and the experience and confidence of the attendant midwife, and may be influenced by the need for the midwife to monitor closely factors such as uterine contraction and blood loss.

Adoption of a dorsal position allows easy palpation of the uterine fundus. However, blood is more likely to pool in the uterus and vagina, thus disguising the true blood loss. Upright, kneeling, squatting and all-fours positions may enhance the effect of gravity and increase intra-abdominal pressure, which may in turn hasten the placental delivery process. Blood loss can be more easily observed as fluids will drain out of the vagina (Fig. 25.8).

Whichever position is adopted, the use of wedges, pillows and physical support from her partner will help to ensure the woman's comfort while completion of the third stage is being accomplished. Some women feel cold and shivery at this time, especially if labour has progressed rapidly. This is usually transient and not abnormal. Additional warmth provided by clean, dry linen, an extra blanket and bed socks help to remedy the situation.

Asepsis

The need for asepsis is even greater now than in the preceding stages of labour. Laceration and bruising of the cervix, vagina, perineum and vulva provide a route for the entry of microorganisms. At the placental site, a raw wound provides an ideal medium for infection. Strict attention to the prevention of sepsis is therefore vital.

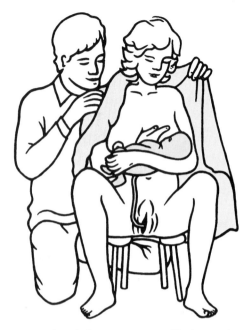

Fig. 25.8 Mother sitting up, supported by her partner. The cord remains unclamped.

The abdomen is draped with a sterile towel and a hand placed lightly on the fundus to monitor progress.

Cord blood sampling

This may be required for a variety of conditions:

- when the mother's blood group is Rhesus negative or as a precautionary measure if the mother's Rhesus type is unknown
- when atypical maternal antibodies have been found during an antenatal screening test
- where a haemoglobinopathy is suspected, e.g. sickle-cell disease.

Using a syringe and needle, the sample should be taken from the fetal surface of the placenta where the blood vessels are congested and easily visible. This must be done before the blood clots, but is a quick procedure if preparation has been made. If the cord has not been clamped prior to placental delivery the fetal vessels will not be congested, but a sample of sufficient volume may still be easily obtained. The appropriate containers should be used for the investigations requested.

These may include the baby's blood group, Rhesus type, haemoglobin estimation, serum bilirubin level, Coombs' test or electrophoresis. Maternal blood for Kleihauer testing can be taken upon completion of the third stage.

COMPLETION OF THE THIRD STAGE

Once the placenta is delivered, the midwife must first check that the uterus is well contracted and fresh blood loss is minimal. Careful inspection of the perineum and lower vagina is important. A strong light is directed onto the perineum in order to assess trauma accurately prior to instigating repair. This should be carried out as gently as possible as the tissues are often bruised and oedematous. Slight lacerations such as damage to the fourchette may be repaired immediately. However, if repair of a more extensive wound such as an episiotomy or a second degree tear is necessary, the mother should be made comfortable by changing soiled bed linen or placing a clean, waterproof-backed pad beneath her buttocks and back whilst the necessary preparations are made (see Ch. 24).

The vulva and perineum are gently cleansed using warm water or an appropriate antiseptic solution, softly dried and a clean pad placed in position. Maternal pulse, blood pressure and temperature are recorded. Once the mother is comfortable, examination of the placenta and membranes is the next priority.

Examination of placenta and membranes

This should be performed as soon after delivery as possible so that if there is doubt about their completeness, further action may be taken before the mother leaves the labour ward or the midwife prepares to leave the home. A thorough inspection must be carried out in order to make sure that no part of the placenta or membranes has been retained. The membranes are the most difficult to examine as they become torn during delivery and may be ragged. Every attempt should be made to piece them together to give an overall picture of completeness. This is easier to see if the placenta is held by the cord, allowing the membranes to hang. The hole through which the baby was de-

livered can then usually be identified and a hand spread out inside the membranes to aid inspection (Fig. 25.9). The placenta should then be laid on a flat surface and both placental surfaces minutely examined in a good light. The amnion should be peeled from the chorion right up to the umbilical cord, which allows the chorion to be fully viewed.

Any clots on the maternal surface need to be removed and kept for measuring. Broken fragments of cotyledon must be carefully replaced before an accurate assessment is possible.

Recent infarctions (areas on the placental surface that indicate deprivation of blood supply) are bright red, old infarctions form grey patches whereas localised calcification can be seen as flattened white plaques feeling gritty to the touch. (None of these is of great significance at this stage, but may provide retrospective evidence of an intrauterine

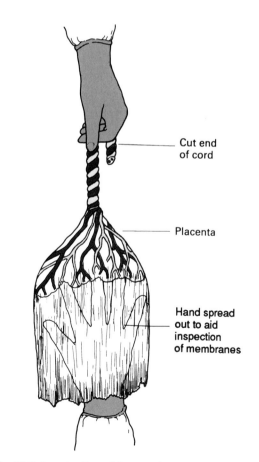

Cut end of cord

Placenta

Hand spread out to aid inspection of membranes

Fig. 25.9 Examination of the membranes.

problem.) The lobes of a complete placenta fit neatly together without any gaps, the edges forming a uniform circle. Blood vessels should not radiate beyond the placental edge. If they do this denotes a succenturiate lobe, which has developed separately from the main placenta (see Ch. 51). When such a lobe is visible there is no cause for concern, but if the tissue has been retained the vessels will end abruptly at a hole in the membrane. On the fetal surface the position of insertion of the cord is noted. This is most commonly central but may be lateral (for abnormal insertion, see Ch. 51). Two umbilical arteries and one vein should be present. The absence of one artery may be associated with congenital abnormality, particularly renal agenesis: the paediatrician should be informed. In some units the placental weight may be recorded. This will vary according to the time of clamping of the cord. Delayed clamping produces a placenta weighing approximately one-sixth of the baby's birthweight, whereas early clamping results in an additional volume of contained blood which increases the weight to nearer one-fifth of the birthweight. The cord length averages 50 cm.

Disposal of placenta

It is important to remember that the placenta is the property of the mother and her wishes regarding its disposal must be solicited and respected. The majority of women will rely on the midwife to undertake this task. It then becomes her responsibility to do so with maximum safety. This does not pose a problem in hospital where incinerators are available; where delivery has taken place in the home, the midwife is best advised to take the placenta to the nearest hospital for incineration. Home delivery packs usually include a plastic bag for this purpose. Disposal by burial is not recommended because of the risk of preying animals.

If there is any suspicion that the placenta or membranes are incomplete, they must be kept for inspection and a doctor informed immediately. Blood loss should be estimated as accurately as possible although Newton et al (1961), Levy & Moore (1985), Duthie et al (1990) and Ravi et al (1996) have demonstrated that the average normal recorded loss of between 150 and 300 ml represents a gross underestimate. Account must be taken of blood which has soaked into linen and swabs as well as measurable fluid loss and clot formation.

Upon completion of the examination, the midwife should return her attention to the mother. The empty uterus should be firmly contracted. If the fundus has risen in the abdomen a blood clot may be present. This should be expelled while the uterus is in a state of contraction by pressing the fundus gently in a downward and backward direction – with due regard to the risk of inversion and acute discomfort to the mother. Force should *never* be used.

Immediate care

It is advisable for mother and baby to remain in the midwife's care for at least an hour after delivery, whether in the home or in a labour ward. Much of this time will be spent in clearing up and completion of records but careful observation of mother and baby is very important. If an epidural cannula is in situ it is usually removed and checked at this time.

Most mothers appreciate being able to either wash or shower at this stage, which can do much to restore comfort and increase a sense of well-being. Cleaning the teeth and the application of lip salve or cream can help relieve the discomfort of a dry mouth and sore lips, especially if inhalational analgesia has been used during labour. The mother should be encouraged to pass urine because a full bladder may impede uterine contraction. She may not actually feel an urge to do so especially if she has passed urine immediately prior to delivery or an effective epidural has been in progress but she should be asked to try. Following use of the bedpan or toilet, the vulva should be douched, dried and a clean pad applied.

Uterine contraction and blood loss should be checked on several occasions throughout this first hour. The mother is left warm and resting comfortably with good pillow support and in a dry bed. Both parents usually welcome a hot drink. If the mother is hungry there is no reason why she should not enjoy a light snack such as toast, but in practice this can often precipitate vomiting especially if pethidine has been given during labour. The choice can be left to her discretion.

Throughout this same period the midwife should pay regard to the baby's general well-being. She should check the security of the cord clamp and observe general skin colour, respirations and temperature. A baby will quickly chill in the comparative cool following birth. She or he needs to be thoroughly dried and then wrapped in a clean, dry towel so that body heat is retained. In many labour wards, electrically warmed cot mattresses and Perspex heat shields are used, but the warmest place for a baby is cuddled close to his mother. At an early stage a full examination of the baby is made in the presence of his parents (see Ch. 35).

Most mothers intending to breast feed will wish to put their babies to the breast during these early moments of contact. This is especially advantageous, as babies are usually very alert at this time and their sucking reflex particularly strong. There is also evidence to suggest that women who breast feed soon after delivery successfully breast feed for a longer period of time (Salariya et al 1979). An additional benefit lies in the reflex release of oxytocin from the posterior lobe of the pituitary gland, which stimulates the uterus to contract. This may result in the mother experiencing a sudden fresh blood loss as the uterus empties and she should be reassured. The desire to feed a newborn baby is a warm, loving and instinctive response and a bottle feed should be available for those who do not wish to breast feed. It may be appropriate for the partner to give part of a bottle feed.

It is important that the midwife allows the new parents a quiet, private time together to admire and inspect their new offspring (Fig. 25.10). She should remain unobtrusively in attendance and this affords the ideal time to complete the labour record.

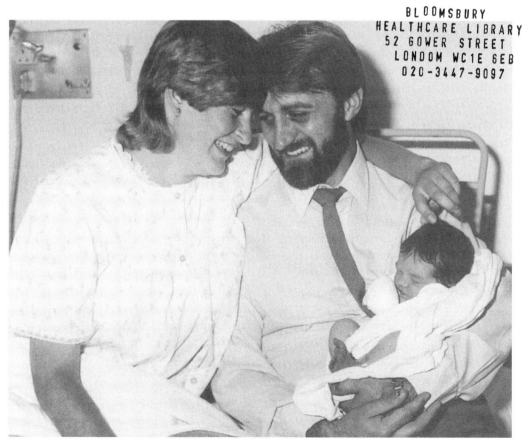

Fig. 25.10 The joy of parenthood.

Records

A complete and accurate account of the labour, including the documentation of all drugs and observations, is the midwife's responsibility. This should also include details of examination of the placenta, membranes and cord with attention drawn to any abnormalities. The volume of blood loss is particularly important. This record not only provides information which may be critical in the future care of both mother and baby but is a legal document which may be used as evidence of the care given. Signatures are therefore essential with co-signatories where necessary. Many mothers now carry their own notes or are supplied with a cooperation card. The completed records are a vital communication link between the midwife responsible for delivery and other caregivers, including the community midwife.

It is usually the midwife who completes the birth notification form. This must be sent within 36 hours to the medical officer of the health district in which the baby was born.

Transfer from the labour ward

The midwife is responsible for seeing that all observations are made and recorded (as specified above) prior to transfer of mother and baby to the postnatal ward or before the midwife leaves the home following the birth.

The postnatal ward midwife should verify these details prior to transfer of mother and baby. Following a domiciliary delivery, the midwife should leave details of a telephone number where she may be contacted should the parents feel any cause for concern.

COMPLICATIONS OF THE THIRD STAGE OF LABOUR

Postpartum haemorrhage

Postpartum haemorrhage is defined as excessive bleeding from the genital tract at any time following the baby's birth up to 6 weeks after delivery. If it occurs during the third stage of labour or within 24 hours of delivery it is termed *primary postpartum haemorrhage*.

If bleeding occurs subsequent to the first 24 hours following birth up until the sixth week postpartum, it is termed *secondary postpartum haemorrhage*.

Postpartum haemorrhage is one of the most alarming and serious emergencies which a midwife may face and is especially terrifying if it occurs immediately following a straightforward delivery. It may also prove a frightening experience for the mother and can undermine her confidence, influence her attitude to future childbearing and delay her recovery. Although the number of maternal deaths from postpartum haemorrhage in the UK has fallen to a very low level (DH et al 1996), this emergency still poses a major threat to the lives of women living in developing countries where conservative estimates of the maternal death rate exceed 600 000 women annually (Adamson 1996).

The midwife is often the first and may be the only professional person present when a haemorrhage occurs, so her prompt, competent action will be crucial in controlling blood loss and reducing the risk of maternal morbidity or even death.

Primary postpartum haemorrhage

Attempts have been made by several authors to define the actual quantity of blood loss to be regarded as excessive during the first hour or two after birth. Fluid loss is extremely difficult to measure with any degree of accuracy, especially when the fluid has soaked into dressings and linen. Several studies have highlighted the resultant gross underestimation, which may represent only 50% of the true blood loss (Levy & Moore 1985, Newton et al 1961, Prendiville et al 1988b). Duthie et al (1990) and Ravi et al (1996) compared laboratory-measured determination of blood loss compared to delivery room visual estimation. Duthie and colleagues reported that 17.7% of the primary postpartum haemorrhages calculated by laboratory measurement had gone unnoticed on visual estimation in a population of women assessed as being at low risk for postpartum haemorrhage.

It should also be remembered that measurable solidified clots only represent about half the total fluid loss. With these factors in mind, the best yardstick is that any blood loss, *however small*, which adversely affects the mother's condition constitutes a postpartum haemorrhage. Much will therefore depend upon the woman's general well-being. In addition, if measured loss reaches 500 ml, it must be treated as a postpartum haemorrhage, irrespective of maternal condition.

There are several reasons why a postpartum haemorrhage may occur.

Atonic uterus

This is a failure of the myometrium at the placental site to contract and retract and to compress torn blood vessels and control blood loss by a living ligature action (see above). When the placenta is attached, the volume of blood flow at the placental site is approximately 500–800 ml per minute. Upon separation, the efficient contraction and retraction of uterine muscle staunches the flow and prevents a haemorrhage which would otherwise ensue with horrifying speed (Box 25.1).

Incomplete placental separation. If the placenta remains fully adherent to the uterine wall it is unlikely to cause bleeding. However, once separation has begun, maternal vessels are torn. If placental tissue remains partially embedded in the spongy decidua, efficient contraction and retraction is interrupted.

Retained cotyledon, placental fragment or membranes will similarly impede efficient uterine action.

Box 25.1 Causes of atonic uterine action

- Incomplete separation of the placenta
- Retained cotyledon, placental fragment or membranes
- Precipitate labour
- Prolonged labour resulting in uterine inertia
- Polyhydramnios or multiple pregnancy causing overdistension of uterine muscle
- Placenta praevia
- Placental abruption
- General anaesthesia especially halothane or cyclopropane
- Mismanagement of the third stage of labour
- A full bladder
- Aetiology unknown

Precipitate labour. When the uterus has contracted vigorously and frequently resulting in a duration of labour that is less than 1 hour, then the muscle may have insufficient opportunity to retract.

Prolonged labour. In a labour where the active phase lasts more than 12 hours uterine inertia (sluggishness) may result owing to muscle exhaustion.

Polyhydramnios or multiple pregnancy. The myometrium becomes excessively stretched and therefore less efficient.

Placenta praevia. The placental site is partly or wholly in the lower segment where the thinner muscle layer contains few oblique fibres: this results in poor control of bleeding.

Placental abruption. Blood may have seeped between the muscle fibres, interfering with effective action. At its most severe this results in a Couvelaire uterus (Ch. 15).

General anaesthesia. Anaesthetic agents may cause uterine relaxation, in particular the volatile inhalational agents, for example halothane.

Mismanagement of the third stage of labour. It is salutary that this factor remains a frequent cause of postpartum haemorrhage. 'Fundus fiddling' or manipulation of the uterus may precipitate arrhythmic contractions so that the placenta only partially separates and retraction is lost.

A full bladder. If the bladder is full, its proximity to the uterus in the abdomen on completion of the second stage may interfere with uterine action. This also constitutes mismanagement.

Aetiology unknown. A precipitating cause may never be discovered.

There are in addition a number of factors which do not directly *cause* a postpartum haemorrhage but they increase the likelihood of excessive bleeding (Box 25.2).

Previous history of postpartum haemorrhage or retained placenta. There is a risk of recurrence in subsequent pregnancies. A detailed obstetric history taken at the first antenatal visit will ensure that arrangements are made for such a mother to give birth in a consultant unit.

High parity. With each successive pregnancy fibrous tissue replaces muscle fibres in the uterus, reducing its contractility and the blood vessels become more difficult to compress. Women who have had five or more deliveries are at increased risk.

Fibroids (fibromyomata). These are normally benign tumours consisting of muscle and fibrous tissue which may impede efficient uterine action.

Anaemia. Women who enter labour with reduced haemoglobin concentration (below 10 g/dl) may succumb more quickly to any subsequent blood loss, however small. Anaemia is associated with debility which is a more direct cause of uterine atony.

Ketosis. The influence of ketosis upon uterine action is still unclear. Foulkes & Dumoulin (1983) demonstrated that in a series of 3500 women, 40% had ketonuria at some time during labour. They reported that if labour progressed well this did not appear to jeopardise either fetal or maternal condition. However, there was a significant relationship between ketosis and the need for Syntocinon augmentation, instrumental delivery and postpartum haemorrhage when labour lasted more than 12 hours. Correction of ketosis is therefore advisable.

Signs of postpartum haemorrhage
These may be obvious such as:

- visible bleeding
- maternal collapse.

However, more subtle signs may present:

- pallor
- rising pulse rate
- falling blood pressure
- altered level of consciousness: may become restless or drowsy
- enlarged uterus as it fills with blood or blood clot. It feels 'boggy' on palpation, i.e. soft and distended and lacking tone. There may be little or no visible loss of blood.

Prophylaxis
By using the above list, it is possible for the midwife to apply some preventive screening in an attempt to identify women who may be at greater risk and to recognise causative factors. During the antenatal period a thorough and accurate history of previous obstetric experiences will identify risk factors such as previous postpartum haemorrhage or precipitate labour. Arrangements can then be made for delivery to take place in a unit where facilities for dealing with emergencies are available. The reasons should be carefully explained. It would be most unwise to book such a woman for delivery at home or in a general practitioner unit. The early detection and treatment of anaemia will help ensure that women enter labour with a haemoglobin level in excess of 10 g/dl. The midwife should check that blood tests are taken regularly and the results recorded. If necessary, action is taken to restore the haemoglobin level before delivery. Women more prone to anaemia should be closely monitored, for example those with multiple pregnancies.

During labour, good management practices during the first and second stages are important to prevent prolonged labour and ketoacidosis. A mother should not enter the second or third stage with a full bladder. Prophylactic administration of an oxytocic agent is recommended for the third stage, either by intramuscular injection or intravenous infusion. Two units of cross-matched blood should be kept available for any woman known to have a placenta praevia.

Treatment of postpartum haemorrhage
Three basic principles apply:

- Call a doctor
- Stop the bleeding
  - rub up a contraction
  - give an oxytocic
  - empty the uterus
- Resuscitate the mother.

Call a doctor.   This is an important initial step so that help is on the way whatever transpires. If the bleeding is brought under control before the doctor arrives, his presence may appear unnecessary, but a mother's condition can deteriorate very rapidly, in which case his assistance will be required urgently. If the mother is at home or in a general practitioner unit, the emergency obstetric unit should be summoned.

Stop the bleeding.   The initial action is always the same, regardless of whether bleeding occurs with the placenta in situ or later.

Rub up a contraction.   The fundus is first felt gently with the fingertips to assess its consistency. If it is soft and relaxed, the fundus is massaged with a smooth, circular motion, applying no undue pressure. When a contraction occurs, the hand is held still.

Give an oxytocic to sustain the contraction. In many instances, Syntocinon 5 units or 10 units or Syntometrine 1 ml has already been administered and this may be repeated. Alternatively, ergometrine 0.25–0.5 mg may be injected intravenously, which will be effective in 45 seconds. No more than two doses of ergometrine should be given (including any dose of Syntometrine) as it may cause pulmonary hypertension. Several reports have described the dramatic haemostatic effects of prostaglandins used in cases of uterine atony but there is no evidence generated from controlled trials (Thiery 1986). Nevertheless, its obvious benefits make it worthy of note for use in this dire emergency. The baby may be put to the breast to enhance the physiological secretion of oxytocin from the posterior lobe of the pituitary gland.

Empty the uterus.   Once the midwife is satisfied that it is well contracted, she should ensure that the uterus is emptied. If the placenta is still in the uterus, it should be delivered; if it has been born,

any clots should be expelled by firm but gentle pressure on the fundus.

Resuscitate the mother.   An intravenous infusion should be commenced while peripheral veins are easily negotiated. This will provide a route for Syntocinon infusion or fluid replacement. As an emergency measure the mother's legs may be lifted up in order to allow blood to drain from them into the central circulation. The foot of the bed should *not* be raised as this encourages pooling of blood in the uterus, which prevents the uterus contracting.

It is usually expedient to catheterise the bladder in order to minimise trauma should an operative procedure be necessary and to exclude a full bladder as a precipitating cause of further bleeding.

On no account must a woman in a collapsed condition be moved prior to resuscitation.

The flow chart (Fig. 25.11) briefly sets out the possible courses of action which may be taken dependent upon whether or not bleeding persists. If the above measures are successful in controlling any further loss, Syntocinon, 40 units in 1 litre of dextrose/saline infused slowly over 8–12 hours, will ensure continued uterine contraction. This will help to minimise the risk of recurrence. Before the infusion is connected, 10 ml of blood should be withdrawn for haemoglobin estimation and for cross-matching compatible blood. If bleeding continues uncontrolled, the choice of further action will depend largely upon whether the placenta remains undelivered.

Placenta delivered.   If the uterus is atonic following delivery of the placenta, light fundal pressure may be used to expel residual clots whilst a contraction is stimulated. If an effective contraction is not maintained, 40 units of Syntocinon in 1 litre of intravenous fluid should be commenced. The placenta and membranes must be re-examined for completeness since retained fragments are often responsible for uterine atony.

Bimanual compression.   If bleeding continues, bimanual compression of the uterus may be necessary in order to apply pressure to the placental site. It is desirable for an intravenous infusion to be in progress. The fingers of the right hand are

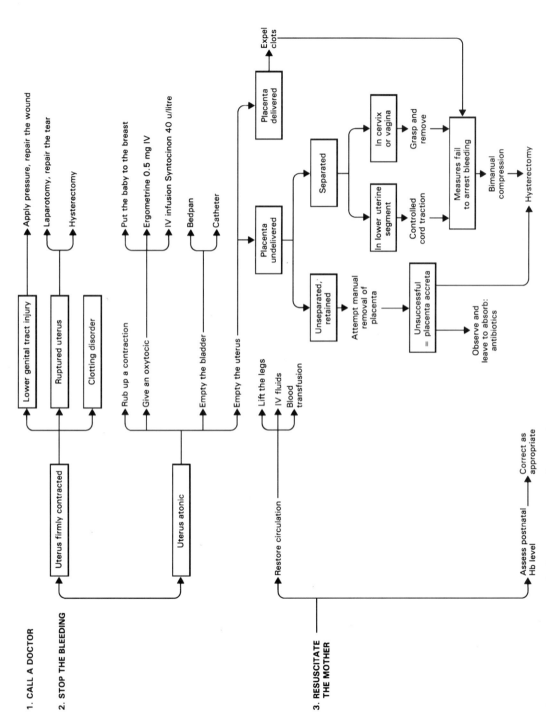

1. CALL A DOCTOR

2. STOP THE BLEEDING

Uterus firmly contracted
- Lower genital tract injury → Apply pressure, repair the wound
- Ruptured uterus → Laparotomy, repair the tear / Hysterectomy
- Clotting disorder

Uterus atonic
- Rub up a contraction
- Give an oxytocic → Put the baby to the breast / Ergometrine 0.5 mg IV / IV infusion Syntocinon 40 u/litre
- Empty the bladder → Bedpan / Catheter
- Empty the uterus

Placenta undelivered
- Separated
  - In cervix or vagina → Grasp and remove
  - In lower uterine segment → Controlled cord traction
- Unseparated, retained → Attempt manual removal of placenta → Unsuccessful = placenta accreta → Observe and leave to absorb: antibiotics

Placenta delivered → Expel clots

Measures fail to arrest bleeding → Bimanual compression → Hysterectomy

3. RESUSCITATE THE MOTHER

Restore circulation
- Lift the legs
- IV fluids
- Blood transfusion

Assess postnatal Hb level → Correct as appropriate

Fig. 25.11 Management of primary postpartum haemorrhage.

inserted into the vagina like a cone; the hand is formed into a fist and placed into the anterior vaginal fornix, the elbow resting on the bed. The left hand is placed behind the uterus abdominally, the fingers pointing towards the cervix. The uterus is brought forwards and compressed between the palm of the left hand and the fist in the vagina (Fig. 25.12). If bleeding persists, a clotting disorder must be excluded before exploration of the vagina and uterus is performed under a general anaesthetic. (See also Ch. 4 for aortic compression.)

Placenta undelivered. The placenta may be partially or wholly adherent.

Partially adherent. When the uterus is well contracted an attempt should be made to deliver the placenta by applying controlled cord traction. If this is unsuccessful a doctor will be required to remove it manually.

Completely adherent. Bleeding does not usually occur if the placenta is completely adherent. However, the longer the placenta remains in situ the greater the risk of partial separation, which may give rise to profuse haemorrhage.

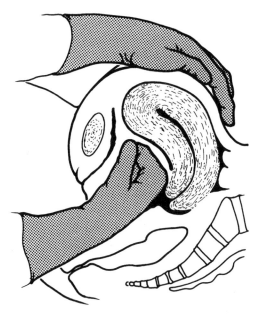

Fig. 25.12 Bimanual compression of the uterus.

Retained placenta

This diagnosis is reached when the placenta remains undelivered after a specified period of time (usually half to 1 hour following the baby's birth). The conventional treatment is to digitally separate the placenta from the uterine wall, effecting a manual removal. Selinger et al (1986) noted that waiting for 1 hour before resorting to this intervention will almost halve the number of women who will require manual removal with its accompanying risks.

Breaking of the cord. This is not an unusual occurrence during completion of the third stage of labour. Before further action, it is crucial to check that the uterus remains firmly contracted. If the placenta remains adherent, no further action should be taken before a doctor is notified. It is possible that manual removal may be indicated. If the placenta is palpable in the vagina, it is probable that separation has occurred and when the uterus is well contracted maternal effort may be encouraged (see expectant management). If there is any doubt, the midwife applies fresh sterile gloves before performing a vaginal examination to ascertain whether this is so. As a last resort, if the mother is unable to push effectively, fundal pressure may be used. An oxytocic must have been given. Great care is exercised to ensure that placental separation has already occurred and the uterus is well contracted. The mother should be relaxed as the midwife exerts downward and backward pressure on the firmly contracted fundus. This method can cause considerable pain and distress to the mother and result in the stretching and bruising of supportive uterine ligaments. If it is performed without good uterine contraction, acute inversion may ensue. This is an extremely dangerous procedure in unskilled hands and is not advocated in everyday practice when alternative, safer methods may be employed.

Manual removal of the placenta

This should be carried out by a doctor. An intravenous infusion must first be sited and an effective anaesthetic be in progress. The choice of anaesthesia will depend upon the mother's general condition. If an effective epidural anaesthetic is already in progress, a top-up may be given in order to avoid the hazards of general anaesthesia. A spinal anaesthetic offers an alternative but otherwise a general anaesthetic will be induced. Details of obstetric anaesthesia are given in Chapter 28.

Management. Manual removal is performed with full aseptic precautions. With the left hand, the umbilical cord is held taut while the right hand is coned and inserted into the vagina and uterus following the direction of the cord. Once the placenta is located the cord is released so that the left hand may be used to support the fundus abdominally, so preventing rupture of the lower uterine segment (Fig. 25.13). The operator will feel for a separated edge of the placenta. The fingers of the right hand are extended and the border of the hand is gently eased between the placenta and the uterine wall, with the palm facing the placenta. With a sideways slicing movement the placenta is carefully detached. When the placenta is completely separated, the left hand rubs up a contraction and expels the right hand with the placenta in its grasp. The placenta should be checked immediately for completeness so that any

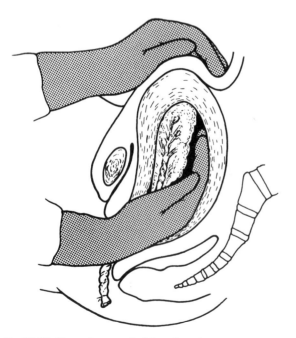

Fig. 25.13 Manual removal of the placenta.

further exploration of the uterus may be carried out without delay. An oxytocic drug is given upon completion.

In very exceptional circumstances when no doctor is available to be called, a midwife would be expected to carry out a manual removal of placenta. Once she has diagnosed a retained placenta as the cause of postpartum haemorrhage the midwife must act swiftly to reduce the risk of onset of shock and exsanguination. It must be remembered that the risk of inducing shock by performing a manual removal of placenta is greater when no anaesthetic is given. In a developed country the midwife is unlikely to find herself dealing with this situation.

At home. If the placenta is retained following a home confinement, the emergency obstetric unit must be summoned. Under no circumstances should a mother be transferred to hospital until an intravenous infusion is in progress and her condition stabilised.

It is best if the placenta can be delivered without moving the mother but if this is not possible, or if further treatment is needed, she should be transferred to a consultant unit. The baby should accompany her.

Morbid adherence of placenta. Very rarely, the placenta remains morbidly adherent: this is known as *placenta accreta*. If it is totally adherent, then bleeding is unlikely to occur and it may be left in situ to absorb during the puerperium. If, however, only part of the placenta remains embedded, the risks of fatal haemorrhage are high and an emergency hysterectomy may be unavoidable.

Trauma as a cause of haemorrhage

If bleeding occurs despite a well-contracted uterus, it is almost certainly the consequence of trauma to the uterus, vagina, perineum or labia, or a combination of these. Poeschmann et al (1991) cautioned that episiotomy may contribute up to 30% of total blood loss; in their study the severity of blood loss was linked to the length of time which elapsed between incision of the perineum and the commencement of repair. Predictably, the longer the wait the greater the blood loss.

In order to identify the source of bleeding, the mother is placed in the lithotomy position under a good directional light. An episiotomy wound or tears to the anterior labia, clitoris and perineum often bleed freely. These external injuries are easily identified and torn vessels may be clamped with artery forceps prior to ligation. Internal trauma to the vagina, cervix or uterus more commonly occurs following instrumental or manipulative delivery. A speculum is inserted to enable the cervix and vagina to be clearly visualised and examined. Tissue or artery forceps may be used to apply pressure prior to suturing under general anaesthesia.

If bleeding persists when the uterus is well contracted and no evidence of trauma can be found, uterine rupture must be suspected. Following a laparotomy, this is repaired, but if bleeding remains uncontrolled, a hysterectomy may become inevitable.

Blood coagulation disorders

As well as the causes already listed above, postpartum haemorrhage may be the result of coagulation failure, which is fully discussed in Chapter 15. The failure of the blood to clot is such an obvious sign that it can be overlooked in the midst of the feverish activity which accompanies torrential bleeding. It can occur following severe pre-eclampsia, antepartum haemorrhage, amniotic fluid embolus, intrauterine death or sepsis. Fresh blood is usually the best treatment as this will contain platelets and the coagulation factors V and VIII. The expert advice of a haematologist will be needed in assessing specific replacement products such as fresh frozen plasma and fibrinogen.

Observation of the mother following postpartum haemorrhage

Once bleeding is controlled the total volume lost must be estimated as accurately as possible. Large amounts appear less than they are in reality. Maternal pulse and blood pressure are recorded quarter-hourly and temperature taken 4-hourly. The uterus should be palpated frequently to ensure that it remains well contracted and lochia lost must be observed. Intravenous fluid replacement should be carefully calculated to avoid circulatory overload. Monitoring the central venous pressure (see Fig. 29.14) will provide an accurate assessment of the volume required, especially if blood loss has been severe. Fluid intake and urinary output are recorded as indicators of renal function. The output should be accurately measured on an hourly basis by the use of a self-retaining urinary catheter.

The woman will usually remain in the labour ward until her condition is stable. This allows her progress to be closely monitored. All records should be meticulously completed and signed as soon as possible. Continued vigilance will be important for 24–48 hours. As this woman will need a quiet period for recuperation, a single room may be offered and visiting may be restricted to close family members. She will not be suitable for early transfer home.

Secondary postpartum haemorrhage

Secondary postpartum haemorrhage is bleeding from the genital tract more than 24 hours after delivery of the placenta and may occur up to 6 weeks later. It is most likely to occur between 10 and 14 days after delivery. Bleeding is usually due to retention of a fragment of the placenta or membranes, or the presence of a large uterine blood clot. The lochia are heavier than normal and will consist of a bright red loss which typically has recurred during the second week. The lochia may also be offensive if infection is a contributory factor. Subinvolution, pyrexia and tachycardia are usually present. As this is an event that is most likely to occur at home, women should be alerted to the possible signs of secondary postpartum haemorrhage prior to discharge from midwifery care.

Management
The following steps should be taken:

- call a doctor
- rub up a contraction by massaging the uterus if it is still palpable
- express any clots
- encourage the mother to empty her bladder

- give an oxytocic drug such as ergometrine maleate by the intravenous or intramuscular route
- keep all pads and linen to assess the volume of blood lost
- if bleeding persists, prepare the woman for theatre.

If the bleeding occurs at home and the woman has telephoned the midwife, she should be told to lie down flat until the midwife arrives (the front door should be left unlocked if the woman is alone). On arrival, the midwife will assess the amount of blood loss and the woman's condition and attempt to arrest the haemorrhage. If the loss is severe or uncontrolled, she will call the emergency obstetric unit and prepare mother and baby for transfer to hospital. The doctor who attends will commence an intravenous infusion and ensure that the mother's condition is stable first.

Careful assessment is usually undertaken prior to the uterus being explored under general anaesthetic. The use of ultrasound as a diagnostic tool is invaluable in minimising the number of mothers who have operative intervention. If retained products of conception cannot be seen on scan, the mother may be treated conservatively with antibiotic therapy and oral ergometrine. The haemoglobin should be estimated prior to discharge. If it is below 9 g/dl, options for iron replacement should be discussed with the woman. The severity of the anaemia will assist in determining the most appropriate care, which may be dependent on whether the woman is symptomatic (e.g. feeling faint, dizzy, short of breath). Management may vary from increased intake of iron-rich foods, iron supplements or, in extreme cases, blood transfusion.

Haematoma formation

Postpartum haemorrhage may also be concealed as the result of progressive haematoma formation. This may be obvious at such sites as the perineum or lower vagina but more difficult to diagnose if it occurs into the broad ligament or vault of the vagina. A large volume of blood may collect insidiously (up to 1 litre). Involution and lochia are usually normal, the main symptom being increasingly severe maternal pain. This is often so acute that the haematoma has to be drained in theatre under a general anaesthetic. Secondary infection is a high possibility.

Care after a postpartum haemorrhage

Whatever the cause of the haemorrhage, the woman will need the continued support of her midwife until she regains her confidence. Her partner may also be fearful of a recurrence and need much reassurance. If the mother is breast feeding, lactation may be impaired but this will only be temporary and she should be encouraged to persevere. The midwife is often the first and may be the only professional person present when a haemorrhage occurs, so her prompt, competent action will be crucial in controlling blood loss and reducing the risk of maternal morbidity or even mortality.

READER ACTIVITIES

1. One simple and effective means of demonstrating the inaccuracy of estimating blood loss to colleagues is to replicate part of the Levy & Moore study (1985).

Four units of expired blood were obtained from the haematology laboratory. These were divided into measured amounts: to each was added citrate to prevent clotting plus 200 ml of normal saline to mimic a moderate quantity of amniotic fluid. The calculated volumes were poured over sets of drapes and pads laid out on trolleys. Staff were then invited to estimate the blood loss, which served to demonstrate gross underestimation.

2. In the unit in which you work search for documents which influence or dictate any aspect of practice related to third stage management. This may include policy statements, guidelines for practice or defined standards of care. When were these documents compiled and by whom? Are any of the recommendations supported by cited research evidence? What can you do to change or improve such statements?

REFERENCES

Adamson P A 1996 Failure of imagination. In: Progress of nations. UNICEF, Wallingford, Oxon, pp 2–9

Begley C M 1990 A comparison of 'active' and 'physiological' management of the third stage of labour. Midwifery 6: 3–17

Bonnar J, McNicol G P, Douglas A S 1970 Coagulation and fibrinolytic mechanisms during and after normal childbirth. British Medical Journal 25 (April): 200–203

Chua S, Shaw S I, Yeoh C L, Roy A C, Ho L M, Selamat N, Aralkamaran S, Ratnam S S 1995 A randomised controlled study of prostaglandin 15 methyl F2alpha compared with Syntometrine for prophylactic use in the third stage of labour. Journal of Australian and New Zealand Obstetrics and Gynaecology 35(4): 413

Department of Health, Welsh Office, Scottish Home and Health Department, Department of Health and Social Services, Northern Ireland 1996 Report on confidential enquiries into maternal deaths in the United Kingdom 1991–1993. HMSO, London

Dombrowski M P, Bottoms S F, Saleb A A A, Hurd W W, Romero R 1995 Third stage of labour: analysis of duration and clinical practice. American Journal of Obstetrics and Gynecology 172: 1279–1284

Dunn P M 1985 Management of childbirth in normal women: the third stage and fetal adaptation. In: Perinatal medicine. Proceedings of the IX European Congress on Perinatal Medicine, Dublin, September 1984. MTP Press, Lancaster, ch 7, pp 47–54

Duthie S J, Ven D, Yung G L K, Dong Z G, Chan S Y W, Ma H-K 1990 Discrepancy between laboratory determination and visual estimation of blood loss during normal delivery. European Journal of Obstetrics, Gynaecology and Reproductive Biology 38: 119–124

El-Refaey H, O'Brien P, Morafa W, Walder J, Rodeck C 1997 Use of oral misoprostol in the prevention of postpartum haemorrhage. British Journal of Obstetrics and Gynaecology 104: 336–339

Inch S 1985 Management of the third stage of labour – another cascade of intervention. Midwifery 1: 114–122

Foulkes J, Dumoulin J G 1983 Ketosis in labour. British Journal of Hospital Medicine 29(6) (June): 562–564

Khan G Q, John I S, Wani S, Doherty T, Sibai B M 1997 Abstract 56: 'Controlled cord traction' versus 'minimal intervention': techniques in the delivery of the placenta: a randomised controlled trial. American Journal of Obstetrics and Gynecology (January)

Khan Q K, John I S, Chan T, Wani S, Hughes A O, Stirrat G M 1995 Abu Dhabi third stage trial: oxytocin versus Syntometrine in the active management of the third stage of labour. European Journal of Obstetrics, Gynaecology and Reproductive Biology 58: 147–151

Ladipo O A 1972 Management of third stage of labour, with particular reference to reduction of feto-maternal transfusion. British Medical Journal 1: 721–723

Levy V, Moore J 1985 The midwife's management of the third stage of labour. Nursing Times 81(5): 47–50

McDonald S J 1996 Timing of interventions in the third stage of labour. In: Management in the third stage of labour. Doctoral Thesis, Faculty of Medicine, Department of Obstetrics and Gynaecology, University Of Western Australia, ch 6

McDonald S J, Prendiville W J, Blair E 1993 Randomised controlled trial of oxytocin alone versus oxytocin and ergometrine in active management of the third stage of labour. British Medical Journal 307: 1167–1171

McDonald S, Prendiville W J, Elbourne D 1997 Prophylactic Syntometrine vs oxytocin in the third stage of labour. In: Neilson J P, Crowther C A, Hodnett E D, Hofmeyr G J, Keirse M J N C (eds) Pregnancy and childbirth module of the Cochrane Database of Systematic Reviews (updated 4 March 1997). Available in the Cochrane Library (database on disk and CD-ROM). (Updated quarterly) The Cochrane Collaboration Issue 2. Update Software, Oxford

Montgomery T L 1960 The umbilical cord. Clinical Obstetrics and Gynaecology 3: 900–910

Newton M, Mosey L M, Egli G E, Gifford W B, Hull C T 1961 Blood loss during and immediately after delivery. Obstetrics and Gynaecology 17: 9–18

Pau-Chen W, Tsu-Shan K 1960 Early clamping of the umbilical cord: a study of its effect on the infant. Chinese Medical Journal 80: 351–355

Peyser R M, Kupfermine M J 1990 Management of postpartum haemorrhage by uterine irrigation with prostaglandin. American Journal of Obstetrics and Gynecology 162(3): 694–696

Poeschmann R P, Docsburg W H, Eskis T K A B A 1991 Randomised comparison of oxytocin, sulprostone and placebo in the management of the third stage of labour. British Journal of Obstetrics and Gynaecology 98: 528–530

Prendiville W, Elbourne D 1989 Care during the third stage of labour. In: Chalmers I, Enkin M, Keirse M J N C (eds) Effective care in pregnancy and childbirth. Oxford University Press, Oxford, pp 1145–1169

Prendiville W, Elbourne D, Chalmers I 1988a The effects of routine oxytocic administration in the management of the third stage of labour: an overview of the evidence from controlled trials. British Journal of Obstetrics and Gynaecology 95: 3–16

Prendiville W J, Elbourne D R, Chalmers I 1988b The Bristol third stage trial: active versus physiological management of the third stage of labour. British Medical Journal 297: 1295–1300

Prendiville W J, Elbourne D, McDonald S 1997 Active versus expectant management of the third stage of labour. In: Neilson J P, Crowther C A, Hodnett E D, Hofmeyr G J, Keirse M J N C (eds) Pregnancy and childbirth module of the Cochrane database of systematic reviews (updated 4 March 1997). Available in The Cochrane Library (database on disk and CD-ROM). (Updated quarterly) The Cochrane Collaboration, Issue 2. Update Software, Oxford

Ravi K, Chua S, Arulkumaran S, Ratnam S S 1996 A comparison between visual estimation and laboratory determination of blood loss during the third stage of labour. Australia and New Zealand Journal of Obstetrics and Gynaecology 36(2): 152–154

Salariya E, Easton P, Cater J 1979 Early and often for best results. Nursing Mirror 148: 15–17

Selinger M, MacKenzie K, Dunlop P, James D 1986 Intraumbilical vein oxytocin in the management of retained placenta. A double blind controlled study. Journal of Obstetrics and Gynaecology 7: 115–117

Thiery M 1986 Prostaglandins for the treatment of hypotonic postpartum haemorrhage. Prostaglandin Perspectives 2: 10

van Selm M, Kanhai H H H, Keiser M I N C 1995 Preventing the recurrence of atonic postpartum haemorrhage: A double-blind trial. Acta Obstetrica et Gynecologia Scandinavica 74: 270–274

Whitfield M F, Salfield S A W 1980 Accidental administration of Syntometrine in adult dosage to the newborn. Archives of Disease in Childhood 55: 68–70

Yao A C, Lind J 1974 Placental transfusion. American Journal of Diseases of Children 127: 128–141

FURTHER READING

Botha M G 1968 The management of the umbilical cord in labour. South African Journal of Obstetrics and Gynaecology 6(2): 30–33

Dahlenburg G W, Burnell R H, Braybrook R 1980 The relation between cord serum sodium levels in newborn infants and maternal intravenous therapy during labour. British Journal of Obstetrics and Gynaecology 87: 519–522

Department of Health, Welsh Office, Scottish Home and Health Department, Department of Health and Social Services, Northern Ireland 1996 Report on confidential enquiries into maternal deaths in the United Kingdom 1991–1993. HMSO, London

Feeney J G 1982 Water intoxication and oxytocin. British Medical Journal 285: 243

Hibbard B 1981 Shock in obstetrics. Nursing Mirror 153(11): ix–xiv

Hibbard B 1981 Complications associated with shock in obstetrics. Nursing Mirror 153(11): xv–xvii

Maine D, Rosenfield A, Wallace M, Kimball A M, Kwast B, Papiernik E, White S 1987 Prevention of maternal deaths in developing countries: program options and practical considerations. Centre for Population and Family Health, University of Colombia, New York

Mulder J I 1985 Amniotic fluid embolism: an overview and case report. American Journal of Obstetrics and Gynecology 152(4): 430–435

Prendiville W, Elbourne D 1989 Care during the third stage of labour. In: Chalmers I, Enkin M, Keirse M J N C (eds) Effective care in pregnancy and childbirth. Oxford University Press, Oxford

Rogers J, Wood J, McCandlish R, Ayers S, Truesdale A, Elbourne D 1998 Active versus expectant management of the third stage of labour: the Hinchingbrooke randomised controlled trial. Lancet 351: 693–699

26

Prolonged pregnancy and disorders of uterine action

Christine V. Shiers

This chapter considers the issues of a pregnancy that continues beyond term, induction of labour and some of the complications that may arise in labour, including abnormal uterine action and obstructed labour.

The chapter aims to:

- discuss the diagnosis and management of a post-term pregnancy taking account of current research and practice

- review the indications for induction of labour and the various methods used

- describe how uterine dysfunction may result in a prolonged labour or one that is precipitate

- consider the serious complication of obstructed labour, which may result in the death of mother and baby, or contribute to long-term morbidity of both

- highlight the importance of the role of the midwife in the care and management of such situations

- emphasise the involvement of the mother and her partner in the care provided.

POST-TERM PREGNANCY

Post-term pregnancy is defined as one that exceeds 294 days, from the first day of the last menstrual period (FIGO 1982). Prolonged pregnancy and post-term pregnancy are used synonymously and relate to the duration of the pregnancy, not a maternal condition. Postmaturity or postmature are terms that relate to the neonate, and refer to features or condition of the baby (Clifford 1954) and should not be used in relation to the duration of pregnancy.

Incidence

The incidence of post-term pregnancy averages 10% (Bakketeig & Bergsjo 1989) falling to 1.1% where accurate dating of the pregnancy takes place (Boyd et al 1988).

Evidence suggests that the duration of pregnancy varies with parity and race. Primigravid women have a longer mean duration of pregnancy, averaging 288 days. Multigravidae average 283 days, the recurrence risk of post-term birth increasing with parity (Bakketeig & Bergsjo 1989). Mittendorf et al (1990) found, in multiracial groups in the US, that gestation amongst black mothers was measured as being 8.5 days shorter than in similar Caucasian women.

Dating

Statistics quoting the incidence of post-term pregnancy have been influenced by the inaccuracies of dating. Pregnancy cannot be said to be prolonged without accurate dating. Term delivery is one that occurs over a range of 5 weeks from 37–42 weeks' gestation. Calculation of the expected date of delivery, using Naegele's rule, gives mothers a single day on which they might be expected to give birth. The accuracy of this depends on the certainty of the woman's memory of her dates and the length of the menstrual cycle. Additional days need to be added if the cycle exceeds 28 days, and subtracted if less than 28. Further to this, the cycle may be influenced by recent use of the oral contraceptive. A significant number of women are uncertain of, or are unable to recall, the date of their last menstrual period (Andersen et al 1981, Hall & Carr Hill 1985).

Estimation of gestational age by clinical assessment can also be flawed. Abdominal examination for fundal height measurements cannot accurately assess gestational age, because of the biological variations in size of the mother and the fetus (Beazley & Kurjak 1979).

Quickening, or the recognition by the mother of fetal movements, may be felt over a range of weeks, primigravidae from 15–22 weeks and multigravidae from 14–22 weeks (O'Dowd & O'Dowd 1985).

Ultrasound scan in early pregnancy can be used to assess duration of pregnancy and fetal age. Measurements taken in the first or second trimesters have been found to be accurate to within 5 days in 95% of cases (Neilson 1990). An increasing number of mothers are offered an early dating scan, in association with haematological screening tests. Early scanning can help reduce the numbers of women who are categorised mistakenly as having a prolonged pregnancy.

Risks and clinical implications of post-term pregnancy

Perinatal mortality is lowest at 40 weeks, rising again after 42 weeks (Crowley et al 1984). The increase in perinatal mortality and morbidity in post-term pregnancy is, however, likely to be a result of labour or birth rather than antenatal events (Crowley 1989).

Post-term pregnancy may be complicated by the condition defined as postmaturity but not in all cases. This condition is marked by characteristics including fetal malnutrition, absence of lanugo and vernix and meconium staining (Clifford 1954). Conversely, macrosomia (birthweight of 4000 g or more) also occurs in 10% of cases, with 1% 4500 g or more. This influences the outcome of pregnancy, by contributing to cephalopelvic disproportion or shoulder dystocia.

The production of amniotic fluid reduces at term, and post-term pregnancy has been linked with oligohydramnios. As one of the primary functions of the liquor is to form a protective cushion for the fetus and the umbilical cord, the reduction in fluid volume can result in both cord compression and reduced placental perfusion. The ensuing fetal hypoxia may lead to passage of meconium. Fetal distress, demonstrated in intrapartum monitoring as decelerations, and meconium aspiration syndrome are also likely to complicate the outcome of a post-term pregnancy (Leveno et al 1984, Usher et al 1988).

Role of the placenta

Placental ageing was once thought to be responsible for fetal and intrapartum complications on the supposition that the demands of the fetus for oxygen and nutrients outstripped the supply and the placenta had come to the end of its functional life (Naeye 1978).

Fox (1991), on the contrary, ascribes the morphological changes attributed to ageing as a maturation process increasing rather than decreasing the efficiency of the villi. The placenta continues to grow up to and beyond term. Post-term pregnancy may be complicated by placental insufficiency but the basis of this will have existed from an early stage in pregnancy, rather than have developed as a consequence of prolongation of pregnancy.

Management of post-term pregnancy

The management of post-term pregnancy has taken account of the increased risk to the fetus as pregnancy lengthens. Two forms of care are offered, expectant management with fetal surveillance or elective induction of labour before 42 weeks of gestation. Both aim to diminish the jeopardy to the fetus.

Antenatal surveillance

Biophysical profile.   Manning and others (1981) identified that scoring combining ultrasound assessment of fetal breathing, fetal movement, fetal tone, reactivity of the heart rate and amniotic fluid volume could be used to predict fetal well-being in a high-risk pregnancy. When used twice weekly with mothers who were post-term, Johnson and colleagues (1986) found that where the score was normal and mothers laboured spontaneously the rate of caesarean section was reduced.

Cardiotocography (CTG).   CTG is also known as non-stress testing (NST). The fetal heart is monitored and the trace is assessed for the presence of reactivity and whether the baseline rate is within the normal range (Phelan 1991). The value of CTG in predicting possible compromise is increased if carried out at least twice weekly, and in conjunction with measurement of amniotic fluid volume (Eden et al 1982). Miyazaki & Miyazaki (1981) found in a study of 125 women, using weekly CTG to monitor fetal well-being, that there was a false-positive rate of 8% with normal CTGs preceding an abnormal outcome.

Amniotic fluid measurement.   Variation in parameters for defining diminished liquor influence the interpretation and thus the decision to induce labour (James 1991). Measurements are taken in several perpendicular planes, to make the diagnosis of oligohydramnios. A range of < 10 mm (Johnson et al 1986) to < 30 mm (Crowley et al 1984) has been used. Where action was instigated if the amniotic fluid volume fell below 30 mm, no perinatal losses occurred.

Doppler ultrasound of umbilical artery.   This is used to assess fetal and uteroplacental blood flow in pregnancies associated with high risk. Study of the umbilical flow velocity wave forms yields information about vascular resistance within the placenta and perfusion within the fetoplacental circulation. Anteby and others (1994) studied a group of 79 mothers with uncomplicated post-term pregnancies and were able to predict a risk of fetal distress in labour from abnormal Doppler assessment.

Elective induction

The active approach to post-term pregnancy, or one approaching the upper limits of term, is for the mother to have labour induced. A statistically significant reduction in perinatal mortality for the normal fetus has been demonstrated where gestation is in excess of 290 days, when this approach is adopted (Crowley 1993).

Hannah and others (1992) published the results of a large multicentre trial comparing induction with antenatal surveillance in post-term pregnancy. Surveillance included twice-weekly cardiotocograph and amniotic fluid volume measurements. Those women who were induced were less likely to have a caesarean section than those who were randomised to the policy of surveillance. There were no major differences in perinatal mortality or neonatal morbidity between the groups.

It is recognised that the administration of endocervical prostaglandins reduces the incidence of caesarean section. Women in the group for induction were thus managed, whereas women in the surveillance group requiring induction did not have prostaglandin. This may have contributed to the elevated rate of caesarean section in the group.

Mother's choice

Women should be given information about the options available to them in a manner that allows them to have informed choice. It is also important that they are aware that management may alter depending on the clinical assessment.

The Confidential Enquiry into Stillbirths and Deaths in Infancy (DH 1995) recommends that consistency is needed in the management of post-term pregnancy, particularly where there are known risk factors. Mothers need to know that management may be reviewed where there is an alteration in clinical signs such as a reduction in fetal movements or onset of abdominal pain.

Summary

• Post-term pregnancy is one that is in excess of 294 days.

• Accurate dating of a pregnancy is essential, as incorrect diagnosis that a pregnancy has gone beyond term may lead to inappropriate or unnecessary intervention.

• Post-term pregnancy is associated with an increase in perinatal mortality and neonatal morbidity rates.

• Possible fetal consequences include macrosomia or postmaturity.

• Prolonged pregnancy is the largest single indication for induction of labour.

INDUCTION OF LABOUR

Induction of labour is the stimulation of uterine contractions before the onset of spontaneous labour. It is an obstetric intervention that should be used when elective birth will be beneficial to mother and baby. The purpose of induction is to effect the birth of the baby, thereby ending the pregnancy. Successful induction depends on adequate contractions which are effective in bringing about progressive dilatation of the cervix. The procedure is more likely to be successful when the cervix is said to be ripe, that is, it has undergone structural changes to produce softening, dilatation, and effacement.

Parents should be partners in the decision-making process, giving their consent based on full information about the alternatives.

Indications for induction

Induction is indicated when the benefits to the mother or the fetus outweigh those of continuing the pregnancy and it is associated with the following maternal and fetal factors.

Maternal indications

1. Prolonged or post-term pregnancy. This is the main indication for induction of labour.

2. Hypertension, including pre-eclampsia. The timing of induction depends on the severity of the symptoms, and the possible consequences on maternal and fetal mortality and morbidity (see Ch. 17).

3. Medical problems. Women with concurrent renal, respiratory or cardiac disease may require induction of labour (see Ch. 16).

4. Placental abruption. Induction may be considered in cases of severe or moderate abruption after the condition of the mother has been stabilised. Caesarean section is more common (see Ch. 15).

5. Obstetric history, such as previous stillbirth.

6. Unstable lie. If placenta praevia and pelvic abnormalities have been excluded, induction may be offered. The lie is corrected to longitudinal but as there remains a possibility of cord prolapse, caesarean section may be preferred.

7. Prelabour rupture of membranes. When rupture occurs at term, spontaneous labour can be anticipated for 60% of mothers within 24 hours and for 90% labour will commence within 72 hours (Grant & Keirse 1989). Delay increases the morbidity to mother and fetus from infection developing.

Results of a study (Hannah et al 1996) indicate that maternal infection (chorioamnionitis and postpartum pyrexia) was reduced where induction with oxytocin followed rupture of membranes.

8. Maternal request. Some women may request to be induced citing social or psychological reasons. Full discussion should take place between the

mother, midwife and obstetrician before a decision is made.

Fetal indications

1. Suspected fetal compromise. Evidence of intrauterine growth retardation, diminished fetal movements or abnormal umbilical artery blood flow detected with Doppler ultrasound may provide indication for induction of labour.

Where compromise is due to Rhesus iso-immunisation, induction may be indicated so that treatment to arrest haemolysis and rectify its effects can be commenced. In cases of fetal compromise the maturity of the fetus needs to be considered with any additional risks associated with preterm birth and vaginal delivery reviewed in conjunction with the risk of continuing the pregnancy.

2. Intrauterine death. Guidance from the Still-birth and Neonatal Death Society (Kohner 1995) reminds professionals that parents may not want to be induced swiftly after diagnosis is made. There is, however, a risk of coagulation defects occurring if the pregnancy continues for a long period after fetal death (Letsky 1989).

Contraindications to induction of labour

1. Placenta praevia
2. Transverse or compound fetal presentation
3. Cord presentation or cord prolapse
4. Cephalopelvic disproportion
5. Severe fetal compromise.

If, in these circumstances, delivery is imperative, it should be effected by caesarean section.

Cervical ripening

The cervix is normally 2 centimetres long, firm and closed throughout pregnancy. Its shape is tubular with a rigid structure designed to retain the fetus within the uterus until term. Maturation of the cervix is the result of the physiological processes that soften, efface and dilate the cervix prior to the onset of labour. This begins as much as 5–6 weeks prior to labour.

Cervical structure

The cervix is composed of dense bundles of collagen fibres, embedded in a protein-based ground substance. These fibres are responsible for the rigidity of the cervix. The cervix also contains elastin fibres, in lesser number. The elastin fibres are thin, running in a line from the internal to the external os. The greatest concentration of elastic fibres is found at the internal os (Leppert 1995). The role of the elastin is to aid expansion in labour and to restore the cervix to pre-pregnant shape (Calder 1994).

The final component of the cervix is smooth muscle fibres, being 10–15% of cervical tissue. During pregnancy they enlarge and become prominent (Leppert 1995). Traditionally viewed as acting as a sphincter, the quantity of muscle is small. Calder (1994) suggests the muscle protects blood vessels and closes the cervix swiftly on completion of labour.

Successful induction occurs when the cervix is favourable or so-called 'ripe'. The cervix is then more compliant, offering less soft tissue resistance to the actions of the myometrium and the presenting part. The muscle, collagen and elastin fibres realign towards term, and water is attracted to the cells of cervix, softening the tissue. Pressure on the cervix from the presenting part helps the process.

With ripening, the ground substance of the cervix changes, cross-linking of fibres occurs and the collagen bundles break down, decreasing in number. There is an increase in the water content of the connective tissue. The process is not dependent on myometrial activity and alters the cervix from one acting as a rigid barrier to a pliant structure (Calder & Greer 1992).

Prostaglandins

The spontaneous changes in the cervix can be replicated by the use of prostaglandin compounds which are available in pharmacological form. They are locally acting chemical compounds derived from fatty acids within cells. Prostaglandins play a significant role in the ripening process and also contribute to the contractibility of the uterus in labour. Although prostaglandins occur throughout the body, specific prostaglandins have been identified as acting on the cervix and the uterus, namely prostaglandin E_2 (PGE$_2$) and F_2 (PGF$_2$). In addition to being produced from the cervix, they are known to be produced by the fetal membranes and the decidua and are detectable in liquor, in increasing quantities before term. PGE$_2$ has been most effective in inducing labour (Keirse 1992c).

Pre-induction prostaglandin can be used to prime or mature the cervix for induction. A low-dose prostaglandin is administered to bring about effacement and dilatation but not to stimulate contractions.

Methods of inducing labour

Prostaglandins and induction

In order to decide on method of induction, assessment of the cervix is required. Prior to prescribing the prostaglandin, the Bishop's score is measured. This is an objective method of assessing whether the cervix is favourable for induction of labour. Key elements in the assessment are dilatation, effacement, position, consistency and station of the presenting part (Bishop 1964). The five different features are considered and each is awarded a score of between 0 and 3. When a total of 6 or over is reached the prognosis for induction is good (Table 26.1).

Prostaglandin is most commonly administered by the intravaginal route, although oral preparations are available. Prostaglandin E$_2$ preparations are available in gel or pessary form, and these are inserted close to the cervix (posterior fornix of the vagina). Prostaglandin E$_2$ administered locally to the cervix is absorbed, resulting in changes which can be assessed on vaginal examination, increasing the Bishop's score.

Prostaglandin produces frequent, but low intensity, contractions of the uterus. These may not be felt by all women and they wear off after 3–4 hours. Labour will result in 30–50% of cases (MacKenzie 1990). Fetal heart rate and uterine contractions should be monitored continuously for 30–60 minutes thereafter. The mother should remain recumbent or resting for 1 hour.

There is a risk of uterine hyperstimulation and, in severe cases, ruptured uterus (DH 1995). Systemic side-effects of prostaglandin include pyrexia, diarrhoea and vomiting.

Sweeping or stripping of membranes

Sweeping the membranes is thought to be an effective method of inducing labour, where there is an uncomplicated pregnancy. Prostaglandins are rapidly produced as the fetal membranes are detached from the decidua. In order to carry out the procedure, a vaginal examination with some cervical stretching is needed. This provides additional stimulus for prostaglandin release.

It could offer an alternative to medical induction in post-term pregnancy (Allott & Palmer 1993, McColgin et al 1990). Further evaluation of the procedure is recommended (Keirse 1992a).

Amniotomy

Amniotomy is the artificial rupture of the fetal membranes resulting in drainage of liquor. It is commonly abbreviated to ARM.

ARM is performed to induce labour when the cervix is favourable or during labour to augment contractions. A well-fitting presenting part is essential, to prevent cord prolapse. ARM may also be carried out to visualise the colour of the liquor or to attach a fetal scalp electrode for the purposes

Table 26.1 Modified Bishop's pre-induction pelvic scoring system

Inducibility features	0	1	2	3
Dilatation of cervix in cm	0	1–2	3–4	5–6
Consistency of cervix	Firm	Medium	Soft	–
Cervical canal length in cm	> 2	1–2	0.5–1	< 0.5
Position of cervix	Posterior	Mid	Anterior	–
Station of presenting part in cm above or below ischial spine	–3	–2	–1, 0	+1, +2

of continuous electronic monitoring of the fetal heart rate. These reasons are not sufficient indications on their own to require ARM.

Rupture of the membranes allows the presenting part to descend, with improved application to the cervical os. This increased stimulation results in stronger contractions, as levels of prostaglandins rise.

ARM is carried out during a vaginal examination using an amnihook, a tool with a small hook at one end, or an amnicot, a glove with a small hook on one finger. Informed maternal consent should be given and reason for the amniotomy clearly stated in the records.

Amniotomy may be used on its own or in association with oxytocin and may be either low, involving rupture of the forewaters, or, less commonly, high, which requires the hindwaters to be ruptured. The latter uses a curved Drew–Smythe catheter and should be reserved for cases of polyhydramnios with a firm indication for induction (Keirse & Chalmers 1989).

Hazards of ARM:

- Intrauterine infection, particularly iatrogenic from digital or instrumental contamination.
- Early decelerations of the fetal heart.
- Cord prolapse.
- Bleeding from the following sources: fetal vessels in the membranes (vasa praevia); the friable vessels in the cervix; or a low-lying placental site (placenta praevia) (Keirse & Chalmers 1989).

Oxytocin

Oxytocin is a hormone released from the posterior pituitary gland. It acts, at cell level, on smooth muscle and is released in a pulsed manner in response to stimulation. Receptors to oxytocin are found in myometrium and increase in number towards term and throughout labour (Fuchs et al 1984).

Oxytocin is used in conjunction with amniotomy and may be commenced at the same time as ARM or after a delay of several hours. Review of trials by Keirse (1992b) found an increased likelihood of delivery within 12 hours if oxytocin and ARM were at the same time. Less analgesia was re-

quired and the rate of postpartum haemorrhage was reduced.

Administration of oxytocin to induce labour

Local policies and protocols should be followed for the administration of oxytocin. Variations occur in the initial dose and the rate of incrementation of oxytocin used for induction of labour (Irons et al 1993). Oxytocin is used intravenously, diluted in an isotonic solution such as normal saline. Dextrose solutions used over long periods, in conjunction with oxytocin, can alter the electrolyte balance because of the mild antidiuretic effect of the hormone (Singhi et al 1985). The infusion should be controlled through a pump to enable accurate assessment of volume and rate. Dosage should be recorded in milliunits per minute. The rate of infusion must be titrated against the assessment of strength and frequency of uterine contractions. The midwife may need to reduce the infusion rate as labour becomes established because the uterus becomes more sensitive to oxytocin as labour progresses. The midwife should aim to administer the lowest dose required to maintain effective, well-spaced uterine contractions, typically occurring every 3 minutes, lasting 45–50 seconds.

Side-effects of oxytocin

1. Hyperstimulation. Oxytocin exposes the mother and fetus to the risk of hyperstimulation of the uterus, which could cause fetal hypoxia and uterine rupture. Hyperstimulation may cause the uterus to contract continuously for several minutes. This is a tonic contraction. The uterus may contract strongly, with the contractions lasting longer than 60 seconds, and more frequently than every 2 minutes. In this case relaxation between contractions is inadequate. The midwife should turn off the infusion and inform the obstetrician in accordance with Midwives Rule 40 (UKCC 1993). The uterus recovers from the hyperstimulation rapidly as the infusion is discontinued, but in some instances salbutamol may be administered, as an inhalation or infusion, to counteract the effect of the oxytocin. Oxytocin should not be

given as a bolus injection during labour because of the risk of hyperstimulation (Seitchik 1987).

2. Prolonged use may contribute to uterine atony postpartum.

3. Water retention, and water intoxication when in prolonged use, due to its antidiuretic effect.

4. Systemic side-effects include direct vascular smooth muscle relaxation leading to transient vaso-dilatation and hypotension where rapid intravenous bolus doses are given (ACOG 1996).

Responsibilities of the midwife and care of a mother for induction of labour

If the reason for induction allows, planning may include a visit to the delivery suite and special care unit, if appropriate, so the woman is familiar with her surroundings. Communication should be clear between personnel with good liaison between midwifery and obstetric and medical teams and the paediatric services to ensure that support and care are available as needed. Mothers and their birth partners should be given factual and unbiased information about induction of labour. Written information should be available as well as an opportunity to discuss issues relating to induction with both medical and midwifery staff. A record of their wishes should be made in the maternity notes.

Care in labour

As with spontaneous labour, all maternal and fetal observations are recorded as contemporaneously as possible on the partogram. A record of discussions and information given during labour is also documented in the mother's notes, with each entry signed and time of entry noted. The midwife caring for the mother should be aware of her local labour ward protocols and policies for induction of labour.

The midwife is monitoring the well-being of the mother and fetus throughout the process of induction. In addition to assessment of progress in labour, observing for signs of the side-effects of oxytocin is essential. For more detailed discussion on care during the first and second stages of labour see Chapters 22 and 24.

Maternal well-being. Observations of maternal pulse rate, blood pressure and temperature are made and recorded on the partogram.

Uterine contractions. Uterine contractions can be felt on palpation and their frequency, duration and strength should be recorded on the partogram every 15–30 minutes. Continuous tocography may be used, in conjunction with monitoring of the fetal heart. The midwife should remain in constant attendance while the rate of oxytocin is increasing, and be able to assess uterine tone both during and after contractions using fingertip palpation (Fig. 26.1).

Fetal well-being. Continuous monitoring is used in conjunction with oxytocin, using an abdominal ultrasound transducer or by applying a fetal scalp electrode. If cardiotocography is not available, the fetal heart rate should be recorded on the partogram every 15 or 30 minutes in accordance with local protocols.

The midwife should be vigilant for signs of fetal distress such as a suspicious or abnormal trace, or signs of meconium-stained liquor (see Ch. 22).

Assessment of pain. The midwife should note the mother's reaction to pain caused by the contractions. With an oxytocin infusion the build-up in frequency and strength of the contractions may be difficult for the woman to cope with. The midwife should be able to give support and encouragement to the woman to help her cope with the

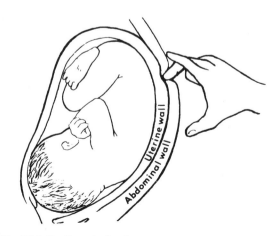

Fig. 26.1 Testing uterine tone.

contractions, and appropriate pain relief should be available if it is required.

Assessment of progress. Before commencing the oxytocin infusion the position of the fetus and relationship of the presenting part to the pelvic brim is assessed by abdominal palpation. A vaginal examination will be performed to assess the length, consistency, position and the dilatation of the cervix. Position and station of the presenting part will also be noted and these observations act as a baseline for assessing progress of the labour. Vaginal examinations are usually carried out 4-hourly, but this may vary if progress is slow, or may be dependent on local policies. If high doses of oxytocin are used, examinations may also be requested more frequently, for example 2-hourly.

When a woman's labour is induced or augmented with oxytocin and there is a previous history of caesarean section, the midwife should be aware of the risk of uterine rupture associated with excessive use of oxytocin (Leung at al 1993). The rate of oxytocin administration should be closely monitored to ensure uterine activity that is adequate to maintain progress in labour.

PROLONGED LABOUR

Prolonged labour has been variously defined from one exceeding 24 hours (Baird 1952) to one exceeding 12 hours of established labour, when labour is actively managed (O'Driscoll et al 1993). Prolonged labour is associated with increasing risks to mother and fetus. The practice of active management and augmentation has been used to reduce the duration of labours, and thus reduce the hazards.

Prolonged labour is most common in primigravidae and may be caused by:

- ineffective uterine contractions
- cephalopelvic disproportion
- occipitoposterior position.

The first stage of labour is divided into a latent and an active phase. During the latent phase the uterus contracts regularly, and the mother experiences discomfort and pain. The cervix effaces and dilatation occurs. The duration of the latent phase

will vary according to each individual and with parity.

Prolonged latent phase

Friedman & Sachtleben (1961) suggested that the average duration of the latent phase in nulliparous women was 8.6 hours and if it lasted 20 hours or more it should be considered as prolonged.

The latent phase of labour is still poorly understood and its duration difficult to define, therefore a diagnosis of a prolonged latent phase may be arbitrary. A prolonged latent phase of labour can be inaccurately diagnosed when the mother is in false labour. It can also be mistakenly considered to be inefficient uterine activity and intervention wrongly occurs.

Prolonged active phase

The active phase is distinguished by an increased rate of dilatation of the cervix, with descent of the presenting part. Slow progress may be defined either in total duration of hours in labour or failure of the cervix to dilate at a fixed rate per hour. A rate of 1 cm per hour is most commonly used (Crowther et al 1989). A prolonged active phase is caused by a combination of factors including the cervix, the uterus, the fetus and the mother's pelvis.

Assessment of the contractions

Clinical assessment by the midwife will give information on the nature of the contractions. Palpation of the fundus during the contraction allows the midwife to assess frequency and duration and gives some indication of the strength. In normal, spontaneous labour this mode of assessment provides adequate information.

External tocographic assessment will show the frequency of the contractions and give some indication of their strength. Strength of the contractions can be difficult to assess because of the size of the abdomen and the contour of the uterus. Assessment of the strength of the contractions can also be made using an internal pressure transducer. Chua et al (1990) reported that no advantage was gained when internal tocography was compared to external monitoring.

Normal uterine action

Normal uterine action is potentiated in labour by increasing levels of prostaglandin and oxytocin receptors. The myometrium contracts and retracts, its efficiency dependent on fundal dominance and polarity between the upper uterine segment and the lower segment. The harmony is facilitated by the appearance in the myometrium towards the end of pregnancy of gap junctions. These gaps play a role in allowing electrical impulses to pass between the muscles (Huszar & Naftolin 1984).

The effectiveness of the contractions is further influenced by resistance, especially from the cervix and other soft tissues, size and position of the fetus and maternal pelvis.

Inefficient uterine action

Slow progress in labour is often attributed to inefficient uterine contractions. In the absence of effective contractions, descent of the presenting part will be delayed, as muscle needs to have an adequate energy supply to contract effectively (Garfield 1987). The practice of restricting food and fluids to labouring mothers may have a detrimental effect on the contractions. The effect of ketones on uterine activity is unclear (Foulkes & Dumoulin 1983). Mothers who are deemed to be at low risk in labour should be encouraged to continue with a light diet (Grant 1990). Alternative approaches and an expectant management suggest that ambulation also produces a return to normal activity. Flynn et al (1978) found that there was a reduced need for oxytocics to improve contractions when mobility was encouraged. The upright position of the labouring mother allows the uterus to fall forward, improves the application of the presenting part onto the cervix and may trigger the neuroendocrine Ferguson reflex. If the mother adopts an upright position, contractions have been found to be less painful although stronger and more efficient than when remaining recumbent (Caldeyro-Barcia 1979a). Stress is known to affect the contractions, and it is possible that less tension, as a result of mobility, enhances the activity (Fenwick & Simkin 1987). The pelvis offers a rigid canal through which the fetus must manoeuvre. Size of the fetus and size of the pelvis have to permit the mechanism of labour.

Where progress is slow, and labour prolonged, consideration of an alternative position may allow the limited opportunity for expansion within the pelvis to be exploited, particularly if there is a malposition of the occiput. Upright positions, or one where the woman adopts a forward-leaning posture, are helpful in encouraging an anterior rotation of the occiput (see Ch. 23, 27). When poor progress of labour is due to hypotonic, inefficient contractions, oxytocin increases the strength and the frequency of the contractions (Gee & Olah 1993). Cephalopelvic disproportion should be excluded before attempts are made to speed up the contractions.

Augmentation of labour

Augmentation of labour occurs to correct slow progress in labour. Correction of ineffective uterine contractions includes amniotomy, amniotomy and administration of oxytocin, or administration of oxytocin in the presence of the previously ruptured membranes. When labour is induced or augmented with oxytocin, the midwife must be vigilant and aware of the risk of hyperstimulation of the uterus.

Active management of labour (see Ch. 22)

The use of active management in preventing prolonged labour and reducing the caesarean section rate is controversial. Analysis of trials show that augmentation with amniotomy and early oxytocin does not improve the caesarean section rates (Thornton & Lilford 1994).

Incoordinate uterine activity

This may be hypertonic and also inefficient. Lacking fundal dominance, the contraction begins and lasts longest in the lower segment. Polarity is reversed. The resting tone of the uterus is raised, the uterus feeling tense on palpation. Pain is intense but out of proportion with the effect on the cervix. This pattern of activity is typically found in association with malposition of the occiput and minor degrees of disproportion.

Where coordination of the contractions is completely lacking, different areas of the uterus contract independently. This is so-called 'colicky' uterus. The mother suffers severe generalised pain, as the resting tone of the uterus is raised. Fetal distress may be the result of diminished placental perfusion.

Constriction ring dystocia

This is a localised spasm of a ring of muscle fibres which occurs at the junction of the upper and lower segments of the uterus. It is rare, affecting less than 1 in 1000 labours and may arise at any stage, although most commonly in the late first or early second stage. It is associated with the use of oxytocin.

Management of prolonged labour

The management of a mother experiencing a prolonged labour will be the responsibility of the obstetric team. Midwives are required to seek medical advice on recognising an aberration from normal (UKCC 1994).

When progress in labour is slow, attempts should be made to determine the cause before deciding on management. Hypotonic uterine activity may be corrected with amniotomy or oxytocin infusion or both. If, however, there have been strong contractions and slow progress, a decision may be made to carry out a caesarean section. Obvious disproportion or malpresentation are indications for caesarean section.

The midwife should ensure the mother's comfort and offer her and her partner support and information about her management and care. Principles of care for a mother in labour are continued as for normal birth but with particular attention to the following:

Informed choice and consent to treatment. As with any situation, the couple should be given as much information as is available to ensure that they understand the events and to obtain consent to all aspects of treatment. Accurate records should be made of discussions and details of any management recorded. Where a mother has previously made a birth plan detailing her wishes, the midwife may need to help her through a change of plan in order to attain a successful outcome.

Comfort and analgesia. Adequate analgesia should be offered to the mother. Where labour is prolonged an epidural block may be beneficial and affords complete pain relief in most cases. Attention should be paid to ensuring that the woman is able to adopt the most comfortable position. General hygiene is important, especially where the membranes have been ruptured, and soiled pads and bed linen should be changed as necessary.

Observations. All observations are recorded on the partogram. Temperature should be taken 4-hourly. Infection may develop where there has been prolonged rupture of membranes. Oral recording of temperature can underestimate maternal pyrexia, owing to the thermometer not being left in long enough for an accurate record (Closs 1987). Vaginal swabs may be taken and broad spectrum antibiotics commenced when infection is suspected.

Pulse and blood pressure are recorded hourly, or more frequently if the woman's condition requires.

Fluid balance. An accurate record should be kept. Note of urinary output is important and the mother is offered the opportunity to empty her bladder every 2 hours. A full bladder may affect the uterine action in labour and if she is unable to void, a catheter should be inserted. A reduction in urinary output may be associated with the antidiuretic effect of oxytocin, be linked with pyrexia and dehydration or be a sign of deterioration of the mother's condition, as in pre-eclampsia. Record of output is important where dextrose 5% is the fluid used to administer oxytocin. Fluid overload can occur which causes hyponatraemia, affecting mother and baby.

Communication should be clear between personnel with liaison between the midwifery and obstetric teams and paediatric services to ensure that support and care are available as needed.

Assessment of progress in prolonged labour. Vaginal examination is carried out, usually on a 4-hourly regimen. Progress is noted by increasing dilatation along with the consistency of the cervix and application of the cervix to the presenting part. Position of the sagittal suture is noted, as is any caput or moulding of the fetal skull. Moulding is an indication that the fetus is experiencing difficulty in negotiating the pelvis. The degree of moulding should be noted and any increase, over successive examinations, reported. Caput succedaneum can develop, particularly if labour is prolonged. This can make position and station difficult to assess, as it masks the sutures and fontanelles.

Descent of the presenting part can be demonstrated by correlating findings from an abdominal examination and station of the presenting part on vaginal examination.

The colour of the amniotic fluid needs to be noted and if meconium is present this should be reported (Mason & Edwards 1993).

Fetal well-being. It is common practice for the fetal heart to be monitored continuously in a prolonged labour. The use of oxytocin and epidural analgesia combined with maternal and fetal indications for induction have been cited as reasons for using electronic monitoring (Steer et al 1985). Fetal blood sampling may be used to support a decision to continue with labour, or intervene (Leveno et al 1986). However, electronic fetal monitoring combined with fetal blood sampling has not been shown to reduce the perinatal mortality rate (Neilson 1994).

The presence of meconium-stained liquor and an abnormal fetal heart tracing is suggestive of fetal hypoxia and, dependent on local policies, fetal blood sampling may be carried out. A paediatrician should be present at the birth and precautions taken to prevent aspiration of meconium.

In the event of the mother being in labour at home, it may be necessary to arrange for her to be transferred into hospital. Advice can be sought from local supervisors of midwives and careful records of discussions made.

Prolonged second stage of labour

Provided that there is evidence of descent of the fetus, in the absence of fetal or maternal distress there is no basis for placing a time limit on the duration of the second stage of labour.

There is no benefit to the mother or fetus in aggressive pushing to speed up this stage of labour (Caldeyro-Barcia 1979b, Thomson 1993).

Adopting an upright position has been found to be advantageous to the mother, although opportunity may be limited by epidural block, infusions or fetal monitors.

Causes of delay in the second stage

Ineffective contractions, poor maternal effort, loss of, or absence of, a desire to push caused by epidural analgesia may all contribute to a lengthy second stage. A full bladder or a full rectum can also impede progress. A large fetus, malpresentation or malposition may account for delay and an assisted birth may be necessary.

A reduced pelvic outlet, in association with an occipitoposterior position, may result in deep transverse arrest. This occurs where advance of the presenting part is prevented as the occipitofrontal diameter becomes caught at the ischial spines.

Management of a prolonged second stage of labour

A vaginal examination should be carried out to confirm position, attitude and station of the presenting part. The fetal heart should be auscultated after every contraction or electronic monitoring used.

In the presence of inefficient uterine contractions an infusion of oxytocin should be commenced. The usual observations for the use of oxytocin apply.

Where there are related factors such as preeclampsia or prematurity, management of the second stage will be assessed constantly.

Where the mother is in labour at home the midwife should arrange for transfer to hospital or seek support via her supervisor of midwives.

Options for birth

Delivery may be expedited where the conditions alter and mother or fetus becomes distressed. The obstetrician will decide on method of delivery. Ventouse or forceps will be utilised where the pelvic outlet is adequate and vaginal birth can be safely carried out. Caesarean section may be necessary where there is evidence of cephalopelvic disproportion.

Cervical dystocia

This occurs rarely and is often acquired as a consequence of scarring of the cervix or a congenital structural abnormality. Despite effective contractions the cervix fails to dilate, although it may efface. Caesarean section is necessary to deliver the baby.

OVER-EFFICIENT UTERINE ACTIVITY (PRECIPITATE LABOUR)

The contractions are strong and frequent from the onset of labour. Resistance from the soft tissue is low, resulting in rapid completion of the first and second stages. The mother may be distressed by the intensity of the contractions and the unexpected speed of the birth. Soft tissue damage of the cervix or perineum may complicate the birth. The uterus may fail to retract during the third stage, leading to retained placenta or postpartum haemorrhage.

Fetal hypoxia may be detected in labour and rapid moulding can occur. The speed of the birth may result in the baby being born in an inappropriate place, and injury from, for example, hard floors or toilets is a risk.

Precipitate labour tends to recur and the woman may be offered the opportunity to be admitted to hospital in subsequent pregnancies.

TRIAL OF LABOUR

A trial of labour is offered to mothers when, in the presence of a minor degree of cephalo-pelvic disproportion, there is concern as to the outcome of labour. The outcome of any labour is dependent on:

- the effectiveness of uterine contractions
- the 'give' of the pelvic joints
- flexion of the fetal head
- the degree of moulding of the fetal head.

These factors are unpredictable until labour is established hence the reason for the trial of labour.

Review of place of birth may be necessary, as care should be offered in a unit which is fully equipped and staffed for operative procedures. The woman will continue her pregnancy until term and may enter labour spontaneously. However, in the presence of other obstetrical indicators, labour may be induced.

Trial of labour will be carried out when the presentation is cephalic and, although the head is likely to be non-enagaged, there should be no major disproportion. The position of the fetus and degree of flexion of the head should be noted on abdominal examination and the findings can be correlated with those confirmed by vaginal examination. Progress is recorded on a partograph and any failure to progress is reported. Ambulation and upright positions can be adopted to promote effective uterine contractions, cervical dilatation and flexion of the head. Continuous fetal monitoring is used to assess fetal well-being. If, despite good uterine contractions, cervical dilatation is slow and the head fails to descend, the outlook for vaginal delivery is poor and the decision must be made whether or not to allow labour to continue.

If at any stage during this labour the mother or fetus are under stress a caesarean section will be performed. Labour should not be permitted to continue until signs of maternal and fetal distress are displayed. The aim is to ensure a successful outcome of a live mother and child who have sustained minimal trauma.

OBSTRUCTED LABOUR

Labour is said to be obstructed when there is no advance of the presenting part despite strong uterine contractions. The obstruction usually occurs at the pelvic brim but may occur at the outlet, for example deep transverse arrest in an android pelvis.

Causes of obstructed labour

- Cephalopelvic disproportion or disparity between the size of the mother's pelvis and the fetus that precludes vaginal birth is the most common cause of obstructed labour. The fetus may be large in relation to the pelvis, or the pelvis may be contracted (see Ch. 49).

• Deep transverse arrest, an outcome of an occipitoposterior position, can cause obstructed labour (see Ch. 27).

• Malpresentation. Vaginal birth is impossible in cases of shoulder or brow presentation, or in persistent mentoposterior position (see Ch. 27).

• Pelvic mass. Fibroids located in the lower segment or on the cervix can prevent descent of the fetal head, causing obstructed labour. Ovarian tumours or rare tumours of the bony pelvis may also prevent the head from entering the pelvis.

• Fetal abnormalities. Abnormalities such as hydrocephalus resulting in disparity between the size of the fetus and the pelvis may cause obstruction. Conjoined twins, or locked twins, are a rare cause.

Signs of obstructed labour

The presenting part does not enter the pelvic brim despite good contractions. The midwife should exclude reasons such as a full bladder, loaded rectum, or excessive liquor volume as factors contributing to the failure in descent.

As the presenting part is unable to descend, cervical dilatation is affected and dilatation is slow. The cervix is described as hanging loosely like 'an empty sleeve' as the presenting part is not applied to it. The uterine contractions exert pressure on the membranes that are over the cervix, which may result in early rupture or the formation of a large elongated sac of forewaters.

Late signs of obstructed labour

These arise in a badly managed or neglected labour and the diagnosis of obstructed labour should be made before these signs are seen. On examination the mother is dehydrated, ketotic and in constant pain. Clinical signs also include pyrexia and a rapid pulse rate. Abdominal palpation is difficult because of maternal distress with the area over the lower segment being particularly tender to the touch. The level of the presenting part may be difficult to assess abdominally but this should be attempted as assessment on vaginal examination is complicated by the presence of caput succedaneum and moulding. Urinary output is poor and haematuria may be present. Evidence of fetal distress may be observed and where the midwife has noted a ma-ternal tachycardia the two rates should be compared. Profound bradycardia or fetal demise may be overlooked as the two rates are misinterpreted.

The uterus becomes moulded round the fetus and it fails to relax properly between contractions. The contractions continue to build in strength and frequency until the uterus is in a continuous state of tonic contraction. The lower segment becomes progressively thinner and longer and the upper segment shorter and thicker. A physiological retraction ring may be seen as an oblique ridge above the symphysis pubis and marks the junction between the upper and lower uterine segment. A visible retraction ring, or Bandl's ring, is similar in appearance to a full bladder. The ridge appears at an oblique angle across the abdomen. Little urine is obtained on catheterisation of the bladder. Uterine exhaustion, in which contractions cease for a while before recommencing with renewed vigour, may occur in a primigravida.

On examination the vagina feels hot and dry, the presenting part is high and feels wedged and immovable. It may be difficult to accurately assess station of the presenting part as there is excessive moulding of the fetal skull and a large caput succedaneum present (Fig. 26.2).

Management of obstructed labour

Management includes prevention of obstructed labour in the first instance. Assessment of the risk within the antenatal period begins with noting any history of prolonged labours or difficult births. Antenatal assessment includes abdominal examination which should alert the midwife to any malpresentation or signs of cephalopelvic disproportion. Appropriate referral can be made prior to the onset of labour and management of the case adjusted to ensure safe delivery. An elective caesarean section may be advocated.

Careful assessment of the progress throughout labour will help detect lack of descent before labour becomes obstructed. Correlation of findings from abdominal examination and vaginal examination helps to confirm descent of the presenting part through the pelvis. This is aided by observation of both maternal and fetal condition and assessment of the length, strength and frequency

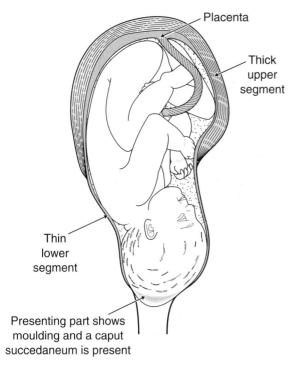

Placenta

Thick upper segment

Thin lower segment

Presenting part shows moulding and a caput succedaneum is present

Fig. 26.2 Obstructed labour. The uterus is moulded around the fetus. The thickened upper segment is obvious on abdominal palpation.

of contractions. If a midwife suspects that labour is obstructed she must seek appropriate medical aid.

An intravenous infusion must be commenced, if not already in progress, to correct dehydration. Blood is taken for cross-matching in case a transfusion is needed. The mother will require treatment with antibiotics, to overcome any infection that may be present. An accurate record of observations of maternal and fetal condition along with any discussions the midwife has with the mother and her family should be made as contemporaneously as possible.

If obstructed labour is recognised in the first stage of labour, as when the head is extended to brow presentation, delivery should be by caesarean section. In the second stage of labour failure to progress and descend may be caused by deep transverse arrest. If the obstruction cannot be overcome by rotation and assisted birth, caesarean section should be performed as soon as possible.

If the mother is labouring at home, arrangements should be made to transfer her to the nearest ma-

ternity unit with facilities for immediate caesarean section and the staff to care for mother and baby. Both may require specialised care. The midwife should take blood for cross-matching and site an intravenous infusion prior to transfer. Detailed records should be kept as previously stated.

If the labour is obstructed and the fetus has died, this will still be the mode of delivery as vaginal birth cannot be achieved. Following the birth of the baby and prior to repair of the uterus and abdomen, the surgeon will check carefully for any indication that the uterus has ruptured.

The fetus is likely to be delivered in a shocked and asphyxiated condition and facilities for resuscitation and expert care should be available. The paediatrician should be present at the birth, and the parents need to be aware that the baby may need special care after birth.

Complications of obstructed labour

Maternal
Trauma to the bladder may occur as a result of pressure from the fetal head during labour or as a result of trauma during delivery. Vesicovaginal fistula is still a common cause of morbidity in women in developing countries. Prolonged compression of the tissues causes necrosis of the bladder and vaginal walls and results in urinary incontinence. Intrauterine infection may follow prolonged rupture of membranes.

Neglected obstruction will result in rupture of the uterus due to thinning of the lower uterine segment. This in turn results in haemorrhage and possible death for the mother and the fetus (see Ch. 29).

Fetal
Intrauterine asphyxia may result in a fresh stillbirth or, if the baby is born alive, permanent brain damage.

Ascending infection can cause neonatal pneumonia which may also develop as a consequence of meconium aspiration.

Refusal of treatment
Where a mother and her partner do not consent to the proposed management this does not absolve

midwives and doctors of their duty towards the client. The midwife is obliged to continue and provide care and support at a level appropriate to her experience while waiting for assistance. If the mother is at home and refuses to be admitted to hospital, the supervisor of midwives should be informed along with the appropriate obstetrician. Records should be kept of treatment offered and received. The consequences of refusal should be made clear to the family and noted (UKCC 1996).

Post-traumatic stress

Untreated distress following a traumatic birth can result in long-term psychological problems. Post-traumatic stress disorder results in the client experiencing flashbacks, avoidance to prevent memories and an increased level of anxiety when in similar situations. Opportunities need to be given to the mother and her family to talk through their experience. Labour needs to be explained to help the mother understand and interpret events (Allott 1996). The psychological trauma is caused by pain, a sense of powerlessness and loss of control over events. Lack of information and failure to consent to management add to the sense of disempowerment. The attitude of midwives and obstetricians also contributes to the distress if they are perceived as unsympathetic and uncaring. Debriefing and follow-up support by midwives or trained counsellors has been successful in overcoming stress caused by a traumatic labour or delivery. (See also Ch. 31.)

Mortality

Obstructed labour is a major contributor to maternal mortality figures worldwide, being responsible for the death of approximately 40 000 women each year. It is a major problem in those countries where women may labour without the help of trained attendants (Kwast 1994). As part of the Safe Motherhood Initiative the World Health Organization has developed and introduced a partograph for use in developing countries. The aim is to increase the detection of women with prolonged or obstructed labour and improve the management of labour. The partograph alerts carers to those women with abnormal progress and enables action to be taken. Maternal and fetal morbidity is thus reduced (Kwast 1994).

READER ACTIVITIES

1. Review the statistics relating to post-term pregnancy in your locality. What form of management is predominant?

Familiarise yourself with the local protocols for care. Collate a package of information that is available for clients in your area on the management of prolonged pregnancy.

2. Reflect on and document a critical incident that illustrates a significant event relating to the use of oxytocin in labour.

3. Compare and contrast the experiences of mothers whom you have cared for during:

   a. labour with spontaneous onset
   b. induction of labour using vaginal prostaglandins
   c. induction of labour with amniotomy and intravenous oxytocin.

4. Consider a case where labour was complicated by dysfunctional uterine activity.

   a. Write down how the case was managed.
   b. What information was needed to make the decisions in this case?
   c. What have you learnt from the experience?
   d. How has your practice been modified as a result of this learning experience?

REFERENCES

ACOG (American College of Obstetricians and Gynecologists) Technical Bulletin 1996 Induction of labor. International Journal of Gynecology and Obstetrics 53: 65–72

Allott H 1996 Picking up the pieces: the post-delivery stress clinic. British Journal of Midwifery 4(10): 534–536

Allott H A, Palmer C R 1993 Sweeping the membranes: a valid procedure in stimulating the onset of labour? British Journal of Obstetrics and Gynaecology 100: 898–903

Andersen H F, Johnson T R B, Barclay M L, Flora J D 1981 Gestational age assessment. 1. Analysis of individual clinical observations. American Journal of Obstetrics and Gynecology 139: 173–177

Anteby E Y, Tadmor O, Revel A, Yagel S 1994 Post-term pregnancies with normal cardiotocograph and amniotic fluid columns: the role of doppler evaluation in predicting perinatal outcome. European Journal of Obstetrics and Gynaecology and Reproductive Biology 54: 93–98

Baird D 1952 The cause and prevention of difficult labor. American Journal of Obstetrics and Gynecology 63: 1200–1212

Bakketeig L S, Bergsjo P 1989 Post term pregnancy, the magnitude of the problem. In: Chalmers I, Enkin M, Keirse M J N C (eds) Effective care in pregnancy and childbirth. Oxford University Press, Oxford, vol 2, ch 46, p 766

Beazley J, Kurjak A 1979 Why palpate a pregnant abdomen? Nursing Mirror 149(6): 35–37

Bishop E M 1964 Pelvic scoring for elective induction. Obstetrics and Gynecology 24(2): 266–268

Boyd M E, Usher R H, McLean F H, Kramer M S 1988 Obstetric consequences of postmaturity. American Journal of Obstetrics and Gynecology 158: 334–338

Calder A A 1994 Prostaglandins and biological control of cervical function. Australian and New Zealand Journal of Obstetrics and Gynecology 34(3): 347–351

Calder A A, Greer I A 1992 Cervical physiology and induction of labour. In: Bonnar J (ed) Recent advances in obstetrics and gynaecology. Churchill Livingstone, Edinburgh, ch 3

Caldeyro-Barcia R 1979a The influence of maternal position on time of spontaneous rupture of the membranes, progress of labor and fetal head compression. Birth and the Family Journal 6(1): 7–15

Caldeyro-Barcia R 1979b The influence of maternal bearing down efforts during the second stage on fetal wellbeing. Birth and the Family Journal 6(1): 17–21

Chua S, Kurup A, Arulkumaran S, Ratnam S S 1990 Augmentation of labor: does internal tocography result in better obstetric outcome than external tocography? Obstetrics and Gynecology 76(2): 164–167

Clifford S H 1954 Postmaturity with placental dysfunction: Clinical syndrome and pathological findings. Journal of Pediatrics 44: 1–13

Closs J 1987 Oral temperature measurement. Nursing Times 83(1): 36–39

Crowley P 1989 Post-term pregnancy: induction or surveillance? In: Chalmers I, Enkin M, Keirse M J N C (eds) Effective care in pregnancy and childbirth. Oxford University Press, Oxford, vol 2, ch 47

Crowley P 1993 Elective induction of labour at or beyond term. In: Enkin M, Keirse M J N C, Renfrew M J, Neilson J P (eds) Pregnancy and childbirth module of the Cochrane Database of Systematic Reviews 1995, issue 1. Update Software, Oxford

Crowley P, O'Herlihy C, Boylan P 1984 The value of ultrasound measurement of amniotic fluid volume in the management of prolonged pregnancies. British Journal of Obstetrics and Gynecology 91: 444–448

Crowther C, Enkin M, Keirse M J N C, Brown I 1989 Monitoring the progress of labour. In: Chalmers I, Enkin M, Keirse M J N C (eds) Effective care in pregnancy and childbirth. Oxford University Press, Oxford, vol 2, ch 53, p 841

Department of Health (DH) 1995 Confidential enquiry into stillbirths and deaths in infancy. Annual Report

January–December 1993. HMSO, London

Eden R D, Gergely R Z, Schifrin B S, Wade M A 1982 Comparison of antepartum testing schemes for the management of post date pregnancy. American Journal of Obstetrics and Gynecology 144: 683–692

Fenwick L, Simkin P 1987 Maternal positioning to prevent or alleviate dystocia in labor. Clinical Obstetrics and Gynecology 30(1): 83–89

FIGO 1982 Report of the Committee following a workshop in monitoring and reporting perinatal mortality and morbidity. FIGO Standing Committee on Perinatal Mortality International Federation Of Gynaecology and Obstetrics. Chameleon Press, London

Flynn A M, Kelly, J, Hollins G, Lynch P F 1978 Ambulation in labour. British Medical Journal 2: 591–593

Foulkes J, Dumoulin J G 1983 Ketosis in labour. British Journal of Hospital Medicine 29(6): 562–564

Fox H 1991 A contemporary view of the human placenta. Midwifery 7: 31–39

Friedman E A, Sachtleben M R 1961 Dysfunctional labor 1. Prolonged latent phase in the nullipara. Obstetrics and Gynecology 17(2): 135–148

Fuchs A R, Fuchs F, Husslein P, Soloff M S 1984 Oxytocin receptors in pregnant human uterus. American Journal of Obstetrics and Gynecology 150: 734–741

Garfield R E 1987 Cellular and molecular bases for dystocia. Clinical Obstetrics and Gynecology 30(1): 3–18

Gee H, Olah K S 1993 Failure to progress in labour. In: Studd J (ed) Progress in obstetrics and gynaecology. Churchill Livingstone, Edinburgh, vol 10, ch 11

Grant J 1990 Nutrition and hydration in labour. In: Alexander J, Levy V, Roch S (ed) Intrapartum care, a research based approach. Macmillan, Basingstoke, ch 4, p 66

Grant J, Keirse M J N C 1989 Prelabour rupture of membranes at term. In: Chalmers I, Enkin M, Keirse M J N C (eds) Effective care in pregnancy and childbirth. Oxford University Press, Oxford, vol 2, ch 64, p 1113

Hall M H, Carr Hill R A 1985 The significance of uncertain gestation for obstetric outcome. British Journal of Obstetrics and Gynecology 92: 452–460

Hannah M E, Hannah W J, Hellmann J, Hewson S, Milner R, Willan A and the Canadian Multicenter Post-term Pregnancy Trial Group 1992 Induction of labor as compared to serial antenatal monitoring in post-term pregnancy. New England Journal of Medicine 326(24): 1587–1592

Hannah M E, Ohlsson A, Farine D et al 1996 Induction of labor compared with expectant management for prelabor rupture of membranes at term. New England Journal of Medicine 334(6): 1005–1010

Huszar G, Naftolin F 1984 The myometrium and uterine cervix in normal and pre-term labor. New England Journal of Medicine 311(9): 571–581

Irons D W, Thornton S, Davison J M, Baylis P H 1993 Oxytocin infusion regimens: time for standardisation? British Journal of Obstetrics and Gynaecology 100: 786–787

James D 1991 Limitation of fetal biophysical assessment. Contemporary Reviews in Obstetrics and Gynaecology 3: 69–74

Johnson J M, Harman C R, Lange I R, Manning F A 1986 Biophysical profile scoring in the management of the post-term pregnancy, an analysis of 307 patients. American Journal of Obstetrics and Gynecology 154: 269–273

Keirse M J N C 1992a Stripping/sweeping the membranes at

term for induction of labour. In: Enkin M, Keirse M J N C, Renfrew M J, Neilson J P (eds) Pregnancy and childbirth module of the Cochrane Database of Systematic Reviews. 1995, issue 1. Update Software, Oxford

Keirse M J N C 1992b Amniotomy plus early versus late oxytocin infusion for induction of labour. In: Enkin M, Keirse M J N C, Renfrew M J, Neilson J P (eds) Pregnancy and childbirth module of the Cochrane Database of Systematic Reviews, 1995, issue 1. Update Software, Oxford

Keirse M J N C 1992c Any prostaglandin/any route for cervical ripening. In: Enkin M, Keirse M J N C, Renfrew M J, Neilson J P (eds) Pregnancy and childbirth module of the Cochrane Database of Systematic Reviews 1995, issue 1. Update Software, Oxford

Keirse M J N C, Chalmers I 1989 Methods for inducing labour. In Chalmers I, Enkin M, Keirse M J N C (eds) Effective care in pregnancy and childbirth. Oxford University Press, Oxford, vol 2, ch 62, pp 1058, 1063

Kohner N 1995 Pregnancy loss and the death of a baby. Guidelines for professionals. SANDS, London, pp 19–20

Kwast B E 1994 World Health Organization partograph in management of labour. Lancet 343: 1399–1404

Leppert P C 1995 Anatomy and physiology of cervical ripening. Clinical Obstetrics and Gynecology 38(2): 267–279

Letsky E A 1989 Coagulation defects in pregnancy. In: Turnbull A, Chamberlain G (eds) Obstetrics. Churchill Livingstone, Edinburgh, ch 38, p 569

Leung A S, Farmer R M, Leung E K, Medearis A L, Paul R H 1993 Risk factors associated with uterine rupture during trial of labor after cesarean delivery: a case-control study. American Journal of Obstetrics and Gynecology 168: 1358–1363

Leveno K J, Quirk J G, Cunningham F G, Nelson S D, Santos-Ramos R, Toofanian A, De Palma R T 1984 Prolonged pregnancy: 1. Observations concerning the causes of fetal distress. American Journal of Obstetrics and Gynecology 150: 465–473

Leveno K J, Cunningham F G, Nelson S et al 1986 A prospective comparison of selective and universal electronic fetal monitoring in 34995 pregnancies. New England Journal of Medicine 315(10): 615–619

McColgin S W, Hampton H L, McCaul J F, Howard P R, Andrew M E, Morrison J C 1990 Stripping membranes at term: can it safely reduce the incidence of post-term pregnancies. Obstetrics and Gynecology 76: 678–680

MacKenzie I A 1990 The therapeutic roles of prostaglandins in obstetrics. In: Studd J (ed) Progress in obstetrics and gynaecology. Churchill Livingstone, Edinburgh, vol 8, ch 11, p 152

Manning F A, Baskett T F, Morrison I, Lange I 1981 Fetal biophysical profile scoring: a prospective study of 1184 high risk patients. American Journal of Obstetrics and Gynecology 140: 289–294

Mason D, Edwards P 1993 Litigation a risk management guide for midwives. Royal College of Midwives, London

Mittendorf R et al 1990 The length of uncomplicated human gestation. Obstetrics and Gynecology 75(6): 929–932

Miyazaki F S, Miyazaki B A 1981 False reaction non stress test in post-term pregnancies. American Journal of Obstetrics and Gynecology 140: 269–276

Naeye R L 1978 Causes of perinatal mortality excess in prolonged gestations. American Journal of Epidemiology 108(5): 429–433

Neilson J P 1990 The measurement of fetal growth. In: Chamberlain G (ed) Modern antenatal care of the fetus. Blackwell Scientific, Oxford, ch 5

Neilson J P 1994 Fetal blood sampling as adjunct to heart rate monitoring. In: Enkin M, Keirse M J N C, Renfrew M J, Neilson J P (eds) Pregnancy and childbirth module of the Cochrane Database of Systematic Reviews 1995, issue 1. Update Software, Oxford

O'Dowd M J, O'Dowd T M 1985 Quickening – a re-evaluation. British Journal of Obstetrics and Gynaecology 92: 1037–1039

O'Driscoll K, Meagher D, Boylan P 1993 Active management of labour. The Dublin experience, 3rd edn. Mosby, London

Phelan J P 1991 Tests of fetal well-being using the fetal heart rate. In: Spencer J D (ed) Fetal monitoring. Physiology and techniques of antenatal and intrapartum assessment. Oxford University Press, Oxford, ch 11, pp 60–63

Seitchik J 1987 The management of functional dystocia in the first stage of labor. Clinical Obstetrics and Gynecology 30(1): 42–49

Singhi S, Chookang E, Hall J, Kalghatgi S 1985 Iatrogenic neonatal and maternal hyponatraemia following oxytocin and aqueous glucose infusion during labour. British Journal of Obstetrics and Gynaecology 92: 356–363

Steer P, Carter M C, Beard R W 1985 The effect of oxytocin infusion on uterine activity levels in slow labour. British Journal of Obstetrics and Gynaecology 91: 1120–1126

Thomson A M 1993 Pushing techniques in the second stage of labour. Journal of Advanced Nursing 18: 171–177

Thornton J G, Lilford R J 1994 Active management of labour: current knowledge and research issues. British Medical Journal 309: 366–369

United Kingdom Central Council for Nursing, Midwifery and Health Visiting (UKCC) 1993 Midwives rules. UKCC, London

United Kingdom Central Council for Nursing, Midwifery and Health Visiting (UKCC) 1994 The midwife's code of practice. UKCC, London

United Kingdom Central Council for Nursing, Midwifery and Health Visiting (UKCC) 1996 Guidelines for professional practice. UKCC, London

Usher R H, Boyd M E, McLean F H, Kramer M S 1988 Assessment of fetal risk on post-date pregnancy. American Journal of Obstetrics and Gynecology 158(2): 259–264

Malpositions of the occiput and malpresentations

Terri Coates

27

CHAPTER CONTENTS

Malpositions and malpresentations present the midwife with a challenge of recognition and diagnosis both in the antenatal period and during labour.

The chapter aims to:

- outline the causes of these positions and presentations
- discuss the midwife's diagnosis and management
- describe the possible outcomes.

OCCIPITOPOSTERIOR POSITIONS

Occipitoposterior positions are the most common type of malposition of the occiput and occur in approximately 10% of labours. A persistent occipitoposterior position results from a failure of internal rotation prior to delivery. This occurs in 5% of deliveries (Pearl et al 1993).

The vertex is presenting, but the occiput lies in the posterior rather than the anterior part of the pelvis. As a consequence, the fetal head is deflexed and larger diameters of the fetal skull present (Fig. 27.1).

Causes

The direct cause is often unknown, but it may be associated with an abnormally shaped pelvis.

In an android pelvis the forepelvis is narrow and the occiput tends to occupy the roomier hindpelvis. The oval shape of the anthropoid pelvis, with its narrow transverse diameter, favours a direct occipitoposterior position.

Antenatal diagnosis

Abdominal examination

On inspection. There is a saucer-shaped

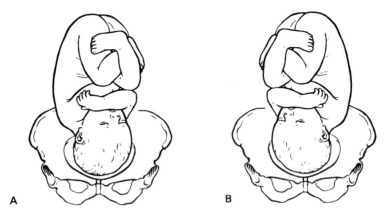

Fig. 27.1 (A) Right occipitoposterior position. (B) Left occipitoposterior position.

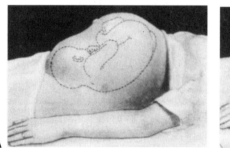

Fig. 27.2 Comparison of abdominal contour in (A) posterior and (B) anterior positions of the occiput.

depression at or just below the umbilicus. This dip is created by the 'dip' between the head and the lower limbs of the fetus. The outline created by the high, unengaged head can look like a full bladder (Fig. 27.2).

On palpation. Whilst the breech is easily palpated at the fundus the back is difficult to palpate as it is well out to the maternal side, sometimes almost adjacent to the maternal spine. Limbs can be felt on both sides of the midline.

The head is usually high, a posterior .position being the most common cause of non-engagement in a primigravida at term. This is because the large presenting diameter, the occipitofrontal (11.5 cm), is unlikely to enter the pelvic brim until labour begins and flexion occurs. Flexion allows the engagement of the suboccipitofrontal diameter (10 cm).

The occiput and sinciput are on the same level (Figs 27.3 and 27.4).

The cause of the deflexion is a straightening of the fetal spine against the lumbar curve of the

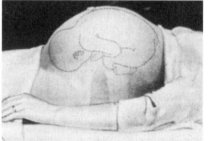

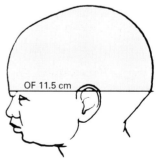

Fig. 27.3 Engaging diameter of a deflexed head: occipitofrontal (OF) 11.5 cm.

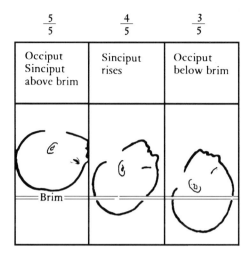

Fig. 27.4 Flexion with descent of the head.

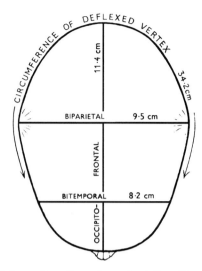

Fig. 27.5 Presenting dimensions of a deflexed head.

maternal spine. This makes the fetus straighten his neck and adopt a more erect attitude.

On auscultation. The fetal back is not well flexed so the chest is thrust forward, therefore the fetal heart can be heard in the midline. However, the heart may be heard more easily at the flank on the same side as the back.

Antenatal preparation

There is anecdotal evidence to suggest that active changes of maternal posture may help to achieve an optimal fetal position before labour (El Halta 1995, Sutton 1996). It may be possible that rotation to an anterior position may be achieved by the mother adopting a knee–chest position several times a day; however, this possibility needs to be researched.

Diagnosis during labour

The woman may complain of continuous and severe backache worsening with contractions. The absence of backache does not necessarily indicate an anteriorly-positioned fetus (Biancuzzo 1993).

The large and irregularly shaped presenting circumference (Fig. 27.5) does not fit well onto the cervix. Therefore the membranes tend to rupture spontaneously at an early stage of labour and the contractions may be incoordinate. Descent of the head can be slow even with good contractions. The woman may have a strong desire to push early in labour because the occiput is pressing on the rectum.

Vaginal examination

The findings (Fig. 27.6) will depend upon the degree of flexion of the head; locating the anterior fontanelle in the anterior part of the pelvis is diagnostic but this may be difficult if caput succedaneum is present. The direction of the sagittal suture or location of the posterior fontanelle will help to confirm diagnosis.

Management of labour

Labour with a fetus in an occipitoposterior position can be long and painful. The deflexed head does not fit well onto the cervix and therefore does not produce optimum stimulation for uterine contractions.

First stage of labour

The woman may experience severe and unremitting backache which is tiring and can be very demoralising especially if the progress of labour is slow. Continuous support from the midwife will help the mother and her partner to cope with the labour (Thornton & Lilford 1994) (see Chs 21

ANTERIOR

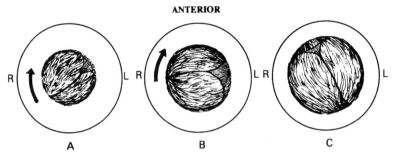

A   B   C

Fig. 27.6 Vaginal touch pictures in a right occipitoposterior position. (A) Anterior fontanelle felt to left and anteriorly. Sagittal suture in the right oblique diameter of the pelvis. (B) Anterior fontanelle felt to left and laterally. Sagittal suture in the transverse diameter of the pelvis. (C) Following increased flexion the posterior fontanelle is felt to the right and anteriorly. Sagittal suture in the left oblique diameter of the pelvis. The position is now right occipitoanterior.

and 23). The midwife can help to provide physical support such as massage and other comfort measures and suggest changes of posture and position. The all-fours position may relieve some discomfort: anecdotal evidence suggests that this position may also aid rotation of the fetal head.

Labour may be prolonged and the midwife should do all she can to prevent the mother becoming dehydrated (see Ch. 21).

Incoordinate uterine action or ineffective contractions may need correction with a Syntocinon infusion (see Ch. 26).

The woman may experience a strong urge to push long before her cervix has become fully dilated. This is due to the pressure of the occiput on the rectum. If the woman pushes at this time, the cervix will become oedematous and this would delay the onset of the second stage of labour. The urge to push may be eased or controlled by a change in position and the use of breathing techniques or Entonox to enhance relaxation. The woman's partner and the midwife can assist throughout labour with massage and physical support and suggestions for alternative methods of pain relief (see Ch. 23). The mother may choose a range of pain control methods throughout her labour depending on the level and intensity of pain that she is experiencing at that time.

Second stage of labour

Full dilatation of the cervix may need to be con-

firmed by a vaginal examination because moulding and formation of a caput succedaneum may bring the vertex into view while an anterior lip of cervix remains. If the head is not visible at the onset of the second stage, then the midwife could encourage the woman to remain upright (see Ch. 23). This position may shorten the length of the second stage and may reduce the need for operative delivery (Nicodem 1995). In some cases where contractions are weak and ineffective a Syntocinon infusion may be commenced to stimulate adequate contractions and achieve advance. As with any labour the maternal and fetal conditions are closely observed throughout the second stage. The length of the second stage of labour is increased when the occiput is posterior and there is an increased likelihood of operative delivery (Gimovsky and Hennigan 1995, Pearl et al 1993).

Mechanism of right occipitoposterior position (long rotation) (Figs 27.7–27.10)

- The lie is longitudinal.
- The attitude of the head is deflexed.
- The presentation is vertex.
- The position is right occipitoposterior.
- The denominator is the occiput.
- The presenting part is the middle or anterior area of the left parietal bone.
- The occipitofrontal diameter, 11.5 cm, lies in the right oblique diameter of the pelvic brim. The

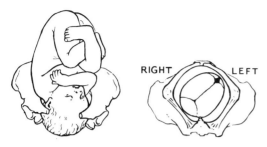

Fig. 27.7 Head descending with increased flexion. Sagittal suture in right oblique diameter of the pelvis.

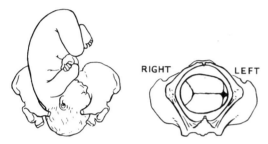

Fig. 27.8 Occiput and shoulders have rotated 1/8 of a circle forwards. Sagittal suture in transverse diameter of the pelvis.

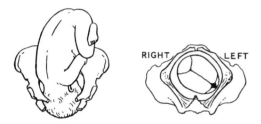

Fig. 27.9 Occiput and shoulders have rotated 2/8 of a circle forwards. Sagittal suture in the left oblique diameter of the pelvis. The position is right occipitoanterior.

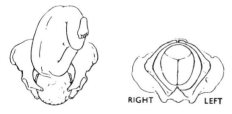

Fig. 27.10 Occiput has rotated 3/8 of a circle forwards. Note twist in neck. Sagittal suture in the anteroposterior diameter of the pelvis.

Figs 27.7–27.10 Mechanism of labour in right occipitoposterior position.

occiput points to the right sacroiliac joint and the sinciput to the left iliopectineal eminence.

Flexion. Descent takes place with increasing flexion. The occiput becomes the leading part.

Internal rotation of the head. The occiput reaches the pelvic floor first and rotates forwards 3/8 of a circle along the right side of the pelvis to lie under the symphysis pubis. The shoulders follow, turning 2/8 of a circle from the left to the right oblique diameter.

Crowning. The occiput escapes under the symphysis pubis and the head is crowned.

Extension. The sinciput, face and chin sweep the perineum and the head is born by a movement of extension.

Restitution takes place and the occiput turns 1/8 of a circle to the right and the head rights itself with the shoulders.

Internal rotation of the shoulders. The shoulders enter the pelvis in the right oblique diameter, the anterior shoulder reaches the pelvic floor first and rotates forwards 1/8 of a circle to lie under the symphysis pubis.

External rotation of the head. At the same time the occiput turns a further 1/8 of a circle to the right.

Lateral flexion. The anterior shoulder escapes under the symphysis pubis, the posterior shoulder sweeps the perineum and the body is born by a movement of lateral flexion.

Possible course and outcomes of labour

As with all labours, complicated or otherwise, the mother should be kept informed of her progress and proposed interventions so that she can make informed choices and give informed consent, ensuring the optimum outcome for herself and her baby.

Long internal rotation

This is the commonest outcome, with good uterine contractions producing flexion and descent of the head so that the occiput rotates forward 3/8 of a circle as described above.

Short internal rotation – persistent occipitoposterior position
(Figs 27.11 and 27.12)
The term 'persistent occipitoposterior position' indicates that the occiput fails to rotate forwards. Instead the sinciput reaches the pelvic floor first and rotates forwards. The occiput goes into the hollow of the sacrum. The baby is born facing the pubic bone (face to pubis).

Cause:

Failure of flexion. The head descends without increased flexion and the sinciput becomes the leading part. It reaches the pelvic floor first and rotates forwards to lie under the symphysis pubis.

Diagnosis:

In the first stage of labour signs are those of any posterior position of the occiput, namely a deflexed head and a fetal heart heard in the flank or in the midline. Descent is slow.

In the second stage of labour delay is common. On vaginal examination the anterior fontanelle is felt behind the symphysis pubis, but a large caput succedaneum may mask this. If the pinna of the

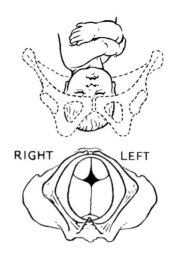

Fig. 27.12 Persistent occipitoposterior position after short rotation: position direct occipitoposterior.

ear is felt pointing towards the mother's sacrum, this indicates a posterior position.

The long occipitofrontal diameter causes considerable dilatation of the anus and gaping of the vagina while the fetal head is barely visible and the broad biparietal diameter distends the perineum and may cause excessive bulging. As the head advances, the anterior fontanelle can be felt just behind the symphysis pubis; the baby is born facing the pubis. Characteristic upward moulding is present with the caput succedaneum on the anterior part of the parietal bone (Fig. 27.13).

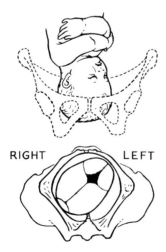

Fig. 27.11 Persistent occipitoposterior position before rotation of the occiput: position right occipitoposterior.

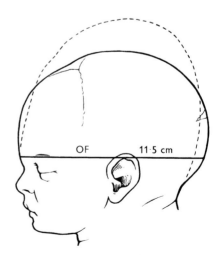

Fig. 27.13 Upward moulding (dotted line) following persistent occipitoposterior position. OF = occipitofrontal.

Management of delivery (Figs 27.14–27.17). The sinciput will first emerge from under the symphysis pubis as far as the root of the nose and the midwife maintains flexion by restraining it from escaping further than the glabella, allowing the occiput to sweep the perineum and be born. She then extends the head by grasping it and bringing the face down from under the symphysis pubis. Owing to the larger presenting diameters, perineal trauma is common and the midwife should watch for signs of rupture in the centre of the perineum ('button-hole' tear). An episiotomy may be required.

Undiagnosed face to pubis. If the signs are not recognised at an earlier stage, the midwife may first be aware that the occiput is posterior when she sees the hairless forehead escaping beneath the pubic arch. She may have been misguidedly extending the head and should therefore now flex it towards the symphysis pubis.

Deep transverse arrest

The head descends with some increase in flexion. The occiput reaches the pelvic floor and begins to rotate forwards. Flexion is not maintained and the occipitofrontal diameter becomes caught at the narrow bispinous diameter of the outlet. Arrest may be due to weak contractions, a straight sacrum or a narrowed outlet.

Diagnosis. The sagittal suture is found in the transverse diameter of the pelvis and both fontanelles are palpable. Neither sinciput nor occiput leads. The head is deep in the pelvic cavity at the level of the ischial spines although the caput may be lower still. There is no advance.

Management. The mother must be kept informed of progress and participate in decisions. If an operative delivery is required for the safe delivery of a healthy baby then the mother's informed consent is required.

Pushing at this time may not resolve the problem; the midwife and the woman's partner can help by encouraging SOS breathing (Ch. 45); a change of position may help to overcome the urge to bear down.

The procedure would be undertaken under local, regional or more rarely general anaesthesia (Ch. 28). The considerations are the choice of the mother and the condition of the mother and fetus.

Vacuum extraction has been associated with lower incidence of trauma to both the mother and the infant (Pearl et al 1993) (see Ch. 28). The doctor may choose to use forceps to rotate the head to an occipitoanterior position before delivery. Whichever procedure is undertaken, the mother should first be given adequate analgesia or anaesthesia.

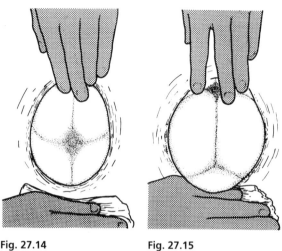

Fig. 27.14   **Fig. 27.15**

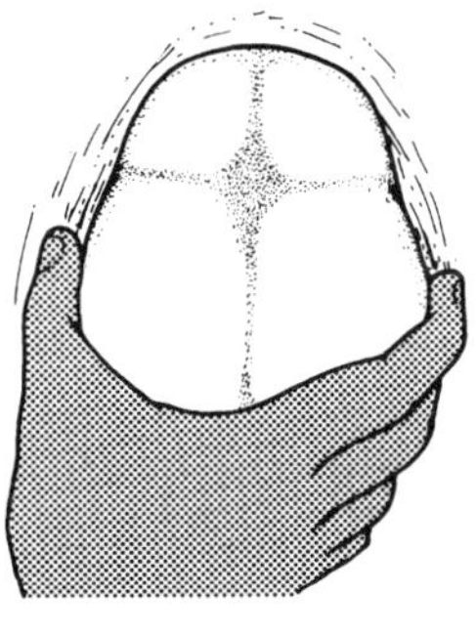

Fig. 27.16   **Fig. 27.17**

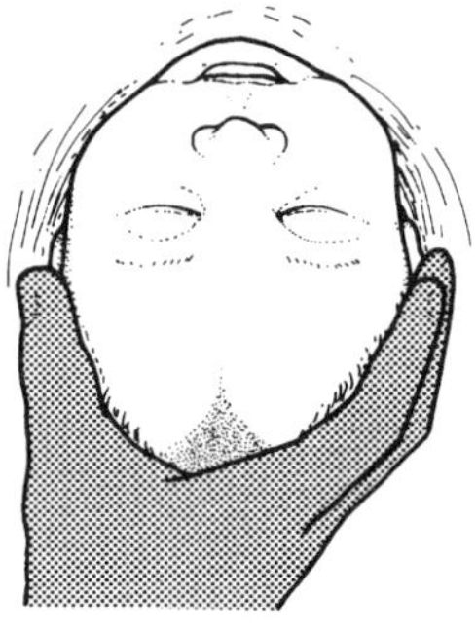

Fig. 27.14 Allowing the sinciput to escape as far as the glabella.
Fig. 27.15 The occiput sweeps the perineum, sinciput held back to maintain flexion.
Fig. 27.16 Grasping the head to bring the face down from under the symphysis pubis.
Fig. 27.17 Extension of the head.

Figs 27.14–27.17 Delivery of head in a persistent occipitoposterior position.

Conversion to face or brow presentation

When the head is deflexed at the onset of labour, extension occasionally occurs instead of flexion. If extension is complete, a face presentation results, but if incomplete, the head is arrested at the brim, the brow presenting. This is a rare complication of posterior positions, and is more commonly found in multiparous women (see also below).

Complications associated with occipitoposterior positions

Apart from prolonged labour with its attendant risks to mother and fetus (see Ch. 26) and the increased likelihood of instrumental delivery, the following complications may occur.

Obstructed labour (see Ch. 29)

This may occur when the head is deflexed or partially extended and becomes impacted in the pelvis.

Maternal trauma

Forceps delivery may result in perineal bruising and trauma. Delivery of a fetus in the persistent occipitoposterior position, particularly if previously undiagnosed, may cause a third-degree tear (Pearl et al 1993).

Neonatal trauma

Neonatal trauma occurring following delivery from an occipitoposterior position has been associated with forceps or Ventouse delivery. The outcome for a neonate delivered from an occipitoposterior position is comparable to that expected for an infant delivered from an occipitoanterior position (Gimovsky & Hennigan 1995, Pearl et al 1993).

Cord prolapse (see Ch. 29)

A high head predisposes to early spontaneous rupture of the membranes which, together with an ill-fitting presenting part, may result in cord prolapse.

Cerebral haemorrhage (see Ch. 40)

The unfavourable upward moulding of the fetal skull, found in an occipitoposterior position, can cause intracranial haemorrhage, due to the falx cerebri being pulled away from the tentorium cerebelli. The larger presenting diameters also predispose to a greater degree of compression. Cerebral haemorrhage may also result from chronic hypoxia which may accompany prolonged labour.

FACE PRESENTATION

When the attitude of the head is one of complete extension, the occiput of the fetus will be in contact with its spine and the face will present.

The incidence is about 1 : 500 and the majority develop during labour from vertex presentations with the occiput posterior; this is termed *secondary face presentation*. Less commonly the face presents before labour; this is termed *primary face presentation*. There are six positions in a face presentation (Figs 27.18–27.23); the denominator is the mentum and the presenting diameters are the submentobregmatic (9.5 cm) and the bitemporal (8.2 cm).

Causes

Anterior obliquity of the uterus. The uterus of a multiparous woman with slack abdominal muscles and a pendulous abdomen will lean forward and alter the direction of the uterine axis. This causes the fetal buttocks to lean forwards and the force of the contractions to be directed in a line towards the chin rather than the occiput, resulting in extension of the head.

Contracted pelvis. In the flat pelvis, the head enters in the transverse diameter of the brim and the parietal eminences may be held up in the obstetrical conjugate; the head becomes extended and a face presentation develops. Alternatively, if the head is in the posterior position, vertex presenting, and remains deflexed, the parietal eminences may be caught in the sacrocotyloid dimension, the occiput does not descend, the head becomes extended and face presentation results. This is more likely in the presence of an android pelvis in which the sacrocotyloid dimension is reduced.

Polyhydramnios. If the vertex is presenting and

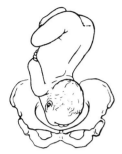

Fig. 27.18 Right mentoposterior.

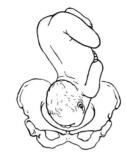

Fig. 27.19 Left mentoposterior.

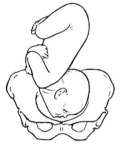

Fig. 27.20 Right mentolateral.

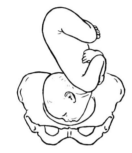

Fig. 27.21 Left mentolateral.

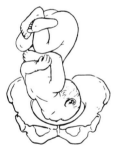

Fig. 27.22 Right mentoanterior.

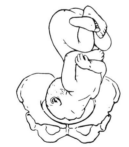

Fig. 27.23 Left mentoanterior.

Figs 27.18–27.23 Six positions of face presentation.

the membranes rupture spontaneously, the resulting rush of fluid may cause the head to extend as it sinks into the lower uterine segment.

Congenital abnormality. Anencephaly can be a fetal cause of a face presentation. In a cephalic presentation, because the vertex is absent, the face is thrust forward and presents. More rarely a tumour of the fetal neck may cause extension of the head.

Antenatal diagnosis

Antenatal diagnosis is rare since face presentation develops during labour in the majority of cases. A cephalic presentation in a known anencephalic fetus may be presumed to be a face presentation.

Intrapartum diagnosis

On abdominal palpation

Face presentation may not be detected especially if the mentum is anterior. The occiput feels prominent, with a groove between head and back, but it may be mistaken for the sinciput. The limbs may be palpated on the side opposite to the occiput and the fetal heart is best heard through the fetal chest on the same side as the limbs. In a mentoposterior position the fetal heart is difficult to hear because the fetal chest is in contact with the maternal spine (Fig. 27.24).

On vaginal examination

The presenting part is high, soft and irregular. When the cervix is sufficiently dilated, orbital ridges, eyes, nose and mouth may be felt. Confusion between mouth and anus could arise. The mouth may be open, and the hard gums are diagnostic. The fetus may suck the examining finger. As labour

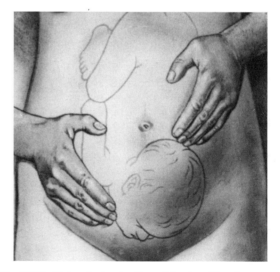

Fig. 27.24 Abdominal palpation of the head in a face presentation. Position right mentoposterior.

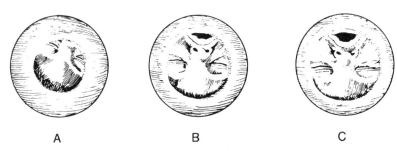

A   B   C

Fig. 27.25 Vaginal touch pictures of left mentoanterior position. (A) Mentum felt to left and anteriorly. Orbital ridges in left oblique diameter of the pelvis. (B) Following increased extension of the head, the mouth can be felt. (C) Face has rotated 1/8 of a circle forwards. Orbital ridges in transverse diameter of the pelvis. Position direct mentoanterior.

progresses the face becomes oedematous, making it more difficult to distinguish from a breech presentation. To determine position the mentum must be located and if it is posterior, the midwife should decide whether it is lower than the sinciput; if so, it will rotate forwards if it can advance. In a left mentoanterior position, the orbital ridges will be in the left oblique diameter of the pelvis (see Fig. 27.25). Care must be taken not to injure or infect the eyes with the examining finger.

Mechanism of a left mentoanterior position

* The lie is longitudinal.
* The attitude is one of extension of head and back.
* The presentation is face (Fig. 27.26).
* The position is left mentoanterior.
* The denominator is the mentum.
* The presenting part is the left malar bone.

Extension. Descent takes place with increasing extension. The mentum becomes the leading part.

Internal rotation of the head occurs when the chin reaches the pelvic floor and rotates forwards 1/8 of a circle. The chin escapes under the symphysis pubis (Fig. 27.27A).

Flexion takes place and the sinciput, vertex and occiput sweep the perineum; the head is born (Fig. 27.27B).

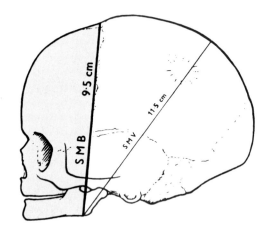

Fig. 27.26 Diameters involved in delivery of face presentation. Engaging diameter, submentobregmatic (SMB) 9.5 cm. The submentovertical (SMV) diameter, 11.5 cm, sweeps the perineum.

Restitution occurs when the chin turns 1/8 of a circle to the woman's left.

Internal rotation of the shoulders. The shoulders enter the pelvis in the left oblique diameter and the anterior shoulder reaches the pelvic floor first and rotates forwards 1/8 of a circle along the right side of the pelvis.

External rotation of the head occurs simultaneously. The chin moves a further 1/8 of a circle to the left.

Lateral flexion. The anterior shoulder escapes under the symphysis pubis, the posterior shoulder

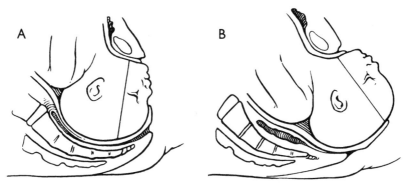

Fig. 27.27 Birth of head in mentoanterior position. (A) Chin escapes under symphysis pubis. Submentobregmatic diameter at outlet. (B) Head is born by a movement of flexion.

sweeps the perineum and the body is born by a movement of lateral flexion.

Possible course and outcomes of labour

The mother should be kept informed of her progress and any proposed intervention throughout labour.

Prolonged labour

Labour is often prolonged because the face is an ill-fitting presenting part and does not therefore stimulate effective uterine contractions. In addition the facial bones do not mould and, in order to enable the mentum to reach the pelvic floor and rotate forwards, the shoulders must enter the pelvic cavity at the same time as the head. The fetal axis pressure is directed to the chin and the head is extended almost at right angles to the spine, increasing the diameters to be accommodated in the pelvis.

Mentoanterior positions

With good uterine contractions, descent and rotation of the head occurs (see above) and labour progresses to a spontaneous delivery.

Mentoposterior positions

If the head is completely extended, so that the mentum reaches the pelvic floor first, and the contractions are effective, the mentum will rotate forwards and the position becomes anterior.

Persistent mentoposterior position

In this case the head is incompletely extended and the sinciput reaches the pelvic floor first and rotates forwards 1/8 of a circle which brings the chin into the hollow of the sacrum (Fig. 27.28). There is no further mechanism. The face becomes impacted because in order to descend further, both head and chest would have to be accommodated in the pelvis. Whatever emerges anteriorly from the vagina must pivot around the subpubic arch; if the chin is posterior this is impossible because the head can extend no further.

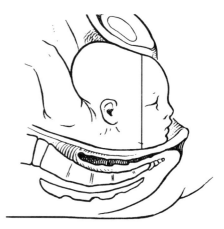

Fig. 27.28 Persistent mentoposterior position.

Reversal of face presentation

A face presentation in a persistent mentoposterior position may, in some cases, be manipulated to an occipitoanterior position using bimanual pressure (Gimovsky & Hennigan 1995, Neuman et al 1994). This method was developed to reduce the likelihood of an operative delivery for those women who refused caesarean section. Using a ritodrine bolus to relax the uterus, the fetal head is disengaged using upward transvaginal pressure. The fetal head is then flexed with bimanual pressure under ultrasound guidance to achieve an occipitoanterior position.

Management of labour

First stage

When she diagnoses a face presentation, the midwife should inform the doctor of this deviation from the normal. Routine observations of maternal and fetal conditions are made as in normal labour (see Ch. 22). A fetal scalp electrode must not be applied, and care should be taken not to infect or injure the eyes during vaginal examinations.

Immediately following rupture of the membranes, a vaginal examination should be performed to exclude cord prolapse as such an occurrence is more likely because the face is an ill-fitting presenting part. Descent of the head should be observed abdominally, and a vaginal examination performed every 2–4 hours to assess cervical dilatation and descent of the head.

In mentoposterior positions the midwife should note whether the mentum is lower than the sinciput, since rotation and descent depend on this. If the head remains high in spite of good contractions, caesarean section is likely. The woman may be prescribed oral ranitidine, 150 mg 6-hourly throughout labour, if it is considered that an anaesthetic may be necessary.

Delivery (Fig. 27.29)

When the face appears at the vulva, extension must be maintained by holding back the sinciput and permitting the mentum to escape under the symphysis pubis before the occiput is allowed to sweep the perineum. In this way the submentovertical diameter (11.5 cm) distends the vaginal

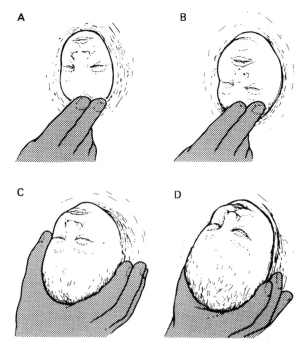

Fig. 27.29 Delivery of face presentation. (A) Sinciput held back to increase extension until the chin is born. (B) Chin is born. (C) Flexing the head to bring the occiput over the perineum. (D) Flexion completed. The head is born.

orifice instead of the mentovertical diameter (13.5 cm). Because the perineum is also distended by the biparietal diameter (9.5 cm), an elective episiotomy may be performed to avoid extensive perineal lacerations.

If the head does not descend in the second stage, the doctor should be informed. In a mentoanterior position it may be possible for him to deliver the baby with forceps; when rotation is incomplete, or the position remains mentoposterior, a rotational forceps delivery may be feasible. If the head has become impacted, or there is any suspicion of disproportion, a caesarean section will be necessary.

Complications

Obstructed labour (see Ch. 29)

Because the face, unlike the vertex, does not mould, a minor degree of pelvic contraction may result in obstructed labour. In a persistent mentoposterior position the face becomes impacted and caesarean section is necessary.

Cord prolapse (see Ch. 29)

A prolapsed cord is more common when the membranes rupture because the face is an ill-fitting presenting part. The midwife should always perform a vaginal examination when the membranes rupture in order to detect such an occurrence.

Facial bruising

The baby's face is always bruised and swollen at birth with oedematous eyelids and lips. The head is elongated (Fig. 27.30) and the baby will initially lie with his head extended. The midwife should warn the parents in advance of the baby's 'battered' appearance, reassuring them that this is only temporary; the oedema will disappear within 1 or 2 days, and the bruising will usually resolve within a week.

Cerebral haemorrhage

The lack of moulding of the facial bones can lead to intracranial haemorrhage caused by excessive compression of the fetal skull or by rearward compression in the typical moulding of the fetal skull found in this presentation (see Fig. 27.30).

Maternal trauma

Extensive perineal lacerations may occur at delivery due to the large submentovertical and biparietal diameters distending the vagina and perineum. There is an increased incidence of operative delivery, either forceps delivery or caesarean section, both of which increase maternal morbidity.

BROW PRESENTATION

In the brow presentation the fetal head is partially extended with the frontal bone, which is bounded by the anterior fontanelle and the orbital ridges, lying at the pelvic brim (Fig. 27.31). The presenting diameter is the mentovertical (13.5 cm; Fig. 27.32), which exceeds all diameters in an average-size pelvis. This presentation is rare, with an incidence of approximately 1 in 1000 deliveries.

Causes

These are the same as for a secondary face presentation (see above); during the process of extension from a vertex presentation to a face presentation,

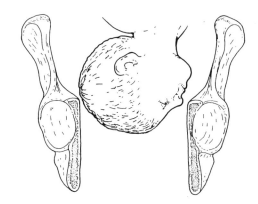

Fig. 27.31 Brow presentation.

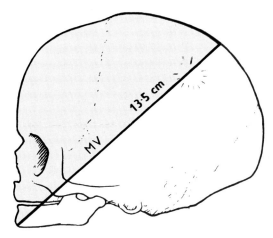

Fig. 27.32 Brow presentation. Mentovertical (MV) diameter, 13.5 cm, lies at the pelvic brim.

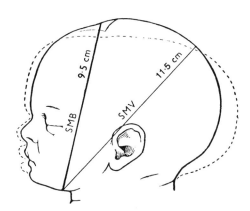

Fig. 27.30 Moulding in a face presentation (dotted line). SMB = submentobregmatic; SMV = submentovertical.

the brow will present temporarily and in a few cases this will persist.

Diagnosis

Brow presentation is not usually detected before the onset of labour.

On abdominal palpation. The head is high, appears unduly large and does not descend into the pelvis despite good uterine contractions.

On vaginal examination. The presenting part is high and may be difficult to reach. The anterior fontanelle may be felt on one side of the pelvis and the orbital ridges, and possibly the root of the nose, at the other (Fig. 27.33). A large caput succedaneum may mask these landmarks if the woman has been in labour for some hours.

Management

The doctor must be informed immediately this presentation is suspected. Vaginal delivery is extremely rare and obstructed labour usually results. It is possible that a woman with a large pelvis and a small baby may deliver vaginally. When the brow reaches the pelvic floor the maxilla rotates forwards and the head is born by a mechanism somewhat similar to that of a persistent occipitoposterior position. The midwife should never expect such a favourable outcome. The mother should be warned about the

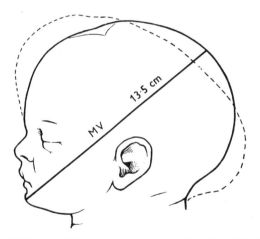

Fig. 27.33 Moulding in a brow presentation (dotted line). MV = mentovertical.

possible course of labour and that a vaginal delivery is unlikely.

If there is no fetal distress, the doctor may allow labour to continue for a short while in case further extension of the head converts the brow presentation to a face presentation. Occasionally spontaneous flexion may occur, resulting in a vertex presentation. If the head fails to descend and the brow presentation persists, a caesarean section is performed, with maternal consent.

Complications

These are the same as in a face presentation, except that obstructed labour requiring caesarean section is the probable rather than a possible outcome.

BREECH PRESENTATION

The fetus lies longitudinally with the buttocks in the lower pole of the uterus. The presenting diameter is the bitrochanteric (10 cm) and the denominator the sacrum. This presentation occurs in approximately 3% of pregnancies at term. In midtrimester the frequency is much higher because the greater proportion of amniotic fluid facilitates free movement of the fetus.

Types of breech presentation and position

There are six positions for a breech presentation, illustrated in Figures 27.34–27.39.

Breech with extended legs (frank breech)
(Fig. 27.40)
The breech presents with the hips flexed and legs extended on the abdomen. 70% of breech presentations are of this type and it is particularly common in primigravidae whose good uterine muscle tone inhibits flexion of the legs and free turning of the fetus.

Complete breech (Fig. 27.41)
The fetal attitude is one of complete flexion, hips and knees both flexed and the feet tucked in beside the buttocks.

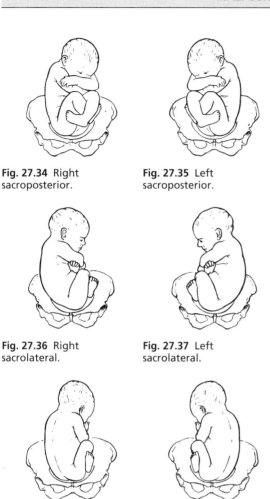

Fig. 27.34 Right sacroposterior.

Fig. 27.35 Left sacroposterior.

Fig. 27.36 Right sacrolateral.

Fig. 27.37 Left sacrolateral.

Fig. 27.38 Right sacroanterior.

Fig. 27.39 Left sacroanterior.

Figs 27.34–27.39 Six positions in breech presentation.

Footling breech (Fig. 27.42)

This is rare. One or both feet present because neither hips nor knees are fully flexed. The feet are lower than the buttocks, which distinguishes it from the complete breech.

Knee presentation (Fig. 27.43)

This is very rare. One or both hips are extended, with the knees flexed.

Causes

Often no cause is identified but the following circumstances favour breech presentation.

Extended legs

Spontaneous cephalic version may be inhibited if the fetus lies with the legs extended, 'splinting' the back.

Preterm labour

As breech presentation is relatively common before 34 weeks' gestation, it follows that breech presentation is more common in preterm labours.

Multiple pregnancy

Multiple pregnancy limits the space available for each fetus to turn, which may result in one or more fetuses presenting by the breech.

Polyhydramnios

Distension of the uterine cavity by excessive amounts of amniotic fluid may cause the fetus to present by the breech.

Hydrocephaly

The increased size of the fetal head is more readily accommodated in the fundus.

Uterine abnormalities

Distortion of the uterine cavity by a septum or a fibroid may result in a breech presentation.

Placenta praevia

Some authorities believe that this may be a cause of breech presentation but there is some disagreement on this.

Antenatal diagnosis

Abdominal examination

Palpation.   In primigravidae, diagnosis is more difficult because of their firm abdominal muscles. On palpation the lie is longitudinal with a soft presentation which is more easily felt using Pawlik's grip. The head can usually be felt in the fundus as a round hard mass which may be made to move independently of the back by ballotting it with one or both hands. If the legs are extended, the feet may prevent such nodding. When the breech is anterior and the fetus well flexed, it may be

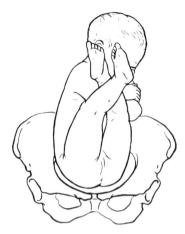

Fig. 27.40 Frank breech.

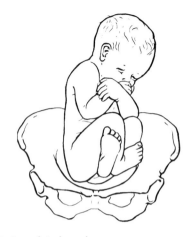

Fig. 27.41 Complete breech.

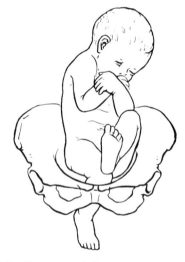

Fig. 27.42 Footling presentation.

Figs 27.40–27.43 Types of breech presentation.

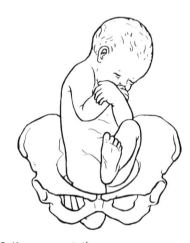

Fig. 27.43 Knee presentation.

difficult to locate the head but use of the combined grip in which the upper and lower poles are grasped simultaneously may aid diagnosis. The woman may complain of discomfort under her ribs, especially at night, due to pressure of the head on the diaphragm.

Auscultation. When the breech has not passed through the pelvic brim the fetal heart is heard most clearly above the umbilicus. When the legs are extended the breech descends into the pelvis easily. The fetal heart is then heard at a lower level.

Ultrasound examination

This may be used to demonstrate a breech presentation.

X-ray examination

Although largely superseded by ultrasound, X-ray has the added advantage of allowing pelvimetry to be performed at the same time.

Diagnosis during labour

A previously unsuspected breech presentation may

not be diagnosed until the woman is in established labour. If the legs are extended, the breech may feel like a head abdominally and also on vaginal examination if the cervix is less than 3 cm dilated and the breech is high.

Abdominal examination

Breech presentation may be diagnosed on admission in labour.

Vaginal examination

The breech feels soft and irregular with no sutures palpable, although occasionally the sacrum may be mistaken for a hard head and the buttocks mistaken for caput succedaneum. The anus may be felt and fresh meconium on the examining finger is usually diagnostic. If the legs are extended (Fig. 27.44) the external genitalia are very evident but it must be remembered that these become oedematous. An oedematous vulva may be mistaken for a scrotum.

If a foot is felt (Fig. 27.45), the midwife should differentiate it from the hand. Toes are all the same length, they are shorter than fingers and the big toe cannot be opposed to other toes. The foot is at right angles to the leg, and the heel has no equivalent in the hand.

Presentation may be confirmed by ultrasound scan or X-ray.

Antenatal management

If the midwife suspects or detects a breech presentation at 36 weeks' gestation or later, she should refer the woman to a doctor. The presentation may be confirmed by ultrasound scan or occasionally

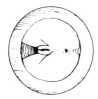 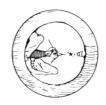

Fig. 27.44 No feet felt. Legs extended.

Fig. 27.45 Feet felt. Complete breech presentation.

Figs 27.44 & 27.45 Vaginal touch pictures of left sacrolateral position.

by abdominal X-ray. There are differing opinions amongst obstetricians as to the management of breech presentation during pregnancy and a decision on management is usually deferred until near term.

External cephalic version

External cephalic version (ECV) is the use of external manipulation on the mother's abdomen to convert a breech to a cephalic presentation. The Royal College of Obstetricians and Gynaecologists (1993) recommend that ECV should be offered at term by a practitioner skilled and experienced in the procedure. The success of the procedure not only depends upon the skill and experience of the operator, but also the position and engagement of the fetus, liquor volume and maternal parity (Hofmeyr 1997).

It has been demonstrated that ECV can reduce the number of babies presenting by the breech at term by two-thirds and therefore reduce the caesarean section rate for breech presentations (Hofmeyr 1997).

Turning the fetus from a breech to a cephalic presentation before 37 weeks' gestation does not reduce the incidence of breech birth or rate of caesarean section as it is likely to turn itself back spontaneously (Zhang et al 1993).

The reasons for attempting ECV and the procedure itself should be explained to the woman so that she can give her informed consent to have ECV performed.

Method. An ultrasound scan is performed to localise the placenta and to confirm the position and presentation of the fetus.

If the procedure is to be performed under tocolysis then a cannula will be sited to allow venous access. A 30-minute CTG is performed to establish that the fetus is not distressed at the start of the procedure and maternal blood pressure and pulse are recorded.

The woman is asked to empty her bladder. The midwife then assists the woman into a comfortable supine position. The foot of the bed may be elevated to help free the breech from the pelvic brim. The abdomen is usually dusted with talcum powder to prevent pinching of the mother's skin during the procedure. Whilst ECV may be uncomfortable for the mother it should not be painful. The breech is displaced from the pelvic brim towards an iliac fossa. Simultaneous force is then used as with one hand on each pole the operator makes the fetus perform a forward somersault (Figs 27.46–27.48). If this is not successful then a backward somersault can be attempted.

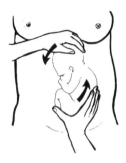

Fig. 27.46 Right hand lifts breech out of pelvis. Left hand makes head follow nose. Flexion of head and back maintained throughout.

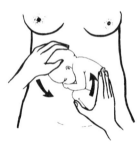

Fig. 27.47 Flexion is continued. Left hand brings head downwards. Right hand pushes breech upwards.

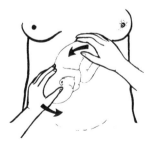

Fig. 27.48 Pressure is exerted on head and breech simultaneously until head is lying at the pelvic brim.

Figs 27.46–27.48 External cephalic version.

If the fetus does not turn easily, then the procedure is abandoned but may be tried again in a few days.

The fetal heart should be auscultated after the procedure, or a CTG performed.

If the woman is Rhesus negative an injection of anti-D immunoglobulin is given as prophylaxis against iso-immunisation caused by any placental separation. If the version is performed immediately prior to the onset of labour, this can be delayed until after delivery when the blood group of the baby is known. In this case if anti-D is needed, it must be given within 72 hours of the version.

Complications:

Knotting of the umbilical cord should be suspected if bradycardia occurs and persists. The fetus is immediately turned back to a breech presentation. The woman is admitted for observation and, if necessary, caesarean section.

Separation of the placenta. The midwife should ask the woman to report pain or vaginal bleeding during and after the procedure.

Rupture of the membranes. If this occurs the cord may prolapse because neither the head nor the breech is engaged.

Relative contraindications. The presence of a uterine scar was previously thought to be an absolute contraindication to performing an ECV. Recent evidence suggests that it is a safe and effective procedure used selectively in those women who have previously had a caesarean section (Flamm et al 1991, Shalev et al 1993).

Contraindications:

- *Pre-eclampsia or hypertension* because of the increased risk of placental abruption.
- *Multiple pregnancy.*
- *Oligohydramnios* because too much force has to be applied directly to the fetus and the version is likely to be unsuccessful.
- *Ruptured membranes.*
- *A hydrocephalic fetus.* If a vaginal delivery is contemplated in preference to a caesarean section, the second stage is managed more easily when the fetus presents by the breech.

- Any condition which would require delivery by caesarean section.

Persistent breech presentation

When external version has been unsuccessful or has not been attempted, a decision should be made before the onset of labour as to whether to perform an elective caesarean section or to attempt a vaginal delivery.

Assessment for vaginal delivery. Any doubt as to the capacity of the pelvis to accommodate the fetal head must be resolved before the buttocks are delivered and the head attempts to enter the pelvic brim. At this point the fetus begins to be deprived of oxygen and a last-minute decision to perform caesarean section may be too late.

Fetal size, especially in relation to maternal size, can be assessed on abdominal palpation but is more accurately judged in association with an ultrasound examination.

Pelvic capacity can be judged on vaginal assessment (see Ch. 13), but it is usual to perform a lateral pelvimetry. This will show the shape of the sacrum and give accurate measurements of the anteroposterior diameters of the pelvic brim, cavity and outlet. No studies have confirmed the value of this procedure in selecting women who are likely to succeed in achieving a vaginal delivery of a breech or in improving perinatal outcome (Hannah 1994). In a multigravida, information about the type of delivery and the size of previous babies when compared with the size of the present fetus can be helpful.

Mechanism of left sacroanterior position

- The lie is longitudinal.
- The attitude is one of complete flexion.
- The presentation is breech.
- The position is left sacroanterior.
- The denominator is the sacrum.
- The presenting part is the anterior (left) buttock.
- The bitrochanteric diameter, 10 cm, enters the pelvis in the left oblique diameter of the brim.

- The sacrum points to the left iliopectineal eminence.

Compaction. Descent takes place with increasing compaction, owing to increased flexion of the limbs.

Internal rotation of the buttocks. The anterior buttock reaches the pelvic floor first and rotates forwards 1/8 of a circle along the right side of the pelvis to lie underneath the symphysis pubis. The bitrochanteric diameter is now in the antero-posterior diameter of the outlet.

Lateral flexion of the body. The anterior buttock escapes under the symphysis pubis, the posterior buttock sweeps the perineum and the buttocks are born by a movement of lateral flexion.

Restitution of the buttocks. The anterior buttock turns slightly to the mother's right side.

Internal rotation of the shoulders. The shoulders enter the pelvis in the same oblique diameter as the buttocks, the left oblique. The anterior shoulder rotates forwards 1/8 of a circle along the right side of the pelvis and escapes under the symphysis pubis, the posterior shoulder sweeps the perineum and the shoulders are born.

Internal rotation of the head. The head enters the pelvis with the sagittal suture in the transverse diameter of the brim. The occiput rotates forwards along the left side and the suboccipital region (the nape of the neck) impinges on the undersurface of the symphysis pubis.

External rotation of the body. At the same time the body turns so that the back is uppermost.

Birth of the head. The chin, face and sinciput sweep the perineum and the head is born in a flexed attitude.

Management of labour

Vaginal delivery should be presented to the woman as the norm for breech delivery (MIDIRS 1997) but it should be made clear that there is a risk of delivery by caesarean section.

In a retrospective study of breech births the outcome for breech presentation diagnosed in labour has been shown to be as good, in all respects, as for those who were selected as suitable for a vaginal birth.

If vaginal delivery is selected with a breech presentation there is approximately a 50% chance of a successful vaginal delivery (Hofmeyr 1989).

The choice of place of confinement is ultimately the mother's decision. With a high risk of delivery by caesarean section she may choose to deliver in a consultant unit.

First stage

Basic care during this stage is the same as in normal labour (see Ch. 22). Although the breech with extended legs fits the cervix quite well, the complete breech is a less well-fitting presenting part and the membranes tend to rupture early. For this reason there is an increased risk of cord prolapse, and a vaginal examination is performed to exclude this as soon as the membranes rupture. If they do not rupture spontaneously at an early stage, it is considered safer to leave them intact until labour is well established and the breech at the level of the ischial spines. Meconium-stained liquor is sometimes found due to compression of the fetal abdomen and is not always a sign of fetal distress.

Analgesia. (See Ch. 23 for analgesia and Ch. 22 for support in labour.) An epidural block may be offered to a woman with a breech presentation as it inhibits the urge to push prematurely. There is no evidence to suggest that this is indicated. Epidural analgesia has been associated with prolongation of the second stage of labour and has not been associated with any unique advantages for a woman delivering a breech at term (Chadha et al 1992) (see also Ch. 28).

Second stage

Full dilatation of the cervix should always be confirmed by vaginal examination before the woman commences active pushing. This is because in a footling presentation a foot may appear at the vulva when the cervix is only partially dilated; or when the legs are extended, particularly if the fetus is small, the breech may slip through an incompletely dilated cervix. In either case, the head may be trapped by the cervix when the fetus is partially delivered.

If the delivery is taking place in hospital it is usual to inform the obstetrician of the onset of the second stage; a paediatrician should be present for delivery and it is usual to inform the anaesthetist in case a general anaesthetic is required. Active pushing is not commenced until the buttocks are distending the vulva. Failure of the breech to descend onto the perineum in the second stage despite good contractions may indicate a need for caesarean section.

Types of delivery

Spontaneous breech delivery. The delivery occurs with little assistance from the attendant.

Assisted breech delivery. The buttocks are born spontaneously, but some assistance is necessary for delivery of extended legs or arms and the head.

Breech extraction. This is a manipulative delivery carried out usually by an obstetrician and is performed to hasten delivery in an emergency situation such as fetal distress.

Management of delivery. The midwife should discuss this with the woman beforehand so that she understands the need for the attendance of the doctors. The delivery is explained in order to help her to appreciate the importance of not pushing until full dilatation of the cervix has been confirmed.

When the buttocks are distending the perineum, the woman is placed in the lithotomy position (unless an upright position is chosen – see below) and the vulva is swabbed and draped with sterile towels. The bladder must be empty and it is usually catheterised at this stage. If epidural analgesia is not being used, the perineum is infiltrated with up to 10 ml of 0.5% plain lignocaine prior to an episiotomy being performed. (Pudendal block is sometimes used by a doctor.)

The woman is encouraged to push with the contractions and the buttocks are delivered spontaneously. If the legs are flexed, the feet disengage at the vulva and the baby is born as far as the umbilicus. A loop of cord is gently pulled down to avoid traction on the umbilicus. Spasm of the cord vessels can be caused by manipulating the cord or by stretching it. If the cord is being nipped behind the pubic bone it should be moved to one side. The midwife should feel for the elbows which are usually on the chest. If so, the arms will escape with the next contraction. If the arms are not felt, they are extended (see below).

Delivery of the shoulders. The uterine contractions and the weight of the body will bring the shoulders down onto the pelvic floor where they will rotate into the anteroposterior diameter of the outlet.

It is helpful to wrap a small towel around the baby's hips, which preserves warmth and improves the grip on the slippery skin. The midwife now grasps the baby by the iliac crests with her thumbs held parallel over his sacrum and tilts the baby towards the maternal sacrum in order to free the anterior shoulder.

When the anterior shoulder has escaped, the buttocks are lifted towards the mother's abdomen to enable the posterior shoulder and arm to pass over the perineum (Fig. 27.49). As the shoulders are born the head enters the pelvic brim and descends through the pelvis with the sagittal suture in the transverse diameter. The back must remain lateral until this has happened but will afterwards be turned uppermost. If the back is turned upwards too soon, the anteroposterior diameter of the head will enter the anteroposterior diameter of the brim and may become extended. The shoulders may then become impacted at the outlet and the extended head may cause difficulty.

Delivery of the head. When the back has been turned the infant is allowed to hang from the vulva without support. His weight brings the head onto the pelvic floor on which the occiput rotates forwards. The sagittal suture is now in the anteroposterior diameter of the outlet. If rotation of the head fails to take place, two fingers should be placed on the malar bones and the head rotated. The baby can be allowed to hang for 1 or 2 minutes. Gradually the neck elongates, the hairline appears and the sub-occipital region can be felt. Controlled delivery of the head is vital to avoid any sudden change in intracranial pressure and subsequent cerebral haemorrhage. There are three methods used.

Forceps delivery. Most breech deliveries are performed by an obstetrician, who will apply forceps to the after-coming head to achieve a controlled delivery.

Burns Marshall method. The midwife or doctor stands facing away from the mother and, with the left hand, grasps the baby's ankles from behind with forefinger between the two (Fig. 27.50). The baby is kept on the stretch with sufficient traction to prevent his neck from bending backwards and being fractured. The suboccipital region, and not the neck, should pivot under the apex of the pubic arch or the spinal cord may be crushed. The feet are taken up through an arc of 180° until the mouth and nose are free at the vulva. The right hand may guard the perineum in order to prevent sudden escape of the head. An assistant may now clear the airway and the baby will breathe. The mother should be asked to take deliberate, regular breaths which allow the vault of the skull to escape gradually, taking 2 or 3 minutes.

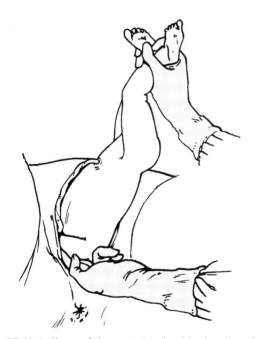

Fig. 27.49 Delivery of the posterior shoulder in a breech presentation.

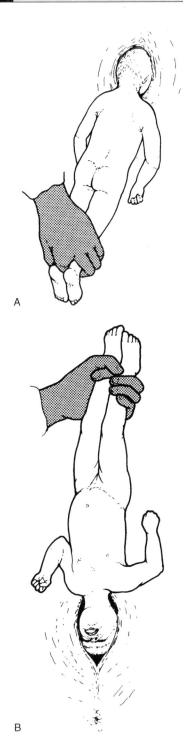

A

B

Fig. 27.50 Burns Marshall method of delivering the after-coming head of a breech presentation. (A) Baby grasped by the feet and held on the stretch. (B) Mouth and nose are free. Vault of the head is delivered slowly.

Mauriceau–Smellie–Veit manoeuvre (jaw flexion and shoulder traction; Fig. 27.51). This is mainly used when there is delay in descent of the head because of extension. Excessive shoulder traction may cause Erb's palsy.

The baby is laid astride the right arm with the palm supporting the chest. Two fingers are inserted well back into the mouth to pull the jaw downwards and flex the head. (If they can be accommodated, two fingers may be placed on the malar bones with the middle finger in the mouth.) Two fingers of the left hand are hooked over the shoulders with the middle finger pushing up the occiput to aid flexion. Traction is applied to draw the head out of the vagina and, when the suboccipital region appears, the body is lifted to assist the head to pivot around the symphysis pubis. The speed of delivery of the head must be controlled so that it does not emerge suddenly like a cork popping out of a bottle. Once the face is free, the airways may be cleared and the vault is delivered slowly.

Alternative positions. When the woman has chosen to deliver in an alternative position, it is the upright or supported squat which is the most suitable. The delivery techniques described above will be adapted accordingly and the midwife will observe and encourage the spontaneous mechanism of delivery.

Use of oxytocics for third stage. These are withheld until the head is delivered.

Delivery of extended legs. The frank breech descends more rapidly during the first stage of labour. The cervix dilates more quickly and there is a risk of the cord becoming compressed between the legs and the body. Cord prolapse is less likely than in other breech presentations because the frank breech is a better-fitting presenting part. Delay may occur at the outlet because the legs splint the body and impede lateral flexion of the spine.

The baby can be born with his legs extended but assistance is usually required. When the popliteal fossae appear at the vulva, two fingers are placed along the length of one thigh with the fingertips in the fossa. The leg is swept to the side of the abdomen (abducting the hip) and the knee is flexed by

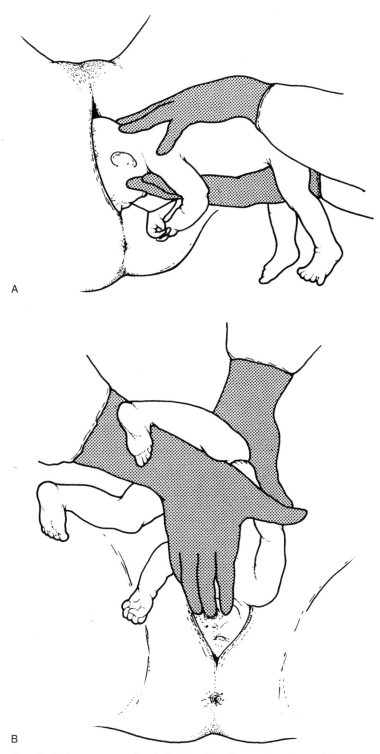

A

B

Fig. 27.51 Mauriceau–Smellie–Veit manoeuvre for delivering the after-coming head of breech presentation (see text). (A) Hands in position before the body is lifted. (B) Extraction of the head.

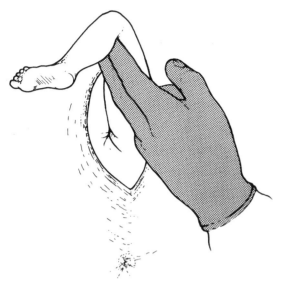

Fig. 27.52 Assisting delivery of extended leg by pressure on popliteal fossa.

the pressure on its under surface. As this movement is continued the lower part of the leg will emerge from the vagina (Fig. 27.52). This process should be repeated in order to deliver the second leg. The knee is a hinge joint which bends in one direction only. If the knee is pulled forwards from the abdomen, severe injury to the joint can result.

Delivery of extended arms. Extended arms are diagnosed when the elbows are not felt on the chest after the umbilicus is born. Prompt action must be taken to avoid delay and consequent hypoxia. This may be dealt with by using the Løvset manoeuvre (Figs 27.53 and 27.54). This is a com-

bination of rotation and downward traction which may be employed to deliver the arms whatever position they are in. The direction of rotation must always bring the back uppermost and the arms are delivered from under the pubic arch.

When the umbilicus is born and the shoulders are in the anteroposterior diameter, the baby is grasped by the iliac crests with the thumbs over the sacrum. Downward traction is applied until the axilla is visible.

Maintaining downward traction throughout, the body is rotated through half a circle, 180°, starting by turning the back uppermost. The friction of the posterior arm against the pubic bone as the shoulder becomes anterior sweeps the arm in front of the face. The movement allows the shoulders to enter the pelvis in the transverse diameter.

The arm which is now anterior is delivered. The first two fingers of the hand which is on the same side as the baby's back are used to splint the humerus and draw it down over the chest as the elbow is flexed.

The body is now rotated back in the opposite direction and the second arm delivered in a similar fashion.

Delay in delivery of the head:

Extended head. If, when the body has been allowed to hang, the neck and hair-line are not visible, it is probable that the head is extended. This may be dealt with by the use of forceps or the Mauriceau–Smellie–Veit manoeuvre. If the head is trapped in an incompletely dilated cervix, an air channel can be created to enable the baby to breathe pending intervention. This is done by inserting two fingers or a Sim's speculum in front of the baby's face and holding the vaginal wall away from the nose. Moisture is mopped away and the airways are cleared. Attempts to release the head from the cervix result in high fetal morbidity and mortality. The McRoberts manoeuvre has been suggested as a method to facilitate the release of the fetal head (Shushan & Younis 1992). The McRoberts manoeuvre requires the woman to lie flat on her back and bring her knees up to her abdomen with hips abducted. This manoeuvre, more commonly used to relieve shoulder dystocia, is described in detail in Chapter 29.

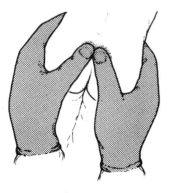

Fig. 27.53 Correct grasp for Løvset manoeuvre.

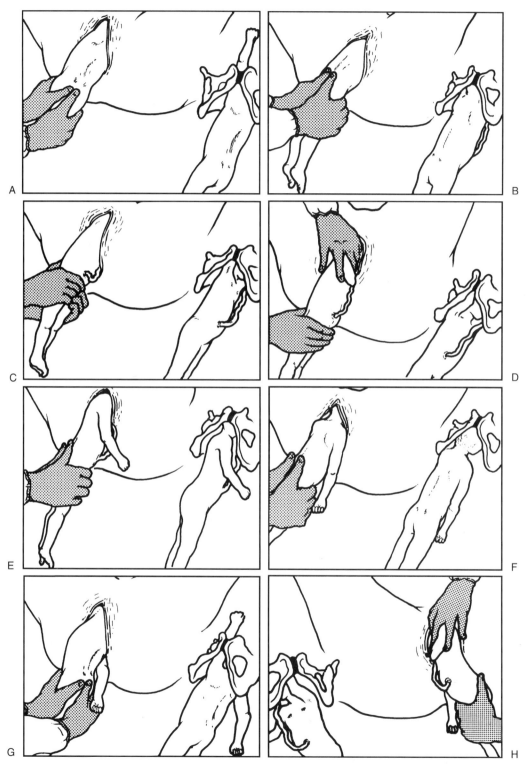

Fig. 27.54 Løvset manoeuvre for delivery of extended arms (see text).

Posterior rotation of the occiput. This mal-rotation of the head is rare and is usually the result of mismanagement, for the back should be turned upwards after the shoulders are born.

To deliver the head with the occiput posterior, the chin and face are permitted to escape under the symphysis pubis as far as the root of the nose and the baby is then lifted up towards the mother's abdomen to allow the occiput to sweep the perineum.

Complications of breech presentation

Apart from those difficulties already mentioned, other complications can arise, most of which affect the fetus. Many of these can be avoided by allowing only an experienced operator, or a closely supervised learner, to deliver the baby.

Impacted breech
Labour becomes obstructed when the fetus is disproportionately large for the size of the maternal pelvis.

Cord prolapse (see Ch. 29)
This is more common in a flexed or footling breech, as these have ill-fitting presenting parts.

Birth injury

Superficial tissue damage. The midwife must warn the mother and her partner of the bruising that may be expected following delivery. Oedema and bruising of the baby's genitalia may be caused by pressure on the cervix. In a footling breech a prolapsed foot which lies in the vagina or at the vulva for a long time may become very oedematous and discoloured.

If the delivery is performed correctly the following are less likely to occur:

Fractures of humerus, clavicle or femur or dislocation of shoulder or hip caused during delivery of extended arms or legs.

Erb's palsy caused by the brachial plexus being damaged by twisting the neck.

Trauma to internal organs especially a ruptured liver or spleen produced by grasping the abdomen.

Damage to the adrenals by grasping the baby's abdomen, leading to shock caused by adrenaline release.

Spinal cord damage or fracture of the spine caused by bending the body backwards over the symphysis pubis while delivering the head.

Intracranial haemorrhage caused by rapid delivery of the head which has had no opportunity to mould. *Hypoxia* may also cause intracranial haemorrhage.

Fetal hypoxia
This may be due to cord prolapse or cord compression or to premature separation of the placenta.

Premature separation of the placenta
Considerable retraction of the uterus takes place while the head is still in the vagina and the placenta begins to separate. Excessive delay in delivery of the head may cause severe hypoxia in the fetus.

Maternal trauma
The maternal complications of a breech delivery are the same as found in other operative vaginal deliveries (see Ch. 29).

SHOULDER PRESENTATION

When the fetus lies with its long axis across the long axis of the uterus (transverse lie) the shoulder is most likely to present. Occasionally the lie is oblique but this does not persist as the uterine contractions during labour make it longitudinal or transverse.

Shoulder presentation occurs in approximately 1 : 300 pregnancies near term. Only 17% of these cases remain as a transverse lie at the onset of labour; the majority are multigravidae (Gimovsky & Hennigan 1995). The head lies on one side of the abdomen, with the breech at a slightly higher level on the other. The fetal back may be anterior or posterior (see Figs 27.55 and 27.56).

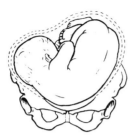

Fig. 27.55 Shoulder presentation, dorsoanterior.

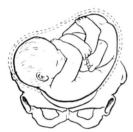

Fig. 27.56 Shoulder presentation, dorsoposterior.

Causes

Maternal

Before term, transverse or oblique lie may be transitory, related to maternal position or displacement of the presenting part by an overextended bladder prior to ultrasound examination (Hofmeyr 1989). Other causes are described below.

Lax abdominal and uterine muscles. This is the most common cause and is found in multigravidae, particularly those of high parity.

Uterine abnormality. A bicornuate or subseptate uterus may result in a transverse lie as, more rarely, may a cervical or low uterine fibroid (see Ch. 15).

Contracted pelvis. Rarely, this may prevent the head from entering the pelvic brim.

Fetal

Preterm pregnancy. The amount of amniotic fluid in relation to the fetus is greater, allowing the fetus more mobility than at term.

Multiple pregnancy. There is a possibility of polyhydramnios but the presence of more than one fetus reduces the room for manoeuvre when amounts of liquor are normal. It is the second twin which more commonly adopts this lie after delivery of the first fetus.

Polyhydramnios. The distended uterus is globular and the fetus can move freely in the excessive liquor.

Macerated fetus. Lack of muscle tone causes the fetus to slump down into the lower pole of the uterus.

Placenta praevia. This may prevent the head from entering the pelvic brim.

Diagnosis

Antenatal

On abdominal palpation. The uterus appears broad and the fundal height is less than expected for the period of gestation. On pelvic and fundal palpation, neither head nor breech is felt. The mobile head is found on one side of the abdomen and the breech at a slightly higher level on the other.

Ultrasound may be used to confirm the lie and presentation.

Intrapartum

On abdominal palpation the findings are as above but when the membranes have ruptured the irregular outline of the uterus is more marked. If the uterus is contracting strongly and becomes moulded around the fetus, palpation is very difficult. The pelvis is no longer empty, the shoulder being wedged into it.

On vaginal examination. *This should not be performed without first excluding placenta praevia.* In early labour the presenting part may not be felt. The membranes usually rupture early because of the ill-fitting presenting part with a high risk of cord prolapse.

If the labour has been in progress for some time

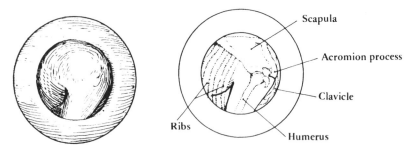

Fig. 27.57 Vaginal touch picture of shoulder presentation.

the shoulder may be felt as a soft irregular mass. It is sometimes possible to palpate the ribs, their characteristic grid-iron pattern being diagnostic (Fig. 27.57). When the shoulder enters the pelvic brim an arm may prolapse; this should be differentiated from a leg. The hand is not at right angles to the arm, the fingers are longer than toes and of unequal length and the thumb can be opposed. No os calcis can be felt and the palm is shorter than the sole. If the arm is flexed, an elbow feels sharper than a knee.

Possible outcome
There is no mechanism for delivery of a shoulder presentation. If this persists in labour, delivery must be by caesarean section to avoid obstructed labour and subsequent uterine rupture (see Ch. 29).

Whenever the midwife detects a transverse lie she must obtain medical assistance.

Management

Antenatal
A cause must be sought before deciding on a course of management. Ultrasound examination can detect placenta praevia or uterine abnormalities, whilst X-ray pelvimetry will demonstrate a contracted pelvis (see Ch. 49). Any of these causes requires elective caesarean section. Once they have been excluded, external version (see above) may be attempted. If this fails, or if the lie is again transverse at the next antenatal visit, the woman is admitted to hospital while further investigations into the cause are made. She frequently remains

there until delivery because of the risk of cord prolapse if the membranes rupture.

Intrapartum
If a transverse lie is detected in early labour while the membranes are still intact, the doctor may attempt an external version followed, if this is successful, by a controlled rupture of the membranes. (This may be considered before labour in some cases (Hofmeyr 1997).) If the membranes have already ruptured spontaneously, a vaginal examination must be performed immediately to detect possible cord prolapse.

Immediate caesarean section must be performed:

- if the cord prolapses
- when the membranes are already ruptured
- when external version is unsuccessful
- when labour has already been in progress for some hours.

Complications

Prolapsed cord (see Ch. 29)
This may occur when the membranes rupture.

Prolapsed arm
This may occur when the membranes have ruptured and the shoulder has become impacted. Delivery should be by immediate caesarean section.

Neglected shoulder presentation
The shoulder becomes impacted, having been forced down and wedged into the pelvic brim. The membranes have ruptured spontaneously and if

the arm has prolapsed it becomes blue and oedematous. The uterus goes into a state of tonic contraction, the overstretched lower segment is tender to touch and the fetal heart may be absent. All the maternal signs of obstructed labour are present (see Ch. 26) and the outcome, if not treated in time, is a ruptured uterus and a stillbirth.

With adequate supervision both antenatally and during labour this should never occur.

Treatment. An immediate caesarean section is performed under general anaesthetic regardless of whether the fetus is alive or dead, as attempts at manipulative procedures or destructive operations can be dangerous for the mother and may result in uterine rupture.

UNSTABLE LIE

The lie is defined as unstable when after 36 weeks' gestation, instead of remaining longitudinal, it varies from one examination to another between longitudinal and oblique or transverse.

Causes

Any condition in late pregnancy that increases the mobility of the fetus or prevents the head from entering the pelvic brim may cause this.

Maternal causes:

- Lax uterine muscles in multigravidae
- Contracted pelvis.

Fetal causes:

- Polyhydramnios
- Placenta praevia.

Management

Antenatal

It may be advisable for the woman to be admitted to hospital to avoid unsupervised onset of labour with a transverse lie. An alternative is for the woman to admit herself to the labour ward as soon as labour commences. Risk associated with the possibility of rupture of membranes and cord prolapse should be emphasised if the mother chooses to remain at home.

Ultrasonography is used to rule out placenta praevia.

Attempts will be made to correct the abnormal presentation by external version. If unsuccessful, caesarean section is considered.

Intrapartum

Many obstetricians induce labour after 38 weeks' gestation, having first ensured that the lie is longitudinal. This may be performed by commencing an intravenous infusion of Syntocinon to stimulate contractions. A controlled rupture of the membranes is performed so that the head enters the pelvis.

The midwife should ensure that the woman has an empty rectum and bladder before the procedure, as a loaded rectum or full bladder can prevent the presenting part from entering the pelvis. She should palpate the abdomen at frequent intervals to ensure that the lie remains longitudinal and to assess the descent of the head. Labour is regarded as a trial (see Ch. 26).

Complications

If labour commences with the lie other than longitudinal, the complications are the same as for a transverse lie.

COMPOUND PRESENTATION

When a hand, or occasionally a foot, lies alongside the head, the presentation is said to be compound. This tends to occur with a small fetus or roomy pelvis and seldom is difficulty encountered except in cases where it is associated with a flat pelvis. On rare occasions, head, hand and foot are felt in the vagina, a serious situation which may occur with a dead fetus.

If diagnosed during the first stage of labour, medical aid must be sought. If, during the second stage, the midwife sees a hand presenting alongside the vertex, she could try to hold the hand back.

READER ACTIVITIES

1. Examine the heads of newborn babies who have been delivered with a large caput succedaneum and/or moulding. Practise defining the sutures and fontanelles you are feeling. Try the same exercise with your eyes closed.

2. Learn to differentiate by feel, with your eyes shut, a baby's hand from his foot, and his elbow from his knee.

3. Practise the different mechanisms and methods for breech delivery using a doll and pelvis.

4. Work with a colleague and try the position for the McRoberts manoeuvre.

5. Ascertain the ECV rate in your unit.

6. Evaluate the effectiveness of various methods of pain control that have been used by women in your care who have complained of backache during labour.

7. Compare the length of labour and the outcome for a primigravida with a fetus presenting as breech and one with a cephalic presentation. Repeat the exercise with two multiparous women.

REFERENCES

Biancuzzo M 1993 How to recognise and rotate an occiput posterior fetus. American Journal of Nursing 93(3): 38–41

Chadha Y C, Mahmood T A, Dick M J 1992 Breech delivery and epidural analgesia. British Journal of Obstetrics and Gynaecology 99(2): 96–100

El Halta V 1995 Posterior labour: a pain in the back. Midwifery Today 36: 19–21

Flamm B L, Fried M, Lonky N M, Giles W A 1991 External cephalic version after previous cesarean section. American Journal of Obstetrics and Gynecology 165(2): 370–372

Gimovsky M, Hennigan C 1995 Abnormal fetal presentations. Current Opinion in Obstetrics and Gynecology 7(6): 482–485

Hannah W J 1994 The Canadian consensus on breech management at term. Society of Obstetricians and Gynaecologists of Canada policy statement. Journal of the Society of Obstetricians and Gynaecologists of Canada 16(6): 1839–1848

Hofmeyr G J 1989 Breech presentation and abnormal lie in late pregnancy. In: Chalmers I, Enkin M W, Keirse M J N C (eds) Effective care in pregnancy and childbirth. Oxford University Press, Oxford, pp 653–665

Hofmeyr G J 1997 External cephalic version at term. In: Neilson J P, Crowther C A, Hodnett E D, Hofmeyr G J, Keirse M J N C (eds) Pregnancy and childbirth module of the Cochrane Database of Systematic Reviews (updated 05 December 1996). Available in the Cochrane Library (database on disk and CD-ROM). (Updated quarterly) The Cochrane Collaboration; Issue 1. Update Software, Oxford

MIDIRS 1997 Informed choice for professionals. Number 9 Breech Presentation – options for care. MIDIRS and The NHS Centre for Reviews and Dissemination, Bristol

Neuman M, Beller U, Lavie O 1994 Intrapartum bimanual tocolytic-assisted reversal of face presentation: preliminary report. Obstetrics and Gynecology 84(10): 146–148

Nicodem V C 1995 Upright vs recumbent position during first stage of labour. In Enkin M W, Keirse M J N C, Renfrew M J, Neilson J P (eds) Pregnancy and childbirth module of the Cochrane Database of Systematic Reviews, 1995 (updated 24 February 1995). Available from BMJ Publishing Group, London

Pearl M L, Roberts J M, Laros R K, Hurd W W 1993 Vaginal delivery from the persistent occiput posterior position. Influence on maternal and neonatal morbidity. Journal of Reproductive Medicine 38(12): 955–961

Royal College of Obstetricians and Gynaecologists 1993 Effective procedures in obstetrics suitable for audit. RCOG, Medical Audit Unit, Manchester, p 2

Shalev E, Battino S, Giladi Y 1993 External cephalic version at term using tocolysis. Acta Obstetrica et Gynecologica Scandinavica 72(6): 455–457

Shushan A, Younis J S 1992 McRoberts manoeuvre for the management of the aftercoming head in breech deliveries. Gynecology and Obstetric Investigations 34(3): 188–189

Sutton J 1996 Birth: medical emergency or engineering miracle? A midwifery approach to keeping birth normal. MIDIRS Digest 6(2): 170–173

Thornton J G, Lilford R J 1994 Active management of labour: current knowledge and research issues. British Medical Journal 309(6951): 366–369

Zhang J, Bowes W A, Fortney J A 1993 Efficacy of external cephalic version: a review. Obstetrics and Gynecology 82(2): 306–312

FURTHER READING

Ben-Arie A, Kogan S, Schachter M 1995 The impact of external cephalic version on the rate of vaginal and cesarean breech deliveries: a 3-year cumulative experience. European Journal of Obstetrics and Gynecology and Reproductive Biology 63(2): 125–129

Calhoun B C, Edgeworth D, Brehm W 1995 External cephalic version at a military teaching hospital: predictors of success. Australian and New Zealand Journal of Obstetrics and Gynaecology 35(3): 277–279

Gardberg M, Tuppurainen M 1994 Anterior placental location predisposes for occiput posterior presentation near term. Acta Obstetrica et Gynecologica Scandinavica 73(2): 151–152

Gifford D S, Keeler E, Kahn K L 1995 Reductions in cost and cesarean section rates by routine use of external cephalic version: a decision analysis. Obstetrics and Gynecology 85(6): 930–936

Megory E, Ohel G, Fisher O 1995 Mode of delivery following external cephalic version and induction of labour at term. American Journal of Perinatology 12(6): 404–406

Royal College of Obstetricians and Gynaecologists 1995 Caesarean for breech as a percentage of total number of babies delivered. In annual statistical return report taken from the 1993 statistics. RCOG, London, p 7

Teoh T 1996 Outcome of external cephalic version: our experience. Journal of Obstetrics and Gynaecology Research 22(4): 389–394

28

Obstetric anaesthesia and operations

Ruth Bevis

Complications may arise in any labour. The aim of this chapter is to give a concise, factual overview of anaesthetic and obstetric procedures, to help the midwife become a knowledgeable, competent member of the team in an emergency. For detailed information on the effects of anaesthetic and analgesic drugs on the fetus see Reynolds (1993).

The chapter:

- distinguishes between anaesthesia and analgesia
- discusses the problems and risks of general anaesthesia with particular emphasis on the prevention of problems
- describes regional techniques in obstetric anaesthesia
- describes the different types of operative delivery, explaining why each may be needed and the possible complications
- provides information as appropriate on the care and support of the mother.

OBSTETRIC ANAESTHESIA

Some definitions
It is important to distinguish between anaesthesia and analgesia. These terms are defined as follows:

Anaesthesia means absence of sensation and therefore implies freedom from pain.

Analgesia means freedom from pain.

Anaesthesia may be described under the headings of:

General anaesthesia when a state of unconsciousness is induced, but which may also involve giving some analgesia.

Regional anaesthesia when a group of nerves is anaesthetised, so giving an area of anaesthesia.

Local anaesthesia when a small specific area is anaesthetised.

Anaesthesia will now be discussed under these general headings.

GENERAL ANAESTHESIA IN OBSTETRICS

For more detailed information on the following topics the reader is referred to Moir & Thorburn (1986), Morgan (1987).

General anaesthesia for the woman in the second and third trimesters of pregnancy, or who is newly delivered, carries certain risks and is dangerous in unskilled hands. Factors connected with general anaesthesia have been a significant cause of maternal deaths in otherwise healthy women until very recently.

In the period 1991–1993 there were eight deaths associated directly with anaesthesia, and a further six in which anaesthetic factors contributed to the death (DH et al 1996). The reports on confidential enquiries into maternal deaths have repeatedly recommended more efficient consultant involvement in obstetric anaesthesia, but the report for 1991–1993 (DH et al 1996) recommends that the anaesthetist's assistant should be 'an appropriately trained operating department practitioner, operating department assistant or a specifically trained anaesthetic nurse'. The recommendations go on to define this as a nationally recognised qualification and not a local training. The midwife should not therefore be directly involved in assisting the anaesthetist, for example in performing cricoid pressure (see below), but it is essential for her to be aware of the risks involved and why they occur, so that she may give intelligent help as a part of the team if required.

Problems in obstetric anaesthesia

The problems which arise in obstetric anaesthesia are due to:

- the effects of progesterone on the mother
- the pressure from the gravid uterus
- the presence of two patients rather than one.

Mendelson's syndrome

The effect of progesterone on the gastrointestinal tract is commonly said to cause delayed emptying of the stomach at term, particularly in the woman in labour. Crawford (1987) states that during advanced labour there may be a 'modest reduction' in gastric emptying time, but that the evidence for this is weak. He had investigated a very small sample of 12 women in 1956 (Crawford 1956) and found normal gastric emptying in active labour in 10 of them. (His sample was too small for credibility, and his method would be unacceptable in the 1990s, since he passed nasogastric tubes on women in labour and aspirated the stomach contents.)

Narcotic analgesics such as pethidine given in labour cause significant delay in gastric emptying (Morgan 1987). Because the stomach contents are static, the pH is raised; fasting also causes stasis with similar results (Roberts & Shirley 1976). Some authorities therefore advocate encouraging women in labour who are considered low risk to eat a light, low-fibre diet (Crawford 1987, Johnson et al 1989).

Pressure from the gravid uterus at term readily causes reflux of stomach contents, especially when the woman lies recumbent. When general anaesthesia is induced, *silent regurgitation* may easily occur unnoticed and if acid stomach contents are then aspirated into the lungs, a condition known as Mendelson's syndrome results. Acid aspiration causes a chemical pneumonitis, damaging the alveoli so that gaseous exchange is impaired; if this is severe it is impossible to oxygenate the woman adequately and death may result.

Prevention

Antacid therapy. In order to try to prevent this condition occurring, women in labour who are deemed 'high risk' in terms of likelihood of instrumental or operative delivery (and who might thus require general anaesthesia) are given regular antacid therapy throughout labour. It is common to give an H_2 antagonist such as ranitidine in order to inhibit production of gastric hydrochloric acid. These drugs do not neutralise the existing acid contents, so any woman who is about to undergo general anaesthesia will be given an oral antacid preparation such as sodium citrate, which has an immediate but short-lived effect. The anaesthetist will give ranitidine prior to general anaesthesia if the woman has not received it regularly throughout labour.

'Rapid sequence induction'. This is the procedure used when giving general anaesthesia to an unprepared patient, for example the victim of a road traffic accident whose surgery cannot be delayed. Because even the prepared obstetric patient is liable to have acid stomach contents, the same technique is employed. Rapid sequence induction always includes endotracheal intubation with the use of cricoid pressure. A cuffed tracheal tube protects the lungs; even if silent regurgitation occurs, the acid contents cannot be aspirated past the cuff into the lungs.

Cricoid pressure is a technique which utilises pressure on the one complete ring of tracheal cartilage, the cricoid cartilage (Fig. 28.1), to occlude the oesophagus, so preventing acid reflux. The anaesthetist will require his assistant to maintain cricoid pressure until the tracheal tube is in position and he has been able to check that the seal provided by the cuff is effective. The correct application of cricoid pressure is essential, and may prevent a mother's death.

Failed intubation

This is more likely to occur in the pregnant woman, particularly if she has pregnancy-induced hypertension, when there may be some laryngeal oedema. Anatomical factors such as poor mouth opening, a fat or stiff neck or large breasts may also contribute to difficulty with intubation since the anaesthetist may have difficulty visualising the vocal cords and introducing the endotracheal tube. Incorrect application of cricoid pressure may compound the problem. Because the woman has been given a muscle relaxant in order to intubate the trachea, she cannot be oxygenated while attempts to intubate continue. Her oxygen needs are increased by the presence of the fetus, so that repeated, prolonged attempts to intubate may prove fatal to both.

Problems with the airway and aspiration of stomach contents continue to be hazards of anaesthesia and should be prevented (DH et al 1996).

Prevention

It is now common practice to 'pre-oxygenate' every pregnant woman prior to induction of anaesthesia. This procedure prolongs significantly the period of time which the anaesthetist may spend attempting to intubate her without cyanosis ensuing.

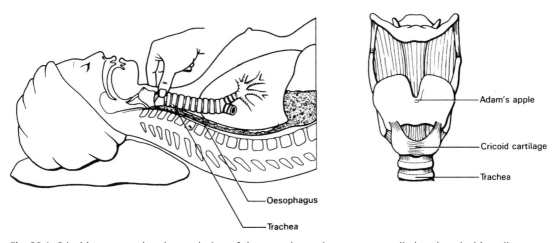

Fig. 28.1 Cricoid pressure, showing occlusion of the oesophagus by pressure applied to the cricoid cartilage.

Pre-oxygenation involves giving oxygen by face mask for an uninterrupted period, usually about 4 minutes. Some women, already stressed by the thought of an emergency caesarean section, find this procedure difficult to tolerate, as they may feel stifled by the mask, but calm careful explanation will help to allay their fears and many anaesthetists will allow the woman to hold the mask herself.

Pre-oxygenation also causes stress in the obstetrician, particularly if there is severe fetal distress, and delivery is an urgent procedure. It may feel like an unnecessary waste of time.

Correct application of cricoid pressure is essential and the midwife should not be afraid to ask the anaesthetist for help if she is asked to assist him in this way but feels uncertain of her ability to perform the technique.

It is usual to have a *failed intubation drill*. Various factors will influence the anaesthetist's decision. If he is able to maintain a clear airway, he may proceed using a face mask and Guedel airway with his assistant maintaining cricoid pressure throughout the anaesthetic. Spinal anaesthesia, after waking the mother, is another possibility. Epidural anaesthesia is not considered to be an option in this situation since if the stressed anaesthetist were unfortunate enough to perform an inadvertent *total spinal block* he would need to intubate the trachea in order to prevent maternal death (see below). The midwife working in the operating theatre must understand clearly the failed intubation drill and the rationale behind it. Failed intubation is an emergency situation demanding prompt, appropriate action; a significant number of maternal deaths due directly to anaesthesia have been caused by a misplaced tracheal tube (DH et al 1991, 1994).

Aortocaval occlusion

This is sometimes referred to as *supine hypotensive syndrome* but this can be misleading, since a fall in blood pressure may be a later sign of the problem and is often preceded by compromise of placental perfusion.

The problem is caused by the weight of the gravid uterus partially occluding the inferior vena cava. Venous return is then reduced, followed by a fall in cardiac output. This sequence of events is not only associated with general anaesthesia but may occur at any time in late pregnancy or during labour. It will always occur if the woman lies supine in late pregnancy. Fortunately most women at term do not find it comfortable to lie flat but the midwife must take steps to ensure that the woman in labour does not do so. If emergency caesarean section is being performed because of fetal distress, aortocaval occlusion will increase the fetal distress and cause further fetal hypoxia.

Prevention

Whenever the woman in labour needs to lie flat the midwife should ensure that she is tilted laterally, either by means of a small rubber wedge under the mattress or by placing a folded blanket under one buttock. It is usual to tilt the woman to the left and an angle of 15° is sufficient. Most modern delivery beds and chairs have this facility, as does every operating table. The ideal means of prevention is to encourage the woman in labour to be upright as much as possible.

Maternal awareness

Most of the drugs given to the mother during general anaesthesia (except the muscle relaxants) will cross the placental barrier and affect the fetus, if only for a short time. In order to prevent a sleepy baby being delivered the anaesthetist will give the mother as light an anaesthetic as possible. The woman's level of consciousness may sometimes become sufficiently light for her to recall events which occurred during the operation but because she is paralysed, in order to allow the light level of anaesthesia, she is unable to give any indication of this. (With this light level of anaesthesia the obstetrician would experience difficulty with access to the abdominal cavity without muscle relaxation, and tracheal intubation is better tolerated.) Many women who have suffered awareness have not recalled pain but have recounted accurate details of conversations held in the operating theatre. This is a terrifying experience for the woman, who may well have opted for general rather than epidural anaesthesia because she wanted to know nothing of what was happening. The anaesthetist will make every effort to prevent awareness in the mother, but it does still occur occasionally.

Prevention

Awareness may occur if the inhalational anaesthetic agent is nitrous oxide alone; adding a volatile agent, which is common practice, should prevent this occurring. The anaesthetist also gives the woman an opioid drug by intravenous injection as soon as the baby is delivered. He can also increase the amount of nitrous oxide given at this stage, as the woman's oxygen requirements are reduced when the baby is born.

The well-being of the fetus is of vital importance during caesarean section and the anaesthetist has to remember this as he treats the mother. In summary, the most important points are prevention of maternal and therefore fetal hypoxia, prevention of Mendelson's syndrome and aortocaval occlusion and avoidance of too deep or too light a level of anaesthesia in the mother.

REGIONAL ANAESTHESIA

Epidural block

For more detailed information on the following topics see Moir & Thorburn (1986), Morgan (1987), Reynolds (1990).

Epidural block was introduced in the 1970s with the expectation that it would provide widely available pain-free labour and delivery (Doughty 1987, Reynolds 1990). Initially, attention was focused on development of the technique itself, but the dissatisfaction of women, midwives and obstetricians soon became evident. The only drugs available at this time were local anaesthetic solutions; bupivacaine and lignocaine were the most commonly used in the UK. These gave the required sensory block, but also blocked motor and sympathetic nerves, causing significant loss of bladder sensation and function, loss of feeling for second stage, complete numbness of the legs and significant hypotension. Women disliked this immobility, and midwives and obstetricians objected to

the perceived rise in instrumental delivery. Unless hypotension was prevented or treated promptly and effectively, fetal distress could ensue as a result of reduced placental perfusion. The combined motor and sensory block resulted in loss of Ferguson's reflex so that the natural bearing down sensation was absent. It is difficult for the woman to direct her pushing effectively without some sensation. Another reason for an increase in instrumental delivery was that relaxation of the pelvic floor musculature removed the 'gutter effect', which encourages the fetal head to rotate anteriorly as it descends. A greater proportion of occipitoposterior and occipitotransverse positions therefore required increased rates of obstetric intervention. Doughty (1987) considered that midwives were not receptive of the new technique for these reasons. They saw the epidural as the cause of a forceps delivery and so manipulated events in order to protect the women. He reported a similar lack of enthusiasm among obstetricians.

Although all the side-effects described in the preceding paragraph still occur to some extent, ongoing research and refinement of obstetric and anaesthetic techniques and management have reduced their frequency.

The ideal epidural is now defined as providing rapid onset of reliable analgesia while allowing retention of:

- awareness of contractions without pain
- bladder sensation and function
- mobility of the legs
- sensation of rectal pressure in the second stage and therefore some urge to bear down
- spontaneous vaginal delivery.

There should be freedom from unwanted effects on either mother or baby (Morgan & Kadim 1994, O'Sullivan 1997).

The unwanted effects should also take account of the psychological sequelae, and maternal satisfaction after the event is as important as physical safety, though often under-regarded. Control is an important element in satisfaction, even if labour did not proceed as anticipated, and a pain-free labour is not necessarily the most satisfactory. Morgan et al (1982) and also Simkin (1991) showed that maternal involvement and choice are important elements in post-delivery satisfaction (Belbin 1996).

The search for the ideal epidural resulted in a review of the length of second stage, and a change in approach. The addition of opioid drugs to local anaesthetic agents reduced motor blockade. Some anaesthetists combined spinal and epidural anaesthesia to give rapid onset of pain relief and to aim to maintain mobility (Morgan & Kadim 1994).

Epidural analgesia may be described as lumbar or caudal, depending on the site used when approaching the epidural space.

The epidural space is situated around the dura mater and contains blood vessels and fatty tissue, as well as the spinal nerves which pass through it. Because of the generalised venous engorgement which occurs in pregnancy, the space tends to be rather smaller in the pregnant woman than it is in other adults and during a uterine contraction, when the veins become more engorged, the space is even further reduced. (For more detail see Gaynor (1990).) The aim of the anaesthetist performing epidural anaesthesia is to introduce local anaesthetic solution into the epidural space so that it will surround the fibres of specific spinal nerves and anaesthetise them, so achieving a selective block, ideally to the level of T10 for labour and to T4 for caesarean section.

Lumbar epidural block

This is the commonest type of approach and there are different techniques which may be used. The anaesthetic is introduced between lumbar vertebrae 3 and 4 or 2 and 3.

A *single shot epidural* is one where the local anaesthetic is introduced using a Tuohy needle, but no catheter is inserted for 'top-up' purposes.

When *continuous technique* is used, a very dilute solution of local anaesthetic is infused via the epidural catheter using an intravenous infusion line attached to an infusion pump. The advantage of this is that inadvertent introduction of the local anaesthetic solution into the subarachnoid space is likely to have less sudden or dramatic results. (Complications of epidural block are discussed in more detail below.)

An *intermittent technique* is one where a fine polyethylene or nylon catheter is inserted into

the epidural space, so that further 'top-up' doses of local anaesthetic may be given when required.

The *'mobile epidural'* was developed in order to provide the 'ideal epidural' (Morgan 1995). It is a combined epidural–spinal technique (see below), thus giving rapid onset of pain relief. An opioid drug is mixed with a dilute solution of local anaesthetic.

Caudal epidural block
(See also Meehan (1987).)

This technique is not popular in obstetric practice in the UK. It is less easy to secure an epidural catheter safely and comfortably. A large amount of local anaesthetic solution is required in order to give effective analgesia and it is not easy to obtain a predictable, selective block; there have been some reports of fetal bradycardia (E. Whitehead, personal communication, 1997). The woman may be required to lie in the knee–chest position during the procedure itself, which is uncomfortable and impractical for a woman in labour. The epidural needle is introduced between the sacral vertebrae and the coccyx, through the sacral hiatus. The complications which may be seen are similar to those in lumbar epidural block but because higher doses of local anaesthetic solution are required, toxicity is more likely.

Indications for epidural analgesia

Maternal request is probably the commonest indication for epidural analgesia. Many consultant obstetric units in the UK are now able to offer an epidural service to all or most mothers who wish to have this form of pain relief. Safety must always be the first consideration and if there are not sufficient anaesthetists for an experienced person to be readily available to the obstetric unit the epidural service will be restricted (House of Commons 1980).

Although epidural analgesia is never performed without the mother's consent and it is unwise to persuade a reluctant subject, there are certain medical and obstetric conditions where an epidural block may be advised.

Malposition. For the woman with an occipitoposterior position where a long, exhausting labour is anticipated, an epidural block may be the ideal form of analgesia, although it may occasionally be difficult to relieve the severe backache completely.

Malpresentation. Epidural analgesia is particularly valuable in a breech presentation when the obstetrician requires a well-relaxed mother if he has to perform an assisted breech delivery. Because she will usually be completely free of pain, this is also ideal from the mother's point of view. When an assisted breech delivery is anticipated, the epidural is 'topped up' so that anaesthesia is more profound than for a normal vaginal delivery. An effective epidural block may also be augmented sufficiently to perform caesarean section, if required, without undue delay.

Multiple pregnancy. An epidural block is advantageous for the woman with a twin pregnancy because of the possibility of manipulative delivery.

Pregnancy-induced hypertension. Epidural analgesia is advised in this situation but *not* for the hypotensive side-effect. Pain and tension will tend to exacerbate the hypertension and effective analgesia is an important part of the woman's treatment. The hypertension is treated with specific hypotensive agents such as hydralazine (see Ch. 17).

Effective analgesia. The woman who is not obtaining adequate pain relief from other analgesic methods, and who is tense and distressed, may need gentle guidance and the suggestion of an epidural block. Maternal distress and tiredness are known to have adverse physiological effects, leading to reduced uterine efficiency and fetal acidosis.

Contraindications

The main contraindications to epidural analgesia are usually cited as maternal reluctance, bleeding disorders, any infection near the site of the epidural, or any systemic infection. A coagulation disorder could give rise to a haematoma within the epidural space, which could then cause spinal cord compression and serious neurological sequelae. Any local or general sepsis could lead to menin-

gitis. Existing central nervous system disease such as multiple sclerosis has often been cited as a relative contraindication. This is not because it has any known adverse effect on the disease, but because any exacerbation suffered by the woman may cause her to regret her decision. MacDonald (1990) considers that provided the woman is counselled wisely during the pregnancy, the benefits may outweigh the risks. Abnormalities of the spine may make it very difficult for the anaesthetist to perform the epidural block, and it may not be fully effective.

Complications

Hypotension. Local anaesthetic solution blocks transmission of nervous impulses along motor and sensory nerves and also has an effect on the sympathetic nervous system. The vasodilatation resulting from this will lead to a fall in blood pressure unless this is prevented by giving a rapid infusion of intravenous fluid prior to establishing the block. This rapid infusion is commonly known as a *preload*; the anaesthetist may give between 500 and 1000 ml of Hartmann's solution, but this topic is open to debate (Scott 1993). A functioning intravenous infusion is essential before epidural analgesia can be commenced in order to prevent hypotension.

Hypotension may need to be treated with a vasoconstrictor such as ephedrine, which must always be readily available, and midwives should be aware of its use.

Dural tap. If the anaesthetist inadvertently punctures the dura mater this is known as a *dural tap*. It is usually recognised when a few drops of cerebrospinal fluid (CSF) leak through the Tuohy needle. It is essential that this problem is recognised promptly (see below).

The anaesthetist will normally resite the epidural catheter in an adjacent space. The obstetrician is informed and a forceps delivery may be planned in order to prevent the woman from pushing and possibly forcing more CSF through the dural puncture. A reduction in volume of CSF usually results in a headache which is often severe and distressing. Another measure designed to minimise leakage of CSF is to leave the epidural catheter in position and infuse normal saline through it with the help of an infusion pump. This is normally continued for 24 hours and it is usual to keep the woman lying flat.

A headache resulting from a dural tap will resolve spontaneously within about a week but will be incapacitating. Lying flat will give considerable if not complete relief, but this does not help the woman to enjoy her baby and the headache may be a lasting memory in place of what should have been a happy experience. The anaesthetist may therefore decide to perform a 'blood patch'. This involves taking between 10 and 20 ml of venous blood from the woman's antecubital vein, under strict asepsis, and introducing it into the epidural space via the intervertebral space nearest the dural puncture. Two anaesthetists will normally perform this procedure together. This treatment often has dramatic results, and the headache is cured almost immediately. The woman is asked to rest quietly for an hour or two, to avoid disturbing the blood clot which has sealed the dural puncture. Some anaesthetists will not carry out this procedure immediately, as there is some risk of infection. The success rate is reported to be approximately 90% on the first occasion and 98% if the procedure has to be repeated.

Total spinal block. This is a rare complication but is seen if a dural puncture is not recognised and the anaesthetist proceeds to inject the local anaesthetic solution. The result will be a profound and rapid motor and sensory block with a dramatic fall in blood pressure. The mother collapses and cardiac arrest often follows. Immediate resuscitation is essential and ventilatory support is required. If maternal hypoxia can be prevented and normal blood pressure restored quickly, the baby may later be delivered unscathed.

Very occasionally this effect may be seen following a later *top-up* and not during the initial stages of the epidural analgesia. The reasons for this are largely unclear but in some cases the epidural catheter is thought to have 'migrated'. The midwife who tops up an epidural must therefore be vigilant and must be aware of the possible complications, their detection and immediate treatment.

Bloody tap. If the anaesthetist punctures one of the epidural veins, blood is seen in the epidural cannula or in the catheter and this is known as a *bloody tap*. The epidural catheter is resited in order to prevent accidental intravenous injection of local anaesthetic solution. If local anaesthetic solution does enter the circulation, toxicity may result. The woman may complain of tingling or numbness of the mouth and tongue and of dizziness; her speech may become slurred and finally she may have a convulsion.

Patchy block. An epidural block may sometimes be more effective on one side of the body or it may be completely unilateral, for no obvious reason. Sometimes it may be impossible to provide analgesia for one particular area. The anaesthetist should always be informed if this occurs since adjustment or resiting of the epidural catheter may be effective.

Disadvantages

During labour the woman may find the reduction of sensation and motor function in her legs unpleasant, although with the use of lower concentrations of local anaesthetic solution she may not be aware of this effect until she tries to lift her legs or walk.

She may not be aware if her bladder becomes full and may find it difficult or impossible to pass urine, although this is common in the later stage of any labour.

The aim is to achieve a spontaneous delivery whenever possible, in the interests of reducing complications for both mother and baby and to give the mother the satisfaction she will enjoy following a normal delivery. Since time constraints on the duration of the second stage have been modified, the woman is not encouraged to bear down until she feels the urge to do so or until the presenting part distends the perineum (Walkinshaw & Crosfill 1990). This makes normal delivery more likely. It is probable that maintaining an adequate level of analgesia (without profound motor block) rather than withholding top-ups during the second stage is more likely to allow the woman a normal delivery (Carli 1990, Morgan 1995).

Certain symptoms which occur in the postnatal

period may be attributed to the epidural block; MacArthur et al (1990) consider these to be under-researched and not adequately acknowledged. They include:

- impaired bladder function
- marked perineal pain
- backache which may be due in part to local bruising where the Tuohy needle was introduced, especially if the anaesthetist had difficulty locating the epidural space.

(See also Clark & McQueen (1993), Russell et al (1993).)

Drugs used in epidural analgesia

Local anaesthetics:

Bupivacaine (Marcain). The local anaesthetic drug most commonly used in the UK is bupivacaine (Marcain). It is marketed in strengths of 0.25% and 0.5% and these concentrations are modified in practice as required by dilution with normal saline. (0.75% bupivacaine is also available but is no longer licensed for use in obstetrics in the UK following maternal deaths from cardiotoxicity after inadvertent intravenous injection (O'Sullivan 1997).)

Bupivacaine is effective within 10–20 minutes of administration and the effect lasts for about 2 hours during labour. The total dose given is therefore not excessive, unless labour is unduly prolonged, and toxicity is not common. The drug does cross the placenta but there are no reported gross effects on the fetus (Kuhnert et al 1984, Reynolds 1989, 1993).

Bupivacaine is available with added adrenaline and this preparation is sometimes used in obstetrics.

Lignocaine. This is also available for epidural administration. It gives effective anaesthesia in a short time but has a short duration of action. This makes it unsuitable for use throughout labour since a large total dose would be required and toxicity is therefore a risk. However, if a woman is very distressed it may be used for the initial dose, with bupivacaine being used thereafter.

Toxicity. If the woman has received a large total dose of local anaesthetic solution or if some of the solution has passed directly into the circulation, she may complain of tingling or numbness of the mouth and tongue, dizziness and tinnitus. This may be followed by drowsiness, muscle twitching and slurring of the speech. Finally, convulsions may occur, with cardiac arrest ensuing.

Ropivacaine (Naropin). This is a more recently developed local anaesthetic agent, licensed for use in the UK in February 1997. It is reported to give good analgesia in lower concentrations with minimal and non-progressive motor block and is suitably long acting for use in labour (O'Sullivan 1997).

Opioid drugs. Several of the opioid drugs have been used in the epidural space including diamorphine, morphine, pethidine and fentanyl. They give good postoperative analgesia without motor or sympathetic block and do not produce hypotension to any extent. They are not as effective as might be expected in relieving the pain of labour but are used by many anaesthetists following caesarean section. There is some risk of respiratory depression (Woods 1993) but this is not thought by the majority to be as great a risk in the young, fit woman as in the elderly patient following surgery (MacLeod 1993). The use of opioids in the epidural solution may be contraindicated if systemic opioids have already been given during labour because of the risk of cumulative effects. Drugs such as diamorphine produce a pleasant feeling of relaxation and well-being.

Combined local anaesthetic agents and opioids. Epidural opioids used alone give disappointing results in labour, but a combination has been found to be very effective.

The greatest advantage is a marked reduction in motor blockade, as only a dilute solution of local anaesthetic, usually bupivacaine, is needed to give good analgesia.

The opioid most commonly used is fentanyl, and this has not been shown to have any adverse effects on the fetus or newborn baby (Murphy et al 1991). There is interest in other similar drugs, but their effect on the baby has not yet been investigated fully.

Preparation of the mother

The woman and her partner should receive information about epidural analgesia during the antenatal period so that they have time to consider this option and to ask any questions.

The woman in labour who opts for epidural analgesia in desperation, rather than as a planned measure, should be given as much information as she can absorb but she must be informed of the risks involved. She must then give her consent to the procedure, although whether or not she is in a position to give informed consent is questionable (Gild 1989).

An intravenous infusion is established, using a wide-bore cannula so that fluid may be infused quickly if necessary. The midwife measures and records the woman's blood pressure. She should also monitor the fetal heart throughout the procedure.

The procedure

The woman is positioned either on her left side or sitting upright with her buttocks on the edge of the bed nearest the anaesthetist.

The skin of the lumbar area is cleaned with a preparation such as chlorhexidine in spirit.

The anaesthetist 'scrubs up' and puts on sterile gown and gloves. He places a sterile towel over the lumbar area, exposing the intervertebral space which he intends to use and infiltrates the skin and deeper tissues with local anaesthetic solution.

When this is effective he introduces the Tuohy needle. He advances the needle cautiously. It passes through the tough ligamentum flavum before reaching the epidural space (Fig. 28.2). Pressure within the epidural space is atmospheric or slightly negative and so he tests for 'loss of resistance' by injecting normal saline or air to check if the needle has passed through the ligamentum flavum. Even slight movement by the woman at this stage may result in dural puncture and she must remain still.

Once the tip of the Tuohy needle lies in the epidural space the anaesthetist threads the epidural catheter through the needle, which is then withdrawn.

He introduces a test dose of 3–4 ml of local anaesthetic solution; its purpose is to ensure that the solution is not in the subarachnoid space (see below).

The epidural catheter is secured firmly with adhesive tape and an antibacterial filter attached to the distal end. The woman is positioned as requested by the anaesthetist. The blood pressure is recorded 5 minutes after the test dose was given.

If this reading is satisfactory and no motor block has developed, the remainder of the first full dose is given. The blood pressure is usually recorded every 5 minutes for 20 minutes, then 15 minutes later. Between top-up doses of local anaesthetic solution or during continuous infusion, half-hourly recordings are usually sufficient.

After about 20 minutes, when the local anaesthetic solution is likely to have settled, the woman may be helped to find a comfortable position.

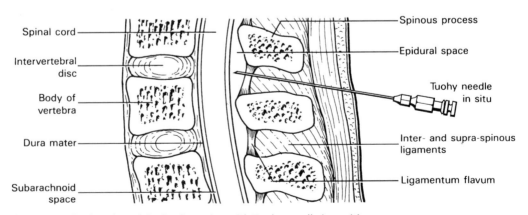

Fig. 28.2 Sagittal section of the lumbar spine with Tuohy needle in position.

Subsequent care

The anaesthetist takes overall responsibility for the establishment of the epidural block but he will then delegate certain aspects of its maintenance to the midwife.

She is responsible for ensuring that adequate analgesia is maintained, whether or not she tops up the epidural block herself. She should report any hypotension, any areas of unsatisfactory analgesia and any symptoms of excessive block or of toxicity. She has a responsibility to ensure that she is adequately trained to care for a woman with an epidural block and she must follow hospital procedures and policies (UKCC 1993, 1994).

She must give particular attention to bladder care during labour. If the legs are relatively immobile they must be moved and positioned with care, in order to avoid nerve damage and pressure.

The epidural top-up

The midwife may be trained to top up the epidural block by giving a further dose as prescribed by the anaesthetist. The prescription should indicate clearly the dosage and frequency of the drugs to be given, and the positioning of the woman. The midwife is personally responsible for ensuring that she is competent to carry out the procedure (UKCC 1992, 1994). The same observations are made as with the initial dose. She should be aware of the possible dangers and complications and their immediate and subsequent treatment. It is important to prevent aortocaval occlusion since this would compound the effect of any hypotension occurring as a result of the epidural block.

Continuous epidural infusion (see above)

Good analgesia is afforded by continuous infusion of dilute local anaesthetic solution, with or without opiates. This is given by infusion pump into the epidural catheter. Top-up doses may be given if needed but generally this technique avoids the peaks and troughs of analgesia afforded by the intermittent top-up technique. The midwife must still observe the woman carefully.

There has been some research in the USA into giving women some control over their epidural infusion – patient-controlled epidural analgesia or

PCEA (Fontenot et al 1993). Certain restraints are built in, just as with patient-controlled intravenous analgesia.

Epidural anaesthesia for caesarean section

Epidural anaesthesia for caesarean section must be more profound and more extensive than for labour. Sensation should be blocked to the level of the nipples (T4), and a good block is required in the pelvic area. If the motor block rises above the level of T4 the woman may have difficulty breathing.

Attaining this extensive block necessitates the use of a larger volume of the stronger local anaesthetic solution (commonly 0.5% bupivacaine). The risk of hypotension is therefore greater and a preload of at least 1 litre of intravenous fluid (usually Hartmann's solution) is required. Hypotension may still occur and ampoules of ephedrine should be ready for immediate use. Some women experience uncontrollable shivering during induction of epidural anaesthesia and this may be due in part to the rapid infusion of intravenous fluid. Some women dislike the complete motor block of the legs.

The greatest advantage for the woman is being able to see and cuddle the baby immediately. In many centres her partner can also be present. The mother does not have to recover from the effects of general anaesthesia and she is up and about very quickly in the postoperative period, especially if epidural opiates are used for postoperative analgesia.

The woman is not exposed to the risks of general anaesthesia, although there is always the possibility that general anaesthesia may have to be induced at some stage if the epidural block is not satisfactory. The anaesthetist is always prepared for this, and women should be warned that it is occasionally necessary. If a woman is slightly apprehensive about having an epidural for caesarean section, she may be relieved to know this.

Spinal anaesthesia

Spinal anaesthesia must be distinguished from epidural anaesthesia.

Spinal anaesthesia is a technique by which local

anaesthetic solution is injected into the subarachnoid space, that is, into the cerebrospinal fluid. It is quick and relatively easy to perform and is almost always completely effective. The onset of anaesthesia is almost immediate. The approach is similar to that for performing lumbar puncture.

A continuous or intermittent technique is not considered practicable by many anaesthetists and its greatest use is for shorter procedures such as manual removal of the placenta, suturing of a third-degree perineal tear or forceps delivery.

It is possible to perform caesarean section using spinal anaesthesia, but there is a risk that the anaesthetic will be wearing off before the end of the procedure, especially if some unexpected complication occurs. In developing countries, the obstetrician may have to rely solely on spinal anaesthesia, which he performs himself prior to delivering the baby by caesarean section. In this situation the obstetrician may also use local anaesthetic solution for infiltration over the incision site (Barth 1992).

The needle used for spinal anaesthesia is very fine so that leakage of CSF is minimal and in recent years variations in design have been refined with the same objective, so as to reduce the incidence of post-spinal headache.

A very small amount of local anaesthetic solution is required. Between 1.5 and 2 ml is usually sufficient to give anaesthesia. Owing to the fact that the drug is being injected into another fluid its location of action can be influenced by two factors:

• Use of a hyperbaric or 'heavy' solution. If the drug being injected has a specific gravity greater than that of the CSF it will settle at the lowest possible point within the subarachnoid space. Hyperbaric bupivacaine is used in the UK; heavy cinchocaine and amethocaine are used elsewhere in the world.
• Positioning the woman. If a hyperbaric solution is used and the woman is positioned carefully, a specific block may usually be obtained without difficulty. Position is also important when an isobaric solution is used (that is, one with a specific gravity similar to that of the CSF).

The woman will have total motor and sensory block over and below the anaesthetised area. It may be difficult to control the level of the block.

There is a risk of hypotension with spinal as with epidural block. The blood pressure is monitored carefully, and prophylactic ephedrine is often given. Care of the bladder is also important in this instance.

Combined spinal and epidural anaesthesia (CSE)

This technique is more widely used now that there is less risk of post-spinal headache. It is used because there is a risk that spinal block will not be sustained throughout caesarean section if the procedure is prolonged for any reason, and so that effective postoperative analgesia may be given via the epidural catheter. Rapid onset of anaesthesia is obtained by spinal blockade. The Tuohy needle may be used as an introducer for the spinal needle; once the spinal solution is given the Tuohy needle is withdrawn slightly, the epidural catheter is passed into the epidural space and the epidural solution is given. Alternatively, the Tuohy needle and epidural catheter are inserted in an adjacent intervertebral space and local anaesthetic solution is injected as necessary in order to maintain anaesthesia and provide postoperative pain relief.

Long-term sequelae
Research undertaken into long-term health problems following childbirth (MacArthur et al 1991) has revealed that the number of women who suffer from backache after epidural or spinal anaesthesia is almost double the number who do so after a normal delivery. This backache may be accompanied by shoulder ache, limb weakness or tingling in the limbs. It is postulated that the cause may be positional and care should therefore be taken to vary the position of the mother from time to time and to help her keep her legs in an anatomically correct position.

Pudendal block

This is a technique used to anaesthetise the specific area served by the pudendal nerve (Ostheimer & Leavitt 1992).

Local anaesthetic solution is injected adjacent

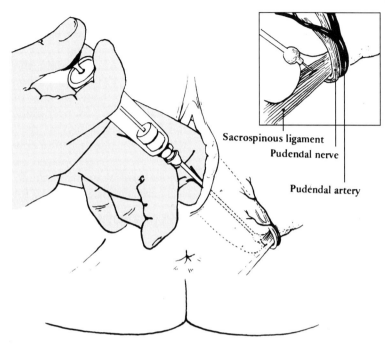

Sacrospinous ligament
Pudendal nerve

Pudendal artery

Fig. 28.3 Locating the pudendal nerve per vaginam.

to the pudendal nerves as they pass close to the ischial spines. The pudendal nerves are sensory nerves serving the lower vagina, the perineum and vulva. Pudendal block is notoriously unreliable and often does not give adequate analgesia. It may be more effective on one side than the other.

A guarded needle such as the Oxford needle is used. The more common approach is transvaginal (Fig. 28.3). The ischial spines are palpated and the injection made on each side. The transperineal approach may be used if the presenting part is very low.

Paracervical block

In this technique the paracervical plexuses are blocked. This gives pain relief for the first stage of labour but each injection is only effective for about 3 hours. The local anaesthetic solution is injected using a guarded needle to prevent deep penetration of the tissues. The uterine artery passes close to the nerve plexus and inadvertent intra-arterial injection of even a small amount of local anaesthetic solution may lead to fetal bradycardia or possibly intrauterine death (Ostheimer 1992). The technique is not popular in the UK although it may be more widely used elsewhere (Ranta et al 1995).

LOCAL ANAESTHESIA

Perineal infiltration

This is the most common instance of use of local anaesthesia for the midwife, who may undertake it herself prior to performing or repairing an episiotomy.

The midwife should be aware of safe dosages and possible side-effects of the drug she is using (UKCC 1992).

The drug in most common use is lignocaine. There is a real risk of toxic reaction if more than 200 mg is given to the woman (the equivalent of 20 ml of 1% solution). For this reason the amount that the midwife may use on her own responsibility is considerably less than this.

The technique used will depend on the type

of episiotomy favoured and on local policy and practice. The principles involved are:

• giving effective analgesia
• minimising the risk of intravenous injection.

It is therefore common practice to insert the needle, aspirate to ensure that the tip of the needle is not in a blood vessel, and inject the local anaesthetic solution as the needle is withdrawn. This may be repeated to give either a fan-shaped or a star-shaped pattern of infiltration (see also Ch. 24).

OBSTETRIC OPERATIONS

Forceps delivery

(See also Llewellyn-Jones (1994), Vacca & Keirse (1989), O'Brien & Cefalo (1991).)

Forceps delivery is a means of extracting the fetus with the aid of obstetric forceps when it is inadvisable or impossible for the mother to complete the delivery by her own effort. Forceps can also be used to assist the delivery of the after-coming head of the breech and on occasion to withdraw the head up and out of the pelvis at caesarean section.

Formerly forceps deliveries were classified by the level of the head at the time the forceps were applied, i.e. high-cavity, mid-cavity or low-cavity. The last one of these is now the only one frequently performed as caesarean section is usually preferred to the more traumatic high- and mid-cavity operations.

Low-cavity forceps deliveries can be divided into rotational and non-rotational. The former refers to a manoeuvre of the fetal head from a malposition into a more favourable position with the aid of specially designed forceps, usually Kielland's. In unskilled hands this is a dangerous procedure and some obstetricians prefer to rotate the head manually prior to applying conventional forceps for the delivery.

Types of obstetric forceps

Obstetric forceps consist of two separate blades, each with a handle. Each blade is marked 'L' (left) or 'R' (right). They are inserted separately either side of the fetal head and locked together by means of the English or Smellie lock. (Rotational forceps have a sliding lock.) The blades are spoon-shaped to accommodate the baby's head, but fenestrated, to minimise trauma and for lightness. The spoon shape of the blades is called the 'cephalic curve'. In most modern obstetric forceps the blade is attached to the handle at an angle which corresponds to the pelvic curve. When the blades are correctly placed on the fetal head the handles will be neatly aligned.

There is a wide variety of forceps designs.

Non-rotational. Some examples are:

• Wrigley's forceps: short, stubby-handled forceps used for very low forceps deliveries, for the after-coming head of a breech delivery or at caesarean section.
• Simpson's forceps: standard, low-cavity forceps.
• Neville–Barnes', Haig Ferguson's, Milne Murray and Anderson's forceps: these were all originally designed for high- and mid-cavity forceps deliveries and have axis traction handle attachments to allow downward traction of a high head into the pelvis. These attachments are rarely, if ever, used and the forceps are used for low-cavity deliveries.

Rotational. One design is in common use:

• Kielland's forceps: for use when the head is in an occipitolateral or occipitoposterior position. Since the blades are applied to the head which is then rotated to an occipitoanterior position, they have no pelvic curve because this could cause trauma to the birth canal. In malposition there may also be asynclitism and their sliding lock allows this to be corrected. When the Kielland's forceps are applied there is a gap between the handles. There is a danger that if they are squeezed together pressure can be applied to the fetal head. Some operators like to rotate the head with the Kielland's forceps and deliver with non-rotational forceps.

Prerequisites for forceps delivery

There are certain conditions which must exist before forceps delivery can be performed:

• full dilatation of the cervix
• ruptured membranes

- positive identification of presentation and position
- no appreciable cephalopelvic disproportion
- definite engagement of the head.

Preparation of the woman

A woman who is to be delivered with forceps will often be relieved to know that her baby is about to be born. The woman and her partner should have been fully informed throughout labour of progress and developments and her care should have been discussed with them. Ideally she should be prepared in advance for the possibility of a forceps delivery if this looks likely. Full explanation of the procedure itself and the need for it is likely to result in greater retrospective satisfaction.

Once the joint decision has been made, adequate and appropriate analgesia must be offered.

When such analgesia has been instituted and the obstetrician is ready to proceed the woman's legs are placed in the lithotomy position. Both legs must be positioned simultaneously to avoid strain on the woman's lower back and hips. This is an undignified and uncomfortable position, especially for a tired woman with a weighty gravid uterus who is in advanced labour. Both medical staff and midwives should try to minimise the woman's loss of dignity when they perform what is, for them, a routine procedure. The woman's legs should not be placed in the stirrups for longer than is necessary, and the vulval area should remain covered whenever possible. The minimum number of staff should be present, and interruptions should be discouraged. The woman will find it helpful to realise that the staff are aware of her probable discomfort and embarrassment.

She should be tilted towards the left at an angle of 15° to prevent aortocaval occlusion. (This is usually achieved by the use of a rubber wedge under the mattress; an operating table has the facility for lateral tilt.)

Preparations must also have been made for the baby and resuscitation equipment checked and in working order. In many centres the paediatrician will be present.

Procedure

The woman's vulval area is thoroughly cleaned and draped with sterile towels using aseptic technique; the bladder is emptied with a Jaques catheter. The obstetrician will perform a vaginal examination in order to confirm the station and exact position of the fetal head. It is usual to positively identify the forceps blades (as left and right) by assembling them briefly before proceeding.

Positioning the forceps. The aim in positioning the forceps is to place them alongside the head over the ears. Myerscough (1982) describes this as being along an imaginary line running from the point of the chin to a point on the sagittal suture near the posterior fontanelle. The left blade is passed gently between the perineum and the fetal head with the first two fingers of the operator's right hand lying alongside the fetal head protecting the maternal tissue (Fig. 28.4). The tip of the forceps blade slides lightly over the head, into the hollow of the sacrum and is then 'wandered' to the left side of the pelvis where it should sit alongside the head. The procedure is repeated with the right blade until it sits on the right of the pelvis (Fig. 28.5). It should then be easy to lock the two blades and there should be little or no gap between

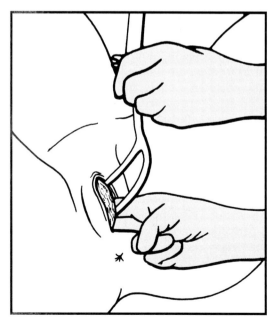

Fig. 28.4 Left blade being inserted. The fingers of the right hand guard the vaginal tissue.

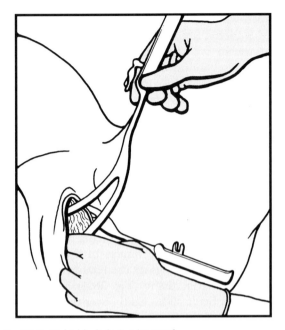

Fig. 28.5 Right blade being inserted.

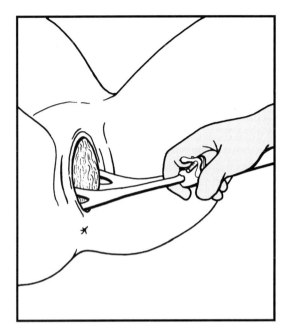

Fig. 28.6 Traction of the head is downwards until this point; when the head is low, the direction of pull is outward, towards the operator.

the handles. A significant gap suggests that the forceps are wrongly positioned and they should be reapplied after carefully checking the position of the head.

During this time the woman needs the full attention and support of the midwife whom she has already come to know during her labour. The fetal heart rate is monitored throughout. As soon as the operator is ready and the uterus contracts the woman is encouraged to push; to supplement her expulsive effort the obstetrician exerts steady, downward traction on the forceps (Fig. 28.6). Traction is released between contractions. The fetal heart is monitored carefully throughout. Intermittent traction is continued in a downward and backward direction until the occiput can be felt below the symphysis pubis. When the head distends the perineum, an episiotomy is performed. Most obstetricians deliver the head using the forceps (Fig. 28.7), as they feel this gives greater control, while others prefer to remove them and control delivery of the head as in a normal delivery. Once the body is delivered, unless the baby requires active resuscitation, he is handed straight to his mother and is dried thoroughly to prevent chilling.

After completion of the second and third stages the episiotomy is sutured as quickly as possible and the woman made comfortable.

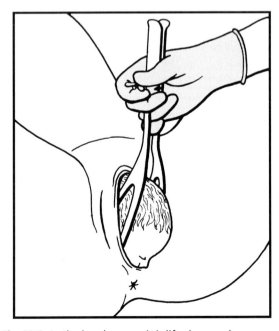

Fig. 28.7 As the head crowns it is lifted upwards.

Manual rotation of the fetal head. Some obstetricians prefer to rotate the fetal head manually in cases of occipitoposterior position, as this is likely to be less traumatic than instrumental rotation. The exact position of the fetal head must be determined. The obstetrician grasps the head, usually by the sinciput, and rotates it, encouraging flexion. It may be possible to lodge a finger on the edge of the anterior fontanelle or the over-riding bone on the frontal suture and apply gentle, steady pressure to rotate the head. One disadvantage is that upward displacement of the head may be necessary in many instances in order to grasp it, but there is then no facility for downward traction. A large hand will take up more space within the birth canal than a pair of obstetric forceps.

Indications for forceps delivery

- Fetal distress in the second stage of labour
- Delay in the second stage of labour
- Malposition: occipitolateral, occipitoposterior positions
- Maternal exhaustion or distress
- Breech presentation: forceps are usually used to deliver the after-coming head in a controlled fashion
- Preterm delivery: this is still a matter of debate, but some obstetricians and paediatricians like to protect the fetal head, with its soft skull bones, if delivery occurs before about the 36th week of gestation
- Conditions in which pushing is undesirable, such as dural tap, some cardiac conditions or moderate to severe hypertension.

Complications

Failure. Undue force should never be used. If the head does not advance with steady traction, the attempt is abandoned and the baby is delivered by caesarean section.

In the infant:

Bruising. Severe bruising will cause marked jaundice which may be prolonged. (Forceps marks are almost always present on the face: parents may be reassured that although these will become more florid in the first few hours of life they will then fade uneventfully over some months.)

Cephalhaematoma. See Chapter 40.

Cerebral irritability. A traumatic forceps delivery may cause cerebral oedema or haemorrhage (see Ch. 40).

Tentorial tear. This may result from compression of the fetal head by the forceps. The compression causes elongation of the head and consequent tearing of the tentorial membrane.

Facial palsy. Occasionally the facial nerve may be damaged since it is situated near the mastoid process where it has little protection.

In the mother:

Bruising and trauma to the urethra. This may cause dysuria and occasionally haematuria or a period of urinary retention or incontinence.

Vaginal and perineal trauma. The vaginal wall may be torn during forceps delivery and the vagina must be inspected carefully, using a good light, prior to perineal repair. The episiotomy may extend or be accompanied by a further perineal tear and these must be repaired with care. As with any damaged perineum there may be bruising, oedema or occasionally haematoma formation.

Vacuum extraction (Ventouse delivery)

(See also Rosevear & Stirrat (1996), Vacca (1992), Vacca & Keirse (1989).)

The Ventouse or vacuum extractor consists of a cup which is attached to the fetal scalp by suction, and the means of providing the vacuum. Its advantages are that it does not add to the presenting diameters and, if correctly positioned, it brings about flexion of the head and natural rotation. Some authorities state that full dilatation of the cervix is not an absolute necessity (Rosevear & Stirrat 1996), but Vacca (1992) refutes this. The implication would seem to be that vaginal delivery with some cervix palpable should only be attempted on rare occasions, and in carefully selected cases. Other considerations would be parity, the amount and consistency of the cervix and the station and position of the fetal head.

The main drawback of this form of delivery is that the operator may be too hasty in applying traction before the suction has been built up, so that the cup comes off. It is useful in remote areas and midwives working in developing countries without medical support perform vacuum extractions.

The equipment

The original vacuum extractors were of a very simple design, with a device similar to a bicycle pump being used to obtain the vacuum. Modern vacuum extractors use an electrical pump, which has much more sensitive controls. The vacuum is built up steadily and is maintained more efficiently so that the cup is less likely to come off.

A metal or Silastic (firm rubber) cup is applied to the fetal head; a vacuum is created inside this cup, which is connected to the pump by rubber tubing, and traction is then applied. Inside the rubber tubing is a metal chain designed to take the strain of traction, with a metal handle to give the operator a good grip. There are various sizes of cup; two different types have been developed for use with an anterior and/or a posterior position. This allows for more precise positioning of the cup with fewer failures (Vacca 1992).

It is possible to apply it to the breech but this is rarely seen in the UK.

Indications

- Mild fetal distress
- Delay in the second stage of labour or late first stage
- Malposition: occipitolateral and occipitoposterior positions
- Maternal exhaustion.

The procedure

The prerequisites are as for forceps delivery. The head must be engaged. The operator must be completely familiar with the technique appropriate to the particular cup design.

The woman is positioned and prepared as for forceps delivery (see above).

The position of the fetal head is determined and an appropriate size and type of cup selected (Vacca 1992). The cup is placed against the fetal head as near to the occiput as possible, ensuring that no cervix is trapped beneath it. Partial pressure of 0.2 kg/cm^2 is attained.

The vacuum is then built up to a negative pressure of 0.8 kg/cm^2 in one step. Once this pressure has been obtained, the operator waits 1–2 minutes for a chignon to form (Fig. 28.8), then exerts steady, gentle traction on the fetal head, in conjunction with uterine contractions and the mother's expulsive efforts (A. Vacca, personal communication, 1994).

With descent of the head, rotation to an occipitoanterior position may be effected if necessary. Because there is no part of the instrument between the head and the vaginal wall an episiotomy may

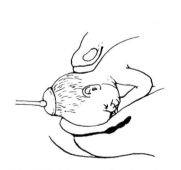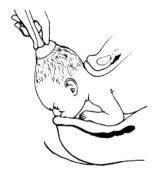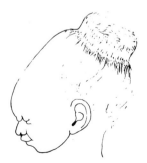

Fig. 28.8 Diagrams showing the application of the Ventouse cup and the chignon which usually results.

not always be judged necessary and vaginal trauma should not occur. As with a forceps delivery, traction is exerted in the direction of the curve of Carus and the head is controlled carefully at crowning. Traction should not be maintained for too long a period but a Ventouse delivery may take slightly longer than a forceps delivery, because of the time required to build up the vacuum.

Complications

Failure. An attempted vacuum extraction may be unsuccessful. Exerting too much traction will result in the cup coming off. In unskilled or impatient hands, the cup is also likely to come off.

Maternal. Trauma to the mother is rare, if the cup is applied carefully.

Fetal. The most common complication of Ventouse delivery is trauma to the fetal scalp and some obstetricians prefer not to use it for this reason.

'Chignon'. Because the vacuum cup is applied to the slightly mobile scalp, all babies delivered with the Ventouse will have a 'chignon'. This is an area of oedema and bruising where the cup was applied. These normally subside uneventfully but they may occasionally become infected.

Cephalhaematoma. Some babies will develop a cephalhaematoma.

Cerebral trauma. A few babies will suffer some degree of cerebral trauma, such as tentorial tear.

Caesarean section

(See also Depp (1991), Francome et al (1993).)

There are two types of caesarean section: lower segment and classical.

The lower segment of the uterus forms after about 32 weeks' gestation and is less muscular than the upper segment of the uterus. In a lower segment caesarean section a transverse incision is made in the lower segment; this heals more rapidly and successfully than an incision in the upper segment of the uterus. There is less muscle and more fibrous tissue there, which reduces the risk of rupture in a subsequent pregnancy.

Classical caesarean section is rarely performed. Indications for this approach are gestation of less than about 32 weeks before the lower segment has formed, placenta praevia which is anteriorly situated, in order to avoid incision of the placenta, and hour-glass contraction (constriction ring).

A longitudinal midline abdominal incision does not necessarily imply a longitudinal uterine incision. A lower segment caesarean section is most commonly performed through a transverse incision, the Pfannenstiel or 'bikini-line' incision, but on occasions a midline incision may be preferred. A classical caesarean section is always performed through a midline incision.

Indications for caesarean section

Elective caesarean section. The term *elective* indicates that the decision to deliver the baby by caesarean section has been made during the pregnancy and before the onset of labour. While some indications are absolute, others will depend on a combination of factors and on the views of the obstetrician concerned. Definite indications include:

- cephalopelvic disproportion
- major degrees of placenta praevia
- multiple pregnancy with three or more fetuses.

  Possible indications include:

- the primigravida and often the multigravida with a breech presentation
- moderate to severe pregnancy-induced hypertension
- diabetes
- intrauterine growth retardation
- antepartum haemorrhage.

If the indication for caesarean section pertains specifically to one pregnancy, such as placenta praevia, vaginal delivery may be expected on subsequent occasions. Certain conditions, however, warrant repeated caesarean section. Cephalopelvic disproportion due to contracted pelvis will recur and a uterus which has been scarred twice or more carries a greater risk of uterine rupture.

Emergency caesarean section is performed when

adverse conditions develop during labour. Definite indications include:

- cord prolapse
- uterine rupture (dramatic) or scar dehiscence (may be less acute)
- cephalopelvic disproportion diagnosed in labour
- fulminating pregnancy-induced hypertension
- eclampsia
- failure to progress in the first or second stage of labour
- fetal distress, if delivery is not imminent.

Psychological preparation of the mother

Some women welcome caesarean section as a means of escaping the rigours of labour; others feel disappointed that they have not had the experience of a normal delivery and have not enjoyed the accompanying sense of achievement.

Different women require differing levels of information. While some feel reassured by a detailed description of what is to happen, others find it distressing and prefer to leave everything in the hands of the professionals.

The midwife must be sensitive in her dealings with women, whether in a group situation or in speaking to individuals. If a woman is to have an elective caesarean section, it may be helpful to give information in stages. She should certainly be given the opportunity to ask whatever questions she wishes and should not be made to feel ridiculous in any way. Women are likely to have friends or relatives who have had caesarean sections, and this usually helps to reduce anxiety. It may be helpful for a woman to meet another person who has had the same experience recently.

If the possibility of caesarean section arises during labour, the midwife should begin to prepare the woman for this eventuality. The couple should be kept fully informed of events and progress during labour and should be given every opportunity to ask questions.

Physical preparation

Antacid therapy.   It is now common practice in the UK for women with any risk factors to receive regular antacid therapy throughout labour (see above). If this has not been given it should certainly be prescribed and administered once the decision to proceed with caesarean section has been made. Antacid preparations such as sodium citrate are effective in neutralising the stomach acid for a short period but do not prevent its secretion. In order to minimise production of gastric acid the anaesthetist may also prescribe a preparation such as ranitidine. The woman who is likely to need a caesarean section should only be permitted clear fluids in labour.

Intravenous infusion.   If an intravenous infusion has not already been established or is not running freely, it is sited or resited.

Pubic shave.   This is still usually considered necessary, though research suggests that tiny skin cuts predispose to infection. The use of a depilatory cream is likely to become more common.

Bowel care.   If caesarean section is elective, it is usual to give two glycerine suppositories the evening before operation in order to empty the rectum.

Bladder care.   The bladder must be empty prior to caesarean section. This may be achieved by passing a catheter which is then removed, or by inserting an indwelling catheter into the bladder. This may be done before or after induction of anaesthesia; if epidural block is used the woman will be less distressed if the catheter is passed after the block has become effective.

Clothing and valuables.   The woman is dressed in a clean operation gown and any valuables are placed in safe keeping according to hospital policy. Any rings or bracelets which cannot be removed are covered with adhesive strapping.

Anatomy

If the midwife is to assist at caesarean section as scrub nurse, it is important that she should understand the anatomy involved.

The most confusing aspect of the layers involved is the presence of two layers of peritoneum. The non-pregnant uterus is a pelvic organ and is closely covered by a layer of pelvic peritoneum. When the pregnant uterus grows up into the abdomen this peritoneum rises up with the uterus and comes into contact with the abdominal peritoneum. Each of these must be incised and repaired separately. The abdominal peritoneum is situated below the abdominal muscle layer.

The anatomical layers are:

- skin
- fat
- rectus sheath
- muscle (rectus abdominis)
- abdominal peritoneum
- pelvic peritoneum (perimetrium)
- uterine muscle.

The surgeon usually incises the rectus sheath, but divides the rectus muscle digitally. Care is taken to avoid trauma to the bladder and the ureters. The scrub nurse must avoid contamination of the sterile field and keep close account of all swabs, instruments and needles.

When the uterine cavity is opened, the amniotic fluid escapes and is aspirated. The baby is delivered in much the same way as in a vaginal delivery but through the uterine incision; obstetric forceps are often used to extract the head from the pelvis. When the baby is born, an oxytocic drug is administered before the placenta and membranes are delivered. If she is having general anaesthesia the mother may now be given a slightly deeper anaesthetic and the operation proceeds at a more leisurely pace. The uterus bleeds freely at this stage and the surgeon will quickly apply the special haemostatic Green-Armytage forceps. The uterine muscle is sutured in two layers, the second of which tends to align or include the cut edges of the pelvic peritoneum. Some obstetricians prefer to suture the pelvic peritoneum as a distinct layer, followed by the abdominal peritoneum. Repair of the rectus sheath also brings the rectus abdominis into alignment. Sometimes the subcutaneous fat is sutured and finally the skin is closed with sutures or clips. A vacuum drain, such as a 'Redivac' drain, may be inserted beneath the rectus sheath to prevent the formation of a haematoma.

Immediate postoperative care

The care of the woman who has had a caesarean section is the same as that following any major abdominal surgery with one or two added considerations.

Observations. The blood pressure and pulse are recorded every quarter-hour in the immediate recovery period. The temperature is recorded every 2 hours. The wound must be inspected every half-hour to detect any blood loss. The lochia are also inspected and drainage should be small initially. Following general anaesthesia the woman is nursed in the left lateral or 'recovery' position until she is fully conscious, since the risks of airway obstruction or regurgitation and silent aspiration of stomach contents are still present.

Analgesia is prescribed and is given as required. If the mother intends to breast feed, the baby should be put to the breast as soon as possible. This can usually be achieved with minimal disturbance to the mother.

Care following regional block. Following epidural or spinal anaesthesia the woman may sit up as soon as she wishes, provided her blood pressure is not low. All observations are recorded as described in the previous paragraph. Fluids are introduced gradually followed by a light diet. Although the woman may feel very hungry, there is a risk of paralytic ileus due to handling of the bowel and food is not permitted until bowel sounds are heard. The intravenous infusion remains in progress for the same reason. Care must be taken to avoid any damage to the legs which will gradually regain sensation and movement. Postoperative analgesia may be given in a variety of ways:

- an epidural opioid
- rectal analgesia, such as diclofenac
- intramuscular analgesia (though this is never given in conjunction with epidural opioids because of the risk of cumulative effects).

As it is possible that an opiate administered via the epidural route may cause some respiratory depression, the woman's respiratory rate must be recorded. This means of pain relief offers the advantage of excellent analgesia without motor block and also seems to give a feeling of well-being. Women are usually able to become mobile very quickly which reduces the risk of deep vein thrombosis.

Ideally the baby should remain with his mother and they should be transferred to the postnatal ward together as soon as possible.

Care in the postnatal ward. When mother and baby are transferred to the postnatal ward, the blood pressure, temperature and pulse are usually checked every 4 hours. The intravenous infusion will continue, and the urinary catheter will remain in the bladder until the woman is able to get up to the toilet. The wound and lochia must be observed at least hourly initially. The baby should remain with his mother, and the midwife should offer extra help to ensure that the mother has adequate rest. The mother is encouraged to move her legs and to perform leg and breathing exercises. The physiotherapist will usually teach these and may give chest physiotherapy. Prophylactic low-dose heparin and TED antiembolism stockings are often prescribed. The woman is helped to get out of bed as soon as possible following caesarean section, and is encouraged to become fully mobile (see also Ch. 45).

Urinary output must be monitored carefully both before and after removal of the urinary catheter; women may have some difficulty with micturition initially and the bladder may be incompletely emptied. Any haematuria must be reported to the doctor.

Women who have had a general anaesthetic for caesarean section may feel very tired and drowsy for hours or even days. A woman may complain of a feeling of detachment and unreality and may feel that she does not relate well to the baby. The woman who is concerned should be reassured and be given the opportunity to talk freely.

Appropriate analgesia must be given as frequently as necessary (see above). It is usual to give intramuscular opiates for up to 48 hours and then to give oral analgesics.

The mother must be encouraged to rest as much as possible and tactful advice may need to be given to her visitors. If the mother becomes too tired, help is needed with care for the baby. This should preferably take place at the mother's bedside and should include support with breast feeding.

Some women may have a lingering feeling of failure or disappointment at having had a caesarean section and may value the opportunity to talk this over with a sympathetic listener.

Destructive operations (embryotomy)

It may occasionally be necessary, in the interests of saving the mother's life, to destroy the fetus.

In the UK these drastic measures will only be undertaken if there is gross fetal abnormality causing fetopelvic disproportion. The alternative is caesarean section but although this is a relatively safe procedure in the 1990s, it still carries attendant risks and vaginal delivery may be preferred. The fetus may be equally difficult to deliver abdominally and may still need to be destroyed first. Whatever the situation, it is traumatic for all concerned and calls for sensitive support of both the family and the staff.

In developing countries, these distressing procedures may have to be performed because of the non-availability or refusal of a caesarean section. A uterine scar carries a risk of uterine rupture in a subsequent pregnancy which may be fatal in an area remote from obstetric help. A uterine scar may be culturally unacceptable (Schott & Henley 1996). The woman may present with exhaustion from prolonged or obstructed labour or may have a uterine infection; the fetus may have been dead for some time.

The instruments used for destructive operations are of necessity brutal and must be used with great care to avoid injuring the mother.

Craniotomy is probably performed most commonly for hydrocephalus. Release of cerebrospinal fluid and brain tissue causes collapse of the skull bones and allows vaginal delivery. If fetal death has already occurred, craniotomy may be used to overcome disproportion due to a brow presentation. In the case of hydrocephalus it is often sufficient to perforate the head and allow escape of CSF; forceps may be applied if the fetus does not deliver spontaneously. If more drastic measures are required, instruments such as the cranioclast and cephalotribe may be used to crush and then deliver the head. A blunt hook, known as a crotchet, may be used to extract the after-coming head of the breech.

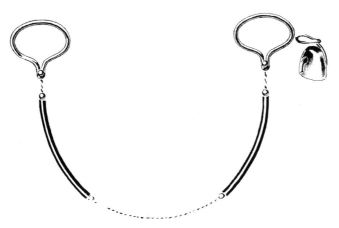

Fig. 28.9 Blond Heidler wire saw decapitator (reproduced by courtesy of Down Bros. and Mayer and Phelps Ltd, Mitcham, Surrey).

Decapitation may be necessary when a shoulder presentation has become impacted. The Blond Heidler wire saw and thimble is usually used (Fig. 28.9). There are also various types of decapitating hooks and knives which may be encountered (Fig. 28.10).

Cleidotomy. In this procedure the clavicles are cut to reduce the width of the shoulder girdle. Heavy, long, straight scissors are used.

Evisceration. It may be necessary to remove the abdominal or thoracic contents in some cases of gross fetal abnormality. If the presentation is cephalic this is difficult but it is more feasible in a breech presentation. The abdomen or chest is opened using a perforator and the contents removed manually.

Supporting the family

It is impossible to summarise this briefly since cultural factors and expectations play an important part in the reactions to the loss of a child. In a developing country, attitudes are very different from those in the West and it may be accepted as a normal life event with very little grief apparent (Schott & Henley 1996). In countries where infant survival is taken for granted, parents are likely to be devastated and the process of grieving should be encouraged (Murray-Parkes 1986). Many questions will be asked and opportunities for free discussion should be given. Parents will question their own actions and may feel intensely guilty at producing an abnormal fetus or perhaps refusing antenatal care or a termination earlier in the pregnancy. A feeling of anger is a normal part of the grieving process and parents should be allowed to express it (Kohner & Henley 1991). Midwives should not feel threatened by this, unless of course there is some justification. Referral to an organisation such as the 'Compassionate Friends' may be helpful in the long term; such a traumatic experience may cause great stress in the couple's relationship (see also Ch. 33).

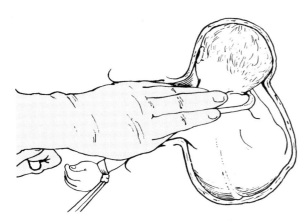

Fig. 28.10 Jardine's decapitation hook round the neck of the fetus. Traction on an arm by an assistant brings the neck within reach and fixes the head and trunk.

Symphysiotomy

This procedure enables a vaginal delivery in cases of minor cephalopelvic disproportion in areas of the world where caesarean section is not an option or a woman is not likely to seek obstetric care in a future pregnancy. The woman is usually primigravid and the operation is performed late in labour.

Both the pubic area and the perineum must be infiltrated with local anaesthetic as a generous episiotomy will be needed to avoid excessive pressure by the fetal head on the urethra and bladder. A firm catheter is inserted into the bladder to allow it to empty. It is held to one side during the incision so as to protect the urethra.

The fibrocartilage is incised over the centre of the symphysis pubis while two assistants hold and abduct the legs. A vacuum extractor is often used to facilitate delivery.

Following the operation broad strips of Elastoplast are applied around the pelvis to give support and the legs are usually bandaged together. A self-retaining catheter remains in position for 4 to 5 days because the area is usually oedematous.

The woman may have backache and experience difficulty in walking but in most cases the pelvic girdle regains its stability.

READER ACTIVITIES

1. Epidural analgesia was once seen by women as heralding a new era of painless labour for all mothers (Morgan 1987).

Prepare a discussion considering the following points:

   a. What were the flaws in this supposition?
   b. To what extent do women expect or want a painless labour today?
   c. Do we give appropriate preparation for labour pain in the antenatal period; if not how could we improve on this?

2. Prepare a leaflet for women who are likely to have a caesarean section, which they could read in the antenatal period. Include:

   a. what will happen in the ward and the anaesthetic room beforehand
   b. a description (at an appropriate level) of induction of general and regional anaesthesia – find out and discuss how these procedures feel
   c. a discussion of how women feel about caesarean section afterwards – consult women who have had the experience, and find some appropriate research papers.

3. It is sometimes said that giving a woman epidural analgesia results in a 'cascade of intervention'.

   a. Discuss this statement with colleagues on the labour ward.
   b. Are there ways of minimising this effect?
   c. How can midwives influence the outcome of such a labour to the woman's benefit?

REFERENCES

Barth W H 1992 Local infiltration for cesarean delivery. In: Ostheimer G W (ed) Manual of obstetric anesthesia, 2nd edn. Churchill Livingstone, New York

Belbin A 1996 Power and choice in birthgiving; a case study. British Journal of Midwifery 4(5): 264–267

Carli F 1990 With-holding top-ups in second stage is barbaric – arguments for. In: Morgan B M (ed) Controversies in obstetric anaesthesia, no 1. Edward Arnold, London

Clark V A, McQueen M A 1993 Factors influencing backache following epidural analgesia in labour. International Journal of Obstetric Anesthesia 2(4): 193–196

Crawford J S 1956 Some aspects of obstetric anaesthesia Part III. British Journal of Anaesthesia 28: 201–208

Crawford J S 1987 Pre-operative oral fluids. Anesthesia and Analgesia 66: 914–915

Department of Health, Welsh Office, Scottish Home and Health Department, Department of Health and Social Services, Northern Ireland 1991 Report on confidential enquiries into maternal deaths in the United Kingdom 1985–1987. HMSO, London

Department of Health, Welsh Office, Scottish Home and Health Department, Department of Health and Social

Services, Northern Ireland 1994 Report on confidential enquiries into maternal deaths in the United Kingdom 1988–1990. HMSO, London

Department of Health, Welsh Office, Scottish Home and Health Department, Department of Health and Social Services, Northern Ireland 1996 Report on confidential enquiries into maternal deaths in the United Kingdom 1991–1993. HMSO, London

Depp R 1991 Cesarean delivery and other surgical procedures. In: Gabbe S G, Niebyl J R, Simpson J L (eds) Obstetrics: normal and problem pregnancies, 2nd edn. Churchill Livingstone, Edinburgh

Doughty A 1987 Landmarks in the development of regional analgesia in obstetrics. In: Morgan B M (ed) Foundations of obstetric anaesthesia. Farrand Press, London

Fontenot R J, Price R L, Henry A et al 1993 Double-blind evaluation of patient-controlled epidural analgesia during labor. International Journal of Obstetric Anesthesia 2(2): 73–77

Francome C, Savage W, Churchill H, Lewison H 1993 Caesarean birth in Britain. Middlesex University Press, NCT, London

Gaynor A 1990 The lumbar epidural region. In: Reynolds F (ed) Epidural and spinal blockade in obstetrics. Baillière Tindall, London

Gild M W 1989 Informed consent: a review. Anesthesia and Analgesia 68: 649–653

House of Commons 1980 Second report from the Social Services Committee on perinatal and neonatal mortality (Chairman Renee Short). HMSO, London

Johnson C, Keirse M J N C, Enkin M, Chalmers I 1989 Nutrition and hydration in labour. In: Chalmers I, Enkin M, Keirse M J N C (eds) Effective care in pregnancy and childbirth. Oxford University Press, Oxford, vol 2

Kohner N, Henley A 1991 When a baby dies. SANDS, London

Kuhnert B R, Harrison M J, Linn P L et al 1984 Effects of maternal epidural anaesthesia on neonatal behavior. Anesthesia and Analgesia 63: 301–308

Llewellyn-Jones D 1994 Fundamentals of obstetrics and gynaecology: volume 1, obstetrics, 6th edn. Mosby, London

MacArthur C, Lewis M, Knox E G et al 1990 Epidural anaesthesia and longterm backache after childbirth. British Medical Journal 301: 9–12

MacArthur C, Lewis M, Knox E G 1991 Health after childbirth. HMSO, London

MacDonald R 1990 Indications and contraindications for epidural blockade in obstetrics. In: Reynolds F (ed) Epidural and spinal blockade in obstetrics. Baillière Tindall, London

MacLeod K 1993 Epidural opiates should be abandoned in obstetric patients – arguments against. In: Morgan B M (ed) Controversies in obstetric anaesthesia, no 2. Edward Arnold, London

Meehan F P 1987 Historical review of caudal epidural analgesia in obstetrics. Midwifery 3(1): 39–45

Moir D D, Thorburn J 1986 Obstetric anaesthesia and analgesia. Baillière Tindall, London

Morgan B M (ed) 1987 Foundations of obstetric anaesthesia. Farrand Press, London

Morgan B M 1995 Protocol for mobile epidural analgesia. Queen Charlottes and Chelsea Hospital, Goldhawk Road, London W6 0XG, UK

Morgan B M, Kadim M Y 1994 Mobile regional analgesia in labour. British Journal of Obstetrics and Gynaecology 101: 839–841

Morgan B M, Bulpitt C J, Clifton P et al 1982 Analgesia and satisfaction in childbirth (the Queen Charlottes 1000 mother survey). Lancet ii: 808–810

Murphy J D, Henderson K, Bowden M I et al 1991 Bupivacaine versus bupivacaine plus fentanyl for epidural analgesia: the effect on maternal satisfaction. British Medical Journal 302(6776): 564–567

Murray-Parkes C 1986 Bereavement: studies of grief in adult life, 2nd edn. Tavistock Publications, London

Myerscough P R 1982 Munro Kerr's operative obstetrics, 10th edn. Baillière Tindall, London

O'Brien W F, Cefalo R C 1991 Labor and delivery. In: Gabbe S G, Niebyl J R, Simpson J L (eds) Obstetrics: normal and problem pregnancies, 2nd edn. Churchill Livingstone, Edinburgh

Ostheimer G W 1992 Paracervical block. In: Ostheimer G W (ed) Manual of obstetric anesthesia, 2nd edn. Churchill Livingstone, New York

Ostheimer G W, Leavitt K A 1992 Pudendal nerve block and local infiltration for vaginal delivery. In: Ostheimer G W (ed) Manual of obstetric anesthesia, 2nd edn. Churchill Livingstone, New York

O'Sullivan G 1997 Epidural analgesia in labour: recent developments. British Journal of Midwifery 5(9): 555–556

Ranta P, Jouppila P, Spalding M et al 1995 Paracervical block – a viable alternative for labor pain relief? Acta Obstetrica et Gynecologica Scandinavica 72(2): 122–126

Reynolds F 1989 Epidural analgesia in obstetrics; pros and cons for mother and baby. British Medical Journal 299: 751–752

Reynolds F 1990 Epidural and spinal blockade in obstetrics. Baillière Tindall, London

Reynolds F 1993 Effects on the baby of maternal analgesia and anaesthesia. W B Saunders, London

Roberts R B, Shirley M A 1976 The obstetrician's role in reducing the risk of aspiration pneumonitis. American Journal of Obstetrics and Gynecology 124: 611–617

Rosevear S K, Stirrat G M 1996 Handbook of obstetric management. Blackwell Science, Oxford

Russell R, Groves P, Taub N et al 1993 Assessing longterm backache after childbirth. British Medical Journal 306(6888): 1299–1303

Schott J, Henley A 1996 Culture, religion and childbearing in a multiracial society. Butterworth Heinemann, Oxford

Scott D 1993 Pre-loading prior to regional block is an old wives tale – arguments for. In: Morgan B M (ed) Controversies in obstetric anaesthesia, no 2. Edward Arnold, London

Simkin P 1991 Just another day in a woman's life? Women's longterm perceptions of their first birth experience. Birth 18(4): 203–210

United Kingdom Central Council for Nursing, Midwifery and Health Visiting (UKCC) 1992 Standards for the administration of medicines. UKCC, London

United Kingdom Central Council for Nursing, Midwifery and Health Visiting (UKCC) 1993 Midwives rules. UKCC, London

United Kingdom Central Council for Nursing, Midwifery and Health Visiting (UKCC) 1994 The midwife's code of practice. UKCC, London

Vacca A 1992 Handbook of vacuum extraction in obstetric practice. Edward Arnold, London

Vacca A, Keirse M J N C 1989 Instrumental vaginal delivery.

In: Chalmers I, Enkin M and Keirse M J N C (eds)
Effective care in pregnancy and childbirth. Oxford
University Press, Oxford, vol 2
Walkinshaw S A, Crosfill F 1990 Labour with epidural
analgesia: second thoughts about the second stage. Journal

of Obstetrics and Gynaecology 10(6): 499–502
Woods S 1993 Epidural opiates should be abandoned in
obstetric patients – arguments for. In: Morgan B M (ed)
Controversies in obstetric anaesthesia, no 2. Edward
Arnold, London

FURTHER READING

Association of Anaesthetists of Great Britain and Ireland and
The Obstetric Anaesthetists Association 1988 Anaesthetic
services for obstetrics: a plan for the future. Association of
Anaesthetists of Great Britain and Ireland, 9 Bedford
Square, London WC1B 3RA and The Obstetric
Anaesthetists Association, London

Bevis R 1984 Anaesthesia in midwifery. Baillière Tindall,
London

Bevis R 1997 Drugs in labour. In: Moore S (ed)
Understanding pain and its relief in labour. Churchill
Livingstone, Edinburgh

Bevis R 1997 Regional analgesia. In: Moore S (ed)
Understanding pain and its relief in labour. Churchill
Livingstone, Edinburgh

Carrie L E S 1987 Regional techniques in obstetrics.
In: Wildsmith J A W, Armitage E N (eds) Principles and
practice of regional anaesthesia. Churchill Livingstone,
Edinburgh

Chamberlain G, Wraight A, Steer P 1993 Pain and its relief in
childbirth: the National Birthday Trust Fund survey.
Churchill Livingstone, Edinburgh

Dickersin K 1989 Pharmacological control of pain during
labour. In: Chalmers I, Enkin M and Keirse M J N C (eds)
Effective care in pregnancy and childbirth. Oxford
University Press, Oxford, vol 2

Kitzinger S 1987 Some women's experiences of epidurals; a
descriptive study. National Childbirth Trust, London

Llewellyn-Jones D 1986 Fundamentals of obstetrics and
gynaecology, 4th edn. Faber & Faber, London

Mander R 1992 The control of pain in labour. Journal of
Clinical Nursing 1: 219–223

Mander R 1993 Epidural analgesia 1: recent history. British
Journal of Midwifery 1(6): 259–263

Mander R 1994 Epidural analgesia 2: research basis. British
Journal of Midwifery 2(1): 12–16

Morgan B M 1993 Mobile epidurals: combined
spinal/epidural analgesia in labour. MIDIRS Midwifery
Digest 3(3): 312–313

Reynolds F 1993 Pain relief in labour. British Journal of
Obstetrics and Gynaecology 100: 979–983

Thorp J A, McNitt J D, Leppert P C 1990 Effects of epidural
analgesia: some questions and answers. Birth 17(3): 157–162

29

Midwifery and obstetric emergencies

Christine V. Shiers   *Terri Coates* (Section on 'Shoulder dystocia')

CHAPTER CONTENTS

The immediate management of the emergencies discussed in this chapter is dependent on the prompt action of the midwife. The speed of this action while calling for medical aid will often help to determine the outcome for the mother or the baby. Recognition of the problem and the instigation of emergency measures allow time for help to arrive.

The chapter aims to:

- describe emergency situations including vasa praevia, cord prolapse and shoulder dystocia, with discussion on possible causes and action to be taken

- consider the rare conditions of uterine rupture and acute inversion, neither of which need occur with good management

- discuss amniotic fluid embolism, which remains an unpredictable catastrophe in which prompt action is needed to preserve the mother's life

- recommend strongly the practising of procedures for basic resuscitation on a regular basis

- provide information on shock, focusing on the conditions of hypovolaemic shock and septic shock, both of which may be seen in midwifery practice.

The midwife should remain alert to the possibility that the emergency, as in the case of sudden collapse, may not be directly associated with the mother's pregnancy. Basic life-support measures are included in this chapter.

VASA PRAEVIA

This term is used when a fetal blood vessel lies over the os, in front of the presenting part. This occurs when fetal vessels from a velamentous insertion of the cord cross the area of the internal os to the placenta. The fetus is in jeopardy, owing to the risk of rupture of the vessels, which could lead to exsanguination.

Vasa praevia may sometimes be palpated on vaginal examination when the membranes are still intact. It may also be visualised on ultrasound. If it is suspected a speculum examination should be made.

Ruptured vasa praevia

When the membranes rupture in a case of vasa praevia, a fetal vessel may also rupture. This leads to exsanguination of the fetus unless birth occurs within minutes.

Diagnosis

Slight fresh vaginal bleeding, particularly if it commences at the same time as rupture of the membranes, may be due to ruptured vasa praevia. Fetal distress disproportionate to blood loss may be suggestive of vasa praevia.

Management

The midwife should call for assistance, requesting urgent medical aid. The fetal heart rate should be monitored. If in the first stage of labour and the fetus is still alive, an emergency caesarean section is carried out. If the mother is in the second stage of labour, delivery should be expedited and a vaginal birth may be achieved. Caesarean section may be carried out but mode of delivery will be dependent on parity and fetal condition.

A paediatrician should be present at delivery and, if the baby is alive, haemoglobin estimation will be necessary after resuscitation. The baby will require a blood transfusion but there is a high mortality associated with this emergency.

PRESENTATION AND PROLAPSE OF THE UMBILICAL CORD (Box 29.1)

Predisposing factors

These are the same for both presentation and prolapse of the cord. Any situation where the presenting part is neither well applied to the lower

---

> **Box 29.1** Definitions
>
> **Cord presentation**
> This occurs when the umbilical cord lies in front of the presenting part, with the fetal membranes still intact.
>
> **Cord prolapse**
> The cord lies in front of the presenting part and the fetal membranes are ruptured (Fig. 29.1).
>
> **Occult cord prolapse**
> This is said to occur when the cord lies alongside, but not in front of, the presenting part.
>
> Prolapse of the umbilical cord is associated with increases in fetal mortality and morbidity.

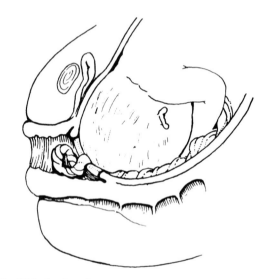

Fig. 29.1 Cord prolapse.

uterine segment nor well down in the pelvis may make it possible for a loop of cord to slip down in front of the presenting part. Such situations include:

- high or ill-fitting presenting part
- high parity
- prematurity
- multiple pregnancy
- malpresentation
- polyhydramnios (Mesleh et al 1993, Murphy & MacKenzie 1995).

High head. If the membranes rupture spontaneously when the fetal head is high, a loop of cord may be able to pass between the uterine wall and the fetus, resulting in it lying in front of the presenting part. As the presenting part descends the cord becomes occluded.

Multiparity. The presenting part may not be engaged when the membranes rupture and malpresentation is more common.

Prematurity. The size of the fetus in relation to the pelvis and the uterus allows the cord to prolapse. Babies of very low birthweight, less than 1500 g, are particularly vulnerable (Mesleh et al 1993).

Malpresentation. Cord prolapse is associated with breech presentation, especially complete or footling breech. This relates to the ill-fitting nature of the presenting parts and also the proximity of the umbilicus to the buttocks. In this situation the degree of compression may be less than with a cephalic presentation but there is still a danger of asphyxia.

Shoulder and compound presentations and transverse lie carry a high risk of prolapse of the cord, occurring with spontaneous rupture of the membranes.

Face and brow presentations are less common causes of cord prolapse.

Multiple pregnancy. Malpresentation, particularly of the second twin, is more common in multiple pregnancy.

Polyhydramnios. The cord is liable to be swept down in a gush of liquor if the membranes rupture spontaneously. Controlled release of liquor during artificial rupture of the membranes is sometimes performed to try to prevent this.

Murphy & MacKenzie (1995) found in 55 cases out of a total 132 that none of the above factors could be attributed as the reason for cord prolapse.

Cord presentation

This is diagnosed on vaginal examination when the cord is felt behind intact membranes. It is, however, rarely detected but may be associated with aberrations in fetal heart monitoring, such as decelerations.

Management
Under no circumstances should the membranes be ruptured. The midwife should discontinue the vaginal examination, in order to reduce the risk of rupturing the membranes. Help should be summoned, including medical aid. If continuous electronic fetal monitoring is available, a recording may be commenced to assess fetal well-being. The mother should be helped into a position that will reduce the likelihood of cord compression. In the absence of continuous fetal monitoring the fetal heart should be auscultated as continuously as possible, particularly during contractions.

Caesarean section is the most likely outcome.

Cord prolapse

Diagnosis
The diagnosis of cord prolapse is made when the cord is felt below or beside the presenting part on vaginal examination. Whenever there are factors present which predispose to cord prolapse, a vaginal examination should be performed immediately on spontaneous rupture of membranes. An abnormal heart rate, particularly bradycardia, may indicate cord prolapse.

A loop of cord may be visible at the vulva. The cord is more commonly felt in the vagina or, in cases where the presenting part is very high, it may be felt in the cervical os.

Immediate action
Where the diagnosis of cord prolapse is made, the midwife should call for urgent assistance. The midwife should explain her findings to the mother and her birth attendants and the emergency measures that will be needed.

If an oxytocin infusion is in progress this should be stopped. The midwife carries out a vaginal examination and assesses the degree of cervical dilatation. She identifies the presenting part and station. The time should also be noted. If the cord can be felt pulsating, it should be handled as little as possible. Spasm of the cord may occur through handling or due to reduction in temperature. If the cord lies outside the vagina, then it should be gently replaced to try to maintain

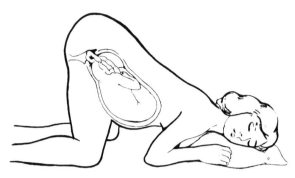

Fig. 29.2 Knee–chest position. Pressure on the umbilical cord is relieved as the fetus gravitates towards the fundus.

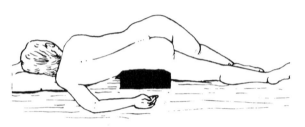

Fig. 29.3 Exaggerated Sims' position. Pillows or wedges are used to elevate the woman's buttocks to relieve pressure on the umbilical cord.

temperature. An assistant should be asked to auscultate the fetal heart and a record of the fetal heart rate is made.

Pressure on the cord must be relieved. In order to do this the midwife keeps her fingers in the vagina and, especially during a contraction, holds the presenting part off the umbilical cord. The mother is helped to change position so that her pelvis and buttocks are raised. The knee–chest position causes the fetus to gravitate towards the diaphragm, relieving the compression on the cord (Fig. 29.2). Alternatively the mother can be helped to lie on her left side, with a wedge or pillow elevating her hips (Fig. 29.3). The foot of the bed may be raised. These measures need to be maintained until the delivery of the baby, either vaginally or by caesarean section.

Management
The risks to the fetus are hypoxia and death as a result of cord compression. The risks are greatest with prematurity and low birthweight (Murphy

& MacKenzie 1995). Delivery must be expedited with the greatest possible speed to reduce the mortality and morbidity associated with this condition. Caesarean section is the treatment of choice in those instances where the fetus is still alive and delivery is not imminent, or vaginal birth cannot be indicated.

In the second stage of labour the mother may be able to push and the midwife may perform an episiotomy to expedite the birth. This may be possible with a multiparous mother. Where the presentation is cephalic, assisted birth may be achieved through ventouse or forceps.

If cord prolapse occurs in the community and the fetus is thought to still be alive, emergency transfer to hospital is essential. The midwife should carry out the same procedures to relieve the compression on the cord, with the mother adopting a left lateral position, with buttocks elevated (exaggerated Sims' position). Consultant unit staff should be informed and be prepared to perform an emergency caesarean section on arrival.

SHOULDER DYSTOCIA

Definition
The term 'shoulder dystocia' is used in this chapter to describe failure of the shoulders to spontaneously traverse the pelvis after delivery of the head (Smeltzer 1986). However, a universally accepted definition of shoulder dystocia has yet to be produced (Roberts 1994).

The anterior shoulder becomes trapped behind or on the symphysis pubis, whilst the posterior shoulder may be in the hollow of the sacrum or high above the sacral promontory (Fig. 29.4). This is, therefore, a bony dystocia, and traction at this point will further impact the anterior shoulder, impeding attempts at delivery.

Incidence
Shoulder dystocia is not a common emergency: the incidence is reported as varying between 0.37% and 1.1% (Bahar 1996).

Risk factors
Whilst it would be useful to identify those women

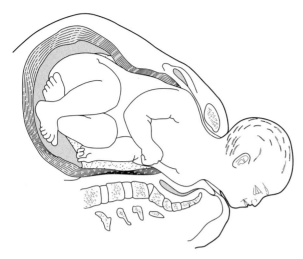

Fig. 29.4 Shoulder dystocia.

at risk from a delivery complicated by shoulder dystocia, most risk factors can only give a high index of suspicion (Al-Najashi et al 1989). Antenatally these risk factors include post-term pregnancy, high parity, maternal age over 35, and maternal obesity (weight over 90 kg at delivery).

Fetal macrosomia (birthweight over 4000 g) has been associated with an increased risk of shoulder dystocia, the incidence increasing as birthweight increases (Acker et al 1985, Delpapa & Mueller-Heubach 1991, Hall 1996). However, ultrasound scanning for prediction of macrosomia to prevent shoulder dystocia has a poor record of success (Combs et al 1993, Hall 1996).

Maternal diabetes and gestational diabetes have been identified as important risk factors (Bahar 1996, Benedetti & Gabbe 1978, Gross et al 1987, Spellacy et al 1985).

In diabetic women a previous delivery complicated by shoulder dystocia increases the risk of recurrence to 9.8%; this compares with a risk of recurrence of 0.58% in the general population (Smith et al 1994).

In labour, risk factors that have been consistently linked with shoulder dystocia include oxytocin augmentation, prolonged labour, prolonged second stage of labour and operative deliveries (Acker et al 1986, Al Najashi et al 1989, Bahar 1996, Benedetti & Gabbe 1978, Keller et al 1991).

Warning signs and diagnosis

The delivery may have been uncomplicated initially (Morris 1955), but the head may have advanced slowly and the chin may have had difficulty sweeping over the perineum. Once the head is delivered it may look as if it is trying to return into the vagina, which is caused by reverse traction.

Shoulder dystocia is diagnosed when manoeuvres normally used by the midwife fail to accomplish delivery (Resnik 1980).

Management

Upon diagnosing shoulder dystocia the midwife must summon help immediately. An obstetrician, an anaesthetist and a person proficient in neonatal resuscitation should be called.

Shoulder dystocia is a frightening experience for the mother, for her partner and for the midwife. The midwife should keep calm and try to explain as much as possible to the mother to ensure her full cooperation for the manoeuvres that may be needed to complete the delivery.

The purpose of all these manoeuvres is to disimpact the shoulders and accomplish delivery. The principle of using the most simple manoeuvres first should be applied.

The midwife will need to make an accurate and detailed record of the type of manoeuvre(s) used and the time taken, the amount of force used and the outcome of each manoeuvre attempted.

Non-invasive procedures

Change in maternal position. Any change in the maternal position may be useful to help release the fetal shoulders. However, certain manoeuvres have proved useful and are described below. It is anticipated that following the use of one or more of these manoeuvres the midwife should be able to proceed with the delivery.

The McRoberts manoeuvre. This manoeuvre involves helping the woman to lie flat and to bring her knees up to her chest as far as possible (Fig. 29.5).

This manoeuvre will rotate the angle of the symphysis pubis superiorly and use the weight of the mother's legs to create gentle pressure on her abdomen, releasing the impaction of the anterior

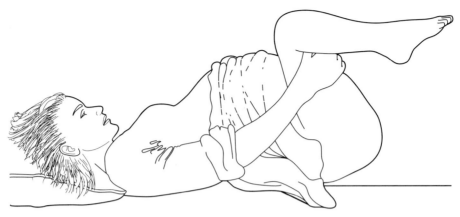

Fig. 29.5 The McRoberts manoeuvre position.

shoulder (Gonik et al 1983, Gonik et al 1989). This manoeuvre is associated with the lowest level of morbidity and requires the least force to accomplish delivery (Bahar 1996, Gross et al 1987, Nocon et al 1993).

Suprapubic pressure.   Pressure should be exerted on the side of the fetal back and towards the fetal chest. This manoeuvre may help to adduct the shoulders and push the anterior shoulder away from the symphysis pubis (Fig. 29.6).

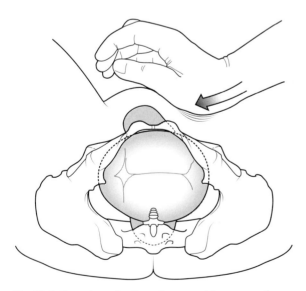

Fig. 29.6 Correct application of suprapubic pressure for shoulder dystocia. (Based on Pauerstein C (ed) 1987 with kind permission.)

Manipulative procedures
Where non-invasive procedures have not been successful, direct manipulation of the fetus must now be attempted.

Positioning of the mother. The McRoberts position as detailed above can be used, or the mother could be placed in the lithotomy position with her buttocks well over the end of the bed so that there is no restriction on the sacrum. If neither the McRoberts nor lithotomy positions are appropriate, then the all-fours position may prove useful. Any of the following manoeuvres can be undertaken with the mother in one of these positions.

Episiotomy. It must be remembered that the problem facing the midwife is an obstruction at the pelvic inlet and is a bony dystocia, not an obstruction caused by soft tissue. Whilst episiotomy will not help to release the shoulders per se, the midwife should perform one (see Ch. 24) to gain access to the fetus without tearing the perineum and vaginal walls.

Rubin's manoeuvre. This manoeuvre (Rubin 1964) requires the midwife to identify the posterior shoulder on vaginal examination, then to push the posterior shoulder in the direction of the fetal chest, thus rotating the anterior shoulder away from the symphysis pubis. By adducting the shoulders this manoeuvre reduces the 12-cm bisacromial diameter (Fig. 29.7).

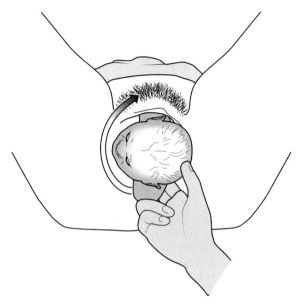

Fig. 29.7 The Rubin manoeuvre.

Woods' manoeuvre. Woods' (1943) manoeuvre requires the midwife to insert her hand into the vagina and identify the fetal chest. Then, by exerting pressure onto the posterior fetal shoulder, rotation is achieved. Whilst this manoeuvre does abduct the shoulders it will rotate the shoulders into a more favourable diameter and enable the midwife to complete the delivery (Fig. 29.8).

Delivery of the posterior arm. To deliver the posterior arm the midwife has to insert her hand into the vagina making use of the space created by the hollow of the sacrum. Then, two fingers splint the humerus of the posterior arm, flex the elbow, and sweep the forearm over the chest to deliver the hand (Fig. 29.9) (O'Leary 1992). If the rest of the delivery is not then accomplished, the second arm can be delivered following rotation of the shoulder using either Woods' or Rubin's

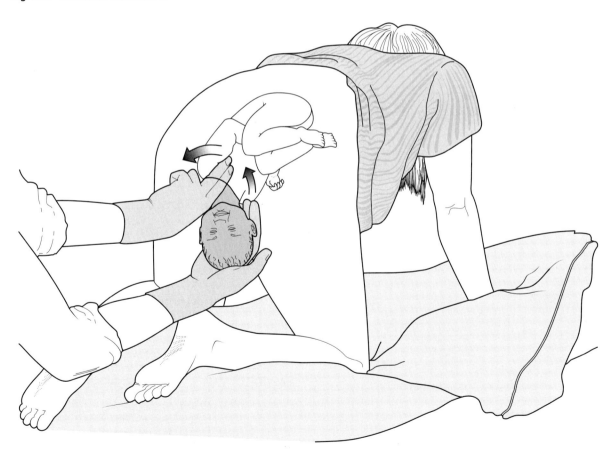

Fig. 29.8 The Woods manoeuvre. (Based on Sweet & Tiran 1996, p. 664, with kind permission.)

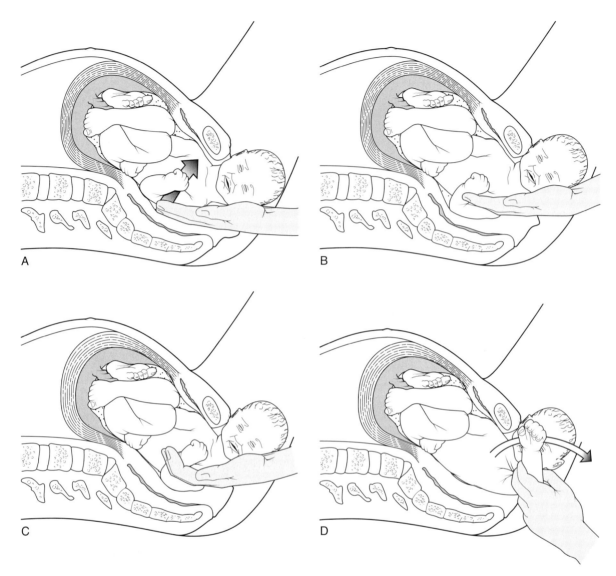

Fig. 29.9 Delivery of the posterior arm: (A) location of the posterior arm; (B) directing the arm into the hollow of the sacrum; (C) grasping and splinting the wrist and forearm; (D) sweeping the arm over the chest and delivering the hand.

manoeuvre or by reversing the Lovset manoeuvre (Ch. 27).

Zavanelli manoeuvre. If the manoeuvres described above have been unsuccessful, the obstetrician may consider the Zavanelli manoeuvre (Sandberg 1985) as a last hope for delivery of a live infant.

The Zavanelli manoeuvre requires the reversal of the mechanisms of delivery so far and reinsertion of the fetal head into the vagina. Delivery is then completed by caesarean section.

Method. The head is returned to its pre-restitution position (Fig. 29.10A). Pressure is then exerted onto the occiput and the head is returned to the vagina (Fig. 29.10B). Prompt delivery by caesarean section is then required.

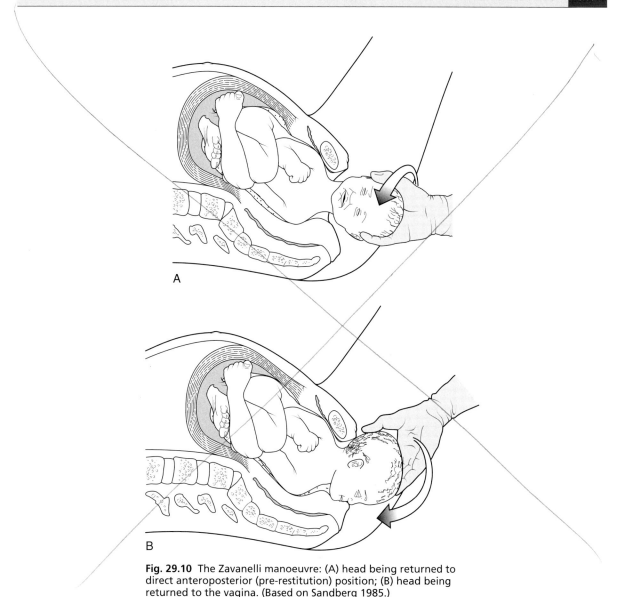

Fig. 29.10 The Zavanelli manoeuvre: (A) head being returned to direct anteroposterior (pre-restitution) position; (B) head being returned to the vagina. (Based on Sandberg 1985.)

Outcomes following shoulder dystocia

Maternal outcome

Approximately two-thirds will have a blood loss of more than 1000 ml from injury associated with the delivery (Benedetti & Gabbe 1978). Maternal death from uterine rupture has been reported following the use of fundal pressure (Seigworth 1966) and from haemorrhage during and following the delivery (O'Leary 1992).

Fetal outcome

Neonatal asphyxia may occur following shoulder dystocia in 5.7% to 9.7% of cases (Acker et al 1985, Modanlou et al 1980, Naef & Morrison 1994).

Brachial plexus injury with damage to cervical nerve roots 5 and 6 may result in an Erb's palsy (see also Ch. 40). This is commonly associated with shoulder dystocia when the head and neck have been twisted (Ubachs et al 1995).

Neonatal morbidity may be as high as 42%

following shoulder dystocia. Fetal damage may occur even with excellent management using appropriate obstetric manoeuvres (Naef & Morrison 1994). Shoulder dystocia remains a cause of intrapartum fetal death.

RUPTURE OF THE UTERUS

This is one of the most serious complications in midwifery and obstetrics. It is often fatal for the fetus and may also be responsible for the death of the mother. With effective antenatal and intrapartum care this complication should be avoided but it remains a significant problem worldwide.

Rupture of the uterus is defined as being complete or incomplete.

Complete rupture involves a tear in the wall of the uterus with or without expulsion of the fetus.

Incomplete rupture involves tearing of the uterine wall but not the perimetrium.

Life of both mother and fetus may be endangered in either situation.

Dehiscence of an existing uterine scar may also occur. This involves rupture of the uterine wall but the fetal membranes remain intact. The fetus is retained within the uterus and not expelled into the peritoneal cavity (Cunningham et al 1993).

Overall the risk of uterine rupture is said to be 1 in 1424 deliveries (Eden et al 1986). When the mother has a trial of labour following a previous caesarean section the risk of rupture of the uterus is 0.87% (Flamm et al 1994, Leung et al 1993).

Three deaths occurred in the UK during the period 1991–1993 as a result of spontaneous rupture of the uterus. One mother died in the same period from traumatic rupture. This constitutes 3.1% of the direct deaths reported in the UK during 1991–1993, a slight increase on the previous report. Evidence of substandard care is cited as contributing to the deaths (DH et al 1996).

Causes of rupture of the uterus
Spontaneous rupture of the uterus can be precipitated in the following circumstances:

• high parity

• injudicious use of oxytocin, particularly where the mother is of high parity
• obstructed labour: the uterus ruptures owing to excessive thinning of the lower segment
• neglected labour, where there is previous history of caesarean section
• extension of severe cervical laceration upwards into the lower uterine segment – this may be the result of trauma during an assisted birth (DH et al 1996)
• trauma, as a result of a blast injury or an accident (Awwad et al 1993)
• perforation of the non-pregnant uterus may result in rupture of the uterus in a subsequent pregnancy; perforation and rupture occur in the upper segment (Howe 1993)
• antenatal rupture of the uterus may occur where there has been a history of previous classical caesarean section.

Cases of spontaneous rupture of an unscarred uterus in primigravid mothers are reported in the literature (Guirgis & Kettle 1989, Roberts & Trew 1991).

Signs of intrapartum rupture of the uterus
Complete rupture of a previously non-scarred uterus may be accompanied by sudden collapse of the mother, who complains of severe abdominal pain. Maternal pulse rate increases. Simultaneously, alterations of the fetal heart may occur, including the presence of variable decelerations (Flannelly et al 1993, Phelan 1990). Heart sounds may be lost (Rachagan et al 1991). There may be evidence of fresh vaginal bleeding. The uterine contractions may stop and the contour of the abdomen alters. The fetus becomes palpable in the abdomen as the presenting part regresses. The degree and speed of the mother's collapse and shock depend on the extent of the rupture and the blood loss.

Incomplete rupture of the uterus

Incomplete rupture may have an insidious onset or be silent, found only after delivery or during a caesarean section. This is more commonly associated with previous caesarean section. Blood loss associated with dehiscence, or incomplete rupture, can be scanty, as the rupture occurs along the fibrous scar tissue (O'Connor & Gaughan 1993).

Incomplete rupture may also be manifest as a cause of postpartum haemorrhage following vaginal birth. Whenever shock during the third stage is more severe than the type of delivery or blood loss warrants or the mother fails to respond to treatment given, the possibility of incomplete rupture should be considered.

Management

An immediate caesarean section is performed, in the hope of delivering a live baby. Following the delivery of the fetus and placenta the extent of the rupture can be assessed. The options to perform a hysterectomy or to repair the rupture depend on the extent of the trauma and the mother's condition. Further clinical assessment will include evaluation of the need for blood replacement and management of any shock.

The mother will be unprepared for the events that have occurred and therefore may be totally opposed to hysterectomy. Reports of successful pregnancy following repair of uterine rupture are available (O'Connor & Gaughan 1993).

AMNIOTIC FLUID EMBOLISM

This rare but potentially catastrophic condition occurs when amniotic fluid enters the maternal circulation via the uterus or placental site. The body responds in two phases. The initial phase is one of pulmonary vasospasm causing hypoxia, hypotension and cardiovascular collapse. The second phase sees the development of left ventricular failure, with haemorrhage and coagulation disorder followed by pulmonary oedema. Mortality and morbidity are high (Clark 1990).

The traditional view is that the amniotic fluid forms an embolus which obstructs the pulmonary arterioles or alveolar capillaries. Following the establishment of a national registry in the United States of America a review of cases suggests that the presence of amniotic fluid in the maternal circulation triggers an anaphylactoid response and that the term embolus is a misnomer (Clark et al 1995).

Predisposing factors

Amniotic fluid embolism can occur at any gestation. It is mostly associated with labour and its immediate aftermath but cases in early pregnancy and postpartum have been documented. There is no evidence to suggest that parity places mothers at any increased risk nor can the condition be attributed to the use of oxytocics (Clark 1990, Clark et al 1995, Morgan 1979).

The risk of amniotic fluid infusion is associated with the exposure of the maternal circulation to even small quantities of amniotic fluid. Transfer of amniotic fluid from the uterus to the maternal circulation can be insidious, associated with a tear in the membranes. Chance entry of amniotic fluid into the circulation under pressure may occur, although the hypertonic uterine activity seen in some cases may be a consequence of uterine hypoxia that occurs in the first phase rather than as a precursor to the condition. Uterine hypertonus protects against liquor transferring into the maternal circulation rather than being responsible for pumping liquor across (Clark et al 1995).

The barrier between the maternal circulation and the amniotic sac may be breached in the presence of a placental abruption, when the placental bed is disrupted. Procedures such as insertion of an intrauterine catheter and artificial rupture of membranes are also associated.

Amniotic fluid embolism can occur during a caesarean section and is not prevented by performing a caesarean section. It may also occur in association with a perforated or ruptured uterus. Trauma may occur during an intrauterine manipulation, such as internal podalic version. The opportunity for amniotic fluid to enter the mother's circulation may also occur during termination of pregnancy.

It is a condition that is difficult to predict and equally difficult to prevent. Amniotic fluid embolism has been associated with a high maternal mortality rate, with little alteration in the total numbers of deaths attributed to it in the UK over the last two decades. 10% of the direct deaths in 1991–1993 were from amniotic fluid embolism.

Clinical signs and symptoms

There is sudden onset of maternal respiratory distress. The woman becomes severely dyspnoeic and cyanosed. There is maternal hypotension and uterine hypertonia. The latter will induce fetal distress and is in response to uterine hypoxia. Cardiopulmonary arrest follows quickly. Minutes only may elapse before arrest. There is evidence that many mothers present with convulsions immediately preceding the collapse (Clark 1990).

Blood coagulopathy develops following the initial collapse, if the mother survives. Where cases have been confirmed, mortality within 1 hour from onset is 50% (Chatelain & Quirk 1990).

Emergency action

Any one of the above symptoms is indicative of an acute emergency. As the mother is likely to be in a state of collapse resuscitation needs to be commenced at once. An emergency team should be called, since the midwife responsible for the care of the mother requires immediate help.

If collapse occurs in a community setting, basic life support should be commenced prior to the arrival of emergency services.

Despite improvements in intensive care the outcome of this condition is poor. Specific management for the condition is life support and high levels of oxygen are required. Mothers who survive are likely to have suffered a degree of neurological impairment (Clark et al 1995).

Complications of amniotic fluid embolism

Disseminated intravascular coagulation (DIC) is likely to occur within 30 minutes of the initial collapse. In some cases the mother bleeds heavily prior to developing amniotic fluid embolism which contributes to the severity of her condition. It has also been reported that the amniotic fluid has the ability to suppress the myometrium, resulting in uterine atony. This further compounds the haemorrhage (Courtney 1970).

Acute renal failure is a complication of the excessive blood loss and the prolonged hypovolaemic hypotension. The mother will require continuous assessment of urinary output, using an indwelling catheter. Accurate records of fluid intake and urinary output and urinalysis should be maintained by the midwife. A urinary output of less than 30 ml per hour should be reported, as should the presence of proteinuria. Transfer to an intensive therapy unit for specialised nursing care is indicated.

Effect of amniotic fluid embolism on the fetus

Perinatal mortality and morbidity are high, where amniotic fluid embolism occurs before the birth of the baby. Delay in the time from initial maternal collapse to delivery needs to be minimal, if fetal compromise or death is to be avoided. However, maternal resuscitation may, at that time, be a priority.

ACUTE INVERSION OF THE UTERUS

This is a rare but potentially life-threatening complication of the third stage of labour. It occurs in approximately 1 in 2500 births (Brar et al 1989).

In the most serious cases the inner surface of the fundus appears at the vaginal outlet. In less severe cases the fundus is dimpled.

A midwife's awareness of the precipitating factors enables her to take preventive measures to avoid this emergency.

Classification of inversion

Inversion can be classified according to severity as follows:

First degree. The fundus reaches the internal os.

Second degree. The body or corpus of the uterus is inverted to the internal os (Fig. 29.11).

Third degree. The uterus, cervix and vagina are inverted and are visible.

Classification is also given according to timing of the prolapse:

Acute. Prolapse occurs immediately after delivery, with the placenta still attached.

Subacute and chronic inversion occur after the first 24 hours.

It is the former, acute inversion, that the remainder of this section considers.

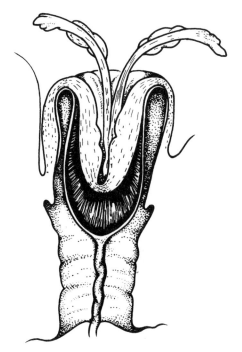

Fig. 29.11 Second degree inversion of the uterus.

Causes

Causes of acute inversion are associated with uterine atony and cervical dilatation:

- mismanagement in the third stage of labour, involving excessive cord traction
- combining fundal pressure and cord traction to deliver the placenta
- use of fundal pressure while the uterus is atonic, to deliver the placenta
- pathologically adherent placenta (Kitchin et al 1975)
- spontaneous occurrence, the cause being unknown
- primiparity (Brar et al 1989, Platt & Druzin 1981)
- fetal macrosomia (Brar at al 1989)
- short umbilical cord (Kitchin et al 1975)
- sudden emptying of distended uterus.

Careful management of the third stage of labour is needed to prevent inversion. Palpation of the fundus to confirm that contraction has taken place, prior to controlled cord traction, is essential.

Recognition

The major sign of acute inversion is haemorrhage which occurs in 94% of documented cases. The loss is in a range of 800–1800 ml (Platt & Druzin 1981, Watson et al 1980).

Shock and sudden onset of pain is seen in 40% of affected mothers. The pain is thought to be caused by the stretching of the peritoneal nerves and the ovaries being pulled as the fundus inverts. Bleeding may or may not be present, depending on the degree of placental adherence to the uterine wall. The cause of the symptoms may not be readily apparent.

The fundus will not be palpable on abdominal examination and diagnosis may be missed if inversion is incomplete and therefore the fundus not visible at the introitus. A mass may be felt on vaginal examination.

Immediate action

A swift response is needed to reduce the risks to the mother.

1. Help is summoned, including appropriate medical support.

2. The midwife in attendance should immediately attempt to replace the uterus. This may be achieved by pushing the fundus with the palm of the hand, along the direction of the vagina, towards the posterior fornix. The uterus is then lifted towards the umbilicus and returned to position with a steady pressure (Johnson's manoeuvre). This, if successful, will reduce the risk to the mother.

3. An intravenous cannula should be inserted and fluids commenced. Blood should be taken for cross-matching prior to starting the infusion.

4. If the placenta is still attached, it should be left in situ as attempts to remove it at this stage may result in uncontrollable haemorrhage.

5. Once the uterus is repositioned, the operator should keep the hand in situ until a firm contraction is palpated. Oxytocics should be given to maintain the contraction (Shah-Hosseini & Evrard 1989).

If manual replacement fails, then medical or surgical intervention is required. The use of the hydrostatic method of replacement involves the instillation of warm saline infused through a giving set into the vagina. The pressure of the fluid builds up as several litres are run into the vagina and restores the uterus to the normal position, while the operator seals off the introitus by one hand inserted into the vagina.

Medical management

If the inversion cannot be manually replaced, it may be due to the development of a cervical constriction ring. Drugs can be utilised to relax the constriction and facilitate the return of the uterus to its normal position.

Throughout the events the mother and her partner should be kept informed of what is happening. Assessment of vital signs, including level of consciousness, is of utmost importance.

BASIC LIFE-SUPPORT MEASURES

Standards of basic life support have been agreed for health professionals and lay people throughout Europe. Basic life support refers to the maintenance of an airway and support for breathing, without any specialist equipment, other than possibly a pharyngeal airway.

The basic principles are:

A – airway
B – breathing
C – circulation.

1. The level of consciousness is established by shaking the mother's shoulders and enquiring whether she can hear.

2. Assistance is called for by ringing the emergency bell or asking the partner to call for help and then return to the midwife who must remain with the mother.

3. The mother is laid flat, removing pillows.

4. The airway is cleared of any mucus or vomit and any dentures removed.

5. The head is tilted back and the chin lifted upwards to improve the patency of the airway (Fig. 29.12).

6. The chest is observed for signs of respiratory effort. The midwife listens for breath sounds and

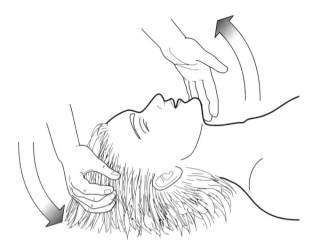

Fig. 29.12 Airway is opened by tilting the head backwards and lifting the chin upwards.

feels for breath being exhaled from the mouth and nose. An airway is inserted if available.

7. The pulse is palpated if necessary at the carotid artery. This is felt in the neck at the side of the mother's larynx.

8. If no breathing is detected the midwife will pinch the nose closed, take a deep breath in and exhale into the mother's mouth, so that her chest can be seen to rise. The air is then allowed to escape. The action is continued repeatedly. If available, a moulded face mask can be used or a rebreathing bag (Ambu-bag) attached to oxygen is used.

9. If there is no pulse, a precordial thump is delivered centrally to the sternum. A short, sharp blow is administered, using the fist. The blow should start from a height of 15 cm. The fist is removed quickly and the pulse is rechecked to see whether the blow has been effective in restarting the heart.

10. If the precordial thump is unsuccessful, the mother appears to be in cardiac arrest. External cardiac massage is needed. The xiphisternum is located. The hands are placed palm downwards on top of one another with the fingers interlinked. The heel of the lower hand is positioned on the lower two-thirds of the sternum. With arms straight, the operator leans onto the sternum depressing it 4–5 cm and releases it slowly at the same rate as compression. The action should be repeated 80 times a minute. The midwife may need to kneel

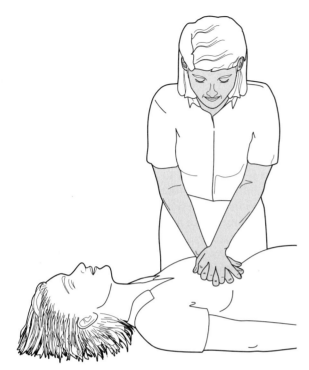

Box 29.2 Summary of basic life-support guidelines

1. Shake and shout
2. Call for help
3. Check breathing
4. Check pulse
5. Cardiac arrest – precordial thump to chest
6. Check pulse
7. 2 breaths to 15 compressions
8. Continue until help arrives

Fig. 29.13 Chest compression. Lean well over the patient, with arms straight. Hands are on top of each other with fingers interlinked. The heel of the hand is used to compress the chest.

over the mother or find something to stand on to ensure that she is suitably positioned to carry out resuscitation (Fig. 29.13). The surface under the mother must be firm for the manoeuvre to succeed.

11. Chest compression and ventilation should be continued until help arrives and until those experienced in resuscitation are able to take over. A rate of 15 chest compressions to 2 breaths is carried on if only one person is present; if two people are available, the rate is 5 compressions to 1 breath (European Resuscitation Council 1996).

These measures are summarised in Box 29.2.

SHOCK

Shock is a complex syndrome involving a reduction in blood flow to the tissues with resulting dysfunction of organs and cells. It entails progressive

collapse of the circulatory system and, if left untreated, can result in death. Shock can be acute but prompt treatment results in recovery, with little detrimental effect on the mother. However, inadequate treatment or failure to initiate effective treatment can result in a chronic condition ending in multisystem organ failure, which may be fatal.

Shock can be classified as follows:

1. *hypovolaemic* – the result of a reduction in intravascular volume
2. *cardiogenic* – impaired ability of the heart to pump blood
3. *distributive* – an abnormality in the vascular system that produces a maldistribution of the circulatory system; this includes septic and anaphylactic shock (Rice 1991).

This section deals with the principles of hypovolaemic shock and septic shock, either of which may develop as a consequence of events of childbearing.

Hypovolaemic shock

This is caused by any loss of circulating fluid volume that is not compensated for, as in haemorrhage, but may also occur when there is severe vomiting. The main causes and management of both these conditions are dealt with elsewhere.

The body reacts to the loss of circulating fluid in stages as follows:

Initial stage. The reduction in fluid or blood decreases the venous return to the heart. The ventricles of the heart are inadequately filled, causing a reduction in stroke volume and cardiac output. As cardiac output and venous return fall, the blood pressure is reduced. The drop in blood pressure decreases the supply of oxygen to the tissues and cell function is affected.

Compensatory stage. The drop in cardiac output produces a response from the sympathetic nervous system through the activation of receptors in the aorta and carotid arteries. Blood is redistributed to the vital organs. Vessels in the gastrointestinal tract, kidneys, skin and lungs constrict. This response is seen by the skin becoming pale and cool. Peristalsis slows, urinary output is reduced and exchange of gas in the lungs is impaired as blood flow diminishes. The heart rate increases in an attempt to improve cardiac output and blood pressure. Pupils of the eyes dilate. The sweat glands are stimulated and the skin becomes moist and clammy.

Adrenaline is released from the adrenal medulla and aldosterone from the adrenal cortex. Antidiuretic hormone is secreted from the posterior lobe of the pituitary. The combined effect is to cause vasoconstriction, an increased cardiac output and a decrease in urinary output. Venous return to the heart will increase but, unless the fluid loss is replaced, will not be sustained.

Progressive stage. This stage leads to multisystem failure. Compensatory mechanisms begin to fail, with vital organs lacking adequate perfusion. Volume depletion causes a further fall in blood pressure and cardiac output. The coronary arteries suffer lack of supply. Peripheral circulation is poor, with weak or absent pulses.

Final, irreversible stage of shock. Multisystem failure and cell destruction are irreparable. Death ensues.

Effect of shock on organs and systems

The human body is able to compensate for loss of up to 10% of fluid volume, principally by vasoconstriction. When loss reaches 20–25%, the compensatory mechanisms begin to decline and fail.

Brain. Level of consciousness deteriorates as cerebral blood flow is compromised. The mother will become increasingly unresponsive. She may not respond to verbal stimuli and there is a gradual reduction in the response elicited from painful stimulation.

Lungs. Gas exchange is impaired as the physiological dead space increases within the lungs. Levels of carbon dioxide rise and arterial oxygen levels fall. Ischaemia within the lungs alters production of surfactant and, as a result of this, alveoli collapse. Oedema in the lungs, due to increased permeability, exacerbates the existing problem of diffusion of oxygen. Atelectasis, oedema and reduced compliance impair ventilation and gaseous exchange, leading ultimately to respiratory failure. This is known as adult respiratory distress syndrome and features in some of the cases discussed in the 'Report on Confidential Enquiries into Maternal Deaths in the United Kingdom 1991–1993' (DH at al 1996).

Kidneys. The renal tubules become ischaemic, owing to the reduction in blood supply. As the kidneys fail, urine output falls to less than 20 ml per hour. The body does not excrete waste products such as urea and creatinine, so levels of these in the blood rise.

Gastrointestinal tract. The gut becomes ischaemic and its ability to function as a barrier against infection wanes. Gram-negative bacteria are able to enter the circulation.

Liver. Drug and hormone metabolism ceases, as does the conjugation of bilirubin. Unconjugated bilirubin builds up and jaundice develops. Protection from infection is further reduced as the liver fails to act as a filter. Metabolism of waste products does not occur, so there is a build up of lactic acid and ammonia in the blood. Death of hepatic cells releases liver enzymes into the circulation.

Management of shock

Urgent resuscitation is needed to prevent the mother's condition deteriorating and causing irreversible damage.

The priorities are to:

1. *Maintain the airway.* If the mother is severely

collapsed she should be turned onto her side and 40% oxygen administered at a rate of 4–6 litres per minute. If she is unconscious an airway should be inserted.

2. *Replace fluids.* Blood should be taken for cross-matching prior to commencing intravenous fluids. A plasma expander or fresh frozen plasma is given until whole blood of the correct match is available.

3. *Avoid warmth.* Constriction of the peripheral blood supply occurs in response to the shock and keeping the mother warm may interfere with this response, causing further deterioration in her condition.

Assessment of clinical condition

Once the mother's immediate condition is stable, the midwife should assess the mother's condition constantly. An interprofessional team approach to management should be adopted, to ensure that the correct level of expertise is available. A clear protocol for the management of shock should be used, with the midwife fully aware of key personnel required.

Clinical observations for the mother in shock

1. Assessment of level of consciousness. Any signs of restlessness or confusion should be noted.

2. Continuous monitoring of blood pressure, or at least every 30 minutes, with note taken of any drop in blood pressure.

3. Cardiac rhythm may be monitored continuously.

4. Measurement of urine output hourly, using indwelling catheter.

5. Assessment of skin colour, core and peripheral temperature hourly.

6. Haemodynamic measures of pressure in right atrium (central venous pressure) to monitor infusion rate and quantities. Fluid balance is maintained accurately (see below).

7. Observation for the occurrence of further bleeding, including oozing from wound or puncture sites.

Detailed observation charts should be accurately maintained. The extent of the mother's illness may require her transfer to a critical care unit.

Central venous pressure

In the presence of acute peripheral circulatory failure which accompanies severe shock the monitoring of central venous pressure (CVP) aids assessment of blood loss and indicates the fluid replacement required. In such a situation it is extremely dangerous to base an intravenous regimen on guesswork. Hyper- or hypovolaemia, cardiac and renal failure may result. CVP is the pressure in the right atrium or superior vena cava. It is an indicator of the volume of blood returning to the heart and reflects the competence of the heart as a pump and the peripheral vascular resistance.

Normal pressure varies between 5 and 10 cmH$_2$O. In shock the pressure will be persistently low, i.e. below 5 cm, and may even register a negative reading, indicating hypovolaemia. The correct volume of replacement fluids may then be assessed with greater accuracy.

Method of measuring CVP

A catheter is inserted into a major vein such as the subclavian or external jugular vein and advanced into the right atrium. The catheter is then connected to a manometer and an intravenous infusion using a three-way tap.

To take a manometer reading, the mother should be lying flat and the base of the manometer should be calibrated to measure 0 cm of water when aligned with the level of the right atrium. This point is level with a mid-axillary line for most people. The three-way tap is opened and filled with intravenous fluid. The fluid will fall and rise with respiratory effort and should be allowed to stabilise before a reading is taken. The highest level the fluid reaches is used for the CVP measurement. Once the reading is completed the tap is returned to the infusion position (Fig. 29.14).

A baseline observation is taken when the CVP catheter is inserted and the position in which the mother was lying is noted. Minor changes in position should be noted, as they may alter the CVP reading.

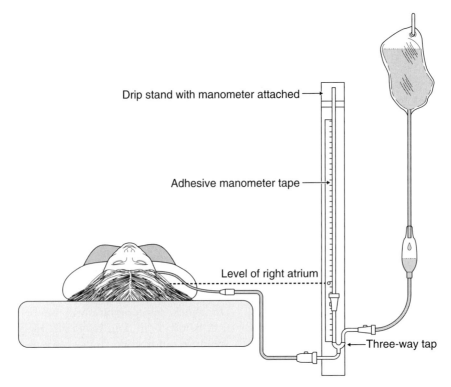

Drip stand with manometer attached

Adhesive manometer tape

Level of right atrium

Three-way tap

Fig. 29.14 Monitoring central venous pressure.

Principles of care of CVP lines

1. Prevention of infection. Insertion of the catheter requires strict asepsis. The site should be inspected regularly for signs of infection and precautions taken to protect against inadvertent contamination during clinical procedures.

2. Maintaining a closed system. The mother will bleed profusely if the catheter becomes disconnected, or incur a possible air embolus. Connections in particular should be checked (Ostrow 1981).

3. Maintaining patency of the catheter by preventing clot formation. Positive pressure of the infusion should be maintained.

Additional complications include pneumothorax, hydrothorax, trauma to lung or veins and cardiac arrhythmias during and due to insertion.

Septic shock

This is a distributive form of shock, where an overwhelming infection develops, commonly from Gram-negative organisms such as *Escherichia coli*, *Proteus* or *Pseudomonas pyocyaneus*. These organisms are common pathogens in the female genital tract and have endotoxins present in their cells. Endotoxins release components that trigger the body's immune response. Septic shock can less commonly be caused by Gram-positive bacteria, viral or fungal infection. In 20–30% of cases the infection is from multiple organisms, making treatment more complex.

The placental site is the main point of entry for an infection associated with pregnancy and childbirth. This may occur following septic abortion, prolonged rupture of fetal membranes, obstetric trauma or in the presence of retained placental tissue.

Clinical signs of septic shock

The mother may present with a sudden onset of tachycardia, pyrexia, rigors and tachypnoea. The mother may also exhibit a change in her mental state. Signs of shock, including hypotension, develop in septic shock as the condition takes hold.

Haemorrhage may be present. This could be a direct result of events due to childbearing, but it occurs in septic shock because of disseminated intravascular coagulation.

The body responds to septic shock in the following way. The primary responses to the infection are alterations in the peripheral circulation. Cells damaged by the infecting organism release histamine and enzymes that contribute to vasodilatation and increased permeability of the capillaries. Mediators are also produced that have the opposite action and vasoconstrict. The overall response, however, is one of vasodilation which reduces the systemic vascular resistance. Cardiac output remains elevated.

Vasodilation and continued hypotension lead to kidney damage, with reduced glomerular filtration, acute tubular necrosis and oliguria.

Adult respiratory distress syndrome occurs in many cases. Disseminated intravascular coagulation is also a feature of septic shock.

Multisystem organ failure will result as an effect of the continued hypotension and myocardial depression. Failure of the liver, brain and respiratory systems follows, and death.

Management of septic shock

This is based on preventing further deterioration by restoring circulatory volume and eradication of the infection. Replacement of fluid volume will restore perfusion of the vital organs. Satisfactory oxygenation is also needed.

Measures are needed to identify the source of infection and to protect against reinfection by maintaining high standards of care in clinical procedures. A full infection screening should be carried out including a high vaginal swab, midstream specimen of urine and blood cultures. Infusion sites and indwelling catheters should be checked for signs of contamination and changed as appropriate. Rigorous treatment with intravenous antibiotics, after blood cultures have been taken, is necessary to halt the illness.

Retained products of conception can be detected on ultrasound, and these can then be removed.

In situations where the mother requires to be transferred for critical or intensive care, relatives should be kept informed of progress. The midwife may be the person with whom the relatives have formed a relationship and therefore is relied on to give information.

The emergency situations included in this chapter are rare, but the actions of the midwife are fundamental to the well-being of mother, baby and also the partner. Awareness of local emergency procedures and knowledge of correct use of any supportive equipment is essential.

READER ACTIVITIES

1. Work through the scenario from diagnosis of cord prolapse to birth of the baby. With a colleague, practise positioning the 'mother' in knee–chest and exaggerated Sims' positions.

Consider the procedure in both a home and a hospital setting.

2. Practise the manipulative procedures described for shoulder dystocia using a doll and pelvis. It may be easier to work with a colleague.

Commit to memory a series of manoeuvres which may relieve shoulder dystocia.

Ensure that you are aware of the arrangements within your unit for obtaining rapid assistance for a case of shoulder dystocia.

3. Discover how often workshops are available for basic resuscitation training in your area. Plan to attend one if you have not updated your skills for the last 6 months. If workshops are not available, try your local libraries for training videos on basic life support.

4. Develop a care plan for a mother recovering from uterine inversion.

REFERENCES

Acker D B, Sachs B P, Friedman E A 1985 Risk factors for shoulder dystocia. Obstetrics and Gynecology 66(6): 762–768

Acker D B, Sachs B P, Friedman E A 1986 Risk factors for shoulder dystocia in the average weight infant. Obstetrics and Gynecology 67(5): 614–618

Al-Najashi S, Al-Suleiman S A, El-Yahia A, Raman M S, Raman J 1989 Shoulder dystocia – a clinical study of 56 cases. Australian and New Zealand Journal of Obstetrics and Gynecology 29: 129–131

Awwad J T, Azar G B, Aswad N K, Suidan F J, Karam K S 1993 Uterine rupture in pregnancy caused by blast injury with fetal survival. Journal of Obstetrics and Gynaecology 13(6): 448

Bahar A M 1996 Risk factors and fetal outcome in cases of shoulder dystocia compared with normal deliveries of a similar birthweight. British Journal of Obstetrics and Gynaecology 103: 868–872

Benedetti T J, Gabbe S G 1978 Shoulder dystocia: a complication of fetal macrosomia and prolonged second stage of labour with mid pelvic delivery. Obstetrics and Gynecology 52(5): 526–529

Brar H S, Greenspoon J S, Platt L D, Paul R H 1989 Acute puerperal uterine inversion. New approaches to management. Journal of Reproductive Medicine 34(2): 173–177

Chatelain S M, Quirk J G 1990 Amniotic and thromboembolism. Clinical Obstetrics and Gynecology 33(3): 473–481

Clark S L 1990 New concepts of amniotic fluid embolism: a review. Obstetrical and Gynecological Survey 45(6): 360–368

Clark S L, Hankins G D V, Dudley D A, Dildy G A, Porter T F 1995 Amniotic fluid embolism: an analysis of the national registry. American Journal of Obstetrics and Gynecology 172(4 Part 1): 1158–1169

Combs C A, Singh N B, Khoury J C 1993 Elective induction versus spontaneous labour after sonographic diagnosis of fetal macrosomia. Obstetrics and Gynecology 81(4): 492–496

Courtney L D 1970 Coagulation failure in pregnancy. British Medical Journal 1: 691

Cunningham F G, MacDonald P C, Gant N F, Leveno K J, Gilstrap L C 1993 Williams obstetrics, 19th edn. Prentice Hall, London, ch 23, pp 544–545

Delpapa E, Mueller-Hubach E 1991 Pregnancy outcome following ultrasound diagnosis of macrosomia. Obstetrics and Gynecology 78(1): 340–343

Department of Health, Welsh Office, Scottish Home and Health Department, Department of Health and Social Services, Northern Ireland 1996 Report on confidential enquiries into maternal deaths in the United Kingdom 1991–1993. HMSO, London

Eden R D, Parker R T, Stanley S A 1986 Rupture of the uterus: a 53 year review. Obstetrics and Gynecology 68: 671–674

European Resuscitation Council 1996. Guidelines for resuscitation. ERC, Antwerp

Flamm B L, Goings J R, Liu Y, Wolde-Tsadik G 1994 Elective repeat cesarian delivery versus trial of labor: A prospective multicenter study. Obstetrics and Gynecology 83: 927–932

Flannelly G M, Turner M J, Rassmussen M J, Stronge J M 1993 Rupture of the uterus in Dublin: an update. Journal of Obstetrics and Gynaecology 13: 440–443

Gonik B, Allen Stringer C, Held B 1983 An alternate maneuver for management of shoulder dystocia. American Journal of Obstetrics and Gynecology 145: 882–883

Gonik B, Allen R, Sorab J 1989 Objective evaluation of the shoulder dystocia phenomenon: effect of maternal pelvic orientation on force reduction. Obstetrics and Gynecology 74(1): 44–48

Gross S J, Shime J, Forrine D 1987 Shoulder dystocia: predictors and outcome. A five year review. American Journal of Obstetrics and Gynecology 56(2): 334–336

Guirgis R R, Kettle M J 1989 Uterine rupture in a primigravid patient. Journal of Obstetrics and Gynaecology 9(3): 214–215

Hall M 1996 Guessing the weight of the baby. British Journal of Obstetrics and Gynaecology 103: 734–736

Howe R S 1993 Third trimester uterine rupture following hysteroscopic uterine perforation. Obstetrics and Gynecology 81(5, Part 2): 827–829

Keller J D, Lopez J A, Dooley S L, Socol M L 1991 Shoulder dystocia and birth trauma in gestational diabetes: a five year experience. American Journal of Obstetrics and Gynecology 165: 928–930

Kitchin J D, Thiagarajah H, May H V, Thornton W N 1975 Puerperal inversion of the uterus. American Journal of Obstetrics and Gynecology 123(1): 51–58

Leung A S, Leung E K, Paul R H 1993 Uterine rupture after previous cesarean delivery: maternal and fetal consequences. American Journal of Obstetrics and Gynecology 169: 945–950

Mesleh R, Sultan M, Sabagh T, Algwiser A 1993 Umbilical cord prolapse. Journal of Obstetrics and Gynaecology 13(1): 24–28

Modanlou H D, Dorchester W L, Thorosian A, Freeman R K 1980 Macrosomia – maternal fetal and neonatal implications. Obstetrics and Gynecology 55(4): 420–424

Morgan M 1979 Amniotic fluid embolism. Anaesthesia 34: 20–32

Morris W I C 1955 Shoulder dystocia. Journal of Obstetrics and Gynaecology of the British Empire 62: 302–306

Murphy D J, MacKenzie I Z 1995 The mortality and morbidity associated with umbilical cord prolapse. British Journal of Obstetrics and Gynaecology 102: 826–830

Naef R W, Morrison J C 1994 Guidelines for management of shoulder dystocia. Journal of Perinatology 15(6): 435–441

Nocon J J, McKenzie D K, Thomas L J, Hansell R S 1993 Shoulder dystocia: An analysis of risk and obstetric maneuvers. American Journal of Obstetrics and Gynecology 168(6): 1732–1739

O'Connor R A, Gaughan B 1993 Rupture of the gravid uterus and its management. Journal of Obstetrics and Gynaecology 13: 29–33

O'Leary J A 1992 Shoulder dystocia and birth injury: Prevention and treatment. McGraw-Hill, New York

Ostrow L S 1981 Air embolism and central venous lines. American Journal of Nursing (November): 2036–2038

Pauerstein C (ed) 1987 Clinical obstetrics. Churchill Livingstone, New York

Phelan J P 1990 Uterine rupture. Clinical Obstetrics and Gynecology 33(3): 432–437

Platt L D, Druzin M L 1981 Acute puerperal inversion of the uterus. American Journal of Obstetrics and Gynecology 141(2): 187–190

Rachagan S P, Raman S, Balasundram G, Balakrishnan S 1991 Rupture of the uterus – a 21 year review. Australian and New Zealand Journal of Obstetrics and Gynaecology 31(1): 37–40

Resnik R 1980 Management of shoulder girdle dystocia. Clinical Obstetrics and Gynecology 23(2): 559–564

Rice V 1991 Shock, a clinical syndrome: an update Part 1. An overview of shock. Critical Care Nurse 11(4): 20–27

Roberts L 1994 Shoulder dystocia. In: Studd J (ed) Progress in obstetrics and gynaecology. Churchill Livingstone, Edinburgh, vol 11, ch 12, pp 201–216

Roberts L, Trew G 1991 Uterine rupture in a primigravida. Journal of Obstetrics and Gynaecology 11(4): 261–262

Rubin A 1964 Management of shoulder dystocia. Journal of the American Medical Association 189: 835

Sandberg E C 1985 The Zavanelli maneuver: a potentially revolutionary method for the resolution of shoulder dystocia. American Journal of Obstetrics and Gynecology 152: 479–487

Seigworth G R 1966 Shoulder dystocia: review of five years experience. Obstetrics and Gynecology 25(6): 764–767

Shah-Hosseini R, Evrard J R 1989 Puerperal uterine inversion. Obstetrics and Gynecology 73(4): 567–570

Smeltzer J S 1986 Prevention and management of shoulder dystocia. Clinical Obstetrics and Gynecology 29(2): 299–308

Smith R B, Lane C, Pearson J F 1994 Shoulder dystocia: what happens at the next delivery? British Journal of Obstetrics and Gynaecology 101: 713–715

Spellacy W N, Miller S, Winegar A, Peterson P Q 1985 Macrosomia maternal characteristics and infant complications. Obstetrics and Gynecology 66(2): 158–161

Sweet B R, Tiran D 1996 Mayes' Midwifery. Baillière Tindall, London

Ubachs J M H, Slooff A C J, Peeters L L H 1995 Obstetric antecedents of surgically treated obstetric brachial plexus injuries. British Journal of Obstetrics and Gynaecology 102: 813–817

Watson P, Besch N, Bowes W A 1980 Management of acute and subacute puerperal inversion of the uterus. Obstetrics and Gynecology 55(1): 12–16

Woods C E 1943 A principle of physics as applied to shoulder delivery. American Journal of Obstetrics and Gynecology 45: 796–805

FURTHER READING

Allott H 1994 A grief shared. British Medical Journal 308: 602

Coates T 1995 Shoulder dystocia. In: Alexander J, Levy V, Roch S (eds) Aspects of midwifery practice. Macmillan, Basingstoke, ch 4, pp 69–94

Coates T 1997 Shoulder dystocia: diagnosis, prediction and risk factors. Modern Midwife 7(8): 12–14

Coates T 1997 Manoeuvres for the relief of shoulder dystocia. Modern Midwife 7(9): 15–19

Coates T 1997 Shoulder dystocia outcome and education. Modern Midwife 7(10): 12–14

O'Leary J A 1992 Shoulder dystocia and birth injury: prevention and treatment. McGraw-Hill, New York

The puerperium

Physiology, complications and management of the puerperium

30

Liz Hynes (née Spruce)

CHAPTER CONTENTS

Effective postnatal care by the midwife, in partnership with the woman, is a vital component of the puerperium. Physiology and psychology are closely interrelated and the woman should be cared for holistically. However, in order to assist the development of knowledge and understanding of these two vital constituents of the puerperium, this chapter will concentrate on the normal physiological adaptation and associated complications, midwifery care and management. The psychological response to motherhood and postnatal mental illness is addressed in Chapter 31, which will conclude by discussion of the '6 week examination' thus reintegrating biological and behavioural components of the puerperium.

The chapter aims to:

- consider the role and responsibilities of the midwife throughout the postnatal period

- use the daily postnatal assessment examination as basis for exploring normal physiology and potential complications, thereby assisting the midwife to look at this aspect of practice in a logical way and to facilitate understanding of recognition of deviation from the normal physiological response

- discuss each element of the assessment procedure, integrating technique, physiology and management.

The puerperium is a period of approximately 6 weeks which commences following completion of the third stage of labour. During this time, the woman recovers from the stresses of pregnancy and delivery and the physiological adaptations which occurred during pregnancy subside, facilitating the restoration of the non-pregnant state. The new mother usually assumes responsibility for the care and nurture of her baby and lactation becomes established in women who choose to breast feed.

It is also a time of psychological adjustment during which the new parents experience a period of transition from their previous life to the assumption of the joys and responsibilities of family life.

THE MIDWIFE'S ROLE AND RESPONSIBILITIES DURING THE POSTNATAL PERIOD

The role of the midwife during the postnatal period is to provide care and support at a level determined in partnership with the woman. The postnatal period is defined as 'not less than ten and not more than 28 days after the end of labour, during which the continued attendance of a midwife on the mother and baby is requisite' (UKCC 1993).

The care which mothers and babies require is based upon four main principles:

- promoting physical and psychological well-being of the mother, her baby and the family unit
- the identification of deviation from normal physiological or psychological progress (see Ch. 31), with appropriate prompt referral where required
- encouraging sound methods of infant care and feeding (see Ch. 36) and promoting the development of effective parent–infant relationships
- supporting and strengthening the woman and her partner's confidence, thus facilitating their transition to the parenting role within their particular family and cultural environment.

NB: appropriate adaptation of these principles will be required for certain groups of women, for example following the loss of a baby.

The midwife should monitor maternal and infant progress remembering that women vary in their needs, expectations and attitudes and babies vary in their developing patterns of feeding and sleeping. A standard routine approach to care will not meet every woman's requirements and it is vital that care is adapted to meet developing needs. The promotion of a relaxed environment is conducive to the establishment of effective communication

networks between the woman, her family and the health professionals involved. The midwife must be non-judgemental in approach, offering guidance, advice and, when necessary, acting as an empathetic counsellor. It is not the midwife's role to make decisions on behalf of the woman nor to convey disapproval of a mother's decisions.

The midwife should promote breast feeding whenever possible but must respect individual choice and support the mother in whatever decision she makes concerning method of feeding (see Ch. 36). If the mother decides to use artificial feeding, the midwife must give advice and guidance on the preparation of artificial feeds and sterilising of equipment (see Ch. 36).

READER ACTIVITY

How flexible is the philosophy of care for your client group? List aspects which you think require development and discuss these with your peers and colleagues. Where appropriate, incorporate the consumer view in any proposed changes.

THE MANAGEMENT OF POSTNATAL CARE

The management of postnatal care begins in the delivery suite and extends throughout the postnatal period. The majority is generally undertaken within the home environment, regardless of place of birth. Ideally, the midwife who provides postnatal care will be known to the mother, having developed a relationship during pregnancy, labour and delivery. Many maternity service providers are offering continuity of care and carer in the form of caseload or team midwifery practice in response to the recommendations of the 'Changing Childbirth' report of the expert maternity group (DH 1993). If no such scheme is available, it is important that all midwives involved in postnatal care cooperate in providing consistency of advice and continuity of contact, whilst maintaining the woman as the central focus. Whenever practicable, a named midwife should be allocated with responsibility for a small group of postnatal women throughout their hospital stay.

Hospital birth – transfer within the hospital or transfer home

Hospital layouts vary from combined antenatal, labour and postnatal wards to separate specified areas. Once a newly delivered mother and her baby are ready to be transferred from the delivery area, the midwife should endeavour to arrange for a bed to be prepared in a quiet area so that the mother will be able to recover from the birth. It may be helpful if all women delivered by caesarean section are in close proximity to each other in order to provide peer support and facilitate consistency in advice from the same named midwife. Similarly, mothers may be roomed together according to their chosen method of infant feeding.

When transfer of care to a different midwife is necessary, the delivering midwife should ensure that adequate handover and appropriate introductions occur. The conditions of both mother and baby should be stable prior to transfer. Clinical observations should be recorded for maternal temperature, pulse and blood pressure. The uterus should be well contracted, the lochia not excessive and the woman should have passed urine since delivery. Any trauma or repair (see Ch. 24) to the perineum should be checked. It should be ascertained whether the new family have been able to spend some time alone together (the fourth stage of labour – see Ch. 31). If this has not taken place, then the parents should be left quietly alone together to explore their emotions and get to know their baby. The midwife should also enquire as to whether the baby has been put to the breast or been bottle fed and if he has passed meconium and urine. The temperature of the baby should also be recorded. Identification of both mother and infant must be confirmed and security labels checked.

The baby should remain by the mother's bedside. This approach to care is known as 'rooming-in' and enhances maternal–infant interaction (Prodromidis et al 1995). However, rooming-in at night should not be allowed to conflict with the mother's need for adequate rest and sleep. A separate nursery area remains an asset to enable new mothers to have an undisturbed sleep, and they should not be made to feel guilty for exercising such a choice. Extreme tiredness is known to increase the incidence of postnatal emotional disturbance (see Ch. 31). Once settled, the mother should then be offered food and drink as required and encouraged to rest. If the mother and baby are being transferred home, appropriate transport arrangements should be made, according to local policy.

If the receiving midwife is not already familiar with the woman's obstetric, relevant medical and family history, particular note should be taken of the following:

- age and parity
- blood group and Rhesus factor; if Rh negative, confirm that cord and maternal blood samples have been sent for analysis
- the most recent estimation of maternal haemoglobin
- any significant antenatal events such as pre-eclampsia, any regular medication or risk factors such as those for depression
- the events of labour and delivery, including the amount of blood loss, any trauma sustained and the nature of analgesia given
- current physical and psychological status of the woman
- the baby's condition at birth and on transfer, the birthweight and initial physical examination findings
- the chosen method of infant feeding and whether yet fed
- results of any screening tests undertaken, those required and affirmation of informed parental consent
- the mother's social and family needs and any particular requests made on the birth plan, or advice given, relevant to the postnatal period
- if in hospital, the mother's wishes about the length of stay; where practicable, a flexible approach should be adopted.

Relevant notes must always be transferred with the woman to ensure continuity of care and advice. If transfer is from hospital to home, it is important that the named or allocated midwife in the community is informed in advance and also the general practitioner, where appropriate.

Home birth

The delivering midwife is usually already known to the woman and will be responsible for the majority of the postnatal care. Where the named midwife is unavailable, handover and priorities are as above. The woman must always know how to contact a midwife for advice, both day and night. The general practitioner may also be involved in the care and good communications should be established between all concerned.

Caesarean section

Women delivered by caesarean section will require a degree of postoperative nursing skills in addition to normal midwifery postnatal care. If an emergency caesarean section was performed, particularly if following a long and difficult labour, the woman may be further debilitated by the stress of two major events. There may also have been anxiety regarding potential risks to the baby or indeed maternal health. In some cases, such as multiple birth, vaginal delivery may have occurred for twin one but an emergency caesarean for twin two. In this case, there may also be perineal trauma, with pain in the genital tract in addition to an abdominal wound.

In a comparative study involving 619 women over a 1-year period, Hillan (1995) reported an increased incidence of intrauterine, urinary tract and/or chest infections in women following emergency caesarean section over those who had been elected for surgery prior to labour. Overall, it appeared that both groups suffered a greater level of morbidity during the postnatal period than women delivered vaginally. Therefore, although the principles of care are similar for all postnatal women, midwives should be particularly vigilant when involved in the care of postoperative women in order to recognise early signs of infection, anaemia or other potential problems.

For specific postoperative care of the woman following general, epidural or spinal anaesthesia for caesarean section, see Chapter 28.

During the first 24 hours, the major physical needs are for adequate relief of pain and for maintenance of fluid intake. The first is achieved by giving the prescribed postoperative drug dependent on local policies and preferences. This may be pethidine 100 mg intramuscularly or morphine 120 mg in 60 ml of saline via patient-controlled analgesic pump (PCA), which may be a portable unit allowing mobility (O'Keefe et al 1994). Diclofenac sodium (Voltarol) 100 mg suppository may be combined with the PCA to facilitate its discontinuation after 12–24 hours. Dependent on pain level and threshold, oral analgesia may be given. Fluid intake is normally maintained initially by intravenous infusion until the woman is able to take oral fluids and her observations are stable. It is common for a self-retaining catheter to be left on free drainage until the woman is mobile. This not only avoids the discomfort of manoeuvring on bedpans but also allows the bladder and sphincter muscles a period of recovery. Once bowel sounds are heard, a light diet may be commenced. A soluble oral analgesic preparation given with hot peppermint water may assist the pain of flatulence many women experience owing to distension of the gut. Deep breathing and leg exercises should be encouraged. Women delivered by caesarean section have an increased risk of developing thrombophlebitis or deep vein thrombosis (see p. 17). Prophylactic antibiotic therapy is used in several units to reduce or prevent postoperative infection (Enkin et al 1995); this trend is supported within the 1991–1993 report into maternal deaths (DH et al 1996).

As soon as her condition allows, often after about 12 hours, the woman should be assisted with mobilisation. A shower is often permitted on the second day, followed by removal of any dressing. Sutures or clips are removed according to the instructions of the obstetrical surgeon. It is important that the mother is able to see and touch her baby and be assisted into a comfortable position for feeding, if she wishes. Once appropriate, the mother should be encouraged to undertake as much of the care of her baby as she feels able. It must be remembered that lifting a baby is painful for a woman with an abdominal wound and she should not be left to cope on her own until she feels fully able to do so. Emotionally, the opportunity to debrief following the birth experience is beneficial (see Ch. 31).

Mothers of babies who are sick or premature, stillborn or die in the early neonatal period

A mother whose baby has died or is being cared for in a special unit should be offered the opportunity for a single room if possible, but her preference should not be presumed. If a baby requires special or intensive care, the mother is likely to be extremely anxious and should be enabled to spend as much time as possible involved in the care of or near to her baby. When a baby has died, the mother and her partner should be encouraged to express their feelings and to spend as much time as they wish with their baby. The midwife requires particular skills to facilitate the grieving process (see Ch. 33). It is important that the normal postnatal care for both of these groups of mothers is not overlooked; in addition, the midwife should be particularly alert for signs of psychological distress (see Ch. 31). Flexibility in relation to the length of stay is important and continuity of care and carer should be provided. The partner and other close family members should be closely involved and also offered support.

READER ACTIVITY

Check the guidelines and resources available to assist with the care of parents whose baby has died or is requiring intensive or special care. What support mechanisms are available for:

a. parents?
b. staff?

PLANNING POSTNATAL CARE

If the woman already knows the midwife, preliminary plans for postnatal care may have been made during the antenatal period. Once the woman has spent time with her baby and rested

from the immediate effects of labour and delivery, her expectations for the postnatal period should be discussed in partnership with her named midwife. A plan identifying the main aspects of required care should be developed and agreed, meeting the individual woman and her baby's holistic needs. This should accommodate the individual social, psychological and demographic needs and family circumstances. The agreed plan should be clearly recorded in the woman's notes in such a way that other health professionals who may be involved in the care of the mother and baby can have easy access to relevant information. Some units utilise certain models (Henderson 1990) around which care may be individually tailored. When a model is used, it must be flexible enough to accommodate the varied and developing ability of women to take full responsibility for both their own care needs and those of their babies.

The framework of the plan should be based on the identified principles (p. 590), particularly taking into account:

- the mother's perception of her degree of experience and confidence in the care of her newborn baby
- any care required as a result of problems identified during pregnancy or labour, such as anaemia, pre-eclampsia (see Ch. 17), trauma or excessive blood loss sustained during the delivery
- any special needs of unsupported mothers, those whose babies are to be adopted or those with more than normal anxiety about the baby, for instance those who have experienced a previous miscarriage, stillbirth or neonatal death
- cultural, language or religious needs
- special needs due to physical, sensory or learning disability
- emotional needs (see Ch. 31)
- if the mother is Rhesus negative or known to have developed antibodies (see Ch. 42)
- maternal or neonatal screening tests required, e.g. maternal haemoglobin estimation and neonatal metabolic tests (see Chs 35 and 43)
- the needs of the family such as the partner's ability to visit, work issues or the care of other siblings.

DAILY POSTNATAL EXAMINATION AND ASSESSMENT OF NEEDS

The named midwife should carry out regular assessment examinations of the mother during the postnatal period, observing and noting her physical and emotional well-being. This provides an opportunity for the midwife to discuss with the woman her needs and those of her baby, as well as for the identification of deviation from normal progress. Whether delivery has occurred within the hospital or at home, a thorough postnatal examination is usually carried out daily, with a second lesser assessment later each day for at least the first 3 postnatal days. Once the condition of both mother and infant is stable, a more flexible pattern may be arranged in agreement with the woman. It may be more effective to miss out a day if all is going well and arrange an extra visit later on when the mother has been managing the baby herself for a while. The woman must always know how to contact a midwife should she need advice in between visits. In the majority of areas, visiting is carried out for at least 10 postnatal days. Following this and dependent on maternal and infant condition, the midwife may discharge the mother and her baby to the care of the health visitor. In some areas, midwives may visit for longer, up to 28 days, particularly for women who are breast feeding or who have specific identified needs. Any concerns the midwife may have in relation to the length of postnatal visiting should be addressed to the appropriate supervisor of midwives or head of midwifery as: 'clarification may be necessary to determine appropriate local policy' (RCM 1994). A final examination should occur prior to discharge from midwifery care and a comprehensive handover should take place between the midwife and health visitor.

Full and accurate records must be kept by the midwife throughout the postnatal period, in accordance with rule 42 (UKCC 1993) and to facilitate continuity of advice between health professionals.

The content of the daily postnatal assessment has remained largely unchanged for many years. Information gathered during a 4-year descriptive survey by the National Perinatal Epidemiology Unit included an analysis of this procedure. It appeared that midwives varied in what items they included in the examination and Marchant (1995) questioned whether a conflict was occurring between continuance of ritualistic practice and the desire to offer individually focused postnatal care. A study looking specifically at postnatal care in the community also discussed variations inherent within midwifery postnatal care (Murphy-Black 1994). It is imperative that the postnatal period is not treated with complacency as it is a time of great significance for the future well-being of mother, infant and family. Practice should be based on sound knowledge of physiology and current research and the midwife should take this into account in parallel with the needs of the individual.

READER ACTIVITY

Critically reflect on the components included within your own daily assessment examination of postnatal women. If possible, observe different midwives and draw up a comparative list of any apparent variation discovered – remembering to maintain confidentiality. Are all women being offered equal care?

After expulsion of the placenta, the circulating levels of human chorionic gonadotrophin, human placental lactogen, oestrogen and progesterone fall rapidly, bringing about a number of physiological changes. The most significant of these result from the fall in oestrogen with reversal of the circulatory haemodilution, and restoration of normal blood viscosity and respiratory function. The fall in circulating progesterone allows its relaxant effects upon the smooth muscle fibres of the pelvic floor, perineum, vagina and bowel to subside. This aids recovery of normal muscle tone and of the ligaments of the uterus. It is a gradual process which is aided by early ambulation, postnatal exercises, and by the avoidance of constipation.

To ensure that no aspect is overlooked and that deviation from normal postnatal progress is detected promptly, it is advisable to undertake the physical aspect of the maternal examination as a 'top-to-toe' assessment. It should always be preceded by explanation and discussion with the mother, involving the partner when appropriate. Certain women, such as those of differing cultural or religious backgrounds or those with sensory or physical disability may have anxieties or particular needs during the puerperium (see p. 610). It is vital that midwives respect individual differences, resist generalist opinions and remember that the woman 'is always the expert on [her] own life, wishes and needs' (Schott & Henley 1996).

THE 'TOP-TO-TOE' POSTNATAL ASSESSMENT EXAMINATION

Figure 30.1 provides a diagrammatic summary of the 'top-to-toe' postnatal assessment examination.

Communication

Effective interpersonal skills are vital for the midwife. Communication must be a two-way process involving the mother and midwife equally. The postnatal examination should utilise all the senses to facilitate the composition of a thorough assessment:

- observation – body language, eyes, skin condition and colour
- active listening
- informing
- touch
- smell.

The mother should be greeted and asked how she is feeling. It is important to pose this as an open question, accompanied by an attentive posture with eye level either equal to or below that of the woman. The midwife should actively listen in an encouraging way in order to facilitate confidence and trust. Additional open questions should be posed as appropriate to draw relevant information. During this exchange, the midwife can form a general impression of the woman's physical and emotional well-being. Awareness of body posture, amount of eye contact, ease of expression, skin condition and colour can all provide valuable cues for further investigation. As the examination proceeds, touch and smell can extend this portfolio of knowledge.

The midwife should take particular note if the

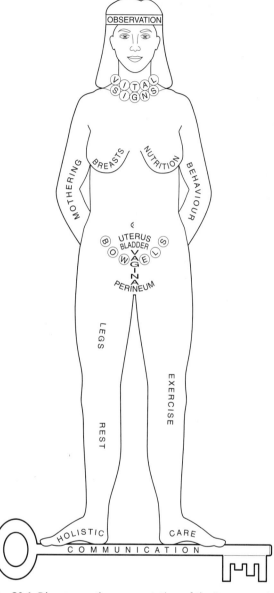

Fig. 30.1 Diagrammatic representation of the 'top-to-toe' postnatal assessment examination.

mother complains of feeling unduly tired. Many women feel tired following delivery but if this persists, it should be explored further. It is useful also to observe the interaction between the mother and her baby (see Ch. 31). Allowing a night of undisturbed sleep may be all that is required to facilitate a normal recovery period and enable coping skills to return. If necessary, a mild sedative may be useful. Undue fatigue can lead to depression and the woman should be given an opportunity to discuss her feelings and be provided with extra help until she feels more able to cope. If a woman is feeling generally unwell, this may be a sign of anaemia or a developing infection. Any pointers such as this should be explored in greater depth as the assessment progresses.

Following this initial exchange of information, the physical assessment should proceed, remembering the aspects of effective communication as a continuum. This is also a valuable opportunity for the offering of consistent advice and education. Hallgren et al (1995), in their analysis of in-depth interviews with 11 primigravid women, found consideration of individual needs and avoidance of conflicting information to be the most important issues for the women.

Appropriate documentation must be maintained.

Clinical observations (vital signs)

The temperature may be labile during the first few days following delivery as a normal physiological response. Puerperal pyrexia arises from infection of the genital or urinary tract, the breasts, or inflammation within the venous system. Mild transient pyrexia may be associated with physiological vascular and/or milk engorgement of the breasts on days 3–4 or with intercurrent infections such as the common cold. As a guide, the temperature should not exceed 37.4°C on more than three occasions, or 38°C on more than one occasion. However, this should not be viewed in isolation but in comparison with the holistic impression.

The adult resting pulse rate is normally between 70 and 80 beats per minute. Any tachycardia may be indicative of excessive bleeding or of a developing puerperal infection. A rising pulse rate which is due to excessive bleeding will usually be accompanied by a fall in the blood pressure and the midwife must check the state of the uterus and lochia in order to identify postpartum haemorrhage (see Ch. 25). A raised temperature accompanied by a rising pulse rate is a cardinal sign of puerperal infection. In some cases tachycardia may be the primary indicator.

On suspicion of infection, the midwife's examination of the woman should be directed toward locating the site of infection. This should include appropriate questioning to elicit any symptoms the woman may be experiencing such as headache, sneezing, coughing, burning on micturition, painful breasts or legs. Subject to local policy, the midwife may proceed to collect laboratory specimens such as throat swab, high vaginal swab and midstream specimen of urine but must inform the doctor if pyrexia persists or other symptoms are apparent. The use of antibiotics has greatly reduced the number of deaths due to puerperal infection but health professionals must not become complacent about this condition and overlook its potential danger. During the triennium 1991–1993 in the UK, nine women died of genital tract sepsis in the puerperium, five of them following caesarean section. Onset can be insidious but rapidly progress to fulminating septicaemia (DH et al 1996). Causative organisms will be discussed later in the chapter (p. 608).

The blood pressure should be recorded within the first 24 hours of birth in the normotensive woman but if the woman has suffered from pre-eclampsia, gestational or essential hypertension or a period of hypotension, it should be measured regularly until satisfactory. The blood pressure should also be recorded for a longer period following caesarean section, other surgical intervention or if excessive bleeding has occurred. It is now recognised that recovery from pre-eclampsia is not immediate and that the potential for eclampsia and maternal death persists during the early puerperium (DH et al 1996, Ferrazzani et al 1994, Usta & Sibai 1995). It has been recommended for high-risk women to remain in hospital for at least 5 postpartum days (C. Redman, personal communication, 1996).

Physiologically, the respiratory rate should return to the pre-pregnant level as the circulatory haemodilution of pregnancy subsides, and with the release of the upward pressure on the diaphragm following delivery of the baby. The respiratory rate can be altered, however, because of muscular strain, postanaesthetic complications such as atelectasis or bronchopneumonia or as a response to infection, severe haemorrhage affecting the circulatory volume, or thromboembolic disorders such as pulmonary embolism (see p. 607). The midwife should be aware of the woman's respiratory function but it is not usually necessary to routinely count and record the actual rate. It should also be remembered that upper respiratory tract infection may occur in any person at any time. Ideally, staff suffering from such infections should endeavour to avoid close contact with mothers and babies during the acute phase. Methicillin-resistant *Staphylococcus aureus* (MRSA) has become a problem in many general hospital wards and, in some units, both patients and staff are routinely screened. Healthy women are considered to be at low risk of MRSA affecting either themselves, their fetuses or their babies. Caesarean section and perineal wounds are sites which may attract the bacteria and there is a potential risk of cross-infection if student midwives are working on an affected general ward prior to a maternity placement and this should be considered. Tea tree oil is currently undergoing trials as it appears it may provide an effective challenge to MRSA.

There is some debate about the necessity of taking the temperature and pulse routinely; the midwife should utilise her clinical judgement and refer to current research and unit policy.

Breasts

The breasts should be examined daily, regardless of the chosen feeding method. Following enquiry as to any discomfort or concerns and with consent of the woman, the midwife should inspect the breasts for areas of redness, then proceed to gently palpate the breasts to exclude areas of heat, hardness or pain. It must be remembered that in a woman whose baby has died, postnatal breast changes and preparation for lactation will still occur and it is important that the midwife deals with this in a sensitive manner. Pharmacological preparations, such as cabergoline, for suppression of lactation may be of value (Enkin et al 1995). The woman should be made aware of what to expect and offered advice similar to that given to a mother who has elected not to breast feed.

Vascular engorgement and the subsequent milk engorgement around the third day inevitably cause considerable discomfort (see Ch. 36). Milk production gradually subsides owing to the absence of tactile stimulation of the nipples, which is needed to elicit contraction of the myoepithelial cells. Circulating levels of oxytocin and prolactin gradually fall. If milk production is particularly high in a mother who has elected not to breast feed, the midwife could discuss with the woman whether she may reconsider. Analgesia or mild night sedation may be necessary at the peak of engorgement for those women who do not wish to alter their decision.

Anatomy and physiology of the breasts and lactation, care of the breasts, significance of abnormal findings on inspection, support and complications of breast feeding are discussed in Chapter 36.

Breast infections are a serious and painful complication of the puerperium (see Ch. 36). The organisms causing breast infections are often passed between baby and mother, therefore preventive education is vital. Scrupulous attention to hand washing and hygiene by mothers and anyone handling neonates or assisting with breast feeding will both lower the incidence of infection among babies and reduce the risk of breast infection in mothers. Rooming-in (see p. 591) has the effect of partially isolating the mother and baby together.

The midwife may consider it appropriate to interweave discussion related to postnatal maternal diet and fluid intake into this part of the assessment.

Nutrition

The diet of a puerperal woman should be nourishing, varied and balanced. It should include adequate protein to aid tissue renewal and milk production, iron and vitamins to counteract anaemia, fibre to aid excretion and improve muscle tone. It is now considered that calorific and fluid intake should be controlled by the natural hunger and thirst of the individual woman (RCM 1991).

Uterus and involution

If delivery was by caesarean section, the midwife should first inspect the scar to review healing and to exclude signs of inflammation or infection. The wound should be kept clean and dry and sutures removed subject to local practice. Regardless of route of delivery, the uterine fundus should be carefully palpated each postnatal day to exclude any complication, ideally by the woman's named midwife to maintain consistency. It is helpful if the woman has emptied her bladder prior to the palpation as a full bladder may make the uterine fundus appear high and deviated to one side. At the completion of labour the uterus weighs approximately 1 kg and the fundus can be palpated at or just below the mother's umbilicus. By the end of the puerperium it has usually returned to its non-pregnant weight of 60 g. This physiological phenomenon is known as involution. It is brought about by a process known as autolysis, during which proteolytic enzymes digest the collagen muscle fibres which have increased during pregnancy to 10 times their normal length and five times their normal thickness. The end products of autolysis are removed by the phagocytic action of polymorphs and macrophages in the blood and lymphatic systems and subsequently excreted via the renal system in the urine. This process is further assisted by the continued contraction and retraction of the uterine muscles under the influence of oxytocin, which is secreted by the posterior pituitary gland, reducing the placental site and assisting haemostasis. This results in compression of the blood vessels and reduction of uterine blood supply producing a relative state of ischaemia. The site is gradually covered by granular tissue and later by endometrium.

In women who choose to breast feed, the suckling of the infant stimulates further secretion of oxytocin, as well as facilitating milk expulsion. This expedites involution and can cause quite painful uterine contractions known as 'afterpains'. In multiparous women the uterus tends to be more flaccid than that of a primipara, and they frequently suffer from afterpains during the first 2 or 3 postnatal days. Analgesia such as a diclofenac sodium (Voltarol) 100 mg suppository once daily, co-codamol or paracetamol 500 mg to 1 g, according to unit policy, may be helpful once deviation from the normal has been excluded.

The most marked reduction in size of the uterus takes place during the first 10 days of the puerperium, but involution is not complete until

Table 30.1 Progression of change in the uterus after delivery (approximate)

	Weight of uterus	Diameter of placental site	Cervix
End of labour	900 g	12.5 cm	Soft, flabby
End of 1 week	450 g	7.5 cm	2 cm
End of 2 weeks	200 g	5.0 cm	1 cm
End of 6 weeks	60 g	2.5 cm	A slit

approximately 6 weeks later. On palpation, the uterus should feel evenly contracted, smooth, firm and central and it should not be painful. The rate of reduction in fundal height varies in different women, but involution should follow a progressive pattern (see Table 30.1 for approximate rate of change). It is usually more rapid in women who breast feed and in primigravidae. Specific daily measurement of fundal descent either by tape measure or manual palpation is of questionable value (Montgomery & Alexander 1994). A small study, involving 13 midwives and 24 postnatal women, concluded that tape measurement of symphysis pubis to fundal height is: 'insufficiently precise to detect abnormally slow daily changes' (Cluett et al 1995, p. 182). Whilst further research may be warranted, midwives should concentrate on developing the skills required to recognise clinical signs of abnormality. Sub-involution is identified if the uterus remains the same size for several days. A bulky uterus may be due to a full rectum or indicate the presence of retained products of conception or blood clots. Uterine fibroids could also lead to delayed involution. Tenderness of the uterus is suggestive of infection. The midwife should look for further indicative signs and must report such findings to a doctor.

Signs and symptoms of genital tract infection

Pyrexia is usually the first sign, accompanied by a rising pulse rate. The onset may be sudden and accompanied by rigor or may be more gradual with the temperature and pulse rate rising each day. The pulse rate is significant and in the case of infection by haemolytic streptococci a rising pulse rate may be the first sign, occurring before pyrexia is manifest. In some cases of infection by haemolytic streptococci, no marked rise in the temperature is seen. The uterus will be tender on palpation. The lochia (see p. 600) may be offensive and suppuration of lacerations and of the suture line may be visible. In the case of infection by haemolytic streptococci, the lochia will be scanty only 24 hours after delivery and may not be at all offensive initially. There may be little sign of external infection and indeed the woman may develop serious pelvic infection or septicaemia whilst the perineum continues to heal. In the case of infection with *Clostridium welchii*, the onset may be heralded by collapse, haematuria and a developing jaundice.

Effects of genital tract infection

Localised infection is seen in infected wounds or the formation of abscesses.

Pelvic infection occurs as a result of ascending spread of infection from the perineum, vagina or cervix to the uterine cavity. From there it may spread to the uterine tubes causing salpingitis and possible blockage of the tubes. It may also spread into the peritoneal cavity. A woman who develops salpingitis or peritonitis becomes severely ill, with a thready pulse, pain on abdominal palpation, vomiting and diarrhoea leading to rapid dehydration. Lateral spread invades the parametrium and leads to pelvic cellulitis. A virulent strain of haemolytic streptococcus A may rapidly infect the entire peritoneal cavity and gain access to the systemic circulation via the placental site causing septicaemia and haemolytic anaemia. The woman becomes acutely ill, suffering rigors and persistent high fever, due to the toxins produced by the organism. The pericardium, pleura and even the synovial membranes of the joints may be involved.

Any pyrexia following birth or miscarriage which persists for 24 hours should be regarded as an infection of the genital tract until proved otherwise. A doctor must be informed and appropriate records maintained.

Investigation and management of genital tract infection

A full general examination is made by the doctor, who will request a high vaginal swab and mid-stream specimen of urine to be sent for bacterial analysis. This is to establish the source and cause of the infection and the sensitivity of the causative organisms to various antibiotics. In taking a high vaginal swab, a speculum should be used to distend the vagina and enable the sample to be taken as high in the vagina and as near to the cervix as possible. No antiseptic lotion or cream should be applied and the midwife or doctor must use sterile gloves. Culture of the organisms may take 48 hours and the doctor may prescribe a broad-spectrum antibiotic in the meantime.

Antibiotic therapy should be commenced as soon as possible. If the woman is severely ill and has been dehydrated, an intravenous infusion may be necessary. Fluid intake and output records should be kept. Analgesics may be given to relieve pain.

The woman's haemoglobin estimation should be checked to exclude anaemia as a predisposing or complicating factor. Where anaemia is present, appropriate treatment should be commenced and in cases of serious infection a blood transfusion may be given.

The midwife requires competent nursing skills in caring for the woman. Regular bathing or sponging to reduce pyrexia and increase comfort may be necessary. Vulval pads must be changed frequently. A light nourishing diet and plenty of fluids should be encouraged. The midwife should endeavour to protect the woman from any unnecessary stress and adequate undisturbed sleep should be promoted. The baby should not be removed from the mother's bedside unless she is severely ill but should be cared for by the midwife or appropriate other, until the mother can resume self-care. Women diagnosed as suffering from puerperal infection are normally isolated from other mothers until such time as the cause has been identified, treatment commenced and the temperature returned to normal. The length of isolation will depend upon the severity of the infection and the causative organism (see p. 609). Every effort must be made to prevent cross-infection and in some cases it will be necessary to institute barrier nursing techniques.

When uninterrupted involution occurs, the uterine fundus should be palpable just above the symphysis pubis at approximately 1 week after vaginal delivery. By the 10th or 12th day it has usually descended into the pelvic cavity. Involution tends to take a little longer following delivery by caesarean section because the scar tissue retards the process.

Cervix

The cervix is soft and vascular immediately after delivery and on inspection may be seen protruding into the vagina. It loses its vascularity rapidly and normally regains its hard consistency within 2 or 3 days of the delivery. The external cervical os also reduces in size and 10 days after delivery has a width of approximately 1 cm.

Lochia

Lochia is the term used to describe the discharges from the uterus during the puerperium and the term is plural. Lochia have an alkaline reaction in which organisms can flourish more rapidly than in the normally acid secretions of the vagina. The odour of normal lochia is heavy but not offensive, and the amount can vary in individual women. The lochia undergo sequential changes as involution progresses:

• Red lochia (lochia rubra) – are usually red in colour, consisting of blood from the placental site, debris arising from the decidua and chorion and are shed during the first 3–4 days of the puerperium.
• Serous lochia (lochia serosa) – are pink in colour and discharged during the next 5–9 days. The lochia now have less blood and more serum and contain leucocytes from the placental site.
• White lochia (lochia alba) – are paler, creamy-brown in colour, and contain leucocytes, cervical mucus and debris from healing tissues.

Some evidence of bloodstained discharge may continue to be seen for a further 2 or 3 weeks.

The midwife should enquire as to the quantity, colour and odour of the lochia daily. A slight increase in the amount or in the blood content may be seen when the mother becomes more active and also during breast feeding. The presence of small blood clots may be normal during the first 24 hours, especially in multiparous women, but if this continues or is accompanied by pain, it suggests that products of conception may not have been fully expelled. There is a slightly increased risk of haemorrhage from the placental site during the first 48 hours after delivery by caesarean section and the midwife must advise the woman to report any excessive blood loss. For aetiology and management of secondary postpartum haemorrhage, see Chapter 25.

Offensive lochia may indicate poor vulval hygiene or contamination by faecal debris and the midwife should sensitively ensure the woman is confident in using the bidet, if available, and in attending to her personal hygiene needs. If the lochia remain offensive or are scanty, this may be indicative of infection of the genital tract, possibly of the uterus itself (see above). Findings should be looked at in context with the condition of the uterus and other clinical observations and reported to a doctor as appropriate.

If a woman had a lowered antenatal haemoglobin (Hb) level, excessive blood loss at delivery or the lochia are heavy, Hb estimation may be undertaken early in the puerperium to exclude anaemia. The blood sample should not be taken less than 24 hours after completion of the delivery or it may be inaccurate due to the effect of blood loss upon the volume of haemoglobin. Hb estimation may also be indicated if the woman complains of constant tiredness or has a tachycardia.

Postnatal anaemia

In developed countries anaemia is judged to be present when the concentration of haemoglobin is less than 9–10 g/dl or when it continues to fall after 30 weeks' gestation (Chamberlain 1995). Up until this point there is a normal physiological lowering of the Hb concentration (see Ch. 11).

Even a moderate blood loss at delivery may reduce the haemoglobin to less than 10 g/dl, if the concentration before delivery was assessed at 11–12 g/dl. Any degree of anaemia will reduce the body's resistance to infection and its capacity for healing. It is important, therefore, that symptoms of anaemia are identified promptly and reported to a doctor for investigation and appropriate treatment. Methods of treating anaemia are identical to those used in pregnancy (see Ch. 16). Most cases can be corrected with a course of oral iron.

Perineum and external genitalia

For examination procedure and technique for repair refer to Chapter 24. Tears of the perineum are graded according to their severity (for classification refer to Ch. 24).

Increased vascularity of the vagina and vulva during pregnancy and the pressure exerted during delivery on these soft tissues frequently causes some degree of bruising and oedema. The excess fluid is usually reabsorbed by the third or fourth day of the puerperium. Other areas of trauma may be the cervix or extended tears deep within the vagina, neither of which may be readily visible (see Ch. 25). Minor trauma to the cervix does not usually cause complications but larger tears give rise to persistent bleeding. A cervical tear may be diagnosed when the woman continues to bleed per vaginam even when the uterus is well contracted. Such bleeding can lead to hypovolaemic shock, so the condition requires prompt attention. Vaginal tears cause considerable pain although the amount of subsequent blood loss is variable. However, a deep vaginal haematoma can sometimes develop, possibly as an extension from a vulval haematoma with the appearance of a tender purple swelling (see Fig. 30.2). These cause extreme pain which may worsen when standing and may lead to shock, becoming a puerperal emergency (Ridgway 1995). They require exploration and evacuation under general anaesthetic. If the bleeding vessel can be found it is ligatured. Firm pressure is put on the area. When severe bleeding has occurred a blood transfusion may be necessary. The repair of any perineal tear requires skilled technique (see Ch. 24) if permanent damage is not to be sustained. Scar tissue may cause pain during coitus and predispose to further tears in subsequent labours.

Management of trauma

Following discussion related to discomfort and the amount of lochia, the midwife should inspect the perineum and vulva to ensure that any trauma is healing satisfactorily and to exclude any signs of infection. Disposable gloves should be worn when handling vulval pads and aseptic technique must be adhered to when applying any treatment or removing sutures. The midwife should discuss the prevention of cross-infection and the importance

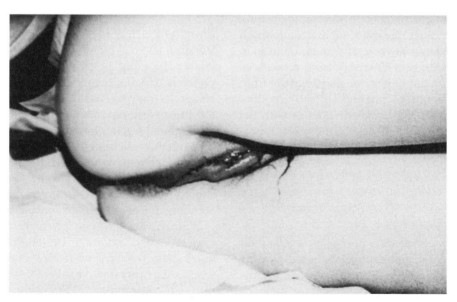

Fig. 30.2 Extensive bruising of the vulva, vagina and perineum following evacuation of a vulvovaginal haematoma.

of changing pads frequently so that the perineum is kept free from stale lochia. Frequent hand washing should be advised, and a daily bath or shower encouraged in addition to use of the bidet or careful vulval cleansing following micturition or defaecation. This promotes the healing of trauma, offers relief from discomfort and reduces the risk of genital or urinary tract infection. Care should be taken to dry the perineum after bathing and sanitary pads should be changed frequently. Genital tract infection is more common in women who have suffered tears or abrasions to the vulva, vagina and perineum. Bruising reduces the tissues' resistance to infection and there is danger that ascending infection may involve the uterus and the placental site (see p. 597).

Trauma may be particularly marked when manipulation of the fetus has been necessary. There is now significant evidence that Ventouse (vacuum extraction) delivery involves less trauma to both the maternal soft tissues and to the infant, than the use of forceps (Meniru 1996). All soft tissue trauma produces devitalised tissue which provides an ideal environment for pathogenic organisms and this may lead to puerperal infection. Trauma also increases the likelihood of clot formation and thromboembolic disorders.

When feeding the baby, mothers may find that lying on one side is the most comfortable position as sitting can cause pressure on the traumatised area. Soft cushions may be useful and mobilisation should be encouraged. There are various methods for the management of perineal pain, varying from topical applications to pharmaceutical remedies. The midwife should discuss the options with the woman and they should decide the most appropriate strategy together.

Topical and complementary methods for the management of perineal pain and healing (see also Chs 44, 45)

The properties of water are now acknowledged for the management of pain during labour and soaking in a warm bath may be also be effective for the relief of perineal pain. Complementary methods of perineal pain management (Harrison 1995) are increasingly popular. Oils such as lavender or tea

tree added to the bath or applied as compresses have been found to be beneficial, having antiseptic and healing properties. Homeopathic remedies can be taken orally or by application. Arnica is believed to be of general benefit for the promotion of healing (Castro 1990). Calendula and Bellis Perennis are more specifically advocated for wound healing (Cummings 1994). Midwives must refer to paragraphs 34 and 35 of their Code of Practice (UKCC 1994) and the Midwives Rules (UKCC 1993) concerning the administration of medicines, and also any local policy, prior to involvement in the use of complementary medicines.

Local anaesthetic spray or gel, such as 5% lignocaine, may be effective and give relief over a longer period of time. Steroid preparations should be avoided.

Physiotherapy (see Ch. 45)

In recent years the application of Megapulse (pulsed electromagnetic energy), infrared heat and ultrasound have been used by physiotherapists to relieve pain and promote healing. Research evidence is inconclusive to support the cost-efficiency of these techniques. An intensive programme of pelvic floor exercises appears to result in reduced pain (Enkin et al 1995).

Pharmaceutical methods

Voltarol 100 mg by suppository once daily, preferably at night, is often effective and used in preference to oral preparations. The following oral analgesics may be useful and are considered safe for breast-feeding mothers (Briggs et al 1990): paracetamol 1 g; ibuprofen 200–400 mg; or soluble preparations such as co-codamol (paracetamol 500 mg, codeine phosphate 8 mg) dissolved in hot peppermint water can also be effective. Women should be made aware, however, that the codeine component can exacerbate constipation.

Women who have sustained third degree tears may experience severe or prolonged pain and require dietary advice to reduce interference with the healing process and to avoid further discomfort through constipation. They may be offered a low-residue diet initially, followed by a glycerine suppository around the third day. It is usual thereafter to encourage a high-residue diet in order to produce a bulky stool which is easier to expel. Lactulose may also be useful.

Disruption of the healing process

If the perineal or abdominal wound becomes infected or if sloughing appears, it may be necessary to remove some of the sutures to allow any pus or fluid to drain. Areas may be cleansed with chlorhexidine or a solution of hydrogen peroxide applied (refer to local policy). When healing is disrupted, the woman will need reassurance and careful attention for some time. The wound may still heal spontaneously but take a number of weeks to do so. Alternatively, resuturing may be required under general anaesthetic. If this occurs it is usual to wait for the resolution of any infection before the scar is incised, and the tissues realigned and resutured. The main danger of a third degree tear is the formation of a rectovaginal fistula, leading to the expulsion of faeces per vaginam. This is not a common occurrence in the western nations. The formation of a fistula is more likely in debilitated or malnourished women and once developed it is extremely difficult to heal, causing considerable distress. In certain cultures it may lead to rejection and isolation of the woman.

Female genital mutilation

Female genital mutilation is still practised in certain cultures, particularly in central Africa. Whilst the practice is deemed illegal in the UK, women may still present for delivery having undergone a degree of this procedure. Restoration to the infibulated state is illegal in the UK (Schott & Henley 1996), and the woman may be extremely anxious postnatally about the reactions of her partner or family and indeed she may herself feel incomplete. Sensitive understanding is essential and the opportunity for education and discussion of this issue is vital between the midwife, doctors, the woman and her family. Midwives working in areas with a multiracial population should endeavour to familiarise themselves with local cultural and religious practices in order to facilitate a relationship of trust with all families.

Bladder and urinary tract

The midwife should establish whether the woman is experiencing any discomfort or difficulty in passing urine postnatally. The withdrawal of oestrogen allows a diuresis to take place, rapidly reducing the plasma volume to normal proportions. This action takes place within the first 24–48 hours following the birth of the baby. During this time, copious amounts of urine will be passed. The falling progesterone level helps to reduce fluid retention inherent in increased vascularity of the tissues which occurred during pregnancy, together with that of oedema due to trauma during delivery of the baby. The dramatic fall in circulating progesterone reverses the haemodilution of pregnancy and renal action is accelerated with urine output further increased as a result of the autolysis of the uterine muscle fibres.

It is not necessary to measure urine output but if a woman expresses difficulty in emptying her bladder, the reason must be sought. Initially, this may be due to oedema at the base of the bladder causing suppression of detrusor activity (Llewellyn-Jones 1994) or spasm of the sphincter muscle induced by pressure of the descending fetus during delivery. Also during labour the bladder is displaced into the abdomen, stretching the urethra to a considerable degree and this frequently leads to bruising of the urethra and loss of muscle tone in the bladder. Micturition may be painful and the bladder can easily become overdistended. Bruising or lacerations can occur to the external orifice of the urethra and surrounding labia which can also be quite painful and induce fear of passing urine. If the problem is not resolved early, retention of urine may occur. It is important for the midwife to explain the relevant physiology and to reassure the woman; remedies which may be tried include the sound of running water or sitting in a warm bath. Where retention does occur it leads to continuing loss of muscle tone, back pressure on the ureters and pelves of the kidneys and increased likelihood of urinary tract or renal infection. This situation can be prevented by encouraging regular micturition and by ensuring that the bladder completely empties on each occasion. A study of 528 women attending a gynaecological clinic found that, through fear of cross-infection, 85% adopted a crouching position when voiding in a public toilet (Moore et al 1991). This position involves contraction of the adductor muscles thereby preventing relaxation of the pelvic floor during micturition; also women may not be able to crouch for a sufficient length of time to permit full emptying of the bladder. Educating women to sit down on toilet seats and to lean slightly forward during voiding (A. Rane, personal communication, 1997), with reassurance relating to cross-infection status, may help avoid further complications.

Catheterisation should be regarded as a last resort and, if undertaken, strict asepsis is mandatory owing to the increased risk of associated infection. Depending on local policy, this may be an isolated procedure purely to relieve the retention, with the expectation that subsequently the woman will be able to micturate spontaneously, or it may involve use of a self-retaining catheter. The latter will be required if the woman remains unable to void urine. In this case, the catheter is often left on free drainage for 24 hours to allow recovery from initial oedema and trauma, then removed. Accurate records must be made including a fluid intake and output chart. Micturition may be painful after removal of the catheter but the woman should be encouraged to pass urine frequently in order to maintain the regained tone and prevent further retention. It is important for the midwife to offer explanation and reassurance, as the woman may fear that she has lost control over her bladder, and it must be remembered that the psychological and reflex control of micturition is as important as the physical control. Mobilisation and fluid intake should be encouraged. Once micturition has been achieved it usually proceeds normally thereafter but the midwife should establish whether it continues to be pain free, that adequate amounts of urine are being passed and that the bladder is not palpable, which would indicate residual urine.

Urinary tract infection

Women remain prone to urinary tract infection during the early puerperium. Its cause lies in the stasis of urine which occurs during pregnancy, encouraging the formation of a reservoir of organisms. Trauma during labour or inadequate vulval hygiene leading to an ascending infection predisposes to its recurrence during the puerperium. It is vital that early recognition occurs, as delay can lead to chronic pyelonephritis and permanent damage in the kidney (see Ch. 16).

Signs and symptoms of urinary tract infection

Mild infection gives rise to malaise, aches and pains in the back and loins and, in some cases, pain on micturition. Pyrexia is not always present. More severe infection may consist of either acute cystitis characterised by scalding on micturition or pyelonephritis, which causes a pyrexia, pain over the kidney and haematuria. If the midwife suspects the woman may be developing a urinary tract infection, a doctor must be informed immediately.

Investigation and management of urinary tract infection

A midstream specimen of urine is obtained for bacteriological investigation. An appropriate antibiotic may be commenced based on clinical findings alone (refer to local protocol). The most common causative organism, *Escherichia coli* (see p. 609), thrives in acid urine and a useful method of additional treatment is the oral administration of potassium citrate mixture which makes the urine alkaline, thereby inhibiting bacterial growth. An increased fluid intake is also beneficial in expediting elimination of the organism.

Other related considerations

Prolonged bladder distension places strain upon the internal sphincter muscles, predisposing to chronic urinary incontinence. It is estimated that 10% of women suffer from stress incontinence at some stage during the puerperium (Llewellyn-Jones 1994). In some, this may continue for much longer. The midwife should take the opportunity, when discussing micturition, to advise and educate concerning the function of the pelvic floor muscles. This set of muscles is probably the least considered of the human body and during vaginal delivery they become stretched and put under considerable pressure. It is important to exercise these muscles, as with all other muscles, in order for them to function efficiently. An extensive literature review has reported on studies which debated the relationship between perineal muscle integrity and resultant urinary incontinence. Whilst data in some instances conflict, there is evidence: 'that a weakened pelvic structure has an impact on the woman's ability to maintain a continent state' (Morin 1994, p. 45). This would support the value of encouraging women to undertake pelvic floor exercise (see Ch. 45) regularly throughout life, but in particular, following vaginal delivery.

Severe prolonged pressure of the presenting part on the pelvic floor musculature or direct injury during instrumental vaginal delivery may lead to necrosis of the internal tissues and cause the formation of a vesicovaginal fistula. This results in urinary incontinence and leakage via the genital tract with increased risk of genitourinary infections. Whilst this is extremely rare in the western world, it remains a high cause of morbidity in women where obstetric facilities are deficient (Chamberlain 1995).

Bowels

The midwife should enquire as to the woman's bowel function postnatally, as some women continue to experience constipation during the period in which circulating hormone levels subside. This can be complicated by any pain due to trauma following delivery and women can become quite anxious and fearful of defaecation. It is important to reassure women that damage will not be caused to any perineal repair or abdominal wound. Dietary advice should be offered, bearing in mind the potential effects on the baby of certain foods if the mother is breast feeding; plenty of roughage and fluids should be encouraged. A mild aperient may be necessary by the second postnatal night and, if bowel function is not resumed, glycerine suppositories may be offered. Usually, a normal pattern will re-establish by the end of the first week.

Women who have undergone repair or structural damage involving the anal sphincter muscles will require particular dietary advice. In some cases, where the internal sphincter is compromised,

faecal incontinence may result (Kamm 1996), and specialist help will be required.

Haemorrhoids

Haemorrhoids which have developed during pregnancy usually resolve spontaneously postnatally but this will not be immediate. Local application of creams such as Anusol or Lasonil, diluted essential oils of cypress, juniper or frankincense (Davis 1988) or oral analgesia may be helpful prior to attempting defaecation.

Legs

Women who suffer from haemorrhoids may also have varicosities of the legs. The midwife should observe and examine the woman's legs for any areas of redness, heat or tenderness which might suggest thrombosis of the superficial or deep veins. The physiological changes which occur during pregnancy (see Ch. 11) followed by the effects of delivery, put women at increased risk of thrombosis postnatally. Refer to Chapter 15 for a full explanation of the normal coagulation process.

THROMBOEMBOLISM

Predisposing factors

Thrombosis and thromboembolism remain the leading cause of maternal death in the UK, with an increase in postpartum deaths over the previous triennium to 17 during 1991–1993 (DH et al 1996, see also Ch. 48). It is vital, therefore, that the midwife is aware of women at increased risk (Box 30.1).

In women whose history suggests that they may be particularly at risk of thrombosis, prophylactic treatment with low doses of anticoagulants may be given and continued during the puerperium. In addition, general avoidable factors should be borne in mind, such as smoking or trauma to the legs.

Prevention of thrombosis

During labour, exhaustion and dehydration should have been avoided. Care should have been taken

Box 30.1 Factors associated with an increased risk of thrombosis and thromboembolism (adapted from: Chamberlain 1995, DH et al 1996)

- A past or family history of thrombosis
- Immobility due to disablement, paralysis or medical condition
- Pre-eclampsia
- Postoperatively, in particular following emergency caesarean section
- Following epidural anaesthesia where the legs have been immobile
- Antiphospholipid syndrome, cardiolipin antibody or lupus anticoagulant
- Congenital deficiency of antithrombin III, protein C, some sickle cell anaemias
- Obesity, age > 35, parity > 4
- Severe varicose veins
- Current other infection or illness

to avoid trauma to the veins of the legs by careless handling or by pressure from the stirrups used to hold the legs in lithotomy position. No woman should be placed in the lithotomy position unnecessarily nor left there longer than is absolutely essential. It is particularly important that care is taken to avoid bruising the legs of an unconscious or heavily sedated woman when moving her from the trolley to the theatre table or delivery bed and that the legs or feet of an unconscious woman are not allowed to lie heavily upon one another. Thromboembolic disease stockings (TEDS) are useful when correctly fitted, offering venous support and a degree of protection.

Mobilisation increases muscle tone and venous return from the legs and lower abdomen and should be encouraged as soon as possible after delivery. Women who had a forceps delivery or suffered marked bruising of the perineum may find walking difficult at first but should be encouraged to persevere as the consequent increase in venous return helps to reduce oedema and bruising. Increasing amounts of exercise should be taken each day and it is important that women are encouraged to walk about and not just sit by the bedside, as this will help them to feel better emotionally and physically. Postnatal exercises help to increase muscle tone and are usually commenced during the first 3 days after delivery. Further information on exercise and back care will be found in Chapter 45.

There are two main types of thrombosis during the puerperium:

- superficial thrombophlebitis
- deep vein thrombosis.

Superficial thrombophlebitis

Thrombophlebitis affects the superficial veins of the legs and is characterised by swelling, hardness and redness of the affected vein. There may be a slight pyrexia, most commonly from the fourth to tenth day (Chamberlain 1995). This form of thrombophlebitis mainly affects varicose veins, which will be tender. It does not normally lead to pulmonary embolism and may be more common in women who are overweight (James & Stirrat 1988). It is important that the diagnosis of superficial thrombophlebitis does not obscure the possibility that such women may also develop deep vein thrombosis. The midwife should, therefore, examine the legs carefully to exclude signs of deeper thrombosis and inform a doctor. Reassurance should be offered and TED stockings or a supportive bandage may be beneficial. Redness and pain may be reduced by the application of hamamelis (witch hazel) or arnica ointment (Castro 1990). Some midwives favour Lasonil or the more traditional glycerine and ichthammol paste, although research is not available to predict the efficacy of these differing practices. Exercise should be encouraged and the legs elevated when the woman is sitting. The midwife should also advise against crossing the legs as this can interfere with venous return.

Deep vein thrombosis (DVT)

Thrombosis of the deep veins of the calf, thigh or pelvis may predispose to pulmonary embolism and should be suspected if there is any tenderness or pain on walking or when the deep veins in the calf of the leg are pressed. Clinical signs depend upon the extent of the thrombosis and whether or not phlebitis is also present. If the clot or thrombus is not obstructing the blood vessel there may be no clinical signs at all. Unfortunately, it is this type of thrombus which is most likely to become detached.

DVT is usually manifest during the first 2 weeks after delivery. There may be some swelling of the area and this can be monitored by taking daily measurements around the affected leg, which may be 2 or 3 centimetres larger than the non-affected leg. The temperature may be raised and the midwife must inform a doctor of indicative findings. Dorsiflexion of the foot, 'Homan's sign', may demonstrate an increase in calf or thigh pain. However, some view this procedure as potentially harmful and it has been superseded by Doppler ultrasonography, which offers a conclusive diagnosis. Blood samples should be taken for full screening including prothrombin time.

Management and treatment of DVT

The midwife should measure the woman's legs for TED stockings as correct sizing is vital to ensure adequate compression. Mobilisation may be restricted to reduce the risk of detachment of the thrombus until the prothrombin time has shown signs of improvement and any swelling has subsided. This will, however, depend upon consultant opinion and the severity of the condition.

Treatment is usually by anticoagulant therapy which acts by preventing clot extension. Intravenous heparin at 40 000 units per day may be administered continuously using a pump or intermittently by bolus injection for 5–10 days, followed by lower-dose subcutaneous heparin (preparations include Fragmin, Tenzaparin and Calciparine) or oral warfarin to maintain the activated thromboplastin time (APTT), usually until the end of the puerperium (Barbour 1996, Chamberlain 1995). The use of anticoagulants must be carefully controlled. There is a potential danger of haemorrhage occurring from the placental site and of the formation of haematomas. If this occurs, anticoagulant therapy must be stopped. The effect of heparin can be reversed by an intravenous injection of protamine sulphate. The effect of warfarin can be reversed by an infusion of fresh frozen plasma (FFP). Vitamin K (Konakion) has the same effect but can complicate future therapy (Chamberlain 1995). The midwife should advise the woman to report any bleeding or vulval pain. Explanation of the condition and reassurance is important.

Pulmonary embolism

Pulmonary embolism occurs when part of a clot breaks away from a vessel wall and enters the systemic circulation. It causes an obstruction once it reaches a vessel with a lumen smaller than itself, usually a pulmonary artery.

Signs and symptoms of small pulmonary emboli

- Chest pain
- Dyspnoea, coughing, slight haemoptysis
- Pyrexia, tachycardia.

Any such symptoms, however slight, must be reported at once to a doctor. The woman should be offered reassurance and oxygen if required, until medical assistance is obtained. The size of the artery blocked determines the effect.

Signs and symptoms of major pulmonary embolism

- Sudden acute chest pain
- Marked distress, shock or sudden collapse
- Dyspnoea, cyanosis
- Pyrexia, tachycardia/bradycardia, hypotension.

This constitutes an obstetric emergency.

If a major pulmonary supply artery becomes blocked, sudden acute chest pain will occur, immediately followed by respiratory collapse and possibly death.

Management and treatment

Emergency medical aid must be summoned. Oxygen should be given and intravenous heparin administered as soon as possible and continued by infusion. Pain may be relieved by intravenous morphine or diamorphine and the woman's condition will usually improve within a few hours. Treatment should then continue as for DVT (see above). However, if the woman does not respond to this therapy, the advice of a vascular specialist will be sought. Surgical embolectomy, alteplase (Gulba et al 1994), streptokinase or other thrombolytic agent may be effective, but the latter is inadvisable before the tenth postnatal day owing to the high haemorrhage risk (Barbour 1996).

It should be remembered that events such as embolism and haemorrhage may act as triggers to the development of disseminated intravascular coagulation (DIC). Further information can be found in Chapter 15.

THE NEONATE

The midwife should remember to address issues relating to the baby, where appropriate, during the postnatal assessment examination. Advice based on current research related to safety issues such as positioning of the baby and optimum room temperature should be offered. The subject of the neonate is fully covered in Chapter 35 and this should be referred to in conjunction with this chapter in order that the mother and baby can be viewed as an integral unit. The midwife should also remember to undertake neonatal screening tests with informed parental consent (see Ch. 43).

Birth registration

The midwife must inform the parents of their responsibility to register the birth within 42 days (21 in Scotland) and, if they default in this duty, anyone present at the birth, including the midwife, may be called upon to register the birth (see Ch. 48).

RECORD-KEEPING

The maintenance of accurate records is an essential part of the midwife's role. These should reflect the wishes and needs of the individual woman and be clear but concise and enable care to be continued by any health professional. Following each postnatal assessment examination, subsequent care should be reassessed in the light of each day's progress or any change in the mother's wishes and be recorded.

READER ACTIVITY

Reflect on the elements of the postnatal assessment examination. Is sufficient time allocated to this important process? Is the work organised in such a way that it prohibits efficient allocation of time? Draw up a proposal for review by peers and colleagues.

OVERVIEW OF PUERPERAL INFECTION AND CAUSATIVE ORGANISMS

The development of a pyrexia during the puerperium is relatively common. Sites of infection include the endometrium, breast tissue, perineal or abdominal wounds and the venous system. It is essential to undertake a thorough eliminative examination to locate the source. In doing this it is important to consider the history, nature of delivery and any other events which may appear relevant. Puerperal infection arises as a result of the invasion, incubation and multiplication of an organism. The timing of the onset of symptoms (Box 30.2) will depend upon the virulence of the causative organism and the individual's degree of resistance.

Endometritis is of significantly increased risk subsequent to caesarean section. The potential for MRSA (see p. 597) should be considered and necrotising fasciitis of which, whilst extremely rare, two cases were reported in the 1991–1993 triennium (DH et al 1996) and early recognition is vital. The effects which an infection has will depend greatly on prompt diagnosis, appropriate

---

Box 30.2 Common times after delivery of onset of overt symptoms (adapted from Calhoun & Brost 1995)

- Up to 6 hours – early streptococcal infections, transfusion reactions, thyroid crisis
- Up to 48 hours – atelectasis (respiratory origin)
- Up to 72 hours – urinary tract infection, pneumonia
- 3–5 days – wound infection, breast engorgement, necrotising fasciitis
- 3–7 days – mastitis, septic thrombophlebitis
- 7–14 days – abscess
- After 2 weeks – mastitis, pulmonary embolism

antibiotic therapy and the general condition of the woman.

Causative organisms

These are classified into two groups:

• endogenous organisms
• exogenous organisms.

Endogenous organisms are those which are naturally resident in regions such as the lower intestine, the vagina and the perineum, where they do no harm provided they remain within their specific environment where they have a role to play in normal ecology. They include coliform organisms such as *Escherichia coli* and *Streptococcus faecalis* which reside in the lower intestine and anus.

Certain organisms are capable of proliferation in the absence of oxygen; these are known as anaerobic organisms. The presence of bruised, lacerated and oedematous tissue therefore provides an ideal environment for organisms such as anaerobic streptococci or clostridia. For this reason puerperal infection is most likely to occur in women who have had a difficult forceps delivery or an emergency caesarean section and in those who are debilitated or anaemic.

Exogenous organisms, as their name implies, come from sources outside the body and are usually transmitted by another person, which may include members of the health care team, other women or visitors. These organisms are spread by touch, droplet infection or hospital dust, which is known to contain certain bacteria such as group A haemolytic streptococcus. Along with staphylococci, this organism is often found in the nose and throat of those with colds and can also be present when the individual exhibits no obvious symptoms. Both of these organisms have developed considerable resistance to antibiotics in recent years and can lead to severe infection for the woman or the baby.

Puerperal infection remains a cause of worldwide maternal mortality although its incidence is less frequent in developed countries. The strict adherence to policies concerning reduction of cross-infection is vital, as is correct aseptic technique for appropriate procedures.

ADDITIONAL POSTNATAL ISSUES

Sexuality and contraception

Sexuality may be the last thing on a woman's mind following the experience of birth but it is, nevertheless, a significant issue and one that is often afforded little attention. Timing of discussion is important and an appropriate moment during the postnatal period should be found. It should be remembered that sexual intimacy between a couple is an important part of their relationship and distress associated with this aspect of their lives could have long-term sequelae for the family unit. Numerous emotions may present including fear, embarrassment, confusion, jealousy and pain and, if left unvoiced, these may fester and create barriers. If the partner has been present at delivery, he may need to explore his response to the experience and his ability to detach the mothering role of the woman from her previous loving sexual role. The new father may feel unable to participate in the close mother–infant relationship and may try to compete by becoming either 'sexually demanding or aloof and distant' (Walton 1994).

The woman herself may need to reflect and re-evaluate her function within the relationship. She may feel unattractive and no longer a sexual being. The couple may feel that the woman's body now belongs to the baby on a nurturing continuum and indeed may feel inhibited by the presence of the baby, especially if during pregnancy intercourse was either limited or omitted owing to potential risk or fear of damaging the baby within the womb.

The midwife may find this a difficult subject to approach and will depend upon several factors including personal awareness of sexuality and rapport with the couple. It may be helpful to utilise a discussion about contraception to provide an opportunity for sexual issues to be raised. There may be additional concerns to be considered if the woman or her partner is HIV positive. Liaison with or referral to the general practitioner or specialist advisors should be offered. For further information on contraceptive advice refer to Chapter 32.

It is no longer uncommon for lesbian couples (see Ch. 2) to seek motherhood and the midwife needs to be aware of the differing needs of these women and their female partners (Wilton 1996), adapt advice accordingly and not form prejudiced attitudes if certain individual beliefs fall outside of personal values.

Culture and religion

In many non-western cultures, complete rest is still considered a vital aspect of postnatal care. The belief that prevention of certain rituals can adversely affect the future well-being of the woman and her child remains an important consideration for many groups wherever they may reside. The midwife should endeavour to familiarise herself with the cultural, language and religious needs of the local population in order that understanding can develop prior to involvement with care. However, the woman may not necessarily conform to the norms of her particular societal group and should always be treated as a unique individual and offered holistic care.

Physical or sensory disability

Women with a physical or sensory disability may have overcome numerous access, communication and prejudice obstacles during pregnancy. Once delivered, they are faced with the challenges of motherhood and the adaptation to this new role is as for any woman. In addition, they may require specialist advice on how to overcome specific difficulties presented by the demands of the baby. The midwife must become aware of the individual strengths and abilities of the woman and should not attempt to undermine her by taking over aspects of self or infant care. Taking responsibility for her baby is important to the woman no matter how slow or comparably less efficient than other mothers she may appear. Praise and encouragement is essential and the woman should not be made to feel inadequate in her new role. To facilitate the development of safe and effective mothering skills, a relationship of trust between the midwife and the woman with continuity of care and carer are particularly valuable. Liaison with outside agencies such as the Disabled Living Foundation or the National Childbirth Trust (Campion 1990), may help with the provision or adaptation of nursery and other equipment. Women with sensory deficiencies may also require special devices such as sound-activated visual indicators so that the deaf mother can know when her baby is crying (Nolan 1994).

It is vital that whatever the disability may be, it does not obscure the physiological and psychological care needs common to all women during the puerperium.

Promoting adequate rest and sleep

In addition to the rapid and wide-ranging physiological changes of the puerperium, this is also a time of major psychological adjustment. Sufficient rest and sleep are essential for physical and psychological well-being, and their promotion is a vital part of postnatal care. The healing of trauma is aided by physical rest, and sleep deprivation can trigger an adverse psychological response. This is dealt with fully in the next chapter. Caring for a small baby brings busy days and broken nights and achieving sufficient rest is not easy. Hospital wards are full of bustle and eager visitors and staff members may not always appreciate the mother's need for peace and quiet. It is helpful for a particular period of each day to be set aside as a rest period, when activity in the ward is kept to a minimum and visitors discouraged. When the woman returns home, the need for adequate rest should be emphasised and the family encouraged to take over the care of the baby for a period of time to allow the continuance of her pattern of resting at least once during the day.

Puerperal skeletal changes: back care

As the circulatory levels of progesterone fall, the loosening effect on the interconnecting ligaments within the pelvis and spine gradually lessens. It is important that the woman is educated in correct lifting techniques and back care (see Ch. 45).

Remaining endocrine changes

The functional cessation of the additional endocrine gland of pregnancy, the placenta, heralds the restoration of the pre-pregnant hormonal balance.

Oestrogen and progesterone fall to basal levels by the seventh postpartum day, resuming the pattern of the normal menstrual cycle unless affected by the process of lactation (see Ch. 36). Human placental lactogen (HPL) is undetectable by the second postnatal day and human chorionic gonadotrophin (HCG) by the tenth day. The effects of postnatal hormonal alterations have already been discussed under the relevant headings.

SUMMARY

This chapter has presented the main components required for the delivery of safe, effective postnatal care in order to promote physical and emotional health for the woman, her baby and the family. The process of adjustment to motherhood continues throughout the puerperium and beyond it. Many women may take several months before becoming really confident in their mothering role. Midwives working in hospital and in the community have a unique opportunity to assist in this adjustment process by their competence, skill and sensitivity to the needs and expectations of individual women and their families. It is important that the woman's full physical and psychological recovery from the effects of pregnancy, labour and delivery is confirmed by a medical examination at the end of the puerperium (see Ch. 31).

READER ACTIVITIES

1. Use the following question in order to test one aspect of your knowledge. If you choose to undertake it as a revision question, allow yourself 1 hour:

Consider and analyse the care requirements during the first 48 hours for a woman who has been delivered by lower segment caesarean section.

2. Prepare a reference guide which could be used as the basis for discussing and planning postnatal care in partnership with:

   a. a woman who intends to breast feed her second baby having previously given formula milk to her first baby
   b. a woman who is registered blind
   c. a woman who is hemiplegic.

What facts would you need to know in order to assess individual needs?

What choices and patterns of care would you wish to offer?

What outside agencies could you liaise with for additional help?

3. Undertake a literature search on postnatal maternal physiological morbidity. Make short notes on available material and share these in discussion at a journal club with peers and colleagues.

ACKNOWLEDGEMENTS

The help of the midwives of The James Paget Hospital, Great Yarmouth, Norfolk, is gratefully acknowledged.

USEFUL ADDRESSES

Disabled Living Foundation
380–384 Harrow Road
London W9 2HU

National Childbirth Trust (NCT)
Alexandra House
Oldham Terrace
London W3 6NH

Association for Improvements in the Maternity Services (AIMS)
40 Kingswood Avenue
London NW6 6LS

The Maternity Alliance
45 Beech Street
London EC2P 2LX

REFERENCES

Barbour L A 1996 Thromboembolism In: Queenan J T, Hobbins J C (eds) Protocols for high-risk pregnancies, 3rd edn. Blackwell, Oxford, ch 34, pp 229–234

Briggs G G, Freeman R K, Yaffe S J 1990 Drugs in pregnancy and lactation, 3rd edn. Williams & Wilkins, London

Calhoun B C, Brost B 1995 Emergency management of sudden puerperal fever. In: Martin J (ed) Intrapartum and postpartum obstetric emergencies. Obstetric and Gynecology Clinics of North America 22(2): 357–367

Campion M J 1990 The baby challenge – a handbook on pregnancy for women with a physical disability. Routledge, London pp 203–205

Castro M 1990 The complete homeopathy handbook. Macmillan, London

Chamberlain G V P (ed) 1995 Obstetrics by ten teachers, 16th edn. Arnold, London

Cluett E R, Alexander J, Pickering R M 1995 Is measuring postnatal symphysis–fundal distance worthwhile? Midwifery 11: 174–183

Cummings B 1994 Using homeopathy in midwifery practice. Modern Midwife 4(11): 17–20

Davis P 1988 Aromatherapy an A–Z. Daniel, Saffron Walden

Department of Health 1993 Changing childbirth: report of the expert maternity group. HMSO, London, part 1

Department of Health, Welsh Office, Scottish Home and Health Department, Department of Health and Social Services, Northern Ireland 1996 Report on confidential enquiries into maternal deaths in the United Kingdom 1991–1993. HMSO, London

Enkin M, Keirse M J N C, Renfrew M, Neilson J 1995 A guide to effective care in pregnancy and childbirth, 2nd edn. Oxford University Press, Oxford

Ferrazzani S, De Carolis S, Pomini F, Testa A C, Mastromarino C, Caruso A 1994 The duration of hypertension in the puerperium of pre-eclamptic women: relationship with renal impairment and week of delivery. American Journal of Obstetrics and Gynecology 171(2): 506–512

Gulba D C, Schmid C, Borst H G et al 1994 Medical compared with surgical treatment for massive pulmonary embolism. Lancet 343(8897): 576–577

Hallgren A, Kihlgren M, Norberg A, Forslin L 1995 Women's perceptions of childbirth and childbirth education before and after education and birth. Midwifery 11(3): 130–137

Harrison J 1995 The use of complementary medicine in postnatal care. British Journal of Midwifery 3(1): 31–34

Henderson C 1990 Models and midwifery. In: Salvage J, Kershaw B (eds) Models for nursing 2. Scutari, London, ch 7

Hillan E M 1995 Postoperative morbidity following caesarean delivery. Journal of Advanced Nursing 22(6): 1035–1042

James D K, Stirrat G M 1988 Pregnancy and risk: the basis for rational management. Wiley, Chichester, p 52

Kamm M 1996 Special focus conference report by Scowen P: childbirth and continence: 2. Professional Care of Mother and Child 6(5): 119–123

Llewellyn-Jones D 1994 Fundamentals of obstetrics and gynaecology, 6th edn. Mosby, London, p 86

Marchant S 1995 What are we doing in the postnatal check? British Journal of Midwifery 3(1): 34–38

Meniru G I 1996 An analysis of recent trends in vacuum extraction and forceps delivery in the UK. British Journal of Obstetrics and Gynaecology 103(2): 168–170

Montgomery E, Alexander J 1994 Assessing postnatal uterine involution: a review and a challenge. Midwifery 10: 73–76

Moore K H, Richmond D H, Sutherst J R et al 1991 Crouching over the toilet seat: prevalence among British gynaecological outpatients and its effect upon micturition. British Journal of Obstetrics and Gynaecology 98: 569–572

Morin K H 1994 Urologic consequences of childbirth: a review of the literature. Urologic Nursing 14(2): 41–47

Murphy-Black T 1994 Care in the community during the postnatal period. In: Robinson S, Thomson A M (eds) Midwives, research and childbirth. Chapman & Hall, London, vol 3, ch 6, pp 120–146

Nolan M 1994 Care for the deaf mother. Modern Midwife 4(7): 16

O'Keefe D, O'Herlihy C, Gross Y, Kelly J G 1994 Patient-controlled analgesia using a miniature electrochemically driven infusion pump. British Journal of Anaesthetics 73(6): 843–846

Prodromidis M, Field T, Arendt R, Singer L, Yando R, Bendell D 1995 Mothers touching newborns: a comparison or rooming-in versus minimal contact. Birth: Issues in Perinatal Care and Education 22(4): 196–203

Ridgway L E 1995 Puerperal emergency: vaginal and vulvar haematomas. Obstetric and Gynaecology Clinics of North America 22(2): 275–282

Royal College of Midwives 1991 Successful breastfeeding, 2nd edn. Churchill Livingstone, Edinburgh, pp 45–46

Royal College of Midwives 1994 RCM standing practice group paper 2: community postnatal visiting. Midwives Chronicle and Nursing Notes (June): 231

Schott J, Henley A 1996 Culture, religion and childbearing in a multiracial society – a handbook for health professionals. Butterworth-Heinemann, Oxford, p 16

Usta I M, Sibai B M 1995 Emergent management of puerperal eclampsia. Obstetric and Gynaecology Clinics of North America 22(2): 315–335

Walton I 1994 Sexuality and motherhood. Books for Midwives Press, Hale, Cheshire, p 105

Wilton T 1996 Caring for the lesbian client: homophobia and midwifery. British Journal of Midwifery 4(3): 127

United Kingdom Central Council for Nursing, Midwifery and Health Visiting (UKCC) 1993 Midwives rules. UKCC, London, pp 8, 21

United Kingdom Central Council for Nursing, Midwifery and Health Visiting (UKCC) 1994 The midwife's code of practice. UKCC, London, p 14

FURTHER READING

Alexander J, Levy V, Roch S (eds) 1990 Postnatal care: a research-based approach. Macmillan, Basingstoke

Ball J A 1989 Postnatal care and adjustment to motherhood. In: Robinson S, Thomson A M (eds) Midwives, research and childbirth. Chapman & Hall, London, vol 1

Bryar R M 1995 Theory for midwifery practice. Macmillan, Basingstoke, *explores philosophies and models for developing midwifery postnatal care (see pp 112–118, 159–163, 173–199)*

Hamadeh G, Dedmon C, Mozley P 1995 Postpartum fever. American Family Physician 52(2): 531–538

Laryea M 1989 Midwives' and mothers' perceptions of motherhood. In: Robinson S, Thomson A M (eds) Midwives, research and childbirth. Chapman & Hall, London, vol 1

Llewellyn-Jones D 1994 Infections of the genital tract. In: Fundamentals of obstetrics and gynaecology, 6th edn. Mosby, London, ch 35

Morkved S, Bo K 1996 The effect of post-natal exercises to strengthen the pelvic floor muscles. Acta Obstetrica et Gynecologica Scandinavica 75(4): 382–385

Paterson J A, Davis J, Gregory M et al 1994 A study on the effects of low haemoglobin on postnatal women. Midwifery 10: 77–86

Royal College of Midwives 1987 Towards a healthy nation: a policy for the maternity services. RCM, London

Smith J A, Mitchell S 1996 Debriefing after childbirth: a tool for effective risk management. British Journal of Midwifery 4(11): 581–586

World Health Organization Safe motherhood newsletter of worldwide activity. WHO, Geneva, published quarterly

31

The postnatal emotional and psychological response

Liz Hynes (née Spruce)

Psychological health in the early postnatal period tends to be overshadowed by the preoccupation with physiological health. However, although physiological events are usually more overt, the midwife should remember that psychological illness may have longer-term sequelae. Simkin (1991) found that women retained deep memories of their birth experiences and believes that 'Anything remembered so vividly must influence the person'. There is also increasing evidence that postnatal depression may adversely affect the quality of interaction between mother and baby and subsequent childhood development (Beck 1995, Murray 1988). It is vital, therefore, that the midwife is able to promote psychological health and recognise deviation from normal emotional response during the puerperium. The assessment of psychological health is an integral part of postnatal care and therefore this chapter should be viewed in conjunction with the preceding chapter.

The chapter aims to:

- stress the need for emotional support in the immediate postnatal period

- highlight the role of the midwife in fostering confidence in the mother and good infant–parent relationships

- examine the different types of psychological disturbance seen in the puerperium, with particular emphasis on the recognition and management of puerperal psychosis and postnatal depression

- discuss the 6-week postnatal examination.

THE NORMAL EMOTIONAL RESPONSE TO PARENTHOOD

Whilst the addition of a new family member may

have been planned and greatly desired, the initial reality of the persistent demands exerted by a baby on energy, time and emotions can seem overwhelming. New parents may feel that they have relinquished control to this tiny bundle of formidable rapture. The emotional reactions experienced can vary between love and extreme joy, to panic, guilt and fear. Preparation for becoming parents varies but no matter how much attention has been afforded to this new role, the reality, once presented, may appear very different from the perceived, perhaps idealistic expectation. Adaptation to the demands of parenthood takes time, and modification of all aspects of previous life is inevitable. As with any change that occurs, the way in which it is managed will affect both the parents' ability to adapt and the consequence of the adjustment. This scenario is also affected by the structure of the family within contemporary society. Few new western parents have the help and support of an extended family, as with certain other cultural groups such as Chinese, South Asian, or African–Caribbean families who tend to have a strong matriarchal family structure (Schott & Henley 1996).

A baby also places new demands financially which may lead to unexpected alterations in lifestyle in addition to those anticipated. Psychological adjustment to parenthood is a varied and gradual process that requires time and patience from all involved, the woman, her partner, siblings, the midwives and other health professionals involved in the partnership of care. The parenting role is a complex experience, accompanied by a number of conflicting reactions and feelings, some of which may be unexpected. The mother must learn to care for her new baby during the time in which she is still recovering from the physical stress of pregnancy, labour and delivery. The partner and any siblings must learn to share love and attention with this newcomer.

The puerperium spans the transitional period during which the parents adjust their patterns of living to meet the needs of a small infant. Many new mothers have little or no experience of caring for a newborn infant and may feel overwhelmed by the responsibility. They will be very sensitive to any suggestion that they are not coping well and

be easily confused and distressed by conflicting or ill-considered advice. The patterns of mothering which develop will depend partly upon the mother's degree of experience in caring for babies, but much more upon her expectations, self-esteem, natural personality and her psychological strengths. This will also be affected by the quality of the support she receives from her partner, family and friends, her midwife and other members of the health care team within the cultural constraints of the society within which she resides.

READER ACTIVITY

If you are a mother, reflect back on how you felt during the early days of new motherhood. If you are not a mother, talk to family or friends about the early feelings of mothering and try to build this into your understanding when with postnatal women.

Self-esteem and body image

The value we allot to ourselves, our self-esteem, may alter at different stages in our lives and indeed over different areas of our lives. For example, prior to childbirth a woman may have believed herself to be proficient at managing her life, with a positive self-image and high self-esteem. However, as a new mother, she may feel completely inadequate to care for her baby and self-esteem may take a dramatic fall.

Body image may have altered considerably during pregnancy, thus affecting the woman's self-image. Societal portrayal of women emphasises the aesthetic 'slim' outward figure rather than that of the functional body. Following delivery, body shape rarely returns quickly to a non-pregnant contour and the woman's self-esteem may be reduced by the realisation that her body may appear fat and unattractive. This is further compounded if the new mother is excessively fatigued following delivery and coping with the demands of her infant (Price 1996). Likewise, to a greater or lesser degree, the new father may also suffer from lowered self-esteem. This will be dependent on his expectations, the relationship between the couple and his preparedness for the inevitable changes in their roles. Existing siblings may also feel their role is threatened by this new family member and they may need reassurance of their parents' continued love and support. Within the partnership of care, it is important that the midwife facilitates the enhancement of confidence and self-esteem within the new family unit.

THE ROLE OF THE MIDWIFE IN THE PROMOTION OF POSTNATAL PSYCHOLOGICAL HEALTH

Giving birth is the culmination of many hopes and fears and heralds not only the beginning of a new individual but also enormous change to a couple's future family life. Caring for a newborn infant is a demanding 24-hour-a-day commitment which is rarely represented accurately within the media. It is an enormously emotional event and both parents, but particularly the mother, need to be supported during a period of acclimatisation. The secret of providing emotional support is to have an encouraging, empathetic attitude, facilitating confidence in the new mother's ability to care for her baby, thus preventing her from feeling unable to fulfil her new role.

Building confidence

Each mother should be helped to realise her unique and inestimable worth in providing for the welfare of her baby, and the attitudes of midwives and other health workers should convey their respect for her. The mother's role as a woman must also be recognised; she is not only a mother but also a person of value in her own right and should be encouraged to take time for herself and to resume some social contacts. It can also be helpful to suggest that the couple endeavour to arrange some time alone together as soon as possible after the birth.

The midwife can facilitate the building of the mother's confidence by giving clear and careful instructions and by providing opportunities for the mother to ask questions and to discuss any concerns she may have. It may be necessary to repeat explanations on a number of occasions and the midwife must be patient in teaching and encouraging those mothers who are particularly anxious. Together with the mother, the midwife should draw up a plan to meet individual learning needs and where feasible the partner should be involved with these sessions. These may include:

- feeding issues including sterilisation methods if bottle feeding with formula milk
- hygiene needs of the baby including dealing with sore buttocks, skin rashes, etc.
- positioning of the baby and prevention of sudden infant death syndrome (SIDS)
- the crying baby including possible reasons and remedies
- discussion relating to the emotional needs of parents and other family members
- the role of the health visitor and the ongoing support mechanisms such as mother and baby clinics, postnatal support groups
- the purpose and importance of postnatal examination
- family planning advice (see Ch. 32).

The sessions should be spread over a period of time and, ideally, be with the mother's named midwife to maintain consistency of advice. Conflicting advice is a potent cause of discouragement and those most vulnerable to emotional distress tend to blame themselves for being unable to understand what the midwife is advising them to do. This is particularly true when a mother is feeding her baby, whether by breast or bottle, because she is doing far more than providing nourishment; she is communicating her love and care to her baby, and is rewarded by contented satisfaction following the feed. This is of much greater significance than the level of skill displayed and midwives should recognise that it is the mother who is the most important person in her baby's life. The maternal–infant relationship must not be impaired by the skilled midwife usurping the mother's role. Some mothers will be highly competent and irritated by receiving too much advice and help, while others may feel foolish if they cannot cope as well as they feel they should.

It is important that the woman is encouraged to participate actively in teaching sessions and that praise and encouragement is offered frequently.

The midwife should provide help, encouragement and advice and should praise the mother for her achievements, both in the act of giving birth and in mothering her infant. The role of the midwife is to nurture the mother and her self-confidence. In this way, the maternal–child relationship can be enriched. Where the midwife has developed a good rapport with the woman during pregnancy and labour, her individual needs may be clearly known and assist the midwife's judgement of the focus of learning required. In the promotion of successful relationships between parents and their baby, nothing succeeds like success and the couple should be congratulated for their achievements in a non-condescending manner. Advice and support should be offered sensitively for tasks that they may find more difficult initially and they should not be criticised or made to feel inadequate. Also, it is important that comparisons are not drawn between the competence of different mothers, and midwives should discourage a woman from comparing her ability in infant care with that of other mothers. Routine patterns of care, particularly within the hospital environment, should be avoided whenever possible, in order that mothers sharing rooms do not feel that they are in competition with each other.

Learning is a gradual process related to individual ability, physical and emotional well-being. Taking increasing responsibility for the care of the baby should be staged and the mother enabled to build upon the successful completion of one aspect of care before being expected to master another. Thus, one mother may feel ready and eager to bath her baby at an early stage, while another may not feel sufficiently confident in handling her small charge safely until the baby is a week old. It should also be remembered that women may have differing postnatal needs according to their cultural or religious background. Midwives should endeavour to ascertain any potential areas of difficulty such as language comprehension and facilitate, where possible, the requirement for certain rituals to be followed. Jewish women, for example, are expected to rest completely for the first 10 postnatal days cared for by female family and friends. They must have no physical contact with their husbands and take a ritual bath at the end of this period. Inability to fulfil their beliefs may lead to extreme anxiety or distress.

READER ACTIVITY

Reflect on your own style of learning. What assists your comprehension of a topic? Do your peers agree? Try to put yourself in the place of new mothers, who not only have differing learning needs and styles, but are also in a situation which may feel alien to them, whether at home or in hospital. How can you help them to learn?

Within the home environment, the midwife should try to ensure that family and friends understand the woman's needs and offer help readily without taking over or undermining confidence. The importance of adequate rest and sleep should be emphasised in order that no unreasonable demands are placed upon the new mother. The woman also needs to have time for relaxation and appropriate postnatal exercise and should be encouraged to spend some time each day on herself.

In the past, assumptions have sometimes been made about potential emotionally damaging effects of unrealistic expectations of both childbirth and motherhood. In a prospective study of 825 women from six units across southeast England, Green et al (1990) concluded that 'it was women with low expectations who were more likely to have poor psychological outcomes'. This would indicate that having high expectations may, in fact, assist women to believe in themselves and act in a positive way even when reality does not echo that which was anticipated. The study also challenged other frequently assumed stereotypes, finding that less well-educated women were not necessarily more likely to want to hand over control to the midwives. It is important that each midwife is aware of her own values and preconceptions and does not inflict these on the women with whom she is involved. It is also important to foster flexibility throughout the process, in particular in the interpretation of the word 'control'. Giving women control does not mean that they become totally responsible for every decision related to their care and 'control' may mean something very different from one woman to the next. It is vital that midwives treat each woman as an individual and not categorise by reference to age, ability, employment, race, culture, religion or class. This is particularly important for women with physical or sensory disability. Implementation of caseload midwifery and continuity of contact between women and a named midwife throughout the childbirth process should facilitate increased insight into the normal personality and needs of individual women. This will not only assist the recognition of deviation from normal psychological health but may also provide a closer relationship between the midwife and the woman in which communication of feelings may be enhanced.

READER ACTIVITY

Imagine you are a new mother who, because of either language or hearing difficulty, cannot understand what is being spoken around and to her. What would help your understanding? It may be useful to enact this as a role play with a colleague and discuss strategies for assisting comprehension. Remember to debrief after any role play.

Debriefing and special groups

It is important for women to be able to debrief following the birth experience, preferably with the midwife who was present during delivery. Ideally, this should happen early during the postnatal period after the woman has had time to rest and recover from the birth.

This is particularly important for special groups such as following late miscarriage, stillbirth, termination for abnormality, or traumatic delivery (see Chs 48 and 33). It is also important for mothers separated from their baby by a requirement for special or intensive care due to prematurity, birth asphyxia or medical problems such as unstable blood glucose subsequent to maternal diabetes. These mothers will feel anxious and may be very distressed about the well-being of their babies and their inability to undertake full infant care. It is vital that as much contact as possible is maintained and that involvement in feeding and general care

of the baby is encouraged. Photographs for the parents to keep with them are also helpful. If the baby is critically ill, many hospitals now have the facility to allow parents to stay together close to the care unit. This enables them to be involved in the care of their baby while offering each other support. Couples will need counselling, with the opportunity to discuss their feelings. Hospital padres often are very helpful and can assist with this role regardless of religious persuasion.

Special consideration will be required for mothers positive for human immunodeficiency virus (HIV), who may need extended support during the months of waiting to discover if this has been transmitted to the baby. Mothers who have been alcohol or drug abusers during pregnancy may experience guilt and extreme anxiety if they see that the baby has been affected in utero and will require sensitive support. The midwife should also remember that a mother who is relinquishing her baby for adoption or whose baby is being taken into care will need particular understanding as she may experience symptoms of grief and be at increased risk of depression if her feelings are suppressed. Parents who have suffered previous loss may also require additional support and time to discuss their concerns. Some may need this opportunity repeated on more than one occasion, allowing time for reflection and for the formulation of further questions which they may have. Whilst the responsibility of the midwife lies primarily with the mother and baby, it is important that the partner's psychological needs are not overlooked. Ultimately, the emotional health of either partner can affect maternal or infant morbidity as well as the family relationship.

It is important for midwives to be able to distinguish between distress which may be considered a natural postnatal response and symptoms of deviation from psychological health. Enhanced knowledge of the woman and her family may assist the decision-making process, but whenever doubt exists, advice should be sought from specialist professional colleagues. Reassurance and additional support may be all that is required for many women. There is a natural empathy between a mother and her baby and this grows into a strong and mutually enriching relationship as the two spend time with each other. Mothers who are well cared for are able to enjoy caring for the baby. The midwife should seek to foster the growth of a strong relationship by building the mother's confidence, preventing or alleviating physical discomfort and ensuring that the mother is protected from unnecessary stress and anxiety. Midwives need to be aware of differing needs and seek to inform, thereby empowering all women to achieve their own optimum attainment level. In this way the groundwork can be laid for a healthy emotional response to childbirth.

All events, advice or instructions given throughout the midwife's involvement in care should be clearly documented as contemporaneously as possible within the woman's records in order that any other midwife or member of the health care team may provide continuity of care and advice. This is also vital for reference during any subsequent pregnancy.

THE MATERNAL–INFANT RELATIONSHIP (see also Ch. 34)

The maternal–infant relationship begins at different times for each woman; it may be around the time of the first scan or when fetal activity becomes evident. However, if the pregnancy is long awaited, some women may feel this bond almost from conception or, alternatively, women who have previously experienced miscarriage, stillbirth or neonatal death, may not allow acknowledgement of the unborn baby until late pregnancy or even birth. The father may not begin to develop a relationship with his baby until he holds it in his arms, but some men may also feel a developing bond during their partner's pregnancy, especially if closely involved during ultrasonography and other events.

The fourth stage of labour

The time immediately following delivery of the baby is a most important time for the fostering of good parent–infant relationships and has been referred to as the fourth stage of labour (Ball 1994). Once safety is assured, the mother and father should be left alone with their baby to explore and enjoy this new experience. The mother should be encouraged to offer the baby a feed soon after birth, either at the breast or by bottle, dependent on her choice. This facilitates early eye contact and appears to be emotionally healthy for both mother and baby. Touch and eye contact between parents and infant are particularly important during the first hour following birth when the newborn infant is often particularly alert. Ideally, this fourth stage of labour should be viewed as an integral part of the birth process or early puerperal care and not as an optional extra when considered convenient. However, the midwife should bear in mind that not all parents may take this opportunity and they should not be made to feel uncomfortable if they do not feel ready to explore their emotions. A great deal has been written and debated about theories of bonding and attachment between the mother and her baby but it is generally accepted that early and consistent close contact enriches the developing relationship between them (Inch 1989, Raphael-Leff 1991). It is important that women are assured that maternal feelings vary in their development. Many women feel an immediate and overwhelming rush of love for their baby as soon as it is born but others may need time for feelings to manifest. Parents should be reassured that failure to experience immediate love for their baby is not unusual and the midwife should ensure that close and intimate contact is not being restricted.

PSYCHOLOGICAL PUERPERAL HEALTH

With rapid physiological and psychological change occurring during the first week of the puerperium it is not surprising to find that many women experience emotional lability during the first 3 or 4 days. The preceding events of pregnancy, labour and delivery together with the peak experience of giving birth all contribute to a mixture of emotional reactions.

There are three distinctive types of psychological disturbance seen in the puerperium: postnatal or 'third day' blues; psychosis; and postnatal depression. Whilst the first can be considered a common and arguably normal response, boundaries between the three states can become blurred and it is vital that the midwife can clearly distinguish symptoms and recognise deviation from normal psychological health.

A fourth category of psychological disorder is beginning to appear on the postnatal agenda, that of post-traumatic stress disorder. Whilst a relatively new concept, there appears to be growing interest in the condition.

Third or fourth day 'maternal postnatal blues'

The transient condition the 'blues' occurs during the early puerperium, is widely acknowledged as a normal reaction to new motherhood and causes few problems, lasting 24–48 hours. Incidence is high: in a study of 68 primigravid women, 69% experienced the 'blues' during the first postnatal week (McIntosh 1986). This study involved too small a cohort to achieve significance, but others have reported similar or even higher levels (Kumar 1984, Raphael-Leff 1991). Incidence is increased by fatigue and any undue stress or anxiety arising from family tensions or insensitive handling by those responsible for caring for the mother. Anxiety about her ability to cope with the demands of the baby may also add to the mother's transient distress. Symptoms vary in severity but commonly include rapid mood changes with crying or laughing for no apparent reason. Women frequently apologise for these responses and feel that they should be able to control these emotional reactions. Current knowledge does not appear to suggest a link to age, parity, social class or traumatic birth experience. There is some evidence to support a link with the dramatic fall in circulating blood levels of progesterone following expulsion of the placenta (Dalton 1996, Harris et al 1996). However, when one considers the events occurring around the time of onset, it seems likely that it is the result of a combination of factors. The stress of hospitalisation may also be a contributory factor but as yet the incidence of the 'blues' following home birth has not been documented. Timing is compounded by the onset of lactation, the extreme tiredness often felt in the early days of motherhood and the fact that many women are discharged from hospital before the third postnatal day to face the responsibility and demands that a new baby brings.

It is important not to trivialise the condition, but to assure a woman that this emotional reaction is normal and is often the best and only treatment required. For some new mothers, however, this distress may last longer than usual and the midwife must be alert in order to distinguish the transitory state from symptoms displayed in women who may be developing a psychosis or early postnatal depression.

PSYCHIATRIC DISORDERS OF THE PUERPERIUM

There are two distinct types of psychiatric disorder associated with the puerperium:

- puerperal psychosis
- postnatal depression.

Puerperal psychosis

The onset of puerperal psychosis is usually rapid, occurring within the first few days of delivery and rarely beyond the first 2–3 weeks. The midwife is therefore likely to be the lead professional in partnership with the woman and her family during this time. It is vital that this extreme illness is recognised promptly, in order to facilitate early intervention and thus expedite recovery.

Puerperal psychosis has been documented in Greek history as far back as 400 BC by Hippocrates. 19th century pioneers in the field included Louis Marcé, who in 1858 wrote a detailed description of psychotic illness during the puerperium. Since then and until very recently, limited research has been undertaken into this rare but extreme puerperal illness. This appears to be partly due to debate over psychiatric classification of the disease and partly to the social stigma attached to mental illness.

READER ACTIVITY

Examine your own attitudes toward mental illness. How have these developed? How do the media represent mental health? How can you, as a midwife, help families address these issues?

Incidence

Puerperal psychosis is of relatively low incidence – 1 : 450; it is more common in primiparous women (Kendall et al 1987). However, Brockington (1992) has reported an incidence as high as 1 : 5 in women who have suffered a previous psychosis either during childbirth or otherwise. No defined cause has yet been isolated.

Recognition

An acute onset of puerperal psychosis with a florid presentation is hard to miss, but sometimes this illness develops more gradually.

> A woman may appear to be experiencing normal emotional adaptive responses to childbirth, and may exhibit similar symptoms to those of maternal blues. Acutely or gradually, these become more profound with extreme mood swings during which feelings of guilt or anxiety may be expressed. A degree of euphoria is often apparent, especially in first time mothers, but in a woman developing a psychosis, this will appear extended or exaggerated. The onset of these symptoms may be heralded by a time of acute restlessness and inability to sleep. The woman is likely to suffer insomnia unassociated with disturbance by her baby. Subsequently, the behaviour of the woman may become bizarre; she may do or say inappropriate things or react out of character; relatives may recognise this and express concern. During the period of bizarre behaviour, the woman may be experiencing delusions or hallucinations and have become temporarily detached from the reality of her situation. She may state that her baby is abnormal, and may believe it to be possessed, but may not express this vocally; instead she may avoid the baby. The woman may also have episodes of lucidity where her behaviour reverts to apparent normality. At times she may appear depressed or weepy; at the early stage she may ask for help or state how she feels to someone, not necessarily to a health professional. If the woman does care for her baby, she may take longer than expected to do simple tasks such as nappy changing or she may forget when her baby was last fed. The woman may experience other thoughts and feelings which cannot be seen by an observer, such as suicidal impulses or desires to harm her baby; she may appear confused or distant at times interspersed with periods of hyperactivity (Spruce 1994).

Suicidal or infanticidal impulses are not unknown, but are rarely enacted. In the period 1989–1992, there were 13 reported cases of infanticide (Dalton 1996). The Infanticide Act was passed in 1939, when it became recognised in British law that a woman's mind may be so unbalanced during the first postnatal year that she may kill her baby. The Act was set up to protect the woman from a conviction of murder of her own baby but she could be convicted of the lesser offence, infanticide, which equates to manslaughter.

Guidelines to help in deciding what action to take if puerperal psychosis is suspected are given in Box 31.1.

READER ACTIVITY

Find out your unit protocol related to referral route for puerperal psychosis. What resources are available in your area for women diagnosed with this illness?

Treatment

Because of the extreme nature of the symptoms, medical help is usually summoned as a matter

---

Box 31.1 Guidelines to assist the action decision

- If it is suspected that a woman may be developing puerperal psychosis, it is important to keep her under constant observation until appropriate help is obtained. Wherever possible, this observation should be by the midwife or other health professional.
- If the midwife is unsure of the symptoms or of the best action to take and if a local liaison agreement is in place, informal advice may be sought from a member of the psychiatric team.
- Dependent on unit protocol, a senior member of the obstetric team or the general practitioner (GP) should be contacted directly, informed of the midwife's suspicions, and requested to seek urgent psychiatric referral.
- If the appropriate psychiatric referral is not being made, the midwife should clearly restate the concerns and try to insist that a psychiatric opinion is sought, refer to the next senior member of the obstetric team or contact a supervisor of midwives.
- Remember – the sooner the woman receives the correct psychiatric assistance, the sooner she will recover (Spruce 1994).

of urgency but there may be some reluctance to involve the psychiatrist. Occasionally heavy sedation at the time of onset has been known to be effective but early intervention with antipsychotic drugs is known to be beneficial. Pharmacological treatment varies according to the presenting symptoms and should be managed under the care of the psychiatric team, but may include lithium and/or electroconvulsive therapy. However, even when treatment is initiated promptly, 'psychosis can persist for 8 or more weeks, especially when the patient has a pre-existing history of schizophrenia or manic depressive illness' (Schorr & Richardson 1995). Admission to a psychiatric unit is usually essential, ideally with a dedicated mother and baby unit. Unfortunately, owing to inadequate resources, these are rare and at the acute stage of the illness it is of questionable value to maintain maternal–infant contact. It is, however, important to reintroduce the mother and baby as soon as it is considered appropriate and safe to do so. The advantages of joint admission are:

- re-establishment of the maternal–infant relationship
- the opportunity to observe the interaction between mother and baby with the opportunity for exploration of feelings
- to rebuild self-esteem by encouraging care of the baby within a safe environment.

The midwife should continue to visit both mother and baby to undertake the non-psychiatric aspects of postnatal care. Family support also needs consideration.

Whilst complete recovery is often achieved, it is possible that further episodes of the illness will occur throughout the woman's life and there is an increased risk of recurrence in subsequent pregnancies. The midwife needs to be able to offer advice and support to women during subsequent pregnancies and to liaise with the psychiatric team when appropriate, in order to initiate prompt referral should it become necessary.

Postnatal depression

Postnatal depression has an incidence of at least 1 : 10 with a further similar figure developing considerable emotional distress (Cox 1992, Dalton 1996, Richards 1990). With an estimated annual birthrate of 600 000, at least 60 000 families will be affected every year in the UK. Onset tends to be gradual, developing after the second postnatal week, often coinciding with the reduction in professional involvement. The condition may last for 3–6 months and in some cases it will persist throughout the first year of the baby's life. Such depression is disabling for the mother and causes considerable disruption of family life and maternal–child relationships. There is some evidence that depression in the mother has an adverse effect upon her baby's performance in developmental tests (Beck 1995, Murray 1988).

Causes

Postnatal depression is a reactive illness. Its causes are complex but possibly provoked by *demand overload*. Despite a vast amount of research and debate, there remains no consistent opinion as to its specific aetiology. It appears to be more prevalent in women who have experienced other stress-inducing life events around the time of the birth, such as moving house, bereavement or relationship disharmony. Low self-esteem, lack of close support networks and stress associated with certain aspects of postnatal care are also contributory factors (Ball 1994). The dramatic fall in the circulating hormones progesterone and oestrogen following expulsion of the placenta have been proposed as causative with a potential link between severe 'maternal blues' and later development of depression. Harris et al (1996) undertook a prospective study involving 120 primiparous women and concluded that they could not support the progesterone theory. They did, however, find an association between lowered evening cortisol levels from before delivery until 10 days postpartum in women diagnosed as depressed at 6 weeks. Women's own perceptions of cause commonly include the demands of motherhood, poor support and loss of personal freedom (McIntosh 1993). Indeed, it has also been proposed that many cases may in fact be a misdiagnosis of maternal distress brought about by the 'normal' changes occurring in the life of the new mother (Barclay & Lloyd 1996).

Recognition

Symptoms of postnatal depression are similar to those of depression occurring at any other time. During the puerperium, however, the woman may complain of numerous indefinable physical symptoms or appear overanxious about her baby in spite of evidence that the infant is well and thriving. The baby may be irritable or show signs of failing to thrive as a response to or effect of the condition of the mother. The main difference from other depression is that in postnatal depression there is the tendency to experience difficulty falling asleep, but once asleep, the woman will sleep for long periods. Women suffering postnatal depression often feel well in the morning but deteriorate as the day goes on. In most other depression, early waking is reported with symptoms more acute in the morning but improving as the day goes on. The postnatally depressed woman may feel constantly tired in spite of adequate periods of rest and be unable to cope with the needs of her baby and other family members. She is likely to feel a failure as a mother and, because of this, be afraid to admit her feelings. Some women have been able to conceal their depression so well that the condition has remained undiagnosed for months. Sensory, language or cultural barriers may make it particularly difficult for women to communicate their feelings. Awareness of body language and knowledge of the individual woman may help the midwife to identify potential risk. It is important that each woman is seen as an individual as 'assumptions about women of minority groups can also create powerful barriers and can interfere with health professionals' ability to recognise symptoms of postnatal depression' (Schott & Henley 1996).

READER ACTIVITY

Ask a friend or colleague to observe your body language over a short period. Then, observe someone else. Try to become more in touch with the silent signals we portray.

The Edinburgh Postnatal Depression Scale (Cox et al 1987) has been designed to assist the recognition of women who may be at risk of development of postnatal depression. This has been a significant move forward but is primarily for use by health visitors and at a stage beyond the normal midwifery remit. Good communication among the health care team, in particular between midwives and health visitors, is essential in order to alert professional colleagues to women who may be considered to be at increased risk. A strategy group in Oxford has successfully developed a multidisciplinary approach, with involvement of local media, purchasers, GPs and psychiatric services as well as midwives and health visitors. The main aim is to raise awareness of postnatal depression and ultimately reduce morbidity associated with the illness. Evaluative audit of the strategy is ongoing (McClarey & Stokoe 1995). Once diagnosed, treatment depends on stage and severity of the depression.

Management and treatment

As with puerperal psychosis, early detection and initiation of appropriate treatment brings the best prognosis and therefore the midwife must be alert for signs that may put a woman at increased risk of development of depression. If the midwife suspects a woman is depressed, this should be reported to a medical practitioner in accordance with The Midwife's Code of Practice (UKCC 1994). In less severe cases, treatment with mild sedation or antidepressants may be prescribed and further support given by the community psychiatric nurse. A trial using transdermal oestrogen patches has reported some success with a cohort of 34 women suffering from major depression which commenced during the first 3 months following childbirth (Gregoire et al 1996). Counselling is known to be helpful, particularly if initiated at an early stage (Holden 1990). Involvement of the partner and other close family members may also be advantageous. The midwife may be able to arrange local groups facilitated by members of the health care team – midwives, health visitors and, where appropriate, community psychiatric nurses or social workers. It may be helpful to encourage peer support for unsupported or otherwise vulnerable mothers by putting them in contact with women in similar circumstances. Women with disabilities may require additional emotional and practical support whilst adapting to the additional needs of their babies, with referral to other agencies if necessary. Also, those with varying cultural or religious needs may require individual help or advice. Whilst mothers with differing needs may not necessarily develop psychological health problems, additional awareness and support may reduce the risk. Information should be offered about how to contact groups and organisations, such as the Meet-a-mum Association (MAMA) or the Marcé Society, to those women who develop depression or are recovering from psychosis or severe depression.

When the depression is more advanced, admission to a local psychiatric hospital, where possible with a mother and baby unit, may be necessary. It should be remembered that untreated or undiagnosed clinical depression can evolve into a psychotic illness.

Whenever depression has occurred, the information must be recorded in the woman's obstetric notes to ensure the opportunity for planning increased support and early alleviation of symptoms in any subsequent pregnancy.

Prevention

Progesterone is thought by some to be an important responsible factor in the prevention of recurrence of postnatal depression. Dalton (1996) recommends that a '100 mg injection of natural progesterone is administered daily for 7 days following delivery, followed by a dose of 400 mg to be given by suppository twice daily until the return of menstruation'. Insufficient research has been undertaken to establish the efficacy of this strategy and there are mixed opinions amongst professionals. There have also been some reported cases of women undertaking placentophagy as a preventive measure, believing that the ingestion of the placenta allows a more gradual subsidence of hormone levels. If a woman believes strongly enough that a particular remedy is likely to prevent her from developing postnatal depression, it is important that this is given full consideration and, where available, appropriate research evidence is sought.

Post-traumatic stress disorder

Unlike the preceding disorders, this condition is not specific to women or to childbirth. It has be-come a widely publicised phenomenon, commonly triggered by an individual or group of individuals having experienced a major traumatic event such as the Hillsborough football stadium disaster or the Gulf War. It appears to affect participants, observers and, possibly, close relatives of victims who may not necessarily have witnessed the event. More recently, it is being linked to any traumatic event that has a major effect on an individual, or a subsequent traumatic event which causes a 'flashback' to the emotions of a previous traumatic event which has been unresolved and 'filed away', similar to unresolved grief. These 'flashbacks' may occur repeatedly in the form of dreams or nightmares, or may be relatively dormant until triggered by a further traumatic experience.

It is thought that in some cases, childbirth could be a primary trigger but previous sexual abuse may lead to the re-emergence of extreme distress during childbirth, due perhaps to the woman feeling that she is not in control. The key factor appears to be that 'it is the woman's *experience* of the event which is the aetiological agent, and not the event itself as perceived by the care-givers' (Crompton 1996). Research is required before a definitive link can be proven. The midwife should be aware of the disorder and consider it as a possible contributory factor when caring for a woman who is suffering from obvious psychological disturbance during the puerperium.

With appropriate knowledge, time and skills the midwife can do a great deal to facilitate a healthy psychological response to motherhood. Through early recognition of deviation from the normal, with initiation of prompt referral and appropriate treatment, the midwife can be instrumental in reducing psychological morbidity for postnatal women.

The midwife's role in caring for the mother and baby normally comes to an end with the transfer of care to the health visitor.

THE 6-WEEK POSTNATAL EXAMINATION

It has been standard practice in the UK and other countries such as America and Australia, over the past 50 years or more, for women to attend for a medical examination at 6 weeks postnatally. The reasoning behind the timing for this appears unclear, but it is assumed to be linked to the discovery in the 1930s that it takes approximately 6 weeks for complete regeneration of the endometrium following healing of the placental site (Sharif & Jordan 1995). The content of the examination generally involves discussion and assessment of the woman's general physical and emotional health with particular attention to any symptoms of anaemia, urinary tract infection or of emotional distress or depression. This is usually followed by an assessment that the physiological changes which occurred during pregnancy have reverted to the non-pregnant state. Health status is checked with weight, blood pressure, pulse and urine measurements. A physical examination is carried out of the breasts, abdomen and pelvis including vaginal examination to ensure that involution is complete and any trauma which was sustained during delivery is fully healed. The integrity and muscular function of the pelvic floor should be assessed and the woman asked directly if she has any dribbling of urine or stress incontinence. A cervical smear is usually taken for cytology. The return of the normal menstrual cycle will be discussed, also issues regarding sexual activity and whether she experiences any dyspareunia during sexual intercourse. Contraceptive practices should have been resumed prior to sexual activity and will have been addressed earlier. If the mother is breast feeding, this will be discussed with explanation as required related to the effect of lactation on the menstrual cycle (see Ch. 32). When the breasts are examined the woman is instructed in self-examination. If any deviations from the normal are identified during the examination, appropriate referral or treatment can be initiated to facilitate optimal physical and emotional health. The baby may also be examined during this visit with discussion as to continuing care.

Whilst it is important that the mother's full recovery from the effects of pregnancy, labour and delivery is ascertained, the timing and most appropriate health professional to undertake the examination has been questioned (Bick & MacArthur 1994, Sharif & Jordan 1995). In the late 1980s,

MacArthur et al (1991) analysed questionnaires returned from 11 701 women related to various aspects of postnatal health. At least one symptom not previously experienced and which had occurred within 3 months of delivery, persisting for longer than 6 weeks, was reported by 46% (5457) respondents. The symptoms reported included frequent headaches (419), various muscular aches, back pain, extreme tiredness, depression or anxiety (1065) and stress incontinence (1782). There were 83.1% (9722) women who reported at least one symptom occurring at some time during the period following delivery. In concluding, it was suggested that in order to reduce the long-term morbidity for a large number of women, further postnatal examination should occur at around 6 months after delivery. Studies undertaken more recently in Scotland and Birmingham have supported these findings and their authors believe that measures to reduce maternal morbidity must be sought as a matter of urgency (Bick & MacArthur 1995, Glazener et al 1995).

In the majority of cases the 6-week postnatal examination is carried out by the general practitioner although mothers who have experienced a difficult labour or had a caesarean section may be offered their postnatal examination from the hospital consultant. Since the implementation of the recommendations of the 'Changing Childbirth' report (DH 1993), continuity of care and carer by a named midwife or doctor is available in many areas. The role of the midwife usually terminates at 28 days following delivery, often sooner. As midwives are the lead professionals involved with care for the majority of women during the childbirth process, it would seem appropriate that they offer a routine postnatal consultation at 3 or 6 months with referral to professional colleagues as necessary (Bick & MacArthur 1994). However, with the economic climate of internal marketing, difficulties with resource allocation would have to be resolved in order to maintain such a service. Unfortunately, longer-term morbidity issues associated with childbirth often receive scant resources even though prompt resolution of complications could prove cost-effective ultimately.

Within the confines of current maternity service provision, the midwife must offer advice and care as appropriate with referral to other agencies if it is anticipated that longer-term follow-up would be beneficial. It is important that the midwife and/or health visitor should encourage each mother to attend for whatever programme of postnatal examination is offered within her particular area. Ideally any woman who does not attend as arranged should be visited at home to ascertain if this is because she does not understand the purpose of the examination or because she is having difficulty coping and may be depressed.

The midwife may have the opportunity to meet the mother and baby again if the general practitioner invites her to attend the surgery to assist with the postnatal examination. Also, the midwife may be involved with a postnatal reunion group for mothers who attended parentcraft classes, in order that they may share experiences and provide mutual support. Midwives and health visitors often share these sessions to provide a link between past and future care and this can be a valuable experience for both the parents and the health professionals.

> Postnatal midwifery care is complex and the importance of it is not yet fully comprehended, though there is potential for the midwifery profession, through provision of sensitive puerperal care and support, to have a dynamic effect on the health of the nation (Magill-Cuerden 1996).

READER ACTIVITIES

1. Use the following question in order to test your knowledge. You may undertake it in the form of a researched assignment, or as a revision examination question, in which case, allow yourself 1 hour.

Society expects a newly delivered mother to be joyous and full of love for her baby.

Discuss this statement related to how the midwife can assist a healthy psychological transition to motherhood.

2. Contact your local community psychiatric team and find out how often they encounter mental illness in postnatal women. Seek their opinions and advice concerning referral patterns and local incidence.

3. Undertake a literature search on postnatal depression and puerperal psychosis. Make short notes on recent research and share these in discussion at a journal club with colleagues.

4. In your local hospital, is there a flexible approach to postnatal care? Are mothers able to rest and to access drinks when desired? If you discover routine procedures inhibit this, try to find out the reason behind this and consider the development of a strategy to introduce greater flexibility.

USEFUL ADDRESSES

Association for Postnatal Illness
25 Jerdan Place
Fulham
London SW6 1BE

The Marcé Society
Secretary Dr T. Friedman, Department of Psychiatry
Leicester General Hospital
Leicester LE5 4PW

The Meet-a-Mum Association (MAMA)
14 Willis Road
Croydon CR0 2XX

Health Information Service – information about health service and support groups
Freephone 0800 665544

REFERENCES

Ball J A 1989 Postnatal care and adjustment to motherhood. In: Robinson S, Thomson A M (eds) Midwives, research and childbirth. Chapman & Hall, London

Ball J A 1994 Reactions to motherhood – the role of postnatal care, 2nd edn. Books For Midwives, Cheshire
Barclay L M, Lloyd B 1996 The misery of motherhood:

alternative approaches to maternal distress. Midwifery 12: 136–139

Beck C T 1995 The effects of postpartum depression on maternal–infant interaction: a meta-analysis. Nursing Research 44(5): 298–304

Bick D E, MacArthur C 1994 Identifying morbidity in postpartum women. Modern Midwife 4(12): 10–13

Bick D E, MacArthur C 1995 The extent, severity and effect of health problems after childbirth. British Journal of Midwifery 3(1): 27–31

Brockington I F 1992 Conference proceedings: notes 6th Marce Society biennial conference 2nd–4th Sept, Heriot-Watt University, Edinburgh

Cox J L 1992 Depression after childbirth. In: Paykel E S (ed) Handbook of affective disorders, 2nd edn. Churchill Livingstone, Edinburgh, ch 36

Cox J L, Holden J M, Sagovsky R 1987 Detection of postnatal depression: development of the Edinburgh postnatal depression scale. British Journal of Psychiatry 150: 782–786

Crompton J 1996 Post-traumatic stress disorder and childbirth. British Journal of Midwifery 4(6): 290–294

Dalton K 1996 Depression after childbirth. Oxford University Press, Oxford, pp 93, 150

Department of Health 1993 Changing childbirth: report of the expert maternity group. HMSO, London

Glazener C M, Abdalla M, Stroud P et al 1995 Postnatal maternal morbidity: extent, causes, prevention and treatment. British Journal of Obstetrics and Gynaecology 102(4): 282–287

Green J M, Coupland V A, Kitzinger J V 1990 Expectations, experiences and psychological outcomes of childbirth: a prospective study of 825 women. Birth 17(1): 23

Gregoire A J P, Kumar R, Everitt B et al 1996 Transdermal oestrogen for treatment of severe postnatal depression. Lancet 347: 930–933

Harris B, Lovett L, Smith J et al 1996 Cardiff puerperal mood and hormone study III: postnatal depression at 5 to 6 weeks postpartum and its hormonal correlates across the peripartum period. British Journal of Psychiatry 168: 739–744

Holden J M 1990 Emotional problems associated with childbirth. In: Alexander J, Levy V, Roch S Midwifery practice: postnatal care. Macmillan, Basingstoke

Inch S 1989 Birthrights: a parents' guide to modern childbirth. Green Print, London

Kendall R E, Chalmers J C, Platz C 1987 Epidemiology of puerperal psychosis. British Journal of Psychiatry 150: 662–673

Kumar R 1984 Motherhood and mental illness: the role of the midwife in prevention and treatment. Midwives Chronicle & Nursing Notes (March 1984): 70–74

MacArthur C, Lewis M, Knox E G 1991 Health after childbirth. HMSO, London

McClarey M, Stokoe B 1995 A multi-disciplinary approach to postnatal depression. Health Visitor 68(4): 141–143

McIntosh J 1986 Postnatal blues: a bio-social phenomenon? Midwifery 2: 187–192

McIntosh J 1993 Postpartum depression: women's help-seeking behaviour and perceptions of cause. Journal of Advanced Nursing 18: 178–184

Magill-Cuerden J 1996 Postnatal potential: editorial comment. Modern Midwife 6(11): 4–5

Murray L 1988 Effects of postnatal depression on infant development: the contribution of direct studies of early mother–infant interaction. In: Kumar R, Brockington I (eds) Motherhood and mental illness 2. John Wright, London

Price B 1996 Changing body image. Modern Midwife (6)4: 12–15

Raphael-Leff J 1991 Psychological processes of childbearing. Chapman & Hall, London

Richards J P 1990 Postnatal depression: a review of recent literature. British Journal of General Practice 40: 472–476

Schorr S J, Richardson D 1995 Psychiatric emergencies. In: Martin J (ed) Intrapartum and postpartum obstetric emergencies. Obstetrics and Gynecology Clinics of North America 22(2): 369–383

Schott J, Henley A 1996 Culture, religion and childbearing in a multiracial society: A handbook for health professionals. Butterworth-Heinemann, Oxford, p 175

Sharif K, Jordan J 1995 The 6-week postnatal visit: are we doing it right? British Journal of Hospital Medicine 54(1): 7–10

Simkin P 1991 Just another day in a woman's life? Women's long-term perceptions of their first birth experience. Part 1. Birth 18(4): 203

Spruce E M 1994 Puerperal psychosis: a descriptive study addressing the nature of the illness with an analysis of midwives awareness related to: recognition of onset and appropriate initial action. Unpublished MSc dissertation, University of Surrey, Guildford

United Kingdom Central Council for Nursing, Midwifery and Health Visiting (UKCC) 1994 The midwife's code of practice. UKCC, London

---

FURTHER READING

Department of Health 1993 The health of the nation: key area handbook: mental illness. HMSO, London, pp 119–120

Matlin M 1993 The psychology of women, 2nd edn. Harcourt Brace Jovanovich, College

Nicholson P 1990 Understanding postnatal depression: a mother centred approach. Journal of Advanced Nursing 15: 689–695

Niven C A 1992 Psychological care for families: before, during and after birth. Butterworth-Heinemann, Oxford

Simkin P 1996 The experience of maternity in a woman's life. Journal of Obstetric, Gynecologic and Neonatal Nursing 25(March/April): 247–252

32

Family planning

Jocelyn Franey

CHAPTER CONTENTS

Contraception plays an important role in many women's lives. It has been argued that control of their own fertility is the largest single factor affecting the independence of women during this century (Roberts 1981).

The benefits of fertility regulation have been recognised by people living in varied social circumstances, with different needs and perspectives. Contraception should also be viewed in the wider context of sexual and reproductive health; the capacity to enjoy and control sexual and reproductive behaviour is a key element of sexual health (WHO 1992), but at the same time it is accepted that birth intervals of at least 2 years improve maternal and infant mortality (Wang & Fraser 1994). Worldwide, concern continues over population levels and the problems of maintaining a sustainable environment.

In the UK, the Government's white paper 'Health of the Nation' (DH 1992) focused attention on the rising number of unintended pregnancies, highlighting the need to improve access to family planning services for all women, particularly the young (Kishen & Presho 1996).

The chapter aims to:

- consider the role of the midwife regarding family planning and related issues

- review contraceptive methods

- explore the provision of family planning services.

THE ROLE OF THE MIDWIFE IN FAMILY PLANNING AND RELATED ISSUES

The role of the midwife in family planning is acknowledged by the World Health Organization,

International Confederation of Midwives, International Confederation of Gynaecologists and Obstetricians and the EC Midwives Directives (UKCC 1994). She or he must be able to facilitate client knowledge and choice by providing valid, current information in a way which is easily understood by the woman and possibly her partner. The midwife's counselling skills, attributes such as being non-judgemental and positive listening skills are thus paramount.

READER ACTIVITY

Before reading on, you may find it useful to consider why the midwife is well placed to initiate such intimate discussion with women.

Ideally, the midwife would be 'with woman' for about 1 year, throughout preconception, pregnancy and delivery and the postnatal period. During this time she will hopefully come to know the woman and her family well. Discussions regarding family planning may well be appropriate at all stages. Preconceptionally, for example, contraception is advocated for 1 month after rubella vaccination (see Ch. 10). Antenatally, the woman and her partner may wish to have information on which to base future choices; whilst following delivery their opinions may change or they may require further information.

A mother who has chosen not to breast feed will need to commence contraception so that it is effective before postpartum ovulation, which occurs on average between 40 and 50 days after delivery (Wang & Fraser 1994). Furthermore, Sleep et al (1984) demonstrated that 32% of women resume intercourse during the first postnatal month, a time when the midwife will be in frequent contact with the new mother. However, Laryea (1980) found that whilst primiparous women would have welcomed discussion concerning resumption of intercourse, they waited for the midwives to initiate it. Midwives thought it an intrusion into the mother's private relationship for them to broach the subject and thus an impasse arose. Talking with a mother about pelvic floor exercises may lead naturally to the subject of intercourse. This will allow the midwife to indicate that intercourse

may be resumed as soon as the couple desire and to initiate discussion regarding methods of contraception. This may also be the ideal opportunity for the midwife to promote issues such as breast awareness, cervical screening and safer sex. The midwife should also be able to sensitively explore with the woman the effect of pregnancy and childbirth on sexuality and sexual relationships (ENB 1994). Such discussions will be more difficult if the midwife does not know the woman well, or if her knowledge is not up to date. The midwife should consider how she intends to ensure that the information she imparts to clients and colleagues remains current, valid and reliable.

The midwife needs to be aware that general factors governing individual contraceptive choices vary enormously and can include religion and culture, relationships, age, motivation to avoid pregnancy, lifestyle and socioeconomic considerations. After childbirth these may be compounded by issues such as breast feeding (for nursing mothers, their chosen method of contraception must not adversely affect lactation or health of their baby), body image, possible loss of libido and the adjustment to motherhood, together with physical factors such as perineal discomfort, vaginal dryness or fatigue. Individuals may well be able to add more to this list.

The midwife will also need to be aware of the family planning services available in the area in which she practises. Additionally, she should know how to refer clients to practitioners with specialist training if appropriate.

READER ACTIVITY

Just consider for a moment what attributes the ideal contraceptive would have.

Guillebaud (1993) suggests that the ideal contraceptive would be 100% effective, perfectly safe, and painlessly reversible. There would be no interruption of spontaneity, no mess, unpleasant odour or taste. It would be easy to use, cheap, not reliant on the user's memory and independent of the medical profession. The method would also need to be culturally acceptable to its users. Needless to say it will probably never exist, but if the midwife is aware of what issues are important to the woman and her partner, then she may be able to facilitate the most suitable choice.

For most contraceptive methods discussed below, the failure rate is given per 100 woman years (HWY) of use. This is the number who would become pregnant if 100 women used the method for 1 year. It is important to note that this rate does not reflect the fact that fertility decreases with age and may be suppressed during lactation; and that the success of a method is partially dependent on motivation, experience in using the method, and the teaching received. It is also noteworthy that unprotected intercourse in women results in 80–90 pregnancies per HWY, and not 100. Bounds (1994) suggests that it is important to relate failure rates to a specific period of time, such as in the 'first year of use' since, with most methods, the risk of failure decreases with time. When discussing failure rates with women, it may be more relevant to give individualised advice, which takes into account such factors as their age, whether they are breast feeding, how often they have intercourse and how important it is for them not to become pregnant.

CONTRACEPTIVE METHODS

Hormonal methods

Combined oral contraceptive pill

The combined oral contraceptive pill ('the pill') contains synthetic steroid hormones oestrogen and progestogen in varying amounts depending on which preparation is prescribed. There are currently 26 different pills available in the UK, of which the most commonly used are monophasic pills which contain a constant dose of steroids throughout the packet. 'Everyday' pills contain 28 pills in the packet, 21 of which are active monophasic pills whilst the seven remaining pills contain no hormones and are thus inactive.

Also available are biphasic and triphasic pills in which the dose of steroids administered varies in two or three phases throughout the packet to mimic the natural fluctuations of the hormones during the menstrual cycle. Guillebaud (1995) states

that although a more normal-looking endometrium is demonstrated histologically with triphasic pill usage, there is no good evidence of better cycle control over long-term use. This, together with the problems associated with giving advice regarding missed pills and delaying withdrawal bleeds, explains why these pills are less commonly used.

The pill is a popular method of contraception chosen by 25% of British women, although usage differs with age and marital status. In the UK it is most popular with women under 24 years of age and with those who are single or cohabiting, rather than married (Wellings et al 1994).

Mode of action. Oestrogen and progestogen suppress follicle-stimulating hormone and luteinising hormone production so that the ovaries go into a resting state, ovarian follicles do not mature and ovulation does not normally take place. Progestogen also causes cervical mucus to thicken, making penetration by spermatozoa difficult. The use of the pill also renders the endometrium unreceptive to implantation by the blastocyst. These actions provide additional contraception in the event of breakthrough ovulation occurring. Guillebaud (1995) suggests that effects on the uterine tubes to impair sperm migration and ovum transport are of doubtful importance.

Failure rate. Provided the pill is taken correctly and consistently, is absorbed normally and interaction with other medication does not affect its metabolism, the pill's reliability is nearly 100% (Guillebaud 1995). Studies point to failure rates of 0.2–3 per HWY, depending on the population reviewed (Guillebaud 1993).

Important considerations. The pill is an easy to use, reliable method of contraception which is independent of intercourse and has many advantages and some drawbacks to its use.

READER ACTIVITY

You may already be aware of some of the advantages and disadvantages of the pill and you might like to think of or list them, with rationales, before reading on.

Your list of advantages may have included:

• Regular, lighter, less painful periods – as the body's own menstrual cycle is inhibited and the usual proliferation of the endometrium does not occur
• Possible reduction in premenstrual symptoms – again because the menstrual cycle is inhibited
• Protection against pelvic inflammatory disease (PID) – because of the thickened cervical mucus
• Decreased incidence of ectopic pregnancy as ovulation is inhibited.

Other advantages include protection against ovarian and endometrial cancers (Thorogood & Villard-Mackintosh 1993), and prevention of ovarian cysts and fibroids (Szarewski & Guillebaud 1994).

Over recent years the steroid dosage of all oral contraceptives has been greatly reduced or modified in order to minimise the disadvantages of the pill. However, many of the metabolic effects of the pill result in potential drawbacks to use and your list may have included the following:

• Venous or arterial thrombosis – as clotting factors and platelet function are modified (Thorogood & Villard-Mackintosh 1993). The risk of venous thrombosis is greatest in women with a body mass index over 30, those with a family history of venous thrombosis, and those who are immobile.
• Hypertension – the pill causes a slight rise in blood pressure in most users, but some women may develop a greater degree of hypertension which could increase the potential for haemorrhagic strokes (Guillebaud 1993).

Following reanalysis of worldwide epidemiological data, it appears that women using the pill either currently or within the last 10 years are at a slightly increased risk of developing breast cancer (Collaborative Group on Hormonal Factors in Breast Cancer 1996). It is also possible that pill use is associated with an increased risk of cervical cancer. However, because of the effects of confounding factors such as sexually transmissible diseases (STD), conclusive findings are awaited. Cigarette smoking is known to potentiate most risks associated with pill use.

Pill use may also lead to other side-effects such as breast tenderness, nausea, weight increase, depression and loss of libido. These effects often diminish with continued use, or may improve with a change of pill.

Contraindications to pill use include:

• pregnancy
• history of arterial or venous thrombosis, or predisposing factors such as immobility
• hypertension
• focal or crescendo migraines
• current liver disease
• undiagnosed abnormal vaginal bleeding
• hydatidiform mole (until serum HCG is no longer detectable)
• smoking if the woman is over 35 years old.

This is not an exhaustive list and, as the pill is not suitable for everyone, any woman wishing to consider using this form of contraception should have a full history taken and recorded and be fully informed and counselled regarding possible side-effects. Any woman using the pill should be informed to stop taking the pill and seek urgent medical advice if any of the following occur:

• sudden, severe chest pain
• sudden breathlessness
• severe, unilateral calf pain
• severe stomach pain
• unusual, severe, prolonged headache (BMA & RPS 1996).

Using the pill. When initially commencing the pill, the very first pill is usually taken on the first day of the menstrual period (for postpartum use, see later). If a 21-day pill has been prescribed, contraceptive effect is immediate, providing of course that the remainder of pills in the packet are taken correctly. If the pill is initially commenced on any day other than the first day of the period, additional means of contraception (such as a condom) should be used in conjunction with the pill for the first 7 days. One pill is taken every day for 21 days, then no pills for the next 7 days. Vaginal bleeding due to hormone withdrawal usually occurs within the 7-day break before the next packet of pills is commenced.

If an everyday pill is being used, at the initial commencement of the medication, inactive pills are taken first and thus the contraceptive effect does not begin until the 15th day after the very first pill has been taken. It is important, therefore, to advise the use of additional contraceptive measures, such as condoms, for the first 14 days. Thereafter with an everyday pill, one pill is taken daily, with care being taken to take them in the correct order. Vaginal bleeding will usually occur during the time the inactive pills are taken, usually denoted by a red coloured section on the pill packet.

It is important to emphasise the importance of taking the pill at an easily remembered time each day. If a pill is forgotten, the woman will then have some idea of when the previous pill was taken and thus how late she is in taking the next pill. If the woman is less than 12 hours late in taking a pill, she can take the pill straight away and carry on as normal. If the pill is forgotten by more than 12 hours, the advice given in Figure 32.1 should be followed.

It is a popular thought that pills missed at the beginning or the end of the packet do not matter. This is a mistaken belief, for if these pills are forgotten, the pill-free period is lengthened and ovulation may be more likely to occur (Guillebaud

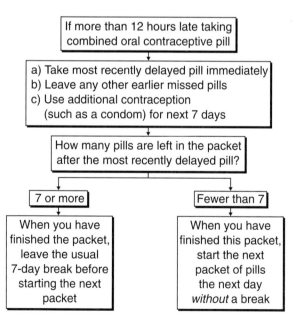

Fig. 32.1 Advice regarding missed combined 21-day oral contraceptive pills over 12 hours late (adapted from Guillebaud 1993).

1995). If a woman is concerned about a missed or late pill, it is always worth contacting the local family planning clinic or GP for reassurance or advice, as emergency contraception may be indicated (see later).

Other factors which may render the pill less effective are bouts of severe diarrhoea, vomiting within 3 hours of taking the pill and interactions with other medications. The advice given in cases of vomiting and diarrhoea is similar to that in Figure 32.1, with additional contraception recommended during the illness and for 7 days afterwards.

Medications which may hinder the effectiveness of the pill include broad-spectrum antibiotics (such as ampicillin or cefaclor) and enzyme-inducing drugs, such as rifampicin and some anticonvulsants or hypnotics. It is important that women are made aware of such possible interactions and appreciate the need to inform the medical practitioner that the pill is used for contraception, so that individual advice may be given if any other medications are prescribed.

Preconception considerations. As the pill disrupts vitamin and mineral metabolism, some authorities advise stopping the pill 2–3 months before attempting to conceive. However, Guillebaud (1995) suggests that there is no objective evidence to support this, although it would certainly do no harm. As the pill causes folic acid levels to fall, it is worthwhile ensuring that any woman planning conception is aware of the recommendation to take folic acid supplements (see Ch. 10). Any woman who does conceive whilst taking the pill may be reassured that studies appear to conclude that the incidence of birth defects following periconception exposure to the pill is no greater than to be expected among any group of women expecting a planned baby (Guillebaud 1995).

For conceptions occurring after the pill has been discontinued, there is no evidence of increased risk of miscarriage, ectopic pregnancy or stillbirth, or of any adverse effects on the fetus (Guillebaud 1995).

Postpartum considerations. The combined oral contraceptive pill reduces milk supply, particularly if lactation is not well established and is therefore not recommended for use in the early months if the mother is breast feeding (Tankeyoon et al 1988). If the mother is bottle feeding, the pill may be commenced 21 days postpartum. Such timing allows for the high oestrogen levels of pregnancy to fall before introducing the pill (Guillebaud 1993). This will reduce the risk of thromboembolism, but allow contraceptive effect to be initiated before ovulation resumes.

The pill can be commenced immediately following spontaneous or therapeutic termination of pregnancy. However, because of the risk of thromboembolism, the pill should be stopped 4 weeks before major surgery and not recommended until 2 weeks following full mobilisation.

There are other postpartum considerations for the midwife to discuss with the mother regarding use of the pill. These may include exploration of whether remembering to take the pill will fit into her busy lifestyle or if she can easily access a clinic or surgery. This will be necessary for review and regular blood pressure recordings, which will usually be required at 3- to 6-monthly intervals. If this proves difficult for the woman, referral to a domiciliary family planning service, if available, may be appropriate.

Also some women may experience an increased awareness of their own mortality once they experience motherhood and given the rare, but potentially catastrophic side-effects of the pill, may need facilitation to explore these aspects in greater depth.

Progestogen-only methods

Progestogen-only methods of contraception were introduced partly to avoid the side-effects of oestrogen in the combined pill as discussed above. They also offer increased choice for women and their partners. Progestogen can be administered in several formats for contraceptive purposes. Currently available in the UK are progestogen-only pills, two kinds of intramuscular injection, depot medroxyprogesterone acetate (DMPA or 'Depo-provera') and norethisterone enanthate (NET-EN or 'Noristerat'), and subdermal implants (such as Norplant). Also available are progestogen-releasing intrauterine systems (IUS), which combine both the contraceptive effects of progestogen and an IUCD (see later). The dose of progestogen administered varies with each method, as shown in Figure 32.2. Future developments may include the use of progestogen-releasing vaginal rings.

The longer-acting progestogen-only methods,

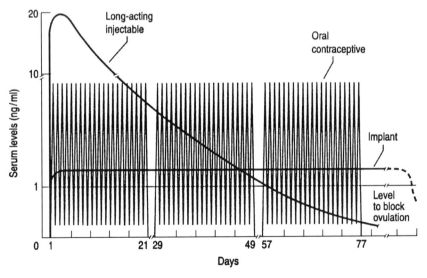

Fig. 32.2 The different blood serum levels of progestogen resulting from progestogen-only methods of contraception (reproduced by kind permission from Szarewski 1991).

such as implants and injectables, have raised issues of concern, mainly regarding informed consent, amongst some consumer and feminist groups (Fraser 1995, Mangla & Mangla 1993).

Mode of action.   As progestogens have many actions within the body, Fraser (1995) suggests that the importance of each contraceptive action is likely to depend on the type of progestogen and the dose. The main actions of the progestogen-only pill are thought to involve the thickening of cervical mucus to provide a barrier to spermatozoa and the modification of the endometrium to prevent implantation (Guillebaud 1991). The contraceptive action of the progestogen-only pill does not rely on prevention of ovulation, although there is some suppression of follicle-stimulating hormone and luteinising hormone release. However, it is thought that follicular development and ovulation is effectively suppressed in some other progestogen-only methods, such as the injection, because of the higher dose of progestogen (Fraser 1995).

Important considerations.   Again, progestogen-only methods of contraception have both general advantages and drawbacks to their use. Each individual progestogen-only method also has pros and cons to its specific use; these will be considered after the use of each method has been discussed.

READER ACTIVITY

You may already be aware of some of the issues surrounding these methods of contraception, and it may be useful to reflect on these before continuing.

General advantages to progestogen-only use include:

- progestogen produces fewer metabolic side-effects than oestrogen and progestogen combined, therefore these methods may be useful in cases where the combined pill is contraindicated
- it can be used during lactation (see below)
- probable reduction in premenstrual symptoms (Newton 1993)
- protection against PID.

Other advantages include possible protection against endometrial and ovarian cancers (Fraser 1995).

Drawbacks to use include:

- Menstrual disturbances, encompassing erratic, sometimes prolonged, bleeding; oligomenorrhoea or amenorrhoea. Fraser (1995) comments that little is known about the mechanism which causes such disturbances which most users experience to some degree. Newton (1993) comments that menstrual disruption is the most common reason for women to discontinue using progestogen-only methods. This illustrates the need for careful explanation to potential users.
- Functional ovarian cysts: an increased prevalence has been demonstrated in women using progestogen-only methods (Newton 1993).

Contraindications to use include:

- pregnancy
- undiagnosed abnormal vaginal bleeding
- severe arterial disease
- hydatidiform mole (until serum HCG is no longer detectable).

Caution should be exercised when using the progestogen-only pill in women who have had a previous ectopic pregnancy. This is because of the possible inhibition of uterine tube motility (Chi et al 1992). This is not a problem with other progestogen-only methods as they usually inhibit ovulation.

Antibiotics do not adversely affect progestogen-only methods, but women should be advised to consult the doctor regarding possible interactions if any other medications (especially enzyme inducers such as rifampicin) are prescribed.

General preconception considerations.   Fraser (1995) reports that there is no evidence of significant increase in congenital abnormalities in fetuses conceived whilst the mother is using progestogen-only contraception or immediately after discontinuing its use.

General postpartum considerations.   The use of progestogen-only methods for contraception in the puerperium has been associated with an increased incidence of vaginal bleeding. Current recommendations of when to start postnatally vary for each method as the dose of progestogen differs.

Generally progestogen has either no effect, or a slightly enhancing effect, on breast milk volume (Foxwell & Howie 1995). Therefore these methods are usually recommended for breast-feeding mothers who cannot, or do not wish to use non-hormonal methods. However, transmission of the steroid to the infant via breast milk may concern some mothers. Studies by the WHO (1994) have demonstrated that such transmission and absorption by the neonate is minimal and does not affect the short-term growth and development of infants. Nevertheless, some authors (Diaz & Croxatto 1993, Pardue 1994) comment that the long-term potential effects have not been fully evaluated. For this reason several authorities (IPPF 1990, WHO 1994) advocate that progestogen-only methods, particularly the higher dose varieties, are not commenced until 6 weeks postpartum. This delay avoids early, unnecessary exposure of the infant to the hormone. Because of this concern, the mother may choose to use the progestogen-only pill, rather than other progestogen-only methods, as it provides a lower dose of steroid.

Progestogen-only methods can be used immediately following spontaneous or therapeutic termination.

Using the progestogen-only pill

When initially commencing this method, if the first tablet is taken on the first day of the menstrual period, contraceptive effect is immediate. If the medication is commenced any later in the cycle, then an additional form of contraception (such as a condom) should be used for 7 days. Normally one tablet is taken every day, there are no pill-free days and thus tablets are taken throughout periods.

If a progestogen-only pill is forgotten, the woman has only 3 hours in which to remember to take it. This is because the effect on cervical mucus is at its maximum between 4 and 22 hours after the tablet has been taken. For this reason, it is also recommended that the daily tablets are taken about 4 hours before the usual time of intercourse and taken at the same time each day. If the woman is over 3 hours late in taking a tablet, then additional contraception will be needed for 7 days, as with the combined pill. Similarly, following vomiting or severe diarrhoea, additional contraception should be used until 7 days after the illness ceases. If a woman is concerned about a missed or late progestogen-only pill, she should be advised to contact her family planning clinic or GP as emergency contraception may be indicated (see later).

Failure rate. The effectiveness of the progestogen-only pill is dependent upon meticulous compliance with tablet taking. Vessey et al (1985) found that the failure rate of this method is clearly related to age, with failure rates ranging from 3 per HWY in a population aged 25–29 compared with only 0.3 per HWY in women aged 40 years or over.

Although the suggestion that failure is more common in overweight women has not been substantiated (Fraser 1995), some practitioners may suggest an increase in dose for women weighing over 70 kilograms.

Specific considerations. As success of this method depends on very precise compliance, it may not be suitable for those with a poor memory or hectic lifestyle.

Preconception considerations. As above.

Postpartum considerations. Early postnatal use of the progestogen-only pill is associated with breakthrough bleeding (BMA & RPS 1996). The FPA (1995a) recommend that women begin this method 21 days after delivery (although some authorities, such as the IPPF (1990) would say to wait until 4–6 weeks).

As the progestogen-only pill is considered less effective in non-lactating women, it may be suggested that women change to a more effective method of contraception at the time of weaning (Chi et al 1992).

READER ACTIVITY

You may wish to reflect on other postpartum considerations for the midwife to discuss with the woman. Factors such as remembering to take the tablets, or being able to access a clinic for review, are similar to those associated with the combined pill.

Progestogen injections

Although in the UK less than 1% of women using contraception use this method (Guillebaud 1993), worldwide over 6 million women use it, and in some countries it is the most commonly used reversible method (Newton 1993).

The two contraceptive progestogen injections currently available in the UK are depot medroxy-progesterone acetate (DMPA or 'Depo-provera') and norethisterone enanthate (NET-EN or 'Noristerat'); both are given by deep intramuscular injection. DMPA is usually given in a dose of 150 mg at 12-week intervals and NET-EN in a dose of 200 mg normally given at 8-week intervals.

Failure rates. Large-scale studies have quoted failure rates of below 0.5 per HWY for DMPA, whilst the failure rate for NET-EN appears slightly higher, although still below 1 per HWY (Fraser 1995).

Using injectable progestogen. The initial injection is usually given within the first 5 days of the menstrual period. If given on day 1, contraceptive effect is immediate, but if the injection is given at any other time, additional contraception should be used for 7 days (FPA 1995b). (For postpartum use see below.)

Specific considerations. Progestogen injections are highly effective methods of contraception and do not rely on the woman remembering to take a tablet every day, only to attend regularly for injections. This method is irreversible for the term of action, therefore any side-effects may also be present until the injection wears off. Such side-effects may include breast discomfort, nausea and vomiting and depression or mood swings. The major side-effect is often menstrual irregularities, although amenorrhoea becomes prominent with long-term DMPA use (Fraser 1995).

Other disadvantages to use include weight gain and a possible link with loss of bone density which is yet to be resolved (Fraser 1995).

Specific preconception considerations. Return of fertility is slow once the injection is stopped, especially with DMPA. The median delay to conception following the presumed end of contra-

ceptive effect is 5–7 months (IPPF 1988). Therefore injectable progestogen is not recommended as contraception for women who plan to conceive soon after its use.

Postpartum considerations. Early postpartum use of progestogen injections is associated with heavy, irregular vaginal bleeding (BMA & RPS 1996) so current recommendations advocate use of this method from 5–6 weeks following delivery. This is also consistent with advice to limit early infant exposure to the steroid as discussed above. Thus an alternative form of contraception may be needed in the interim and for 7 days following the injection.

Subdermal implants

These have been used internationally for a number of years. 'Norplant' was licensed for use in the UK in 1993.

Using implants. Implants are capsules containing progestogen which are inserted subdermally into the inner aspect of the upper arm under local anaesthetic (see Fig. 32.3). The steroid is released into the body at a constant rate (slightly higher during the first year of use) and the steady circulating blood level of steroid gives high contraceptive efficacy (Smith 1994).

Ideally, the implants are inserted on the first day of the menstrual period, otherwise additional contraception is required for 7 days (Smith 1994). The implants then remain in place and are effective from 2–5 years, depending on the preparation used. Currently available in the UK is 'Norplant', which consists of six capsules and is effective for

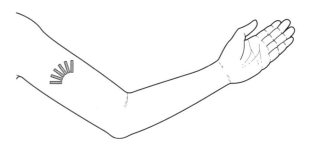

Fig. 32.3 Subdermal implants.

5 years. A version using two capsules, to last 3 years, is currently being developed, and work is progressing on a version using natural progesterone which would be preferable for use in breast-feeding mothers (Davies & Newton 1991).

Failure rate. Studies demonstrate a failure rate of 0.7 per HWY (Newton 1993).

Specific considerations. As implants are generally advocated for long-term use, women should be carefully counselled to ensure such use is suitable for them. Additionally, the incidence of irregular vaginal bleeding, especially in the first year, is high (Davies & Newton 1991). Women choosing to use this method will need to undergo surgical procedures to both insert and remove the implants.

Preconception considerations. Preinsertion fertility is regained within 48 hours of removal of the implants (Smith 1994).

Postpartum considerations. Implants can be inserted 21 days after delivery (BMA & RPS 1996), although a delay until 5–6 weeks postpartum may be preferable if the mother is breast feeding.

Intrauterine contraceptive device (IUCD)

As the name suggests, this is inserted into the uterus, as illustrated in Figure 32.4. All standard IUCDs currently available in the UK contain copper, which increases contraceptive efficacy. About 7% of women in the UK use an IUCD (Bromham 1993), whereas worldwide it is the second most popular, reversible method after the pill (Drife 1995).

Mode of action. The IUCD causes an inflammatory response, with the increased number of leucocytes destroying spermatozoa and ova. Gamete viability is further impaired by alteration of uterine and tubal fluids (Drife 1995). Copper affects endometrial enzymes, glycogen metabolism and oestrogen uptake, thus rendering the endometrium hostile to implantation.

Failure rate. The failure rate is less than 1–2 per HWY (FPA 1995c).

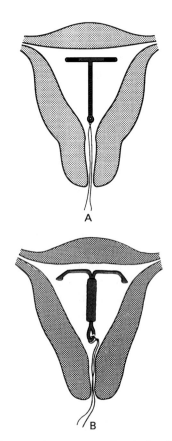

Fig. 32.4 Intrauterine contraceptive devices (both are radio-opaque). After insertion through the cervix, the device assumes the shape shown; the threads attached to it protrude into the vagina. (A) Copper-carrying device. (B) Levonorgestrel-releasing system.

Using the IUCD. Some practitioners prefer to insert an IUCD towards the end of or just after menstruation, although it can be fitted at any point of the menstrual cycle as long as the chance of pregnancy has been excluded (Bromham 1993). The woman may experience some discomfort during the procedure which should be performed using aseptic techniques.

The IUCD may be left in place for 5 years and longer in some instances; for example, if a woman over 40 years of age has an IUCD fitted, it may remain in place until the menopause. Once fitted, the IUCD requires little action on behalf of the user and does not interfere with intercourse. Women are usually taught to feel for the threads of the IUCD as reassurance that it remains in place and they are generally reviewed annually. Side-effects may include menorrhagia and, as with implants, the woman will need to consult with a doctor before discontinuing use.

The suggestion that IUCDs promote pelvic inflammatory disease (PID) has been refuted, although there is evidence to suggest infection may be introduced at the time of insertion (Bromham 1993). This author comments that other risk factors, such as multiple sexual partners, are of greater importance in the causation of PID than the use of an IUCD.

IUCDs are associated with a decreased risk of ectopic pregnancies because of their effectiveness. However, the ratio of ectopic to intrauterine pregnancies is greater among women using IUCDs as, in general, IUCD use prevents more intrauterine pregnancies than ectopic pregnancies (Ross & Frankenburg 1993). Thus a woman who has an IUCD inserted should be counselled to seek early medical advice should she suspect that she is pregnant.

Should pregnancy occur, there is an increased risk of spontaneous abortion. If the pregnancy continues, most obstetricians advise removal of the device to reduce the risk of septic abortion. There is also an increased risk of premature labour, but no evidence of teratogenicity (Szarewski & Guillebaud 1994).

Postpartum considerations. It is recommended that the IUCD is inserted 6–8 weeks after delivery to minimise the risks of expulsion and uterine perforation. The ordinary IUCD has no effect on lactation. Insertion is possible immediately following termination of pregnancy, but may be associated with an increased incidence of expulsion (Drife 1995).

Future developments include the development of modified shapes, with the aim of reducing side-effects such as pain, bleeding and expulsion. Frameless devices, with copper tube threaded onto a string which is embedded into the endometrium are also being researched (FPA 1995c)

Progestogen-releasing intrauterine systems (IUS)

These were developed to try to overcome some of the problems associated with conventional IUCDs and vaginal bleeding. The device consists of a small plastic 'T'-shaped frame carrying a Silastic sleeve containing levonorgestrel (see Fig. 32.4). It is inserted into the uterus and the steroid hormone is released gradually. Both the steroid and the IUCD acting as a carrier have contraceptive properties as discussed above. The system is usually initially fitted within the first 7 days of the menstrual period. Contraceptive effect is immediate and remains effective for 3–5 years depending on the type of IUS used.

Failure rate.   Failure rates of less than 0.1 per HWY have been reported (Fraser 1995).

Specific considerations.   Irregular vaginal bleeding is common initially, then gradually ceases. The menstrual bleeding is lighter than with conventional IUCDs, with possible amenorrhoea.

Barrier methods

Barrier methods prevent spermatozoa from coming into contact with the ovum and comprise male and female condoms and diaphragms, usually used with spermicides.

READER ACTIVITY

You are probably already aware of the advantages and drawbacks of the use of barrier methods and you may like to consider these before reading on.

General advantages include the easy availability of condoms and the fact that the use of barrier methods (once a diaphragm has been fitted) is independent of professional intervention and they are only used when needed. As condoms afford some (although not absolute) protection against sexually transmissible diseases (STD), including human immunodeficiency virus (HIV), concurrent use of condoms and another method, such as the pill, is becoming more popular. Barrier methods also confer some protection against cervical cancer (Ross & Frankenburg 1993). The possible interruption to intercourse may constitute a drawback for some couples.

General consideration for use. It is good practice to ensure that anyone choosing to use barrier methods is aware of the availability of emergency contraception (see below), and how to access it should the need arise.

Condom (or sheath)

Condom use has increased in recent years in response to publicity given to HIV infection. In their study of sexual attitudes in the UK, Wellings et al (1994) found that over 25% of women and 36.9% of men had used a condom in the previous year, with use being more prevalent in younger age groups.

Many varieties of condom are available, including hypoallergenic. They are available free from family planning clinics, and can be purchased by mail order and from retailers such as chemists, supermarkets and vending machines, but they are not available on prescription.

Using a condom. This thin tube of latex rubber is rolled onto the erect penis. It must be applied before any genital contact occurs as some semen may escape prior to ejaculation. About 1 cm of air-free space must be left at the tip to accommodate the ejaculate, otherwise the condom may burst. (Some designs incorporate a teat end for this purpose.) Care should be taken when handling the condom to prevent tearing. The condom must be held in place during withdrawal of the still erect penis so that it does not slip off. The condom should only be used once and disposed of responsibly.

Some sheaths may already be impregnated with spermicides (see below) which increases the efficacy. The lubrication afforded by this may be helpful in cases of vaginal dryness, which is not uncommon postnatally. Water-based lubricants should be advocated if needed, as oil-based lubricants will damage the rubber.

Failure rate. This is given as 2–15 per HWY (FPA 1995d), although it is dependent on the age and experience of the user.

Important considerations. If available, only condoms with a CE Mark, as indication that the product has met stringent quality requirements, should be used. The condom should not be used past its expiry date which should also be visible on the packet. They should be stored away from extremes of heat, light and damp.

Future developments for the UK include a polyurethane condom, which is already available in America. Polyurethane is stronger than latex, less sensitive to heat and humidity and is not affected by oil-based lubricants (FPA 1995c).

Female condom

This consists of a polyurethane sheath which is inserted into the vagina. The closed inner end is anchored in place by a polyurethane ring, whilst the open outer edge lies flat against the vulva (see Fig. 32.5). This is not currently available on prescription, but is available free of charge from some family planning clinics and may be purchased from chemists. Despite its expense, it may be popular as no contact with professionals is needed. Some studies however (Bounds et al 1992, Ford & Mathie 1993) have questioned its acceptability to users.

Failure rate. Preliminary findings suggest that efficacy is comparable to other barrier methods (FPA 1995d).

Diaphragm

This is a thin rubber dome with a circumference of metal to help maintain its shape. It is available in a range of types and sizes and the woman is individually fitted. About 2% of women in Britain use this method (Szarewski & Guillebaud 1994).

Cervical and vault caps cover only the cervix, adhering to it by suction. Their use is similar to that of the diaphragm. Although less common, they may be useful for women who have suffered a vaginal prolapse.

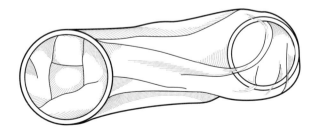

Fig. 32.5 Female condom: 'Femidom'.

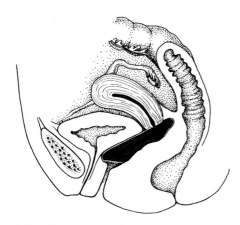

Fig. 32.6 The diaphragm in place.

Using the diaphragm. When in place, the rim of the diaphragm should lie closely against the vaginal walls and rest in the posterior fornix and against the back of the symphysis pubis (see Fig. 32.6). Before insertion, spermicide should be applied to the upper surface (some authorities say to the lower surface also). After insertion, the woman must check that her cervix is covered. In order to preserve spontaneity during intercourse, the woman may decide to insert her diaphragm every evening as a matter of routine. This should be done after bathing, if applicable, rather than before.

If intercourse occurs more than 3 hours after the diaphragm was inserted, additional spermicide is required. The diaphragm must be left in place for 6 hours after the last intercourse, but ideally for no longer than 30 hours (FPA 1995e). On removal, the diaphragm should be washed with a mild soap, dried, and inspected for any damage. A new diaphragm should be fitted annually and following any alteration in weight by more than 3 kilograms.

Failure rate depends on age and experience of use, but is between 4 and 18 per HWY (FPA 1995e).

Important considerations. In order to feel confident in using this method, the woman must feel comfortable in touching her own genitalia. She will also need the physical ability to do this. If she is unable, for any reason, perhaps her partner could be involved in positioning the diaphragm.

The woman will also need privacy and access to water to clean the diaphragm.

Cystitis may be a problem for some users, owing to pressure on the urethra from the rim of the diaphragm. This may be remedied by a change in size or type of diaphragm.

Postpartum considerations. After delivery, the woman should not rely on her previous diaphragm but have its size checked 5–6 weeks postpartum when the vagina and pelvic floor muscles will have regained some of their tone, and any repairs will have healed. Size should also be checked following spontaneous or therapeutic termination of pregnancy.

Future developments include new designs to cover the cervix more closely, and polymer caps which release spermicide (FPA 1995c).

Spermicidal creams, jellies, aerosols, films, vaginal tablets and pessaries

These preparations kill spermatozoa, but as they are not able to penetrate the cervical mucus and are thus probably only active in the vagina, they are not recommended for use on their own (Gebbie 1995). They must be applied immediately before, or in the case of pessaries, 10 minutes before intercourse. Allergy can occur, but as there are many different preparations of different consistency and odour, the couple may need to experiment to find the most suitable. Some spermicides are available free from family planning clinics and on prescription, or they may be bought from chemists.

Spermicides may offer some protection against HIV, gonorrhoea and syphilis (Ross & Frankenburg 1993). Concern has been expressed about possible teratogenicity if spermicides are used around the time of conception, but most studies are reassuring (Guillebaud 1993).

Failure rate. When used alone the failure rate of spermicides is 4–25 per HWY (Chantler 1992).

Natural methods

Natural methods of family planning (NFP) are based on observations of naturally occurring signs and symptoms of the fertile and infertile phases of the menstrual cycle with abstention from intercourse during fertile phases (WHO 1988). These methods are attractive to those who, for any reason, cannot or do not wish to use mechanical or hormonal methods of contraception.

Advantages of NFP methods include the absence of physical side-effects, the use of fertility awareness to avoid or plan a pregnancy, and freedom from dependence on medically qualified personnel (WHO 1988). However, it is imperative that users are adequately taught the methods by experienced, qualified personnel, which may take about 3 months. Such instruction is beyond the scope of most midwives and family planning clinics but can be obtained from the relevant addresses given at the end of the chapter.

As NFP involves abstention from intercourse around the time of ovulation, the commitment and cooperation of both partners are essential. The communication between a couple which is necessary to use these methods effectively may enhance the quality of their relationship. Women may also feel empowered by further knowledge of their own bodies.

Awareness of physiological signs of fertility may include the following methods.

Observation of cervical mucus (also called Billings or ovulation method)

In order to use this method the woman needs to learn to identify the characteristic changes that occur in the cervical mucus throughout the menstrual cycle.

Following menstruation thick mucus blocks the cervical canal, acting as a barrier to spermatozoa. The woman is thus aware of dryness at the vulva. As oestrogen levels rise, the mucus absorbs water and nutrients, softens and begins to flow. At this stage the mucus is opaque, white or creamy and gives a sensation of stickiness.

Around the time of ovulation and the peak of fertility, the mucus becomes transparent and slippery with the appearance of egg white. At this stage the mucus is capable of considerable stretching between finger and thumb, a property known as spinnbarkeit. This occurs as the molecules become parallel to one another to facilitate

the passage of spermatozoa. Progesterone subsequently causes the mucus to thicken and the sensations of stickiness followed by dryness then return.

Observations of the cervical mucus are made throughout the day. The fertile phase begins when mucus is first noticed and ends 4 days after the last day of 'fertile' mucus. The presence of semen can make interpretation difficult, therefore in the preovulatory infertile phase, it is recommended that intercourse takes place only on alternate days. Some suggest that there must be abstinence from intercourse during menstruation because if any mucus were to be produced it might not be noticed. Mucus interpretation may also be difficult if the woman has a vaginal infection. It will also be greatly hindered by the presence of spermicide if a couple choose to use barrier methods of contraception, rather than abstain from intercourse.

Postpartum considerations. Daily observation of mucus and charting should be commenced 3 weeks postpartum. As lactation suppresses ovarian activity, Foxwell & Howie (1995) suggest that observations are made for 2 weeks to find the basic infertile pattern. Henceforth any change in this pattern may signal ovarian activity and the return of fertility. Once the basic infertile pattern is recognised, intercourse may take place on alternate nights. Abstinence should follow any change in the basic infertile pattern for 4 days from the last day of the change.

Observation of body temperature

The woman is taught to take her temperature in a consistent manner immediately on waking each day (if she has had to get up during the night, the woman must have been resting in bed for at least 2 hours before taking her temperature). After ovulation, secretion of progesterone by the corpus luteum causes body temperature to rise by about 0.2°C and to remain at the higher level until menstruation. Hence the postovulatory infertile phase of the menstrual cycle is said to begin on the third day after the temperature shift has been observed (WHO 1988). Factors such as illness, stress, alcohol consumption or a late night may affect temperature and therefore great care should be taken when interpreting charts.

Postpartum considerations. For practical reasons, it may be difficult for a mother to adhere to the recommendations for accurate temperature recording.

Palpation of the cervix

Changes in the cervix occurring throughout the menstrual cycle can be detected by daily palpation by the woman or her partner. After menstruation, the cervix is low in the pelvis and easily felt. The cervix feels firm and dry and the os is closed. Around the time of ovulation the cervix shortens, softens and dilates slightly under the influence of oestrogen.

Postpartum considerations. The hormonal changes of pregnancy, which may take around 6 weeks to resolve, may affect this method.

Calendar or rhythm method

This is used to calculate the probable fertile days by estimating them from records of the woman's previous 6–12 menstrual cycles. The remainder of the cycle used to be called the 'safe period'.

The first fertile day is computed by subtracting 20 days from the length of the woman's shortest cycle: and her last fertile day is calculated by subtracting 11 days from the length of her longest cycle (Foxwell & Howie 1995). For example, if a woman's cycle varies from 25 to 31 days, using this method, she would be fertile between days 5 and 20.

As this method provides only an estimate of the fertile time, the calendar method is rarely used on its own.

Symptothermal method

This method combines temperature charting with observation of cervical mucus to identify the beginning of the fertile phase. Other physiological symptoms of ovulation, such as breast tenderness, ovulation pain and cervical changes may also be recorded.

When a couple are using this method to avoid pregnancy, they abstain from intercourse from the appearance of wet cervical mucus until the third day of elevated temperature or the fourth day after the peak day of mucus, whichever comes later (WHO 1988). Using more than one indicator increases accurate identification of the fertile time, thus reducing the length of abstinence required (Foxwell & Howie 1995).

Failure rate of NFP. This is hotly debated. Reports range from 2–30 per HWY (WHO 1988), and are dependent upon factors such as motivation, teaching and periodic abstinence from intercourse.

Personal system of contraception

This system, which was launched in the UK in October 1996 under the name of 'Persona', comprises a small monitor and urine test sticks. The urine test sticks, which are used when indicated by the monitor, determine urine levels of an oestrogen and luteinising hormone. The woman checks the monitor daily and coloured lights indicate whether she is in a fertile phase or not. This is an individualised system and is not available on prescription. The manufacturers claim the system to be 93–95% effective.

Postpartum considerations. The monitor is not recommended for use during lactation. Following delivery or after cessation of breast feeding, the manufacturer recommends that a woman should wait until she has had at least two natural, consecutive monthly cycles (each lasting 23–35 days) before using the monitor with the beginning of the third period.

The contraceptive effect of breast feeding

Before modern forms of contraception, lactation, with its inhibitory action on ovulation, was a major factor in ensuring adequate intervals between births (IPPF 1988). Additionally, in some cultures sexual intercourse during lactation is considered taboo.

Mode of action. Full understanding of the process is still incomplete but it is thought that the action of the infant suckling at the nipple causes neural inputs to the hypothalamus, resulting in the inhibition of gonadotrophin release (especially luteinising hormone) from the anterior pituitary gland, leading to suppression of ovarian activity

(Short 1993). The role of high levels of prolactin is unclear (Diaz and Croxatto 1993).

The delay in return of postpartum fertility in lactating mothers varies greatly as it depends on patterns of breast feeding, which are influenced by local culture, custom and socioeconomic status. The time taken for return of ovulation is directly related to suckling frequency, intensity and duration; the maintenance of night-time feeding, and the introduction of supplementary food.

Lactational Amenorrhoea Method (LAM)

Lactation can be considered as a method of family planning when used according to the Bellagio Consensus statement (Saarikoski 1993). This concludes that there is a 98% protection against pregnancy during the first 6 months following delivery if the mother is still amenorrhoeic and fully or nearly fully breast feeding her infant (see Fig. 32.7). Pardue (1994) suggests that even mothers who work outside the home can be considered to be 'nearly fully breast feeding' provided they stimulate the nipples by expressing breast milk several times a day. The LAM is not recommended for use after 6 months postpartum because of an increased tendency to ovulation.

Coitus interruptus (withdrawal)

This involves withdrawal of the penis from the vagina prior to ejaculation and is often referred to as 'being careful'. It necessitates tremendous self-control and both partners may find this interruption of intercourse frustrating. The practice is widely used, especially among young couples; Wellings et al (1994) found it more commonplace than diaphragm use. The failure rate may be as high as 25 per HWY, although it is more effective than no contraception at all.

Vaginal douching

Douching after intercourse will not prevent pregnancy as spermatozoa can reach the internal cervical os within 90 seconds of ejaculation.

Male and female sterilisation

This is the contraceptive choice of approximately

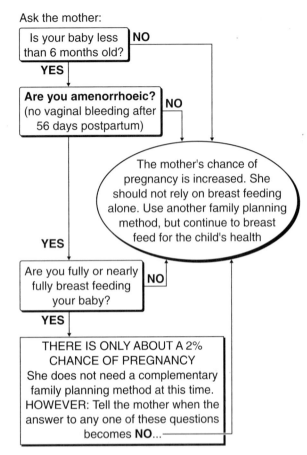

Fig. 32.7 Lactational Amenorrhoea Method of contraception (courtesy Institute for Reproductive Health, Georgetown University Medical Center, under cooperative agreement with the US Agency for International Development, Washington, DC).

25% of couples in the UK (FPA 1995f). Although, technically, sterilisation procedures may be reversible, they should be viewed as permanent. Couples need thorough and careful counselling to ensure that they have completely considered all eventualities, including possible changes in family circumstances, and accept the permanence of the procedures. Although consent of a spouse is not required, joint counselling of both partners is desirable. The operation is available for both sexes under the NHS, but waiting lists may be long. With the commonly used techniques, neither male nor female sterilisation results in any hormonal changes. Diminished libido may result for psychological reasons but some find the freedom from fear of pregnancy very liberating.

Female sterilisation

The passage of ova to uterus is interrupted by occluding the uterine tube by division and ligation, application of clips or rings, diathermy or laser treatment. Modern methods aim at minimal tissue destruction and the isthmus is chosen (for here the tube is of static diameter) so as to increase the chance of a reversal being successful. The operation, performed under either local or general anaesthetic, may be carried out via laparotomy, mini-laparotomy or laparoscopy. Recent possibilities include the use of a hysteroscope, which does not leave a scar (Szarewski & Guillebaud 1994). Attempts are being made to develop non-surgical methods of occluding the uterine tubes.

Failure rate. This is 0.2–0.6 per HWY (FPA 1995g).

Important considerations. The effect is immediate, although the woman may be advised to use contraception until her next menstrual period in case ovulation had already occurred prior to the operation. For this reason, some women are asked to abstain from sexual intercourse for 7 days prior to the procedure being carried out.

In the case of failure, there may be an increased chance of ectopic pregnancy (Glasier 1995). Thus women should be advised to seek medical help urgently if they suspect they may be pregnant following sterilisation.

Postpartum considerations. Hepburn (1995) suggests that immediate postpartum female sterilisation may be associated with increased risk of thromboembolism and regret. This highlights the need for thorough counselling prior to the procedure.

Male sterilisation (vasectomy)

This procedure, usually performed under local anaesthetic, involves occlusion of the vas deferens by division and ligation, diathermy or application of clips. A 'no-scalpel' technique may be used, with a small puncture used instead of a skin incision.

Failure rate. The FPA (1995g) comments that in about 1 in 1000 cases, vasectomy fails within a few months and that, very rarely, late recanalisation can occur.

Important considerations. This procedure is not immediate as it takes some time for spermatozoa to be cleared from the distal part of the vas. Therefore an additional means of contraception must be used until two samples of ejaculate clear of sperm have been verified by laboratory testing. This generally takes up to 30 ejaculations.

Emergency or postcoital contraception

This is reserved for use when contraception was used incorrectly, failed (as in a condom mishap) or was not used at all. Two methods of emergency contraception are commonly used.

Insertion of an intrauterine contraceptive device (IUCD) is the most effective method. If it is inserted within 5 days of the unprotected intercourse or earliest ovulation, implantation of a fertilised ovum can be avoided. If appropriate, it could also be left in place for future contraception.

Alternatively, two high-dose combined pills can be taken within 72 hours of unprotected intercourse, with an identical dose 12 hours later. The pills work by either delaying ovulation or preventing implantation of a fertilised ovum, depending on the stage of the menstrual cycle (Szarewski & Guillebaud 1994).

Nausea can be a problem; therefore it may be helpful to take the pills with food. Additional doses should be taken if the woman vomits within 2 hours of taking either dose of pills. The next period may start earlier or later than expected and follow-up is essential to ensure that the treatment has worked. The risk of teratogenicity is extremely small (Glasier 1995), but must be discussed, as should future contraception. The need to use contraception until the next period should be stressed.

Large doses of the progestogen-only pill may also be used. This method is not widely used or licensed in the UK, but it may be advised if the use of the combined hormonal emergency contraception is contraindicated (see below). It must be initiated within 48 hours of unprotected intercourse.

Failure rate. Failure rates of 0.2–7.4% have been reported for use of combined hormonal emergency contraception in the fertile phase of the cycle (Glasier 1995).

Important considerations. The use of the pills may be contraindicated if there has been more than one episode of unprotected intercourse during the cycle, as the earlier intercourse may already have resulted in a pregnancy. The use of the combined hormonal method is also contraindicated in women who have a history of thrombosis, or those who have a focal migraine at the time they would need to take it (BMA & RPS 1996).

Hormonal emergency contraception may be available from sources such as accident and emergency departments, as well as family planning clinics and GPs. It has been suggested that it should be more easily available from sources such as pharmacists.

READER ACTIVITY

Do you know where hormonal emergency contraception is available in your practice area?

Postpartum considerations. Szarewski & Guillebaud (1994) suggest that it may be safer to avoid oestrogen-containing emergency contraception whilst breast feeding, owing to interference with lactation and possible transmission of steroid to the infant. If necessary, breast milk could be expressed and discarded for 48 hours. An IUCD or progestogen-only method could be used.

Future developments. Studies are ongoing regarding the use of mifepristone (RU 486) as emergency contraception.

FAMILY PLANNING SERVICES

History

The provision of family planning services today owes a great deal to the struggles of pioneers, such as Marie Stopes, who opened the first clinic in 1921. Initially, family planning services were provided by independent agencies, such as the Family Planning Association (FPA). These services were only handed over to the National Health Service (NHS) following the 1973 NHS Reorganisation Act, with family planning supplies and advice available free of charge and irrespective of marital status and age. General practitioners started to provide family planning services under the NHS in 1975.

Services today

READER ACTIVITY

Do you know what family planning services are available in your area?

You may be aware that health authorities or trusts run family planning clinics in most areas. These are often run in premises away from hospital sites, to provide ease of access for the client. The client can usually go along to the clinics without referral, and many have open access without set appointment times, and partners are welcome. The doctors and nurses normally have a specialist interest in family planning and related issues, usually having completed post-basic educational courses in this field.

Clinics may also provide a wide range of services including psychosexual and genetic counselling and well-woman sessions. In the UK, addresses of family planning clinics are available from health centres, community health councils, telephone directories or from the FPA (see addresses at end). Lists of general practitioners (GPs) are kept in libraries, advice centres and are available from family health service authorities. GPs who provide contraceptive advice have the letter 'C' after their names. Clients may choose a GP other than their own to consult for contraceptive services if they wish.

In recent years there has been concern regarding family planning clinic closures (FPA 1995h) although the provision of family planning services by both clinics and GPs is seen as necessary and complementary (FPA 1995h). Clients may choose to attend a family planning clinic for its relative anonymity and specialism of staff; whereas others may consult their GP for reasons of familiarity (Fleissig 1992).

Some health authorities, particularly those in inner city areas, also provide domiciliary family planning services. This may be invaluable for clients who, for a variety of reasons such as physical disability, learning or language difficulties or cultural considerations are unable to access conventional services.

READER ACTIVITY

If your area has a domiciliary family planning service, do you know how referrals are made?

Private services and some run by charitable organisations, such as Brook, also exist. Some useful addresses are given at the end of the chapter.

Additionally, the majority of health authorities now provide clinics and projects specifically for young people. In England and Wales, following the House of Lords' decision in the Gillick case (*Gillick* v. *West Norfolk and Wisbech Area Health Authority* 1985), it is legal for contraceptive advice to be given to young people under 16 years, provided that parental involvement is encouraged and that the client understands the nature and consequences of treatment. The practitioner should also be of the opinion that if contraception were withheld, sexual intercourse would still be likely to take place and the young person's physical and mental health could be compromised. The Northern Ireland Department of Health and Social Services concluded in 1987 that the above guidelines are likely to also be applicable to Northern Ireland (FPA 1995i).

Whoever a woman chooses to consult regarding contraceptive advice, she must be assured of confidentiality.

READER ACTIVITIES

1. Reflect on your awareness of different religious and cultural beliefs with regard to contraception and family planning methods. How can you increase your awareness, and how would this enhance client care?

2. Consider the possible contraceptive needs of your client group. Identify the resources you have available to meet these needs (for example, leaflets in various languages). If necessary, how will you develop these resources?

3. Reflect on how you initiate discussion regarding sexual health and family planning issues with your clients. You may like to share this reflection with a colleague (remember to maintain confidentiality).

ACKNOWLEDGEMENTS

I would like to thank the following people: Andy and Ellie Plane for help and support; Dr Jo Alexander, Dr S. Randall, J. Rea, J. Stosiek, S. Turrell for their helpful comments.

USEFUL ADDRESSES

Brook Advisory Centres
165 Gray's Inn Road
London WC1X 8UD
Tel: 0171 713 9000 (Helpline)

FPA (including Contraceptive Education Service)
2–12 Pentonville Road
London N1 9FP

International Planned Parenthood Federation
Regent's College
Inner Circle
Regent's Park
London NW1 4NS

National Association of the Ovulation Method of Ireland (NAOMI)
16 North Great George's Street
Dublin 1

The Association to Aid the Sexual and Personal Relationships of People with a Disability (SPOD)
286 Camden Road
London N7 OBJ

REFERENCES

Bounds W 1994 Contraceptive efficacy of the diaphragm and cervical caps used in conjunction with spermicides – a fresh look at the evidence. British Journal of Family Planning 20: 84–87

Bounds W, Guillebaud J, Newman G 1992 Female condom (Femidom). A clinical study of its use-effectiveness and patient acceptability. British Journal of Family Planning 18: 36–41

British Medical Association and Royal Pharmaceutical Society of Great Britain 1996 British National Formulary, No 32. BMA and The Pharmaceutical Press, London and Oxon

Bromham D 1993 Intrauterine contraceptive devices – a reappraisal. British Medical Bulletin 49(1): 100–123

Chantler E 1992 Vaginal spermicides: some current concerns. British Journal of Family Planning 17: 118–119

Chi I-C, Robbins M, Balogh S 1992 The progestin-only oral contraceptive: place in postpartum contraception. Advances in Contraception 8: 93–103

Collaborative Group on Hormonal Factors in Breast Cancer 1996 Breast cancer and hormonal contraceptives: collaborative reanalysis of individual data on 53 297 women with breast cancer and 100 239 women without breast cancer from 54 epidemiological studies. Lancet 347: 1713–1727

Davies G, Newton J 1991 Subdermal contraceptive implants – a review: with special reference to Norplant. British Journal of Family Planning 17: 4–8

Department of Health 1992 Health of the nation. Cm 1986. HMSO, London

Diaz S, Croxatto H 1993 Contraception in lactating women. Current Opinion in Obstetrics and Gynaecology 5(6): 815–822

Drife J 1995 Intrauterine contraceptive devices. In: Louden N, Glasier A, Gebbie A (eds) Handbook of family planning and reproductive health care, 3rd edn. Churchill Livingstone, Edinburgh

English National Board for Nursing, Midwifery and Health Visiting 1994 Sexual health education and training. ENB, London

Family Planning Association 1995a Choosing and using the progestogen-only pill. FPA, London

Family Planning Association 1995b Choosing and using injections and implants. FPA, London

Family Planning Association 1995c Factsheet 3A: methods of contraception: past, present and future. FPA, London

Family Planning Association 1995d Choosing and using male and female condoms. FPA, London

Family Planning Association 1995e Choosing and using diaphragms and caps. FPA, London

Family Planning Association 1995f Factsheet 3E: contraceptive usage and trends in the UK. FPA, London

Family Planning Association 1995g Factsheet 3F: sterilisation usage and trends in the UK. FPA, London

Family Planning Association 1995h Factsheet 1B: use of family planning services in the UK. FPA, London

Family Planning Association 1995i Factsheet 1A: family planning services: past, present and future. FPA, London

Fleissig A 1992 Family planning services – use and preference of recent mothers. British Journal of Family Planning 17: 110–114

Ford N, Mathie E 1993 The acceptability and experience of the female condom, Femidom, among family planning clinic attenders. British Journal of Family Planning 19: 187–192

Foxwell M, Howie P 1995 Natural regulation of fertility. In: Louden N, Glasier A, Gebbie A (eds) Handbook of family planning and reproductive health care, 3rd edn. Churchill Livingstone, Edinburgh

Fraser I 1995 Progestogen-only contraception. In: Louden N, Glasier A, Gebbie A (eds) Handbook of family planning and reproductive health care, 3rd edn. Churchill Livingstone, Edinburgh

Gebbie A 1995 Barrier methods. In: Louden N, Glasier A, Gebbie A (eds) Handbook of family planning and reproductive health care, 3rd edn. Churchill Livingstone, Edinburgh

Glasier A 1995 Emergency postcoital contraception. In: Louden N, Glasier A, Gebbie A (eds) Handbook of family planning and reproductive health care, 3rd edn. Churchill Livingstone, Edinburgh

Guillebaud J 1991 The pill. Oxford University Press, Oxford

Guillebaud J 1993 Contraception: your questions answered. Churchill Livingstone, Edinburgh

Guillebaud J 1995 Combined hormonal contraception. In: Louden N, Glasier A, Gebbie A (eds) Handbook of family planning and reproductive health care, 3rd edn. Churchill Livingstone, Edinburgh

Hepburn M 1995 Factors influencing contraceptive choice. In: Louden N, Glasier A, Gebbie A (eds) Handbook of family planning and reproductive health care, 3rd edn. Churchill Livingstone, Edinburgh

International Planned Parenthood Federation 1988 Family planning handbook for doctors. IPPF, London

International Planned Parenthood Federation 1990 New IPPF statement on breastfeeding, fertility and postpartum contraception. IPPF Medical Bulletin 24(2): 2–4

Kishen M, Presho M 1996 Emergency contraception – a prescription for change. British Journal of Family Planning 22: 25–27

Laryea M 1980 The midwife's role in the postnatal care of primiparae and their infants in the first 28 days following childbirth. Unpublished MPhil Thesis, Newcastle upon Tyne Polytechnic, Newcastle upon Tyne

Mangla B, Mangla V 1993 India: family planning project stirs Norplant debate. Lancet 341: 1016

Newton J 1993 Long acting methods of contraception. British Medical Bulletin 49(1): 40–61

Pardue N 1994 On the LAM. Mothering 72: 76–81

Roberts H (ed) 1981 Women, health and reproduction. Routledge and Kegan Paul, London

Ross J, Frankenburg E 1993 Findings from two decades of family planning research. The Population Council, New York

Saarikoski S 1993 Contraception during lactation. Annals of Medicine 25(2): 181–184

Short R 1993 Lactational infertility in family planning. Annals of Medicine 25(2): 175–180

Sleep J, Grant A, Garcia J, Elbourne D, Spencer J, Chalmers I 1984 West Berkshire perineal management trial. British Medical Journal 289: 587-590

Smith C 1994 Norplant: a long term hormonal contraceptive. Prescriber (19 May): 19–20, 23

Szarewski A 1991 Hormonal contraception. Macdonald Optima, London

Szarewski A, Guillebaud J 1994 Contraception: a user's handbook. Oxford University Press, Oxford

Tankeyoon M, Dusitin N, Chalapati S et al 1988 Effects of hormonal contraceptives on breast milk composition and infant growth. Studies in Family Planning 19(6): 361–369

Thorogood M, Villard-Mackintosh L 1993 Combined oral contraceptives: risks and benefits. British Medical Bulletin 49(1): 124–139

United Kingdom Central Council for Nursing, Midwifery and Health Visiting (UKCC) 1994 The midwife's code of practice. UKCC, London

Vessey M, Lawless M, Yeates D, McPherson K 1985 Progestogen-only oral contraception. Findings in a large prospective study with special reference to effectiveness. British Journal of Family Planning 10: 117–121

Wang I, Fraser I 1994 Reproductive function and contraception in the postpartum period. Obstetrical and Gynaecological Survey 49(1): 56–63

Wellings K, Field J, Johnson A, Wadsworth J 1994 Sexual behaviour in Britain. Penguin Books, London

World Health Organization 1988 Natural family planning. WHO, Geneva

World Health Organization 1992 Reproductive health: a key to a brighter future. WHO, Geneva

World Health Organization 1994 Progestogen-only contraceptives during lactation: I. Infant growth. Contraception 50(July): 35–52

FURTHER READING

Family Planning Association 1995 FPA Factfile. FPA, London

Leathard A 1980 The fight for family planning. Macmillan, Basingstoke

Montford H, Skrine R 1993 Contraceptive care: meeting individual needs. Chapman & Hall, London

33

Bereavement and loss in maternity care

Rosemary Mander

This chapter introduces the reader to the issues which those working in the maternity area are likely to have to face in the event of bereavement or loss. It is hoped that it will help the reader to be better able to cope with the situation and, thus, be able to care for those who are more directly involved and affected. Throughout the chapter the assumption is made that care in situations of loss is more likely to be effective if it is research-based.

The chapter aims to:

- consider the meaning of bereavement and loss and their significance in maternity care

- discuss the forms of loss which the midwife may encounter

- draw on the available research to review the care of those who are likely to be affected by the loss.

INTRODUCTION

In our 20th century western society, bereavement has become inextricably linked with loss through death. In this chapter, to make these concepts more relevant to the midwife, I am broadening the focus to include other sources of grief which may impinge on care of the childbearing woman. In widening out the topic, I reflect the original meaning of 'bereavement' which carries connotations of plundering, robbing, snatching or otherwise removing traumatically and without consent. This meaning may appear to conflict with the other part of my title – 'loss' – which is also widely used in this context. Such inconsistency is fallacious because, while the child may be taken in any of a variety of ways, the unspoken hopes and expectations invested in that child remain irretrievably lost.

In many ways loss in childbearing is unique. This uniqueness may be due to the awful contrast between the sorrow of death and the mystical joy of a new life emerging from a mother (see also Ch. 2). Additionally, there is the cruel paradox of simultaneous birth and death; we tend to assume that these events are ordinarily separated by a lifetime and the experience becomes incomprehensible when they become unified (Bourne 1968). Although any perinatal loss is unique, the uniqueness of both the individual's experience and the phenomenon itself must be contrasted with the frequency with which a woman may encounter lesser losses during childbearing. Such lesser losses may include the woman's loss of her previous independence, her loss of her special relationship with her fetus at the birth, or her loss of her expectations for a perfect baby when she comes to recognise that her actual baby is very real (Raphael-Leff 1991).

In this chapter I focus mainly on the reactions of the woman and the care that the midwife provides for her. The midwife is in the privileged position of being able to be with the woman when she first faces such losses. It is the responsibility of the midwife to draw on her theoretical knowledge which, as in any area of her care, should be based as far as possible on research. Such knowledge is utilised in the skilled care of the woman to assist her adjustment to these greater or lesser losses.

GRIEF AND LOSS

Grief, like death and other fundamentally important matters, is a fact of life. It is something which human beings invariably meet in one form or another at a relatively early age. In spite of its universality, a woman in a developed country who loses her baby is likely to be young enough not have previously encountered grief due to death. This is another of the reasons for the uniqueness of loss in childbearing.

Attachment

Our limited understanding of mother–child attachment, sometimes known as 'bonding', for a long time prevented midwives and others from recog-

nising the significance of perinatal loss, resulting in care based largely on incorrect assumptions. The strength of the relationship which develops during pregnancy between the woman and her fetus emerged in a small research project involving bereaved mothers (Kennell et al 1970). This relationship is facilitated by the woman feeling fetal movements and by her experience of pregnancy, as well as by investigations such as ultrasound scans. Ordinarily the process of attachment continues well beyond the birth. The development of attachment during pregnancy does mean, however, that should the relationship not continue, it has to be ended or completed in the same way as any parting. Thus, the reality of the relationship between the mother and the child during pregnancy must be recognised before the loss may be accepted. These processes are crucial to the initiation of healthy grieving.

Grief

It is through grieving that we are able to adjust to the more serious as well as the lesser losses which confront us as we move through life (Marris 1986). Healthy grief means that we are able to move forward, although not invariably directly, from our initial feelings of distraught hopelessness. We eventually achieve some degree of resolution which permits our usual functioning for a large part of our lives; we may even find that in the process we have grown by learning something about ourselves and the resources available to us. Although grief may be viewed as a state of apathetic passivity, it is better regarded as a time during which people actively strive to complete the emotional tasks facing them; to describe this activity the term 'grief work' has been coined (Engel 1961).

The stages of grief through which the person is likely to have to work have been described in a number of ways, but Kübler-Ross's (1970) account is well known and may be the most useful. These stages (Box 33.1) are not negotiated in a consistent sequential order but there will be individual variation and often the person moves back and forth through them before eventually achieving resolution.

The initial response to learning of a loss comprises a defence mechanism which serves to protect

---

Box 33.1 Stages of grief

Shock and denial

Increasing awareness
- Emotions
  - sorrow
  - guilt
  - anger
- Searching
- Bargaining

Realisation
- Depression
- Apathy
- Bodily changes

Resolution
- Equanimity
- Anniversary reactions

---

from the full impact of the news or realisation. This reaction comprises shock or denial, which helps by providing insulation from the unthinkable reality. This initial response allows the bereaved person a 'breathing space' in which she is able to marshal her emotional resources, which will assist in coping with the eventual realisation.

Denial soon ceases to be effective and awareness of the reality of the loss gradually dawns. Awareness brings with it powerful emotional reactions and their physical manifestations. Feelings of sorrow may be easily apparent but other, less acceptable, emotions may simultaneously overwhelm the bereaved person; such emotions may include guilt and dissatisfaction, as well as compulsive searching and, still more worryingly, feelings of anger. Realisation dawns in waves as the bereaved person tries out various coping strategies to 'bargain' with herself to delay accepting reality.

When such fruitless strategies are exhausted, the despair of full realisation of the loss materialises, bringing with it apathy and poor concentration as well as some bodily changes. At this point in her grief, the bereaved person may show the anxiety and physical symptoms of a true depression.

Eventually, after the loss has been accepted, it is integrated into the person's life. As mentioned already, this process is not straightforward and may involve slow progress and many setbacks. Such uncertain progress has been described in terms of 'oscillation and hesitation' (Stroebe & Stroebe

1987). Although the person is never likely to 'get over' her loss, she will probably eventually be able to integrate it into her experience of life. This ultimate degree of 'resolution' is recognisable in the bereaved person's ability to contemplate realistically and with equanimity the strengths as well as the weaknesses of her lost relationship.

Significance

Healthy grieving matters because of its contribution to the resumption of some degree of balance or homeostasis in the life of the bereaved person. Grief is crucial in helping people to recover from the wounding effects which the greater and the lesser losses of life inflict. The hazards of being unable to grieve healthily have long been recognised in emotional terms, but more recently the association between perinatal loss and the woman's physical ill health has emerged (Ney et al 1994). These researchers emphasise the woman's need for support, regardless of the nature of the loss or the extent to which it is recognised or her grief sanctioned by society.

Culture

I have described a general picture of healthy grieving and mentioned the likelihood of individual variation, which has been shown to be common to people of many ethnic backgrounds (Cowles 1996). It is now necessary to emphasise that the overt manifestations of grief, and the mourning rituals which accompany it, vary even more. These variations are influenced by a number of factors. In her book, Cecil (1996) shows us the massive differences between ethnic groups in their attitudes towards loss in childbearing. In my own research I found that a midwife may encounter difficulty in accepting the different attitudes to loss in women belonging to cultures other than her own, possibly illustrating the fundamental nature of these feelings (Mander 1994). The extent to which midwives are able to work through such feelings, to permit them to fully support women whose attitudes are different, is uncertain.

Closely bound up with culture, and certainly influencing mourning behaviour, is the religious persuasion of the grieving person. These aspects may be difficult to dissociate from the influence of social class and the prevalent social attitudes.

Despite the huge variations in the manifestation of grief, the underlying purpose of mourning is universal. It serves to establish support for those most closely affected, by strengthening the links between those who remain. In perinatal loss the midwife initially provides this support; the role of the midwife is to be with the woman at the time when she is beginning to realise the extent of her loss and to ensure that nothing is allowed to interfere with the mother's healthy initiation of her grieving.

FORMS OF LOSS

As I have mentioned already, the terms 'loss' and 'bereavement' may be applied to a wide range of experiences, which vary considerably in their severity and effects. We must be careful, however, to avoid making assumptions about the meaning of a childbearing loss to a particular woman. It is difficult, if not impossible, for anybody else to understand the significance of a pregnancy or a child to another person; this is because childbearing carries with it a huge range of immensely deep feelings, which include unspoken hopes and expectations based on personal as well as cultural value systems. It is necessary to accept that, as has been said in the context of pain, sorrow 'is what the person experiencing it says it is' (McCaffery 1979).

I mention here some of the situations in which we may expect to encounter grief. I have to emphasise, however, that this list is in no way exclusive; there may well be situations of grief which are not included here and, in the same way, some of the situations mentioned may not invariably engender grief.

Perinatal loss

When loss in childbearing is mentioned, loss in the perinatal period comes quickly to mind. This includes babies who are stillborn (that is, in the UK, who show no sign of life after complete expulsion from the mother after 24 weeks' gestation) and babies who die in the first week of life (sometimes referred to as early neonatal deaths).

Attempts have been made to compare the severity of the grief reaction which follows loss at different stages, perhaps to demonstrate that certain women deserve more sympathy or care. A study which investigated this point, however, showed no significant differences in the grief response between mothers losing a baby by miscarriage, stillbirth or neonatal death (Peppers & Knapp 1980). This study serves to emphasise the crucial role of the mother's developing relationship with her fetus, knowledge of which has facilitated great improvements in care of the grieving mother.

Stillbirth

The long-term recovery of the mother from the experience of stillbirth was the subject of a recent study which was undertaken in Sweden. Rådestad and colleagues (1996a) were able to compare the recovery of 380 women who had given birth to a stillborn baby with the health of 379 women who had borne a healthy child. Judging from the 84% response rate, the mothers were comfortable to be involved in this study. These researchers found that the bereaved mother made a better recovery if she was able to decide how long to keep her baby with her after the birth and if she was able to keep tokens or mementoes of her baby's birth. The mother who was less likely to make a good recovery was the one in whom there was some delay between her realisation of fetal demise and the birth of the baby. Clearly, these findings have important implications for the midwifery care as well as the obstetric care of the mother (see below). Additionally, they emphasise that stillbirth may be 'known', when the mother realises in advance of the birth that her baby has died. This situation has been known in the past as 'intrauterine death' or 'IUD'. Alternatively, the loss may be unexpected. While avoiding any comparison of the two mothers' grief, it is understandable that the mother who knows that she is to give birth to a dead baby carries a particular emotional burden. This may be compounded by the process of maceration having changed the baby's appearance.

Grieving early neonatal death

Grieving the loss of a baby who has lived independently, albeit briefly, may be facilitated by three factors. The first is that the mother is likely to have been able to see and hold her real live baby, thus giving her a genuine memory of her experience. Second is the legal requirement that a baby who dies neonatally must have both his/her birth and death registered, providing written evidence of his/her being. The third factor relates to the investment of the staff in their care of this dying baby which, Littlewood (1992) suggests, increases the likelihood of them providing good support for the parents.

Accidental loss in early pregnancy: miscarriage

Early pregnancy loss may be due to one of a number of pathological processes, such as ectopic pregnancy or spontaneous abortion. The word 'abortion' is avoided in this context, because it carries with it connotations of deliberate interference, which may be unacceptable to a grieving mother. The term 'miscarriage' is preferable to include all of these spontaneous forms of loss. The grief of miscarriage has been ignored in the past, largely owing to the frequency with which it happens. This has been estimated at up to 31% of pregnancies in USA (Bansen & Stevens 1992), though the figure may be higher in the UK (Oakley et al 1990).

Understanding of the woman's experience of miscarriage was sought through a qualitative research project (Bansen & Stevens 1992). Among the 10 mothers whom they interviewed 2–5 months after the miscarriage, these researchers identified profound grief, which was associated with anger that their bodies had allowed them to miscarry, and anxiety about their future childbearing. Far from being an insignificant event, these mothers were so ill during the miscarriage that they became fearful that they might die. Although each mother found reassurance in the conception of the pregnancy which was lost, each had lost confidence in her fertility. As may happen in other forms of childbearing loss, each mother found difficulty in locating suitable support and had to face comments which belittled her loss and denigrated its significance.

It may be necessary to seek the cause of a woman's miscarriage, especially if it happens repeatedly. Miscarriage has been found to be significantly correlated with stressful life events (O'Hare & Creed 1995). Unfortunately these researchers were unable to identify whether stressful events are actually the cause of the miscarriage. It may be that both the woman's stressful life event and her miscarriage are caused by some other factor, such as her environment, her lifestyle or her personality characteristics.

The former lack of recognition of miscarriage is now being addressed, and women are encouraged to create their own rituals to assist their grieving. Speakman (1996) discusses the helpful nature of a religious service, of suitable photographs or of communicating sorrow through writing a poem or a letter.

Infertility

The grief associated with involuntary infertility is less focused than that experienced when grieving for a particular person and it has been likened to 'genetic death' (Crawshaw 1995). In this situation the couple grieve for the hopes and expectations which are integral to the conception of a baby. The realisation of their infertility, and the grief which it brings, is aggravated by the widespread assumption of the easiness of childbearing; this is sufficiently prevalent for the emphasis, in society in general and in health care in particular, to be on the prevention of conception. The complex investigations and prolonged treatment associated with infertility result in a 'roller-coaster' of hope and despair.

As with any grief, the woman and the man in the infertile relationship are likely to grieve differently, giving rise to tensions. The announcement of a diagnosis or cause of the couple's infertility may resolve some of their uncertainty about themselves and their predicament but it also raises other difficulties. These may include the problems associated with one partner being 'labelled' as infertile and, hence, the cause of the couple's difficulty. A complex spiral of blame and recrimination may develop to further damage what may already have become an unstable relationship.

It is clear that counselling an infertile couple must differ markedly from counselling those who are bereaved through death and that, because of the nature of our society, infertility counselling focuses on the woman (Crawshaw 1995). Bearing in mind the limited success of assisted reproduction techniques, it follows that part of the role of the infertility counsellor lies in encouraging the couple to contemplate their continuation of investigations or treatment, as well as the other options which are open to them in the creation of their family.

Relinquishment for adoption

Although it has long been widely accepted that relinquishment is followed by grief (Sorosky et al 1984) the view still persists among some health care personnel that, because of relinquishment's voluntary nature, grief is unlikely (Mander 1995). Each mother in this study was quite clear that her relinquishment was in no way a voluntary action and that she was presented with no alternative but to give up her baby for adoption. These mothers really were bereaved in the original meaning of the word (see above).

The grief of relinquishment differs from the grief of death in certain crucial ways. First, following relinquishment grief is likely to be delayed. This is partly because of the nature of the woman's lifestyle at the time of her loss and partly because of the secrecy which her family in particular and society in general imposes on the woman who does not mother her baby in the conventional way. Second, the grief of relinquishment is unable to be resolved in the short or medium term. This is because, ordinarily, the acceptance of the loss is fundamental to the resolution of grief. Following relinquishment such acceptance is impossible because of the likelihood that the one who was relinquished will seek to make contact with her mother when she is legally permitted to do so. The possibility of being reunited with the relinquished one was fundamentally important to the mothers who spoke with me. The words of Rosa reflected what many mothers said to me: 'I'd be delighted if she would turn up on the doorstep'.

Termination of pregnancy

Grief associated with elective termination of a normal pregnancy (TOP) is problematic and it may be for this reason that it tends not to be included in the literature on grief. The experience of grief following TOP for fetal abnormality and guilt following TOP do, however, tend to be recognised and accepted. In view of the frequency with which TOP happens and the grief which is likely to be engendered, it may deserve more attention.

TOP for fetal abnormality (TFA)

The package of investigations which is available to the pregnant woman and has become known as 'prenatal diagnosis' may ultimately lead to the mother's decision to undergo TFA. Although it may be assumed that the mother's reaction is solely one of relief at avoiding giving birth to a baby with a handicap, Iles (1989) suggests several reasons why this mother may experience conflicting emotions which may impede her grieving:

- the pregnancy is likely to have been wanted
- the TFA is a serious event in both physiological and social terms
- the reason for the TFA may arouse guilty feelings
- the recurrence risk may constitute a future threat
- the woman's biological clock will be ticking away
- her failure to achieve a 'normal' outcome may engender guilt.

Interventions have been introduced to facilitate the grieving of the mother who has undergone TFA. These may involve the creation of memories, which is attempted in other forms of childbearing loss (see below), and counselling. A study of the effectiveness of psychotherapeutic counselling in such mothers with no other risk factors was undertaken in the form of a randomised controlled trial (Lilford et al 1994). This study suggests that bereavement counselling does not make a difference in terms of the difficulty or duration of grieving and, additionally, these researchers go on to conclude that mothers who attend for counselling would probably have resolved their grief more satisfactorily than the other group anyway.

TOP for other reasons

The non-recognition of grief associated with TOP may be partly because the mother who decides to have her pregnancy ended may be regarded as 'undeserving' of the luxury of grief. Additionally, this may be aggravated by her being held responsible or blamed for her situation (Hey 1996). Research on the psychological sequelae of TOP has focused largely on the guilt of having decided to end the pregnancy, as opposed to grief reactions; it may be that such a focus is associated with the current abortion debate. Thus, the 'post-abortion blues' have been identified, presenting as grief, regret and tearfulness and have been linked with feelings of 'feminine inadequacy' (Raphael-Leff 1991). This researcher suggests that these reactions may be prevented by counselling prior to as well as after the TOP.

On the basis of the limited material on grief following TOP, it is necessary to question the extent to which grief is still regarded as a luxury in which people may allow themselves to wallow or whether it is a painful way of coming to terms with a traumatic experience.

The baby with a handicap

For a variety of reasons a baby may still be born with a handicap, which may or may not be expected. The possible handicaps vary hugely in their severity and in their implications for the future of the baby. It may be that a mother will have to adjust to the possibility of her baby not surviving, but some conditions will certainly be compatible with the continuation of life.

The mother's reaction to the birth of a baby with a handicap will involve some elements of grief. This is particularly true if the condition was unexpected, as the mother will have to begin her grieving for the expected baby before she is able to embark on her relationship with her real baby.

The mother may be shocked to find herself thinking that her baby might be better off if it did not survive (Lewis & Bourne 1989). While the mother may be reassured that she is not unique in experiencing such thoughts, she may find difficulty in completing her grieving.

In the case of a baby being born with an unexpected handicap, the problem of breaking the news emerges. There seem to be no easy answers as to how this may be done with the minimum of trauma, but clear, effective and honest communication is crucial (Crowther 1995).

The inside baby

It may be hard to understand, but even in uncomplicated, healthy childbearing the need for grief may still be present. This is because, in spite of obstetric technology, the mother is unable to see her baby before the birth and inevitably the real baby will be different in some ways from the one with whom she developed a relationship during pregnancy. These differences are likely to be minor, such as hair colour or crying behaviour. Lewis (1979) coined the term 'inside baby' to denote the one whom she came to love during pregnancy and who was perfect. The 'outside baby' is the real one, for whom she will care and who may have some imperfections, such as being of the wrong sex. Clearly the mother may have a few moments of regret, during which she must grieve the loss of her fantasy baby, while at the same time forming her relationship with her real baby.

CARE

In considering the care which midwives provide in the event of loss, we encounter difficulties in deciding where to begin. Thus, I have organised this section by focusing first on those who are involved and/or affected and then on other crucial issues. From this material will emerge the principles on which our care in this situation is based. While I recognise the artificiality of distinguishing care for individuals in such a complex situation, this approach may help us to consider the different needs among people affected by a single event.

The baby

It is particularly hard to separate the care of the baby from the care of those who are grieving, because much of our care comprises the creation of memories of the baby which will facilitate the grieving (see Box 33.2).

We may think of the care of the baby beginning

Box 33.2 Creating memories

Midwifery activities
- Information giving
- Taking photographs
- Cutting a lock of hair
- Taking a footprint
- Giving a cot card or name band

Parental activities
- Naming baby
- Seeing baby
- Holding baby
- Caring for baby
  – bathing
  – dressing
- Taking photographs

Other activities
- Writing in a book of remembrance
- Service/funeral/burial
- Tree planting
- Writing a letter
- Writing a poem

before the actual birth by considering the presence of the cot in the labour room (Mander 1994). Although the presence of the cot may cause the staff some discomfort, it may serve to remind all concerned of the reality of the baby.

If possible, that is if the loss is known, the midwife discusses with the parents prior to the birth the contact which will be made with the baby. This contact may take any of a number of forms, beginning with just a sight of the wrapped baby. Contact with the baby has been shown to resolve some of the confusion which may surround the experience of the birth and mothers who do choose to make some contact do not regret their decision (Kellner & Lake 1986). The midwife has to decide whether and how much encouragement she will give to the mother to make contact with her baby, drawing on her knowledge of its beneficial effect on grief (Mander 1995). This decision is not an easy one, but midwives tend to be over-cautious in helping the mother to make contact with her baby; this was one of the findings from an important study of the views of 380 mothers who had experienced perinatal loss (Rådestad et al 1996b). These researchers found that one-third of the mothers would have appreciated more encouragement to make contact with their babies.

The mother may choose to have considerable contact with her baby, perhaps keeping the baby with her for some time. During this time the mother may wish to have her baby baptised which, as well as its religious significance, serves to emphasise the reality of the baby. This simple act, which may be undertaken by the midwife, additionally presents an opportunity to name the baby. The mother may also during this time take advantage of other opportunities to create memories of her experience; these include doing some of the things which a mother ordinarily does for her baby, such as bathing and dressing her. Whether or not the mother feels able to make contact with her baby immediately, it is usual to collect certain mementoes at the time of the birth, such as a lock of hair, a footprint or photographs. If she chooses no contact at the time of birth she may, at a later date, avail herself of these mementoes. Taking photographs which are of a suitable quality may present a challenge to the midwife who is not skilled in using a camera, giving rise to dissatisfaction (Rådestad et al 1996b). The photographs in Figures 33.1 and 33.2 show the way in which different aspects of the baby have been made

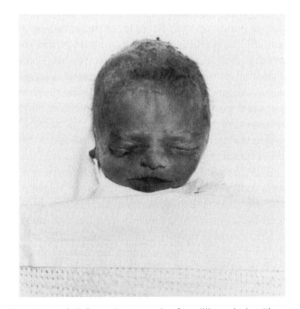

Fig. 33.1 A full-face photograph of a stillborn baby. The impression is rather 'clinical' as the cot sheet is straight and there has been no attempt to hide bruises on the baby's face.

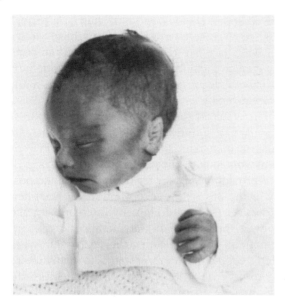

Fig. 33.2 Another photograph of the same baby as in Figure 33.1. In this photograph the baby's head has been turned to the side to hide bruising. Additionally the fold in the cot sheet and the baby's hand being exposed give a more 'natural' impression.

apparent by a medical photographer, Shamus K Reddin at Peterborough District Hospital. Thus, the mother who declines immediate contact may choose, later, that which is most appropriate. Alternatively, the parents may decide that a photograph should be taken of them holding their baby; this would be like ordinary parental behaviour.

In the hope of preventing a future loss, the parents may be advised that the baby should have a postmortem examination. This raises many difficult issues for parents, who may consider that their baby has suffered enough already.

The funeral serves a multiplicity of purposes, including a demonstration of community support as well as establishing the reality of the loss. A young woman who has no experience of death may have difficulty imagining how such a ritual could possibly be beneficial. She may be helped, though, by being reminded how cemetery and crematorium staff are becoming more sensitive to the need to provide a suitable ceremony and a suitable environment in which the child may subsequently be remembered. In some situations, such as early miscarriage, a funeral might not be appropriate.

The mother may find that an impromptu service is helpful near the time of her loss or, later, she may create her own memorial by writing a letter to her lost baby or by planting a tree.

The mother

Much of the midwife's care of the grieving mother comprises helping her to make some sense of the incomprehensible experience which has happened to her. As I have mentioned already, the mother may need help to recognise that she has given birth and that she no longer has that baby. Integral to this is assisting her realisation that she is a mother, which may be achieved through our midwifery care.

The mother may start to make sense of her loss by talking about it. Although this may sound simple enough, 'opening up' may present the mother with a number of challenges. For example, she may have little experience of and be uncomfortable talking about such profound feelings. Further, she may have difficulty finding a suitable and willing listener at the time when she feels ready to talk. The problem of her finding a listener was identified in a research project which showed that senior hospital staff appear too busy and other staff insufficiently experienced for her to unburden herself (Lovell et al 1986). Family members who might be expected to help by listening have been shown to have their own difficulties in coping, which makes them less than receptive to the mother's needs (Rajan 1994).

In a situation involving loss, any of us may feel that our control over our lives is slipping away. Such feelings of losing control may be exacerbated when the loss involves a physiological process such as childbearing, which a large number of people seem to achieve successfully and effortlessly. As midwives we are able to help the mother to retain some degree of, or at least some sense of, control. This is by giving her accurate information about the choices open to her and on which she is able to base her decision-making.

The reality of the grieving mother's control over her care was the subject of Gohlish's research (1985). She met with 15 mothers of stillborn babies and asked them to identify the 'nursing' behaviours which they had found to be most helpful. This study clearly showed the importance which the grieving mother attaches to assuming control over her environment.

The difficulty, mentioned already, which the mother experiences in identifying a suitable listener may be associated, more generally, with the support which she is able to locate. Support and counselling following perinatal bereavement was researched by Forrest and colleagues (1982) using a randomised controlled trial. The experimental group, comprising 25 bereaved mothers, received ideal supported midwifery care together with counselling; whereas the control group comprised another 25 bereaved mothers who received the standard care. Unlike Lilford's more psychotherapeutically oriented study (see above), Forrest found that the well-supported and counselled group recovered from their grief more quickly than the mothers in the control group. It is unfortunate that both of these studies encountered difficulty in retaining contact with the grieving mothers.

The benefits of support in facilitating grieving have been established by Forrest and colleagues (1982) and the mother may find support in any of a number of people, who may provide it on a more formal or less formal basis. While we may assume that identifying support is easy, research has shown that, like finding a suitable listener, locating support may be problematic for this mother (Rådestad et al 1996b). These researchers found that in just over one-quarter of bereaved mothers their support lasted for less than 1 month; while for just over one-quarter, their support was non-existent. Of particular significance to midwives is the contribution of the lay support groups, who may be organised on a self-help basis. My own research showed that midwives are generally happy to recommend that a mother may find a support group, such as the Stillbirth and Neonatal Death Society (SANDS) helpful. Unfortunately, little is known about the effectiveness of such groups or about the experience of those who attend (Mander 1994).

The family

While the mother is clearly most intimately involved and likely to be most affected by a perinatal loss, to a greater or lesser extent those close to her will share her grief. In this context, as well as the conventional family members, I include in the family a wide range of non-blood and non-marital relationships.

The effect of the loss on the father may in the past have been underestimated. This may be partly because men tend to show their grief differently from women and partly because they are socialised into providing support for their womenfolk, possibly at the cost of their own emotional well-being (Kowalski 1987). Additionally, men are less likely to avail themselves of the therapeutic effects of crying and communicating their sorrow in words. Men's coping mechanisms may also involve resorting to other less healthy grieving strategies which may include an early return to work and the use of potentially harmful substances, such as nicotine or alcohol.

Possibly in association with their different patterns of grieving, the parental relationship is likely to change following perinatal loss (Kowalski 1987). Whether the couple find that their relationship is strengthened or otherwise is hard to predict.

Perhaps because they are less closely involved, the grandparents may be disproportionately adversely affected by the loss. This may be due to their inability to protect their children (the bereaved parents) from their painful loss. Inevitably and additionally they will experience their own sense of loss at the threat to the continuity of their family and what it means to them.

The effects of perinatal loss on a sibling may be problematic because of uncertainty about the (probably young) child's understanding of the event. This difficulty is compounded by the parents' limited ability to articulate their pain in a suitable form. The parents may seek to solve these problems by 'protecting' their other child or children from the truth, little knowing that such protection may only create a pattern of unhealthy grieving, which may leave the family with a legacy of dysfunctional relationships (Dyregrov 1991).

Although my own research found that midwives tend to assume that the family are the best people to support a grieving mother (Mander 1994), it has been found that family responses may not invariably be healthy or helpful (Kissane & Bloch 1994).

The caregivers

The difficulty that staff face in caring for a grieving mother has been linked with their own personal reactions to the loss of a baby (Bourne 1968). This may be part of the reason for the longstanding neglect of this mother in particular and this topic in general. Additionally, the loss of a baby may represent all too clearly the failure of the health care system, and those who work in it, to provide the mother with a successful outcome to her pregnancy. The fear of failure may in turn engender a cycle of avoidance, which may serve to continue the neglect of this mother.

While, as mentioned already, this vicious cycle has been interrupted to the extent that the care of the mother has been changed, it is necessary to question whether the care of staff has kept pace. The emotional costs of providing care are now being recognised increasingly. Phillips (1996) describes how, in a nursing context, the devaluation of the emotional component of care is associated with increasing use of the medical model. This devaluation may contribute to the increasing recognition of the phenomenon which is sometimes known as 'burnout'. The remedy has been identified in a midwifery setting to comprise support in the form of development of 'team spirit' (Foster 1996). The education of staff for their counselling role is a further solution, which is enhanced by the availability of a counsellor for the counsellors themselves. The role of the midwife manager in creating a suitably supportive environment for staff working in stressful situations should not be underestimated. The midwife may also be able to locate support in other personnel alongside whom she works, such as the hospital minister or chaplain. Additionally, the National Association for Staff Support (address at end of chapter) is an example of a potentially helpful outside body.

The extent of the involvement of staff in the mother's grief raises some difficult questions. First is the helpfulness or otherwise of the midwife sharing the tears of the bereaved mother. While some midwives may be prepared to cry alongside the mother, others feel that such behaviour is 'unprofessional' and would not be comfortable shedding even a few tears. The midwives in my research told me that, on the whole, crying was not a problem, but that any loss of control which impeded their ability to provide care needed to be avoided at all costs (Mander 1994). A further difficult decision relates to whether the staff should attend the funeral for the baby. Some of the midwives with whom I spoke had found this helpful and they had not been uncomfortable being present. It is easy to imagine circumstances, however, in which this might not apply.

Other aspects of care

Because of the possibility of their impeding the initiation of grieving, otherwise insignificant aspects of care assume greater importance.

Formalities

Her record-keeping is at all times a fundamental part of the midwife's role, but in the event of loss it becomes even more significant. This is because of the importance of communication in ensuring consistent care which will facilitate the mother's grieving. While far from ideal, it may be difficult to avoid a number of staff being involved in this mother's care. Thus, it is crucial that each midwife should be able to learn from her records what decisions and actions have been taken. A checklist may be helpful to ensure good continuity but we are warned that such devices may serve as an impediment to individualised care at the time of this most individual of experiences (Leon 1992).

The statutory documentation relating to a stillborn baby, who is born after 24 weeks of pregnancy and shows no sign of life after complete expulsion, and to a baby who dies neonatally, having been born alive, are specific to the countries of the UK (McDonald 1996). Additionally, other documents have been devised to meet the needs of those whose baby is lost before 24 weeks or in other circumstances; these include the book of remembrance, which remains in the maternity unit.

Long-term care

As mentioned already, ongoing support for the grieving mother may be provided by a number of different sources. This support may be unrelated to when she decides to transfer home from the maternity unit. Although midwives tend to assume that the mother grieves more healthily in her own surroundings, and early transfer home following perinatal loss is widespread, the research evidence is ambiguous (Mander 1996). The midwife continues to provide care and support for the woman until 10 days after the birth.

The suppression of lactation may need particular attention in the case of the grieving mother.

The principles of care

The standard of care available to the grieving mother is unaffected by the situation of loss; if anything, a higher standard of care is appropriate for this more vulnerable mother, who is at risk of serious emotional consequences in the event of less than ideal care. In a large and authoritative study, however, the care of bereaved mothers was reported to fall below this standard (Rådestad et al 1996b). Nearly 40% of the mothers experienced sorrow, deep hurt or anger in relation to the behaviour of those providing care.

Because of this mother's unique experience of loss, it is particularly important that her care should be individualised. As argued by Leon (1992), there is a tendency to apply interventions following perinatal death in a mechanistic way, without considering the needs of the individual mother and without true empathy. This tendency, he maintains, must be avoided at all costs.

Underpinning our care of this mother is the need to facilitate her healthy grieving. We aim to achieve this in a number of ways, such as by creating memories, by recognising the reality of the baby, by helping her to make sense of the loss, by helping her to retain a sense of control and by assisting her in finding support.

CONCLUSION

I have shown in this chapter that the midwife's care of the mother grieving a loss in childbearing requires research-based knowledge. Although undertaking such research is not easy for any who are involved, it is only by obtaining and using such knowledge that we are able to give this mother care which is of the highest standard. In this way the midwife facilitates healthy grieving in the mother, having avoided any impediments which may interfere with or complicate her grief and prevent its resolution.

In this most human of situations we must remember that 'being nice' is not enough; we need to ensure that our care is based on strong evidence if the woman is eventually to come to terms with her loss.

READER ACTIVITIES

Questions for contemplation or debate:

1. What are the benefits of telling the parents if their baby has a condition which may cause disability, or if their baby has died in utero? Under what circumstances should such 'bad news' be broken?

2. What advice should the midwife give to parents who are trying to decide what contact they should have with their baby who has died or who has a condition which may cause disability?

3. How should the midwife behave when she is caring for a couple whose baby has died or whose baby is lost? What should she say? What should she not say?

4. How may a midwife care for a woman of a different cultural background from her own, who has lost her baby?

5. Where is the best place to care for a woman who does not have her baby with her?

USEFUL ADDRESS

National Association for Staff Support (NASS)
9 Caradon Close
Woking
Surrey
GU21 3DU

REFERENCES

Bansen S, Stevens H 1992 Women's experience of miscarriage in early pregnancy. Journal of Nurse Midwifery 37(2): 84–90

Bourne S 1968 The psychological effects of stillbirth on women and their doctors. Journal of the Royal College of General Practitioners 16: 103–112

Cecil R 1996 The anthropology of pregnancy loss: comparative studies in miscarriage, stillbirth and neonatal death. Berg, Oxford

Cowles K 1996 Cultural perspectives of grief: an expanded concept analysis. Journal of Advanced Nursing 23(2): 287–294

Crawshaw M 1995 Offering woman-centred counselling in reproductive medicine. In: Jennings S (ed) Infertility counselling. Blackwell Science, Oxford

Crowther M 1995 Communication following a stillbirth or neonatal death: room for improvement. British Journal of Obstetrics and Gynaecology 102(12): 952–956

Dyregrov A 1991 Grief in children: a handbook for adults. Kingsley, London

Engel G C 1961 Is grief a disease? A challenge for medical research. Psychosomatic Medicine 23: 18–22

Forrest G, Standish E, Baum J 1982 Support after perinatal death: a study of support and counselling after perinatal bereavement. British Medical Journal 285: 1475–1479

Foster A 1996 Perinatal bereavement: support for families and midwives. Midwives 109(1303): 218–219

Gohlish M 1985 Stillbirth. Midwife Health Visitor and Community Nurse 21(1): 16

Hey V 1996 A feminist exploration. In: Hey V, Itzin C, Saunders L, Speakman A (eds) Hidden loss: miscarriage and ectopic pregnancy, 2nd edn. The Women's Press, London

Iles S 1989 The loss of early pregnancy. In Oates M R (ed) Psychological aspects of obstetrics and gynaecology. Baillière Tindall, London, ch 5

Kellner K, Lake M 1986 Grief counselling. In: Knuppel R A, Drukker J E (eds) High risk pregnancy. W B Saunders, Philadelphia

Kennell J, Slyter H, Klaus M 1970 The mourning response of parents to the death of newborn infant. New England Journal of Medicine 283(7): 344–349

Kissane D, Bloch S 1994 Family grief. British Journal of Psychiatry 164: 728–740

Kowalski K 1987 Perinatal loss and bereavement. In: Sonstegard L, Kowalski K, Jennings B (eds) Women's health: crisis and illness in childbearing. Grune & Stratton, Orlando

Kübler-Ross E 1970 On death and dying. Tavistock Publications, London

Leon I G 1992 Choreographing loss on the obstetric unit. American Journal of Orthopsychiatry 62: 7–8

Lewis E 1979 Mourning by the family after a stillbirth or neonatal death. Archives of Disease in Childhood 54: 303–306

Lewis E, Bourne S 1989 Perinatal death. In: Oates M (ed) Psychological aspects of obstetrics and gynaecology. Baillière Tindall, London

Lilford R, Stratton P, Godsil S, Prasad A 1994 A randomised trial of routine versus selective counselling in perinatal bereavement from congenital disease. British Journal of Obstetrics and Gynaecology 101(4): 291–296

Littlewood J 1992 Aspects of grief: bereavement in adult life. Tavistock/Routledge, London

Lovell H, Bokoula C, Misra S, Speight N 1986 Mothers' reactions to perinatal death. Nursing Times 82(46): 40–42

McCaffery M 1979 Nursing management of the patient with pain. Lippincott, Philadelphia

McDonald M 1996 Loss in pregnancy: guidelines for midwives. Baillière Tindall, London

Mander R 1994 Loss and bereavement in childbearing. Blackwell Scientific, Oxford

Mander R 1995 The care of the mother grieving a baby relinquished for adoption. Avebury, Aldershot

Mander R 1996 The grieving mother: care in the community? Modern Midwife 6(8): 10–13

Marris P 1986 Loss and change. Routledge Kegan Paul, London

Ney P, Tak F, Wickett A, Beaman-Dodd C 1994 The effects of pregnancy loss on women's health. Social Science and Medicine 38(9): 1193–1200

Oakley A, McPherson A, Roberts H 1990 Miscarriage. Penguin, London

O'Hare T, Creed F 1995 Life events and miscarriage. British Journal of Psychiatry 167(6): 799–805

Peppers L, Knapp R 1980 Maternal reactions to involuntary fetal/infant death. Psychiatry 43: 55–59

Phillips S 1996 Labouring the emotions: expanding the remit of nursing work? Journal of Advanced Nursing 24(1): 139–143

Rådestad I, Steineck G, Nordin C, Sjogren B 1996a Psychological complications after stillbirth. British Medical Journal 312(7045): 1505–1508

Rådestad I, Nordin C, Steineck G, Sjogren B 1996b Stillbirth is no longer managed as a non-event: a nationwide study in Sweden. Birth 23(4): 209–216

Rajan L 1994 Social isolation and support in pregnancy loss. Health Visitor 67(3): 97–101

Raphael-Leff J 1991 Psychological processes of childbearing. Chapman & Hall, London

Sorosky A D, Baran A, Pannor R 1984 The adoption triangle. Anchor, New York

Speakman M A 1996 Letting go and holding on. In: Hey V, Itzin C, Saunders L, Speakman M A (eds) Hidden loss: miscarriage and ectopic pregnancy, 2nd edn. The Women's Press, London

Stroebe W, Stroebe M S 1987 Bereavement and health: the psychological and physical consequences of partner loss. Cambridge University Press, Cambridge

FURTHER READING

Jones A 1996 Psychotherapy following childbirth. British Journal of Midwifery 4(5): 239–243

Schott J, Henley A 1996 Childbearing losses. British Journal of Midwifery 4(10): 522–526

The newborn baby

SECTION CONTENTS

The baby at birth

Maureen M. Michie

The newborn baby's survival is dependent on his ability to adapt to his extrauterine environment. This involves adaptations in cardiopulmonary circulation and other physiological adjustments to replace placental function and maintain homeostasis. Continued dependence on the mother for nutrition and safety necessitates the establishment of an emotional relationship which is initiated at the time of birth.

The chapter aims to:

- describe the physiological changes taking place at birth

- discuss the care of the baby during and immediately after birth

- consider the early responses of both parents and baby, identifying steps that can be taken to promote good parent–baby relationships

- identify factors to be considered when the baby fails to establish respirations at birth and describe the principles of neonatal resuscitation.

The transition from intrauterine to extrauterine existence is a dramatic one and demands considerable and effective physiological alterations by the baby in order to ensure survival. The fetus leaves an environment which has been completely life sustaining where his needs for oxygenation, nutrition, excretion and thermoregulation have been met with minimal effort on his part. The aquatic amniotic sac has permitted movement but freedom to extend his limbs has been limited towards the end of pregnancy as his size has increased in relation to the capacity of the uterus. Though the fetus is sensitive to sound, the uterine environment has dulled the impact of the noises of the outside world where daylight also contrasts sharply with the dim interior of the uterus.

Subjected to intermittent diminution of his

oxygen supply during uterine contractions, compression followed by decompression of his head and chest, and extension of his limbs, hips and spine during delivery, the baby emerges from his mother to encounter light, noises, cool air, gravity and tactile stimuli for the first time. Simultaneously he has to make major adjustments in his respiratory and circulatory systems as well as control his body temperature. These initial adaptations are crucial to his subsequent well-being and should be facilitated by the midwife at the time of birth.

Respiratory and cardiovascular changes are interdependent and concurrent.

ADAPTATION TO EXTRAUTERINE LIFE

Onset of respiration

The initiation and establishment of respiration is of paramount importance to the survival of the neonate. Most infants achieve sustained regular respiration within 60 seconds of complete expulsion from the mother, many taking their first breath as soon as the head is delivered.

Effective establishment of respirations tests the integrity of the respiratory, cardiovascular and central nervous systems of the neonate and is best achieved when these systems are both structurally and functionally normal. A patent airway is necessary to enable ventilation of the lungs. The episodic shallow fetal breathing movements must be replaced by regular rhythmic respirations following lung expansion, and an increased pulmonary blood flow is required to facilitate gaseous exchange in the alveoli and the removal of lung fluid.

At term approximately 20 ml/kg of lung fluid is present within the respiratory tract (Blackburn & Loper 1992). Some fluid absorption is initiated in the lungs prior to the onset of labour and is believed to be essential to facilitate initiation of normal ventilation at birth (Lowe & Reiss 1996). Fluid absorption is assisted by alteration in the pressure gradient between the alveoli, interstitial tissue, and capillaries (Perry 1995). During delivery compression of the chest wall assists in the expulsion of some of the remaining fluid; however, the majority is absorbed by the pulmonary circula-

tion and lymphatic system after birth. Infants delivered by caesarean section are denied the benefits of chest compression and therefore expression of lung fluid. Residual lung fluid may contribute to transient tachypnoea of the newborn (Box 34.1).

Box 34.1 Transient tachypnoea of the newborn

This condition is characterised by rapid respirations of up to 120 per minute. The baby may be cyanosed but maintains normal blood gases apart from pO_2. Little or no recession of the rib cage is evident and there is minimal, if any, grunt on expiration. The respiratory rate may remain elevated for up to 5 days. Treatment consists of oxygen therapy to maintain adequate oxygenation and tube feeding to prevent aspiration of feeds. It is essential that other causes of respiratory distress are excluded, especially infective causes (which mimic this condition) and respiratory distress syndrome (see also Ch. 39).

The presence of surfactant in the lungs reduces surface tension. This assists expansion and prevents adherence of the walls of the alveoli following expiration (see Ch. 39).

The first breath which the infant takes is stimulated by the effect of cool air on his face. Initial heat loss by evaporation from the skin at birth is thought to provide some continuing stimulus to respiratory efforts.

Compression of the chest wall during delivery followed by elastic recoil of the thorax as the body is delivered stimulates stretch receptors in the lungs. Considerable negative intrathoracic pressure of up to 9.8 kPa (100 cm water) is exerted as the first breath is taken. The effectiveness of the first breath is enhanced by a pulmonary reflex which stimulates additional inspiratory effort prior to exhalation (Blackburn & Loper 1992). Pressures exerted to effect inhalation diminish with each breath taken until only 5 cm water pressure is required to inflate the lungs. This is as a result of surfactant lowering surface tension thus permitting residual air to remain in the alveoli between breaths.

Compression and decompression of the baby's head during delivery are thought to stimulate the respiratory centre in the brain which in turn maintains the stimulus to respiratory effort. The role of chemoreceptors in stimulating the onset of respiration is not clear though it is suggested that the alteration in the blood gas state of the fetus during labour is influential. Carotid baroreceptors, sensitive to changes in pressure, may also contribute to respiratory stimulus by their response to the circulatory changes which take place when the placental circulation ceases.

Tactile stimulus is considered to be of minimal importance. However, pain caused by extension of the hitherto flexed limbs, joints and spine is thought to contribute to the initial responses of the infant to extrauterine life. The sensations of cold, gravity, noise, light and odours have also been suggested as significant, though less critical, sensory stimuli.

Sustained regular respirations are established normally within 60 seconds of delivery and are accompanied by simultaneous changes occurring in the cardiovascular system.

Circulatory changes

Separated from his life-support system, the placenta, the baby must make major adjustments within his circulatory system in order to divert deoxygenated blood to the lungs for reoxygenation. This involves several mechanisms which are influenced by the clamping of the umbilical cord and also by the lowered resistance in the pulmonary vascular bed.

During fetal life (see Ch. 52) only approximately 10% of the cardiac output is circulated to the lungs through the pulmonary artery. With the expansion of the lungs and lowered pulmonary vascular resistance, virtually all of the cardiac output is sent to the lungs. Oxygenated blood returning to the heart from the lungs increases the pressure within the left atrium. At almost the same time, pressure in the right atrium is lowered because blood ceases to flow through the cord. As a result, a functional closure of the foramen ovale is achieved. During the first days of life this closure is reversible and reopening may occur if pulmonary vascular resistance is high, for example when crying, resulting in transient cyanotic episodes in the baby (Perry 1995). The septa usually fuse within the first year of life forming the interatrial septum, though in some individuals perfect anatomical closure may never be achieved.

The ductus arteriosus, which is nearly as wide in lumen as the aorta, provides a diversionary route to bypass the lungs of the fetus. Contraction of its muscular walls occurs almost immediately after birth. This is thought to occur because of sensitivity of the muscle of the ductus arteriosus to increased oxygen tension and reduction in circulating prostaglandin (Heyman 1989). As a result of altered pressure gradients between the aorta and pulmonary artery, a temporary reverse left-to-right shunt through the ductus may persist for a few hours though there is usually functional closure of the ductus within 8–10 hours of birth. Intermittent patency has been demonstrated in most healthy infants in the first 3 days of life (Lim et al 1992). Anatomical closure with the formation of the ligamentum arteriosum takes several months. Persistence or reopening of the ductus, with associated cyanosis or cyanotic attacks, may occur if pulmonary vascular resistance is high or hypoxia is present. This is a common problem in preterm infants with respiratory distress syndrome (see Ch. 39). Persistence of the foramen ovale and/or ductus arteriosus may be life-saving in some forms of congenital heart abnormality (see Ch. 41).

The remaining temporary structures of the fetal circulation – the umbilical vein, ductus venosus and hypogastric arteries – close functionally within a few minutes after birth and clamping of the cord. Anatomical closure by fibrous tissue occurs within 2–3 months, resulting in the formation of the ligamentum teres, ligamentum venosum and the obliterated hypogastric arteries. (The proximal portions of the hypogastric arteries persist as the superior vesical arteries.)

The interdependent cardiopulmonary adaptations which take place at birth are essential to survival. Failure to establish respirations and satisfactory tissue oxygenation presents a life-threatening situation and is exacerbated by hypothermia.

Thermal adaptation

Vacating a thermoconstant environment of 37.7°C the baby enters a much cooler atmosphere at delivery. A delivery room temperature of 21°C contrasts sharply with intrauterine temperature and causes rapid cooling of the infant as amniotic fluid evaporates from his skin. Each millilitre which

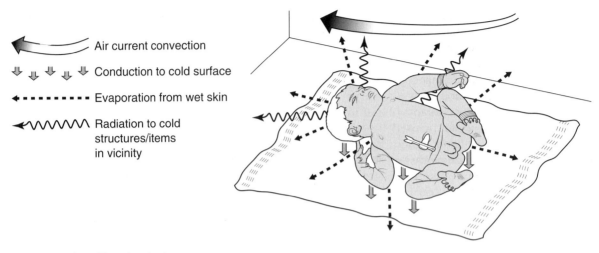

Air current convection

Conduction to cold surface

Evaporation from wet skin

Radiation to cold structures/items in vicinity

Fig. 34.1 Modes of heat loss in the neonate.

evaporates removes 560 calories of heat (Rutter 1992). The infant's large *surface area:body mass* ratio potentiates heat loss, especially from his head which comprises 25% of his size. His subcutaneous fat layer is thin and provides poor insulation, allowing rapid transfer of core heat to the skin and to the environment and also cooling of his blood. In addition to heat loss by *evaporation*, further heat will be lost by *conduction* when the baby is in contact with cold surfaces, by *radiation* to cold objects in the environment, and by *convection* caused by currents of cool air passing over the surface of his body (Fig. 34.1) (Brueggemeyer 1993, Greer 1988, Rutter 1992, Thomas 1994).

The heat-regulating centre in the baby's brain has the capacity to promote heat production in response to stimuli received from thermoreceptors. However, this is dependent on increased metabolic activity, compromising the baby's ability to control his body temperature, especially in adverse environmental conditions. The baby has a limited ability to shiver and is unable voluntarily to increase his muscle activity in order to generate heat. This means that he must depend on his ability to produce heat by metabolism which in turn requires an increase in oxygen consumption.

The normal neonate, in common with some other young mammals, is endowed with brown adipose tissue which assists in the rapid mobilisation of heat resources, namely free fatty acids and glycerol, in times of cold stress. This mechanism is called non-shivering thermogenesis (Dawkins & Hull 1964). Brown adipose tissue is found in the mediastinum, around the nape of the neck, between the scapulae, along the spinal column and suprarenally (Fig. 34.2). These deposits of brown fat have rich vascular and nerve supplies and are capable of increasing heat by up to 100%. Reserves of brown fat, however, are depleted rapidly with cold stress. Continued cold stress results in increased oxygen consumption as the infant strives

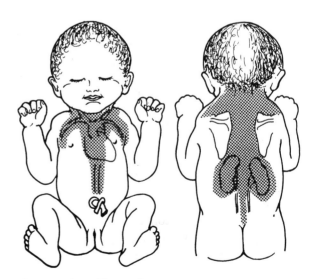

Fig. 34.2 Sites of brown fat.

to maintain sufficient heat for survival. Brown fat uses up to three times that of other tissue (Wong 1995). This has the undesired effect of diverting oxygen and glucose from vital centres, such as the brain and cardiac muscle. Vasoconstriction occurs also, thus reducing pulmonary perfusion, and respiratory acidosis develops as the pH and pO_2 of the blood decrease and the pCO_2 increases. This, together with the reduction in pulmonary perfusion, may result in the reopening or maintenance of the right-to-left shunt across the ductus arteriosus. Anaerobic glycolysis (i.e. the metabolism of glucose in the absence of oxygen) resulting in the production of acids compounds the situation by adding a metabolic acidosis. Protraction of cold stress, therefore, should be avoided.

The peripheral vasoconstrictor mechanisms of the baby are unable to prevent the fall in core body temperature which occurs during the first few hours after birth. It is important, therefore, for the midwife to ensure that she employs measures to minimise heat loss at delivery (Dahm & James 1972, Rutter 1992).

IMMEDIATE CARE OF THE BABY AT BIRTH

The midwife's knowledge of the baby's transitional requirements and capabilities enables her to make appropriate preparations for his reception into the world. Heat loss by convection, radiation and evaporation are very high at birth (Rutter 1992). Whether the baby is born at home or in hospital, it is important that the midwife endeavours to provide a delivery room temperature in the range 21–25°C. It is accepted that, in some remote parts of the world, and in emergency situations, this may not be possible. However, within controlled circumstances, provision of an optimal thermal environment is a paramount consideration in facilitating a successful transition to extrauterine life. Switching off fans prior to delivery helps to minimise heat loss by convection; delivery rooms without external windows help to reduce heat loss by radiation which, unlike other methods of heat loss, is unaffected by ambient temperature. Reduction of radiant heat loss to windows is assisted

by closing curtains (Karlsson 1996). Prevention of heat loss after delivery remains important throughout, and after, the initiation and establishment of respirations at birth.

Initial care

As the baby's head is born, excess mucus may be wiped gently from his mouth. Care must be taken to avoid touching the nares as such action may stimulate reflex inhalation of debris in the trachea. Gentle handling during the delivery is essential, the baby being drawn up towards and, if wished by the parents, onto the mother's abdomen. (Maternal posture during delivery may necessitate modification of this manoeuvre.) The time of birth and sex of the baby are noted and recorded once the baby has been completely expelled from his mother.

Clearing the airway
Although fetal pulmonary fluid is present in the mouth, most babies will achieve a clear airway unaided. Mechanical clearing of the baby's airway can interfere with normal physiology and can be considered to constitute an assault on the baby. If necessary, the airway can be cleared with the aid of a mucus extractor or soft suction catheter attached to low pressure (10 cm water) mechanical suction. It is important to aspirate the oropharynx prior to the nasopharynx so that, when the baby gasps as his nasal passages are aspirated, mucus or other material is not drawn down into the respiratory tract. Deep suction is neither necessary nor desirable as trauma or laryngospasm and bradycardia may result.

Cutting the cord
Separation of the infant from the placenta is achieved by dividing the umbilical cord between two clamps which should be applied approximately 8–10 cm from the umbilicus. Application of a gauze swab over the cord while cutting it with scissors will prevent blood spraying the delivery field. *The cord should not be cut until it has been clamped securely. Failure to comply with this procedure will result in exsanguination of the baby.*

The timing of clamping of the cord is not crucial

unless asphyxia, prematurity or Rhesus incompatibility is present (see Ch. 39 and Ch. 42). Some centres advocate delay until respirations are established and cord pulsation has ceased, thus ensuring that the infant receives a placental transfusion of some 70 ml of blood. This view is countered by those who maintain that the placental transfusion so acquired may predispose to neonatal jaundice (see Ch. 42). Prior to clamping the cord, if the infant is held above the level of the uterus, blood will gravitate to the placenta and, if the infant is held below the level of the uterus, an increased placental transfusion will result. The ensuing anaemia in the former instance and polycythaemia with increased viscosity of the blood, increased blood volume and systolic blood pressure in the latter, can compromise the cardiopulmonary status of the infant.

It is the practice in many units to apply name bands to the infant *before* the cord is cut.

Identification

Within the baby's own home, unless he is a twin, identification does not present a problem. However, when babies are born in hospital, it is essential that they are readily identifiable from one another. Various methods of indicating identity can be employed, for example name bands or china bead necklets. In the UK name bands are applied, usually one on the infant's wrist and one on the ankle, each of which should indicate *legibly* in indelible pen the family name, sex of the infant and date and time of birth. In some centres, the name bands are number coded with the infant's case records, in others the number coding corresponds with that of the mother. The amount of informa-

tion written on the name bands may vary slightly according to local policy. The mother and/or father should verify that the information on the bands is correct prior to their being applied to the baby. The midwife should ensure that the name bands are fastened securely and are neither too tight impeding circulation or likely to excoriate the skin, nor too loose risking loss of the means of identification which should remain on the baby until his discharge from hospital.

Assessment of the baby's condition

Provided the baby is seen to be making some respiratory effort, the midwife can proceed to dry the infant gently (to minimise evaporative heat loss) while attending also to the foregoing procedures. At 1 minute after the baby's birth, she will make an assessment of his general condition and will repeat this assessment at 5 minutes. This involves consideration of five signs and the degree to which they are present or absent. The factors assessed are heart rate, respiratory effort, muscle tone, reflex response to stimulus, and colour. A score of 0, 1 or 2 is awarded to each of the signs in accordance with the guidelines in Table 34.1. This scoring system, the Apgar score (Apgar 1953) is recognised and used universally. Of the five signs the heart rate and respiratory effort are the most important. Colour is least important and some centres have discontinued recording this part of the score, making the maximum score 8 rather than 10. Documentation of use of this modified system requires to be indicated in the baby's birth record, for example 'Apgar minus colour score = 7'. The colour of babies with pigmented

Table 34.1 The Apgar score. The score is assessed at 1 minute and 5 minutes after birth. Medical aid should be sought if the score is less than 7. 'Apgar minus colour' score omits the fifth sign. Medical aid should be sought if the score is less than 6

Sign	Score		
	0	1	2
Heart rate	Absent	Less than 100 bpm	More than 100 bpm
Respiratory effort	Absent	Slow, irregular	Good or crying
Muscle tone	Limp	Some flexion of limbs	Active
Reflex response to stimulus	None	Minimal grimace	Cough or sneeze
Colour	Blue, pale	Body pink, extremities blue	Completely pink

skin is best assessed by inspecting the colour of the mucous membranes. A normal infant in good condition at birth will achieve an Apgar score of 7–10. Continued vigilance with regard to thermal adaptation is essential.

Prevention of heat loss

The baby's temperature can drop by as much as 3–4.5°C within the first minute (Dahm & James 1972, Greer 1988, Sinclair 1992, Thomas 1994). Drying the baby at delivery helps to minimise heat loss by evaporation. It is important to ensure that the wet towel is removed prior to wrapping the baby in dry prewarmed towels. Skin-to-skin contact with the mother assists the baby to conserve heat although transfer of heat from the mother to the baby is not of major significance and continued considerable heat loss by convection, conduction, and radiation persists from exposed areas of the baby's skin (Karlsson 1996). This can be minimised by covering the baby with an insulating blanket. Loose clothing, swaddling and cuddling of the baby all help to maintain body heat. Covering of the baby's head is of particular importance. Insulated (multilayered) fabric hats have been shown to be more efficient than stockinette caps in preventing heat loss (Greer 1988). In some hospitals, the provision of overhead radiant heaters within labour rooms has helped to avoid hypothermia, the heater being placed above the baby while he is in his cot or in his mother's arms covered with a blanket. Care must be taken to avoid overheating when using radiant heaters. Electric heating pads within babies' cots must be used with care to avoid burning and hot water bottles used to prewarm cots must be removed before the baby is placed in the cot.

After a period of rest, in his cot or in his mother's arms, preliminary care of the baby is continued.

Continued early care

Prior to leaving the mother's home, or transferring the baby to the ward with his mother, the midwife undertakes a detailed examination of the baby to detect any major abnormalities. She replaces the initial cord clamp with another method of securing haemostasis by applying a disposable plastic clamp (or rubber band or three cord ligatures) approximately 2–3 cm from the umbilicus and cutting off the redundant cord. Depending on local policy, vitamin K 1 mg I.M. may be given as prophylaxis against bleeding disorders (see Ch. 40). In some centres this is given orally *provided* the preparation is licensed in that country (see Tyler 1996). The baby's temperature is recorded and he is then dressed and wrapped warmly (without constraining movement).

Instillation of eyedrops as prophylaxis against gonococcal infection is not practised in the UK. Drops or antibiotic ointment may be instilled in other parts of the world (Wong 1995). It is suggested that, to be effective, such treatments should be administered within 1 hour of birth (Tyson 1992). Localised reactions to silver nitrate drops have been shown to impair eye-to-eye contact with the mother and it has been noted that this may interfere with early mother–baby relationships (de Château 1987).

The air-conditioning systems in some modern delivery suites can compromise the infant's ability to maintain his body temperature without effort. Early transfer of the baby to a postnatal ward or nursery has been advocated as a means of minimising this problem. This raises concern regarding separation from the mother. It is preferable that transfer to the nursery or ward should be at the same time as the mother with the baby in a warmed cot or cuddled in the mother's arms to prevent heat loss while passing through corridors. The first bath and other non-urgent procedures may be deferred in order to minimise thermal stress. (Further care is discussed in Ch. 35.)

The baby should remain with his mother during the first few hours of life whenever possible, that is, providing both mother and baby are in good condition, as this is the time when parent–infant interactions are initiated and the reality of parenthood begins.

EARLY PARENT–INFANT RELATIONSHIPS

The safe delivery of a healthy baby engenders considerable emotion in most parents and indeed in attendants at the birth. The efforts of the preceding hours are temporarily forgotten as the mother sees her baby for the first time. Characteristically her first query relates to the sex of the infant speedily followed by an anxious enquiry about the infant's state of health – 'Is he all right?'. Reassured on these points, a mother progresses to an examination of her baby, which follows a fairly predictable pattern unless the condition of either the mother or the baby has been affected adversely by the process of labour or by narcotic drugs. Fathers too are involved in this early exploration of the newborn infant. The response of both parents is coloured not only by their prenatal understanding and previous experiences with babies but also by the appearance, behaviour and responses of their baby who takes an active part in the proceedings (Salariya 1990, Williams 1995, White & Woollet 1987). Cultural background may also play a part in parental behaviours at this time (Callister 1995).

The mother.   The first hour after birth is a time of particular sensitivity for the mother. Close contact with her baby during this time facilitates the attachment process.

Regardless of age, parity or marital status, mothers are likely to display a similar behavioural pattern when touching their babies for the first time. This sequence of touching behaviour is enhanced if the baby is naked. The mother begins her examination of her baby by exploring his extremities and head with her fingertips. Thereafter, she caresses her baby's body with her entire hand before gathering her baby in her arms often in the *en face* position where eye-to-eye contact can be established. She talks to her baby in a high pitched voice commenting on his appearance and behaviour to him, her partner and other birth attendants (Klaus et al 1975).

Her emotions at this time may be mixed. She may display great excitement and happiness – laughing, talking or even crying with joy. She may feel too tired to react positively towards her baby or may display disappointment or even anger towards her baby, showing disinclination to touch him. Factors which may predispose to this latter reaction include prolonged labour, instrumental

delivery, baby of the 'wrong' sex or congenital abnormality. Lack of support from partner or parents may influence the behaviour of an unmarried mother and for some mothers high parity may dampen their response. Childhood deprivation can inhibit some women from reacting in the anticipated manner.

For some mothers, the sight of an unwashed, wet and sometimes bloody infant is profoundly distasteful and they are not appreciative of skin-to-skin contact with a baby in this condition. A good midwife will ascertain the mother's attitude during pregnancy or early labour. This will allow her to modify her delivery technique and immediate care of the baby to meet the mother's wishes and so assist the mother to feel comfortable at her first meeting with her baby.

Some, though not all, mothers are keen to encourage their babies to suckle at birth. This practice should be facilitated and encouraged by the midwife as it is known to promote good mother–baby relationships and also good lactation (Salariya et al 1979). (See also Ch. 36.)

The father.   Many fathers are surprised at their profound emotional response to the birth of their babies. Sometimes a man's reactions are stronger than those of his wife or partner who may be rather tired initially. The father feels a sense of deep satisfaction and self-esteem and is elated and keen to touch and hold his baby and his partner and share his excitement (Bedford & Johnson 1988, Wildman 1995).

Intimacy shared between the father and mother at this time is extended to include their new baby within an exclusive family group, often oblivious to their surroundings.

The baby.   The baby at birth is alert and wakeful, reactive to his surroundings. His rounded, soft features provide an appealing image to which other human beings react protectively. The reaction of his parents is increased by their emotional ties with their baby.

Having accomplished his immediate physiological adaptations of respiration and circulation, the baby displays interest in sound, light and nutrition, responding to his mother's voice by moving his limbs in synchrony. His response to touch is illustrated in his grasp reflex and in his suckling of the breast if offered – or his own fist. He appears to focus on his mother's face at a distance of 20 cm and responds to movement of bright shiny objects, such as his mother's eyes, by tracking them visually. These responsive behaviours evoke reinforcing responses from his parents, thus promoting the interactions essential to his survival which is dependent on good parenting. A slightly darkened delivery room encourages the baby to open his eyes widely and look around him, whereas bright lights cause him to frown. The midwife's understanding of these responses allows her to create optimum conditions for interaction to occur.

Promotion of parent–baby interaction

The term 'bonding' has been used to describe the establishment of parent–baby relationships in the early neonatal period. The implication of the desirability to feel instant love for one's child can lead to feelings of guilt in some parents who do not identify a strong emotional tie with their baby at birth. It is important to recognise that, as individuals, parents develop a loving relationship with their child at their own pace, some taking longer than others – days, weeks or months. Parents should feel able to express their disappointments as well as their joys without fear of being thought a 'bad' parent (Herbert & Sluckin 1985, Parkinson & Harvey 1987, Sluckin et al 1984).

A good rapport between the parents and the midwife should enable the development of their love for their baby to progress happily and at its own speed. However, the midwife must be alert to report and document marked negative reactions from either or both parents as this may be an early sign of future parenting difficulties. Adverse behaviours of note include hostile verbal or non-verbal attitude, lack of supportive interaction between the parents, disinclination to touch or hold the baby, disparaging remarks about the baby or marked disappointment about the sex of the baby.

Involvement of the father in the delivery of the baby's body, clamping of the cord, and early bathing have been introduced in some centres to help to promote father–baby relationships. The midwife can do much to promote the beginnings of loving relationships by encouraging both parents to handle and examine their baby, by her positive comments about the baby and by examining the baby beside the parents.

Privacy to talk, touch and be alone together with their baby is a privilege which most parents should be able to enjoy whether their baby is born at home or in hospital. The midwife should be sensitive to this often unexpressed need and leave the family alone together for some time before progressing with further care of the baby.

The opportunity for this initial intimate family moment is dependent on the baby's condition being satisfactory. A baby whose Apgar score is below 7 requires some form of resuscitation which may necessitate his speedy removal to a special resuscitation area. It is essential that parents receive a reassuring explanation and adequate information about the need for this separation which can be totally unexpected and therefore very frightening.

FAILURE TO ESTABLISH RESPIRATIONS AT BIRTH

Although the majority of infants gasp and establish respirations within 60 seconds of birth, some do not. Failure to initiate and sustain respiration at birth necessitates prompt and effective intervention. The midwife must therefore be aware of the predisposing factors and causes of respiratory depression and be proficient in the resuscitative measures which can be employed in the absence of medical aid. Mild hypoxia is thought to be one of the factors involved in initiating respiration. Prolonged hypoxia predisposes to asphyxia (hypoxia, hypercarbia and acidaemia) (Roberton 1992).

Intrauterine hypoxia

Oxygenation of the fetus is dependent on oxygenation of the mother, adequate perfusion of the placental site, placental function, fetoplacental circulation and adequate fetal haemoglobin. Absence or impairment of any of these factors will result in a reduction of oxygen supply to the fetus (Fig. 34.3).

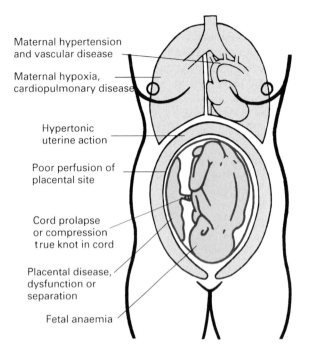

Maternal hypertension
and vascular disease

Maternal hypoxia,
cardiopulmonary disease

Hypertonic
uterine action

Poor perfusion of
placental site

Cord prolapse
or compression
true knot in cord

Placental disease,
dysfunction or
separation

Fetal anaemia

Fig. 34.3 Factors predisposing to intrauterine hypoxia.

Oxygenation of the mother may be impaired as a result of cardiac or respiratory disease, an eclamptic fit, or during induction of general anaesthesia if difficulties arise during intubation. Perfusion of the placental site is dependent on satisfactory blood supply. This may be reduced in the presence of maternal hypertension or if hypotension occurs in response to haemorrhage, shock or aortocaval occlusion. Hypertonic uterine action, when uterine resting tonus is elevated, will impede the blood supply to the placental site. This is sometimes due to hyperstimulation of the uterus by Syntocinon and necessitates discontinuation of the oxytocic agent to allow the uterus to relax, thus restoring circulation to the placental bed. The umbilical cord transports oxygenated blood to the fetus. If prolapsed outside the uterus (causing vasoconstriction) or if compressed, fetal oxygenation will be reduced. The transport of oxygen within the fetus necessitates the availability of adequate haemoglobin which may be reduced if Rhesus incompatibility is present. Abnormal fetal cardiac function may also diminish the supply of oxygen to the fetal brain.

The fetus responds to hypoxia by accelerating his heart rate in an effort to maintain supplies of oxygen to the brain. If hypoxia persists, glucose depletion will stimulate anaerobic glycolysis resulting in a metabolic acidosis. Cerebral vessels will dilate and some brain swelling may occur. Peripheral circulation will be reduced. As the fetus becomes acidotic and cardiac glycogen reserves are depleted, bradycardia develops, the anal sphincter relaxes and the fetus may pass meconium into the liquor. Gasping breathing movements triggered by hypoxia may result in the aspiration of meconium-stained liquor into the lungs, which presents an additional problem after delivery.

Auscultation of the fetal heart, use of cardiotocography and observation of meconium staining of the liquor draining per vaginam alert the midwife to fetal distress (see Ch. 22). Subsequent fetal blood sampling by the doctor may confirm a compromised fetus by revealing acidosis. However, Apgar scores do not always correlate with these findings (Jacobs & Phibbs 1989, Silverman et al 1985).

The length of time during which the fetus or neonate is subjected to hypoxia determines the outcome. It is considered that the human neonate responds to hypoxia in a similar manner to other young mammals (Roberton 1992). This involves an initial response of gasping respirations followed by a period of apnoea lasting 1–1½ minutes – *primary apnoea* – which, if not resolved by intervention techniques, is followed by a further episode of gasping respirations which accelerate while diminishing in depth until, approximately 8 minutes after birth, respirations cease completely – *terminal apnoea*. This suggests that it should be possible to determine the degree of hypoxia by assessment of the infant's condition at birth. The Apgar score provides a guide to the general condition of the infant but does not provide information about his metabolic status. It is therefore not *diagnostic* of asphyxia. This presents a dilemma for the birth attendant who may be uncertain as to whether primary or secondary (terminal) apnoea is present at birth (Table 34.2).

Respiratory depression by fetal hypoxia is an important cause of neonatal respiratory depression. However, it is only one factor to be considered when the baby does not breathe at birth.

Table 34.2 Degrees of respiratory depression

Mildly depressed	Severely depressed
Heart rate not severely depressed (60–80 bpm)	Slow feeble heart rate (less than 40 bpm)
Short delay in onset of respiration	No attempt to breathe
Good muscle tone	Poor muscle tone
Responsive to stimuli	Limp, unresponsive to stimuli
Deeply cyanosed	Pale, grey
Apgar score 5–7	*Apgar score less than 5*
No significant deprivation of oxygen during labour (Primary apnoea)	Oxygen lack has been prolonged before or after delivery, circulatory failure is present, baby is shocked (Secondary apnoea)

Respiratory depression

Obstruction of the baby's airway by mucus, blood, liquor or meconium, is one of the most common reasons for a baby failing to establish respirations. Depression of the respiratory centre may be due to the effects of drugs administered to the mother, for example narcotic drugs, diazepam or chlormethiazole (Heminevrin), or to cerebral damage during labour or traumatic delivery. Immaturity of the infant causes mechanical dysfunction because of underdeveloped lungs, lack of surfactant and a soft pliable thoracic cage. Intranatal pneumonia can inhibit successful establishment of respirations and should be considered, especially if the membranes have been ruptured for some time. Severe anaemia, caused by fetomaternal haemorrhage or Rhesus incompatibility, diminishes the oxygen-carrying capacity of the blood. Respiratory function may be compromised by major congenital abnormalities such as congenital heart defects, abnormalities of the central nervous system or abnormalities within the respiratory tract, for example hypoplastic lungs coexisting with diaphragmatic hernia or renal agenesis. Rarely, a congenital abnormality such as choanal or tracheal atresia may be present. (Choanal atresia should be suspected when an infant is pink when crying but becomes cyanosed at rest.)

Failure to establish respirations compounds hypoxia as previously described. It is necessary therefore to be able and prepared to undertake specific resuscitative measures for any infant who has difficulty establishing respirations at birth.

RESUSCITATION OF THE NEWBORN

Though the need for resuscitation can be anticipated in some situations, there are occasions when a baby is born in poor condition without forewarning. It is essential that resuscitation equipment (see Box 34.2) is always available and in working order and that personnel in attendance

---

Box 34.2 Resuscitation equipment

- Resuscitaire with overhead radiant heater (switched on) and light, piped oxygen, manometer, suction and clock timer. The shelf should provide a firm surface and enable a 15° head tilt to be achieved.
- Two straight-bladed infant laryngoscopes, spare batteries and bulbs
- Neonatal endotracheal tubes (with shoulders) 2.5, 3.0, and 3.5 mm and connectors
- Neonatal airways sizes 0, 00, 000
- Mucus extractors
- Suction catheters sizes 6, 8, 10 FG
- Neonatal bag and mask and face masks of assorted sizes (circular, soft masks)
- Syringes 5 ml and 2 ml and assorted needles
- Drugs
  - naloxone hydrochloride 1 ml ampoules 400 micrograms/ml (adult Narcan)
  - THAM (tris-hydroxymethyl-amino-methane) 7%
  - sodium bicarbonate 8.4%, 7.5% and 4.2%
  - dextrose 10% and 5%
  - vitamin K_1 1 mg ampoules
  - normal saline
- Stethoscope
- Cord clamps
- Warmed dry towels
- Adhesive tape for tube fixation

at the delivery of a baby are familiar with the equipment, resuscitation techniques, and local policies regarding the provision of medical aid.

In some units resuscitation of babies is undertaken in a specific area, whereas in others each delivery room is equipped to deal with this emergency. Whenever problems are anticipated, such as preterm delivery, instrumental or breech delivery, or fetal distress, it is desirable that a paediatrician, paediatric nurse or midwife experienced in resuscitation techniques is present at the delivery. (In some centres an anaesthetist may be the person responsible for neonatal resuscitation.) At home the midwife is the responsible person.

The aims of resuscitation are:

- to establish and maintain a clear airway, ventilation and oxygenation
- to ensure effective circulation
- to correct acidosis
- to prevent hypothermia, hypoglycaemia and haemorrhage.

As soon as the baby is born, the clock timer should be started. The Apgar score is assessed in the normal manner at 1 minute. In the absence of any respiratory effort, resuscitative measures are not delayed, however. The baby's upper airways should be cleared by gentle suction of the oro- and nasopharynx and the presence of an apex beat verified. The baby is dried quickly and transferred to a well-lit resuscitation area where he should be placed on a flat, firm surface at a comfortable working height and under a radiant heat source to prevent hypothermia. The baby's shoulders may be elevated on a small towel to straighten the trachea by slight extension of the head. Hyperextension is not necessary and may cause airway obstruction owing to the short neck of the neonate and large, ill-supported tongue. It is not desirable to hold the baby upside down as this causes a sharp rise in intracranial pressure, hyperextends and stretches the spine and hips which is painful, and risks the infant being dropped.

Stimulation

Rough handling of the infant merely serves to increase shock and is unnecessary. Gentle stimulation by drying the baby and clearing the airway should suffice. Directing a low flow (2–4 litres/min) of oxygen over the baby's face may stimulate a gasp reflex.

Warmth

Hypothermia exacerbates hypoxia as essential oxygen and glucose are diverted from the vital centres in order to create heat for survival. Wet towels should be removed and the baby's body and head should be covered with a prewarmed blanket leaving only the chest exposed. NB: It is hazardous to use a silver swaddler under a radiant heater because it could cause burning.

Clearing the airway

The oro- and nasopharynx are cleared by suction as previously described. Mechanical suction, if used, should not exceed 10 cm water pressure and should be applied in short 10-second periods as the catheter is withdrawn. Side hole catheters minimise the risk of trauma (Young 1995). No force should be exerted while passing the catheter as this could cause trauma to the mucosa predisposing to oedema, bleeding and increased secretions. If meconium is present in the airway, suction under direct vision should be performed by passing a laryngoscope and visualising the larynx (Roberton 1992). Care should be taken to avoid touching the vocal cords as this may induce laryngospasm, apnoea and bradycardia. Thick meconium may require to be aspirated out of the trachea through an endotracheal tube.

Ventilation and oxygenation

If the baby fails to respond to clearing of his airway, assisted ventilation is necessary. This can be achieved in a variety of ways.

Neonatal bag and mask. A close-fitting mask is applied over the baby's nose and mouth taking care not to encroach on his eyes. Oxygen or air is blown through the mask by means of a bag which has a self-limiting pressure valve of 2.9 kPa (30 cm water), for example Ambu or Cardiff bag. The baby's jaw must be held forward and supported to maintain the airway. Insertion of a neonatal airway helps to prevent obstruction by the baby's tongue. Note that overextension of the baby's head causes airway obstruction. Ventilation at a rate of 40 respirations per minute is applied by squeezing the bag. A longer inspiration phase improves oxygenation. Higher inflation pressures may be required to produce chest movement (Milner 1991). If the infant is attempting to breathe out, his efforts at expiration may be foiled as the operator inflates the chest with positive pressure. This technique therefore requires a skilled operator to achieve success. Used correctly this method can avoid the need for endotracheal intubation (Palme-Kilander 1992).

Endotracheal intubation. If the baby fails to

respond to intermittent positive pressure ventilation (IPPV) by bag and mask, or if bradycardia is present, an endotracheal tube should be passed without delay. Intubating a baby is different from intubating an adult and requires special skill which, once acquired, must be practised to be retained. The midwife can learn this skill by practice on models. (Practising resuscitation techniques on stillborn infants, while realistic, poses ethical questions, especially with regard to parental consent (Carlisle 1992).)

Technique of intubation (Fig. 34.4). The blade of the laryngoscope is introduced over the baby's tongue into the pharynx until the epiglottis is seen. Elevation of the epiglottis by the tip of the

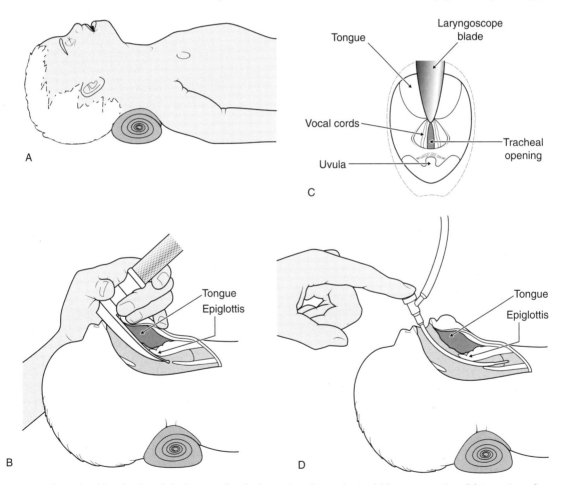

Fig. 34.4 Endotracheal intubation. (A) Place small rolled towel under neck. Avoid hyperextension. (B) Insertion of laryngoscope blade over tongue. (C) Tip of laryngoscope elevates epiglottis against tongue, revealing vocal cords. (D) Endotracheal tube in position.

laryngoscope reveals the vocal cords. Any mucus, blood or meconium which is obstructing the trachea should be cleared by careful suction prior to passing the endotracheal tube a distance of 1.5–2 cm into the trachea. (Pressure on the cricoid cartilage may facilitate visualisation of the larynx. Intubation may be easier if a cold tube which has been in the refrigerator is used.) After the laryngoscope is removed, oxygen is administered by IPPV to the endotracheal tube via the Ambu bag or Y-piece connector attached to the manometer. A maximum of 30 cm water pressure should be applied as there is risk of rupture of alveoli or tension pneumothorax if higher pressure is applied. The rise and fall of the chest wall should indicate whether the tube is in the trachea. This can be confirmed by auscultation of the chest. Distension of the stomach indicates oesophageal intubation necessitating resiting of the tube.

Mouth-to-face resuscitation. In the absence of specialised equipment, assisted ventilation can be achieved by mouth-to-face resuscitation. With the baby's head in the 'sniffing' position the operator places her mouth over the infant's mouth and nose and, using only the air in her buccal cavity, breathes gently into the baby's airway at a rate of 20 breaths per minute, allowing the infant to exhale between breaths. It may be easier with larger babies to use mouth-to-nose resuscitation (Tonkin et al 1995).

External cardiac massage

If bradycardia persists or the heart rate is less than 40 beats per minute, external cardiac massage may be applied. The most effective way of achieving this is by encircling the baby's chest with the fingers on the spine and thumbs on the lower mid-sternum (Fig. 34.5) (David 1988, Graves 1988, Milner 1991, Roberton 1992) and depressing the chest at a rate of 100–120 times per minute. (Excessive pressure over the lower end of the sternum may cause rib, lung or liver damage.)

Use of drugs

If the baby's response is slow or he remains hypotonic after ventilation is achieved, consideration

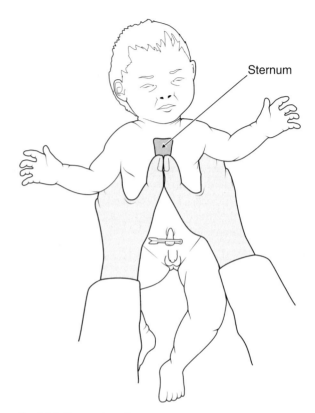

Fig. 34.5 External cardiac massage.

will be given to the use of drugs. In specialist obstetric units pulse oximetry (see Ch. 39) may be employed to monitor hypoxia (Letko 1996) and blood obtained through the umbilical artery or vein to ascertain biochemical status (Harris et al 1996). Results will enable appropriate administration of sodium bicarbonate or THAM to correct acidosis. In some centres these more intensive aspects of care are deferred until transfer of the intubated infant to the neonatal unit (see below).

Naloxone hydrochloride. This is *not* an emergency drug per se and should be used with caution and only in specific circumstances. It is a powerful anti-opioid drug used to reverse the effects of maternal narcotic drugs given in the preceding 3 hours. Ventilation should be established prior to its use. **It must not be given to apnoeic infants.** A dose of up to 40 micrograms (or approximately 10 micrograms/kg bodyweight) may be administered intravenously (through the umbilical vein). It may be repeated after 2–3 minutes. Alternatively, 200 micrograms (approximately 60 micrograms/kg bodyweight) may be given intramuscularly for a more prolonged action. As opioid action may persist for some hours the midwife must be alert for signs of relapse when a repeat dose may be required. NB: It should not be administered to infants of narcotic-addicted mothers as this may precipitate acute withdrawal (Gibbs et al 1989). The use of the 20 micrograms/ml preparation is no longer recommended because of the risk of fluid overload (Reynolds 1996). Policies relating to dosage and route of administration may vary in different hospitals.

Sodium bicarbonate.   6–8 mmol/kg of 4.2%, 7.5% or 8.4% solution given intravenously assists in the correction of metabolic acidosis. It should be administered slowly (for example at a rate of 1 ml per minute) in order to avoid rapid elevation of serum osmolality with the attendant risk of intracranial haemorrhage (Howell 1987). **It should not be given prior to ventilation being established**. THAM may be used in preference to sodium bicarbonate (Roberton 1992).

Dextrose.   5 ml of 5% or 10% solution may be given intravenously to correct or prevent hypoglycaemia.

Konakion (vitamin K₁).   Up to 1 mg may be given intramuscularly to reduce the risks associated with haemorrhage.

Dexamethasone.   1–2 mg may be given intravenously or intramuscularly to minimise the risk of cerebral oedema if severe asphyxia is present.

NB: Sodium bicarbonate and THAM are normally administered by medical staff and dexamethasone only on prescription.

Observations and after-care

Throughout the resuscitation procedure the baby's response should be monitored and recorded. A full narrative description of the baby's behaviour is desirable, making special note of the time when spontaneous respirations are established (Roberton 1992). The endotracheal tube may be left in place for a few minutes after the baby starts to breathe spontaneously. Suction may be applied through the endotracheal tube as it is removed. Careful documentation of all drugs given and of serial Apgar scores is essential. A baby whose Apgar score was less than 6 at 5 minutes, or who was slow to respond to resuscitation, and babies requiring continued ventilatory assistance should be transferred to the neonatal unit for a period of observation in order to monitor behaviour and enable early detection of post-asphyxial encephalopathy (see Ch. 39).

Explanation about the resuscitation and the need for transfer to hospital (if born at home) or to the special care nursery must be given to the parents and, providing the baby's condition permits, the mother should have the opportunity to see and hold her baby prior to being separated from him. This assists the attachment process previously described. Babies who respond quickly to resuscitation can be reunited with their parents, remaining in the delivery room until the usual transfer time to the postnatal ward where their care continues as normal.

The principles of resuscitation of the newborn are applicable wherever and whenever apnoea occurs. The midwife must be able to implement emergency care whilst awaiting medical assistance (Box 34.3).

It can be seen that the midwife's role at the time of delivery is both one of privilege and of immense responsibility. Her wish to meet the psychological needs of the parents and the baby must be tempered with the need to accommodate the infant's necessary adaptations at the time of birth and to institute emergency care when required. Continued care of the newborn takes the history of the baby's condition at delivery into account and is discussed in Chapter 35.

Box 34.3 Resuscitation action plan		
A Anticipation	assessment (Apgar)	airway – clear debris
B Breathing	bag + mask	endotracheal tube
C Circulation	cardiac massage	caring – warmth, comfort
D Doctor	drugs	documentation
E Explanation		
F Follow-up care		

READER ACTIVITIES

Repeating each of the following activities more than once will add to the information and experience gained.

1. Observe and record the time of the first gasp and onset of spontaneous breathing in babies delivered:

a. by spontaneous vertex delivery
b. by forceps delivery
c. by caesarean section.

Compare the responses of these babies.

2. When you are present at a birth but are not delivering the baby, record the Apgar score of the newborn. Compare your score with that awarded by the midwife and discuss your findings with her.

3. Observe the interactions between a mother and father and their baby at and just after birth. Compare the reactions and behaviour of the mother with those of the father. Do reactions of first-time parents differ in any way from those of experienced parents?

4. Observe a baby during the first hour of life. Consider what factors may influence behaviour, such as handling, maternal sedation during labour or other factors.

5. Compare the skin temperature of the baby after birth with the temperature recorded 1 hour, then 2 hours, later.

6. Attend the resuscitation of a baby by a paediatrician or a specialist midwife. Record the baby's response to treatment. Review the labour record to find out whether signs of hypoxia were observed before birth.

7. Familiarise yourself with the Resuscitaire, its equipment, and its functioning.

8. Familiarise yourself with the resuscitation policy manual in your place of work.

9. If available in your area, view a video recording of resuscitation of the newborn.

10. Using a model, practise mouth-to-face resuscitation; bag and mask resuscitation; intubation and intermittent positive pressure ventilation. This experience will stand you in good stead when, under supervision, you undertake the resuscitation of an infant with respiratory depression.

11. Monitor the subsequent behaviour of a baby who required resuscitation. Compare this with the observations of normal behaviour that you made earlier.

12. Make a plan of action for your emergency resuscitation of a baby born at home or other given situation, for example a baby found apnoeic in his cot.

REFERENCES

Apgar V 1953 A proposal for a new method of evaluation of the newborn infant. Current Research in Anaesthesiology and Analgesics 40: 340
Bedford V, Johnson N 1988 The role of the father. Midwifery 4: 190–195
Blackburn S T, Loper D L 1992 Maternal, fetal, and neonatal physiology: a clinical perspective. W B Saunders, Philadelphia, chs 5, 6, 7
Brueggemeyer A 1993 Neonatal thermoregulation. In: Kenner C, Brueggemeyer A, Gunderson L P (eds) Comprehensive neonatal nursing: a physiologic perspective. W B Saunders, Philadelphia

Callister L C 1995 Cultural meanings of childbirth. Journal of Obstetric, Gynecologic, and Neonatal Nursing 24(4): 327–331
Carlisle D 1992 A secret procedure? Nursing Times 88(35): 16–17
Dahm L S, James L S 1972 Newborn temperature and calculated heat loss in the delivery room. Pediatrics 49(4): 504–513
David R 1988 Closed chest cardiac massage in the newborn infant. Pediatrics 81(4): 552–554
Dawkins M, Hull D 1964 Brown adipose tissue in the response of newborn rabbits to cold. Journal of Physiology 172: 215–238

de Château P 1987 Promotion of mother–infant relationship during delivery. In: Harvey D (ed) Parent–infant relationships. Wiley series on perinatal practice. John Wiley, Chichester, vol 4

Gibbs J, Newson T, Williams J, Davidson D C 1989 Naloxone hazards in infants of opioid abusers. Lancet 2(8655): 159–160

Graves B 1988 Challenges of neonatal resuscitation for nurse-midwives. Journal of Nurse-Midwifery 33(5): 217–224

Greer P S 1988 Head coverings for newborns under radiant warmers. Journal of Obstetric, Gynecologic, and Neonatal Nursing 17: 265–271

Harris M, Beckley S L, Garibaldi J M, Keith R D F, Greene K R 1996 Umbilical cord blood analysis at the time of delivery. Midwifery 12(3): 146–150

Herbert M, Sluckin A 1985 A realistic look at mother–infant bonding. In: Chiswick M (ed) Recent advances in perinatal medicine 2. Churchill Livingstone, Edinburgh

Heyman M 1989 Arachidonic acid derivatives in the perinatal period. In: Barness L, De Vivo D, Morrow G, Oski F, Rudolph A (eds) Advances in pediatrics 36. Year Book Medical, Chicago, pp 151–176

Howell J 1987 Sodium bicarbonate in the perinatal setting – revisited. Clinics in Perinatology 14(4): 807–816

Jacobs M, Phibbs R 1989 Prevention, recognition and treatment of perinatal asphyxia. Clinics in Perinatology 16(4): 785–807

Karlsson H 1996 Skin to skin care: heat balance. Archives of Disease in Childhood 75(2): F130–132

Klaus M H, Trause M A, Kennell J H 1975 Does human maternal behaviour after delivery show a characteristic pattern? In: CIBA Foundation Symposium 33, parent–infant interaction. Associated Scientific, Amsterdam

Letko M D 1996 Understanding the Apgar score. Journal of Obstetric, Gynecologic, and Neonatal Nursing 25(4): 299–303

Lim M K, Hanretty K, Houston A B, Lilley S, Murtagh E P 1992 Intermittent ductal patency in healthy newborn infants: demonstration by colour Doppler flow mapping. Archives of Disease in Childhood 67(10): 1217–1218

Lowe N K, Reiss R 1996 Parturition and fetal adaptation. Journal of Obstetric, Gynecologic, and Neonatal Nursing 25(4): 339–349

Milner A D 1991 Resuscitation of the newborn. Archives of Disease in Childhood 66(1): 66–69

Palme-Kilander C 1992 Methods of resuscitation in low-Apgar-score newborn infants – a national survey. Acta Paediatrica 81: 739–744

Parkinson C E, Harvey D 1987 Child development and the maternal-infant relationship. In: Harvey D (ed) Parent–infant relationships. Wiley series on perinatal practice. John Wiley, Chichester, vol 4

Perry S E 1995 The newborn. In: Bobak I M, Lowdermilk D L, Jensen M D (eds) Maternity nursing, 4th edn. Mosby, St Louis

Reynolds J E (ed) 1996 Martindale: the extra pharmacopoeia, 31st edn. Royal Pharmaceutical Society, London, pp 986–987

Roberton N R C 1992 Resuscitation of the newborn. In: Roberton N R C (ed) Textbook of neonatology. Churchill Livingstone, Edinburgh

Rutter N 1992 Temperature control and its disorders. In: Roberton N R C (ed) Textbook of neonatology. Churchill Livingstone, Edinburgh

Salariya E 1990 Parental–infant attachment. In: Alexander J, Levy V, Roch S (eds) Postnatal care – a research based approach. Macmillan, Basingstoke

Salariya E, Easton P, Cater J 1979 Early and often for best results. Nursing Mirror 148(22): 15–17

Silverman F, Suidan J, Wasserman J, Antoine C, Young B 1985 The Apgar score: is it enough? Obstetrics and Gynaecology 66: 331–336

Sinclair J C 1992 Management of the thermal environment. In: Sinclair J C, Bracken M B (eds) Effective care of the newborn infant. Oxford Medical Publications, Oxford University Press, Oxford

Sluckin W, Sluckin A, Herbert M 1984 On mother-to-infant bonding. Midwife, Health Visitor and Community Nurse 20(11): 404–407

Thomas K 1994 Thermoregulation in neonates. Neonatal Network 13(2): 15–22

Tonkin S L, Davis S L, Gunn T R 1995 Nasal route for infant resuscitation by mothers. Lancet 345(8961): 1353–1354

Tyler S 1996 Catching up with vitamin K. Midwives 109(1305): 273

Tyson J E 1992 Immediate care of the newborn infant. In: Sinclair J E, Bracken M B (eds) Effective care of the newborn infant. Oxford Medical Publications, Oxford University Press, Oxford

White D G, Woollet E A 1987 The father's role in the neonatal period. In: Harvey D (ed) Parent–infant relationships. Wiley series on perinatal practice. John Wiley, Chichester, vol 4

Wildman J 1995 Is this finally it? New Generation 14(2): 5

Williams R P 1995 Family dynamics after childbirth. In: Bobak I M, Lowdermilk D L, Jensen M D (eds) Maternity nursing, 4th edn. Mosby, St Louis

Wong D L (ed) 1995 Whaley and Wong's nursing care of infants and children, 5th edn. Mosby, St Louis

Young J 1995 To help or to hinder: endotracheal suction and the intubated neonate. Journal of Neonatal Nursing 1(4): 23–28

FURTHER READING

American Academy of Pediatrics Committee on Fetus and Newborn 1986 Use and abuse of the Apgar score. Pediatrics 78(6): 1148–1149

Brant H 1985 Childbirth for men. Oxford Medical, Oxford

Harvey D (ed) 1987 Parent–infant relationships. Wiley series on perinatal practice. John Wiley, Chichester, vol 4

Hey E 1996 Principles of resuscitation at birth, 5th edn.

Northern Neonatal Network, Hudson Print, Newcastle-upon-Tyne

Hull J, Dodd K 1991 What is birth asphyxia? British Journal of Obstetrics and Gynaecology 98(10): 953–955

Josse E, Connelly J 1988 Mucus extractors: an infection risk? Nursing Times 84(9): 84

London M L 1993 Resuscitation and stabilisation of the

neonate. In: Kenner C, Brueggemeyer A, Gunderson L P
(eds) Comprehensive neonatal nursing: a physiologic
perspective. W B Saunders, Philadelphia

Peliowski A, Finer N 1992 Birth asphyxia in the term infant.
In: Sinclair J C, Bracken M B (eds) Effective care of the
newborn infant. Oxford Medical, Oxford University Press,
Oxford

Richards S R, Britton D T, Donohoe T, Monk S, Shipley
A D C 1994 Mouth-operated mucus extractors: safe to
use? British Journal of Obstetrics and Gynaecology
101(7): 629–631

Roberton N R C (ed) 1992 Textbook of neonatology, 2nd
edn. Churchill Livingstone, Edinburgh

Sangstad O D 1996 Resuscitation of newborn infants: do we
need new guidelines? Prenatal and Neonatal Medicine
1(1): 26–28

Sharif K, Olah K, Gee H 1993 Umbilical cord blood pH
and base deficit: time-dependent change at room
temperature. Journal of Obstetrics and Gynaecology
13(2): 107–110

Tyson J, Silverman W, Reisch J 1990 Immediate care of the
newborn. In: Chalmers I, Enkin M, Keirse M J N C (eds)
(1989 corrected) Effective care in pregnancy and childbirth.
Vol 2: Childbirth. Oxford University Press, Oxford

Valman H B 1995 The first year of life. BMJ Publishing,
London

Vaughans B 1990 Early maternal–infant contact and neonatal
thermoregulation. Neonatal Network 8(5): 19

Yudkin P L, Johnson A, Clover L M, Murphy K W 1994
Clustering of perinatal markers of birth asphyxia and
outcome at five years. British Journal of Obstetrics and
Gynaecology 101(9): 774–781

35

The normal baby

Maureen M. Michie

The normal neonate continues to adapt to extrauterine life in the first weeks after delivery. He remains vulnerable to airway obstruction, hypothermia, hypoglycaemia and infection. This necessitates the provision of an environment which is optimal in relation to his physiological competence. The provision of this environment, normally by his mother, is enhanced by the developing mother–baby relationship.

The chapter aims to:

- describe the external features of the normal newborn baby

- discuss the functioning of the different body systems in relation to their stage of maturity and the changes taking place at birth

- describe the behaviour of the baby during the first weeks of life

- detail the systematic examination of the baby at birth and the subsequent daily examinations

- discuss the care of the baby and the measures employed to ensure security and safety and promotion of normal growth and development

- highlight the role of the midwife in promoting confidence and competence in the parents and encouraging interaction between them and their baby.

Extrauterine life presents a challenge to the newborn infant. The most important changes, those in the heart and lungs, take place at birth (see Ch. 34). However, continued adaptations are necessary in the first weeks of life as the infant assumes independence from the maternal and placental nurturing which he enjoyed before birth. He remains dependent on his mother or other caregiver for nutrition and protection, but is responsible for his own metabolism and homeostasis among other functions essential to survival.

GENERAL CHARACTERISTICS

Appearance

A normal full-term infant weighs approximately 3.5 kg, when fully extended measures 50 cm from the crown of his head to his heels, and has an occipitofrontal circumference of 34–35 cm. His head comprises one-quarter of his size. He is plump and has a prominent abdomen. He lies in an attitude of flexion – in the supine position with his head turned to one side and one shoulder elevated off the mattress, in the prone position with his buttocks elevated, his knees drawn up under his abdomen, and his head turned to one side. With his arms extended his fingers reach to mid-thigh level.

Vernix caseosa, a white sticky substance, is present on the baby's skin at birth. The amount of vernix is variable. It is thought to have a protective function and is mostly absorbed within a few hours. Residual vernix in the axillae and groin areas predisposes to excoriation of the skin.

The skin

One of the largest organs in the body, the skin has an important role in temperature regulation, protection from infection, reflecting the well-being of the baby, and in facilitating communication. The midwife must be knowledgeable about the normal parameters of neonatal skin which differs somewhat from that of the adult (Michie 1996).

The skin of a newborn baby is thin, delicate, and easily traumatised by friction, pressure or substances with a different pH. This renders the skin prone to blistering, excoriation and infection. Sterile at birth, the skin is colonised by micro-organisms within 24 hours. The low pH of the skin surface (pH < 5) creates an 'acid mantle' which protects against infection.

The umbilical cord's position on the anterior abdominal wall predisposes to its contamination from excreta. The stump is rapidly colonised and necroses and separates by a process of dry gangrene usually within the first 10 days of life.

Downy hair, lanugo, covers the skin and is plentiful over the shoulders, upper arms and thighs. The general colour of the skin depends on the baby's ethnic origin, ranging from pink and white to olive or dark brown. Peripheral cyanosis is common. Pigmentation of nipples and genitalia is deeper in babies with darker skins and a linea nigra may be present. Another feature of racial origin is the Mongolian blue spot which presents as a diffuse bluish-black area usually over the sacral region. Dark-skinned babies become more pigmented in the first weeks of life though the palms of the hands and soles of the feet remain paler than the rest of the body.

A mature baby has plentiful skin creases on the palms of his hands and soles of his feet. His nails are fully formed and adherent to the tips of the fingers, sometimes extending beyond the finger tips. His hair is soft and silky: some babies have virtually no hair and appear somewhat bald, whereas others have plentiful straight or curly hair. Eyebrows and eyelashes present a similar variation. The cartilage of the ears is well formed.

Sebaceous glands, though present in the skin, are relatively inactive. Distended glands, milia, may be present over the nose and cheeks. Sweat glands are present but inactive in the first days of life. The vasoconstrictor mechanism is inefficient because the vascular plexuses are underdeveloped. The infant's poor melanin production renders him vulnerable to sunburn.

Sensitivity to touch and pressure, heat and cold, and pain are mediated through the skin.

Genitalia and breasts

Both boys and girls have a nodule of breast tissue around the nipple. In boys the testicles are descended into the scrotum which has plentiful rugae. The urethral meatus opens at the tip of the penis and the prepuce is adherent to the glans. In girls born at term the labia majora normally cover the labia minora. The hymen and clitoris may appear disproportionately large.

Eyes

Most babies have dark blue-grey eyes. Permanent colouring of the iris is not manifest for weeks, months or even several years. Dark-skinned babies may have brown eyes though this varies according to the racial origins of the parents. The shape of the baby's eyes also reflects racial origin, for instance the epicanthic folds of Oriental babies alter the appearance of the orbital region. No tears are present in the eyes of a newborn baby and they become infected easily.

PHYSIOLOGY

Respiratory system

At birth the respiratory system is developmentally incomplete, growth of new alveoli continuing for several years. The lumen of the peripheral airways is narrow which predisposes to airway obstruction. The baby's short neck and poorly supported tongue predispose to partial airway obstruction when he is in the supine position (Blackburn & Loper 1992). Respiratory secretions are more plentiful than in an adult and the mucous membranes are delicate and sensitive to trauma, the area below the vocal cords being particularly prone to oedema. (See also Ch. 34.)

The normal baby has a respiratory rate of 30–60 breaths per minute. His breathing is diaphragmatic, chest and abdomen rising and falling synchronously. The breathing pattern is erratic. Respirations are shallow and irregular, being interspersed with brief 10- to 15-second periods of apnoea (Perry 1995). This is known as periodic breathing. Apart from the initial profound respiratory efforts at birth, no nasal flaring, sternal or subcostal recession or grunting is present. The pattern of respiration alters during sleeping and waking states. Babies are obligatory nose breathers and do not convert automatically to mouth breathing when nasal obstruction occurs. Respiratory difficulties can occur because of neurological, metabolic, circulatory or thermoregulatory dysfunction as well as infection, airway obstruction or abnormalities of the respiratory tract itself (see relevant chapters).

The baby has a lusty cry which he uses to evoke a response from his attendants with a view to controlling his environment. The cry is normally loud and of medium pitch unless neurological damage, infection or hypothermia is present, when it may be high pitched or weak. Transient cyanosis may arise in the first few days when the baby is crying and altered pressure gradients re-create right-to-left shunts within the heart and great vessels (see Ch. 34).

Cardiovascular system and blood

The changes in the infant's heart at birth have been described in Chapter 34. The heart rate is rapid, 120–160 beats per minute, and fluctuates in accordance with the baby's respiratory function and activity or sleep state. Peripheral circulation is sluggish. This results in mild cyanosis of hands, feet and circumoral areas and in generalised mottling when the skin is exposed. Blood pressure fluctuates according to activity and ranges from 50–55/25–30 mmHg to 80/50 mmHg in the first 10 days of life (Roberton 1996). It is considered that, even at rest, the baby's heart probably functions at full capacity, rendering the infant vulnerable to additional stress (Blackburn & Loper 1992).

The total circulating blood volume at birth is 80 ml/kg bodyweight. However, this may be raised if there is delay in clamping the umbilical cord at birth. The haemoglobin level is high (13–20 g/dl) of which 50–85% is fetal haemoglobin (Blackburn & Loper 1992). Conversion from fetal to adult haemoglobin which commenced in utero is completed in the first 1–2 years of life. Haemoglobin, red cell count ($5–7 \times 10^{12}$/l) and haematocrit (55%) levels decrease gradually during the first 2–3 months of life during which time erythropoiesis is suppressed. The white cell count is high initially (18.0×10^9/l) but decreases rapidly (Perry 1995, Roberton 1992).

Breakdown of excess red blood cells in the liver and spleen predisposes to jaundice in the first week. Because colonisation of the intestine by the bacteria which synthesise vitamin K is delayed until feeding is established, vitamin K dependent clotting factors II (prothrombin), VII, IX and X are low. This inhibits blood clotting during the first week. Platelet levels equal those of the adult but there is a reduced capacity for adhesion and aggregation (Blackburn & Loper 1992).

Temperature regulation

Thermal control in the neonate remains poor for some time. Initial thermal adaptation and modes of heat loss and gain have been described in Chapter 34. Owing to the immaturity of the hypothalamus, temperature regulation is inefficient and the infant remains vulnerable to hypothermia particularly when exposed to cold or draughts, when wet, when unable to move about freely, or when deprived of nutrition. As a baby who is cold is unable to shiver, he will attempt to maintain his body heat by adopting a flexed fetal posture, increasing his respiratory rate and activity. He may also cry. These activities increase calorie consumption and may result in hypoglycaemia which in turn will compound the effects of hypothermia, as do hypoxia, acidosis and hyperbilirubinaemia (see Chs 39 and 42).

The infant's normal core temperature is 36–37°C. A healthy, clothed, term infant will maintain this body temperature satisfactorily provided his environmental temperature is sustained between 18 and 21°C, his nutrition is adequate, and his movements are not restricted by tight swaddling. However, like adults, babies are individuals with differing metabolic rates. This makes finite statements of thermoneutral range difficult (Hull et al 1996a,b). Hyperthermia can occur when the infant is exposed to a radiant heat source. Sweating may occur especially over the forehead, although the neonate's ability to sweat is limited. An unstable temperature may indicate infection.

Renal system

Though the kidneys are functional in fetal life, their workload is minimal until after birth. They are functionally immature. The glomerular filtration rate is low and tubular resorption capabilities are limited. The infant is not able to concentrate or dilute the urine very well in response to variations in fluid intake nor can he compensate well for high or low levels of solutes in the blood. This results in a narrow margin between homeostasis and fluid overload or underload (see Ch. 53). The ability to excrete drugs is also limited and the baby's renal function is vulnerable to physiological stress (Blackburn & Loper 1992, Perry 1995, Roberton 1992). The first urine is passed at birth or within the first 24 hours and thereafter with increasing frequency as fluid intake rises. The urine is dilute, straw coloured and odourless. Cloudiness caused by mucus and urates may be present initially until fluid intake increases. Urates may cause pink staining which is insignificant. Urine is voided by reflex emptying of the bladder. As the neonatal pelvis is small, the bladder becomes palpable abdominally when full.

Gastrointestinal system

The gastrointestinal tract of the neonate is structurally complete though functionally immature in comparison with that of the adult (Blackburn & Loper 1992, Perry 1995, Roberton 1992). The mucous membrane of the mouth is pink and moist. The teeth are buried in the gums and ptyalin secretion is low. Small epithelial pearls are sometimes present at the junction of the hard and soft palates. Sucking pads in the cheeks give them a full appearance. Sucking and swallowing reflexes are coordinated.

The stomach has a small capacity (15–30 ml) which increases rapidly in the first weeks of life. The cardiac sphincter is weak, predisposing to regurgitation or posseting. Gastric acidity, equal to that of the adult within a few hours after delivery, diminishes rapidly within the first few days and by the 10th day the infant is virtually achlorhydric which increases the risk of infection. Gastric emptying time is normally 2.5–3 hours.

In relation to the size of the infant the intestine is long, containing large numbers of secretory glands and a large surface area for the absorption of nutrients. Enzymes are present though there is a deficiency of amylase and lipase, which diminishes the infant's ability to digest compound carbohydrates and fat.

When food enters the stomach a gastrocolic reflex results in the opening of the ileocaecal valve. The contents of the ileum pass into the large intestine and rapid peristalsis means that feeding is often accompanied by reflex emptying of the bowel.

The gut is sterile at birth but is colonised within

a few hours. Bowel sounds are present within 1 hour of birth. Meconium, present in the large intestine from 16 weeks' gestation, is passed within the first 24 hours of life and is totally excreted within 48–72 hours. This first stool is blackish green in colour, is tenacious and contains bile, fatty acids, mucus and epithelial cells. From the third to fifth day the stools undergo a transitional stage and are brownish-yellow in colour. Once feeding is established, yellow faeces are passed. The consistency and frequency of stools reflect the type of feeding. Breast milk results in loose, bright yellow and inoffensive acid stools. The baby may pass eight to ten stools a day or alternatively pass stools as infrequently as every 2 or 3 days. The stools of the bottle-fed infant are paler in colour, semi-formed, less acidic, and have a slightly sharp smell (Roberton 1992). The baby passes four to six stools a day but there is an increased tendency to constipation.

Physiological immaturity of the liver results in low production of glucuronyl transferase for the conjugation of bilirubin. This, together with a high level of red cell breakdown, may result in a transient jaundice which is manifest on the third to fifth days (see also Ch. 42). Glycogen stores are rapidly depleted, so early feeding is required to maintain normal blood glucose levels (2.2–4.4 mmol/l). Feeding stimulates liver function and colonisation of the gut which assists in the formation of vitamin K.

Infant feeding practices are designed to meet the physiological needs and capabilities of the baby and are discussed in Chapter 36.

Immunological adaptations

Neonates demonstrate a marked susceptibility to infections, particularly those gaining entry through the mucosa of the respiratory and gastrointestinal systems. Localisation of infection is poor, 'minor' infections having the potential to become generalised very easily.

The baby has some immunoglobulins at birth but the sheltered intrauterine existence limits the need for learned immune responses to specific antigens (Blackburn & Loper 1992, Crockett 1995, Perry 1995, Stern 1992). There are three main immunoglobulins, IgG, IgA and IgM, and of these only IgG is small enough to cross the placental barrier. It affords immunity to specific viral infections. At birth the baby's levels of IgG are equal to or slightly higher than those of the mother. This provides passive immunity during the first few months of life.

IgM and IgA do not cross the placental barrier but can be manufactured by the fetus. Levels of IgM at term are 20% those of the adult, taking 2 years to attain adult levels (elevation of IgM levels at birth is suggestive of intrauterine infection). This relatively low level of IgM is thought to render the infant more susceptible to enteric infections. IgA levels are very low and increase slowly, although secretory salivary levels attain adult values within 2 months. IgA protects against infection of the respiratory tract, gastrointestinal tract and eyes. Breast milk, and especially colostrum, provides the infant with passive immunity in the form of *Lactobacillus bifidus*, lactoferrin, lysozyme and secretory IgA among others (see Ch. 36).

The thymus gland, where lymphocytes are produced, is relatively large at birth and continues to grow until 8 years of age.

Reproductive system

Spermatogenesis in boys does not occur until puberty but the total complement of primordial follicles containing primitive ova is present in the ovaries of girls at birth. In both sexes withdrawal of maternal oestrogens results in breast engorgement sometimes accompanied by secretion of 'milk' by the fourth or fifth day. Baby girls may develop pseudomenstruation for the same reason. This is short-lived.

Skeletomuscular system

The muscles are complete, growth occurring by hypertrophy rather than by hyperplasia. The long bones are incompletely ossified to facilitate growth at the epiphyses. The bones of the vault of the skull also reveal lack of ossification. This is essential for growth of the brain and facilitating moulding during labour. Moulding is resolved within a few days of birth. The posterior fontanelle closes at 6–8 weeks. The anterior fontanelle remains open until 18 months of age, making assessment of hydration and intracranial pressure possible by palpation of fontanelle tension.

Neurological system

In comparison with the other body systems the nervous system is remarkably immature both anatomically and physiologically at birth. This results in predominantly brain stem and spinal reflex activity with minimal control by the cerebral cortex in the early months though social interaction occurs early. After birth, brain growth is rapid, requiring constant and adequate supplies of oxygen and glucose. The immaturity of the brain renders it particularly vulnerable to hypoxia, biochemical imbalance, infection and haemorrhage. Temperature instability and uncoordinated muscle movement reflect the incomplete state of brain development and incomplete myelination of nerves.

The neonate is equipped with a wide range of reflex activities, the presence of which at varying ages provides indication of the normality and integrity of the neurological and skeletomuscular systems (Gandy 1992, Roberton 1992).

Moro reflex. This reflex occurs in response to a sudden stimulus. It can be elicited by holding the baby at an angle of 45° and then permitting the head to drop 1 or 2 cm. The infant responds by abducting and extending his arms with his fingers fanned, sometimes accompanied by a tremor. The arms then flex and embrace the chest. A similar response may be seen in the legs which, following extension, flex onto the abdomen (Fig. 35.1). The reflex is symmetrical and is present for the first 8 weeks of life. Absence of the Moro reflex may indicate brain damage or immaturity. Persistence of the reflex beyond the age of 6 months is suggestive of mental retardation.

Rooting reflex. In response to stroking of the cheek or side of the mouth the baby will turn towards the source of stimulus and open his mouth ready to suckle.

Sucking and swallowing reflexes are well developed in the normal baby and are coordinated with breathing. This is essential for safe feeding and adequate nutrition.

Gag, cough and sneeze reflexes protect the infant from airway obstruction.

Blinking and corneal reflexes protect the eyes from trauma.

Grasp reflexes. A palmar grasp is elicited by placing a finger or pencil in the palm of the baby's hand. The finger or pencil is grasped firmly. A

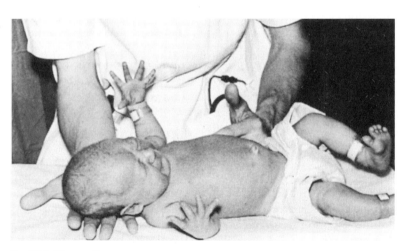

Fig. 35.1 Moro reflex.

similar response can be demonstrated by stroking the base of the toes (plantar grasp).

Walking and stepping reflexes. When supported upright with his feet touching a flat surface the baby simulates walking. If held with the tibia in contact with the edge of a table the infant will step up onto the table (limb placement reflex).

Asymmetrical tonic neck reflex. In the supine position the limbs on the side of the body to which the head is turned extend while those on the opposite side flex.

Muscle tone is reflected in the baby's response to passive movements.

Traction response. When pulled upright by the wrists to a sitting position the head will lag initially (Fig. 35.2) then right itself momentarily before falling forward on to the chest.

Ventral suspension. When held prone, suspended over the examiner's arm, the baby momentarily holds his head level with his body and flexes his limbs (Fig. 35.3).

These reflexes and responses are only a few of the many present at birth and assist in the attachment process to the mother who views these responses as indications of communication by her baby.

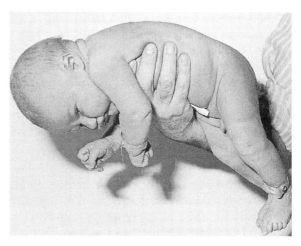

Fig. 35.3 Ventral suspension (reproduced by permission from Gandy 1992).

PSYCHOLOGY AND PERCEPTION

The newborn baby is alert and aware of his surroundings when he is awake. Far from being impassive he reacts to stimuli and begins at a very early age to amass information about his environment (Brazelton 1984).

Special senses

Vision

Though immature, the structures necessary for vision are present and functional at birth. The baby is sensitive to bright lights, which cause him to frown or blink. He demonstrates a preference for bold black and white patterns and the shape of the human face. His focusing distance is 15–20 cm which allows him to see his mother's face when being nursed. He can track a moving object briefly within the first 5 days. His ability to establish eye contact with his mother helps to enhance bonding. By 2 weeks of age he can differentiate his mother's face from that of a stranger. Interest in colour, variety and complexity of patterns develops within the first 2 months of life (Blackburn & Loper 1992, Perry 1995, Roberton 1992).

Hearing

The baby turns his eyes towards sound. On hearing

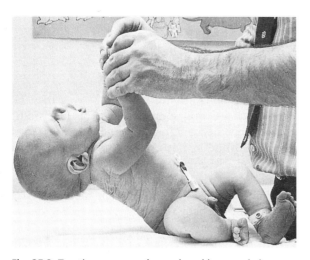

Fig. 35.2 Traction response (reproduced by permission from Gandy 1992).

a high-pitched sound he first stills and then becomes agitated. He is comforted by low-pitched sounds. A sudden sound elicits a startle or blink reflex. He prefers the sound of the human voice to other sounds and within a few weeks the patterns of adult speech are mimicked in his movements. He can discriminate between voices and prefers his mother's (DeCasper & Fifer 1987). This, too, promotes mother–baby interaction.

Smell and taste

Babies prefer the smell of milk to that of other substances and show a preference for human milk. Within a few days the baby can differentiate the smell of his mother's milk from that of another woman (MacFarlane 1975). He prefers the smell of an unwashed breast to that of a washed one (Righard 1995). He turns away from unpleasant smells. His preference for sweet taste is demonstrated by vigorous and sustained sucking and a speedy grimacing response to bitter, salty or sour substances (Blackburn & Loper 1992).

Touch

Infants are acutely sensitive to touch, enjoying skin-to-skin contact, immersion in water, stroking, cuddling and rocking movements (Blackburn & Loper 1992, Perry 1995). A puff of air on his face induces an inspiration or gasp reflex. His curving response to touch and his grasp reflexes enhance his relationship with his mother. The baby withdraws from painful stimuli, bulges his brow and nasolabial furrow and may cry vigorously (Rushforth & Levene 1994).

Habituation

If a stimulus is repeated several times in succession it will eventually fail to elicit a response from the infant unless his responding behaviours are reinforced in some way. It has been suggested that some habituation may be initiated in utero (Damstra-Wijmenga 1991). Babies learn quickly and soon demonstrate individuality in the way they become irritable or can be soothed (Brazelton 1984, Perry 1995). This influences the responses of their parents.

Sleeping and waking

Following the initiation of respiration at birth, the baby remains alert and reactive for a period of approximately 1 hour, after which he relaxes and sleeps. The length of this first sleep varies from a few minutes to several hours and is followed by a second period of reactivity during which mucus accumulation in the oropharynx may occur, causing choking or gagging (Perry 1995). Subsequent sleeping and waking rhythms show marked variations and the baby takes some time to settle into his individual pattern. Initially, waking periods are related to hunger, but within a few weeks the waking periods last longer and meet the need for social interaction.

Sleep states

Two sleep states are identifiable:

• In *deep sleep*, the baby's eyes are closed, respirations are regular, no eye movements are present, response to stimuli is delayed and is quickly suppressed. Jerky movements may occur at intervals.

• In *light sleep*, rapid eye movements are observable through the closed eyelids. Respirations are irregular and sucking movements occur intermittently. Response to stimuli occurs more readily and may result in an alteration of sleep state. Random movements are noted.

Awake states

A wider range of awake states is observed, ranging from drowsiness to crying:

• In the *drowsy state*, the baby's eyes may be open or closed with some fluttering of the eyelids. Smiling may occur. Limb movements are variable, generally smooth, but are interspersed by startle responses. Alteration in state occurs more readily following stimulation.

• In the *quiet alert state*, though motor activity is minimal, the baby is alert to visual and auditory stimuli.

• In the *active alert state*, the baby is generally active and reactive to his environment.

• In the *active crying state*, the baby cries vigorously

and may be difficult to console. Muscular activity is considerable.

The amount of time that the baby spends in each state varies tremendously and influences the way in which he responds to stimuli, whether visual, auditory or tactile (Brazelton 1984).

Crying

The crying repertoire of the baby distinguishes different needs and is the way in which he communicates discomfort and summons assistance. With experience it is possible to differentiate the cry and identify the need, which may be hunger, thirst, pain, general discomfort (for example wanting a change of position or feeling too cold or too hot), boredom, loneliness or a desire for physical and social contact. Maternal anxiety and difficulties related to infant crying can be allayed by information and advice from the midwife. The mother needs to learn how to comfort her baby. Rapid rocking induces sleep, swaddling and an upright position appear to be soothing (Downey & Bidder 1990).

Growth and development

Because of his physiological limitations, the baby is dependent on his mother (or other caregiver) for his continued survival, growth and development. These will progress satisfactorily only if he is physiologically and neurologically normal, he is in a safe environment, his nutritional needs are met, and his psychological development is promoted by appropriate stimulation and loving care. Abnormality of the infant's body systems, inadequate nutrition or emotional deprivation will compromise the baby's ability to grow and develop to his full potential. His relatively immature organ functions and his vulnerability to infection and hypothermia demand that his care must be designed to meet his needs and capabilities.

Normality of the baby is assessed by a variety of means. This assessment begins at birth.

SCREENING PROCEDURES

Some congenital abnormalities are readily identified at birth.

Examination at birth

Following a period of socialisation with his parents, the baby is examined carefully by the midwife to ascertain that, externally at least, the baby is normal. If any defects are identified, medical assistance can be sought early.

Examination of the baby, whenever possible, should be performed beside the parents. The midwife should talk to them as she proceeds, explaining her findings. Prior to examining the baby the midwife should wash her hands to prevent infection. Her hands should be warm to prevent chilling of the infant. During the examination the baby should be naked in a warm, draught-free environment. There should be sufficient light to allow the midwife to see the baby clearly. The examination is performed in an orderly manner from the head of the infant to his feet. Overall symmetry should be verified and skin blemishes or abrasions noted.

Colour and respirations. During quiet breathing the baby breathes through his nose. If one nostril is blocked, occlusion of the other results in cyanosis and unsuccessful attempts to breathe through the mouth, culminating in crying. Bilateral obstruction has the same effect.

Face, head and neck. After a general impression of the facies has been gained, the eyes and mouth of the infant are examined first. Each eye should be visualised to confirm that it is present and that the lens is clear. The baby may open his eyes spontaneously if held in an upright position. Any slight oedema or bruising is noted but may be insignificant. The normal space between the eyes is up to 3 cm.

The mouth can be opened easily by pressing against the angle of the jaw. This allows visual inspection of the tongue, gums and palate. The palate should be high arched, intact and the uvula central. Epithelial pearls may be observed. The midwife uses her little finger to feel the palate for any submucous cleft. A normal baby will respond by sucking the finger. Precocious teeth may protrude through the central part of the lower gum. (Though usually covered by epithelial tissue, such teeth may have erupted and be loose, requiring extraction in the early neonatal period to prevent their inhalation.) A tight frenulum will give the appearance of tongue tie: no treatment is necessary for this. The frenum of the upper lip should be central.

The ears are inspected, noting their position. The upper notch of the pinna should be level with the canthus of the eye. Patency of the external auditory meatus is verified. Accessory auricles, small tags of tissue, are sometimes noted lying in front of the ear.

By palpating the vault of the skull the midwife can determine the degree of moulding by the amount of overriding of the bones at the sutures and fontanelles. The bones should feel hard in a full-term infant. A wide anterior fontanelle and splayed sutures may indicate hydrocephalus or immaturity. The shape of the baby's head as a result of moulding gives indication of the presentation in utero (Fig. 35.4). An oedematous swelling, caput succedaneum, may be noted overlying the part that was presenting. This is a result of pressure from the cervical os and will disappear spontaneously within 24 hours (see Ch. 40).

The short thick neck of the baby must be examined to exclude the presence of swellings and to ensure that rotation and flexion of the head is possible.

Chest and abdomen. Observation of respiratory movement should reveal that chest and abdominal movements are synchronous. The respirations may still be irregular at this stage. Spacing of the

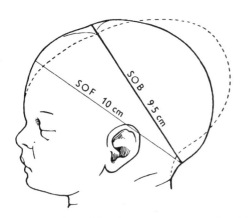

Fig. 35.4 Type of moulding in a vertex presentation. SOB = suboccipitobregmatic; SOF = suboccipitofrontal.

nipples should be noted, widely spaced nipples being associated with chromosomal abnormality.

The shape of the abdomen should be rounded. The midwife notes any variation, including a scaphoid (boat-shaped) abdomen or any protrusions, particularly at the base of the umbilical cord.

The artery forceps securing the umbilical cord should be replaced by a plastic disposable clamp applied approximately 2 cm from the umbilicus. Excess cord is discarded. Normally three cord vessels are present. Absence of one of the arteries is associated with renal or cardiac anomalies and must be brought to the attention of the paediatrician.

Genitalia and anus. The genitalia should be examined carefully. If the sex is uncertain, the paediatrician· will initiate investigations. Depending on local policy, the baby's temperature may be taken rectally to detect any excessive cooling and to confirm patency of the anus.

Limbs and digits. In addition to noting length and movement of the limbs, it is essential that the digits are counted and separated to ensure that webbing is not present. The hands should be opened fully as any accessory digits may be concealed in the clenched fist. The axillae, elbows, groins and popliteal spaces should also be examined. Normal flexion and rotation of the wrist and ankle joints should be confirmed.

Spine. With the baby lying prone the midwife should inspect and palpate the baby's back. Any swellings, dimples or hairy patches may signify an occult spinal defect.

Hips. It is essential that all babies undergo specific examination to detect developmental dysplasia of the hips (Aronsson et al 1994, Beverley & Nathan 1995). In some centres this is performed by the midwife; in others the paediatrician is the person responsible. Care must be taken in order to avoid producing an iatrogenically unstable hip (Beverley & Nathan 1995). The examination should not be undertaken by inexperienced staff. To examine the hips the examiner must place the baby on a firm flat surface at waist height.

Ortolani's test (Fig. 35.5). The baby's legs are grasped with the flexed knees in the palms of the

Preparation for tests
Flex knee and hip at right angles

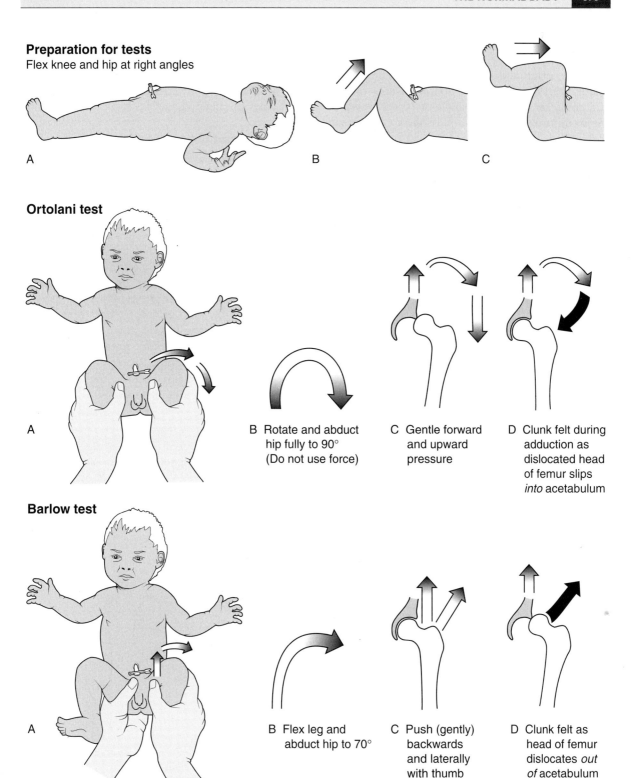

A

B

C

Ortolani test

A

B Rotate and abduct
   hip fully to 90°
   (Do not use force)

C Gentle forward
   and upward
   pressure

D Clunk felt during
   adduction as
   dislocated head
   of femur slips
   into acetabulum

Barlow test

A

B Flex leg and
   abduct hip to 70°

C Push (gently)
   backwards
   and laterally
   with thumb

D Clunk felt as
   head of femur
   dislocates *out
   of* acetabulum

Fig. 35.5 Examination of the hips.

examiner's hands and the femur splinted between the index and middle fingers and the thumb. Both hips are examined simultaneously. The baby's thighs are flexed onto the abdomen and rotated and abducted through an angle of 70–90° towards the examining surface. *No force should be exerted.* If the hip is dislocated a 'clunk' will be felt as the head of the femur slips into the acetabulum during adduction and the dislocation is reduced.

Barlow's test (Fig. 35.5). With the baby's legs flexed (as above), the head of the femur is held between the examiner's thumb and index finger while the other hand steadies the pelvis. Following the initial movement of flexion and rotation, as the hip is abducted to 70° *gentle* pressure is exerted in a backwards and lateral direction. A 'clunk' will be felt as the head of the femur dislocates out of the acetabulum.

In some centres a modified Ortolani/Barlow procedure is followed. This incorporates the essential elements of both of the above manoeuvres (Hall et al 1994).

Early referral to a paediatrician is essential if effective treatment for a dislocated, or dislocatable, hip is to be achieved (see Ch. 41).

Measurements. The baby's head circumference, length and weight are measured to provide parameters against which future growth can be monitored.

The head circumference is measured, encircling it at the occipital protuberance and the supraorbital ridges with a measuring tape. Moulding may reduce this measurement and for this reason this estimate is sometimes delayed until the third day when the head shape has resumed its normal contours.

Accurate measurement of the baby's crown–heel length is extremely difficult and can only be measured accurately using calibrated equipment. In circumstances where this is not available only an approximation of length can be achieved. The midwife should comply with local policy and procedures in this regard.[1] When using calibrated equipment it is essential that the baby's legs are fully extended and that his head and feet are in full contact with the measuring device (Fig. 35.6). This requires assistance from a second person (which may be the mother). The practice of suspending the baby upside down for measuring purposes is outmoded and hazardous for the reasons stated in Chapter 34. It is advisable to record the method by which the baby was measured in order that the validity of this basic parameter can be taken into account if future

---

1. In circumstances where specialised calibrated equipment is not available an approximation of the baby's length can be achieved by using a paper (i.e. non-stretchable) tape measure. The length is calculated in two stages. First, by measuring from the crown of the head to the base of the spine and, second, from that point at the base of the spine to the heels when the baby's legs are fully extended.

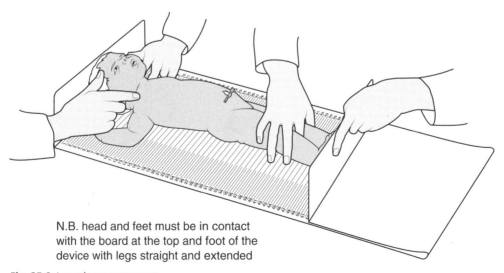

N.B. head and feet must be in contact with the board at the top and foot of the device with legs straight and extended

Fig. 35.6 Length measurement.

assessments reveal a discrepancy. It is suggested that serial length measurements monitoring growth should be made by the same individual to improve reliability (Doull et al 1995).

The baby is weighed and the identity bands are verified as correct prior to his being dressed and wrapped in warm blankets.

Documentation. The midwife records her findings in the case notes and any abnormalities are brought to the attention of the paediatrician (or GP if born at home) and of the receiving midwife in the postnatal ward.

Examination by the paediatrician

All newborn babies should be examined by a paediatrician (or other medical practitioner if a paediatrician is not available) within the first 24 hours of life and again prior to transfer home. Moss et al (1991) assert that a second examination is of little value, apart from a repeat examination of the hips. The mother should be present. Some of the examination duplicates what has been described above and so only the medical aspects are considered here. In some areas the midwife incorporates, and is accountable for, these additional elements of examination following appropriate in-service education (MacKeith 1995, Michaelides 1995, Rose 1994). A general appraisal of the baby's colour, overall appearance, muscular activity, and response to handling is made throughout the examination.

Neurological assessment. The baby's reflex responses are elicited in order to establish normality of the neurological system. These are tested while the baby is in a quiet alert state. Absent or weak responses may indicate immaturity, cerebral damage or abnormality.

Auscultation. The paediatrician listens to the heart and lung sounds. A heart murmur may be present for some days after birth.

Palpation. The abdominal organs, particularly the liver, spleen and kidneys, are palpated, noting any enlargement. Femoral pulses are assessed ensuring that they are full and of equal strength. The hips are re-examined at this juncture (or examined for the first time, see above).

Blood tests

Certain inborn errors of metabolism and endocrine disorders are detected by means of a blood test, for example the Guthrie test. Blood, obtained from a heel prick made with a stilette on the lateral aspect of the heel to avoid nerves and blood vessels, is dripped onto circles on an absorbent card onto which full details of the baby's identity are entered. For detection of phenylketonuria, the baby must have had at least 48 hours of milk feeding and if for any reason the infant is receiving antibiotics himself or via breast milk, this information should be included on the card. The blood collection may be delayed until the sixth or seventh day in order to test for hypothyroidism. Some centres test routinely for galactosaemia as well. (See Ch. 43 for details of these conditions and tests.)

Child health surveillance

Following discharge from the care of the midwife into that of the health visitor, the screening of the baby is continued on a regular basis at the child health clinic (see Ch. 46).

The specific screening procedures described in this section are complemented by the daily care and observations by the midwife during the first 10 days of life.

OBSERVATION AND GENERAL CARE

Identification and security procedures

In hospital, the midwife receiving the baby from the delivery suite staff should verify that the baby's name, sex, date and time of birth on the two name bands match the information in the case notes and are entered onto the cot card. The name bands should remain on the baby until his discharge from hospital. It is recommended that the presence of two legible, matching, correct name bands is verified daily, on transfer to other wards, and on discharge from hospital. If the information becomes illegible, or a name band is lost, new name band(s) should be prepared, verified with the mother *and replaced in her presence*. The replacement of the name bands should be documented in the case notes. In the event of a baby being found without any name bands the midwife must notify the unit manager and comply with local policy and procedures for their replacement. No mother should ever be in any doubt about her baby's identity (Laurent 1992).

Abduction of infants from hospitals has led to the development of security tagging and other monitoring devices being employed in recent years (Day 1995). It is advisable that the mother accompanies her baby at all times and should be able to identify members of staff who are involved in her baby's care. Staff should be alert to movement of babies who are apart from their mothers and not accompanied by a known member of staff.

Rest

Following the necessary administrative procedures, the baby should be warmly dressed and placed in a preheated cot beside his mother to allow him to rest until he awakes to feed. During these first few hours after birth especially, the midwife should observe frequently that the baby's colour remains pink, his airway unobstructed and that the umbilical cord clamp is secure. His temperature should be monitored to ensure that it is maintained within the normal range. The mother's wishes regarding feeding should be determined so that the midwife is aware of her plans for the baby's nutrition (see Ch. 36).

Neonatal care is designed to provide an optimum environment which will promote well-being and prevent complications. These include airway obstruction, haemorrhage, hypothermia, infection, injury and accident. Promotion of parent–baby relationships is integral to all aspects of care.

Prevention of airway obstruction

Choking can occur during feeding if coordination is poor and also following vomiting or regurgitation of mucus or feed. When in his cot, the baby should be laid on his back or side with his feet at the foot of the cot (Fig. 35.7) (Foundation for the Study of Infant Deaths 1996, Lerner 1993). A mucus extractor should be readily available so that aspiration of the baby's airway can be effected quickly.

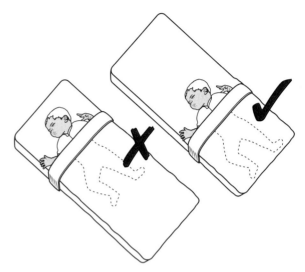

Fig. 35.7 'Feet-to-Foot' sleeping position.

Prevention of haemorrhage

Haemostasis of the umbilical cord is vital. A blood loss of 30 ml from a baby is equivalent to almost half a litre of blood from an adult. In some hospitals prophylactic vitamin K 1 mg is given orally or intramuscularly to promote prothrombin formation (Jørgensen et al 1991, Shearer 1995). This is to prevent bleeding disorders (see Ch. 40).

Prevention of hypothermia

Overexposure of the baby should be avoided to prevent heat loss. Where possible the room temperature should be maintained at 18–21°C. In hospital, and where higher ambient temperatures are able to be maintained, the infant should be dressed in a cotton gown and covered by two cellular blankets. An additional blanket underneath the bottom sheet will provide extra warmth for babies who are having difficulty in maintaining a stable body temperature. At home, or in cold environments, additional clothing including a hat may be required. Bath water should be warm, 37°C, and wet clothing should be changed as soon as possible. It is essential also to avoid overheating (Bacon 1991, Rutter 1992, Thomas 1994). Advice regarding clothing and bedding can only be a guide as infants have marked individual variations in their metabolic rates (Hull et al 1996a). Parents should be advised to take account of environmental temperature when dressing the baby. Swaddling should be loose enough to permit movement of arms and legs, allowing the infant to adjust his posture in response to the need for a change in temperature (Hull et al 1996b).

Prevention of infection

Each baby should be provided with equipment for his sole use. Adequate linen supplies are essential. This is especially important in hospital. The number of people handling the baby should be restricted. Members of staff who are liable to be a source of infection should not handle babies, and friends and relatives who have colds or sore throats (especially children) should not visit. Hand washing before and after handling babies is essential. Cross-infection can be a particular problem in hospitals. For this reason rooming-in and the use of hexachlorophane, Betadine, or chlorhexidine preparations for hand washing by personnel handling babies is recommended. The wearing of gowns when handling babies is not necessary.

The baby's skin is a barrier to infection provided its integrity and pH balance is maintained. By applying her knowledge of the physiology of neonatal skin the midwife can employ appropriate skin care.

Skin care

Promotion of skin integrity is enhanced by avoiding friction against hard fabrics or soiled or wet clothing, and by minimising the length of time the skin is in contact with irritants such as gastric contents, urine and stool. Cleansing of the skin should be carried out gently to prevent damage to the epidermis. Soaps, creams, isopropyl alcohol and other skin care preparations should be used with caution to prevent irritation and disturbance of the skin pH and absorption of topical agents. Baby soaps and other baby washing solutions are usually pH adjusted. Arachis oil and aqueous cream have also been recommended for baby care. In some centres hexachlorophane-based soap or liquid preparations (maximum concentration 3%) are used for cleansing the baby's skin (excluding the face). It is important to remember that these preparations should be rinsed off the skin as the risk of absorption of hexachlorophane has to be considered. The use of biological powders, fabric softeners and starch should be avoided when laundering babies' clothing (Michie 1996).

The timing of the first bath is not critical although it has been suggested that removal of blood and liquor reduces the risk of transmission of HIV and other organisms to staff (Penny-MacGillivray 1996). Bathing should be deferred until the baby's temperature is above 36.5°C. The temperature of the bath water should be 37°C. The hair is washed and dried carefully at the first bath but need not be washed daily. If the baby has been regurgitating mucus, a thin layer of petroleum jelly may be applied to his cheek to prevent soreness. Petroleum jelly applied to the buttocks will prevent meconium adhering to the skin and causing excoriation.

Daily bathing is not essential but the mother should be given sufficient opportunities to bath the baby in order to increase her confidence. 'Topping and tailing' (cleansing the baby's face, skin flexures and napkin area only) may be carried out once or twice a day. It should be noted that greater heat loss may be incurred during this procedure than when the baby is bathed (Perry 1995).

The baby's eyes do not need to be cleansed unless a discharge is present. Attention should be paid to the washing and drying of skin flexures to prevent excoriation. The buttocks must be washed and dried carefully at every napkin change. Sore buttocks may occur if the stools are loose, if there is protracted delay in changing a soiled napkin or if the skin is traumatised by overenthusiastic rubbing. Regular use of a barrier cream is recommended by some people (Jethwa 1994) but may interfere with the 'one-way' membrane in disposable nappies.

Cleanliness of the umbilical cord is essential. Hand washing is required before and after handling the cord. No specific cord treatment is required although a wide variety of preparations have been used to promote early separation. However, it should be noted that topical applications may interfere with the normal process of colonisation and delay separation. Cleansing with tap water and keeping the cord dry have been shown to promote separation (Barclay et al 1994, Mugford et al 1986, Rush 1990, Salariya & Kowbus 1988, Verber & Pagan 1993). It is advisable to ensure that the cord is not enclosed within the baby's napkin where contamination by urine or faeces may occur. The cord clamp is removed on the third day provided the cord is dry and necrosed.

Circumcision

Although not commonly practised in the UK, in other parts of the world neonatal circumcision may be undertaken whilst the baby is in hospital. There is little evidence to support this practice as beneficial; rather it is a traditional cultural custom (Gonik & Barrett 1995). It is recommended that appropriate anaesthesia, dorsal penile nerve block, is used for this procedure and that postoperative analgesia is also prescribed (Rabinowitz & Hulbert 1995). After-care involves the use of a non-adherent dressing, observing for haemorrhage and keeping the area clean and dry.

Vaccination and immunisation

BCG vaccination may be given during the early neonatal period in some areas where early protection is desirable. Vaccination against hepatitis B and poliomyelitis may also be given in some parts of the world (Roberton 1992).

Prevention of injury and accident

Sensible precautions should be observed by all staff in their own practice and explained to the parents. A baby should not be left unattended unless in his cot as vigorous activity may result in his falling off a bed or table. He should be moved from place to place in his cot rather than in arms and the bassinet of the cot should be flat, not elevated, to prevent dropping him if uneven floors are encountered. If in a larger crib, cot sides should be up and secured. The cot design should comply with safety standards. Babies do not require a pillow until the age of 2 years and mothers should be advised that placing a pillow behind the baby's head is unsafe and an unnecessary decoration in pram or cot. Similarly, polythene bags or sheeting should not be used near a baby and waterproof mattress covers should enclose the mattress completely to prevent suffocation of the baby by a loose cover.

The temperature of bath water should be tested prior to immersing the baby to avoid scalding or chilling and the temperature of a bottle feed tested before it is offered to the baby.

If safety pins are used to secure the napkin they should be inserted into the cloth from side to side (not vertically) and with one hand protecting the baby's abdomen to avoid penetration of the skin or genitalia.

If the baby's nails are long or ragged he may scratch his face. Mittens worn to prevent this should be made from cotton material with French seams to prevent loose threads entwining the fingers and occluding the circulation.

Advice should also be given to mothers about safety in the home. This should address such issues as bed-sharing, use of cat-nets, fireguards, cooker guards, stair gates, pram brakes and car seats. 'Back to Sleep' and 'Feet-to-Foot' advice should be reinforced (see above).

Observation of behaviour

Observation of the baby's behaviour provides information about his general well-being.

Feeding

During feeds the midwife should observe the baby's eagerness or reluctance to feed and the co-ordination of his sucking and swallowing reflexes. She should note the frequency with which he demands feeds. While feeding, the baby clenches his fists, tucks them under his chin and wriggles his toes. He may grasp his mother's fingers during feeding. Eye contact also occurs, which enhances communication between mother and baby. Sucking is interspersed with rest periods. (Infant feeding is discussed in Ch. 36.)

Abnormal feeding behaviours may signify cerebral damage, congenital abnormality or illness (see Chs 38, 40, 41).

Excretion

Observation of the phases of the stools and of any vomiting helps to identify abnormalities of the gastrointestinal tract, inborn errors of metabolism and infection.

Sleeping and waking

A newborn baby usually sleeps for most of the time between feeds but should be alert and responsive when awake. Erratic sleep patterns may prove disconcerting to new parents. Undue lethargy or irritability may indicate cerebral damage or sepsis.

Daily examination

Each day, the baby should be examined by a midwife to evaluate his progress and identify problems as they arise. The examination is similar to that undertaken at birth but is now concerned with monitoring daily changes in the baby and detecting any signs of infection.

The skin is a barometer of the baby's hydration and general well-being. The midwife's knowledge of its normal parameters and minor variations assists in the interpretation of her findings.

The examination begins by noting the baby's posture and his colour and respirations. Any cyanosis should be reported to the paediatrician immediately. Jaundice may be noted from the third day and is abnormal if it arises earlier, deepens or persists beyond the seventh day.

Palpation of the head permits assessment of the anterior fontanelle, which should be level, resolution of caput succedaneum and moulding, and identification of any new swellings, for example cephalhaematoma (see Ch. 40).

The baby's eyes and mouth are inspected for signs of infection. Sticky eyes are cleaned with normal saline after obtaining a swab for culture and sensitivity testing. The mouth should be clean and moist. Adherent white plaques indicate oral thrush infection. Sucking blisters on the baby's lips may be observed, especially if he has been fed recently. These do not require any treatment.

As the baby is undressed his response to handling can be observed, his identity bands inspected and his responses to the midwife's voice noted as she talks to him and explains her actions to his mother.

The skin, especially in flexures and between the digits, is inspected for rashes, septic spots, excoriation or abrasions. Skin rashes such as erythema toxicum, a red blotchy rash, are of little significance. Sometimes a harlequin colour change may be noted when the infant is lying on his side, the dependent part of the body appearing pinker than the rest with a clear line of demarcation down the centre of the body. This is caused by vasomotor instability and is of little importance. However, its appearance is startling and can alarm the mother.

The fingertips and toes are examined for ragged nails and paronychia. Septic spots must be differentiated from milia which do not require treatment. Even a few septic spots must be taken seriously. The paediatrician may prescribe topical applications or systemic antibiotics and consider possible isolation of the baby. Areas that rub on cot sheets may become excoriated. If this occurs the affected part should be protected from further friction.

The umbilical cord base is inspected for redness and the mother is reminded about care.

In some areas the baby's temperature is recorded with a low-recording thermometer. This may be taken in the axilla, ear (tympanic membrane), in the groin or rectally. If the rectal route is used it is essential that the baby's legs and the thermometer are held to prevent sudden movement of the baby (which could cause the thermometer to break and perforate the rectum) and that the bulb of the thermometer is inserted no further than 2.5 cm into the rectum. Concern regarding the risk of injury has led to an increased use of alternative methods of measuring infants' temperatures. This concern must be balanced against the need for an accurate estimate of core temperature when babies are ill (Morley 1992). Midwives are advised to identify and abide by local policy in regard to taking temperatures rectally.

The stools are observed and compared with expectations in relation to the baby's age and feeding method. Constipation may be alleviated by offering the baby water between feeds. Loose watery stools may signify sugar intolerance or infection and may cause sore buttocks. Sore buttocks may be treated by exposure to the air but care must be taken to avoid chilling and the infant should be nursed on his side to prevent excoriation of his knees. The frequency of passing urine and stools in the preceding 24 hours should be noted.

Breast engorgement and pseudomenstruation

require no treatment but explanation to the mother is essential. No attempt should be made to express engorged breasts.

If the baby is to be weighed, this is done before he is dressed and the result compared with his birthweight. A common regimen is weighing every third day. Weight loss is normal in the first few days but more than 10% bodyweight loss is abnormal and requires investigation. Most babies regain their birthweight in 7–10 days, thereafter gaining weight at a rate of 150–200 g per week.

All findings at the daily examination are entered in the baby's records and abnormalities reported. Parents can be introduced to the concept of daily examination and gradually assume this responsibility as their confidence increases. This helps to enhance parent–baby interaction.

PROMOTING FAMILY RELATIONSHIPS

Parent–infant attachment

Positive responses from the baby to the attention or care given by the parents reinforce parental attachment and stimulate further interaction. Knowledge of the reflexes, general abilities and sleep and awake states of babies enables the midwife to teach the parents how to take advantage of the occasions when their baby is likely to be most responsive. The resulting interactions continue the process of attachment initiated at delivery (see Ch. 34). Admiration of the baby's best features, use of his given name and requesting the mother's permission to handle the baby help the woman to perceive herself as a mother.

Parents develop their relationship with their babies in individual ways and at their own pace. Some mothers feel somewhat distant from the baby at first; others experience an overwhelming protective urge and intense absorption with their babies (Jowitt 1996). It is important not to overemphasise 'bonding' as this may create non-productive guilt feelings in parents who do not experience instant love for their child and result in negative attitudes towards the baby (Billings 1995, Rutter 1995).

It is suggested that the parents' relationship

with one another is enhanced when the father is encouraged to be involved in discussions, choices and decisions about baby care and to share the responsibility for care. The resultant maternal confidence is reflected in her responsiveness toward her baby, thus promoting the infant's feeling of security (Adams & Cotgrove 1995). The father's reactions to and feelings about his baby should be afforded expression (Heath 1995, McLennan 1995). Parents may express anxiety about the possible reactions of siblings to the new arrival. A positive attitude on the part of the midwife can do much to allay fears which are often unfounded (Gullicks & Crase 1993).

Promoting confidence and competence

It is important that the midwife does not let her own maternal feelings 'take over', thus denying the mother opportunity to provide care for her baby. The father too should be encouraged to share in baby care. Total care should be delegated to the parents as soon as possible. In hospital especially, procedures can be rendered unnecessarily complicated for new mothers, many of whom have had no previous involvement with newborn babies (Thomas 1995). Teaching the principles rather than the minutiae of hospital procedures can help to overcome this. Dressing tips, for instance pulling rather than trying to push an arm through the sleeve of a jacket, are better understood by explaining the baby's response to passive movement.

Promoting communication

The increasing interest in baby massage in recent years capitalises on the knowledge that the baby is sensitive and responsive to touch (Adamson-Macedo 1992, Lim 1996, McLintock 1995). Grapeseed or sweet almond oil is used rather than baby oils which stick to the skin. Aromatherapy oils should not be used as the extent of their absorption is not known (McLintock, personal communication, 1996). The naked baby is stroked and caressed in a leisurely manner using the fingertips and palms of the hands. Throughout this quiet time together eye-to-eye contact is promoted by the close proximity of the baby, and the mother (or father) instinctively interacts with the baby's pleasurable responses. This assists in reinforcing the developing emotional relationship.

By applying her knowledge of the physiological and psychological capabilities and potential complications of the newborn, the midwife can ensure that optimal baby care is planned and provided and can do much to foster happy family relationships.

The foregoing discussions in this chapter have endeavoured to illustrate how the midwife can enhance the parent–baby relationship. Her teaching, support and encouragement of the mother as she learns to provide for her baby's needs is of paramount importance and should culminate in a happy, confident and competent mother being discharged from the midwife's care. The midwife can also do a great deal to encourage a father's interaction with his baby and should take every opportunity to do so. These aspects of midwifery practice are described more fully in Chapter 30.

READER ACTIVITIES

The mother's agreement should be obtained before undertaking these activities. Repeating the activity will help you notice differences between babies.

1. Compare the examination of the baby's head on day 1 and day 4 with regard to:

   a. fontanelle size
   b. overriding of the sutures
   c. measurement of occipitofrontal circumference.

2. Observe a baby who is awake. Is the baby in a drowsy, quiet alert, active alert or active crying state? Relate the awake state to the timing of the last feed or period of handling.

3. Examine a baby in a quiet alert state and endeavour to elicit:

   a. Moro reflex
   b. grasp, stepping and walking reflexes
   c. rooting reflex.

   Involve the mother in your observations.

4. Observe a sleeping baby. Determine whether the sleep is light or deep. Shine a light on the baby's face and observe the response. Repeat the action and note habituation. Repeat the exercise using sound, e.g. clapping your hands. Explain the baby's behaviour to the mother.

5. Keep a detailed record of the umbilical cords of 10 babies (five boys and five girls) with regard to:

   a. treatment – type, frequency, number of persons involved
   b. day of cord separation
   c. mother's reaction to the cord
   d. relevance, if any, of the sex of the baby.

6. Compare five breast-fed and five bottle-fed babies with regard to:

   a. stool pattern – colour, consistency, odour and frequency
   b. sleep/awake pattern
   c. feeding behaviour – sucking pattern, coordination between sucking, swallowing and breathing.

   Does the baby behave in the same way at each feed? Is the baby held in the same way at each feed? Does he have a preference to be held in the mother's right or left arm? How much eye contact is made with the mother?

7. Observe and record the interaction of 10 babies with their parents – five first babies, and five later babies. Note the response of each baby to the mother's voice in comparison with others; observe the baby's visual tracking; compare the patterns of stroking and touching by both parents.

8. Observe sibling reactions to the baby. Note:

   a. age and birth order of sibling(s)
   b. parental reactions to sibling interest/actions.

   Engage the sibling in talking about the new baby.

9. Observe crying babies and note:

a. crying pattern
b. colour
c. mother's reaction.

Does it make a difference if the mother has had a baby before? What strategies appear to soothe babies most? What is your own reaction to persistent crying?

10. Ascertain the addresses of local support groups for mothers of crying babies, e.g. CRY-SIS. Do the mothers in your care know about this help-line?

11. If available in your area, view a video about the capabilities of newborn babies. (Examples of videos are listed at the end of this chapter.)

REFERENCES

Adams L, Cotgrove A 1995 Promoting secure attachment patterns in infancy and beyond. Professional Care of Mother and Child 5(6): 158–160

Adamson-Macedo E 1992 TAC-TIC therapy: the importance of systematic stroking. British Journal of Midwifery 2(6): 244–269

Aronsson D D, Goldberg M J, Kling T F, Roy D R 1994 Developmental dysplasia of the hip. Pediatrics 94(2): 201–208

Bacon C J 1991 The thermal environment of sleeping babies and possible dangers of overheating. In: David T J (ed) Recent advances in paediatrics. Churchill Livingstone, Edinburgh

Barclay L, Harrington A, Conroy R, Royal R, Laforgia J 1994 A comparative study of neonates' umbilical cord management. Australian Journal of Advanced Nursing 11(3): 34–40

Beverley M, Nathan S 1995 Diagnosing developmental dysplasia of the hip (DDH). Maternal and Child Health 20(4): 120, 122–124

Billings J R 1995 Bonding theory – tying mothers in knots? A critical review of the application of a theory to nursing. Journal of Clinical Nursing 4(4): 207–211

Blackburn S T, Loper D L 1992 Maternal, fetal, and neonatal physiology: a clinical perspective. W B Saunders, Philadelphia, chs 5–12

Brazelton T B 1984 Neonatal behavioural assessment scale, 2nd edn. Spastics International Medical Publications, Blackwell Scientific, London

Crockett M 1995 Physiology of the neonatal immune system. Journal of Obstetric, Gynecologic, and Neonatal Nursing 24(7): 627–634

Damstra-Wijmenga S M I 1991 The memory of the newborn baby. Midwives Chronicle and Nursing Notes (March): 66–69

Day M 1995 Babies at risk as maternity units fail to step up security. Nursing Times 91(28): 6

DeCasper A, Fifer W 1987 Of human bonding: newborns prefer their mothers' voices. In: Oates J, Sheldon S (eds) Cognitive development in infancy. Lawrence Erlbaum Associates in association with the Open University, Hove

Doull I J M, McCaughey E S, Bailey B J R, Betts P R 1995 Reliability of infant length measurement. Archives of Disease in Childhood 72: 520–521

Downey J, Bidder R T 1990 Perinatal information on infant crying. Child: Care, Health and Development 16(2): 113–121

Foundation for the Study of Infant Deaths 1996 'Feet to Foot' – a new initiative to reduce sudden infant death. Press release. MIDIRS Midwifery Digest 6(1): 97

Fry T 1994 Monitoring children's growth: introducing the new child growth standards. Professional Care of Mother and Child 4(8): 231–233

Gandy G M 1992 Examination of the neonate including gestational age assessment. In: Roberton N R C (ed) Textbook of neonatology, 2nd edn. Churchill Livingstone, Edinburgh

Gonik B, Barrett K 1995 The persistence of newborn circumcision: an American perspective. British Journal of Obstetrics and Gynaecology 102(12): 940–941

Gullicks J N, Crase S J 1993 Sibling behaviour with a newborn: parents' expectations and observations. Journal of Obstetric, Gynecologic, and Neonatal Nursing 22(5): 438–444

Hall D, Hill P, Elliman D 1994 The child surveillance handbook, 2nd edn. Radcliffe Medical Press, Oxford

Heath T 1995 New fatherhood. New Generation (June): 11

Hull D, McArthur A J, Pritchard K, Goodall M 1996a Metabolic rate of sleeping infants. Archives of Disease in Childhood 75(4): 282–287

Hull D, McArthur A J, Pritchard K, Oldham D 1996b Individual variation in sleeping metabolic rates in infants. Archives of Disease in Childhood 75(4): 288–291

Jethwa K 1994 Nappy rash: a pharmaceutical approach. Professional Care of Mother and Child 4(7): 219–220

Jørgensen F S, Felding P, Vinther S, Andersen G 1991 Vitamin K to neonates. Peroral versus intramuscular administration. Acta Paediatrica 80: 304–307

Jowitt M 1996 Birth and bonding. Midwifery Matters 69(Summer): 3

Laurent C 1992 A mother's nightmare. Nursing Times 88(52): 18

Lerner H 1993 Sleep position of infants: applying research to practice. Maternal and Child Nursing 18(Sept/Oct): 275–277

Lim P 1996 Baby massage. British Journal of Midwifery 4(8): 439–441

MacFarlane A 1975 Olfaction in the development of social preferences in the human neonate. In: Parent–infant interaction. CIBA Foundation Symposium 33, Elsevier, Amsterdam

MacKeith N 1995 Who should examine the 'normal' neonate? Nursing Times 91(14): 34–35

McLennan I 1995 Ian's story. New Generation (June): 13

McLintock F 1995 Baby massage. Connections 26(2): 4–6

Michaelides S 1995 A deeper knowledge. Nursing Times 91(35)(suppl): 59–61

Michie M 1996 A delicate concern: caring for neonatal skin. British Journal of Midwifery 4(3): 159–163

Morley C 1992 Measuring infants' temperatures. Midwives Chronicle and Nursing Notes (Feb): 26–29

Moss G D, Cartlidge P H T, Speides B D, Chambers T L 1991 Routine examination in the neonatal period. British Medical Journal 302: 878–879

Mugford M, Somchiwong M, Waterhouse I 1986 Treatment of umbilical cords: a randomised trial to assess the effect of treatment methods on the work of midwives. Midwifery 2: 177–186

Penny-MacGillivray T 1996 A newborn's first bath: when? Journal of Obstetric, Gynecologic, and Neonatal Nursing 25(6): 481–487

Perry S E 1995 Nursing care of the newborn. In: Bobak I M, Lowdermilk D L, Jensen M D (eds) Maternity nursing, 4th edn. Mosby, St Louis, Ch. 14

Rabinowitz R, Hulbert W C 1995 Newborn circumcision should not be performed without anaesthesia. Birth 22(1): 45–46

Righard L 1995 How do newborns find their mother's breast? Birth 22(3): 174–175

Roberton N R C 1992 Care of the normal term newborn baby. In: Roberton N R C (ed) Textbook of neonatology, 2nd edn. Churchill Livingstone, Edinburgh

Roberton N R C 1996 A manual of normal neonatal care, 3rd edn. Edward Arnold, London

Rose S 1994 Physical examination of the full-term baby. British Journal of Midwifery 2(5): 209–213

Rush J 1990 Care of the umbilical cord. In: Alexander J, Levy V, Roch S (eds) Midwifery practice: postnatal care – a research-based approach. Macmillan, Basingstoke

Rushforth J A, Levene M I 1994 Behavioural response to pain in healthy neonates. Archives of Disease in Childhood 70(3): F174–F176

Rutter N 1992 Temperature control and its disorders. In: Roberton N R C (ed) Textbook of neonatology, 2nd edn. Churchill Livingstone, Edinburgh

Rutter M 1995 Clinical implications of attachment concepts: retrospect and prospect. Journal of Child Psychology and Psychiatry 36(4): 549–571

Salariya E, Kowbus N 1988 Variable umbilical cord care. Midwifery 4: 70–76

Shearer M J 1995 Vitamin K. Lancet 345(8944): 229–234

Stern C M 1992 Neonatal immunology. In: Roberton N R C (ed) Textbook of neonatology, 2nd edn. Churchill Livingstone, Edinburgh

Thomas G 1995 Empowerment. The baby bath demonstration. Midwives 108(1289): 178

Thomas K 1994 Thermoregulation in neonates. Neonatal Network 13(2): 15–22

Verber I G, Pagan F S 1993 What cord care – if any? Archives of Disease in Childhood 68(5)(Fetal and Neonatal edn): 594–596

FURTHER READING

American Academy of Pediatrics 1989 Committee on Fetus and Newborn: report of the ad hoc task force on circumcision. Pediatrics 84: 388

Arbiter E, Sato R, Kolvin I 1995 Cross-cultural differences in mother–infant relationships: implications for a multi-cultural society. Maternal and Child Health 20(10): 336–338

Bobak I M, Lowdermilk D L, Jensen M D (eds) 1995 Maternity nursing, 4th edn. Mosby, St Louis

Bowers-Clarke M 1993 Baby massage. New Generation 12(3): 4–5

Brant H 1985 Childbirth for men. Oxford Medical, Oxford

Condo A S, Nishioka E 1993 Neonatal assessment. In: Kenner C, Brueggemeyer A, Gunderson L P (eds) Comprehensive neonatal nursing: a physiologic perspective. W B Saunders, Philadelphia, ch 17

Croucher C, Azzopardi D 1994 Compliance with recommendations for giving vitamin K to newborn infants. British Medical Journal 308(2 Apr): 894–895

Davies L 1995 Babies co-sleeping with parents. Midwives 108(1295): 384–386

Draper G, Ninch A 1994 Vitamin K for neonates: the controversy. British Medical Journal 308(2 Apr): 867–868

Fowlie P, Forsyth S 1994 Common problems of newborn infants. Modern Midwife 4(12): 16–19

Fowlie P, Forsyth S 1995 Examination of the newborn infant. Modern Midwife 5(1): 15–18

Gelbaum I 1993 Circumcision: refining a traditional surgical technique. Journal of Nurse–Midwifery 38(2)(suppl): 18S–30S

Gordon A 1995 Why do we still circumcise male babies? British Journal of Obstetrics and Gynaecology 102(12): 939–940

Hepper P G, Scott D, Shahidullah S 1993 Newborn and fetal response to maternal voice. Journal of Reproductive and Infant Psychology 11(3): 147–153

Hiley C M H, Morley C 1995 What do mothers remember about the 'Back to Sleep' campaign? Archives of Disease in Childhood 73(6): 496–497

Holditch-Davis D 1993 Neonatal sleep–wake states. In: Kenner C, Brueggemeyer A, Gunderson L P (eds) Comprehensive neonatal nursing: a physiologic perspective. W B Saunders, Philadelphia, ch 49

Kenner C, Brueggemeyer A, Gunderson L P (eds) 1993 Comprehensive neonatal nursing: a physiologic perspective. W B Saunders, Philadelphia

Klaus M H, Kennell J H 1996 Bonding: building the foundations of secure attachment and independence. Cedar, London

Klonoff-Cohen, Edelstein S L 1995 Bed-sharing and sudden infant death syndrome. British Medical Journal 311(Nov 11): 1269–1272

McKenna J J, Moskos S S 1994 Sleep and arousal, synchrony and independence, among mothers and infants sleeping apart and together (same bed): an experiment in evolutionary medicine. Acta Paediatrica Supplement 397: 94–102

O'Kane M 1995 Evaluating cord care. Nursing Times 91(29)(suppl): 57–58

Olds S B, London M L, Ladewig P W 1996 Maternal–newborn nursing: a family centered approach. 5th edn. Addison Wesley, Menlo Park, California, chs 23, 27, 28, 29

Perry S E 1995 The newborn. In: Bobak I M, Lowdermilk D L, Jensen M D (eds) Maternity nursing, 4th edn. Mosby, St Louis, ch 13

Pinyard B J 1994 Infant cries: physiology and assessment. Neonatal Network 13(4): 15–20

Price S, Price L 1995 Aromatherapy for health professionals. Churchill Livingstone, Edinburgh

Rush J, Chalmers I, Enkin M 1990 Care of the new mother and baby. In: Chalmers I, Enkin M, Keirse M J N C (eds) Effective care in pregnancy and childbirth Vol 2 Childbirth. Oxford University Press, Oxford, ch 78

Russell J 1993 Touch and infant massage. Pediatric Nursing 5(3): 8–11

Salariya E 1990 Parent–infant attachment. In: Alexander J, Levy V, Roch S (eds) Postnatal care – a research based approach. Macmillan, Basingstoke

Salariya E M, Robertson C M 1993 The development of a neonatal stool comparator. Midwifery 9(1): 35–40

Scowen P 1996 Safe not sorry: preventing baby and child accidents. Professional Care of Mother and Child 6(2): 47–49

Sheeran M S 1996 Thermoregulation in neonates: obtaining an accurate axillary temperature measurement. Journal of Neonatal Nursing 2(4): 6–9

Sinclair J C 1992 Management of the thermal environment. In: Sinclair J C, Bracken M B (eds) Effective care of the newborn infant. Oxford Medical, Oxford, ch 4

Sluckin W, Sluckin A, Herbert M 1984 On mother-to-infant bonding. Midwife, Health Visitor and Community Nurse 20(2): 404–407

Stratton P (ed) 1982 Psychobiology of the human newborn. Development psychology series. John Wiley, Chichester

Swartz M K 1992 Primary care and differential diagnosis of the newborn: general considerations for the CNM. Journal of Nurse-Midwifery 37(2)(suppl): 18S–26S

Thorpe-Raghdo B 1995 Newborn examinations – another delivery service. MIDIRS Midwifery Digest 5(4): 459

Tuffnell C S, Petersen S A, Wailoo M P 1996 Higher rectal temperatures in co-sleeping infants. Archives of Disease in Childhood 75(3): 249–250

Tyler S 1996 Catching up with vitamin K. Midwives 109(1305): 273

Walker P 1995 Baby massage. Judy Piatkus Publishers, London

Watson J 1990 Screening for congenital dislocation of the hip. Maternal and Child Health 15(10): 310, 312–314

Weiss M E, Poelter D, Gocka I 1994 Infrared tympanic thermometry for neonatal temperature assessment. Journal of Obstetric, Gynecologic, and Neonatal Nursing 23(9): 798–804

Weiss M E, Richards M T 1994 Accuracy of electronic axillary temperature measurement in term and preterm neonates. Neonatal Network 13(8): 35–40

Wellington N, Rieder M J 1993 Attitudes and practices regarding analgesia for newborn circumcision. Pediatrics 92(2): 541–543

Wells N, King J, Hedstrom C, Youngkins J 1995 Does tympanic temperature measure up? Maternal and Child Nursing 20(2): 95–100

Williams R P 1995 Family dynamics after childbirth. In: Bobak I M, Lowdermilk D L, Jensen M D (eds) Maternity nursing, 4th edn. Mosby, St Louis, ch 17

Wong D L (ed) 1995 Whaley and Wong's nursing care of infants and children, 5th edn. Mosby, St Louis, ch 8

VIDEOTAPES

Gregg C 1979 Getting to know each other. Plymouth Medical Films, Plymouth

Morris D 1992 Babywatching. Lifetime Broadcast, distributed by Polygram Video

Watkins R 1993 Baby massage: a video for parents and carers. From Birth and Beyond, MIDIRS Book Service, Bristol

Feeding

Chloe Fisher

Many hours of the mother's time, day and night for many months, will be spent feeding her baby. She should be supported in the feeding method of her choice and enabled to accomplish it with skill, knowledge, confidence and pleasure. A firm mother–baby attachment can be forged during these frequent encounters, provided that they proceed without anxiety. When breast feeding goes well, there is the added advantage of the mother's sense of achievement and satisfaction. For these reasons alone, breast feeding must be the ideal way to feed a baby.

The chapter aims to:

- describe the structure and function of the female breast

- outline the properties and components of breast milk

- discuss breast feeding with particular emphasis on the role of the midwife in ensuring success for both mother and baby

- consider the different causes of difficulty with breast feeding

- discuss bottle feeding and the various products available.

The World Health Organization's definition of a midwife includes the ability to give skilled supervision, care and advice to the mother during the postpartum period and to give care to the newborn baby and the young infant. Responsibility for the initiation of infant feeding and lactation therefore lies with the midwifery profession. The International Confederation of Midwives adopted a policy about breast feeding in 1984 which clearly defines the midwife's responsibility in this field and describes the 'unique and vital role of the midwife in the promotion of breast feeding' (ICM 1985).

THE BREAST AND BREAST MILK

In developing countries, where the knowledge and skills of breast feeding have been retained within society, women consider it the normal thing to do. In these countries midwives will encourage mothers to breast feed because of the protection against infection conferred on the baby and breast feeding will have an excellent chance of being successful. On the other hand, in the so-called developed world, the midwife should recognise that the majority of women who choose to breast feed do so because they regard it as the fulfilment of motherhood and are less conscious of the benefits of human milk for their babies. Unfortunately, there is currently a high failure rate which must in part be attributed to lack of knowledge and loss of skills. It is most important for midwives to understand the benefits of human milk for human babies because this will help to inspire them in their supportive role (Howie et al 1990, Lucas & Cole 1990). This knowledge should be shared with mothers but should not be used to put undue pressure on them.

Anatomy and physiology of the breast (Fig. 36.1)

The breasts are compound secreting glands, composed mainly of glandular tissue which is arranged in *lobes*, approximately 20 in number. Each lobe is divided into *lobules* that consist of *alveoli* and *ducts*. The alveoli contain *acini cells* which produce milk and are surrounded by *myoepithelial cells* which contract and propel the milk out (Fig. 36.2). The breasts are richly supplied with blood. Small *lactiferous ducts*, carrying milk from the alveoli, unite to form larger ducts; one large duct leaves each lobe and widens to form a *lactiferous sinus* or *ampulla* which acts as a temporary reservoir for milk. A *lactiferous tubule* from each sinus emerges on the surface of the nipple. Each breast functions independently of the other.

The *nipple*, composed of erectile tissue, is covered with epithelium and contains plain muscle fibres which have a sphincter-like action in controlling the flow of milk. Surrounding the nipple is an area of pigmented skin called the *areola* which contains *Montgomery's glands*. These produce a

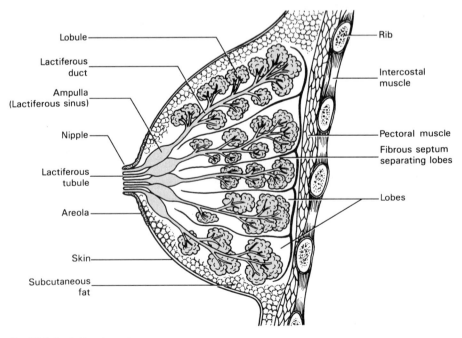

Fig. 36.1 Lactating breast.

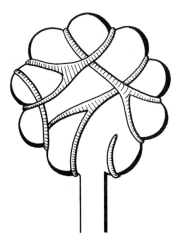

Fig. 36.2 Alveoli surrounded by myoepithelial cells which propel the milk out of the lobule.

sebum-like substance which acts as a lubricant during pregnancy and throughout breast feeding. Breasts, nipples and areolae vary considerably in size from one woman to another.

The breast is supplied with blood from the internal and external mammary arteries and branches from the intercostal arteries. The veins are arranged in a circular fashion around the nipple.

Lymph drains freely between the two breasts and into lymph nodes in the axillae and the mediastinum.

During pregnancy, oestrogens and progesterone induce alveolar and ductal growth as well as stimulating the secretion of *colostrum*. Other hormones are also involved and they govern a complex sequence of events which prepare the breast for lactation. The production of milk is held in abeyance until after delivery, when the levels of placental hormones fall. This allows the already high levels of prolactin to initiate milk production. Continued production of prolactin is caused by the baby feeding at the breast, with concentrations highest during night feeds. Prolactin suppresses ovulation and causes some women to remain anovulatory until lactation ceases, although for others this effect is not so prolonged (Kennedy et al 1989, Ramos et al 1996). If breast feeding (or expressing) has to be delayed for a few days, lactation can still be initiated because prolactin levels remain

high, even in the absence of breast use, for at least the first week (Kochenour 1980).

Prolactin seems to be much more important to the initiation of lactation than to its continuation. As lactation progresses, the prolactin response to suckling diminishes and milk removal becomes the driving force behind milk production (Applebaum 1970). This is in part due to the removal of the autocrine inhibitory factor (sometimes referred to as FIL – feedback inhibitor of lactation) which builds up over time and if not removed (by the baby feeding or breast expression) inhibits further milk synthesis (Daly 1993, Prentice et al 1989).

Milk release is under *neuroendocrine control*. Tactile stimulation of the breast stimulates the production of oxytocin causing contraction of the myoepithelial cells. This process is known as the '*let-down*' or '*milk-ejection*' *reflex* and makes the milk available to the baby. This occurs in discrete pulses throughout the feed and may well trigger the bursts of active feeding. In the early days of lactation this reflex is unconditioned and is therefore unlikely to be inhibited by anxiety. Later it becomes a conditioned reflex responding to the baby's cry (or other circumstances associated with the baby or feeding). At this stage it could be inhibited to some extent by anxiety. Although this may make the feed a little longer, it has no effect on either prolactin levels or the amount of milk the baby receives (Ueda et al 1994) The active removal of milk by the action of the baby's tongue and jaw plays a greater part than milk ejection in determining the quality and quantity of milk the baby receives.

Properties and components of breast milk

Human milk varies in its composition:

- with the time of day
- with the stage of lactation
- in response to maternal nutrition
- because of individual variations.

Fore-milk, at the beginning of the feed, differs from hind-milk, towards the end of the feed. Samples obtained for research may not represent the milk obtained by the baby because of the methods used for collection. Comparison with the milks of other mammals shows human milk to be unique. It meets all the nutritional requirements of the new baby and has many other important properties as well.

Fat provides the baby with more than 50% of his calorific requirements (Helsing & Savage King 1982). The fat content in human milk has diurnal variations, being lowest in the morning and highest in the afternoon. The proportion of fat in the milk increases during the course of the feed, sometimes increasing to five times the initial value. It is utilised very rapidly because of the action of the enzyme *lipase* which is present in the milk in a form which only becomes active in the infant's intestine. Pancreatic lipase is not plentiful in the newborn baby.

Lactose. There is more lactose in human milk than in any other mammalian milk. It is converted into galactose and glucose by the action of the enzyme *lactase* and these sugars provide energy to the rapidly growing brain. Lactose enhances the absorption of calcium and also promotes the growth of lactobacilli which increase intestinal acidity, thus stemming the growth of pathogenic organisms.

Protein. Human milk contains less protein than any other mammalian milk (Akre 1990a) and this accounts in part for its more 'transparent' appearance. Human milk is whey dominant (the whey being mainly alpha-lactalbumin) and forms soft, flocculent curds when acidified in the stomach. This provides a continuous flow of nutrients to the baby.

Colostrum contains nearly three times the amount of protein that is present in mature milk and contains all the essential amino acids. It also contains secretory IgA and *lactoferrin* (see below).

Allergic problems occur less frequently in breast-fed babies than in bottle-fed babies. This may be because the infant's intestinal mucosa is permeable to proteins before the age of 6–9 months and proteins in cow's milk can act as allergens. In particular, beta-lactoglobulin, which has no human milk protein counterpart, is capable of producing antigenic responses in atopic infants (Adler & Warner 1991, Bahna 1987). Bovine serum albumin,

present only in formula, has recently been implicated as the trigger for the development of insulin-dependent diabetes mellitus (Carvahlo et al 1996, Karjalainen et al 1992, Monte et al 1994).

Occasionally a baby may react adversely to substances in his mother's milk which come from her diet. This is rare and can be resolved by the mother identifying and avoiding the foods which cause the trouble so that she may continue to breast feed.

Fat-soluble vitamins

There are four fat-soluble vitamins, A, D, E and K.

Vitamin A. Mature human milk contains 280 international units (IU) of vitamin A, and colostrum contains twice that amount.

Vitamin D. It is now believed that both water-soluble and fat-soluble vitamin D are present in human milk. Provided that the mother's diet is adequate and the baby can be exposed to the sun, the baby's vitamin D status should be satisfactory. The babies of dark-skinned mothers living in temperate zones and preterm babies may be the exceptions, in which case it may be safer to give the supplement to the mother (Pyke 1986).

Vitamin E. Although present in human milk, its role is uncertain. It appears to prevent the oxidisation of polyunsaturated fatty acids and may prevent certain types of anaemia to which preterm infants are susceptible.

Vitamin K. This vitamin is essential for the synthesis of blood-clotting factors. It is present in human milk and absorbed efficiently. Recent research suggests that the breast-fed baby may receive more vitamin K than has previously been demonstrated because it has been discovered that levels are higher in colostrum and, in the early days, in the high-fat hind-milk (Kries et al 1987). Later, levels depend on maternal dietary intake. Babies who are at risk of haemorrhage, such as the preterm and those delivered precipitately or instrumentally, commonly receive a prophylactic dose, usually by intramuscular injection. Many paediatricians currently consider that all breast-fed babies should receive vitamin K soon after birth. After 2 weeks the breast-fed baby's gut flora should be synthesising adequate amounts of vitamin K (Akre 1990b). Colonisation of the gut may be aided by encouraging the mother not to wash her breasts, or otherwise clean them before a feed.

Water-soluble vitamins

Vitamin B complex. All of the B vitamins are present at levels which are believed to provide the baby with his necessary daily requirements.

Vitamin C. Human milk contains 43 mg/100 ml of vitamin C. This vitamin is essential for collagen synthesis.

Unless the mother's diet is seriously deficient, breast milk will contain adequate levels of all the vitamins. Since most vitamins are fairly widely distributed in foods, a diet significantly deficient in one vitamin will be deficient in others as well. Thus an improved diet will be more beneficial than artificial supplements.

Minerals and trace elements

Iron. Normal full-term babies are usually born with a high haemoglobin level (16–22 g/dl) which decreases rapidly after birth. The iron recovered from haemoglobin breakdown is utilised again. They also have ample iron stores, sufficient for at least 4–6 months. Although the amounts of iron are less than those found in formula, the bioavailability of iron in breast milk is very much higher; 70% of the iron in breast milk is absorbed whereas only 10% is absorbed from formula (Saarinen & Siimes 1979). The difference is due to a complex series of interactions which take place within the gut. Babies who are fed fresh cow's milk or formula may become anaemic because of microhaemorrhages of the bowel. Preterm babies do not have good iron stores and may need supplementation with oral iron.

Zinc. This trace mineral is essential to humans. A deficiency may result in failure to thrive and typical skin lesions. Although there is more zinc present in formula than in human milk, the bioavailability is greater in human milk.

Other minerals. Human milk has significantly lower levels of calcium, phosphorus, sodium and potassium than formula. Copper, cobalt and selenium are present at higher levels. The higher bioavailability of these minerals and trace elements ensures that the infant's needs are met whilst also imposing a lower solute load on the neonatal kidney than does formula. If a baby is fed on 'doorstep' milk he may become dehydrated due to hypernatraemia (excess sodium). The breast-fed baby does not ingest an overload of salts and is therefore unlikely to need additional water under most conditions (Almroth 1978, Goldberg & Adams 1983, Sachdev et al 1991).

Anti-infective factors

Leucocytes. During the first 10 days there are more white cells per ml than there are in blood. *Macrophages* and *neutrophils* are amongst the most common leucocytes in human milk and they surround and destroy harmful bacteria by their phagocytic activity.

Secretory IgA and interferon are important anti-infective agents produced in abundance by lymphocytes in human milk.

Immunoglobulins IgA, IgG, IgM and IgD are all found in human milk. Of these the most important is IgA, which appears to be both synthesised and stored in the breast. It 'paints' the intestinal epithelium and protects the mucosal surfaces against entry of pathogenic bacteria and enteroviruses. It affords protection against *Escherichia coli*, salmonellae, shigellae, streptococci, staphylococci, pneumococci, poliovirus and the rotaviruses.

Lysozyme is present in breast milk in concentrations 5000 times greater than in cow's milk. It is a well-known general anti-infective agent and its activity appears to increase during lactation.

Lactoferrin is abundant in human milk but is not present in cow's milk. It affects the absorption of enteric iron, thus preventing pathogenic *E. coli* from obtaining the iron they need for survival.

The bifidus factor in human milk promotes the growth of Gram-positive bacilli in the gut flora, particularly *Lactobacillus bifidus*, which discourages the multiplication of pathogens. Babies who are fed on cow's milk formula have more potentially pathogenic bacilli in their gut flora.

MANAGEMENT OF BREAST FEEDING

Medical involvement in infant feeding is known to have occurred throughout the history of the human race. Modern medicine entered the 'scientific' era early this century and, as a result, many practitioners came to believe that they had knowledge which would enable them to improve upon nature and they applied this belief to the management of breast feeding. Unfortunately, they were unaware of the fact that each mother–baby pair is unique and that the 'rules' that they evolved would be inappropriate for the majority. Another unfortunate fact is that when information is published in a medical textbook, it is repeated in further editions as well as in textbooks by other authors. In this manner, an idea that may have been speculative and never tested soon becomes an accepted 'truth'.

There are many examples of ideas about breast feeding which originated in the first 20 years of this century and were never properly tested. Some were still to be found in textbooks in use in the 1990s. A few *fallacies* will serve to illustrate this point:

• 'During the first few days of breast feeding, the length of the feed should be limited to prevent sore nipples'. (This must have been based on a mistaken belief that the baby fed from the nipple, not the breast.)
• 'Both breasts must be used at each feed'.
• 'The baby should feed for 10 minutes at each breast' or 'feeds should last only 20 minutes'.
• 'The breast must be held away from the baby's nose during a feed'.
• 'The baby should feed at regular intervals'.

These are the most common errors that were perpetuated over a period of more than 60 years. They have been repeated in both medical and midwifery textbooks because the authors relied on the writings of other 'experts' rather than common sense or research evidence. Such evidence is now available.

Antenatal preparation

The majority of women know before they conceive that they want to breast feed their babies (R. Thompson, personal communication). It is, however, important to inform all pregnant women about the benefits of breast feeding. A few may not make a final decision until after giving birth, so it is important that the midwife should have a sensitive approach and not require a definite decision. Time should also be taken during antenatal classes to talk briefly about the day-to-day progress and management of early breast feeding. The woman should at the very least be aware that breast feeding is a learned skill, that it should not hurt and that she may well receive conflicting advice. This does not mean that she will not require to be taught about the major details of management *after* the baby is born as some pregnant women find it difficult to project their thoughts forward to the time beyond the birth.

Breasts and nipples are altered by pregnancy (see Ch. 11). Increased sebum secretion obviates the need for cream to lubricate the nipple. A comfortable brassiere that does not compress the breast may be worn to support the increasing weight but this will not affect the changes in the shape of the breast which occur as a result of pregnancy. Anatomically small nipples cannot be altered by preparation but they are no bar to satisfactory breast feeding. Women who have inverted and non-protractile (flat) nipples often find that they improve spontaneously during pregnancy (Hytten & Baird 1958). If not, help given with attaching the baby to the breast after birth often results in successful breast feeding (Hytten 1954). The wearing of Woolwich shells inside a brassiere and gentle stretching of the breast tissue at the base of the nipple (Hoffmann's exercises) which have both been recommended for many years, are now known to be of no value (Main Trial Collaborative Group 1994).

Education of the mother is better preparation than any physical exercises. If she understands how milk is produced and has an opportunity to observe babies feeding, she will be well on the way to success with feeding her own.

Technique

The commencement of breast feeding

The first feed is a profoundly important experience for the mother and her baby. If it proceeds without pain and if the baby is allowed to terminate the feed naturally, both will have been helped to begin the learning process necessary for good breast feeding in a happy and positive way. This feed should be supervised by the midwife. Unless individual circumstances dictate otherwise, the mother should have her baby with her immediately after birth. Early and extended contact will ensure that the cues that indicate that the baby is ready to feed will not be missed.

Early feeding contributes to the success of breast feeding but the time of the first feed should, to a large extent, depend on the needs of the baby. Some may demonstrate a desire to feed almost as soon as they are born. Many midwives use this as a means to facilitate uterine contractions during the third stage of labour and thereby reduce blood loss. Other babies may show no interest until they are an hour or so old (Righard & Alade 1990, Widström et al 1987). Babies of mothers who have received narcotics during labour may sleep for some time before wanting to feed.

Whenever the first feed takes place, the quality of that experience is of the utmost importance. Mothers who receive the right help and education at the start will require less support and remedial intervention later.

They should be told about the cause, and therefore prevention, of sore nipples (see below). They should be urged to seek help if problems do arise. They should be told about the changes that will take place in their breasts during the next few days. An explanation about the changes in the pattern of feeds and the reasons for the variation in the length of feeds will enable them to greet these changes with confidence. Helping them to understand that breast feeding is a learned, not an instinctive, skill will enable them to be patient with themselves and their babies during this time (Royal College of Midwives 1991).

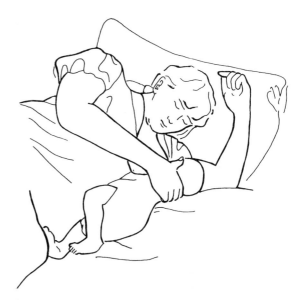

Fig. 36.3 Mother lying comfortably on her side.

Positioning the mother

There are two main positions for the mother to adopt while she is breast feeding. The first is lying on her side and this may be appropriate at different times during her lactation (Fig. 36.3). If she has had a caesarean section, or if her perineum is very painful, this may be the only position she can tolerate in the first few days after birth. She will need assistance in placing the baby at the breast because it will be difficult for her to manipulate him skilfully. When feeding from the lower breast it may be helpful to raise her body slightly by tucking the end of a pillow under her ribs. Later she may choose to feed lying down after she and her baby have learned how to breast feed, either during the day because she finds it more comfortable and restful or at night because it is more convenient.

The second position is sitting up. In the early days it is particularly important that the mother's back is upright and at a right angle to her lap (Fig. 36.4). This is not possible if she is sitting in bed with her legs stretched out in front of her (though she might be able to achieve it by sitting cross-legged) or if she is sitting in a chair with a deep backward-sloping seat and a sloping back.

Both lying on her side and sitting correctly in

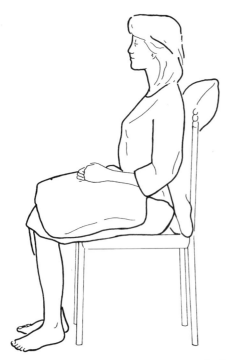

Fig. 36.4 Mother sitting with upright back and flat lap.

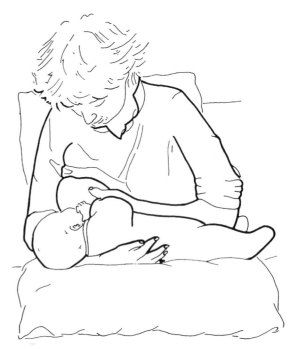

Fig. 36.5 The baby's body turned towards the mother's body.

a chair (with her back and feet supported) enhance the shape of the breast and also allow ample room in which to manoeuvre the baby.

Positioning the baby's body

The baby's body should be turned towards the mother's body (Fig. 36.5). If the baby's nose is opposite the nipple before he is brought to the breast and the neck is slightly extended, the baby's mouth will be in the correct relationship to the nipple (Fig. 36.6).

Attaching the baby to the breast

The baby should be supported across his shoulders, so that the slight extension of the neck can be maintained. The head may be supported by the extended fingers of the supporting hand (Fig. 36.7) or on the mother's forearm (Fig. 36.8). It may be helpful to wrap the baby firmly in a small sheet so that his hands are by his sides (Fig. 36.9). If the baby's mouth is moved gently but persistently against his mother's nipple he will open his mouth

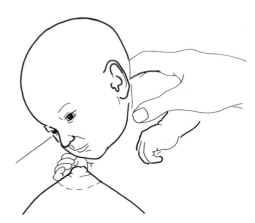

Fig. 36.6 The baby's mouth opposite the nipple, the neck slightly extended.

wide (Fig. 36.10). As he gapes (drops his lower jaw and darts his tongue down and forward) he is moved quickly to the breast. The intention is to aim the bottom lip at least ½ inch (1.5 cm) away from the base of the nipple. This allows the baby to draw breast tissue as well the nipple into his

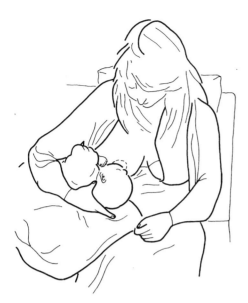

Fig. 36.7 The baby's head supported by the mother's extended fingers.

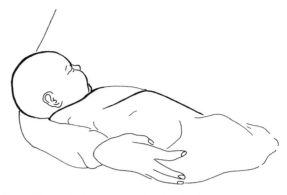

Fig. 36.9 The baby wrapped firmly with hands by sides.

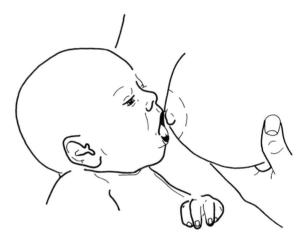

Fig. 36.10 Wide gape, with tongue down and forward.

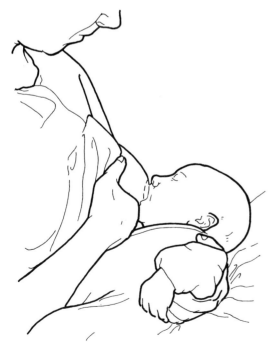

Fig. 36.8 The baby's head supported on the mother's forearm.

mouth with his tongue. If correctly attached, the baby will have formed a 'teat' from the breast and the nipple. The lactiferous sinuses will now be within the baby's mouth (Fig. 36.11) (Woolridge 1986). The nipple should extend as far as the junction of the hard and soft palate. Contact with the hard palate triggers the *sucking reflex*. The baby's lower jaw moves up and down, following the action of the tongue. If the baby is well attached, minimal suction is required to hold the 'teat' within the oral cavity and the tongue can then apply rhythmical cycles of compression so that milk is stripped from the ducts. Although the mother may be startled by the physical sensation, she should not experience pain.

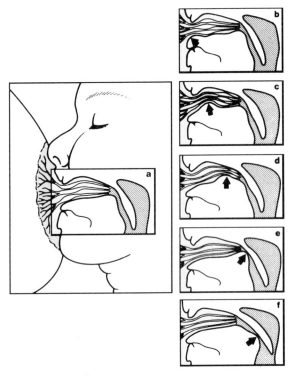

Fig. 36.11 The baby has formed a 'teat' from the breast and the nipple, which causes the nipple to extend back as far as the junction of the hard and soft palates. The lactiferous sinuses are within the baby's mouth. A generous portion of areola is covered by the bottom lip. (Reproduced from Woolridge 1986.)

The role of the midwife

The midwife's role during the first few feeds is twofold. First, she must ensure that the baby is adequately fed at the breast. Second, she must help the mother to develop the necessary skills so that she is able to feed her baby by herself. Some mothers will need more teaching and support than others; even women who have breast fed previously may require help with their new babies. Correct attachment of the baby to the breast prevents many breast-feeding problems.

In practical terms it may be necessary for the midwife to help attach the baby to the breast for several feeds. In this case she should think of her own comfort, as well as that of the mother and her baby, because she will be much less capable of providing skilled help if she is strained and

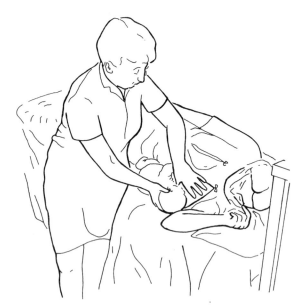

Fig. 36.12 The mother lying on her left side with the midwife helping her baby to feed at the left breast.

uncomfortable. She should also consider which hand guides the baby most skilfully and use it for preference. For example, she may be helping a mother who is lying on her left side and have successfully attached the baby to the left breast with her right hand (Fig. 36.12). Instead of asking the mother to turn on her right side she could raise up the baby on a pillow and attach him to the right breast, again using her right hand (Fig. 36.13). If the mother is sitting up, she could consider placing the baby under the mother's arm on the side she finds less easy (Fig. 36.14). Some midwives feel more comfortable if they stand behind the mother so that they get the same view as she does. Once the baby has fed efficiently he is more likely to do so again and it is from this point that the mother can begin to learn how to feed her baby by herself.

The midwife must give the mother positive, correct advice.

The baby feeds from the breast rather than from the nipple and the mother should guide her baby towards her breast without distorting its shape. *The baby's neck should be slightly extended* and *the chin should be in contact with the breast.* A generous portion of areola should be taken in by the lower

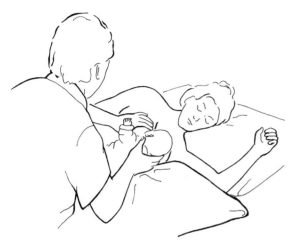

Fig. 36.13 The mother still on her left side with the midwife helping the baby to feed from the right breast.

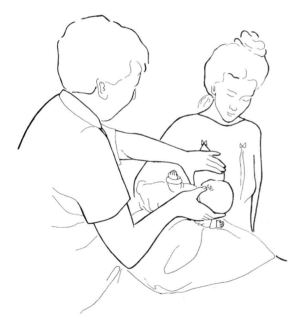

Fig. 36.14 The baby placed under the mother's arm with midwife helping.

jaw but the baby is often unable to draw in the whole of the areola.

Feeding behaviour

When the baby first goes to the breast he feeds vigorously, with few pauses. As the feed progresses, pausing occurs more frequently and lasts longer. Pausing is an integral part of the baby's feeding rhythm and should not be interrupted. The midwife should simply encourage the mother to allow herself to be paced by the baby. The change in the pattern probably relates to milk flow. The *fore-milk* which he obtains first is more generous in quantity but lower in fat than the *hind-milk* delivered at the end, which is thus higher in calories (Woolridge & Fisher 1988).

If the baby receives an excessive quantity of fore-milk (owing to either poor attachment or premature breast switching – see below), it may result in increased gut fermentation causing colic, flatus and explosive stools (Woolridge & Fisher 1988).

This is the commonest cause of colic in breast-fed babies and is resolved by improving attachment. Simethicone preparations which are often prescribed for this condition have been shown to be of no value (Metcalf et al 1994).

Finishing the first breast and finishing a feed

The baby will release the breast when he has had sufficient milk from it. His ability to know this may be controlled either by the calories he has received or by the change in the volume available. The baby should be offered the second breast after he has had the opportunity to bring up wind. Sometimes in the early days the baby will not need to feed from the second breast. Taking the baby off the first breast before he has finished may cause two problems. Firstly, the baby is deprived of the high-calorie hind-milk and secondly, if adequate milk removal has not taken place, milk stasis may occur, leading to mastitis or diminution of secretion. Provided that the baby starts each feed on alternate sides, both breasts will function equally. If the baby does not release the breast or will not settle after a feed, the most likely reason is that he had not been correctly attached to the breast and was therefore unable to strip the milk efficiently.

Other reasons for coming off the breast

- The baby may not have been correctly attached.
- The baby may need to let go and pause if the milk flow is very fast.

- The baby may have swallowed air with the generous flow of milk that occurs at the beginning of a feed and need an opportunity to bring it up.

Timing and frequency of feeds

If the length of the feed is determined by the baby from the beginning, the feed lengths will be fairly long, as will the intervals between. This is described as *baby-led feeding* which is a term preferable to 'demand feeding'. It is not unusual in the first day or two for the baby to have 6- to 8-hour gaps between good feeds (Inch & Garforth 1989, Waldenström & Swensen 1991). This is normal and provides an excellent opportunity for the mother to rest. As the milk volume increases, the feeds become more frequent and a little shorter. It is unusual for a baby to feed less often than six times in 24 hours from the third day. If he demands fewer feeds he may also be taking less than he needs at each feed. Reasons for this include drowsiness, immaturity and illness. Each possibility should be investigated. The feeding technique and the weight should be monitored. Individual mother–baby pairs develop their own unique pattern of feeding and, provided the baby is thriving, there is no need to change it.

Volume of the feed

Well-grown term infants are born with good glycogen reserves and high levels of antidiuretic hormone. Consequently they do not need large volumes of milk or colostrum any sooner than they are made available physiologically. In the first 24 hours the baby takes an average of 5 ml per feed; in the second 24 hours this increases to 14 ml per feed (Moody et al 1996).

No precise information is available on the actual volume of breast milk which an individual baby requires in order to grow satisfactorily. Previous recommendations (150 ml per kg) were based on the requirements of artificially fed babies, and these can therefore be used only as a guideline. If the baby's initial weight loss exceeds 10%, his intake is clearly inadequate and the mother needs help. If the baby has regained his birthweight by the 10th day, this indicates that his intake has been adequate.

Expressing breast milk

Routine expression of the breasts should not be part of the normal management of lactation. Provided that no limitation is placed on either feed frequency or duration and the baby is correctly attached, the volume of milk produced will be in step with the requirements of the baby. This will prevent the occurrence of problems (such as engorgement) that would require artificial removal of milk.

The situations where expressing is appropriate are:

- where there is concern about the interval between feeds in the early newborn period (expressed colostrum should always be given in preference to formula to healthy term babies)
- where there are major problems in attaching the baby to the breast
- where the baby is separated from the mother, owing to prematurity or illness
- later in lactation, when the mother may be separated because of work.

Manual expression of milk. This method has not been commonly practised where electric breast pumps are available but it has several advantages over mechanical pumping and should be taught to all mothers. It costs nothing and can be practised anywhere. It causes a higher level of prolactin release which will help to maintain lactation over a longer period. It is the most efficient method of obtaining colostrum.

Expressing with a breast pump. There are several types:

Electrical. There are several designs. Some pumps provide a regular vacuum and release cycle, with variability in the strength of the suction. Some vary the frequency of the cycle as well. Some simpler models provide only continuous suction, so that the mother has to take her finger off a hole or push a button to release it. Women are very adaptable and can make all of these work. The size of the breast cup may be the determinant of success and it is important to encourage the mother to experiment.

Manually controlled breast pumps. There are many designs. Most manually operated pumps are not efficient enough to allow initiation of full lactation but they can be useful when expressing is necessary in established lactation. It is helpful to mothers to explain that the pumps function most efficiently if the vacuum phase is considerably longer than the release phase.

Care of the breasts

Daily washing is all that is necessary for breast hygiene. The normal skin flora are beneficial to the baby. Brassieres may be worn in order to provide comfortable support and are useful if the breasts leak and breast pads are used. They should be large enough not to compress the breasts.

Action should be taken if the mother complains of sore breasts or nipples.

Breast problems

Sore and damaged nipples

These two conditions occur so commonly in developed countries that many health professionals believe them to be inevitable. The cause is almost always trauma from the baby's mouth and tongue which results from incorrect attachment of the baby to the breast. Correcting this will provide immediate relief from pain and will also allow rapid healing to take place. It is thought that there may be healing properties contained in fresh human milk and saliva which aid this process. 'Resting' the nipple also enables healing to take place but makes the continuation of lactation much more complicated because it would be necessary to express the milk and to use some other means of feeding it to the baby. The use of nipple shields does not solve the problem either, because they do not allow the mother to learn how to feed her baby correctly and the feeds may both continue to be painful and to cause trauma to the nipple. They should never be used before the mother has begun to lactate.

Better understanding of the cause of these problems enables midwives to be proficient at helping women with these distressing conditions.

Other causes of soreness

Infection with *Candida albicans* (thrush) can occur, although it is not common during the first week. The sudden development of pain, when the mother has had a period of trouble-free feeding, is suggestive of thrush. The nipple and areola are inflamed and shiny and pain persists throughout the feed. The baby may show signs of oral or anal thrush. Both mother and baby should receive fungicidal treatment (nystatin: see Ch. 42) and it may take several days for the pain in the nipple to disappear. Thrush seems to be increasing and this may be linked to the widespread use of antibiotics (Amir 1991).

Sensitivity may develop to topical applications such as creams, ointments or sprays. The mother with sore nipples should be questioned about the use of such products.

Feeding difficulties due to the mother

Abnormal nipples

Long nipples. These can lead to poor feeding because the baby is able to latch on to the nipple without drawing breast tissue into his mouth. The mother may need to be shown how to help the baby to draw in a sufficient portion of the breast.

Short nipples. As the baby has to form a teat from both the breast and nipple, short nipples should not cause problems and the mother should be reassured of this.

Abnormally large nipples. If the baby is small, his mouth may not be able to get beyond the nipple and on to the breast. Lactation could be initiated by expressing, although pumps may not be of any use because the nipple may not fit into the breast cup. As the baby grows and the breast and nipple become more protractile, breast feeding may become possible.

Inverted and flat nipples. As stated earlier, there is no clear evidence that physical preparation during pregnancy can effect a change in the nipples. Many babies are able to attach to the breast, even if the nipple is considered to be unfavourable, and are able to feed adequately (Main Trial Collaborative Group 1994). In more difficult cases it may be necessary to initiate lactation by expressing and delay attempting to attach the baby to the breast until lactation is established and the breasts have become soft and the breast tissue more protractile.

Complications of breast feeding

Engorgement

This condition occurs around the third or fourth day postpartum. The breasts are hard (often oedematous), painful and sometimes flushed. The mother may develop a pyrexia. Engorgement is usually an indication that the baby is not in step with the stage of lactation. Research published in the early 1950s demonstrated that the incidence was greatly reduced when restrictions on the duration of the early feeds were removed; early unrestricted feeding thus helps to prevent engorgement (Illingworth & Stone 1952). The condition also occurs when the baby is unable to feed efficiently because he is not correctly attached to the breast.

Management should be aimed at enabling the baby to feed well. Pushing away the oedema by gently manipulating the tissue that lies under the areola may be all that is required. Sometimes a breast pump can be used for the same purpose. Quicker resolution will occur if the baby is allowed to feed completely from the first breast before being offered the other one. In severe cases the only solution will be the gentle use of a pump. This will reduce the tension in the breast and does not cause excessive milk production. The mother's fluid intake should not be restricted, as this has no direct effect on breast function.

Mastitis

Mastitis means inflammation of the breast. In the majority of cases it is the result of milk stasis, not infection, although infection may supervene (Thomsen et al 1984). Typically, one or more adjacent segments are inflamed and appear as a wedge-shaped area of redness and swelling. The woman's pulse and temperature may rise and in some cases flu-like symptoms, including shivering attacks or rigors, may occur.

Non-infective (acute intramammary) mastitis. This condition results from milk stasis. It may occur during the early days as the result of unresolved engorgement or at any time when poor feeding technique results in the milk from one or more segments of the breast not being efficiently removed by the baby. It occurs much more frequently in the breast that is opposite the mother's preferred side for holding her baby (Inch & Fisher 1995). Pressure from fingers or clothing have been blamed for causing the condition, without any supporting evidence.

It is extremely important that breast feeding from the affected breast continues, otherwise milk stasis will increase further and provide ideal conditions for pathogenic bacteria to replicate. An infective condition may then arise which could, if untreated, lead to abscess formation, causing much pain and distress to the mother.

Where close supervision is available, 6–8 hours could be allowed to elapse to ascertain whether the process can be reversed by instructing the mother on good feeding technique and encouraging her to allow the baby to finish the first breast first. If supervision is not available, or if no improvement occurs during that period, antibiotics (e.g. cephalexin, flucloxacillin or erythromycin) should be given prophylactically (RCM 1991).

Infective mastitis. The main cause of superficial breast infection is damage to the epithelium which allows bacteria to enter the underlying tissues. The damage results from incorrect attachment of the baby to the breast which has caused trauma to the nipple. The mother therefore urgently needs help to improve her technique. Multiplication of bacteria may be enhanced by the use of breast pads or shells. In spite of antibiotic therapy, abscess formation may occur. Infection may also enter the breast via the milk ducts if milk stasis remains unresolved.

Breast abscess. A fluctuant swelling develops in a previously inflamed area. Pus may be discharged from the nipple. Simple needle aspiration may be effective or incision and drainage may be necessary (Dixon 1988). It may not be possible to feed from the affected breast for a few days but milk removal should continue and breast feeding should recommence as soon as practicable because this has been shown to reduce the chances of further abscess formation (Benson & Goodman 1970). A sinus which drains milk may form but it is likely to heal in time. Bilateral or multiple abscesses may sometimes occur.

Feeding difficulties due to the baby

Cleft lip

Provided that the palate is intact, the presence of a cleft in the lip should not interfere with breast feeding because the vacuum that is necessary to enable the baby to attach to the breast is created between the tongue and the hard palate, not the breast and the lips.

Cleft palate

Though there are cases documented which suggest that it is possible to breast feed if the baby has a cleft of the palate, a closer look indicates that the babies were able to obtain milk only as the result of the mother's milk ejection reflex. This would suggest that it is rarely likely to be completely successful. Because of the cleft, the baby is unable to create a vacuum and thus form a teat out of the breast and nipple. The use of an orthodontic plate is unlikely to help because the baby is unable to feel the breast against the hard palate and this is necessary to elicit the sucking response.

Many mothers have expressed their milk and used various techniques to feed it to their babies. A device called the Haberman feeder has proved useful. Some mothers have maintained their lactation until the baby has had a surgical repair and have then succeeded in breast feeding.

Blocked nose

Babies normally breathe through their noses. If there is an obstruction, they have great difficulty with feeding because they have to interrupt the process in order to breathe. A blockage caused by mucus may be relieved by instilling drops of normal saline before a feed. Choanal atresia is a rare abnormality causing obstruction to the nasal passage and the baby is unable to feed successfully before corrective surgery.

Down syndrome

Babies with this condition can be successfully breast fed, although extra help and encouragement may be necessary initially.

Prematurity

Preterm infants who are sufficiently mature to have developed sucking and swallowing reflexes may successfully breast feed. Breast feeding has been shown to suit the preterm baby because it is less tiring than bottle feeding and because the milk is adapted to the individual baby in its composition (Meier & Cranston-Anderson 1987). If the reflexes are not strongly developed, the baby may tire before the feed is complete and complementary tube feeding may be necessary.

Less mature babies who are unable to suck or swallow at all will be dependent on artificial methods such as tube feeding and intravenous alimentation.

Illness or surgery

Babies recover quickly following illness or surgery. If they have never been to the breast, or if feeding has been interrupted for a long period, the mother may require skilled help to initiate or re-establish feeding.

Contraindications to breast feeding

Drugs

Breast feeding may have to be suspended temporarily following the administration of certain drugs or following diagnostic techniques which use radioactive isotopes. Some drugs (such as those used to treat cancer) and certain hormones are an absolute contraindication to breast feeding. Most regions have drug centres where advice may be sought about the safety of drugs for lactating women.

Cancer

If the mother has cancer, the treatment she receives will make it impossible to breast feed without harming the baby; though she could express and discard her milk for the duration of the treatment and resume breast feeding later. If she has had a mastectomy, she may feed successfully from the other breast. Following a lumpectomy for cancer she may also be able to breast feed. She should seek advice from her surgeon.

Breast surgery

Neither breast reduction nor augmentation are an inevitable contraindication to breast feeding, but much depends on the techniques used. Where possible, advice should be sought from the surgeon. If the nipple has been displaced, the duct system is not likely to be patent. No harm can result from testing it out by allowing the baby to go to the breast.

Breast injury

Injuries caused by scalding in childhood may cause such severe scarring that breast feeding is impossible. Burns or other accidents may also cause serious damage.

HIV infection

The human immunodeficiency virus (HIV) may be transmitted in breast milk. In developed countries, where artificial feeding is relatively safe, the mother may be advised not to breast feed if she is HIV positive (see Ch. 18). In countries where artificial feeding is a significant cause of infant mortality, breast feeding may be the safer option (Akre 1990c).

Cessation of lactation

Suppression of lactation

If a mother chooses not to breast feed or if she has a late miscarriage or stillbirth, lactation will still begin. The woman may experience discomfort for a day or two but if unstimulated the breasts will naturally cease to produce milk. Very rarely severe discomfort with engorgement occurs. Expressing small volumes of milk once or twice can afford great relief without interfering with the rapid regression of the condition. The mother will be more comfortable if her breasts are supported but it is doubtful if binding the breasts contributes anything towards suppression.

Midwives should resist the temptation to advise restricting fluid intake and should not seek a prescription for a diuretic. These measures merely add to the woman's discomfort by making her thirsty.

Suppression with hormones is effective. Bromocriptine acts as a suppressant for prolactin. It is very expensive and may lead to rebound lactation when it is stopped; it is no longer licensed for this use in the USA. Stilboestrol and related preparations also suppress lactation but are no longer used in the UK because of the risk of thrombosis.

Discontinuation of breast feeding

Stopping lactation abruptly once breast feeding has become established may cause serious problems for the mother. She could develop engorgement or mastitis or even a breast abscess. She should be encouraged to mimic normal weaning by expressing her breasts but reducing the frequency over a few days. The gradual reduction in the volume of milk removed will result in a corresponding diminution in the production of milk. After a few days she should be encouraged to express only if she feels uncomfortable. The most tragic circumstance under which this advice might be required follows the death of a baby.

Weaning from the breast

When the mother or the baby decides to stop breast feeding, feeds should be tailed off gradually. Breast feeds may be omitted, one at a time, and spaced further apart. Adding supplementary foods should not begin until 4–6 months of age.

Complementary and supplementary feeds

Complementary feeds are given after a breast feed. A widely held belief that these feeds were frequently necessary became firmly established over a period of many years. This practice probably had its origin at the turn of the century, when it was recommended that the duration of the early feeds should be severely restricted and that the baby should be given complementary feeds of cow's milk 'until its mother is able to nurse it' (Vincent 1904). Since the advent of baby-led feeding it has become apparent that healthy term babies can safely be left to decide for themselves how much and how often they should feed. The only demonstrable effect of giving complementary feeds in hospitals is to reduce the overall duration of breast feeding (White et al 1992).

If problems arise which make the giving of complementary feeds necessary (the baby is small-for-dates, lethargic, jaundiced or difficult to attach), the mother's own expressed milk should be used.

Alternatively, donor milk from a human milk bank could be used. Donors must have been serologically tested for HIV and a negative result received before their milk can be accepted. There is no evidence that water or glucose solutions are of any value in these circumstances.

Whilst in hospital these feeds should be given by cup rather than in a bottle as this will allow the baby, who will only need small amounts at this stage, to remain more in control of his intake. If the problem (such as attachment difficulty) persists after the mother has left hospital, she may find it quicker and more efficient to give her expressed milk by bottle. She should be reassured that there is no evidence that the baby will subsequently refuse the breast in these circumstances.

The use of formula feeds based on either cow's milk or soya 'milk' should be avoided whenever possible. Their use may cause sensitivity to either product to occur later in the child's life and may cause changes in the flora of the baby's gut which may take some time to revert to the pre-complementary feed status. It also has a damaging effect on the mother's confidence in her ability to feed her baby herself.

Supplementary feeds are given in place of a breast feed. There can be no justification for their use except in extreme circumstances (such as severe illness or unconsciousness) because each breast feed missed by the baby will interfere with the establishment of lactation and damage the mother's confidence.

Return to work

If the breast-feeding mother returns to work, her baby will have to be fed in her absence (unless she is fortunate enough to have a crèche at work

or a child minder close at hand). She may wish her baby to have her own milk at all times and she may express for this purpose. Her baby may refuse milk from a bottle but he can be fed with a cup or spoon. On the other hand, she may find it difficult to provide her own milk and her baby may receive a formula feed while she is away but she may continue to breast feed at all other times. Midwives should help mothers to understand that returning to work does not mean that breast feeding has to be terminated.

ARTIFICIAL FEEDING

The amazing adaptability of the human infant has been demonstrated by the fact that adequate growth and development can take place in spite of being fed on a formula based on the milk of another species, even one which is deficient in many of the properties and components found in human milk.

Most women who artificially feed their babies belong to one of two distinct groups and it is important for midwives to understand the difference. The first group comprises mothers who have chosen to feed their babies this way. Those in the second group wanted to breast feed but have been prevented from doing so, either because breast feeding was contraindicated or because they have had unresolved breast-feeding problems.

Reasons for the primary choice

Women who choose to artificially feed their babies do not do so because they believe it better for their babies, but because they do not want to breast feed (Hally et al 1984). Many will have experienced the disappointment felt by relatives or friends who failed to breast feed because of unresolved problems. Some state that they find the idea of using their breasts for this function repulsive or 'animal-like', others that they would be embarrassed to breast feed in front of relatives or in public. A few may state that their partners do not wish them to breast feed.

Midwives should ensure that the mother is able to make an informed choice and then support her in her choice. It must be accepted that, under the right conditions, formula milk provides a safe alternative to breast feeding.

Cow's milk

The chart in Figure 36.15 shows that, when compared with human milk, unmodified cow's milk contains more protein. It also contains more minerals, less lactose (sugar) and about the same amount of fat.

Cow's milk *protein* contains 90% caseinogen and 10% lactalbumin, whereas human milk contains equal proportions of each. The proportion of amino acids is completely different from that in human milk (Fig. 36.16).

The proportion of *minerals*, compared with human milk, is almost twice the quantity. There is three times as much sodium.

The *fat* in human milk is easily digested because it is accompanied by lipase. *Cow's milk fat* is poorly digested and absorbed. Human milk contains much more cholesterol and it has been speculated that this suppresses the body's own synthesis of

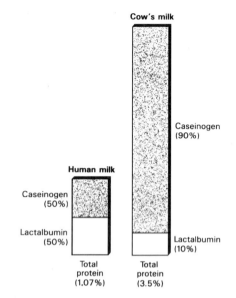

Fig. 36.15 Diagrammatic representation of ratio of caseinogen to lactalbumin in human and cow's milk.

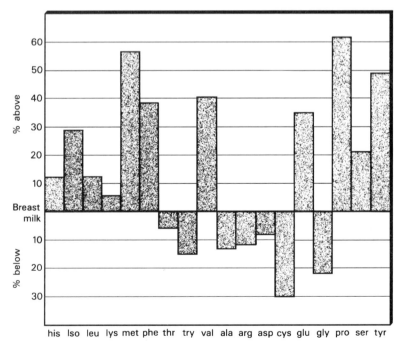

Fig. 36.16 The amino acid profile of cow's milk compared with breast milk (from FAO 1970 and Jelliffe & Jelliffe 1978).

cholesterol, an effect which may last throughout life.

Unmodified cow's milk should not be given to infants under 1 year old because it may lead to anaemia, which is caused by minute haemorrhages in the baby's gut.

Modified cow's milk formulae

Until the early 1970s most infant formulae consisted of crudely modified dried cow's milk with added vitamins. It became evident that their high solute loads contributed to infantile hypocalcaemia and to hypernatraemic dehydration. This led to the development of a new generation of infant formulae and the older types were phased out. This included National Dried Milk which was withdrawn in 1977.

The two main components used are skimmed milk (a by-product of butter manufacture) and whey (a by-product of cheese manufacture). Other substances used are not products of the dairy industry. They include maltodextrin, vegetable oils, animal fats, mineral salts and vitamins. Midwives must be aware that some animal fats may be unacceptable to mothers of certain faiths. In particular Hindus eschew beef fat.

There are now two main types of formula: whey-dominant and casein-dominant.

Whey-dominant formulae. These are recommended for use from birth for the first few weeks. A small amount of skimmed milk is combined with demineralised whey. Added fats are vegetable oils and animal fats. The ratio of proteins in the formulae resembles the ratio of whey protein (lactalbumin) to casein found in human milk. The use of demineralised whey reduces the mineral content which then resembles the concentration found in mature human milk. These feeds are more readily digested than the casein-dominant formulae. This leads to feeding patterns that more closely resemble those of breast-fed babies.

Casein-dominant formulae. These are recommended for use after the first few weeks and the baby should continue to be fed on this type of milk formula until he is about 1 year old, after which household milk can be used. The casein-dominant formulae contain skimmed milk with added carbohydrates and fats and a mixture of vegetable and animal fats.

Non-cow's milk formulae

There are soya-based milk substitutes which approximate to the compositional guidelines for infant formulae and which are suitable as the sole source of nourishment for young infants. They should not be used unless there is a clear indication that a cow's milk formula would be unsuitable for the baby, because babies can become sensitive to soya as well as to cow's milk. They contain only vegetable fats.

Babies intolerant of standard formulae

For the small number of babies who are unable to tolerate either cow's milk or soya-based formulae there are expensive feeds based on protein hydrolysate or comminuted chicken and these are available on prescription.

Preparation of the mother for artificial feeding

All mothers who choose to feed artificially should be shown how to prepare a bottle feed safely. This demonstration should take place in the mother's own home if possible, using her own equipment. If she has her baby in a hospital where ready-to-feed formula is not used, she may be shown there.

Clear instructions about the volumes of powder and water are provided on the container but the midwife should ensure that the mother understands them, as inaccurate measurements occur frequently (Lucas 1991).

Ready-to-feed bottles, as supplied to mothers in many hospitals, should not be used a second time. They are not intended to be resterilised and the measurement marks are not accurate.

In some developed countries formulae come ready made in cans or cartons but most are available in powdered form. The milk must be reconstituted accurately, using the precise amounts of powder and water specified by the manufacturers. It is essential that the water used is free from bacterial contamination and any harmful chemicals.

In some areas of the UK, mothers who are artificially feeding their babies have to be provided with a separate supply of water because the tap water is not suitable for babies' consumption. If bottled water is used, a still, non-mineralised variety suitable for babies must be chosen and it should be boiled as usual. Softened water is usually unsuitable.

Concern has been voiced about the nitrosamine content of rubber teats; in some countries mothers have been urged to boil the teat several times with fresh water before using. Silicone teats are now available but, as these have been known to split, the mother should be urged to check for signs of damage in order to ensure that the baby does not swallow any fragments. The effective cleaning of all utensils used must be demonstrated and the method of sterilisation discussed. If boiling is to be used, full immersion is essential and the contents of the pan must be boiled for at least 5 minutes. If cold sterilisation using a hypochlorite solution is the method of choice, the utensils must be fully immersed in the solution for the recommended time. Where the risk of cross-infection is high, namely in hospitals or in unhygienic home conditions, no rinsing should take place before the equipment is used. Otherwise it is recommended that rinsing with recently boiled water should be carried out. Equipment that sterilises by steam is now available. Microwave (steam) sterilisation is now possible, but the mother should check that the equipment can withstand it.

Mothers should be warned about the dangers of 'bottle propping', and told that the baby must never be left unattended while feeding from a bottle. They should be told about the need of the baby to relate to a small number of caregivers and that he should not be passed from person to person for feeding.

The baby is 'programmed' to feed from a breast and the mother should use the baby's innate skills when bottle feeding. The baby's lips should be touched to elicit a gape and the teat should follow the line of the baby's tongue, so that the baby uses the teat effectively. The mother should try to simulate breast-feeding conditions for the baby by holding him close, maintaining eye-to-eye contact and allowing him to determine his intake.

Modern formulae do not, when correctly prepared, cause hypernatraemia as the older types did. There is therefore no need to give the babies extra water.

The stools and vomit of a formula-fed baby have an unpleasant sour smell. The stools tend to be more formed than those of a breast-fed baby and, unlike a breast-fed baby, there is a real risk that the artificially fed baby may become constipated.

The size of the hole in the teat causes much anxiety to mothers. It is probably a good idea to have several teats with holes of different sizes so that they can be changed throughout the feed as necessary. A useful test for the correct hole size is to turn the bottle upside down; the feed should drip at a rate of about one drop per second.

If an emergency artificial feed has to be prepared from liquid pasteurised (doorstep) milk, it should be made as follows: 2/3 full cream milk; 1/3 water; 1 level teaspoonful of sugar. The milk should be boiled for 2 minutes so as not to overconcentrate it before adding the previously boiled water and the sugar.

Midwives and the WHO Code

In 1981, the combined forces of the World Health Organization (WHO) and the United Nations Children's Fund (UNICEF) produced the WHO International Code of Marketing of Breast Milk Substitutes. This Code was adopted by the Health Assembly of the WHO at its 34th World Health Assembly. The Code has major implications for the work of midwives. Although it is at present a voluntary code in most countries, some countries have implemented their own legal version. The existence of international recommendations for the practice of infant feeding must affect the work of midwives.

Recommendations in the Code include:

• No advertising or promotion directly to the public (this includes posters in hospitals and advertisements in mother-and-baby books).

• No free samples of breast milk substitutes to be given to mothers.

• No free gifts relating to products within the scope of the Code should be given to mothers, including discount coupons or special offers.

• Information provided by manufacturers to health workers should include only scientific and factual material and should not create or imply a belief that bottle feeding is equivalent or superior to breast feeding.

• No financial or material gifts should be given to health workers for the purpose of promoting products.

• Health workers should encourage and protect breast feeding.

The Code does not prevent mothers from bottle feeding but rather seeks to contribute to safe, adequate nutrition for infants and to promote and protect breast feeding.

The Baby Friendly Hospital Initiative

This is an initiative that was launched in 1991 by WHO and UNICEF to encourage hospitals to promote practices that are supportive of breast feeding. It was focused around the 'Ten Steps' with which all hospitals who wish to achieve 'baby friendly' status must comply.

The Ten Steps are:

1. Have a written breast feeding policy that is routinely communicated to all health care staff.
2. Train all health care staff in skills necessary to implement this policy.
3. Inform all pregnant women about the benefits and management of breast feeding.
4. Help mothers initiate breast feeding within half an hour of birth.
5. Show mothers how to breast feed and how to maintain lactation even if they should be separated from their infants.
6. Give newborn infants no food or drink other than breast milk, unless medically indicated.
7. Practice rooming-in: allow mothers and infants to remain together 24 hours a day.
8. Encourage breast feeding on demand.
9. Give no artificial teats or pacifiers (also called dummies or soothers) to breast-feeding infants.
10. Foster the establishment of breast-feeding support groups and refer mothers to them on discharge from hospital or clinic.

READER ACTIVITIES

1. A mother has no access to clocks. How does she know:

   a. When to feed her baby?
   b. When her baby has had sufficient?

Provide at least two factors for each.

2. The baby is not correctly attached to the breast. List at least four problems which might arise:

   a. in the mother
   b. in the baby.

3. Interview a recently delivered mother who is breast feeding. Identify what advice she has received and ascertain, from your own reading, whether it is based on research and knowledge of physiology. If it is not, identify its source if possible. What action could you take?

REFERENCES

Adler B R, Warner J O 1991 Food intolerance in children. Royal College of General Practitioners Members reference book. Campden Publishing, London, pp 497–502

Akre J (ed) 1990a Lactation. In: Infant feeding: the physiological basis. Bulletin of the World Health Organization 67[1989](suppl): 25

Akre J (ed) 1990b The low birth weight infant. In: Infant feeding: the physiological basis. Bulletin of the World Health Organization 67[1989](suppl): 79

Akre J (ed) 1990c Health factors that may interfere with breastfeeding. In: Infant feeding: the physiological basis. Bulletin of the World Health Organization 67[1989] (suppl): 45

Almroth S G 1978 Water requirements of breastfed babies in a hot climate. American Journal of Clinical Nutrition 31: 1154–1157

Amir L H 1991 Candida and the lactating breast: predisposing factors. Journal of Human Lactation 7(4): 177–181

Applebaum R M 1970 The modern management of successful breastfeeding. Paediatric Clinics of North America 17: 203–205

Bahna S L 1987 Milk allergy in infancy. Annals of Allergy 59: 131–136

Benson E A, Goodman M A 1970 An evaluation of the use of stilboestrol and antibiotics in the early management of acute puerperal breast abscess. British Journal of Surgery 57: 258

Carvahlo M R et al 1996 Cell mediated response to beta casein in recent onset insulin dependent diabetes: implications for disease pathogenesis. Lancet 348: 926–928

Daly S 1993 The short term synthesis and infant regulated removal of milk in lactating women. Experimental Physiology 78: 209–220

Dixon J M 1988 Repeated aspiration of breast abscess in lactating women. British Medical Journal 297: 1517–1518

Food and Agriculture Organization (FAO) 1970 Nutritional studies: amino-acid content of foods. FAO/WHO, Rome

Goldberg N M, Adams E 1983 Supplementary water for breastfed babies in a hot dry climate – not really a necessity. Archives of Disease in Childhood 58(January): 73–74

Hally M R, Bond J, Crawley J et al 1984 Factors influencing the feeding of first-born infants. Acta Paediatrica Scandinavica 73: 33–39

Helsing E, Savage King F 1982 Breast-feeding in practice. Oxford University Press, Oxford, p 175

Howie P W, Forsyth J S, Ogston S A et al 1990 Protective effect of breast feeding against infection. British Medical Journal 300: 11–16

Hytten F E 1954 Clinical and chemical studies in human lactation, IX Breast feeding in hospital. British Medical Journal ii: 1447–1452

Hytten F E, Baird D 1958 The development of the nipple in pregnancy. Lancet i: 1201–1204

Illingworth R S, Stone D G H 1952 Self-demand feeding in a maternity unit. Lancet i: 683–687

Inch S, Garforth S 1989 Establishing and maintaining breastfeeding. In: Chalmers I, Enkin M, Keirse M (eds) Effective care in pregnancy and childbirth. Oxford University Press, Oxford, ch 80, p 1364

Inch S, Fisher C 1995 Mastitis in lactating women. The Practitioner 239: 472–476

International Confederation of Midwives 1985 ICM speaks out on breast feeding. Midwifery 1: 47

Jelliffe D B, Jelliffe E F P 1978 Human milk in the modern world. Oxford University Press, Oxford

Karjalainen J et al 1992 A bovine peptide as a possible trigger of insulin dependent diabetes mellitus. New England Journal of Medicine 327: 302–307

Kennedy K I et al 1989 Consensus statement on the use of breastfeeding as a family planning method. Contraception: 439: 477

Kochenour N K 1980 Lactation suppression. Clinical Obstetrics and Gynecology 23: 1052–1059

Kries R V, Shearer M, McCarthy P T et al 1987 Vitamin K_1 content of maternal milk: influence of the stage of lactation, lipid composition, and vitamin K_1 supplements given to the mother. Pediatric Research 22(5): 513–517

Lucas A 1991 Milk for babies and children. Correspondence. British Medical Journal 301: 350–351

Lucas A, Cole T J 1990 Breast milk and neonatal necrotising enterocolitis. Lancet 336: 1519–1523

Main Trial Collaborative Group 1994 Preparing for breastfeeding: treatment of inverted and non-protractile nipples in pregnancy. Midwifery 10: 200–214

Meier P, Cranston-Anderson J 1987 Responses of small preterm infants to bottle and breast-feeding. Maternal–Child Nursing Journal 12: 97–105

Metcalf I J, Irons T G, Lawrence D S, Young P C 1994 Simethicone in the treatment of infant colic: a randomised placebo-controlled multicentre trial. Pediatrics 94: 29–34

Monte C S et al 1994 Bovine serum albumin detected in infant formula is a possible trigger for insulin dependent diabetes mellitus. Journal of the American Dietetic Association 94: 314–416

Moody J, Britten J, Hogg K 1996 Breastfeeding your baby. A National Childbirth Trust guide. HMSO, London

Prentice A M, Addey C V P, Wilde C J 1989 Evidence for local feed-back control of human milk secretion. Biochemical Society Transactions 17: 122, 489–492

Pyke M 1986 Success in nutrition. John Murray, London, pp 134–137

Ramos R, Kennedy K I, Visness C M 1996 Effectiveness of lactational amenorrhoea in prevention of pregnancy in Manila, the Philippines: non-comparative prospective trial. British Medical Journal 313: 909–912

Righard L, Alade M O 1990 Effect of delivery room routines on success of first breast-feed. Lancet 336: 1105–1107

Royal College of Midwives 1991 Successful breastfeeding, 2nd edn. Churchill Livingstone, Edinburgh

Saarinen U M, Siimes M A 1979 Iron absorption from breastmilk, cow's milk and iron supplemented formula: an opportunistic use of changes in total body iron determined by hemoglobin, ferritin and body weight in 132 infants. Pediatric Research 13: 143–147

Sachdev H P S, Krishna J, Puri R K 1991 Water supplementation in exclusively breastfed infants during the summer in the tropics. Lancet 337: 929–933

Thomsen A C, Espersen M D, Maigaard S 1984 Course and treatment of milk stasis, noninfectious inflammation of the breast, and infectious mastitis in nursing women. American Journal of Obstetrics and Gynecology 149: 492–495

Ueda T, Yokoyama Y, Irahara M, Aona T 1994 Influence of psychological stress on suckling-induced pulsatile oxytocin release. Obstetrics and Gynecology 84: 259–262

Vincent R 1904 The nutrition of the infant. Baillière Tindall and Cox, London, p 40

Waldenström U, Swensen Å 1991 Rooming-in at night in the postpartum ward. Midwifery 7: 82–89

Widström A M, Ransjo-Arvidson A B, Christensson K et al 1987 Gastric suction in healthy newborn infants. Acta Paediatrica Scandinavica 76: 566–578

White A, Freith S, O'Brien M 1992 Infant feeding 1990. Survey carried out for the Department of Health by the Office of Population Censuses and Surveys. HMSO, London

Woolridge M W 1986 The 'anatomy' of sucking. Midwifery 2: 164–171

Woolridge M W, Fisher C 1988 'Overfeeding' and symptoms of malabsorption in the breast-fed baby: a possible artefact of feed management? Lancet ii: 382–384

World Health Organization 1981 International code of marketing of breast-milk substitutes. WHO, Geneva

FURTHER READING

Akre J (ed) 1990 Infant feeding: the physiological basis. Bulletin of the World Health Organization 67[1989](suppl)

DHSS 1988 Present-day practice in infant feeding: third report. HMSO, London

Chalmers I, Enkin M, Keirse M J N C (eds) 1989 Effective care in pregnancy and childbirth. Oxford University Press, Oxford

Fisher C 1981 Breast feeding: a midwife's view. Maternal and Child Health 6: 52–57

Fisher C 1984 The initiation of breastfeeding. Midwives Chronicle 97: 39–41

Greaseley V 1986 Breastfeeding. Nursing 3(2): 63–70

Helsing E, Savage King F 1982 Breast-feeding in practice: a manual for health workers. Oxford University Press, Oxford

Henschel D, Inch S 1996 Breastfeeding – a guide for midwives. Books for Midwives Press, Cheshire

Howie P W 1985 Breast feeding: a new understanding. Midwives Chronicle 98: 184–192

Inch S 1990 Postnatal care relating to breastfeeding. In: Alexander J, Levy V, Roch S (eds) Midwifery practice. Postnatal care. A research-based approach. Macmillan Education, Basingstoke

Palmer G 1993 The politics of breastfeeding, 2nd edn. Pandora Press, London

Renfrew M, Fisher C, Arms S 1990 Bestfeeding. Celestial Arts, Berkeley

Woolridge M W 1986 Aetiology of sore nipples. Midwifery 2: 172–176

World Health Organization 1989 Protecting, promoting and supporting breast-feeding: the special role of maternity services. A joint WHO/UNICEF Statement. WHO, Geneva

The healthy low birthweight baby

Annie C. Halliday

The World Health Organization (WHO 1978) optimistically set the targets of 'Health for All by the Year 2000'. In particular, improvements were sought in maternity care provision and a reduction in perinatal mortality rates. The incidence of preterm labours has not reduced but owing to improved neonatal management, increasing numbers of small babies are surviving. As a consequence the UK has lowered the legal age of viability from 28 to 24 weeks' gestation. While it is indisputable that the low birthweight baby is more likely to have problems in the neonatal period there are still a considerable number who successfully circumnavigate the difficulties and problems to which babies of their size are susceptible.

The chapter aims to:

- distinguish between different classes of low birthweight babies

- help the reader to be able to recognise their differing clinical characteristics

- discuss the appropriate care for these babies.

The internationally accepted definition of a low birthweight baby is one whose weight at birth is 2.5 kg or less (WHO 1977). Further subdivisions within this group include the very low birthweight (VLBW) baby weighing 1001–1500 g and the extremely low birthweight (ELBW) baby who weighs 1000 g or less. Considered in isolation, birthweight is an inadequate index for assessing a baby's needs or likely progress. Equally important is assessment of gestational age. A term infant is one born after 37 completed weeks of gestation. A preterm infant is one born before 37 completed weeks of gestation. Where there is doubt, the assessment tool devised by Dubowitz et al (1970) remains the most efficient method of assessing

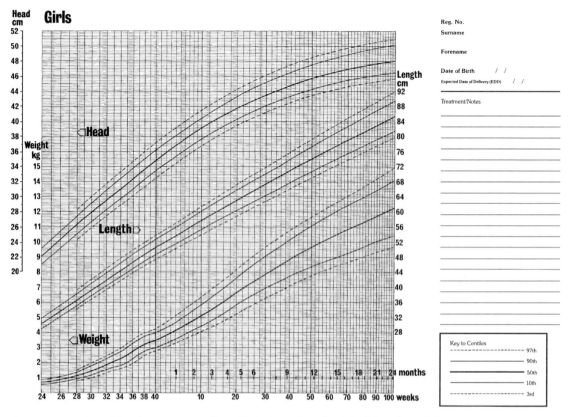

Fig. 37.1 Growth and development chart (female). (Adaptation of original chart by Gairdner D, Pearson J 1971, first published in Archives of Disease in Childhood 46: 783. Reproduced by kind permission of Castlemead Publications. Chart stock reference (GPG3).)

gestational age of the neonate. It consists of two parts. Part 1 is based on a detailed examination of the physical characteristics of the baby (Fig. 37.4), while part 2 deals with the assessment of neurological development (Fig. 37.3 and Box 37.1). The final score is plotted on a graph (Fig. 37.5). This assessment should only be made when the baby has had opportunity to rest following delivery and when he is awake.

It is customary for these two factors, gestational age and birthweight, to be given joint consideration. Centile charts have been devised on which a baby's birthweight is plotted against his gestational age (Fig. 37.1). A baby whose weight lies between the 10th and 90th centile is considered appropriate for gestational age (AGA); if birthweight is greater than the 90th centile this is described as large for gestational age (LGA) and a

baby whose weight is below the 10th centile is described as being small for gestational age (SGA). It follows that a baby who is born at term may be LGA, AGA, or SGA; similarly a preterm baby may be LGA, AGA or SGA. Should the weight be 2.5 kg or less, such a baby would additionally be described as being of low birthweight.

Two very different clinical pictures are presented by the term baby who is small for gestational age and the preterm infant who is appropriate for gestational age. It is important for the midwife to be able to differentiate between the two and tailor management accordingly. Because of improvements in prenatal care there is a group of preterm babies who are not low birthweight but whose needs are substantially the same as many whose birthweight is less than 2.5 kg. For convenience they are included in this chapter.

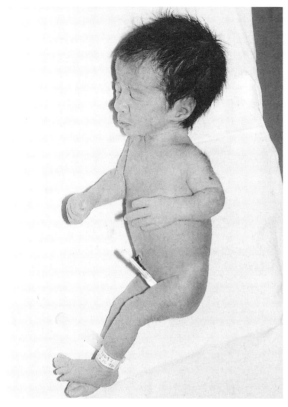

Fig. 37.2 Baby with asymmetrical growth retardation. Note the apparently large head.

SMALL FOR GESTATIONAL AGE TERM INFANT

Clinical appearance

Typically this baby is long and thin with an apparently disproportionately large head (Fig. 37.2). The skin is often dry and peeling, and there are abundant palmar and plantar skin creases. These babies are sometimes described as looking like worried old men. It has been suggested that having been starved in utero they are 'worried' that this pattern is going to continue. In behaviour they are active and indicate from an early age that they are hungry. This group of babies demonstrates an asymmetrical growth pattern. While weight is low for gestational age, length is less affected and occipitofrontal head circumference may well be within the normal range for a term infant.

A second group of babies is apparently small for gestational age but growth retardation is symmetrical. These are likely to be totally normal babies whose size is compatible with ethnic and genetic expectations. Multiple gestation pregnancies not infrequently produce babies who are symmetrically growth retarded.

A third group comprises those whose growth has been stunted in utero by the teratogenic effects of infection, drug or alcohol abuse. All three parameters, weight, length and occipitofrontal circumference, are compromised. This last group is likely to present a variety of problems in the neonatal period and therefore lies outwith the remit of this chapter.

Causes

Factors contributing to intrauterine growth retardation are discussed in previous chapters. These include maternal disease such as hypertensive disorders which lead to poor placental perfusion, reduced availability of nutrients, or placental transfer of inappropriate substances which have a teratogenic effect, for example nicotine, alcohol, cocaine or infective agents. Extremes of maternal age, that is those at either end of the childbearing spectrum, socioeconomic factors, parity and the number of fetuses in utero all may impinge on normal growth pattern. Neonatal management is planned to redress the balance or at best minimise the effects of such intrauterine deprivation.

Management at birth

There is no significant difference in management at delivery from that described for the normal baby, except perhaps that the baby will be more susceptible to hypothermia. Extra care should therefore be taken to ensure that the delivery room is warm and that the baby is dried and wrapped in a warm wrap and blankets.

Nutritional needs

To meet the nutritional needs of a baby who has been starved in utero, early and frequent feeding is called for (often literally). These babies are hungry. Since successful initiation and establishing of lactation operates by the law of supply and demand, a mother choosing to breast feed should encounter few problems. Breast milk from mothers of SGA babies has increased proteins and immunoglobulins for the first few days.

Should the mother choose to offer formula milk, calorie requirements are normally calculated at a higher rate than for an AGA baby. This is because SGA babies have been shown to have a higher metabolic rate and higher total energy expenditure than AGA babies (Davies et al 1996). Lack of subcutaneous fat and liver glycogen stores further compromises their nutritional reserves. Feeds are therefore calculated at a rate of 90 ml/kg/day, increasing by 10–15 ml/kg/day to a maximum of 200 ml/kg/day. Blood sugar levels should be monitored at least 6-hourly for the first 48 hours. These babies lose minimal amounts of weight before gaining weight rapidly.

Temperature control

This baby has a relatively mature temperature control mechanism but his lack of subcutaneous fat makes him more susceptible to hypothermia from fluctuations in environmental temperature. A thermoneutral environment should be provided and his temperature should be monitored regularly. Nursing in suboptimal temperatures will encourage non-shivering thermogenesis by metabolism of areas of brown fat. Once metabolised this cannot be replaced.

Skin care

Particular attention should be given to those babies whose skin is dry and perhaps cracked and peeling. Ensuring that the baby is kept clean and dry will prevent infection. Emollient may be added to bath water or applied to the skin afterwards. Skin massage offers additional benefits of enhancing the mother–baby relationship.

PRETERM BABY

Causes

In many instances the cause of preterm birth re-

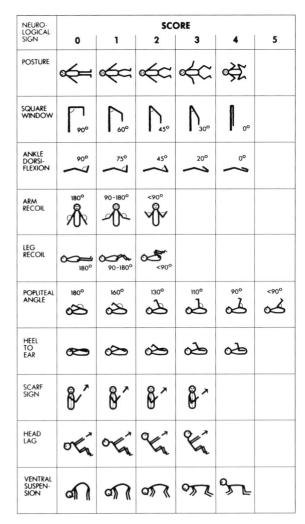

Fig. 37.3 Neurological criteria (Dubowitz et al 1970). (See also Box 37.1.)

mains unknown although there are several factors which are considered to predispose to a shortened pregnancy.

Maternal age
This is not considered to be a major factor in the duration of pregnancy although there does appear to be an increase in premature birth outside the optimum childbearing age range of 20–35 years.

Multiple pregnancy
Overdistension of the uterus not infrequently results in spontaneous preterm labour especially

Box 37.1 Some notes on techniques of assessment of neurological criteria (Dubowitz et al 1970). (See also Fig. 37.3.)

Posture. Observed with infant quiet and in supine position. Score:

0 Arms and legs extended
1 Beginning of flexion of hips and knees, arms extended
2 Stronger flexion of legs, arms extended
3 Arms slightly flexed, legs flexed and abducted
4 Full flexion of arms and legs.

Square window. The hand is flexed on the forearm between the thumb and index fingers of the examiner. Enough pressure is applied to get as full a flexion as possible, and the angle between the hypothenar eminence and the ventral aspect of the forearm is measured and graded according to the diagram. (Care is taken not to rotate the infant's wrist while doing this manoeuvre.)

Ankle dorsiflexion. The foot is dorsiflexed onto the anterior aspect of the leg with the examiner's thumb on the sole of the foot and other fingers behind the leg. Enough pressure is applied to get as full flexion as possible and the angle between the dorsum of the foot and the anterior aspect of the leg is measured.

Arm recoil. With the infant in the supine position the forearms are first flexed for 5 seconds, then fully extended by pulling on the hands, and then released. The sign is fully positive if the arms return briskly to full flexion (score 2). If the arms return to incomplete flexion or the response is sluggish it is graded as score 1. If they remain extended or are only followed by random movements the score is 0.

Leg recoil. With the infant supine, the hips and knees are fully flexed for 5 seconds, then extended by traction on the feet, and released. A maximal response is one of full flexion of the hips and knees (score 2). A partial flexion scores 1, and minimal or no movement scores 0.

Popliteal angle. With the infant supine and his pelvis flat on the examining couch, the thigh is held in the knee–chest position by the examiner's left index finger and thumb supporting the knee. The leg is then extended by gentle pressure from the examiner's right index finger behind the ankle and the popliteal angle is measured.

Heel to ear manoeuvre. With the baby supine, draw the baby's foot as near to the head as it will go without forcing it. Observe the distance between the foot and the head as well as the degree of extension at the knee. Grade according to diagram. Note that the knee is left free and may draw down alongside the abdomen.

Scarf sign. With the baby supine, take the infant's hand and try to put it around the neck and as far posteriorly as possible around the opposite shoulder. Assist this manoeuvre by lifting the elbow across the body. See how far the elbow will go across and grade according to illustrations. Score:

0 Elbow reaches opposite axillary line
1 Elbow between midline and opposite axillary line
2 Elbow reaches midline
3 Elbow will not reach midline.

Head lag. With the baby lying supine, grasp the hands (or the arms if a very small infant) and pull him slowly towards the sitting position. Observe the position of the head in relation to the trunk and grade accordingly. In a small infant the head may initially be supported by one hand. Score:

0 Complete lag
1 Partial head control
2 Able to maintain head in line with body
3 Brings head anterior to body.

Ventral suspension. The infant is suspended in the prone position with examiner's hand under the infant's chest (one hand in a small infant, two in a large infant). Observe the degree of extension of the back and the amount of flexion of the arms and legs, Also note the relation of the head to the trunk. Grade according to diagrams.

If the score for an individual criterion differs on the two sides of the baby, take the mean.

when there are more than two babies (see Ch. 19), otherwise induction of labour is often planned for 38 weeks' gestation.

Social class

There appears to be an increased risk of women in social classes IV and V having a shorter gestation period though there may be other compounding factors present such as maternal illness.

Maternal disease in pregnancy

Pre-eclampsia, infection, or antepartum haemorrhage due to either placenta praevia or placental abruption may prompt the decision to conclude the pregnancy early. Likewise, chronic maternal disease such as hypertension or renal disease may be an indication for obstetric intervention.

EXTERNAL SIGN	SCORE 0	1	2	3	4
OEDEMA	Obvious oedema hands and feet; pitting over tibia	No obvious oedema hands and feet; pitting over tibia	No oedema		
SKIN TEXTURE	Very thin, gelatinous	Thin and smooth	Smooth; medium thickness. Rash or superficial peeling	Slight thickening. Superficial cracking and peeling esp hands and feet	Thick and parchment-like; superficial or deep cracking
SKIN COLOUR (Infant not crying)	Dark red	Uniformly pink	Pale pink: variable over body	Pale. Only pink over ears, lips, palms or soles	
SKIN OPACITY (trunk)	Numerous veins and venules clearly seen, especially over abdomen	Veins and tributaries seen	A few large vessels clearly seen over abdomen	A few large vessels seen indistinctly over abdomen	No blood vessels seen
LANUGO (over back)	No lanugo	Abundant; long and thick over whole back	Hair thinning especially over lower back	Small amount of lanugo and bald areas	At least half of back devoid of lanugo
PLANTAR CREASES	No skin creases	Faint red marks over anterior half of sole	Definite red marks over more than anterior half; indentations over less than anterior third	Indentations over more than anterior third	Definite deep indentations over more than anterior third
NIPPLE FORMATION	Nipple barely visible; no areola	Nipple well defined; areola smooth and flat diameter <0.75 cm.	Areola stippled, edge not raised; diameter <0.75 cm.	Areola stippled, edge raised diameter >0.75 cm.	
BREAST SIZE	No breast tissue palpable	Breast tissue on one or both sides <0.5 cm. diameter	Breast tissue both sides; one or both 0.5–1.0 cm.	Breast tissue both sides; one or both > 1 cm.	
EAR FORM	Pinna flat and shapeless, little or no incurving of edge	Incurving of part of edge of pinna	Partial incurving whole of upper pinna	Well-defined incurving whole of upper pinna	
EAR FIRMNESS	Pinna soft, easily folded, no recoil	Pinna soft, easily folded, slow recoil	Cartilage to edge of pinna, but soft in places, ready recoil	Pinna firm, cartilage to edge, instant recoil	
GENITALIA MALE	Neither testis in scrotum	At least one testis high in scrotum	At least one testis right down		
FEMALES (With hips half abducted)	Labia majora widely separated, labia minora protruding	Labia majora almost cover labia minora	Labia majora completely cover labia minora		

Fig. 37.4 External superficial criteria (Dubowitz et al 1970).

Previous obstetric history

A history of previous mid-trimester miscarriage is not uncommon in women who have a preterm birth. Controversy continues regarding the effect of therapeutic abortion on subsequent pregnancy but in practice a proportion of women who have had a previous termination of pregnancy do experience a preterm birth. It is possible that any interventions relating to the cervix may give rise to cervical incompetence, thereby increasing the risk of preterm labour.

Fetal causes

Instances where the well-being of the fetus may be seriously compromised if the pregnancy were continued include placental insufficiency and Rhesus disease. The presence of congenital abnormalities possibly complicated by growth retardation may also be associated with preterm birth.

Care at birth

In the absence of problems during labour the preterm infant will frequently establish respiration successfully and require no active resuscitation. It is important that optimum conditions surround his immediate care. Transfer to a special care baby unit (SCBU) may be needed in order to maintain his health status.

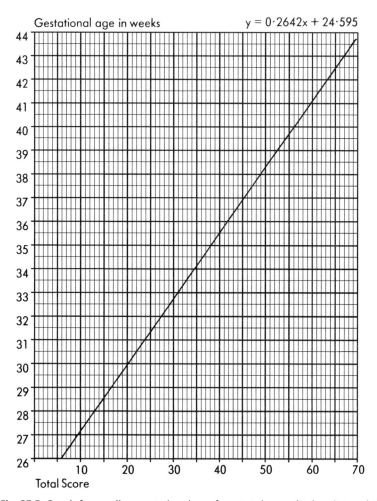

Fig. 37.5 Graph for reading gestational age from total score (Dubowitz et al 1970).

Clinical appearance

Relative to his size the preterm baby has a big head, small thoracic area and large abdomen. Limbs are more or less flexed with reduced muscle tone (Fig. 37.6). The skull bones are soft with wide sutures and large fontanelles. Clinical features vary considerably according to maturity; Figure 37.3 shows the gestational age assessment tool which describes these details.

Nutritional needs

The challenge presented by the preterm baby is to provide the type and amount of nutrients that would best simulate intrauterine growth and development. Midwives have long been encouraged to promote breast feeding. Research evidence abounds to substantiate the claim that breast milk is best; even donor breast milk has an advantage over standard formula milk for preterm babies according to Lucas et al (1994). Donor breast milk does, however, carry the risk of transmission of human immunodeficiency virus (HIV) and as a result is no longer used in many units. The components of breast milk and formula milks are described in detail in Chapter 36 as are the advantages of breast feeding. The rate of growth in a breast-fed baby may not be as rapid as in the baby who is fed formula milk but the specific types of

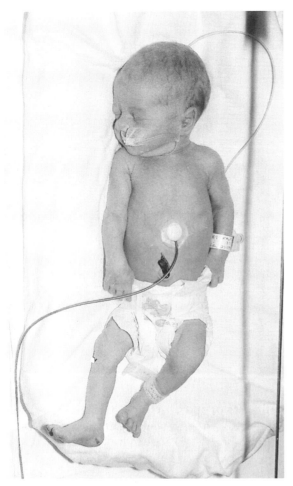

Fig. 37.6 Healthy preterm infant born at 32 weeks' gestation.

fat found in breast milk may be essential for normal neurological development. Formula milks contain the precursor essential fatty acids but immature babies lack the necessary enzymes to convert them to two essential long-chain polyunsaturated acids, arachidonic and docosahexanoic acid. These two substances are necessary for the myelination of cortical nerve fibres and for intracellular components such as mitochondria. Lucas and others (1992) have demonstrated that preterm babies who were breast fed had a higher intelligence quotient (IQ) at age 5 and 8 years than their formula-fed counterparts. A further advantage of breast milk for the preterm baby is described by Ewer et al (1994), namely improved gastric emptying.

For maximum effect, that is nutrition and growth, it is the practice in some units to combine breast milk and preterm formula feeds. Prolactin levels are highest in the night and so one night-time feed or expression is encouraged. Because of the changes in the composition of breast milk as the feed progresses it is recommended by Jones (1994) that a preterm baby be fed hindmilk first. She explains that this may be achieved by expressing the foremilk and then allowing the baby to fix at the breast to access the hindmilk or alternatively both may be expressed and the baby be fed hindmilk first. Hindmilk has a higher fat content than foremilk.

Methods of feeding

Breast feeding

It is acknowledged that the sucking–swallowing reflex is developed by the preterm baby around 34 weeks' gestation but babies must be individually assessed. For babies who are able, direct feeding from the breast is the method of choice. It should be remembered, however, that a preterm baby may tire easily and not be able to sustain the effort long enough to obtain his necessary fluid requirements. In addition, the energy expended in sucking may leave insufficient calories to support growth and development. Weighing the baby daily is the best means of assessing this. Test-weighing before and after every feed is counterproductive since increased maternal anxiety may inhibit lactation.

Successful breast feeding is a two-way process dependent upon competencies of both mother and baby. Any competencies the baby has in relation to feeding at the breast will be enhanced by correct positioning at the breast and by offering the breast regularly and exclusively. It is best to put baby to the breast when he is awake. The optimum position to facilitate a preterm baby in feeding from the breast is shown in Figure 37.7. This allows the mother to support the baby's head and neck, and increases the possibility of eye-to-eye contact with the mother, permitting her to monitor her baby's behavioural responses. This position also maximises the baby's chest expansion. Cradling the baby will only encourage him to fall asleep. Since milk production operates on a supply and

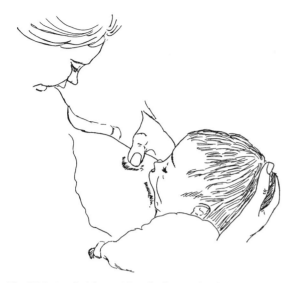

Fig. 37.7 A suitable position for breast feeding.

demand basis, offering the breast regularly will help establish lactation provided this does not overtire the baby. Since the technique of sucking from the breast is different from that of sucking from a bottle, it is preferable to offer complementary and/or supplementary feeds if required from a cup or spoon. Those babies who are too immature to meet their nutritional needs by breast feeding may still be put to the breast for short periods. Non-nutritive sucking gives the baby opportunity to learn the technique and taste and smell breast milk and if this is followed by a gavage (tube) feed an association will be made between the two incidents. It is important that the purpose of non-nutritive sucking is clearly explained to the mother, otherwise she may imagine she is trying but failing to feed her baby. If appropriate support is proffered, she will feel instead that she is able to make some contribution to her baby's care and will doubtless enjoy the experience. This will help her relax and promote the let-down reflex. Jones (1995) and Lawrence (1994) both suggest the use of a supplemental nutritional system when the baby is able to coordinate sucking and swallowing but lactation is not yet established. Such a system consists of a container of expressed breast milk or formula feed being attached to a neck cord and positioned between the mother's breasts. A fine catheter leading from the container is placed alongside the mother's

nipple and allowed to drip milk into the baby's mouth as he suckles. In this way he associates the taste of the milk with sucking and is encouraged to continue to stimulate lactation.

Ways in which the mother's competencies in breast feeding may be enhanced are described in Chapter 36. Additional features in relation to the preterm infant are noted here.

Contact. If unable to put the baby directly to the breast, the mother may improve lactation by expressing milk whilst in close proximity to her baby (McAlpine, personal communication, 1996) or by touching or smelling a toy or blanket belonging to the baby.

Privacy. In a study commissioned by the Department of Health, Ingram and others (1994) demonstrated that privacy is an important factor in encouraging a mother to breast feed or express milk. A quiet room with comfortable furnishings and facilities for refreshments, where the mother and baby can relax together without feeling themselves to be in a goldfish bowl, is conducive to successful breast feeding.

Attitudes of staff. Positive staff attitudes and a willingness to offer consistent advice is particularly important to the mother of a preterm baby who, according to Petit (1992), requires to have a greater degree of commitment to her intention to breast feed than the mother of a healthy term baby.

Cup feeding

Moody (1993) suggests that this method of feeding provides a viable alternative for the baby who is unable, for whatever reason, to suck directly from the breast (see Fig. 37.8). It prevents the baby who will later breast feed from being confused by learning the different technique needed to suck from a bottle. It also provides the baby opportunity to participate by exercising appropriate oral feeding skills. Useful buccal digestive enzyme production is also encouraged.

Naso- or orogastric tube feeding

A size 5 French gauge catheter is suitable for most preterm infants. Measurement should be made

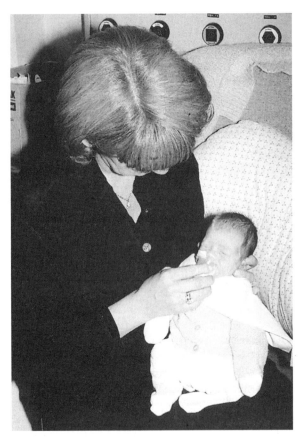

Fig. 37.8 A preterm baby learning the art of cup feeding.

from the root of the nose to the xiphisternum with the baby's head in a position of slight extension plus 2.5 cm. Preference for the oro- or nasogastric route in a healthy baby is one of personal choice. An orogastric tube may be marginally easier to pass but it is also more likely to be dislodged. The tube may be secured by application of hypoallergenic tape. Care should be taken to ensure that the tube is correctly positioned before instilling milk. In some units midwives aspirate the tube and check the acidity of the gastric aspirate with litmus paper in order to demonstrate that the tube is in the stomach. An additional method is the use of marker threads strategically placed around the tube about 2.5 cm from the mouth or nostril to alert the staff if the tube has partly come out.

This route may be used to administer feeds by means of continuous infusion or by 1-, 2- or 3-hourly bolus feeds. It is a technique which may be taught to parents, thus affording them further opportunity of participating in their baby's care. Provided that the baby's position is maintained in a head-up tilt, the baby may be cradled in the mother's arm during the feed.

The midwife should be alert for any behavioural cues such as sucking movements or rooting which may demonstrate that the baby is ready to attempt breast or bottle feeding. This is then introduced gradually according to ability.

Mothers who have chosen to offer their babies formula milk require an equally high level of support while they learn the technique of feeding such a small baby.

Meeting thermal needs

The principles of temperature control are discussed in Chapters 34 and 35 in relation to the full-term infant. The preterm baby is vulnerable to changes in ambient temperature on a number of counts and although he has increasing thermoregulating abilities from 30 weeks onwards they are insufficient to meet his needs. Particular difficulties are:

- large surface area to body mass ratio
- lack of subcutaneous fat
- lack of brown fat deposits – these are normally laid down after 36 weeks
- comparatively thin skin with increase in transepidermal water loss and consequent heat loss from evaporation
- lack of glycogen stores to use in heat generation by increasing metabolic rate
- inability to reduce temperature by sweating.

To preserve and maintain thermal homeostasis, the preterm infant should be nursed in a neutrothermal environment. Failure to do so will cause an increase in metabolic rate, increase oxygen requirements and may lead to respiratory difficulty.

Smaller babies may require to be nursed in an incubator to maintain their temperature within normal limits. Preferably this will be a double-glazed model (Fig. 37.9) which will reduce radiation heat loss. Incoming air is heated and the ambient temperature is maintained by generation of convection currents of warm air around the

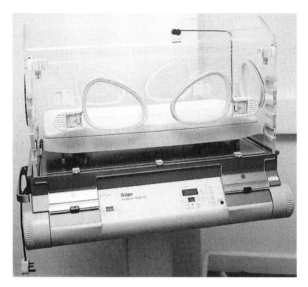

Fig. 37.9 Double-glazed incubator (courtesy of Drager Medical).

baby. Servocontrol mechanisms may be employed which means that the ambient temperature will automatically increase to a preset level, thus counteracting incursions of cooler air when incubator doors are open.

Encouraging the baby to adopt a flexed position, which can be done by the use of nests or boundaries, will reduce heat loss. Although there is a wide range of manufactured aids, rolled blankets or sheets serve the purpose equally well and are less expensive. Sheepskin mats are placed under the babies in some units. Additional aids available are heat shields or plastic bubble wrapping. These are more likely to be used for the very low birthweight or sick baby.

Clothing

Dressing the baby appropriately for either incubator or cot nursing not only keeps him warm but makes him look more attractive. The family can become involved in providing or at least choosing suitable outfits. A woollen hat should be worn and preferably mittens and bootees if the baby can be persuaded to keep them on. Any clothing should be light, warm, not constricting and easily laundered. Swaddling the baby in a flannelette wrap in addition to keeping him warm will also give him a sense of security. If being nursed in a cot, the baby can also be covered with light warm blankets.

It is important to monitor the temperature. This may be carried out using a mercury thermometer and measuring the axillary temperature. This method gives a close approximation to core temperature. (Normal range is 36.5–37°C.) Alternatively a skin probe may be used with or without attachment to servocontrol. (Normal skin temperature is 36–36.5°C.) Rectal temperature measurement is no longer advised because of the risk of damaging rectal mucosa; midwives should identify and abide by local policy.

Preventing infection

The risk of acquiring infection in these otherwise healthy babies is still appreciable. Great care should be taken to minimise risk factors. The simplest and most effective way of doing this is by meticulous attention to hand washing. All carers should be instructed in correct hand washing techniques. The use of bactericidal soaps or antiseptic solutions is recommended. Drying the hands properly is also important.

Encouraging parents to participate in care as soon as possible will cut down the number of people handling the baby and thereby minimise the risk of cross-infection. For the healthy low birthweight baby, enabling the parents to care for their own baby will have the added advantage of facilitating earlier discharge from hospital, thereby reducing the risk of nosocomial infection.

Whilst in hospital, other steps that can be employed include:

- the use of disposable equipment
- as far as possible ensuring that the baby has his own equipment
- drying the bowls used for washing/bathing the baby after use – bacteria thrive in a warm moist atmosphere.

Skin care

Bathing the baby is one of those procedures which traditionally form part of a baby's daily routine. The need for this with regard to prevention of infection is questionable; indeed there is strong argument for not bathing a preterm infant, particularly in the first few days.

Depending on the gestation of the baby the epidermal layer of skin will be more or less keratinised and therefore will afford variable protection against invading organisms. In the neonatal period there is accelerated maturation of the epidermal layer of the preterm baby's skin (Blackburn & Loper 1992). This process of keratinisation may, however, be hampered and inhibited if the baby is regularly immersed in a bath of water and towelled dry, be it ever so gently, leaving a 'soggy' easy portal for infection. Bathing will also alter the naturally low pH of the skin provided by normal skin flora, especially if alkaline or bactericidal soaps are used. Keeping the baby socially clean by removing milk or vomit debris and keeping the napkin area clean and dry will suffice. Occasionally, of course, to limit overexposure bathing is the fastest and best option for ensuring that vomit or faecal matter is removed.

Much discussion has taken place and a great deal of money has been spent on products for ensuring cleanliness of the baby's skin and making sure the baby smells like a baby. The safest, cheapest and best product is plain tap water. The risk of stimulating allergic conditions in a baby whose immune system is immature is thereby avoided as are toxic reactions from absorption of any of the ingredients of the soaps or oils.

Visiting
The advantages of more flexible, baby-friendly visiting policies outweigh the disadvantages of previous 'penal regimes', but anyone with a known or obvious infection should be excluded.

Promoting growth and development

Promotion of growth and development is one of the main objectives in caring for the low birthweight infant. One of the ways in which this can be done is by positioning the baby correctly. In an economy driven by market forces, paying attention to the relatively simple intervention of ensuring correct positioning may be cost-effective. A baby who conserves energy and interacts more positively with his parents will be able to be discharged sooner and save on expensive hospitalisation.

Position
Left to him- or herself the healthy LBW infant is capable of roaming around the incubator and is likely to be found lying across the bottom of the mattress, head against the side and with an arm or leg draped over the edge. Adult carers would spend time and effort righting the deviant's position not just once but often. Incubator design has improved to become more baby-friendly, having Perspex pieces to act as cot bumpers, thereby preventing small heads and limbs from becoming wedged in such awkward positions. Neonatal nurses and midwives are for their part gradually getting the message that their infant charges have been trying to convey: 'Please wrap me up to help me feel secure or at least give me some soft parameters to push against'. Even the less mobile infant will automatically adopt abducted positions if afforded the space an incubator provides. Research by Wolke (1987) and Als et al (1994) has brought into sharper focus the importance of position to the preterm infant. Most of their work has centred on nursing interventions which improve outcomes for the sick baby. The same principles, however, obtain for the well LBW infant and can be implemented more readily since the baby is not trammelled by ventilator tubing and numerous leads from monitoring equipment. The principle behind containment, nesting, or providing boundaries is that of encouraging flexed positions. Reference has already been made to the benefits of the flexed position for conservation of heat. Other benefits derived are adduction of the shoulder girdle which encourages hand-to-mouth behaviours; the pelvic girdle and hips are also supported. Downs et al (1991) claims that internal rotation of the hips and flexing the feet against a boundary provides appropriate sensory information which in turn helps prevent the 'toe-walking' phenomenon seen in some infants who have been born prematurely. A further advantage of containment is that it conserves energy. Calories may be preferentially diverted for necessary growth and development. The 'Back to Sleep' campaign mounted as a result of a report

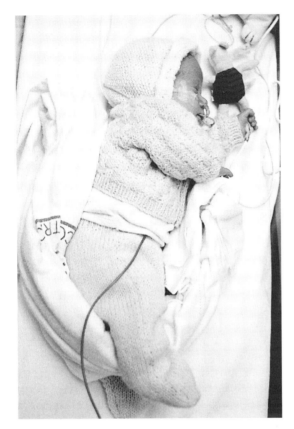

Fig. 37.10 Lateral position with support for hips and pelvic girdle.

from the Department of Health (1993) to help reduce the risk of cot death has highlighted the importance of positioning a baby correctly. A safe alternative to the supine position is the side-lying position (Fig. 37.10). Although babies seem to enjoy lying prone and there is some evidence to suggest that it is beneficial for maintenance of stability, this position should only be allowed in hospital and then only with an apnoea alarm in situ. Not least it is claimed by Warren (1993, p. 453) that the baby's position can affect the parents' perception of and hence their relationship with their baby. 'A comfortably curled baby with hands touching the face looks far more appealing than a flat extended baby.' Young (1996, p. 67) recommends 'frequent changes of position so that weightbearing forces are not permitted to persist for prolonged periods in any one direction'.

Touch

Seeing a baby in such a comfortable posture almost always leads to the involuntary action of stroking. Stroking or caressing the baby is normally the instinctive reaction of parents on being shown their baby after delivery. Such stroking is an expression of love which is invariably accompanied by talking to the baby in characteristically soft, sibilant tones. The baby responds by turning towards the direction of the sound and if held at an appropriate level will open his eyes and look at his mother. The mature baby may hold that gaze for a few seconds. Repetition of the stroking will quickly lead to the baby closing his eyes, relaxing and drifting off to sleep. The preterm infant may focus and hold his mother's face in view for only a fraction of that time but is certainly capable of seeing, hearing and responding to such stimuli. Parents of preterm infants, even those that are well, are often so frightened or dismayed by the baby's size that they will ask questions such as 'Can she really see?' or 'What can he hear?'. The midwife should encourage the parents to interact with the baby and attempt to elicit these positive, reinforcing responses. They will then find it easier to pluck up the courage to pick up and hold their baby.

The therapeutic value of touch therapy, systematic stroking and infant massage have increasingly been discussed over the past 10 years. Touching and Caressing, Tender in Caring (Tac-Tic) is a programme of systematic stroking involving all areas of the baby's body, described by Adamson-Macedo and Attree (1994). The possible beneficial effects of this programme are that production of growth hormone is increased and the immune system is strengthened. They recommend that midwives learn the skill and pass their expertise on to the parents. The pluses for the parents are that they enjoy the contact and feel that they are doing something positive and helpful for the baby. It should be remembered, though, that each baby is an individual and some may be less responsive to this stimulation than others. Close observation is necessary to pick up the behavioural cues that suggest the baby is unhappy.

Kangaroo care

Placing the baby in skin-to-skin contact with his

mother or father (Fig. 37.11), kangaroo care, was first described as an option of care in Bogota, Colombia, in a situation where incubators were at a premium (Whitelaw 1990). The idea has since spread to many other parts of the world. Not every mother would wish to participate in this way but those who do appear to enjoy these skin-to-skin sessions. Wearing only a napkin, the otherwise naked baby is placed against the mother's chest inside her blouse or dress. The baby's back may be covered with a blanket if necessary. Luddington (1990), among others, has investigated the effects of this type of care. She found that both the mother and baby appear to enjoy the experience. The baby relaxes, lulled to sleep by the soporific beat of his mother's heart and the 'see-saw' respiratory movements. It has been shown that the type of sleep the baby engages in is quiet sleep, the most economical in terms of energy expenditure and

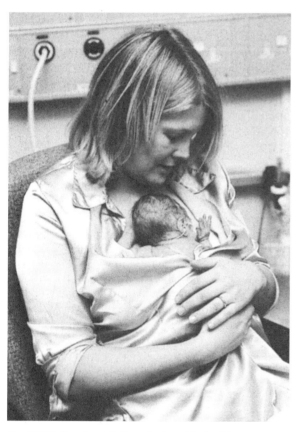

Fig. 37.11 A preterm baby enjoying skin-to-skin contact.

most beneficial for growth and development. The psychological advantages for the mother claimed for this type of care are that she also relaxes and becomes more confident in handling her baby. Being more relaxed improves lactation for women who are breast feeding.

Some disquiet has been voiced in some quarters about the risk of infection for those so vulnerable but it seems that where this type of care is provided infection rates have not risen (Whitelaw 1990).

Noise

Sounds come in various forms, pleasant and unpleasant; soft or loud. Noise bears the connotation of being unpleasant and loud. A low birthweight baby responds to noise in a similar way to a mature baby. Initially there is a startle response with or without crying but once the baby recognises that the noise is non-threatening no further responses will be elicited on repetition of the noise. This is the habituation phenomenon. Neonatal nurseries are not renowned for being quiet. There is a growing body of evidence to suggest that excessive noise is detrimental to the development of normal hearing and particularly stress provoking for the sick baby. De Paul & Chambers (1994) also suggest that 'energy used in noise-induced arousal may decrease the neonate's ability for social interaction'. Perhaps a lesser but nonetheless real problem is that the baby will not only habituate to the noise levels but become dependent on them, requiring a similar environment at home.

The midwife working in a neonatal unit should therefore be aware of these possible deleterious effects and take steps to reduce noise levels where possible. The introduction of the quiet hour is becoming an increasingly popular intervention. If nothing else this practice raises awareness of a potential hazard.

Auditory stimuli are not all bad. It is thought by some that a baby can recognise his mother's voice or other familiar sounds from prenatal intrauterine existence. Some units therefore are encouraging parents to leave tape recordings of themselves reading stories to the baby or tapes of the mother's favourite music.

During periods of quietness it is customary to dim the lights. Research by Mann et al (1986) and Blackburn & Patteson (1991) claims that the benefits to be had from establishing day–night cycles are longer quiet sleep patterns and better weight gain. This pattern of day–night cycles is helpful in preparing the well baby for life at home.

DECIDING THE OPTIMUM PLACE OF CARE

Two categories of neonatal care are described by the British Paediatric Association, intensive care levels 1 and 2 and special care. Intensive care units are labour intensive and expensive to run. Consequently these centres of excellence are restricted in number, strategically placed in cities and frequently form part of a much larger hospital complex. Being without the ability to foretell accurately the outcome of premature labour or of a pregnancy compromised by intrauterine growth retardation, obstetricians and paediatricians are faced with a dilemma. Do they arrange for intrauterine transfer of all such babies so that they are within reach of intensive care facilities or wait to assess the baby's condition after delivery and arrange transfer only if the baby proves to be unwell? In reality, this decision is often made easier by considering the availability or otherwise of beds in a neonatal intensive care unit (NICU) or the mother's medical or obstetric condition. If the birth has occurred in a larger hospital some distance from home, arrangements will be made for transfer back to the smaller unit once it is ascertained that both mother and baby are well.

One of the main concerns of parents, regardless of where the special care baby unit (SCBU) is located, is that they are separated from their baby. In the 1970s and 1980s worries were expressed that such separation resulted in delayed or defective bonding with the parents and in failure in the integration of the baby into the family unit. This in turn was linked with the increasing incidence of child abuse and non-accidental injury. A more realistic view is now taken that such a direct link cannot be assumed and that in truth any failure to bond with the child or integrate him into the family unit is multifactorial. The term low birthweight infant, in the absence of acute problems,

need not be separated from his mother. Blood sugar levels and temperature monitoring may be carried out in the postnatal ward. Single room accommodation can often be arranged that would cater for the baby who required to be kept warm in an incubator.

Transitional care

As a result of such theories the concept of transitional care was born. The philosophy of transitional care is that as soon as the mother is well enough to do so, she rooms in with her baby in a unit which is under the jurisdiction of midwives and nurses from the SCBU. Advantages of such an arrangement are:

- separation from the baby is avoided
- the mother has the opportunity to learn to care for the baby herself
- she is able to assume the role of mother and be seen to be doing so.

In a conventional postnatal ward the feeling of separation is augmented by seeing all the other babies being looked after by their own mothers. Mothers of LBW babies have expressed the feeling that they have only visiting rights and are resentful of strangers being in charge of their baby.

Although the philosophy of transitional care is sound, in practice many areas are unable to provide such a unit. Logistically it may not be possible to locate a transitional care unit close to a SCBU and, if at a distance, deployment of staff to best advantage becomes a problem. Employing additional staff is a luxury in which few hospitals are able to indulge. For either or both of these reasons transitional care has not mushroomed as envisaged. Nevertheless the principles of enabling parents to assume control of the care of their own baby should still be fostered. A compromise version of transitional care is offered in many places. The baby is nursed in the SCBU; the parents visit and participate in the baby's care as and when they are able to do so. When the baby is ready to go home, arrangements are made for the mother to room in for 2 or 3 days to afford her the opportunity of taking responsibility for total 24-hour care. An individualised programme of parenthood education is followed in order that specific needs are met. Feeding, winding and bathing are three areas of care that often present a challenge, especially for first-time parents. Looking after the baby in hospital with the security of knowing that help is at hand if required is one thing; taking the baby home and being alone is particularly daunting for the parents of a preterm baby. Careful preparations are essential to ensure that a smooth transition is effected.

Home

Care in the community is a tenet of health service management for many differing client groups. The same philosophy prevails for the care of the well low birthweight infant. Provided adequate support mechanisms are in place, there are advantages to be had from early discharge. This support can be offered in a number of ways. Primarily, whenever discharge of the baby is considered, the parents should feel happy about taking the baby home and not feel pressurised into doing so.

A domiciliary visit by a community midwife or a member of the neonatal team can be arranged, if necessary, to ensure home conditions are adequate. Paediatric liaison visitors are employed by some hospitals; in others the primary nurse who looked after the baby will continue to visit the family at home.

Points for discussion with parents

Heating. A stable room temperature is preferable to peaks and troughs. It is wise not to have the room too hot. The baby may become overheated and the fuel bills will be exorbitant.

Bedding. Choice of bed and bedding should be discussed. Sleeping bags and baby nests are not recommended for small babies. Lightweight woollen blankets are preferable. The mattress should be firm and conform to British safety standards. No pillows should be used. In an attempt to reduce the possibility of suffocation or of sudden infant death, parents are advised to place the baby on his back with his feet at the foot of the cot as in Figure 35.7.

Feeding. Mothers who are breast feeding should be warned of a possible temporary reduction in milk supply in the first few days because of the change in their routine. Conversely, being able to relax in their own home uninhibited by strangers has been found to improve lactation. Mothers who have chosen to give the baby formula milk should be comfortable about all aspects of preparation of feeds and sterilising of equipment. Vitamin and iron supplements are recommended for these babies regardless of the method of feeding. Parents should be advised in the method of administration of these.

Clothes. Low birthweight babies, particularly those who were growth retarded in utero, tend to gain weight rapidly. Many firms now supply special ranges of clothes for small babies but often these are more expensive than other baby clothes. Having a clothes library for these small babies is an enterprising form of support being offered by some hospitals and is especially helpful to those families struggling on a low income. The advent of a preterm baby may have totally altered a mother's plans for return to work or child care arrangements.

Telephone contact numbers. On discharge, parents should be given the telephone number of the nursery or of the community midwives and reassured that they can make contact at any time if they are concerned.

Support groups. There are many such groups now available to offer help and advice to families with small babies. Contact names and telephone numbers of local branches should be offered. Some hospitals arrange their own parent support group.

All these are ways of helping parents manage a low birthweight baby at home. One of the biggest advantages of being at home is that the risk of hospital-acquired infection is reduced. Shapiro (1995) concluded that early discharge home from the SCBU was cost-effective from a management perspective and, provided the correct support measures are put in place, that mothers express greater satisfaction.

READER ACTIVITIES

1. Watching one of the available videotapes of gestational age assessment will aid recognition of the appearance and capabilities of the preterm infant.

2. Whilst on placement in a special care baby unit, discuss with the parents of the babies in your care how they feel about looking after their LBW baby.

3. Arrange to accompany a paediatric liaison visitor on a domiciliary visit.

4. Present a case history or seminar paper to your peer group on the care of the well LBW baby.

REFERENCES

Adamson-Macedo E N, Attree J L A 1994 Tac Tic therapy: the importance of systematic stroking. British Journal of Midwifery 2(6): 264–269

Als H, Lawhon G, Duffy F H, McAnulty G B, Gibes-Grossman R, Blickman J G 1994 Individualised developmental care for the very low birthweight preterm infant. Journal of the American Medical Association 272(11): 853–858

Blackburn S T, Loper D L 1992 Maternal fetal and neonatal physiology. A clinical perspective. W B Saunders, Philadelphia, ch 11, p 511

Blackburn S, Patteson D 1991 Effects of cycled light on respiratory state and cardiorespiratory function in preterm infants. Journal of Perinatal and Neonatal nursing 4(4): 47–54

British Paediatric Society 1992 Report of working group of the British Association of Perinatal Medicine on categories of babies requiring neonatal care. BPA, London

Davies P S W, Clough H, Bishop N J, Lucas A, Cole J J, Cole T J 1996 Total energy expenditure in small for gestational age infants. Archives of Disease in Childhood 74: F208–210

Department of Health 1993 Report of the Chief Medical Officer's expert group on the sleeping position of infants and cot death. HMSO, London

de Paul D, Chambers S 1995 Environmental noise in the neonatal intensive care unit: implications for nursing practice. Journal of Perinatal and Neonatal Nursing 8(4): 71–76

Downs J A, Edwards A A, McCormick D C, Stewart A L 1991 Effect of intervention on development of hip posture in very preterm babies. Archives of Disease in Childhood 66: 797–801

Dubowitz L M S, Dubowitz V, Goldberg C 1970 Clinical assessment of gestational age in the newborn infant. Journal of Paediatrics 77(1): 1–10

Ewer A K, Durbin G M, Morgan M E I, Booth J W 1994 Gastric emptying in preterm infants. Archives of Disease in Childhood 71: 24–27

Ingram J, Redshaw M, Harris A 1994 Breastfeeding in neonatal care. British Journal of Midwifery 2(9): 412–418

Jones E 1994 Breastfeeding in the preterm infant. Modern Midwife 4(1): 22–26

Jones E 1995 Strategies to promote preterm breastfeeding. Modern Midwife 5(3): 8–11

Lawrence R 1994 Breastfeeding, 4th edn. Mosby, St Louis, ch 17, p 571

Lucas A, Morley R, Cole T J, Lister G, Leeson-Payne G 1992 Breastmilk and subsequent intelligence quotient in children born preterm. Lancet 339: 261–264

Lucas A, Morley R, Cole T J, Gore S M 1994 A randomised multicentre study of human milk versus formula and later development in preterm infants. Archives of Disease in Childhood, Fetal and Neonatal edn 70(2): F141–146

Luddington S M 1990 Energy conservation during skin to skin contact between premature infants and their mothers. Heart and Lung 19(5): 446–451

Mann N P, Haddow R, Stokes L, Goodley S, Rutter N 1986 Effect of night and day on preterm infants in a newborn nursery: randomised trial. British Medical Journal 293(15): 1265–1267

Moody J 1993 A revolution in baby feeding. New Generation 12(2): 9

Petit J 1992 Breastfeeding in special care nursery. Paediatric Nursing 4(7): 24–25

Shapiro C 1995 Shortened hospital stay for low birthweight infants. Nuts and bolts of a nursing intervention project. Journal of Obstetrics, Gynecology and Neonatal Nursing 24(156): 59–62

Warren L 1993 How to place a baby. MIDIRS Midwifery Digest 3(4): 452–453

Whitelaw A 1990 Kangaroo baby care: just a nice experience or an important advance for preterm infants. Pediatrics 85(4): 604–605

Wolke D 1987 Environmental and developmental neonatology. Journal of Reproductive and Infant Psychology 5: 17–42

World Health Organization (WHO) 1978 Health for all by the year 2000. WHO, Geneva

World Health Organization (WHO) 1977 Manual of international statistical classification of diseases, injuries and causes of death. WHO, Geneva, vol 1

Young J 1996 Developmental care of the premature baby. Baillière Tindall, London

FURTHER READING

Buehler D M, Als H, Duffy F H, McAnulty G B, Liederman J 1995 Effectiveness of individualised developmental care for low risk preterm infants. Pediatrics 96(5): 923–932

Dodd V 1996 Gestational age assessment. Neonatal Network 14(1): 27–36

King A, Luke Y W 1994 Unexplained fetal growth retardation: what is the cause? Archives of Disease in Childhood 70: F225–227

Royal College of Midwives 1992 Successful breastfeeding. RCM, London, ch 8, pp 75–76

Russell J 1995 Touch and infant massage. Paediatric Nursing 5(5): 8–11

Turrill J 1992 Supported positioning in intensive care. Paediatric Nursing 4(4): 24–27

Wakefield J 1994 Nasogastric tube feeding and early discharge. Paediatric Nursing 6(9): 18–19

Wyly M V (ed) 1995 Premature infants and their families. Singular Publishing Group, London

Recognising the ill baby

Jean Evelyn Bain

The length of time a mother now spends in hospital with her newborn infant is ever decreasing. The focus of this chapter is to aid the midwife in the early detection of diseases in the neonate, so that appropriate action can be taken as soon as possible. The chapter design takes a systematic approach which can be used in conjunction with the newborn examination, thus allowing the midwife to distinguish the ill baby from the well.

The chapter aims to:

- assist the midwife in the assessment and identification of the ill neonate

- provide an overview of the potential or presenting problems of the neonate

- consider the needs of the family by the integration of family-centred care in the neonatal unit.

INTRODUCTION

The majority of newborn babies are born normal and healthy; they require no intervention after delivery except to be dried with a warm towel and then to be given back to their mothers. However, even though the labour and delivery may have been uneventful, the baby will still need to be observed at this time to ensure that the respirations are normal, that there is good colour, the body temperature is stable and that the baby is active and responsive.

The midwife soon becomes familiar with the appearance and behaviour of the well baby, but must also learn the signs and signals caused by illness, some of which may be subtle and non-specific. The labour and delivery have an obvious effect on the well-being of the infant, but added to this are the genetic background, the mother's illnesses in pregnancy and any drugs she may have taken or received during that period (Black 1972).

Parents welcome the observation of their newborn as it provides an opportunity for them to discuss any concerns they may have and can reassure them that their baby is normal and healthy. If the baby is unwell, this needs to be identified quickly and parents need to be made aware of any problem as soon as possible.

ASSESSMENT OF THE INFANT

Immediately after birth, all infants should be examined for any gross congenital abnormalities or evidence of birth trauma. They should also have their weight and gestational age plotted on a standard growth chart. Infants can then be classified as:

- appropriate for gestational age: between the 10th and 90th centile
- small for gestational age (SGA): below the 10th centile
- large for gestational age (LGA): above the 90th centile
- preterm: born before 37 weeks' gestation.

This classification allows the midwife to assess infants who may require specialised care. Infants who are preterm, SGA or LGA are at an increased risk of respiratory disease, hypoglycaemia, polycythaemia and disturbed thermoregulation. Later, usually within the next 24 hours, a more comprehensive, systematic, physical examination should take place.

Increasingly, it is being recognised that maternal height, ethnic origin, sex of the infant and gestation have important effects on classification, and care must be taken not to wrongly assign infants to a particular category.

Decreasing morbidity and mortality is the goal of all those involved with the care of the newborn infant. The early recognition of existing or potential problems is vital if the appropriate treatment is to be initiated as soon as possible.

Maternal health

Any disease in the mother can have an effect on the pregnancy. Some have more specific effects than others and reviewing the maternal history is an essential starting point in the understanding of the potential or presenting problems of the neonate. Influencing factors include:

- pregnancy-induced hypertension
- a history of epilepsy
- maternal diabetes
- a history of substance abuse
- a history of sexually transmitted diseases.

Fetal well-being and health in pregnancy

The following are examples of significant questions that a midwife may ask herself as they may have a critical influence on the well-being of the infant:

- What was the estimated date of delivery?
- Was this a twin pregnancy?
- Was the baby presenting by the breech?
- Is the baby preterm?
- Is the infant small for gestational age?
- Was there poor growth in utero?
- Was any evidence of congenital abnormalities picked up on the scan, such as enlarged heart, or bowel obstruction?

Perinatal and delivery complications

Labour and delivery may also have an effect on the general welfare of the newborn infant. Listed below are important points that can confirm or rule out fetal compromise:

- prolonged rupture of membranes
- abnormal fetal heart rate pattern
- meconium staining
- difficult or rapid delivery
- caesarean section and the reason for this.

Over a period of a few hours the newborn baby needs to adapt to living without placental support, and it is during this time that some problems may become manifest. The midwife needs to be able to recognise warning signs and initiate prompt action if deterioration of the baby's condition is to be prevented.

PHYSICAL ASSESSMENT

Most of the information the midwife requires for the assessment of an infant's well-being comes from observation. The baby's breathing pattern will alter depending on levels of activity but a respiratory rate above 60 breaths per minute is considered as tachypnoea. Much can be learned by observing the infant's resting position. The normal baby will lie with his limbs partially flexed and active. The skin colour should be centrally pink indicating adequate oxygenation; there should be no rashes or skin lesions. The signs listed in Box 38.1 may indicate an underlying problem.

After the initial observation there usually follows a more systematic examination commencing at the baby's head and working gradually down to the feet.

The skin

The skin of a neonate varies in its appearance and can often be the cause of unnecessary anxiety in the mother and the nursing and medical staff. It is, however, often the first sign that there may be an underlying problem in the baby.

The presence of meconium on the skin, usually seen in the nail beds and around the umbilicus, is frequently associated with infants who have cardio-respiratory problems. More generally, the skin of all babies should be examined for pallor, plethora, cyanosis, jaundice and skin rashes.

Box 38.1 General assessment warning signs

- Pallor
- Central cyanosis
- Jaundice
- Apnoea lasting longer than 20 seconds
- Heart rate less than 110 or more than 180 beats per minute (taken during spells of inactivity)
- Respiratory rate less than 30 or greater than 60 breaths per minute
- Skin temperature less than 36.2°C or above 37.2°C
- Lack of spontaneous movement and responsiveness
- Abnormal lying position either hypotonic or hypertonic
- Lack of interest in surroundings.

Pallor

A pale, mottled baby is an indication of poor perfusion. At birth it can be associated with low circulating blood volume or with circulatory adaptation and compensation for perinatal hypoxaemia. The anaemic infant's appearance is usually pale pink, white or in severe cases where there is vascular collapse, grey. Other presenting signs are tachycardia, tachypnoea and poor capillary refill (to assess capillary refill, press the skin briefly on the forehead or abdomen and observe how long it takes for the colour to return; this should be prompt).

The most likely causes of anaemia in the newborn period are:

- a history in the infant of haemolytic disease of the newborn
- twin-to-twin transfusions in utero (which can cause one infant to be anaemic and the other polycythaemic)
- maternal antepartum or intrapartum haemorrhage.

Pallor can also be observed in infants who are hypothermic or hypoglycaemic.

Problems associated with pallor include:

- anaemia and shock
- respiratory disorders
- cardiac anomalies
- sepsis (where poor peripheral perfusion might also be observed).

Plethora

Babies who are beetroot in colour are usually described as plethoric. Their colour may indicate an excess of circulating red blood cells (polycythaemia). This is defined as a venous haematocrit greater than 70%. Newborn infants can become polycythaemic if they are recipients of:

- twin-to-twin transfusion in utero
- a large placental transfusion.

Contributing factors are delayed clamping of the umbilical cord, or holding the infant below the level of the placenta, thereby allowing blood to flow into the baby and giving a greater circulating blood volume (sometimes occurring in unassisted deliveries). Other infants at risk are:

- small for gestational age babies
- infants of diabetic mothers
- those with Down syndrome.

Hypoglycaemia is commonly seen in plethoric infants because red blood cells consume glucose. The infant can exhibit a neurological disorder; irritability, jitteriness and convulsions can occur. Other problems that may manifest are:

- apnoea
- respiratory distress
- cardiac failure
- necrotising enterocolitis.

Treatment by partial plasma exchange to dilute the red blood cells is recommended if the infant is symptomatic (Leven et al 1987).

Cyanosis

Central cyanosis should always be taken very seriously. The mucous membranes are the most reliable indicators of central colour in all babies and if the tongue and mucous membranes appear blue, this indicates low oxygen saturation levels in the blood, usually of respiratory or cardiac origin. Episodic central cyanotic attacks may be an indication that the infant is having a convulsion. Peripheral cyanosis of the hands and feet is common during the first 24 hours of life; after this time it may be a non-specific sign of illness. *Central cyanosis always demands urgent attention.*

Jaundice

Early onset jaundice (occurring in the skin and sclera within the first 12 hours of life) is abnormal and needs investigating. If a jaundiced baby is unduly lethargic, is a poor feeder, vomits or has an unstable body temperature, this may indicate infection and action should be taken to exclude this (see Ch. 42).

Other factors that affect the appearance of the skin

Preterm infants have thinner skin which is redder in appearance than that of term infants. In post-term infants the skin is often dry and cracked.

The skin is a good indicator of the nutritional status of the infant. The SGA infant may look malnourished and have folds of loose skin over joints, owing to the lack or loss of subcutaneous fat. This can predispose the infant to problems with hypoglycaemia due to poor glycogen stores in the liver and can cause problems with hypothermia.

If the infant is dehydrated, the skin looks dry and pale and is often cool to touch. If gently pinched, it will be slow in retracting. Other signs of dehydration are: pallor or mottled skin, sunken fontanelle or eyeball sockets and tachycardia.

Skin rashes

Skin rashes are quite common in newborn babies but most are benign and self-limiting.

Milia are white or yellow papules seen over the cheeks, nose and forehead. These invariably disappear spontaneously over the first few weeks of life.

Miliaria are clear vesicles on the face, scalp and perineum, caused by retention of sweat in unopened sweat glands. The treatment is to nurse the infant in a cooler environment or remove excessive clothing.

Petechiae or purpura rash can occur in neonatal thrombocytopenia, which is a condition of platelet deficiency and usually presents with a petechial rash over the whole of the body. There may also be prolonged bleeding from puncture sites and/or the umbilicus and bleeding into the gut. Thrombocytopenia may be found in infants with:

- congenital infections, both viral and bacterial
- maternal idiopathic thrombocytopenia
- drugs (administered to mother or infant)
- severe Rhesus haemolytic disease.

Mongolian blue spot is found on the lumbosacral area in infants of races with pigmented skin. The pigmentation may be mistaken for bruising.

Bruising can occur extensively following breech extractions, forceps deliveries and Ventouse extractions. The bleeding can cause a decrease in circulating blood volume, predisposing the infant to anaemia or, if the bruising is severe, hypotension.

Erythema toxicum is a rash that consists of white papules on an erythematous base and occurs in about 30–70% of infants. This condition is benign and should not be confused with a staphylococcal infection which will require antibiotics. Diagnosis can be confirmed by examination of a smear of aspirate from a pustule which will show numerous eosinophils (white cells indicative of an allergic response, rather than infection).

Infectious lesions

Thrush is a fungal infection of the mouth and throat. It is very common in neonates especially if they have been on antibiotics. It presents as white patches seen over the tongue and mucous membranes and as a red rash on the perineum.

Herpes simplex virus, if acquired in the neonatal period, is a most serious viral infection. Transmission in utero is rare; the infection usually occurs during delivery. 70% of affected infants will produce a rash, which appears as vesicles or pustules. Mortality depends on severity of the illness and when treatment commenced (Weston 1985).

Umbilical sepsis can be caused by a bacterial infection. Until its separation, the umbilical cord can be a focus for infection by bacteria that colonise the skin of the newborn. If periumbilical redness occurs or a discharge is noted it may be necessary to commence antibiotic therapy in order to prevent an ascending infection.

Bullous impetigo is a condition which makes the skin look as though it has been scalded and is caused by streptococci or staphylococci. It presents as widespread tender erythema, followed by blisters which break, leaving raw areas of skin. This is particularly noticeable around the napkin area but can also cause umbilical sepsis, breast abscesses, conjunctivitis and, in deep infections, there may also be involvement of the bones and joints.

Respiratory system

Respiratory distress in the newborn can be a presentation of a number of clinical disorders and is the major factor in the morbidity and mortality in the neonatal period.

It is important to observe the baby's breathing when he is at rest and when he is active. The midwife should always start by observing skin colour and then carry out a respiratory inspection, taking into account whether the baby is making either an extra effort or insufficient effort to breathe.

Respiratory inspection

Respirations should be counted by watching the lower chest and abdomen rise and fall for a full minute. The respiration rate should be between 40 and 60 breaths per minute but will vary between levels of activity. The chest should expand symmetrically. If there is unilateral expansion and breath sounds are diminished on one side, this may indicate that a pneumothorax has occurred (Dickason et al 1990).

Increased work of breathing

If the baby's respiratory rate at rest is above 60 breaths per minute, this is described as *tachypnoea*. When observing an infant's respiratory rate the midwife must always take into consideration the environment and the temperature in which the baby is being nursed. Overheating will cause an infant to breathe faster.

Any infant with tachypnoea may be described as having respiratory distress and observations should also be made of the quality of the respirations, noting if there is any inspiratory pulling in of the chest wall above and below the sternum or between the ribs (retraction). If nasal flaring is also present, this may indicate that there has been a delay in the lung fluid clearance, or that a more serious respiratory problem is developing (Dickason et al 1990).

Grunting, heard either with a stethoscope or audibly, is an abnormal expiratory sound. The grunting baby forcibly exhales against a closed glottis in order to prevent the alveoli from collapsing. These infants require help with their breathing, either by intubation or continuous positive airway pressure ventilation (CPAP). See also Chapter 39.

Apnoea

Apnoea is defined as a cessation of breathing for 20 seconds or more. It is associated with pallor, bradycardia, cyanosis, oxygen desaturation or a change in the level of consciousness (Faranoff & Martin 1987). Any baby having apnoeic spells needs to be admitted to a neonatal unit to have his cardiorespiratory system monitored.

The most common cause of apnoea in preterm babies is pulmonary surfactant deficiency (see Ch. 39) or the immaturity of the central nervous system control mechanism.

Other disorders that may produce apnoea in the newborn are:

- hypoxia
- pneumonia
- aspiration
- pneumothorax
- metabolic disorders, e.g. hypoglycaemia, hypocalcaemia, acidosis
- anaemia
- maternal drugs
- neurological problems, e.g. intracranial haemorrhage, convulsions, developmental disorders of the brain
- congenital anomalies of the upper airway.

It is also very important to remember that apnoea may also be induced by stimulation of the posterior pharynx by suction catheters.

Body temperature

Thermoregulation is a critical physiological function that is closely related to the survival of the infant. It is therefore essential that all those caring for newborn infants are aware of the importance of the thermal environment and understand the need for maintenance of normal body temperature (Merenstein & Gardner 1993).

A neutral thermal environment is defined as the ambient air temperature at which oxygen consumption or heat production is minimal with body temperature in the normal range.

The normal body temperature range for term infants is (Mayfield et al 1984):

Axillary   36.5–37°C
Rectal (core temperature)   36.7–37.2°C.

Environments that are outside the neutral thermal environment may result in the infant developing hypothermia or hyperthermia. Babies who are too cold or too warm will try and regulate their temperature and this action, especially in the preterm and small for gestational age infant, can have a detrimental effect. See also Chapter 35.

Hypothermia

Hypothermia is defined as a core temperature below 36°C (Morris 1994). When the body temperature is below this level the infant is at risk from cold stress. This can cause complications such as increased oxygen consumption, lactic acid production, apnoea, decrease in blood coagulability and, the most commonly seen, hypoglycaemia. In preterm infants, cold stress may also cause a decrease in surfactant secretion and synthesis.

Letting infants get cold increases mortality and morbidity.

After delivery an infant's body temperature falls very quickly. The healthy full-term infant will try to maintain his temperature within the normal range. If, however, the infant is compromised at birth by any of the following conditions, the added stress of hypothermia can be disastrous:

- severe asphyxia
- extensive resuscitation
- delayed drying at birth
- respiratory distress
- hypoglycaemia
- sepsis – septic infants often have hypothermia rather than hyperthermia
- being preterm or small for gestational age – these infants have poor glucose stores, decreased subcutaneous tissue and little or no brown fat stores.

When a neonate is exposed to cold he will at first become very restless, then, as his body temperature falls, he adopts a tightly flexed position to try to conserve heat. The sick or preterm infant will tend to lie supine in a frog-like position with all his surfaces exposed, which maximises heat loss (Roberton 1993).

Adults can generate heat from shivering whereas neonates perform non-shivering thermogenesis utilising their brown fat stores. During brown fat metabolism, oxygen is consumed and this may cause an alteration in the respiratory pattern, usually by increasing the rate. Added to this, the baby often looks pale or mottled and may be uninterested in feeding. Hypoglycaemia is a common feature of infants with increased energy expenditure associated with thermoregulation and this can cause the infant to have jittery movements of the limbs, even though he is quiet and often limp.

Hyperthermia

Hyperthermia is defined as an axillary temperature above 37.5°C (Woods Blake & Murray 1993). The usual cause of hyperthermia is overheating of the environment but it can also be a clinical sign of sepsis, brain injury or drug therapy. If an infant is too warm, he/she becomes restless and may have bright red cheeks. Hyperthermia has a similar effect on the body to that of hypothermia and is equally detrimental. An infant will attempt to regulate his/her temperature by increasing his/her respiratory rate and this can lead to an increased fluid loss by evaporation through the airways. Other problems caused by hyperthermia are: hypernatraemia, jaundice and recurrent apnoea.

Variability in body temperature, either high or low, may be the first and only sign that a baby is unwell.

Cardiovascular system

The normal heart rate of a newborn is (Korones 1986):

Term infants   120–160 bpm
Preterm infants   130–170 bpm.

Heart rates persistently outwith this range may suggest an underlying cardiac problem.

Cardiovascular dysfunction should be suspected in infants who commonly present with lethargy and breathlessness during feeding. It is often the baby's mother who first expresses concern: her baby may be slow with his feeds, she may say he looks pale at times or that he feels very sweaty or has fast or laboured breathing.

It can be very difficult to identify infants with congenital heart disease because the clinical picture of tachycardia, tachypnoea, pallor or cyanosis may be suggestive of a respiratory problem or sepsis (Dickason et al 1990).

Problems that occur in neonatal cardiovascular function are usually caused by either congenital defects or by a failure of the transition from fetal to adult circulation. Persistent pulmonary hypertension of the newborn is usually seen in term or post-term infants who have a history of hypoxia or asphyxia at birth. The infants are slow to take their first breath or are difficult to ventilate. Respiratory distress and cyanosis are seen before 12 hours of age. Hypoxaemia is usually profound and may suggest cyanotic heart disease. See Chapter 41.

Risk factors include meconium-stained amniotic fluid, nuchal cord, placental abruption, acute blood loss and maternal sedation.

Congenital heart disease affects just under 1% of newborn infants, many of whom will be asymptomatic in the neonatal period (Fowlie & Forsyth 1995). Infants who appear breathless but have little or no rib recession, are not grunting and have only a moderately raised respiratory rate may have heart disease.

Cyanosis can be a prominent feature in some cardiac defects, but not all. Box 38.2 lists signs that may be indicative of congenital heart disease.

Cardiac failure may be rapid in onset and the earlier it presents, the more sinister the cause. Delays in recognising and treating heart failure may lead to a rapid deterioration and cardiogenic shock. Cardiac shock may resemble early septicaemia, pneumonia or meningitis (Qureshi 1989). The first indication of an underlying cardiac lesion may be the presence of a murmur heard on routine

---

Box 38.2 Warning signs suggestive of congenital heart disease

- Cyanosis (often the cyanosis is out of proportion to the degree of respiratory distress)
- Persistent tachypnoea
- Persistent tachycardia at rest
- Poor feeding: infants may be breathless and sweaty during the feed or after feeding; they may not complete their feeds and subsequently fail to thrive
- A sudden gain in weight leading to clinical signs of oedema; this is usually noted as the baby having puffy feet or eyelids and, in males, the scrotum being swollen
- A very loud systolic murmur is invariably significant
- Evidence of cardiac enlargement on X-ray, persisting beyond 48 hours of age
- Enlargement of the liver

examination. However, a soft localised systolic murmur with no evidence of any symptoms of cardiac disease is usually of no significance.

Central nervous system

Assessment of an infant's neurological status is usually carried out on a baby who is awake but not crying. Abnormal postures which include neck retraction, frog-like postures, hyperextension or hyperflexion of the limbs, jittery or abnormal involuntary movements, high-pitched or weak cry could be indicative of neurological impairment and need investigation (Halliday et al 1989). It is often useful to draw up a list of signs if it is suspected that there may be a problem.

Normal behaviour

After birth, there is a distinct pattern of normal behaviour. During the first hour of life, the newborn appears alert and interested in his/her surroundings, will cry lustily and is keen and eager to feed. Following this period of activity he/she will then sleep for 2–4 hours. During this time, all the vital signs of temperature, heart rate and respiration rate will be within the normal range. After sleeping the baby will awaken, begin rooting for food and have a strong suck–swallow reflex (Dickason et al 1990).

Neurological disorders

Neurological disorders found at or soon after birth may be either prenatal or perinatal in origin. They include:

- congenital abnormalities: hydrocephaly, microcephaly, encephalocele, chromosomal anomalies
- hypoxic–ischaemic cerebral injuries
- birth traumas: skull fractures, spinal cord and brachial plexus injuries, subdural and subarachnoid haemorrhage
- infections passed on to the fetus (toxoplasmosis, rubella, cytomegalovirus (CMV), syphilis).

Neurological disorders that appear in the neonatal period need to be recognised promptly in order to minimise brain damage. These include:

- infection: meningitis, herpes simplex, viral encephalitis
- hypoxia: birth asphyxia, respiratory distress, apnoeic episodes
- metabolic: acidosis, hypoglycaemia, hyponatraemia, hypernatraemia, hypothermia, hypocalcaemia, hypomagnesaemia
- drug withdrawal: narcotics, barbiturates, general anaesthesia
- intracranial haemorrhages/intraventricular haemorrhage (IVH)
- secondary bleeding: intracranial haemorrhage from thrombocytopenia or disseminated intravascular coagulation.

Cerebral hypoxia and bacterial infections are of prime importance. Of these, cerebral hypoxia is more common and more difficult to diagnose (Halliday et al 1989).

Terminology

Terminology that describes abnormal movement in babies is very variable and includes 'fits', 'convulsions', 'seizures', 'twitching', 'jumpy' and 'jittery'. In contrast, a baby with poor muscle tone is described as floppy. It is often very difficult to distinguish a seizure from jitteriness or irritability. The jittery baby has tremors, rapid movement of the extremities or fingers that are stopped when the limb is held or flexed. Jitteriness can be normal but is more often seen in infants who are affected by drug withdrawal or in infants with hypoglycaemia.

Seizures

Seizures in the newborn period can be extremely difficult to diagnose as they are often very subtle and easily missed (Table 38.1).

The most common causes of seizure activity are:

- asphyxia
- metabolic disturbance
- intracranial/intraventricular haemorrhage
- infection
- malformation/genetic defect.

Hypotonia (floppy infant)

The term hypotonia or floppy baby describes the loss of body tension and tone. As a result, the infant

Table 38.1 Neonatal seizure chart (after Volpe & Hill 1987)

Type	Affected infants
Subtle Apnoea usually seen with abnormal eye movements, tonic horizontal deviation, blinking, fluttering eyelids, jerking, drooling, sucking, tonic posturing or unusual movements of limbs (rowing, pedalling or swimming)	Most frequent type and most common in preterm infants
Clonic Jerking activity Multifocal: movements of one body part followed by another	Full-term infants: hypoxic–ischemic encephalopathy or inborn errors of metabolism
Focal: movement of one part	Disturbance of the entire cerebrum
Tonic Posturing similar to decerebrate posture in adults	Preterm infants with intraventricular haemorrhage
Myoclonic Single or multiple jerks of upper and lower extremities	Possible prediction of myoclonic spasms in early infancy

adopts an abnormal posture which is noticeable on handling.

Preterm infants below 30 weeks' gestation have a resting position that is usually characterised as hypotonic. By 34 weeks their thighs and hips are flexed and they lie in a frog-like position, usually with their arms extended. At 36–38 weeks' gestation, the resting position of a healthy newborn baby is one of total flexion with immediate recoil. Hypotonia in a full-term infant is not normal and requires investigation. It is also important to determine whether the hypotonia is associated with weakness or normal power in the infant's limbs.

The causes of hypotonia include:

- maternal sedation
- birth asphyxia
- prematurity
- infection
- Down syndrome
- metabolic problems, e.g. hypoglycaemia, hyponatraemia, inborn errors of metabolism
- neurological problems, e.g. spinal cord injuries (sustained by difficult breech or forceps delivery), myasthenia gravis related to maternal disease, myotonic dystrophy
- endocrine, e.g. hypothyroidism
- neuromuscular disorders.

Renal/genitourinary system

Urinary infections in the newborn period are quite common, especially in males. The baby typically presents with lethargy, poor feeding, increasing jaundice and vomiting. Urine that only dribbles out, rather than being passed forcefully, may be an indication of a problem with posterior urethral valves. Urine that is cloudy in appearance or smelly, may be an indication of a urinary tract infection.

The genitourinary tract has the highest percentage of anomalies, congenital or genetic, of all the organ systems. Prenatal diagnosis is possible with ultrasound and aids the early assessment and intervention which is essential if kidney damage is to be prevented. Renal problems may present as a failure to pass urine. The normal infant usually passes urine 4–10 hours after birth (Dickason et al 1990). Normal urine output for a term baby in the first day of life should be 2–4 ml/kg/h. Urine output of less than 1 ml/kg/h (oliguria) should be investigated (Halliday et al 1989).

Urinalysis using reagent strips will give information that may be helpful in diagnosis (Table 38.2).

Common causes of reduced urine output include:

- inadequate fluid intake

Table 38.2 Information obtainable from urinalysis with reagent strips

Test	Significance
Urine pH	Failure to acidify the urine may indicate a dysfunction of the renal tubular system, which plays a primary role in the regulation of bicarbonate concentration
Specific gravity	Indicates urine concentration
Blood	Is suggestive of trauma or inflammation of the genitourinary tract
Protein	May suggest renal disease

- increased fluid loss due to hyperthermia, use of radiant heaters and phototherapy units
- birth asphyxia
- congenital abnormalities
- infection.

Care should be taken, of course, that urine output does not go unnoticed by the midwife when the infant is on the labour ward or elsewhere.

Gastrointestinal tract

Some congenital abnormalities of the gastrointestinal tract can now be diagnosed antenatally by ultrasound. This knowledge allows for time to prepare for an affected infant, which is vital when dealing with exposed organs as in the disorder of gastroschisis or omphalocele. Parents can also have a clear understanding of the condition and are able to prepare themselves for the events that will follow after the birth. Other defects, however, may not be suspected until the infant becomes unwell.

Structural deformities of the oesophagus or intestine can be life-threatening in the newborn period. Oesophageal atresia can be diagnosed antenatally, because the fetus is unable to swallow the amniotic fluid, giving rise to polyhydramnios in the mother. If, however, the condition is not identified antenatally, the infant usually presents with copious saliva, which causes gagging, choking, pallor or cyanosis. In infants who are inadvertently

fed milk this may cause a severe respiratory arrest due to milk aspiration.

Intestinal obstructions may be caused by atresias, malformations or structural damage anywhere below the stomach. In the newborn period, gastrointestinal disorders often present with vomiting, abdominal distension, a failure to pass stools, or diarrhoea with, or without, blood in the stools.

However, vomiting in the postnatal period can be caused by factors other than gastrointestinal obstructions. The midwife should distinguish between posseting that occurs with winding and overhandling after feeding and vomiting due to overfeeding, infection or intestinal abnormalities. Early vomiting may be caused by the infant swallowing meconium or maternal blood at delivery. This can cause a gastritis which will eventually settle. Some infants may require a gastric lavage if the symptoms are severe.

All vomit should be checked for the presence of bile or blood. Observe the infant for other signs such as abdominal distension, watery or blood-stained stools and temperature instability.

The normal full-term infant usually passes about eight stools a day. Breast-fed babies' stools are looser and more frequent than those of bottle-fed infants and the colour varies more and sometimes appears greenish. The infant who has an infection can often display signs of gastrointestinal problems, usually poor feeding, vomiting and/or diarrhoea. Diarrhoea caused by gastroenteritis is usually very watery and may sometimes resemble urine. The cause is either bacterial or viral. Infants with this condition must be isolated and scrupulous hand washing adhered to (Halliday et al 1989). Loose stools can also be a feature of infants being treated for hyperbilirubinaemia with phototherapy.

Some of the more commonly seen gastrointestinal problems include: duodenal atresia, malrotation of the gut, volvulus, meconium ileus, necrotising enterocolitis, imperforate anus, rectal fistulas and Hirschsprung's disease.

Duodenal atresia

Duodenal atresia usually presents with bile-stained vomiting within 24 hours of birth. Abdominal distension is not usually present, but often visible peristalsis is seen over the stomach. Insertion of a nasogastric tube may reveal a large amount of bile in the stomach and there is usually a history of polyhydramnios and a delay in passing meconium. Antenatal diagnosis is possible. The most commonly associated anomaly is Down syndrome which occurs in 30% of cases (Davis & Young 1992).

Malrotation of the gut

Malrotation may present as a mechanical bowel obstruction caused by the abnormal attachments (Ladd's bands). The infant usually has no problems in the first few days of life, then presents with bilious vomiting and abdominal distension.

Volvulus

Volvulus can occur in infants who have an incomplete rotation of the gut. Diagnosis can be delayed because the obstruction is intermittent, twisting enough to cause obstruction, then untwisting causing relief. As a result of venous impairment and mucosal injury, there may be blood passed per rectum. Bilious vomiting also occurs. These infants are commonly gravely ill.

Meconium ileus

The infant with meconium ileus often has cystic fibrosis. Clinical signs include marked abdominal distension. Meconium is not passed, but occasionally small pellet-type stools, pale in colour, are mistakenly identified as bowel action. Vomiting gradually increases, mainly gastric secretions and feed, but later becomes bilious.

Necrotising enterocolitis (NEC)

NEC is an acquired disease of the small and large intestine caused by ischaemia of the intestinal mucosa. It occurs more often in premature babies, but may also occur in term infants who have been asphyxiated at delivery or infants with polycythaemia and hypothermia (commonly found in SGA infants). NEC may present with vomiting or, if gastric emptying is being monitored, the aspirate is large and bile stained. The abdomen becomes distended, stools are loose and may have blood in them. In the early stages of NEC, the infant can display non-specific signs of temperature instability, unstable blood sugars, lethargy and poor peripheral circulation. As the illness progresses, the infant becomes apnoeic and bradycardic and may need ventilating.

Imperforate anus

All infants should be checked at birth for this.

Rectal fistulas

The midwife should look for the presence of meconium in the urine, or in female infants, meconium being passed per vaginam.

Hirschsprung's disease

Hirschsprung's disease should be suspected in term infants with delayed passage of meconium, certainly outwith the first 24 hours of life. It is caused by an absence of ganglion cells in the distal rectum. The area of aganglionosis varies and may include the lower rectum, colon and small intestine. An incomplete obstruction occurs above the affected segment. Abdominal distension and vomiting are clinical signs, with the vomit becoming bile stained if meconium is not passed.

Metabolic disorders

Metabolic disorders, such as galactosaemia and phenylketonuria, present in the newborn period with vomiting, weight loss, jaundice and lethargy.

MEETING THE NEEDS OF THE ILL BABY AND THE FAMILY

The baby

The admission of a newborn infant to a neonatal unit interrupts the normal course of events that surrounds a birth. Instead of the parents providing love, warmth and food and taking responsibility for their baby, the task is taken on by professionals. This leaves the parents with an unidentified role which can seriously damage the parent–infant bond.

The neonatal unit is noisy, hot and brightly lit, and is not the normal environment that is usually provided for the newly born infant. Babies are subjected to multiple carers who interrupt their sleep–wake cycles, carry out painful, intrusive, invasive procedures and separate them from their loved ones (Gorski 1991).

It should be the aim of all neonatal units to try to normalise the environment as much as possible. This should begin with the reduction of excess stimuli and noise.

Minimal handling

Care should be individualised for each baby and not be performed routinely. At the start of each work shift, the midwife should determine what the needs of the infant are and carry out the required care, all at one time, instead of repeatedly disturbing the baby. Questions should be asked about performing unnecessary procedures such as repeated heel stabs. Painful, invasive procedures that are not vital to the individual baby's needs are stress-producing events and should be eliminated. Often the best care for the sick infant is rest (Lester & Tronick 1990).

Reducing noise levels

A lot of noises that occur in neonatal units are unnecessary and could be eliminated if more thought was given. It is important to close incubator doors quietly and avoid banging bottles of milk, stethoscopes and other items of equipment on the top of incubators. Staff should talk in a normal speaking voice and resist the temptation to play loud pop music on radios.

Day and night cycles should be recognised, lights should be dimmed at night-time and noise further reduced, remembering though that it is essential that ill babies are observed, so when monitor alarms are cancelled, they need to be reset.

Parents as partners in care

For parents, the birth of a baby is a mixture of joy, emotional exhilaration and relief. Most newborn infants are normal and healthy and few parents ever expect or consider the possibility of having a baby that is less than perfect (Cameron 1996). Neither will they have considered the implications of separation if their baby were to be admitted to a neonatal unit. So when a baby requires medical assistance, because of prematurity, illness or congenital malformations, the effects on the parents can be devastating and force the family into crisis. The parents' ability to resolve the crisis will depend on how realistically they perceive their infant's problems.

The period immediately after the birth is a very sensitive time for mother and baby where the attachment process, that began during the prenatal period, is built on and strengthened. Separation of mother and baby, even if it is for a short while, may increase the risk of the parents developing parental difficulties, with effects on their pattern of behaviour and general responses towards their baby (Lancaster 1986).

It is therefore of utmost importance that only infants who require specialist medical treatment are admitted to the neonatal unit. Non-symptomatic, small for gestational age infants and those with non-life-threatening abnormalities could, with a little extra care and vigilance, stay beside their mothers on the postnatal ward.

The environment of a neonatal unit, however thoughtful the layout and design, is an alarming place to enter. With the emphasis on modern technology, babies are wired up to machines that bleep and alarm continuously, with nurses in hot pursuit. For many parents entering a neonatal unit following the admission of their baby it is a first-time experience, therefore it is of utmost importance that midwives and nurses learn skills which enable them to reduce the level of anxiety that parents feel and stress the importance of them becoming partners in care.

Neonatal units should be bright, friendly and welcoming. The walls should be decorated with appropriate, coloured pictures. Parents should be encouraged to bring in brightly coloured toys and mobiles for their babies and one or two of them can be placed in the incubator or cot.

In most neonatal units a sitting room, often with kitchen facilities, is provided for the parents and children. This is a place to retreat to, away from the stresses and strains of the busy nurseries. The provision of bedrooms and/or family rooms where parents can stay if their baby is critically ill, or a place were they can be alone with their baby if sadly he has died, is of crucial importance. For some parents this may be the only time they have been a whole family together and it may provide them with some long-lasting and cherished memories.

If it is known in advance that a baby may require admission to the neonatal unit, parents should be given the opportunity to visit and meet with some of the staff. They can be shown the room or area where their baby will be admitted and a brief explanation of the various items of monitoring equipment may help to alleviate some of their fears about what will happen to their baby after it has been born.

Following the delivery and if it is at all possible, the parents should be allowed to hold or touch their baby, even if it is for just a few moments, before he is taken to the neonatal unit.

On admission to a neonatal unit, a photograph should be taken. This photograph must be given to the parents as soon as possible, as this will go some way towards reassuring them that their baby is safe and alive (Slade 1988). Parents should be encouraged to visit their baby in the neonatal unit as soon they are able.

On their first visit, the named nurse should be present to explain the baby's condition and the monitoring equipment being used. Any questions the parents may have should be answered in a positive and realistic manner, however grim the situation might appear. The midwife or nurse needs to be able to provide emotional support and guidance. Often parents experience a feeling of grief and sadness at the loss of their anticipated, perfect child (Grant & Seigal 1978). See Chapter 33.

When discussing the baby with the parents, try always to use the name that they have given their child as this establishes the baby's identity and makes the conversation more personalised.

The premature infant may require a lengthy stay in a neonatal unit, in which case parenting roles may be difficult to establish owing to the physical condition of the baby who may be on a ventilator, being fed intravenously, or be under phototherapy lights. All of these act as a barrier between the infant and the parents and undermine their confidence. The most important visual aid for any infant is the human face, especially the talking face

which stimulates both visual and auditory pathways. Parents and siblings should be encouraged to communicate with their baby even if it has to be through the porthole window of the incubator (Gardner et al 1993).

Involving the parents as partners in care should be encouraged as soon as the baby's condition and tolerance to handling permits. This early involvement will strengthen their understanding of the baby belonging to them and increase their confidence in their ability to provide care. A supportive environment, in which the parents gain confidence in assuming the role of caregivers, is of fundamental importance to the general well-being of the baby.

In order to reinforce the parents' involvement in the care of their baby, it is important to discuss whether the baby is to be breast or bottle fed. Most neonatal units encourage mothers to breast feed their babies, or to express their breast milk, as it provides a greater protection against infection. Breast feeding or expressing milk may help the mother feel closer to her baby and also make her feel that she is contributing to her baby's care in a way that nobody else can. Support and encouragement should, however, be given whatever method of feeding is chosen; putting mothers under pressure to provide breast milk for their babies will only produce a feeling of guilt and failure.

Parents should be allowed to hold and cuddle their babies as soon as possible, with this decision being based on the baby's condition. Skin-to-skin contact (kangaroo care), where the baby is placed naked (apart from a nappy) between the mother's breasts, has been shown to be most beneficial. It can improve oxygenation and breathing rates, have a calming effect and, in the infant, reduce stress levels; it may also increase breast milk supply and boost the mother's confidence (Whitewall et al 1988).

Sibling relationship

Encouraging brothers and sisters to visit their new baby is important. Parents are often anxious about the effect an ill baby may have on the family. However, this may cause anxiety in the siblings and they may feel worried, rejected and left out, causing them to demonstrate behavioural problems.

Discharge home

Effective discharge planning should commence long before the baby is ready for home. Encouraging parents to participate in the care of their baby from the beginning enables them eventually to be the sole caregivers and resume total charge.

Every parent should learn how to feed, bathe, dress and generally care for their child. If the baby has special needs like tube feeding or stoma care, training needs may span several weeks. The parents must feel comfortable about caring for their baby before going home.

READER ACTIVITIES

1. Make a list of possible causes of an increase in the respiratory rate of a newborn infant. When you have completed the list, add, beside each cause, other signs and symptoms the baby may present with.

2. Keep a reflective diary of your experiences of the normal behaviour state of a newborn infant. Compare your observations with infants who are known to have neurological impairment (you

may have to visit the neonatal unit in order to complete this exercise).

3. Observe a baby on the neonatal unit who is receiving kangaroo care from his/her mother. Ask her about how she feels holding her baby this way. Is she more relaxed?

Does she think there is an improvement in her lactation?

REFERENCES

Black J 1972 Neonatal emergencies and other problems. Butterworth, London

Cameron J 1996 Parents as partners in care. British Journal of Midwifery 4(4): 218–219

Davis C F, Young D G 1992 Gastroenterology. In: Roberton N R C (ed) Textbook of neonatology, 2nd edn. Churchill Livingstone, New York

Dickason E J, Schult M O, Silverman B L 1990 Maternal infant nursing care, 4th edn. Mosby, St Louis

Faranoff A A, Martin J M 1987 Neonatal perinatal medicine. Mosby, St Louis, pp 619–620

Fowlie P, Forsyth J S 1995 Examination of the newborn infant. Modern Midwife 4(12): 15–17

Gardner S L, Garland K E, Merenstein S L, Lubchenco O 1993 The neonate and the environment: impact on development. In: Merenstein G V, Gardner S L (eds) Handbook of neonatal intensive care, 3rd edn. Mosby, St Louis

Gorski P A 1991 Developmental interventions during hospitalisation – critiquing the state of the sciences. Pediatric Clinics of North America 38(6): 1469

Grant P, Seigal R 1978 Families in crisis: birth of a sick infant. Perinatal section meeting of the American Academy of Pediatrics, District VIII, April, Scotsdale, Arizona

Halliday H L, McClure G, Reid M 1989 Handbook of neonatal intensive care. Baillière Tindall, London

Korones S B (ed) 1986 High risk newborn infants, 4th edn. Mosby, St Louis

Lancaster J 1986 Impact of intensive care on the parent infant relationship. In: Korones S B (ed) High risk newborn

infants, 4th edn. Mosby, St Louis, pp 407–417

Lester B M, Tronick E Z 1990 Guidelines for stimulation with preterm infants. Clinical Perinatology 17(1): XV–XVII

Leven M I, Tudehope D, Thearle J 1987 Essentials of neonatal medicine. Blackwell Scientific, Oxford

Mayfield S R, Bartia J, Nakamura K T, Rios G R, Bell G F 1984 Temperature measurements in term and preterm neonates. Journal of Pediatrics 104: 271–275

Merenstein G V, Gardner S L 1993 Handbook of neonatal intensive care, 3rd edn. Mosby, St Louis

Morris M 1994 Neonatal nursing. Chapman & Hall, London, ch 5

Qureshi S 1989 Signs of neonatal heart disease. Nursing 3(36): 16–19

Roberton N C R 1993 A manual of neonatal intensive care, 3rd edn. Edward Arnold, London

Slade P 1988 A psychologist's view of a special care baby unit. Maternal and Child Health 13(8): 208–212

Volpe J J, Hill A 1987 Neurological disorders. In: Avery G (ed) Neonatology: pathophysiology of the newborn, 3rd edn. J B Lippincott, Philadelphia

Weston W L 1985 Practical paediatric dermatology, 2nd edn. Little Brown, Boston

Whitewall A, Heisterkemp G, Sleath K 1988 Skin to skin contact for very low birthweight infants and their mothers. Archives of Disease in Childhood 63: 1377–1381

Woods Blake W, Murray J 1993 In: Merenstein G V, Gardner S L (eds) Handbook of neonatal intensive care, 3rd edn. Mosby, St Louis

FURTHER READING

Avery G B 1994 Neonatology: pathophysiology and management of the newborn, 4th edn. J B Lippincott, Philadelphia

Beachy P, Deacon J 1993 Core curriculum for neonatal intensive care nurses. W B Saunders, Philadelphia

Campbell A G M, McIntosh N 1997 Forfar and Arneil's textbook of paediatrics, 5th edn. Churchill Livingstone, Edinburgh

Crawford D, Morris M 1994 Neonatal nursing. Chapman & Hall, London

Forsyth J S 1991 Handbook of neonatal care. Cow & Gate, Trowbridge

Halliday H L, McClure G, Reid M 1989 Handbook of neonatal intensive care. Baillière Tindall, London

Rennie J, Roberton N R C 1998 Textbook of neonatology, 3rd edn. Churchill Livingstone, Edinburgh

Respiratory problems

Alison Livingston

CHAPTER CONTENTS

As a group, respiratory problems are the commonest cause of mortality and morbidity in the neonatal period. Problems can occur in term as well as premature infants. The midwife, in managing labour and giving direct care to the newborn baby, is able to recognise the first signs of respiratory distress. This chapter will assist the midwife in developing her ability to recognise the baby with respiratory problems, and also to identify the 'at-risk' group.

The chapter aims to:

- review the anatomy and physiology of the respiratory system
- describe the clinical signs of respiratory problems
- outline the causes of respiratory problems
- discuss the management of the most common conditions
- consider the principles of caring for a baby with a respiratory problem.

ANATOMY AND PHYSIOLOGY OF THE RESPIRATORY SYSTEM

The development of the lungs in the fetus is described in Chapter 52. The lungs in utero are non-functional as the placenta oxygenates the fetus and carries away waste products (see Ch. 52, 'The fetal circulation').

READER ACTIVITY

Review your knowledge of the fetal circulation:

- Which side of the fetal heart receives oxygenated blood?
- What is the name of the blood vessel that

diverts blood away from the non-functional lungs to the arch of the aorta?

The first breath after birth (see Ch. 52, 'Adaptation to extrauterine life') inflates the lungs with air, and the lungs replace the placenta as the organ of respiration. After birth, the baby develops additional conductive airways and alveoli. The lungs are not fully developed until the age of 8 years.

Differences in anatomy and physiology between the baby and adult

The main differences are as follows.

• The baby is an obligatory nose breather because of the high, anterior position of the larynx, which produces a direct airway to the lungs from the nasal cavity.

• The narrowest part of the baby's airway is below the vocal cords, at the level of the cricoid cartilage, which increases the risk of obstruction. (In adults and older children the narrowest part of the airway is above the vocal cords.)

• The infant's airways are smaller in diameter and become easily blocked by inflammation and secretions.

• The infant has fewer alveoli for the exchange of gases and to maintain air reserves (resting volume) in his lungs – because of the lower resting volumes of air in the lungs a baby has limited respiratory reserves, making him more sensitive to hypoxia.

• The muscles in the chest wall are weak and the ribs are more pliable than in the adult, providing less support to keep the lungs expanded.

• The ribs in a baby are more horizontally placed, so that contraction of the diaphragm in breathing draws in the lower ribs. Also, a baby's breathing movement is diaphragmatic.

• Because of the weaker chest muscles and pliable ribs, the baby is at greater risk of respiratory fatigue than an adult.

• The baby has a higher metabolic rate than an adult. Oxygen consumption in the baby is 6–8 ml/kg/min compared to 3–4 ml/kg/min in the adult.

CLINICAL SIGNS OF RESPIRATORY PROBLEMS

Common signs found in most respiratory difficulties are as follows.

• Increased work of breathing causing:
  – recession of intercostal and subcostal muscles and retraction of the sternum; the chest wall appears to be caving in
  – the chin to appear to tug down, the head to 'bob', and the nostrils to flare as the baby tries to draw in as much air as possible, using accessory muscles in the upper body
  – grunting, caused by the baby breathing out against a partially closed glottis in an effort to keep as much air as possible in the lungs.
• Hypoxia causing pallor or cyanosis of the skin and mucous membrane tissues.
• General appearance and behaviour:
  – because of the increased work of breathing the baby has a tense worried appearance and the chest may appear distorted
  – the baby may be restless and unable to feed adequately because of breathing difficulties
  – the baby will become lethargic with more severe respiratory difficulties in struggling with the effort of breathing. An exhausted baby may become apnoeic, particularly if preterm.
• Tachypnoea – the respiratory effort will become raised in an effort to achieve adequate gaseous exchange. The definition of tachypnoea may vary between different units. Roberton (1993) considers the normal respiratory rate in a newborn baby to be up to 60 breaths per minute when awake.

CAUSES OF RESPIRATORY PROBLEMS

Breathing problems have many causes which are not necessarily respiratory in origin. Causes include:

• infection
• aspiration
• lung immaturity

- transient tachypnoea of the newborn
- pneumothorax
- congenital problems
- central nervous system disorders
- cardiovascular and circulatory problems
- other problems affecting mostly preterm babies.

Infection

Generalised infection

A baby with generalised infection may present showing signs of respiratory distress, that is, he may have a respiratory rate greater than 60 breaths/min and be pale or cyanosed because of hypoxia.

Congenital or acquired pneumonia

A baby may be born with congenital pneumonia that will present immediately or soon after delivery. Once the mother's membranes are ruptured there is a route for infective organisms to affect the fetus. If the membranes have been ruptured for longer than 24 hours, the baby is at greater risk of developing pneumonia.

The midwife needs to be vigilant for signs of sepsis in the mother, such as purulent vaginal discharge, maternal pyrexia, or offensive smelling liquor. Any of these signs will indicate that the baby is at greater risk of developing infection. When maternal sepsis is suspected, there is a case for the administration of intravenous antibiotics to the mother before delivery to prevent serious neonatal infection (Grant & Keirse 1989). In many centres when there have been ruptured membranes for longer than 18–24 hours, the baby is routinely screened for infection, that is, blood cultures, a full blood count and an ear and throat swab are taken. It is the responsibility of the midwife to alert the paediatric staff if there has been prolonged rupture of membranes and to initiate the screening investigations. If these investigations show signs of sepsis, as in a raised or suppressed white cell count, or the baby exhibits signs of infection, such as poor temperature control, poor feeding, respiratory signs, or hypoglycaemia, then intravenous antibiotics may be prescribed. Organisms, such as Group B streptococcus, which may be commensal to the mother's vagina, can cause congenital pneumonia and generalised septicaemia. A baby with severe Group B streptococcal sepsis will be critically ill, and may not survive.

After delivery, the baby is exposed to organisms in the environment, which can cause pneumonia. Again, common organisms that are commensal to the skin of adults, such as *Staphylococcus epidermidis*, can lead to serious respiratory infection in the newborn.

Aspiration

At delivery it is possible for the baby to inhale any of the fluids that are present when he takes his first breath.

Meconium aspiration

During labour, if there is fetal distress, hypoxia can stimulate peristalsis and relaxation of the anal sphincter and meconium is then released into the amniotic fluid. If the fetus becomes very distressed, he may start to make gasping movements in utero before birth, taking in the surrounding amniotic fluid. If the amniotic fluid is heavily stained with thick meconium, this can cause the baby breathing difficulties after delivery. It is for this reason that the midwife caring for a labouring mother with meconium-stained liquor should have staff skilled in neonatal resuscitation present at delivery. In some units the midwife or a neonatal nurse will undertake this role, rather than a paediatrician. The person responsible for resuscitation will visualise the vocal cords using a laryngoscope; if there is no meconium present around the cords, meconium aspiration is unlikely. However, if there is meconium present below the vocal cords, the baby will be intubated and the trachea suctioned to remove any inhaled meconium that is accessible. Because meconium is thick and tenacious, it blocks the airways. Meconium is alkaline and irritant to lung tissues, and can lead to a chemical pneumonitis.

Clinical presentation. Meconium aspiration syndrome is rarely seen in babies of less than 36 weeks. It is typically found in term and post-term infants (particularly the intrauterine growth-restricted group). A baby with meconium aspiration syndrome will present with signs of respiratory distress, which can range from mild to severe (see 'Clinical signs of respiratory problems'). The chest may appear barrel-shaped or hyperinflated. There may also be yellow-green staining of the skin and nail beds. A baby with severe meconium aspiration will need mechanical ventilation, intravenous antibiotics and chest physiotherapy to help clear the lungs.

Other aspiration problems

It is possible for the baby to inhale maternal blood or amniotic fluid at delivery, which can result in similar problems to meconium aspiration. Also, a baby may inhale milk, resulting in aspiration pneumonia. This may be as a result of vomiting, or when there is an abnormal passage between the airway and the oesophagus, as in tracheo-oesophageal fistula (see Chs 38 and 41).

Lung immaturity

Respiratory distress syndrome (RDS)

RDS is the commonest cause of neonatal respiratory disease and is one of the most common causes of neonatal and infant mortality in the UK (Roberton 1993). RDS is sometimes referred to as hyaline membrane disease. Hyaline membrane is made up of proteins that are exuded into the alveoli and airways of a baby with RDS. It is caused by deficiency of surfactant in the baby's lungs (see Ch. 52). Surfactant is made by cells in the alveolar walls. Its production slowly increases from 20 weeks' gestation, with a surge at 30–34 weeks, and at term with the onset of labour.

A number of factors cause surfactant deficiency in the neonate. The main factors are prematurity, perinatal asphyxia, maternal diabetes and delivery by caesarean section. The preterm baby is most at risk of developing RDS at under 34 weeks. However, there are some babies who will develop RDS at term, for reasons that are not fully understood (Roberton 1993). Hypoxia reduces surfactant synthesis, which in the preterm with low reserves of surfactant has more impact than in the healthy term baby. Maternal diabetes is also associated with an increased incidence of RDS. It is thought that surfactant maturation is delayed, particularly when there has been poor antenatal control

of maternal diabetes. Elective caesarean section delivery is also associated with an increased incidence of RDS, presumably because the stimulus of labour has not increased surfactant production and reduced fetal lung fluid.

Of particular relevance to the midwife are antenatal management of diabetic women and the education of pregnant women in being alert for signs of preterm labour.

The incidence and severity of RDS have been greatly influenced in recent years by the introduction of antenatal steroid administration to stimulate surfactant production. Crowley et al (1990) suggest that the use of antenatal steroids reduces the incidence of RDS by 50% and the mortality by 35%. Also, the use of prophylactic artificial surfactant, administered into the baby's lungs after delivery, has been a recent successful advance in the management of RDS (Roberton 1993).

Management of RDS. In RDS the alveoli, depleted of surfactant, collapse, which makes the lungs stiff. A diagnosis of RDS can be made if a baby presents with the following signs within 4 hours of birth and if these symptoms persist:

- recession of the intercostal and subcostal muscles, and retraction of the sternum
- tachypnoea with a breathing rate greater than 60/min
- grunting on expiration.

On X-ray examination the lung field has a white 'ground glass' appearance as the alveoli are collapsed and not filled with air. The main airways that are air-filled stand out as dark areas and the appearance is referred to as an 'air bronchogram'.

In the natural course of RDS, surfactant will start to reappear in the lungs at about 36–48 hours of age. The baby will be at his worst at about 24–36 hours, and then as surfactant is produced by the lungs he will improve. The more preterm or sick the baby is at the onset of RDS, the more complicated his recovery will be.

The overall aim of managing the treatment of RDS is to support the baby's breathing and to maintain the baby in as good a condition as possible. For further details see 'Principles of caring for a baby with a respiratory problem' below.

Transient tachypnoea of the newborn (TTN)

TTN occurs mostly in term infants, although it can affect the preterm group as well. It is thought to be caused by the delayed clearing of lung fluid after birth (Roberton 1993). It is more common in babies born by elective caesarean section. The baby with TTN will present with tachypnoea, sometimes the respiratory rate will be over 100 breaths/min and there will be mild grunting and slight subcostal and intercostal recession. The baby may also be cyanosed in air. If cyanosed, a baby with TTN will need to be supported with oxygen therapy and may even require ventilation if the condition is severe. As it is difficult to differentiate from serious infection, such as Group B streptococcal septicaemia, prophylactic antibiotic therapy is likely to be started. The baby's condition improves as the lung fluid clears, usually within 24 hours.

Pneumothorax

Pneumothorax can occur spontaneously after delivery, or may result from over-vigorous bag-and-mask ventilation. One radiological survey of a group of normal newborn babies showed an incidence of pneumothorax of 1.0–1.5% (Steele et al 1971).

Small tension pneumothoraces may be asymptomatic and resolve without treatment.

Clinical signs of pneumothorax are:

- pallor or cyanosis
- difficulty in breathing
- an asymmetrical appearance to the chest
- the abdomen may appear distended as the pneumothorax can push the diaphragm down
- the breath sounds will not be equal on auscultation.

A diagnosis will be made by chest X-ray or possibly by transilluminating the chest with a fibre-optic light source. The affected side will show the light source clearly, as it is filled with air, not lung tissue.

Treatment may require the pneumothorax to be drained with a chest drain. If the pneumothorax is not severe, and the baby is not too distressed, it may be sufficient to support the baby with oxygen therapy and intravenous fluids until the air from the pneumothorax is reabsorbed.

Pneumothoraces, or air leaks as they are sometimes called, are most common in babies who require mechanical ventilation. This type of air leak may also involve air trapped in the lung tissue and this is known as pulmonary interstitial emphysema.

Congenital problems

There are many congenital problems that can cause respiratory difficulties. These may involve a mechanical obstruction of the respiratory tract, an abnormality of development in the chest and its structures or an abnormality of the central nervous system.

Among these problems are:

Upper airway

- Choanal atresia, nasal obstruction allowing the baby to breathe only through his mouth.
- Cleft palate, which allows the tongue to fall to the back of the pharynx causing obstruction.
- Laryngeal obstruction, e.g. cysts, or laryngomalacia when the baby has a 'floppy larynx' causing laryngeal stridor.

Lower airway and lung

- Tracheo-oesophageal fistula, providing an abnormal passage between the trachea and oesophagus.
- Hypoplastic lungs, lung tissue that has not developed adequately because of lack of amniotic fluid or other problem.
- Diaphragmatic hernia, where the gut herniates up into the chest cavity through a defect in the diaphragm.

Central nervous system disorders

The newborn baby may show signs of respiratory distress with a number of problems affecting the central nervous system. The most common observed by the midwife is hypoglycaemia. This results in deprivation of energy to brain tissues, which can cause convulsions. Apnoea may be the only outward sign of a convulsion in the neonate, as his neurological system is immature.

Intracranial haemorrhage may also result in signs of respiratory distress. This is most common after perinatal asphyxia.

Cardiovascular and circulatory problems

Because of the changes in circulation at birth (see Ch. 52, 'The fetal circulation'), there are a number of cardiovascular problems that will present with some respiratory signs in the neonatal period. Among these cardiovascular problems is congenital heart disease (CHD). The incidence of all CHD is slightly less than 1 in 100 births (Baker 1993).

Among the problems presenting are those which involve failure of the fetal circulation to change fully to the postnatal pattern and congenital malformation of the heart and major blood vessels.

Patent ductus arteriosus (PDA)

In PDA the ductus arteriosus fails to close, causing blood to be diverted from the lungs. In normal neonates the ductus arteriosus is functionally closed by about 12 hours of age. Closure may be delayed by hypoxia, RDS, and cyanotic heart disease. The ductus arteriosus secretes prostaglandins from cells in its walls, which encourage it to stay open in utero. In preterm babies, these cells remain active after delivery and encourage the duct to remain open.

Persistent pulmonary hypertension of the newborn

This condition is also known as persistent fetal circulation. It can present in babies without apparent cause and in babies who have other underlying conditions such as RDS, polycythaemia, hypoglycaemia (particularly if due to maternal gestational diabetes), postmaturity and meconium aspiration syndrome. The treatment of mothers antenatally with prostaglandin inhibitors, such as indomethacin, has been implicated in persistent fetal circulation (Baker 1993).

A baby with persistent pulmonary hypertension will present with signs of respiratory distress and cyanosis in air. The aim of treatment is to maintain the general condition of the baby until the pulmonary vascular resistance falls, allowing normal circulation to be established.

Structural heart defects

A number of congenital heart defects will present in the neonatal period with signs of respiratory distress. Amongst these defects are:

- transposition of the great arteries
- atrial and ventricular septal defects
- valve stenosis
- hypoplastic heart
- coarctation of the aorta.

There are a number of conditions that are a combination of one or more structural defects, such as tetralogy of Fallot. Also, CHD is more common in the presence of other congenital abnormalities such as Down syndrome.

It is possible with good antenatal scanning to recognise some of the structural cardiac defects antenatally. Of importance to the midwife is that the incidence of CHD is increased in babies of diabetic women, maternal systemic lupus or when there is a family history of CHD.

Other problems affecting preterm babies

Some respiratory problems are found mostly in the preterm and may be encountered by the midwife working on a neonatal unit. Alternatively, a mother in her care may have a baby on the neonatal unit who is experiencing one of these problems.

Apnoea of prematurity

Apnoea is a common problem found in babies of less than 34 weeks' gestation. It occurs as a result of immaturity of the respiratory centre in the brain and respiratory fatigue. Cardiorespiratory monitoring and the use of therapeutic respiratory stimulants, such as caffeine, help to prevent prolonged apnoeas. Physical stimulation of the baby when he is apnoeic may be sufficient stimulus to 'remind' him to breathe. Alternatively, if he does not respond to tactile stimulation, a bag and mask can be used to ventilate him until he breathes spontaneously. It may be sufficient to give breaths by bag and mask without oxygen to avoid hyper-oxygenation of the baby.

Bronchopulmonary dysplasia (BPD)

BPD, or what is sometimes referred to as chronic lung disease, has become one of the major problems of neonatal intensive care. As more very low birthweight babies and babies with severe respiratory disease survive, there are more infants with this long-term problem blocking cots on neonatal units. This group of babies is often referred to as 'geriatric neonates'. Roberton (1993) states that as many as 50% of babies weighing less than 1.00 kg develop BPD.

Northway and colleagues (1967) first described the condition and its characteristic clinical and radiological findings. It is diagnosed in babies who remain oxygen-dependent for more than 28 days. The group covers a wide spectrum of severity and this condition is sometimes fatal. Its causes are a combination of barotrauma from mechanical ventilation and toxicity of oxygen to vulnerable lung tissue following RDS. Other contributory causes are recurrent aspiration, apnoea of prematurity and infection. Whatever the cause, the management is similar (Southall & Samuels 1990).

BPD babies require skilled care. The baby with BPD is frequently irritable, because of hypoxia, and requires planned interventions to meet all of his needs. The parents of such a baby need consistent support and education in understanding their baby's condition and management. For further information on the care of a baby with BPD, see Sleath (1995). Some of these babies may be candidates for home oxygen as recommended by the Royal College of Physicians (1992).

PRINCIPLES OF CARING FOR A BABY WITH A RESPIRATORY PROBLEM

The overall aim of caring for a baby with a respiratory problem is to provide support, relieve the work of breathing and detect signs of deterioration.

This section of the chapter covers the principles of caring for a baby with breathing difficulties. Areas covered are:

* positioning
* observation
* oxygenation
* nutrition and hydration
* basic physical care needs
* meeting the emotional and psychological needs of the baby and family.

These principles can be applied by the midwife caring for a baby needing minimal intervention at the mother's bedside or to a neonate undergoing intensive care within a neonatal unit.

Positioning

A baby with breathing difficulties will breathe more easily in the prone position or supported on either side in a symmetrically flexed position and with his head slightly elevated. Because the neonate's neck is short in comparison to that of the adult or older child, he is more likely to block his airway if the chin is too far upwards or downwards.

He should be nursed on a soft sheet or sheepskin to give him tactile warmth and comfort. Newborn babies do not like the feel of wide open spaces and need to feel secure. This can be achieved by providing him with boundaries formed by rolled soft blankets or sheets (Turrell 1992). However, care must be taken that the support does not impede breathing. Also, it is important to emphasise to parents that nursing their baby in the prone or supported side position is contraindicated at home as it is a factor implicated in the occurrence of cot death (Fleming et al 1996).

Observation

A baby with any type of breathing difficulty needs to be closely monitored for signs of deterioration in his condition. It is common for midwives to encounter a baby with noisy breathing after delivery. This is usually caused by secretions in the airway. Provided the baby is not showing signs of respiratory distress (see 'Clinical signs of respiratory problems' above), is kept warm and fed early, the noisy breathing settles as the secretions disperse.

The baby's respiratory rate should be monitored, and rates over 60 breaths/min are indicative of respiratory distress. Colour and the work of breathing should also be noted. Ideally, in a baby showing signs of respiratory distress, continuous cardio-respiratory monitoring should be used. This allows for close monitoring of the baby's condition without disturbing him/her. The baby is then able to rest, conserving energy for breathing. Continuous monitoring of respiration, heart rate, blood pressure, temperature and oxygenation is possible using non-invasive means.

Oxygenation

The baby with breathing difficulties is provided with oxygen according to his needs. His needs are assessed clinically by his colour, rate and work of breathing and measurement of blood oxygenation.

Assessment of oxygen levels

Blood oxygenation can be assessed in the following ways:

Oxygenation saturation. A saturation monitor measures how saturated the haemoglobin is with oxygen. This is a non-invasive, simple form of monitoring. It is inaccurate if the baby is poorly perfused and cold peripherally. Saturations of less than 90% will indicate that a baby may require supplementary oxygen.

Transcutaneous oxygen. It is possible to monitor both oxygen and carbon dioxide levels transcutaneously in the neonate. The monitor probe warms up the skin to a temperature of 42–43°C, allowing the gases to diffuse from the capillaries through the skin to the probe. As the skin is warmed up, the probe needs to be resited 3- to 4-hourly to prevent skin damage. Normal levels of transcutaneous oxygen will vary from unit to unit. In general, levels between 6.5–10.0 kPa will be accepted as normal limits (transcutaneous levels of oxygen are lower than arterial oxygen levels).

Blood gases. Blood gases can be measured using both capillary and arterial oxygen. The most accurate method is arterial. By using an arterial line, either in an umbilical or radial artery, it is possible to take arterial blood easily for measurement of gases. Using the umbilical route, it is possible to measure arterial oxygen levels continuously with an oxygen-sensitive electrode at the tip of the umbilical catheter.

Oxygen provision

Whether or not a baby needs oxygen is determined by the blood gas results and also by the clinical assessment. Oxygen can be provided by the following methods.

Ambient or headbox oxygen. Warmed and humidified oxygen can be provided either into an incubator or enclosed cot or by headbox (a clear Perspex dome that is placed over the baby's head into which oxygen is delivered). It is essential that the concentration of oxygen is assessed accurately by means of an oxygen analyser placed near the baby's face.

Nasal cannulae. Low flows of oxygen can be delivered. The advantage of this method is that it allows the baby to be nursed out of an incubator or headbox and to be handled more easily. This is a good method to use as a baby's condition improves and feeding needs to be established.

Infant flow driver continuous positive airways pressure (CPAP). If a baby needs minimal mechanical ventilatory support, the flow driver CPAP is a non-invasive method. Soft nasal prongs are kept in position by means of a hat and a continuous flow of fresh humidified and warmed gases is delivered at low pressures by the flow driver. The baby's own breathing is supported by the CPAP, helping to prevent his alveoli from collapsing.

Mechanical ventilation requiring intubation is used when a baby is unable to support his own respiratory effort. It is an area of treatment that is rapidly changing as ventilators are developed and different modes of ventilation are evaluated. Neonatal ventilators are in general pressure-controlled (gases are given at a known pressure), and the breath cycle is controlled by time. This mode of ventilation causes a rapid rise in pressure that is maintained for a set time, allowing the lungs to inflate and for gaseous exchange to occur. To remove the waste gases, the pressure is allowed to drop to a preset limit, to prevent alveolar collapse, and a continuous flow of fresh gases pushes out the waste gases.

Ventilation methods:

- intermittent mandatory ventilation (IMV)
- intermittent positive pressure ventilation (IPPV)
- trigger ventilation
- continuous positive airways pressure (CPAP)
- high frequency oscillation ventilation (HFOV).

HFOV is being used in babies with severe respiratory disease. It is thought that the lower volumes of gas given at lower pressures, at rates of 400–1000 or more breaths/min, reduce trauma to vulnerable lung tissue (Clark 1994).

Other techniques that are available in specialist centres are: extracorporeal membrane oxygenation (ECMO) used to treat very severe lung disease; the use of nitric oxide therapy (a vasodilator) combined with mechanical ventilation, in treating persistent pulmonary hypertension; and continuous negative extrathoracic pressure ventilation.

Nutrition and hydration

A baby who has breathing problems will either be unable to feed or find sucking difficult. A full stomach will also impede breathing, and gut peristalsis slows down in a sick infant. If the baby's breathing difficulty is short lived and minimal, it may be possible to meet nutritional and hydration requirements by gastric tube feeding. However, most babies with breathing difficulties will initially require an intravenous infusion of 10% dextrose, calculated according to weight and unit policies.

If the baby's respiratory problem is not predicted to be resolved in 48 hours and if total parenteral nutrition is available, it will be administered until milk feeding can be safely introduced. Total parenteral nutrition is of particular importance for use in the very low birthweight and intrauterine growth restricted baby.

Milk feeding is introduced as early as possible, as it is the most natural form of feeding. Even in the very sick and preterm baby, a small volume, such as 0.5–1.0 ml/hour (preferably mother's expressed breast milk) may be fed by gastric tube to stimulate natural enzyme activity in the gut.

When it is not possible for the baby to suck, he/she can be fed by either orogastric or nasogastric tube. To stimulate sucking, the practice of non-nutritive sucking on either a dummy or finger, as milk is put down the gastric tube, may help to build up the association of sucking with feeding. If the mother is breast feeding, contact with the mother's breast during gastric tube feeding will help to build up sucking abilities and stimulate her milk supply. This can be achieved, even if the baby is ventilated, provided that his condition is stable.

As the baby develops the ability to suck, more sucking feeds can be introduced. In breast-fed babies, cup feeding will help to reduce nipple and teat confusion.

In order to assess the hydration status of a baby with respiratory problems, it is important to maintain an accurate intake and output record. A method of assessing urine output is by weighing nappies before and after the baby has worn them. It is also possible to obtain clean urine samples from cotton wool balls left in the nappy by drawing out the urine using a sterile syringe. Weighing is also an accurate method used in assessing a baby's nutrition and hydration status. In the sick neonate requiring intravenous fluids, it is essential that his blood electrolytes are measured daily.

It is the midwife's role to support and educate the mother in whatever method that she has chosen to feed her baby. If the mother is breast feeding, the midwife will need to teach her to express and store her breast milk. It is not easy for a mother to maintain her milk supply when she is under stress. She will need all possible support and encouragement in expressing her milk.

Basic physical care needs

The baby with a respiratory problem has the same needs as the normal baby (see Chs 35 and 38).

However, in a very preterm baby, there will be

differences in the ability to maintain body temperature. Also, a baby of any gestation who is critically ill has reduced ability to maintain normal temperature. The use of incubators (open or closed), heated cots and added humidity will assist in the maintenance of temperature.

One of the main differences in meeting the basic care needs of a baby with breathing difficulties is that he/she may not tolerate the handling required for simple activities, such as nappy changing. Minimal handling needs to be practised, with the caregivers coordinating activities where possible.

Meeting the emotional and psychological needs of the baby and family

The baby with breathing difficulties who requires admission to the neonatal unit is separated from the family and placed in an environment that can discourage physical contact with the family. If the baby requires the intervention of intensive care, the machinery surrounding him/her imposes a barrier to be overcome by the family. The baby is also deprived of the physical comfort of contact with the mother whenever he/she wants.

The midwife who is involved in caring for a baby and mother in this situation needs to be aware of the impact of separation. Wherever possible, the family should be involved in giving care to the baby. Physical contact should be encouraged between the family and baby. The positive effects of touching, stroking and talking to their baby can be emphasised.

Parents need to be provided with consistent and accurate information about their baby's condition. Families may also benefit from support groups set up for families with babies in a neonatal unit.

READER ACTIVITIES

1. Describe three of the main differences between the neonatal and adult airway. Why is the baby more at risk than an adult of a blocked airway?

2. Name three antenatal factors which are indicative that a baby is at greater risk of developing sepsis.

3. Why is it advisable for a midwife to have staff skilled in neonatal resuscitation present at the delivery of a baby when there has been meconium-stained liquor in labour?

REFERENCES

Baker E 1993 Congenital heart disease in the neonatal period. In: Roberton N R C (ed) A manual of neonatal intensive care, 3rd edn. Edward Arnold, London, ch 11

Clark R 1994 High frequency ventilation. Journal of Pediatrics 124(5): 661–670

Crowley P, Chalmers I, Keirse M 1990 The effect of corticosteroid administration before preterm delivery: an overview of the evidence from controlled trials. British Journal of Obstetrics and Gynaecology 97: 11–25

Fleming P, Blair P, Bacon C, Bensley D, Smith I, Taylor E, Berry J, Golding J, Tripp J 1996 Environment of infants during sleep and the risk of the sudden infant death syndrome: result of 1993–1995 case control study for confidential enquiry into stillbirths and deaths in infancy. British Medical Journal 313: 191–195

Grant J, Keirse M J N C 1989 Prelabour rupture of the membranes at term. In: Chalmers I, Enkin M, Keirse M J N C (eds) Effective care in pregnancy and childbirth. Oxford University Press, Oxford

Northway R, Rosan R C, Porter D Y 1967 Pulmonary disease following respiratory therapy for hyaline membrane disease. New England Journal of Medicine 276: 357

Roberton N R C 1993 Disorders of the respiratory tract. In: Roberton N R C (ed) A manual of neonatal intensive care, 3rd edn. Edward Arnold, London, ch 10

Royal College of Physicians 1992 A report of a working group of the committee on thoracic medicine. Domiciliary oxygen therapy for children. RCP, London

Sleath K 1995 Home oxygenation. In: Crawford D, Morris M (eds) Neonatal nursing. Chapman & Hall, London, ch 18

Southall D, Samuels M 1990 Bronchopulmonary dysplasia: a new look at management. Archives of Disease in Childhood 63: 1377–1381

Steele R W, Metz J R, Bass J W, duBois J J 1971 Pneumothorax and pneumomediastinum in the newborn. Radiology 98: 629–632

Turrell S 1992 Supported positioning in intensive care. Paediatric Nursing 4(May): 24–27

FURTHER READING

Crawford D, Morris M 1995 Neonatal nursing. Chapman & Hall, London

Sparshott M 1997 Pain, distress and the newborn baby. Blackwell Science, Oxford

Trauma during birth, haemorrhage and convulsions

Claire Greig

CHAPTER CONTENTS

This chapter offers the opportunity to learn more about some less frequent complications that can occur in specifically vulnerable babies; it is important that the midwife is aware of this vulnerability so that attempts can be made to prevent such complications. However, if they do occur, the midwife should be able to detect them quickly and facilitate and assist with treatment.

Using a process approach, the chapter aims to:

- give an overview of the trauma which may occur during birth to skin and superficial tissues, muscle, nerves and bones

- consider the major types of haemorrhage in the newborn, due to trauma, hypoxia, coagulopathies and other causes

- discuss convulsions in the newborn

- provide a summary of interventions with parents.

Following reading of this chapter and further exploration of the complications through literature and experiential learning, it is expected that the midwife will be able to:

- employ, when possible, the preventive strategies which will reduce the incidence of these complications

- detect signs of these complications

- facilitate and assist with appropriate, effective and efficient treatment

- understand the possible sequelae of these complications.

TRAUMA DURING BIRTH

Trauma during birth includes:

- trauma to skin and superficial tissues

Table 40.1 Selected diagnoses 1988/1993/1994 in Scotland (information reproduced by courtesy of Mr M. Hollinsworth, Information and Statistics Division, Common Services Agency, Scotland)

Diagnosis	1988	1993	1994
Subdural haemorrhage	No figure	5	2
Subaponeurotic haemorrhage	0	1	2
Fracture of clavicle	20	31	28
Other injuries to skeleton:			
Skull	1	0	1
Femur	1	1	2
Other long bones	3	1	2
Facial nerve injury	37	32	33
Injury to total brachial plexus	N/A	6	9
Erb's palsy	39	63	50
Klumpke's palsy	0	2	3
Intraventricular haemorrhage	No figure	121	147
Subarachnoid haemorrhage	No figure	3	3
Total live births	66 212	63 337	61 656

Source: Scottish Morbidity Record (SMR) 11 and SMR(E)

- muscle trauma
- nerve trauma
- fractures.

Despite the highly skilled midwifery and obstetric care available in developed, western societies and a reduction in the incidence of birth trauma or injury, such trauma does still occur (Table 40.1). It is therefore important that the midwife understands the cause and nature of the main injuries to which a baby can be subjected, in order that attempts can be made to prevent their occurrence either prenatally or intranatally. However, if trauma does occur, the midwife should be able to quickly detect it postnatally and, if necessary, facilitate and assist with appropriate, effective and efficient treatment.

Trauma to skin and superficial tissues

Skin

Damage to the skin is often iatrogenic, resulting for example from forceps blades, vacuum extractor cups, scalp electrodes and scalpels. Poorly applied forceps blades or vacuum extractor cups can result in abrasions of the scalp (Figs 40.1 and 40.2). Forceps blades can cause bruising or superficial fat necrosis. Scalp electrodes cause puncture wounds,

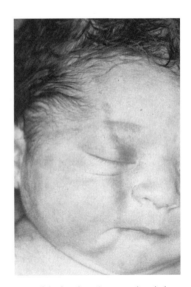

Fig. 40.1 Forceps blade abrasion on cheek (reproduced by permission from Thomas & Harvey 1997).

as can fetal blood sampling techniques. Occasionally, during incision of the uterus at caesarean section, laceration of the baby's skin can occur.

All of these injuries, except superficial fat necrosis, should be detected during the detailed physical examination of the baby immediately after birth.

Superficial fat necrosis does not become evident

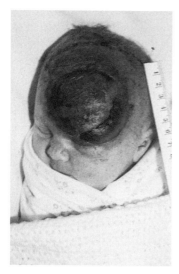

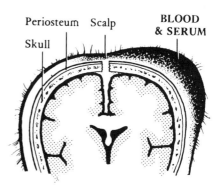

Fig. 40.3 Caput succedaneum.

Fig. 40.2 Scalp abrasion suffered during vacuum extraction; note the chignon (reproduced by permission from Thomas & Harvey 1997).

until several days after the birth when the well-defined areas of induration where pressure was applied should be detected during the baby's daily examination.

Abrasions and lacerations should be kept clean and dry. If there is any indication of infection, medical advice should be sought and antibiotics may be required. Deeper lacerations may require closure with butterfly strips or suture material. There is no specific management for fat necrosis. Healing is usually rapid with no residual scarring.

Superficial tissues

Trauma to soft tissue involves oedematous swellings and/or bruising. During labour the part of the fetus overlying the cervical os can be subjected to pressure, a 'girdle of contact'. This leads to obstruction of the venous blood return and congestion and oedema result. The oedema usually consists of serum and blood (serosanguineous fluid).

Caput succedaneum. If the presentation is cephalic, an oedematous swelling under the scalp is known as a caput succedaneum (Fig. 40.3). In occipitoanterior positions, one caput succedaneum may be present. If the occiput rotates anteriorly in occipitoposterior positions, a second caput

succedaneum can develop. A second caput succedaneum may also form if, during the second stage of labour, the birth of the head is delayed and the perineum acts as another 'girdle of contact'. A 'false' caput succedaneum can also occur if a vacuum extractor cup is used. Because of its distinctive shape, the resulting oedematous deformity is known as a 'chignon' (Fig. 40.2).

A caput succedaneum is present at birth, does not tend to enlarge, can 'pit' on pressure, can cross a skull bone suture line and, if double, is unilateral. It is likely that the baby will experience some discomfort, therefore, although care continues as normal, gentleness when handling or dressing the baby is appropriate. Abrasion of the chignon is possible and the interventions for abrasions (see above) should be employed.

The caput succedaneum usually resolves by 36 hours of life, with no longer-term consequences. An abraded chignon usually heals rapidly if the area is kept clean, dry and is not irritated.

Other injury. The cervical os may restrict venous blood return when the fetal presentation is other than cephalic. If the face is the presenting part, it will become congested and bruised and the eyes and lips oedematous. In a breech presentation the fetus will develop bruising and oedema to the genitalia.

This type of trauma is immediately apparent at birth. As it is very likely that the baby will experience discomfort and pain, extreme care should be taken when handling or dressing the baby. Excoriation of the overlying skin is likely, particularly on the genitalia with the possibility of infection complicating the baby's progress. The need to keep the areas clean and dry is paramount.

Uncomplicated oedema and bruising usually resolve within a few days of life. However, the trauma following a birth by the breech can result in serious complications which require specific treatment and thus take longer to resolve. These complications include excessive red cell breakdown resulting in hyperbilirubinaemia; excessive blood loss resulting in hypovolaemia, shock, anaemia and disseminated intravascular coagulation; and damage to muscles resulting in difficulties with micturition and defaecation.

Muscle trauma

Injuries to muscle can occur when it is torn or when its blood supply is disrupted.

Torticollis

The most commonly damaged muscle is the sternomastoid muscle during the birth of the anterior shoulder when the fetus assumes a vertex presentation, or during rotation of the shoulders when the fetus is being born by the breech. This damage causes torticollis, which means a twisted neck.

Torticollis presents as a small lump (approximately 2 cm diameter) over the sternomastoid muscle on the affected side of the neck. The lump consists of blood and fibrous tissue and appears to be painless for the baby.

Stretching of the muscle can be achieved by laying the baby to sleep on the unaffected side and by using muscle stretching exercises under the guidance of a physiotherapist. The swelling will resolve over several weeks.

Nerve trauma

The most common trauma is to the facial nerve or to the brachial plexus nerves.

Facial nerve

Damage to the facial nerve usually results from its compression against the ramus of the mandible by a forceps blade, resulting in a unilateral facial palsy.

There is a unilateral facial weakness with the eyelid of the affected side remaining open and the mouth drawn over to the normal side (Fig. 40.4). If the baby cannot form an effective seal on the

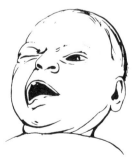

Fig. 40.4 Left-sided facial palsy. Note that the eye is open on the paralysed side and the mouth is drawn over to the non-paralysed side.

nipple or teat, there may be some initial feeding difficulties.

There is no specific treatment. If the eyelid remains open, regular instillation of methyl cellulose eye drops can help lubricate the eyeball. Feeding difficulties are usually overcome by the baby's own adaptation, although alternative feeding positions can be tried. Spontaneous resolution usually occurs within 7–10 days.

Brachial plexus

Trauma to this group of nerves usually results from excessive lateral flexion, rotation or traction of the head and neck during a birth by breech or when shoulder dystocia occurs.

READER ACTIVITY

Avoidance of excessive lateral flexion will prevent the occurrence of such trauma. Recall the effective management techniques for these complications of birth.

There are three main injuries: Erb's palsy; Klumpke's palsy; and total brachial plexus palsy.

Erb's palsy. There is damage to the upper brachial plexus involving the fifth and sixth cervical nerve roots. The baby's affected arm is inwardly rotated, the elbow is extended, the wrist is pronated and flexed and the hand is partially closed. This is commonly known as the 'waiter's tip position'. The arm is limp although some movement of the fingers and arm is possible (Fig. 40.5).

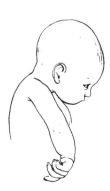

Fig. 40.5 Erb's palsy.

Klumpke's palsy. There is damage to the lower brachial plexus involving the seventh and eighth cervical and the first thoracic nerve roots. The upper arm has normal movement but the lower arm, wrist and hand are affected. There is wrist drop and flaccid paralysis of the hand with no grasp reflex.

Total brachial plexus palsy. There is damage to all the brachial plexus nerve roots. There is complete paralysis of the arm and hand with a lack of sensation and circulatory problems. If there is bilateral paralysis, spinal injury should be suspected.

All types of brachial plexus trauma will require further investigations which are likely to include X-ray and/or ultrasound examination of the clavicle, arm, chest and cervical spine and assessment of the joints. Passive movements of the joints and limb should be initiated under the direction of a physiotherapist.

Spontaneous recovery within days to weeks is expected for the majority of babies, with Erb's palsy tending to resolve more quickly than the other forms. Follow-up is recommended as early surgical repair has been effective in the 5% of babies who do not recover spontaneously within 4–6 months (Brucker et al 1991).

Fractures

Fractures are rare but the most commonly affected bones are the clavicle, humerus, femur and those of the skull. With all such fractures, a 'crack' may be heard during the birth.

READER ACTIVITY

Review the relevant anatomy and the physiological healing process after a fracture.

Clavicle

Fractures can occur if there is shoulder dystocia or during a birth by the breech. The affected bone is usually the one which is nearest the maternal symphysis pubis. It is possible to feel a distortion in the bone and crepitus or callus formation during an examination.

Humerus

Mid-shaft fractures can occur if there is shoulder dystocia or during a birth by the breech when the extended arm is brought down and born. Considerable deformity is evident on examination and the baby will be reluctant to move the arm owing to the pain.

Femur

Mid-shaft fractures can occur during a birth by the breech when the extended legs are brought down and born. Considerable deformity is evident on examination and the baby will be reluctant to move the leg owing to the pain.

In cases of suspected fractures, an X-ray examination can confirm the diagnosis.

The baby is likely to experience pain, therefore careful handling, cleansing and dressing of the baby to reduce discomfort is required. In some babies, mild analgesia in the form of paracetamol (Northern Neonatal Network 1996) may also be appropriate. Positioning the baby on the back or unaffected side is likely to be more comfortable and assist healing.

Fractures of the clavicle require no specific treatment. In fractures of the humerus, immobilisation of the arm is achieved by placing a pad in the axilla and splinting the arm to the chest with a bandage. Application should be firm but should not embarrass respirations. With fractures of the femur, immobilisation of the leg is relatively easy using a splint and a bandage.

Stable union of a fractured clavicle usually occurs in 7–10 days, while the humerus and the femur take 2–3 weeks.

Skull

Although rare, these fractures can occur during prolonged or difficult instrumental births. They are usually linear although depressed fractures are possible. There may be no signs. A cephalhaematoma (see below) can overlie the fracture and a skull fracture may then be detected. Signs of associated complications such as intracranial haemorrhage, raised intracranial pressure, neurological disturbances, leakage of cerebrospinal fluid or seizures can also lead to the detection of a fracture.

X-ray examination can confirm the diagnosis. Linear fractures usually require no treatment. Depressed fractures may require surgical intervention. If there is leakage of cerebrospinal fluid through the ear or nose, antibiotic therapy is indicated. Treatment of the associated complications is necessary.

Linear skull fractures usually heal quickly with no sequelae. Depressed fractures have a similarly optimistic outcome except if complications have occurred, when permanent neurological damage is likely.

HAEMORRHAGE

Haemorrhages can be due to:

* trauma
* hypoxia

or can be related to:

* coagulopathies
* other causes.

Blood volume in the term baby is approximately 80–100 ml/kg and in the preterm baby 90–105 ml/kg bodyweight; therefore even a small haemorrhage can be potentially fatal. Haemorrhage in the newborn can be classified according to the principal cause. In this section haemorrhage due to trauma, hypoxia, coagulopathies and other causes will be discussed. Sub-classifications will be used when necessary.

Haemorrhage due to trauma

Cephalhaematoma

A cephalhaematoma is an effusion of blood under the periosteum which covers the skull bones (Fig. 40.6). During a vaginal birth, if there is friction between the fetal skull and the bones of the maternal pelvis, such as in cephalopelvic disproportion or precipitate labour, the periosteum is torn from the bone, causing bleeding underneath. Because the skull bones are not fused in the newborn and as the periosteum is adherent to the edges of the skull bones, a cephalhaematoma

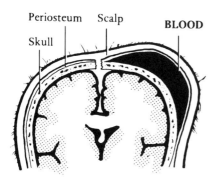

Fig. 40.6 Cephalhaematoma.

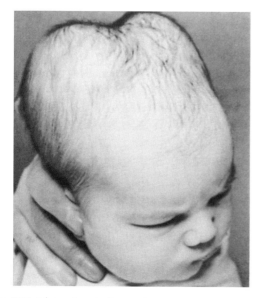

Fig. 40.7 Bilateral cephalhaematoma.

is confined to one bone. However, more than one bone may be affected, therefore multiple cephalhaematomas develop. A double cephalhaematoma is usually bilateral (Fig. 40.7).

A cephalhaematoma is not present at birth but a swelling appears after 12 hours, grows larger over the subsequent few days and can persist for weeks. The swelling is circumscribed, does not pit on pressure and does not cross a suture line.

No treatment is necessary: the blood is absorbed and the swelling subsides. Hyperbilirubinaemia may complicate the baby's recovery. A ridge of bone may later be felt round the periphery of the swelling, owing to the accumulation of osteoblasts.

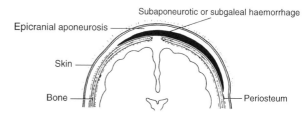

Fig. 40.8 Subaponeurotic haemorrhage.

Subaponeurotic haemorrhage

A subaponeurotic (or subgaleal) haemorrhage is rare. Under the scalp, the epicranial aponeurosis is pulled away from the periosteum of the skull bones and bleeding occurs between with a resultant swelling (Fig. 40.8). It can occasionally result from an otherwise normal birth but more often it is associated with vacuum extraction.

The swelling is present at birth, increases in size and is a firm, fluctuant mass. It can cross suture lines and the swelling can extend into the subcutaneous tissue of neck and eyelids. Bruising may be apparent for days and sometimes weeks. The blood is reabsorbed and the swelling resolves over 2–3 weeks. Normally no treatment is required. Hyperbilirubinaemia may complicate the baby's recovery.

If the haemorrhage is severe, the baby will show signs of shock and supportive care, including blood transfusion, will be required. In rare cases, the haemorrhage is massive and the baby may die.

It is important that the midwife is able to differentiate between subaponeurotic haemorrhage, caput succedaneum, chignon and cephalhaematoma and be able to explain each to parents.

READER ACTIVITY

1. Differentiate between a caput succedaneum, a chignon, a cephalhaematoma and a subaponeurotic haemorrhage with respect to: time of appearance, growth, relationship to sutures, response to pressure, associated complications and eventual resolution.

2. Review the structure and function of the meninges covering the brain and spinal cord: the pia, arachnoid and dura mater. Review the names of the potential spaces between these membranes.

Subdural haemorrhage

A sickle-shaped, double fold of dura mater known as the falx cerebri dips into the fissure between the cerebral hemispheres. Attached at right angles to the falx cerebri, between the cerebrum and the cerebellum, is a horseshoe-shaped fold of dura mater known as the tentorium cerebelli. Within these folds of dura run the large venous sinuses draining blood from the brain.

Normally, moulding of the fetal skull bones and stretching of the underlying structures during birth is well tolerated by the fetus. When there is trauma to the fetal head involving excessive compression, abnormal stretching and eventually tearing of the dura can occur, leading to rupture of the venous sinuses and the development of a subdural haemorrhage. Predisposing traumatic circumstances include those in which the moulding is rapid, abnormal or excessive, such as precipitate labour or rapid birth, malpositions, malpresentations, cephalopelvic disproportion or undue compression during forceps manoeuvres. A tentorial tear is the most common lesion and is most often experienced by term babies (Korones 1986).

A baby who has suffered a large subdural haemorrhage is likely to have severe asphyxia and be difficult to resuscitate. However, if the haemorrhage is initially smaller, the signs can develop over several days. As blood accumulates, the baby develops cerebral irritation, cerebral oedema and raised intracranial pressure. There is likely to be vomiting, non-response, a bulging anterior fontanelle, abnormal eye movements, apnoea, bradycardia and convulsions.

Diagnosis is confirmed by cranial ultrasound (US) scan examination. Supportive treatment is geared towards controlling the consequences of asphyxia and raised intracranial pressure. Subdural taps may be required to drain large collections of blood. This type of haemorrhage can be fatal.

Haemorrhages due to hypoxia

Primary subarachnoid haemorrhage

This haemorrhage occurs when small amounts of capillary or venous bleeding take place in the subarachnoid space. Preterm babies, those who suffer hypoxia at birth and those term babies who suffer traumatic births are vulnerable (Korones 1986, McCulloch 1993).

It often goes undiagnosed as many babies show no signs. If the baby develops signs, there will be generalised convulsions from the second day of life. Preterm babies may have apnoeic episodes. Otherwise the baby appears normal.

Diagnosis is more difficult as a subarachnoid haemorrhage is difficult to see on ultrasound scanning, although computerised tomography (CT) scanning can demonstrate the haemorrhage. If a lumbar puncture is performed, the cerebrospinal fluid will be uniformly bloodstained. Management involves the control of the consequences of asphyxia and the control of convulsions. The condition is usually self-limiting.

Post-haemorrhagic hydrocephalus, demonstrated on serial cranial ultrasound scans, can complicate the baby's recovery. Drainage of the hydrocephaly is usually not required and prognosis for recovery is usually favourable (Levene & Tudehope 1993).

READER ACTIVITY

Review the gross structure of the cerebrum, including the cortex and medulla, and the internal cerebral structure, noting the position and function of the ventricular system.

Parenchymal haemorrhage

This is haemorrhage into the cerebral tissue and is usually secondary to periventricular or intraventricular haemorrhage. It may also occur as a complication of birth asphyxia, coagulopathies or rare central nervous system malformations, when it is considered to be a periventricular haemorrhagic infarction (Horbar 1992).

Both term and preterm babies may be affected and they can show signs of cerebral irritation and/or convulsions. Supportive care is required to help control convulsions and reduce cerebral irritation.

The diagnosis is usually made by US and CT scan. If there is resultant destruction of cerebral tissue, cystic cavities, known as porencephalic cysts, will develop and can be detected by US scan.

Periventricular or intraventricular haemorrhages

These are the most common and serious of all intracranial haemorrhages and primarily affect infants of less than 32 weeks' gestation and those weighing less than 1500 g (Horbar 1992). The infant particularly at risk is one who experiences hypoxia around the time of birth or in the early postnatal period. There may have been birth trauma but most of the multiple associated factors are experienced postnatally and affect cerebral haemodynamics. These include acidosis, hypotension, hypertension, handling, respiratory distress syndrome requiring mechanical ventilation, rapid volume expansion, rapid administration of sodium bicarbonate or other hyperosmolar solution, pneumothorax and patent ductus arteriosus.

The stage of brain development is a crucial factor in the aetiology of periventricular and intraventricular haemorrhages (PVH/IVH). The lateral ventricles are lined with ependymal tissue. Tissue lying immediately next to the ependyma is the germinal matrix, sometimes also known as the subependymal layer. From 8–28 weeks' gestation, the germinal matrix is responsible for producing cells – neuroblasts – which migrate to become the cerebral cortex. During this period, a rich blood supply is provided through fragile capillaries which lack supporting muscle or collagen fibres. These vessels are particularly vulnerable to haemodynamic changes and can easily rupture. After 32 weeks' gestation the germinal matrix becomes less and less active and by term has almost completely involuted. At the same time the capillaries become more stable.

In a baby of less than 32 weeks' gestation, if there is a significant haemodynamic insult, there is rupture of the fragile capillaries and haemorrhage within the germinal matrix. This is a periventricular haemorrhage which is also known by three synonyms: subependymal, germinal matrix and Grade 1 haemorrhage. If there is extension of the haemorrhage into the lateral ventricle(s), this is known as an intraventricular haemorrhage or Grade 2 haemorrhage. The choroid plexus of the lateral ventricles normally produces cerebrospinal fluid (CSF). If there is blockage to the outflow of CSF, post-haemorrhagic hydrocephalus will

Table 40.2 Grades of periventricular/intraventricular haemorrhage

Grade	Location
1	Periventricular, subependymal, germinal matrix
2	Intraventricular with no dilatation of ventricles
3	Intraventricular with dilatation of ventricles
4	Parenchymal extension from a Grade 3 haemorrhage

develop and the ventricles will dilate. This is termed a Grade 3 intraventricular haemorrhage. A subependymal haemorrhage can also extend into the cerebral tissue, giving rise to a parenchymal haemorrhage which is also known as a Grade 4 haemorrhage (Papile et al 1978) (Table 40.2).

A PVH/IVH appears soon after birth, with approximately 50% occurring on the first day and 90% having occurred within 3 days of birth (Horbar 1992). A small periventricular haemorrhage may have no clinical features. If the haemorrhage increases or extends, the clinical features may include apnoeic episodes, which become more frequent and severe, episodes of bradycardia, pallor, metabolic acidosis and convulsions. If the PVH/IVH is large and sudden in onset, the infant may present with apnoea and circulatory collapse.

At-risk babies are usually screened within the first days of life for PVH/IVH using cranial US scan. If a haemorrhage is detected, serial scannings can determine if there is any increase, extension or complication.

Much of the care of the at-risk babies is focused on the prevention of PVH/IVH. The prenatal administration of steroids to the mother to stimulate the maturation of surfactant may also have a neuroprotective effect and when prenatal steroids are followed by the administration of artificial surfactant postnatally, there is a reduction in the incidence of PVH/IVH (Jobe et al 1993).

In order to help the baby to remain haemodynamically stable and reduce the likelihood of a PVH/IVH occurring or extending, the birth should ideally take place in a regional obstetric unit with high grade neonatal facilities. Resuscitation should be efficient and effective and transfer from the delivery suite to the neonatal intensive care unit should be under the care of skilled neonatal staff. Haemodynamic stability will continue to be an aim of all further care, as will be the prevention of the many complications which the preterm baby can develop. Therefore, the baby's needs related to respiration and acid–base balance, circulation, temperature control, nutrition and elimination must be carefully assessed and meticulously met, with continuing evaluation and appropriate adjustments to care. Sophisticated monitoring equipment and the judicious use of analgesic and sedative drugs such as morphine or fentanyl citrate, can assist in achieving and maintaining stability. If the baby is ventilated, muscle relaxants such as pancuronium bromide can facilitate more stable control. Inotropic drugs such as dopamine and dobutamine can also be used to improve cardiac output and stabilise blood pressure (Northern Neonatal Network 1996). If any complications do develop, these should be quickly detected and effectively treated. It is essential that the baby's neurodevelopmental needs are also assessed and met, particularly in relation to supportive positioning, adjustment to lighting, a quiet, undisturbed environment and appropriate interaction with parents and others (Wyly 1995).

In spite of excellent prenatal, intranatal and neonatal care, babies do develop PVH/IVH and the outcome depends on the nature of the haemorrhage. The neurological prognosis for babies with Grade 1 and 2 haemorrhages is usually good. Even if there is ventricular dilatation, a Grade 3 haemorrhage, the ventricular dilatation can resolve spontaneously and the baby will have no long-term consequences. However, if there is a large Grade 3 haemorrhage, the accumulating CSF may have to be drained using ventricular taps as an interim measure. If the accumulation of CSF persists, the baby may require more permanent CSF drainage. This can be achieved by the surgical insertion of a 'shunt'. This usually involves siting a drainage tube into the ventricular system and connecting it to a one-way valve placed subcutaneously behind the ear. The outflow tube from the valve is attached to a catheter which allows drainage of the CSF into a large vein in the neck or into the peritoneum where it is subsequently reabsorbed and eliminated (McCulloch 1993). Babies who suffer a massive

Grade 4 haemorrhage usually die within 48 hours of the onset and those who survive are likely to develop convulsions, cerebral atrophy and rapidly developing hydrocephalus. Long-term neurological follow-up is necessary and parents need much support.

Periventricular leukomalacia

Although not strictly a haemorrhage, periventricular leukomalacia (PVL) has been included as a primary lesion but also because it can complicate PVH/IVH (Armstrong et al 1987). In the baby of less than 32 weeks' gestation, around the area of the lateral ventricles, there is a watershed, a boundary zone, of two of the cerebral arteries. When the fetus or baby suffers hypotension there can be poor perfusion of this particular area of white matter. The ischaemic damage which follows appears as small white spots on US scan and results in softening and necrosis of the tissue and cystic cavities, porencephalic cysts, can develop.

Similar pathogenesis is seen in the older preterm and term baby, but the lesion occurs in the subcortical region rather than the periventricular region. This is because the watershed moves away from the ventricles to the cortex once the germinal matrix involutes. The lesion is then known as subcortical leukomalacia.

Care instituted to reduce the incidence of PVH/IVH can also reduce the incidence of PVL or the severity of the related ischaemic damage. Weindling (1995) emphasises the link between PVL and subsequent neurological impairment, including spastic diplegia.

Haemorrhage related to coagulopathies

These haemorrhages occur as a result of a temporary disruption in the baby's blood clotting abilities.

READER ACTIVITY

Review the sequence of events known as the 'clotting cascade' (Ch. 15).

Haemorrhagic disease of the newborn

This is due to a temporary deficiency of the specific clotting factors, factor II (prothrombin), factor VII (proconvertin), factor IX (plasma thromboplastin component) and factor X (thrombokinase). These factors are proteins which need vitamin K to convert them into active clotting factors.

Vitamin K_1 is poorly transferred across the placenta, therefore the fetus has low stores. Any stores are quickly depleted after birth and, to enable normal clotting to occur, the baby must receive dietary vitamin K_1, absorption of which requires fat and bile salts. Vitamin K_2 is synthesised by normal bowel flora and may also assist in the conversion of the above proteins to active clotting factors. Because the neonate's bowel is sterile, vitamin K_2 production is restricted until colonisation has occurred.

Because of the lack of these active clotting factors, babies are susceptible to haemorrhage. Lane & Hathaway (1985) describe three forms of haemorrhagic disease of the newborn (HDN):

- 'early' (from 0–24 hours)
- 'classical' (from 1–7 days)
- 'late' (from 1–12 months).

Early HDN is rare and principally affects babies born to women who have taken, during pregnancy, warfarin, phenobarbitone or phenytoin for treatment of their medical conditions. To prevent early HDN, these women should take vitamin K_1 supplements during the last 2 weeks of pregnancy (Lane & Hathaway 1985).

The babies who are more susceptible to developing classical HDN are those suffering birth trauma, asphyxia, postnatal hypoxia and those who are preterm, of low birthweight or who are receiving antibiotic therapy. Babies who have been exclusively breast fed or who have been feeding poorly are also considered to be at risk.

After the neonatal period, infants who have liver disease or a condition which disrupts vitamin K's absorption from the bowel, for example cystic fibrosis, are more likely to develop late HDN. This form of HDN is also reported to be more common in babies who are exclusively breast fed.

Bleeding may be evident superficially from the umbilicus, the skin as bruising or puncture sites, the nose and the scalp. Gastrointestinal bleeding is manifested as melaena and haematemesis. In early and late HDN, serious extracranial and intracranial bleeding can also occur. If the haemorrhage is severe, circulatory collapse occurs. Diagnosis is confirmed if blood tests reveal prolonged prothrombin and partial thromboplastin times. The platelet count is normal.

Babies who have HDN require careful investigation and monitoring to assess their need for treatment. With all forms of HDN, the baby will require administration of vitamin K_1, 1–2 mg intramuscularly. In severe cases, when coagulation is grossly abnormal and there is active bleeding into vital structures, replacement of deficient clotting factors is essential and will involve a transfusion of fresh frozen plasma and/or transfusion of the specific clotting factors. If circulatory collapse and severe anaemia have occurred, a transfusion of red cell concentrate will be required in addition to fresh frozen plasma. Affected babies may also require other supportive therapy to assist in their recovery.

The overall incidence of HDN is variously reported as 1 : 12 000 to 1 : 20 000 (McNinch & Tripp 1991), or 1.49 per 100 000 (Jackson 1993). However, it is a potentially fatal condition, therefore prophylactic administration of vitamin K_1, 1 mg intramuscularly, to the majority of babies within the first hour after birth, became routine and effective practice in many countries including the UK, despite some disquiet over the invasive nature of the prophylaxis (Soin & Katesmark 1993).

Controversy over this prophylaxis was heightened when two papers suggested a possible link between intramuscular vitamin K_1 administration and the development of childhood cancers (Golding et al 1990, 1992). This finding has not been confirmed in subsequent studies (Ansell et al 1996, Ekelund et al 1993, Klebanoff et al 1993, von Kries et al 1996), yet doubt persists as a possible link cannot be definitely ruled out. This led to a reassessment of vitamin K_1 prophylaxis and the emergence of a variety of regimens. Vitamin K_1 prophylaxis is essential for the babies particularly at risk of HDN. However, whether vitamin K_1 prophylaxis is necessary for normal babies and by which route remained a dilemma for midwives (Tyler 1996).

A licensed oral preparation of vitamin K_1 became available in August 1996 and can be used as an alternative to the intramuscular injection or the intramuscular preparation being given orally for prophylaxis for normal babies. The Royal College of Midwives (1996) published guidelines to assist midwives to safely and legally administer vitamin K_1.

Despite a lack of research evidence, it is recommended that breast-fed babies have more than one oral dose to ensure prophylaxis, although how many additional doses is uncertain. This recommendation may continue to undermine the efforts of health professionals to promote breast feeding; therefore there is an urgent need to investigate the relationship of breast milk and HDN (Jackson 1993, Tyler 1996).

All parents should be given the opportunity to discuss vitamin K_1 prophylaxis during pregnancy and agree on their choice for their normal baby, as well as understand the difference in prophylaxis if their baby has one or more of the at-risk factors.

Thrombocytopenia

Thrombocytopenia is a low count of circulating platelets, less than 100 000 per mm^3 (Glass 1993), and results from a decreased rate of formation of platelets or an increased rate of consumption. Babies who are at risk of developing thrombocytopenia include those:

- who have a severe congenital or acquired infection, e.g. syphilis, cytomegalovirus, rubella, toxoplasmosis, bacterial infection
- whose mother has idiopathic thrombocytopenia, purpura, systemic lupus erythematosus, thyrotoxicosis
- whose mother takes thiazide diuretics
- who have isoimmune thrombocytopenia
- who have inherited thrombocytopenia.

A petechial rash appears soon after birth presenting in a mild case, with a few localised petechiae. In a severe case there is widespread and serious haemorrhage from multiple sites. Diagnosis is based on history, clinical examination and the presence of a reduced platelet count. It is differentiated from other haemorrhagic disorders because coagulation times, fibrin degradation products and red blood cell morphology are normal. In mild cases no treatment is required. In severe cases where there is haemorrhage and very low platelet counts, a transfusion of platelet concentrate may be required.

Disseminated intravascular coagulation (DIC)

DIC is an acquired coagulation disorder which is associated with the release of thromboplastin from damaged tissue, stimulating abnormal coagulation and fibrinolysis. This has a number of consequences, including widespread deposition of fibrin in the microcirculation and the excessive consumption of clotting factors and platelets.

DIC is a condition secondary to other primary conditions. Maternal causes include pre-eclampsia, eclampsia and placental abruption (see Chs 17, 15). Fetal causes include severe fetal distress, the presence of a dead twin in the uterus and a traumatic birth. Neonatal causes include conditions resulting in hypoxia and acidosis, severe bacterial or viral infections, hypothermia, hypotension and thrombocytopenia.

As the clotting factors and platelets are depleted and fibrinolysis is stimulated, the baby will develop a generalised purpuric rash and will bleed from multiple sites, including pulmonary and intracranial haemorrhage. With stimulation of the clotting cascade, multiple microthrombi appear in the circulation. These can occlude vessels, leading to organ and tissue ischaemia and damage, particularly affecting the kidneys, resulting in haematuria and reduced urine output. The baby will also become anaemic due both to the haemorrhage and to fragmentation of red cells by the fibrin deposits in blood vessels.

As well as the clinical signs, the diagnosis is made from laboratory findings which show a low platelet count, low fibrinogen level, distorted and fragmented red blood cells, low haemoglobin and raised fibrin degradation products (FDPs) with a prolonged prothrombin time (PT) and partial thromboplastin time (PTT).

Treatment includes correction of the underlying cause if possible and full supportive care. To try to control the DIC, transfusions of fresh frozen plasma, cryoprecipitate, concentrated clotting factors and platelets are required. When the baby also has anaemia, transfusions of whole blood or red cell concentrate are required. Occasionally an exchange transfusion of fresh heparinised blood may be performed, removing FDPs while at the same time replacing the clotting factors.

If treatment of the primary disorder and/or replacement of clotting factors does not lead to resolution, heparin can be administered to try to reduce fibrin deposition. An initial dose is given followed by a continuous infusion, the dose of which is titrated to keep a PTT of 60–70 seconds (Glass 1993).

The prognosis depends on the severity of the primary condition as well as of the DIC and the response to treatment.

Inherited coagulation factor deficiencies

The X-linked recessive conditions such as haemophilia (factor VIII deficiency) and Christmas disease (factor IX deficiency) rarely cause problems in the neonatal period but may present with excessive bleeding after birth trauma or surgical intervention, such as circumcision. Diagnosis is confirmed by a prolonged PTT and a normal PT, with decreased levels of the specific factors. Replacement transfusions are required.

An affected baby will require continuing follow-up by haematologists after discharge home. If there is no experience of the condition in the family, there may be a requirement for education, genetic counselling and support.

Haemorrhage related to other causes

Umbilical haemorrhage

This usually occurs as a result of a poorly applied cord ligature. The use of plastic cord clamps has almost eliminated this type of haemorrhage, although care is required in case the clamp catches or pulls. Tampering with partially separated cords before they are ready to come off should be discouraged. Cord haemorrhage is a potential cause of death. A purse-string suture should always be inserted if umbilical bleeding does not stop after 15 or 20 minutes.

Vaginal bleeding

A small temporary discharge of bloodstained mucus occurring in the first days of life and often referred to as pseudomenstruation is due to the withdrawal of maternal oestrogen. Parents need to know that this is a possibility, is normal and is self-limiting. Continued or excessive bleeding warrants further investigation to exclude a pathological cause.

Haematemesis and melaena

These signs usually present when the baby has swallowed maternal blood during delivery or from cracked nipples during breast feeding. The diagnosis must be differentiated from HDN, from other causes of haematemesis which include oesophageal, gastric or duodenal ulceration and from other causes of melaena, which include intestinal duplications, haemangiomas within the gut, necrotising enterocolitis and anal fissures.

If the cause is swallowed blood, the condition is self-limiting, requiring no specific treatment. However, if the cause is cracked nipples, appropriate treatment for the mother must be implemented.

Haematuria

Haematuria can be associated with coagulopathies, urinary tract infections and structural abnormality of the urinary tract. Birth trauma may cause renal contusion and haematuria. Occasionally, after suprapubic aspiration of urine, transient mild haematuria may be observed. Treatment of the primary cause should resolve the haematuria.

Catheters

Umbilical arterial and venous catheters, central venous lines, radial and femoral artery lines and peripheral venous infusion sites all carry the potential danger of severe haemorrhage resulting from dislodgement of the catheter from the vessel or from accidental disconnection of the catheter from the infusion administration set.

Close observation and careful handling of these infants and their lines is imperative to prevent these potentially fatal haemorrhages. If such a haemorrhage does occur, continuous pressure should be applied to the site or, specifically for the umbilicus, it should be squeezed between the fingers until haemostasis occurs naturally or until haemostatic sutures can be applied. A replacement transfusion of whole blood or packed red cells may be required.

CONVULSIONS

A convulsion is a sign of a neurological disturbance rather than a disease. Because the newborn brain lacks organisation and development of neuronal contacts and myelination, convulsions (seizures, fits) can present quite differently in the neonate and can be more difficult to recognise than those of later infancy, childhood or adulthood.

Convulsive movement can be differentiated from jitteriness or tremors in that with the latter two, the movements are rapid, rhythmic, equal movements which are often stimulated or made worse by disturbance and can be stopped by touching or flexing the affected limb. They are normal in an active, hungry baby and are usually of no consequence, although their occurrence should be documented. Convulsive movements tend to be slower, less equal, are not necessarily stimulated by disturbance, cannot be stopped by restraint and are always pathological.

If a baby demonstrates abnormal, sudden or repetitive movements of any part of the body, investigations of possible convulsions should be undertaken. However, Ballweg (1991) suggests that the type of movement a baby has can help classify the convulsion as either subtle, tonic, multifocal clonic, focal clonic or myoclonic. The specific appearance of these convulsions is described as follows.

Subtle convulsions include movements such as blinking or fluttering of the eyelids, staring, clonic movements of the chin, horizontal or downward movements of the eyes, sucking, drooling, sticking the tongue out, cycling movements of the legs and apnoea. Both term and preterm infants can experience subtle convulsions. These movements should be differentiated from the normal movements associated with rapid eye movement sleep.

If the baby has tonic convulsions, there will be extension or flexion of the limbs, altered patterns of breathing and maintenance of eye deviations.

Tonic convulsions are more common in preterm babies.

Multifocal clonic convulsions are demonstrated by term babies and the movements include random jerking movements of the extremities.

Term babies also experience focal clonic convulsions in which localised repetitive clonic jerking movements are seen. An extremity, a limb or a localised muscle group can be affected.

Myoclonic convulsions are the least common but affect both term and preterm babies. The movements are single or multiple flexion jerks of the feet, legs, hands or arms which should not be confused with similar movements which a sleeping baby can demonstrate.

During a convulsion the baby may have tachycardia, hypertension, raised cerebral blood flow and raised intracranial pressure, all of which can predispose to serious complications.

There are many conditions which can result in convulsions in the newborn period and these can be classified into central nervous system causes, metabolic causes, other causes and idiopathic causes (Table 40.3).

Immediate treatment of a convulsion necessitates getting the assistance of a doctor while ensuring that the baby has a clear airway and adequate ventilation either spontaneously or mechanically.

Table 40.3 Selected causes of neonatal convulsions

Category	Selected causes
Central nervous system	Intracranial haemorrhage Intracerebral haemorrhage Hypoxic–ischaemic encephalopathy Kernicterus Congenital abnormalities
Metabolic	Hypo- and hyperglycaemia Hypo- and hypercalcaemia Hypo- and hypernatraemia Inborn errors of metabolism
Other	Hypoxia Congenital infections Severe postnatally acquired infections Drug withdrawal Hyperthermia
Idiopathic	Unknown

It may also involve turning the infant to the semi-prone position, with the head neither hyperflexed nor hyperextended. Gentle oral and nasal suction may be required to remove any milk or mucus. If the baby is breathing but remains cyanosed, facial oxygen is given at a flow rate of 2–3 litres per minute. Resuscitation may be required if apnoea occurs and cyanosis persists. The baby should not be handled unnecessarily. If the baby is nursed in an incubator without covering blankets yet dressed and well supported, observation and maintenance of a neutral thermal environment can be achieved.

It is important that observations of a convulsion are documented, noting the type of movement, the areas affected, the length, any colour change, any change in heart rate, respiratory rate or blood pressure and any immediate sequelae.

If a convulsion is suspected, a complete history and physical and laboratory investigations would be undertaken, related to the possible causes.

READER ACTIVITY

Using the causes of convulsions given above, compile a list of appropriate investigations which should be undertaken.

An electroencephalogram (EEG) can be helpful in detecting the abnormal electrical brain activity associated with convulsions, which can then guide treatment. The primary aims of care are to treat the primary cause and control the convulsions. The pharmacological treatment of convulsions is controversial in respect of which anticonvulsant to use, at what dose and for how long treatment should continue (Anon 1989, Ballweg 1991).

The drug still most commonly used is phenobarbitone which is given as an intravenous injection of 10–20 mg/kg over 20 minutes, followed by a maintenance dose of 3–5 mg/kg/day given intravenously or orally (Northern Neonatal Network 1996).

Phenytoin is also used to control convulsions and is given as an intravenous injection of 10–20 mg/kg over 20 minutes, followed by a maintenance dose of 2.5 mg/kg given 12-hourly intravenously (Northern Neonatal Network 1996).

Other anticonvulsants such as paraldehyde and diazepam have been effective but their side-effects limit their use. Anticonvulsant therapy may be discontinued when convulsions cease, whereas other clinicians prefer to continue therapy for 3–6 months (Anon 1989).

The outcome for babies who have convulsions is also controversial and statistics vary remarkably. Ballweg (1991) suggests that the prognosis depends on the cause of convulsion, the type of convulsion and the EEG tracing. Babies who have congenital malformations of the brain, hypoxic–ischaemic encephalopathy, Grade 3 or 4 PVH/IVH or types of bacterial meningitis tend to have a higher mortality or a poor neurological outcome, whereas babies who have late hypocalcaemia, hyponatraemia or primary subarachnoid haemorrhage are more likely to survive neurologically intact.

Babies who experience subtle, generalised tonic and some myoclonic convulsions tend to have a poorer neurological outcome than babies experiencing the other types of convulsions. Abnormal EEG tracings generally indicate a poor prognosis (Ballweg 1991, Blackburn 1993). The need for well conducted randomised controlled trials to determine the most effective treatment and the outcome is urgent (Anon 1989).

PARENTS

When their baby suffers trauma during birth, or haemorrhage or convulsions, parents are likely to be extremely shocked. Although the care of parents is more comprehensively discussed elsewhere in this text, it is important to summarise their care under these circumstances.

Although the extent of the contact with parents will depend on the nature of the birth injury, all parents are entitled to be given honest, clear information about their baby's condition as soon as is possible after detection. It has been recommended that parents receive this type of bad news when they are together and from someone who is known to them (Richards & Reed 1991). Involvement of the neonatologist is advisable. Uninterrupted time for such information-giving is essential, as is time for questions, which the parents should be encouraged to ask. Follow-up discussions are essential and all verbal interaction should be documented so other staff not intimately involved can understand what the parents have been told and so do not give conflicting information. Involvement in the care of the baby is essential.

Continuing supportive care for parents will be required and additional help may be available from outside agencies if parents consider this helpful to them (Price 1994, Richards & Reed 1991, Sablewicz et al 1994).

READER ACTIVITIES

1. During her pregnancy, you are helping a woman develop her birth plan. She indicates that she is unsure whether to allow her baby to have an injection of vitamin K_1 after he is born. Discuss with an experienced midwife/midwife teacher what information you can discuss with this woman in order that her choice/decision is informed.

2. During your examination of a healthy baby on his third day of life, you detect a soft swelling over his left parietal bone. In order to determine the significance of this swelling:

a. What questions would you ask his mother about her baby?
b. What information would you seek from the mother's and the baby's records?
c. How would you explain to this mother what is the likely cause, treatment and outcome of this swelling?

3. A mother notices a small amount of fresh blood on her 2-day-old daughter's nappy. What is the probable cause and how would you explain the cause, treatment and outcome to the mother?

REFERENCES

Anonymous 1989 Neonatal seizures. Lancet 8655: 135–137
Ansell P, Bull D, Roman E 1996 Childhood leukaemia and intramuscular vitamin K: findings from a case control study. British Medical Journal 313: 204–205
Armstrong D L, Sauls C D, Goddard-Finegold J 1987 Neuropathologic findings in short-term survivors of intraventricular haemorrhage. American Journal of Diseases of Children 141: 617–621
Ballweg D D 1991 Neonatal seizures: an overview. Neonatal Network 10(1): 15–21
Blackburn S T 1993 Assessment and management of neurological dysfunction. In: Kenner C, Brueggemeyer A, Gunderson L P (eds) Comprehensive neonatal nursing. W B Saunders, Philadelphia, ch 29
Blackburn S 1995 Hyperbilirubinaemia and neonatal jaundice. Neonatal Network 14(7): 15–25
Brucker J, Laurent J P, Lee R et al 1991 Brachial plexus birth injury. Journal of Neuroscience Nursing 23(6): 374–380
Campbell J 1993 Making sense of shock. Nursing Times 89(5): 34–36
Crawford D, Morris M (eds) 1994 Neonatal nursing. Chapman & Hall, London
Ekelund H, Finnström O, Gunnarskog J et al 1993 Administration of vitamin K to newborn infants and childhood cancer. British Medical Journal 307: 89–91
Emery M L 1992 Disseminated intravascular coagulation in the neonate. Neonatal Network 11(8): 5–14
Glass S M 1993 Haematological disorders. In: Beachy P, Deacon J (eds) Core curriculum for neonatal intensive care nursing. W B Saunders, Philadelphia, ch 17
Golding J, Patterson M, Kinlen L J 1990 Factors associated with childhood cancer in a national cohort study. British

Journal of Cancer 62: 304–308
Golding J, Greenwood R, Birmingham K, Matt M 1992 Childhood cancer, intramuscular vitamin K and pethidine given during labour. British Medical Journal 305: 341–346
Hollinsworth M 1996 Scottish morbidity record (SMR) 11 and SMR(E). Information and Statistics Division, Common Services Agency, Scotland
Horbar J D 1992 Prevention of periventricular–intraventricular hemorrhage. In: Sinclair J C, Bracken M B (eds) Effective care of the newborn infant. Oxford University Press, Oxford, ch 23
Jackson S 1993 Vitamin K prophylaxis in infancy. British Journal of Midwifery 1(3): 128–132
Jobe A H, Mitchell B R, Gunkel J H 1993 Beneficial effects of the combined use of prenatal corticosteroids and postnatal surfactant on preterm infants. American Journal of Obstetrics and Gynecology 168: 508–513
Klebanoff M A, Read J S, Mills J L, Shiono P H 1993 The risk of childhood cancer after neonatal exposure to vitamin K. New England Journal of Medicine 329(13): 905–908
Korones S B 1986 High-risk newborn infants, 4th edn. C V Mosby, St Louis
Lane P A, Hathaway W E 1985 Vitamin K in infancy. Journal of Pediatrics 106: 351–359
Levene M I, Tudehope D 1993 Essentials of neonatal medicine, 2nd edn. Blackwell Scientific, Oxford
McCulloch M 1993 Neurological disorders. In: Beachy P, Deacon J (eds) Core curriculum for neonatal intensive care nursing. W B Saunders, Philadelphia, ch 20
McNinch A W, Tripp J H 1991 Haemorrhagic disease of the newborn in the British Isles: two year prospective study. British Medical Journal 303: 1105–1109

Northern Neonatal Network 1996 Neonatal formulary. BMJ Publishing, Plymouth

Papile L A, Burnstein J, Burnstein R, Koffler H 1978 Incidence and evolution of subependymal and intraventricular hemorrhage: a study of infants with birth weights less than 1500 gm. Journal of Pediatrics 92: 529–534

Price W R 1994 What do families need and what can we do to meet their needs? Neonatal Network 13(5): 70

Richards C, Reed J 1991 Your baby has Down's syndrome. Nursing Times 87(46): 60–61

Royal College of Midwives (RCM) 1996 Position Paper no 13, The midwife's role in the administration of vitamin K. RCM, London

Sablewicz P, Kershaw B, Mangan P 1994 Breaking bad news: the role of the nurse. Nursing Times 90(11) (unit 2): 5–8

Soin H, Katesmark M 1993 By muscle or mouth. Nursing Times 89(42): 32–33

Thomas R, Harvey D 1997 Colour guide: neonatology, 3rd edn. Churchill Livingstone, Edinburgh

Tyler S 1996 Catching up with vitamin K. Midwives 109(1305): 273

von Kries R, Gobel U, Hachmeister A et al 1996 Vitamin K and childhood cancer: a population-based case-control study in Lower Saxony, Germany. British Medical Journal 313: 199–203

Weindling M 1995 Periventricular haemorrhage and periventricular leukomalacia. British Journal of Obstetrics and Gynaecology 102(4): 278–281

Wyly M 1995 Premature infants and their families. Singular Publishing, San Diego

FURTHER READING

VandenBerg K A 1995 Behaviourally supportive care for the extremely premature infant. In: Gunderson L P, Kenner C (eds) Care of the 24–26 week gestational age infant. Small baby protocol, 2nd edn. NICU INK, Petaluma, ch 6

Volpe J J 1987 Neurology of the newborn, 2nd edn. W B Saunders, Philadelphia

von Kries R 1995 Vitamin K. Annales Nestlé 53: 69–74

Congenital abnormalities

41

Annie C. Halliday

Looking forward to the arrival of a healthy baby is every prospective parent's dream. Sadly for some this dream is shattered when the presence of some form of abnormality is recognised prenatally, at birth or in the neonatal period. According to Modell & Modell (1992) the incidence of major congenital abnormalities is 2–3% of all births. This figure is of course subject to familial, cultural and geographic variations for certain abnormalities. It is therefore very likely that every practising midwife will at some time be confronted with the challenge of providing appropriate care and support for such babies and their families.

The chapter aims to:

- describe and explain specific congenital abnormalities
- explore the complementary roles of the midwife and paediatrician in providing care
- address issues such as who should tell the parents and how and when they should be told
- consider the psychological impact on staff and the strategies that could be put in place to minimise the accompanying stress.

DEFINITION AND CAUSES

By definition, a congenital abnormality is any defect in form, structure or function. Identifiable defects can be categorised in four ways:

- chromosome and gene abnormalities
- teratogenic causes
- multifactorial causes
- unknown causes.

Chromosome and gene abnormalities

Each human cell carries a blueprint for reproduction in the form of 44 chromosomes (autosomes) and two sex chromosomes. Each chromosome comprises a number of genes which are portions of deoxyribonucleic acid (DNA) coded for a particular protein. The fertilised zygote should have 22 autosomes and one sex chromosome from each parent. Should a fault occur in either the formation of the gametes or following fertilisation an excess or deficit of chromosomal material will result. Each abnormal chromosomal pattern has a different clinical presentation. Only the most common of these will be discussed.

Genetic disorders (Mendelian inheritance)

Genes are composed of DNA and each is concerned with the transmission of one specific hereditary factor. Genetically inherited factors may be dominant or recessive.

A dominant gene will produce its effect even if present in only one chromosome of a pair. An autosomal dominant condition can usually be traced through several generations. Achondroplasia, osteogenesis imperfecta, adult polycystic kidney disease, and Huntington's chorea are examples of dominant conditions.

A recessive gene needs to be present in both chromosomes before producing its effect. Examples of autosomal recessive conditions are cystic fibrosis or phenylketonuria.

Teratogenic causes

A teratogen is any agent that raises the incidence of congenital abnormality. The list of known and suspected teratogens is continually growing but according to Levene & Tudehope (1993) currently includes: prescribed drugs, for example anticonvulsants, anticoagulants, preparations containing large concentrations of vitamin A such as those prescribed for the treatment of acne; drugs used in substance abuse such as heroin, alcohol, nicotine; environmental factors such as radiation and chemicals (that is dioxins, pesticides); infective agents, for example rubella or cytomegalovirus; maternal disease, for example diabetes. It should be borne in mind that several factors influence the effect(s) produced by any one teratogen such as gestational age of the embryo or fetus at the time

of exposure, length of exposure, toxicity of the teratogen. Direct cause and effect is sometimes difficult to establish.

Multifactorial causes

These are due to a genetic defect in addition to one or more teratogenic influences.

Unknown causes

In spite of a growing body of knowledge the specific cause of around 80% of abnormalities remains unspecified.

THE ROLE OF PRECONCEPTION ADVICE

Whilst the midwife may advise on modulation of behaviour or diet during pregnancy, by the time the majority of women present for a booking visit the damage has been done. The burden of prevention therefore lies with dissemination of information and appropriate counselling in preconception clinics. The increasing awareness and availability of preconception advice has helped reduce the incidence of some categories of abnormality, notably those associated with poorly controlled diabetes and neural tube defects. Whyte (1995) cites a 72% decrease in neural tube defects as a result of folic acid supplements being taken prior to conception.

PRENATAL SCREENING AND DIAGNOSIS

Improved prenatal screening and diagnostic techniques have led to increased recognition of abnormality, particularly in early pregnancy. This has resulted in some families making the decision to have their pregnancy terminated, whilst allowing many others time to adjust and try to come to terms with the news that their baby will be born with a particular problem. One advantage of prenatal diagnosis is that, if necessary, arrangements can be made for the mother to have prenatal transfer to a unit where neonatal surgical or intensive care facilities are available. The disadvantage of transfer is that the mother may then be separated from family, friends and the support of the midwives she knows best. This makes it all the more imperative that the staff in these units are sensitive to the needs of such women.

BREAKING THE NEWS

It is often the midwife who first notices an abnormality in the baby either during the process of the delivery or during the subsequent examination of the baby. All abnormalities, identified or suspected, should be notified to medical staff but there is sometimes a difference of opinion as to who should break the news to the parents.

There is a very strong argument for suggesting that this should be done by the midwife present at the delivery. The midwife–client relationship is or ought to be one of mutual trust and respect. Honesty is an implicit tenet of such a relationship. It is well recognised that one of the first questions a mother will ask of the midwife after the delivery is 'Is the baby all right?'. For the midwife to be noncommittal or economical with the truth is to betray that trust. It is preferable that the midwife tell the mother (and if possible the father at the same time), albeit sensitively but honestly, and show her any obvious abnormality in the baby.

Where there is doubt in the midwife's mind, for example in cases of suspected chromosomal abnormalities, it could be argued that the issue is less clear cut. Discretion could therefore be exercised in the precise form of words used, but the intention of inviting a second opinion should be made clear to the parents. It is advisable that both the parents and the midwife be present when the paediatrician examines the baby and that the midwife be present during any dialogue between the parents and medical staff so that she is aware of exactly what has been said. She is then in a position to be able to clarify, explain or repeat any points not fully understood. Opportunities for repeat consultation with the paediatrician should be offered as and when the parents desire. Patience, tact and understanding are prerequisites for midwives caring for these families.

Some abnormalities are slight and cause no further problems for the parents or child, while others are profound and cause the subsequent daily care to be fraught with difficulties. Unlike most others, abnormalities involving the face cannot be disguised or hidden and therefore must rate amongst the most distressing for parents. This is confirmed by Wirt and others (1992) who claim that congenital defects of head, face and neck often precipitate a major family crisis. The psychological impact on parents of being told and/or shown that their baby has a congenital abnormality is often not dissimilar to the grieving process discussed in Chapter 33. Great sensitivity is required on the part of the midwife when showing the baby to the parents for the first time.

Since a comprehensive discussion of every abnormality is clearly not possible, selection has been made of those the midwife is most likely to encounter.

FETAL ALCOHOL SYNDROME

This topic has been chosen to open the discussion on congenital abnormalities since the direct link between the abuse of alcohol and this condition is established. Preconception preparation for pregnancy advice on alcohol intake, if heeded, could dramatically reduce the incidence of this phenomenon. Health promotion objectives and successful outcomes are, however, rarely totally synchronous.

The midwife may be alerted to the possibility of a baby being born with this syndrome prenatally if, in addition to psychosocial markers, clinical intrauterine growth retardation is evident. Postnatally the following characteristics are recognisable: a growth-retarded infant with microcephaly, flat facies, close-set eyes, epicanthic folds, small upturned nose, thin upper lip and low-set ears. According to Spohr and others (1993) most of these features become less pronounced as the child grows. Microcephaly, small stature and mental retardation remain. The baby will probably experience acute withdrawal symptoms and require appropriate supportive therapies. The midwife will require to exercise counselling skills to provide much needed support for the mother. Collaboration with social services is usually called for to ensure that the care options decided are in the best interests of the family.

Establishing such a direct link between a teratogen and such a complex clinical pattern is the exception rather than the rule.

GASTROINTESTINAL MALFORMATIONS

Most of the abnormalities affecting this system call for prompt surgical intervention, for example atresias, gastroschisis and exomphalos. Many are likely to be diagnosed prenatally. If prenatal diagnosis has been made, the parents will be at least partially prepared. In this event, where possible, the paediatric surgeon should speak to the parents before delivery of the baby to explain the probable sequence of events. Certainly he should do so once the baby is delivered and prior to obtaining their consent for surgery. If the baby's condition allows, parents should be encouraged to hold the baby even briefly and photographs can be taken.

Gastroschisis and exomphalos

Gastroschisis is a paramedian defect of the abdominal wall with extrusion of bowel which is not covered by peritoneum, thus making it very vulnerable to infection and injury. Surgical closure of the defect is usually possible and the size of the defect will determine whether or not the insertion of a Teflon graft will be necessary to achieve this.

Exomphalos or omphalocele is when the bowel or other viscera protrude through the umbilicus. Very often these babies have other abnormalities, for example heart defects, which could be a contraindication to surgery in the immediate neonatal period. Closure of the defect may consequently be delayed as long as 1 or even 2 years.

Immediate management of both the above conditions is to cover the herniated abdominal contents with warm sterile saline swabs or a sterile Silastic bag. Stomach contents should be aspirated. Transfer of the baby to a surgical unit is then expedited.

Atresias

Oesophageal atresia

Oesophageal atresia occurs when there is incomplete canalisation of the oesophagus in early intrauterine development. It is commonly associated with tracheo-oesophageal fistula which connects the trachea to the upper or lower oesophagus or both. The commonest type of abnormality is where the upper oesophagus terminates in a blind pouch and the lower oesophagus connects to the trachea. This abnormality should be suspected in the presence of maternal polyhydramnios. At birth the baby has copious amounts of mucus coming from the mouth. Early detection is essential. The midwife should attempt to pass an orogastric tube but it may travel less than 10–12 cm. Radiography will confirm the diagnosis. The baby must be given no oral fluid but a wide-bore oesophageal tube should be passed and connected to gentle continuous suction. He should be transferred immediately to a paediatric surgical unit. It may be possible to anastomose the blind ends of the oesophagus. If the distance is too large a series of bouginages can be carried out in an attempt to stretch the ends of the oesophagus, stimulate growth and thereby eventually facilitate repair by end-to-end anastomosis. Alternatively a Teflon graft or transplant of, for example, a section of colonic tissue will be needed at a later date. If the repair is delayed, cervical oesophagostomy may be performed to allow drainage of secretions. Meanwhile the baby will require to be fed via a gastrostomy tube. This method of feeding obviously deprives the baby of oral stimuli. Such a baby may be given 'sham' feeds to allow him to taste the milk and to promote sucking, swallowing and normal development of the mandible.

Duodenal atresia

Atresia may occur at any level of the bowel but the duodenum is the most common site. If this has not already been diagnosed in the prenatal period, persistent vomiting within 24–36 hours of birth will be the first feature encountered. The vomit will often contain bile unless the obstruction is proximal to the entrance of the common bile duct. Abdominal distension may not be present and the baby may pass meconium. A characteristic double bubble of gas may be seen on radiological examination. Treatment is by surgical repair. Prognosis is good if the baby is otherwise healthy but this abnormality is often associated with others (30% of cases occur in children with Down syndrome according to Roberton 1993).

Rectal atresia and imperforate anus

An imperforate anus should be obvious at birth on examination of the baby but a rectal atresia might not become apparent until it is noted that the baby has not passed meconium. Where it is practice to measure temperature by using a rectal thermometer the problem will be noted at an earlier stage. Both situations require that the baby be referred for surgery.

Should a baby fail to pass meconium in the first 24 hours, three other possibilities should be considered:

- malrotation
- cystic fibrosis
- Hirschsprung's disease.

Malrotation

This is a developmental abnormality where incomplete rotation of the gut has taken place, giving rise to signs of obstruction. Surgical correction is necessary.

Cystic fibrosis

This is an autosomal recessive condition affecting 1 in 2500 births. The majority of cases are not diagnosed until later in infancy or childhood when the child fails to thrive or has repeated chest infections but a proportion may present with meconium ileus in the neonatal period. In this condition the meconium is particularly viscous and causes intestinal obstruction. There is accompanying abdominal distension and bile-stained vomiting. Intravenous fluids and a gastrografin enema may relieve the obstruction. Definitive diagnosis will be by identifying a raised immunoreactive trypsin level. Treatment is supportive rather than curative and involves administration of pancreatin and a rigorous programme of chest physiotherapy.

Hirschsprung's disease

In this disease, which has an incidence of 1 in 5000 births, there is an aganglionic section of bowel present. This means that peristalsis does not occur and the bowel therefore becomes obstructed. The baby develops abdominal distension and bile-stained vomiting. Definite diagnosis is made by doing colonic biopsy. Resection of the aganglionic segment of bowel is indicated.

Pyloric stenosis

Pyloric stenosis arises from a genetic defect which causes hypertrophy of the muscles of the pyloric sphincter. The characteristic clinical presentation is projectile vomiting usually around 6 weeks of age but it may occur earlier and hence is included in this section. There is a gender-related predominance in that it is usually boys who are affected. Surgical repair is effected by Ramstedt's operation.

The remaining abnormalities of the gastrointestinal system while amenable to surgery do not necessitate immediate action.

Cleft lip and cleft palate

The incidence of cleft lip occurring as a single deformity is 1.3 per 1000. This defect may be unilateral or bilateral. Since it is very often accompanied by cleft palate both will now be considered.

Clefts in the palate may affect hard palate, soft palate, or both. Some defects will include alveolar margins and sometimes the uvula. It is recommended that during the initial examination of the infant the palate be examined by means of a good light source rather than by digital palpation. The greatest problem for these babies initially is feeding. If the defect is limited to a unilateral cleft lip, there is no reason why the mother who had intended to breast feed may not continue to do so. Where there is the additional problem of cleft palate, arranging for the baby to be fitted with an orthodontic plate may facilitate breast feeding but this obviously does not afford the same stimulus as nipple to palate contact.

Middle ear infection is a concomitant risk for

babies with cleft palate. Repeated infections of this type could impede hearing and subsequent development of speech. Danner (1992) suggests that breast feeding be encouraged since passive immunity may protect these babies from the infections to which they are prone. Expressed breast milk may of course be given. Cup or spoon feeding are alternative methods but for those who wish to bottle feed there is a wide variety of specially shaped teats available to accommodate the different sizes and positions of palate defects. Above everything else, an unending supply of patience is required. The midwife should encourage the mother and father to find the most successful technique rather than 'taking over' since this may compound any feelings of guilt or inadequacy the parents may feel.

Corrective surgery will be carried out at some stage but there is currently some debate as to the most appropriate time to carry out these procedures. Sullivan (1996) examines the arguments for both early and late repair of a cleft lip. He explains that some surgeons advocate effecting closure of the cleft lip within 2 weeks of birth in order to capitalise on the increased tissue-healing properties which are present as a short-lived legacy of intrauterine existence. They also argue that an early repair will be instrumental in encouraging healthy attachment between mother and baby. Advocates of later intervention suggest cleft lip repair at the age of 3–4 months because cleft lip often occurs

as a feature of other medical conditions which may not be detected immediately. Surgery in the early neonatal period for such a baby may be too hazardous. Closure of the palate defect is suggested at around the age of 12–15 months. One of the main reasons for this apparently long delay is to allow normal growth to take place which may result in reducing the size of the defect, thus increasing the possibility of a more satisfactory repair. Some children have a series of cosmetic operations at some time after the initial repairs are carried out. It is often helpful for the midwife to show families 'before and after' photographs of babies for whom surgery has been a success (see Fig. 41.1A and B).

Clearly, although the midwife may offer valuable support in these early days, she is limited in the length of time she is available to help these families. Giving the parents the address of a support group such as the Cleft Lip And Palate Association (CLAPA) is useful.

Pierre Robin syndrome

Pierre Robin syndrome is characterised by micrognathia (hypoplasia of the lower jaw), abnormal attachment of muscles controlling the tongue which allows it to fall backward and occlude the airway, and a central cleft palate. This triad of abnormalities presents a challenge for nursing care. Maintenance of a clear airway is paramount. In order to achieve this the baby will be nursed prone.

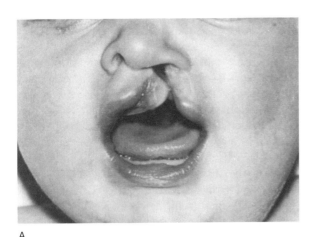

A

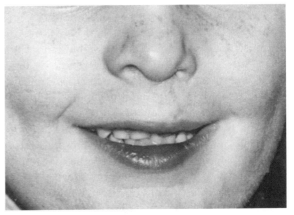

B

Fig. 41.1 (A) Cleft lip and palate; (B) the repaired cleft (reproduced by permission from Raine 1994).

This is one of the few exceptions to the 'Back to sleep' campaign aimed at reducing cot deaths. Feeding can be problematic. There is a high risk of aspiration occurring. Suction catheter and oxygen equipment should be ready to hand. Some of these babies may be fitted with an orthodontic plate to facilitate feeding. The action of sucking will encourage development of the mandible. Parents will need considerable support during what may be for some babies a protracted period of hospitalisation. Discharge will be when the lower jaw has grown sufficiently or when the parents feel comfortable about taking the baby home. Habel and others (1996) suggest that some of these babies can have an earlier transfer home if a shortened endotracheal tube is in place to ensure a patent nasopharyngeal airway. They recommend replacing the tube every 2 weeks until adequate mandibular development takes place.

ABNORMALITIES RELATING TO RESPIRATION

Making a successful transition from fetus to neonate includes being able to establish regular respiration. Any abnormality of the respiratory tract or accessory respiratory muscles is likely to hamper this process.

Diaphragmatic hernia

This abnormality consists of a defect in the diaphragm which allows herniation of abdominal contents into the thoracic cavity. The extent to which lung development is compromised as a result depends on the size of the defect and the gestational age at which herniation first occurred. At birth, the condition may be suspected if the baby is cyanosed and difficulty is experienced in resuscitation. In addition, since the majority of such defects are left-sided, heart sounds will be displaced. The abdomen may have a scaphoid appearance. Chest X-ray will confirm the diagnosis. Continuous gastric suction should be commenced. Immediate surgical repair of the defect is necessary. Prognosis relates to the degree of pulmonary hypoplasia. There is also the possibility of coexistent abnormalities such as cardiac defects or chromosomal anomalies. Incidence is 1 in 2000 births.

Choanal atresia

Choanal atresia describes a unilateral or bilateral narrowing of the nasal passage(s) with a web of tissue or bone occluding the nasopharynx. Tachypnoea and dyspnoea are cardinal features particularly when a bilateral lesion is present. A helpful diagnostic aid is that the baby's colour will improve with crying (Bagwell 1993). Maintaining a clear airway is obviously essential and an oral airway may have to be used to effect this. *A unilateral defect may not be noticed until the baby feeds for the first time. The midwife should therefore bear in mind the possibility of this problem if respiratory difficulty and cyanosis occur at this time.* Surgery will be required to remove the obstructing tissue. The incidence is 1 in 8000. Occasionally choanal atresia is associated with other abnormalities.

Laryngeal stridor

This is a noise made by the baby usually on inspiration and exacerbated by crying. Most commonly the cause is laryngomalacia which is due to laxity of the laryngeal cartilage. Although it sounds distressing, the baby generally is not at all upset. It is the parents who require to be comforted and reassured (often repeatedly). It should be explained to them that the stridor may take some time to resolve, perhaps up to 2 years. If, however, the stridor is accompanied by signs of dyspnoea or feeding problems, further investigations would become necessary to rule out a more sinister cause.

CONGENITAL CARDIAC DEFECTS

Babies born with congenital heart defects comprise the second largest group of babies born with abnormalities, according to Nixon & O'Donnell (1992). Accurate figures are, however, difficult to obtain since many defects, both major and minor, are not identified at birth.

Causes

Approximately 90% of cardiac defects cannot be attributed to a single cause; chromosomal and genetic factors account for 8%, and a further 2% are reckoned to be caused by teratogens. The critical period of exposure to teratogens in respect of embryological development of cardiac tissue is from the third to the sixth week. Cardiac defects are thought to arise as a result of one of two underlying mechanisms:

- abnormal cell migration, for example transposition of the great arteries
- disordered intracardiac blood flow, for example hypoplastic left heart (Rose & Clark 1992).

Prenatal detection

An increasing number of cardiac problems are being identified by means of detailed ultrasound scanning (see Ch. 20). However, the detection of most defects is still dependent upon accurate observations and examination during the neonatal period.

Postnatal recognition

Clinically, babies with cardiac anomalies can be divided into two groups: those with cyanotic heart disease and those with 'acyanotic' heart disease.

Cardiac defects presenting with cyanosis

Defects included in this group are:

- transposition of the great arteries
- total anomalous pulmonary venous drainage
- tricuspid atresia
- Fallot's tetralogy
- pulmonary atresia
- univentricular heart.

The persistence of central cyanosis (that is cyanosis of lips, mucous membranes, trunk), tachypnoea and tachycardia may be the first signs that a cardiac defect is present. If there is cyanosis present, administration of oxygen to these babies will be ineffective in improving their colour. In-deed, giving 100% oxygen may encourage closure of the ductus arteriosus, the patency of which, as Paul (1995) remarks, is literally a lifeline for some of these babies. Chest X-ray should be carried out to exclude abnormalities of the respiratory tract, respiratory disease and diaphragmatic hernia. The precise nature of the cardiac anomaly may be further explored by echocardiography.

The baby with transposition of the great arteries is worthy of special mention since early detection allows intervention which will be life-saving. This is a condition where the aorta arises from the right ventricle and the pulmonary artery from the left ventricle. Consequently, oxygenated blood is circulated back through the lungs and deoxygenated blood back into the systemic circuit. It is apparent therefore that unless there is opportunity for oxygenated blood to access the systemic circulation either by means of a patent ductus arteriosus or accompanying septal defects, such a baby will die.

Prostaglandin infusion may be commenced to maintain patency of the ductus arteriosus and arrangements made to transfer the baby to a unit where a Rashkind septostomy can be performed. This procedure involves creating an atrial septal defect to allow oxygenated blood to access the systemic circulation. Corrective surgery is then carried out at a later date.

Potentially more distressing for the parents are the defects which do not initially present with marked cyanosis. These babies may for a time be considered to be healthy.

'Acyanotic' cardiac defects

Anomalies subsumed under this heading include:

- left heart hypoplasia
- coarctation of the aorta
- patent ductus arteriosus
- atrial or ventricular septal defects.

Close observation of each baby in her care is part of the midwife's role. Astute observers may detect in these babies the first signs of cardiac failure, that is tachypnoea, tachycardia and incipient cyanosis, especially following the exertion of crying or feeding. These signs will become more evident, sometimes dramatically so, with the closure of the ductus arteriosus if either or both of the first two anomalies is present. Detailed examination may disclose heart murmurs and diminution or absence of femoral pulses.

Corrective surgery for coarctation of the aorta is sometimes possible depending on the extent of the stricture. Babies with hypoplastic left heart have a bleak prognosis. The psychological impact on the parents following confirmation of such a diagnosis is substantial and calls for particularly supportive management.

Changing patterns of postnatal care often mean early discharge home. It is essential that each baby is examined by a competent practitioner before dismissal from hospital. It is equally important to realise, however, that not all heart murmurs heard at this time are significant. There is therefore increased responsibility on community midwives to be observant and to communicate effectively with parents. Parents who report any changes in the baby's behaviour such as breathlessness or cyanosis should never be ignored, but rather encouraged to seek medical advice promptly.

CENTRAL NERVOUS SYSTEM ABNORMALITIES

Ingestion of folic acid supplements prior to conception and during the early stages of pregnancy has helped prevent such abnormalities. In addition, the ability to recognise these anomalies prenatally, by means of screening tests such as measuring alpha-fetoprotein levels and detailed ultrasound scanning, has resulted in some parents choosing selective termination of pregnancies where severe neural tube defects are found. All of these measures have combined to reduce the number of babies born with abnormalities of the central nervous system.

Anencephaly

This major abnormality describes the absence of the forebrain and vault of the skull. It is a condition which is incompatible with sustained life but occasionally such a baby is born alive. The midwife

should wrap the baby carefully before showing to the mother. It is recognised that seeing and holding the baby will facilitate the grieving process. It may be beneficial for the parents then to see the full extent of the abnormality, unpleasant though it is. Seeing the whole baby will help them to accept the reality of the situation and prevent imagination of an even more gruesome picture.

Spina bifida aperta

Spina bifida aperta results from failure of fusion of the vertebral column. There is no skin covering the defect which allows protrusion of the meninges, hence *meningocele*. The meningeal membrane may be flat or appear as a membranous sac with or without cerebrospinal fluid but it does not contain neural tissue (Fig. 41.2). *Meningomyelocele* on the

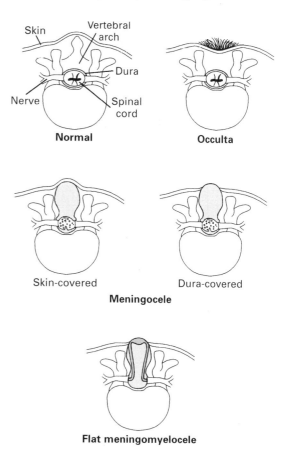

Fig. 41.2 Various forms of spina bifida (based on Wallis & Harvey 1979).

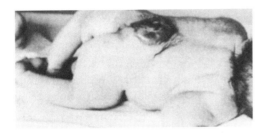

Fig. 41.3 Baby with meningomyelocele.

other hand does involve the spinal cord (Figs 41.2 and 41.3). This lesion may be enclosed or the meningocele may rupture and expose the neural tissue. Meningomyelocele usually gives rise to neural damage producing paralysis distal to the defect and impaired function of urinary bladder and bowel. The lumbosacral area is the most common site for these to present but they may appear at any point in the vertebral column. When the defect is at base of skull level it is known as an *encephalocele*. The added complication here is that the sac may contain varying amounts of brain tissue. Normal progression of labour may be impeded by a large lesion of this type.

Immediate management involves covering open lesions with a non-adherent dressing. Babies with enclosed lesions should be handled with the utmost care in an attempt to preserve the integrity of the sac. This will limit the risk of meningitis occurring. A paediatric surgeon should be contacted. Surgical closure for meningocele carries a high rate of success. Nixon & O'Donnell (1992) suggest that it is no longer necessary to close the back within 24 hours of birth. Following the paediatrician's examination of the baby, discussion with the parents will allow them to make an informed choice about whether or not they wish their baby to have surgery.

Spina bifida occulta

Spina bifida occulta (see Fig. 41.2) is the most minor type of defect where the vertebra is bifid. There is usually no spinal cord involvement. A tuft of hair or sinus at the base of the spine may be noted on first examination of the baby. Ultrasound investigation will confirm the diagnosis and rule out any associated spinal cord involvement.

Parents who have a baby with a neural tube defect should be offered genetic counselling since the risk of recurrence is 1 in 25.

Hydrocephalus

This is a condition which arises from a blockage in the circulation and absorption of cerebrospinal fluid. The large lateral ventricles increase in size and eventually compress the surrounding brain tissue. It is a not infrequent accompaniment to the more severe spina bifida lesions because of a structural defect around the area of the foramen magnum known as the Arnold–Chiari malformation. Consequently, hydrocephaly may either be present at birth or develop following surgical closure of a myelomeningocele. The risk of cerebral impairment may be minimised by the insertion of a ventriculoperitoneal shunt. As the baby grows, this will need to be replaced. Attendant risks with these devices are that the line blocks and that the shunt is a portal for infection leading to meningitis. The midwife must be alert for the signs of increased intracranial pressure:

- large tense anterior fontanelle
- splayed skull sutures
- inappropriate increase in occipitofrontal circumference
- sun-setting appearance to the eyes
- irritability, or abnormal movements.

Microcephaly

This is where the occipitofrontal circumference is more than two standard deviations below normal for gestational age. The disproportionately small head may be the result of intrauterine infection, for example rubella, a feature of fetal alcohol syndrome, or part of a number of defects in some trisomic disorders. Invariably the baby will be mentally impaired.

MUSCULOSKELETAL DEFORMITIES

These range from relatively minor anomalies, for example an extra digit, to major deficits such as absence of a limb.

Polydactyly and syndactyly

Careful examination including separation and counting of the baby's fingers and toes during the initial examination is important, otherwise anomalies such as syndactyly (webbing) and polydactyly (extra digits) may go unnoticed.

Syndactyly more commonly affects the hands. It can appear as an independent anomaly or as a feature of a syndrome such as Apert's syndrome which is a genetically inherited condition in which there is premature fusion of the sutures of the vault of the skull, cleft palate and complete syndactyly of both hands and feet. It would depend on the degree of webbing or fusion as to whether any surgical division was carried out.

In polydactyly the extra digit(s) may be fully formed or simply extra tissue attached by a pedicle. Where there is a rudimentary digit without bone involvement it is common practice to ligate the base of the digit and allow it to necrose; more complex attachments may require surgical removal.

Where there is a family history of either of these defects the mother will be anxious to examine the baby for herself.

Limb reduction anomalies

Over the years various suggestions have been postulated with regard to the cause(s) of limb reduction anomalies. Amniotic band syndrome was the reason most often given for a baby being born with a limb deficit. It was thought that the amnion ruptured, then wrapped itself around a developing limb causing strangulation and necrosis. Although this may account for some instances, it cannot explain all of them. Clustering of cases in certain geographical areas, for example in close proximity to nuclear energy plants, has provoked research in an attempt to identify environmental teratogens, but to no avail. One of the most recent possibilities being mooted is an iatrogenic cause, namely damage inflicted at the time of chorionic villus sampling (Carr & Lui 1994).

Limb reduction defects comprise a wide range of possibilities. In some either a hand or a foot will be completely missing while in others a normal hand or foot will be present on the end of a short-ened limb. Thalidomide, an antiemetic, has been proven to be teratogenic in this context.

Although, as with any deviation from normal, the parents of a child with a limb defect will grieve for the loss of their perfect child, the child is not ill and will not be upset by the defect. Children usually prove themselves to be most adaptable and able to cope (Fig. 41.4). For those who require them, different types of prostheses are available and can be fitted as early as 3 months of age. Innovative surgical techniques such as the transferring of toe(s) to hand to serve as substitute finger(s) are proving successful for some children. Once again one of the most helpful things the midwife can do in these early days of parental adjustment is to offer the address of a support group such as Reach. This appropriately named support group for parents of children with upper limb deformities was first formed in 1978 and now has branches throughout the UK.

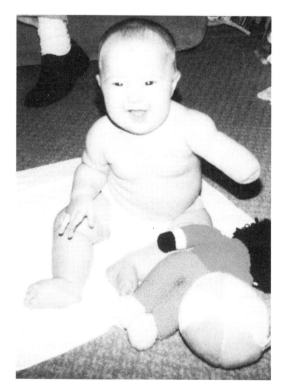

Fig. 41.4 A baby with a limb reduction defect quickly learns to adapt (photograph courtesy of Reach).

Talipes

Talipes equinovarus (TEV) is the descriptive term for a deformity of the foot where the ankle is bent downwards (plantarflexed) and the front part of the foot is turned inwards (adducted). Talipes calcaneovalgus describes the opposite position where the foot is dorsiflexed and everted. It is thought that these deformities are more likely to occur when intrauterine space has been at a premium, for example in multiple pregnancy, macrosomic fetus or oligohydramnios. TEV is also more likely to occur in conjunction with spina bifida deformities. There is in some instances a family history of the defect. Statistically more boys than girls are born with talipes. In the mildest form the foot may easily be turned to the correct position. The midwife should encourage the mother to exercise the baby's foot in this way several times a day. More severe forms will require manipulation, splinting and/or surgical correction. The advice of an orthopaedic surgeon should be sought. Care should be taken to ensure that for babies who have splints applied, the strapping is not too tight and that the baby's toes are well perfused.

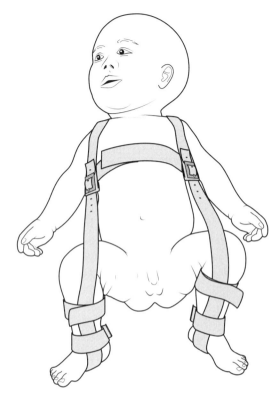

Fig. 41.5 Pavlik harness for congenital dislocation of hip (reproduced with permission from Barr 1992).

Developmental hip dysplasia

Congenital hip dysplasia is an abnormality more commonly found where there has been a history of oligohydramnios or breech presentation. It more often occurs in primigravid pregnancies and there is a higher percentage of girls born with this defect. The left hip is more often affected than the right. The dysplastic hip may present in one of three ways: dislocated, dislocatable or with subluxation of the joint. Prenatal diagnosis by ultrasound is possible; most, however, are diagnosed in the neonatal period. Examination of the hip should be carried out by an experienced practitioner with the baby lying relaxed on a firm surface. It will depend on individual unit policies whether this is a midwife, obstetrician, or paediatrician. Repeated examinations by inexperienced people may compound any pre-existing damage to the joint. Either Ortolani's test or Barlow's test is employed. For a detailed explanation of how to perform these examinations the reader is referred to Chapter 35.

Any abnormal findings should be reported and the baby referred for an ultrasound scan and then to an orthopaedic surgeon. Where the diagnosis is confirmed it is usual for the baby to have a splint or harness such as the Pavlic harness (Fig. 41.5) applied that will keep the hips in a flexed and abducted position of about 60°. The splint should not be removed for napkin changing or bathing (Le Maistre 1991). Parents will require additional support in learning how to handle and care for their baby. Particular attention should be paid to skin care and checking for signs of chafing or excoriation.

Achondroplasia

Achondroplasia is an autosomal dominant condition where the baby is generally small with a disproportionately large head and short limbs. These babies often develop a marked lordosis. Cognitive development is not usually impaired.

ABNORMALITIES OF THE SKIN

Capillary haemangiomata

The most common of these is the simple capillary haemangioma known as the stork mark. These are usually found on the eyelids or at the nape of the neck. They are generally small and will fade. No treatment is necessary. The more significant capillary haemangioma is not noticeable at birth but appears as a red raised lesion in the first few weeks of life. These lesions are particularly common in preterm infants and especially in girls. They can appear anywhere in the body but cause particular distress to the parents when they appear on the face. However, parents may be reassured that although the lesion will grow bigger for the first few months, it will then regress and disappear completely by the age of 5 or 6 years. No treatment is normally required unless the haemangioma is situated in an awkward area where it is likely to be subject to abrasion, such as on the lip. Treatment with steroids or pulsed laser therapy is possible.

Port wine stain

This is a blue–purple capillary haemangioma affecting the face. It occurs in approximately 1 in 3000 births and is twice as common in girls. This type of birthmark does not regress with time. Laser treatment and the skilful use of cosmetics will help to disguise the problem. Parents and later the child herself will need substantial psychological support.

Should the haemangioma appear to mimic the distribution of a branch of the trigeminal nerve it can be suspected that there are further haemangiomata in the meninges. This is known as Sturge–Weber syndrome.

Pigmented naevi

These are brown, sometimes hairy, marks on the skin which vary in size and may be flat or raised. A percentage of this type of birthmark may become malignant. Surgical excision may be recommended to pre-empt this.

It is unlikely that treatment for any of these birthmarks will be carried out in the immediate neonatal period. The midwife's responsibilities are therefore to notify appropriate medical staff and offer parents general emotional support.

GENITOURINARY SYSTEM

At birth the first indication that there is an abnormality of the renal tract may be finding a single umbilical artery in the umbilical cord or alternatively recognising the abnormal facies associated with Potter's syndrome (discussed later). Attention should be paid at the time of delivery to see if the baby passes urine. If no urine is passed within 24 hours or the baby is noted to be dribbling urine constantly, the paediatrician should be informed. Dribbling of urine is a sign of neural damage such as occurs with neural tube defects as previously discussed.

Posterior urethral valve(s)

This is an abnormality affecting boys. The presence of valves in the posterior urethra prevents the outflow of urine. As a result the bladder distends, causing back pressure on the ureters and to the kidneys. This will ultimately cause hydronephrosis. Prenatal diagnosis and intervention by intrauterine fetal catheterisation is possible. Failing this, early diagnosis in the neonatal period is clearly important but severe renal damage may already have been sustained. Different treatment strategies are possible with surgical procedures featuring prominently.

Polycystic kidneys

It is likely that problems may arise in delivering this baby because of increase in abdominal girth. On abdominal examination the kidneys will be palpable. Radiological or ultrasound investigations will be carried out to confirm the diagnosis. Unfortunately the prognosis is poor, with renal failure the likely outcome. The condition has an autosomal recessive inheritance pattern.

Hypospadias

Examination of a baby boy may reveal that the

urethral meatus opens on to the under surface of the penis. It can be at any point along the length of the penis and in some cases will open on to the perineum. This abnormality often coexists with chordee in which the penis is short and bent. It is anticipated that some babies will require surgery in the neonatal period to 'release' the chordee and enlarge the urethral meatus.

Cryptorchidism

This may be unilateral or bilateral. If on examination of the baby after delivery the scrotum is empty, the undescended testes may be found in the inguinal pouch. Sometimes the testis in this position can be manipulated into the scrotal pouch. This augurs well for future normal development. Testes that are found too high in the inguinal canal to manipulate into the scrotum may be malformed. Parents will be encouraged to have the baby examined at regular intervals. If descent of the testis has not occurred by the time the child is approaching school age, arrangements for orchidopexy will be made.

Ambiguous genitalia

Parents are usually invited to identify the baby's sex for themselves at delivery. On some occasions the midwife may be asked to clarify this and be unable to give a definitive answer. Examination of the baby may reveal any of the following: a small hypoplastic penis, chordee, bifid scrotum, undescended testes (careful examination should be made to detect undescended testes in the inguinal canal) or enlarged clitoris, incompletely separated or poorly differentiated labia. Most of these babies are found to be female.

Congenital adrenal hyperplasia

One of the reasons for ambiguous genitalia is an autosomal recessive condition called congenital adrenal hyperplasia. The adrenal gland is stimulated to overproduce androgens because of a deficiency of an enzyme called 21-hydroxylase. If aldosterone production is reduced these babies will rapidly lose salt. Urea and electrolyte levels should be measured and appropriate fluid replace-ments given. In the process of eliminating or confirming this cause a 24-hour urine collection may be requested. The attendant midwife may be of assistance by ensuring that the urine bag is correctly placed to avoid faecal contamination. Placing one end of a catheter or feeding tube in the urine bag and aspirating the contents at regular intervals will help to prevent spillage and the unnecessary trauma to the baby of repeated applications of urine bags. Baby girls with this condition may require later cosmetic surgery. The condition is not always recognised in boys in the neonatal period.

Intersex

This is where the internal reproductive organs are at variance with the external appearance of the genitalia. Ultrasound examination will help identify the nature of internal reproductive organs. True hermaphroditism is extremely rare. Following chromosomal studies to determine genetic make-up, hormone assays and consideration of the potential for cosmetic surgery, the decision of sex attribution is made.

Clearly, this time of waiting for results of investigations is a time of great concern for parents because they cannot tell relatives and friends the sex of the baby. Delay in naming the baby is an additional pressure. Some parents in this invidious position elect to give the baby a name that would suit either a boy or a girl. It is, however, more common for a child of truly ambiguous gender to be raised as a girl.

COMMONLY OCCURRING SYNDROMES

Box 41.1 provides definitions of terms used in this section.

Trisomy 21 or Down syndrome

The classic features of what is now known as Down syndrome were first described in 1866 by physician John Down. He recognised a commonly occurring combination of facial features amongst mentally subnormal individuals. His description included

> **Box 41.1** Glossary of terms
>
> **Karyotyping.** The process of identifying chromosomes by size.
>
> **Meiosis.** The type of cell division which occurs in the formation of gametes when one of each chromosome pair is reduced or 'lost'.
>
> **Mitosis.** The type of cell division in somatic cells.
>
> **Non-disjunction.** Failure of a chromosome pair to separate during meiosis or paired chromatids during mitosis.
>
> **Trisomy.** This describes a situation where a particular chromosome is represented three times in the nucleus.
>
> **Deletion.** Breaking off or loss of part of a chromosome.
>
> **Translocation.** Transfer of material from one chromosome to another of a different kind. Should this occur during mitosis, the result will be a balanced or reciprocal translocation where the total chromosomal complement is normal. This would only be discovered during karyotyping. There is no clinical manifestation. If, however, translocation happens during meiosis an unbalanced translocation will result in either an excess or deficit of chromosomal material in the gamete formed.

features such as widely set and obliquely slanted eyes, small nose and thick rough tongue (Toliss 1995). In addition to these, it is now accepted that other signs are evident: small head with flat occiput; squat broad hands with incurving little finger; wide space between thumb and index finger; single palmar (simian) crease; Brushfield spots in the eyes; and generalised hypotonia. Not all of these manifestations need be present and any of them can occur alone without implying chromosomal aberration. Babies born with Down syndrome also have a higher incidence of cardiac anomalies, leukaemia and hypothyroidism. Intelligence quotient is below average at 40–80.

Although there may be little doubt in the midwife's mind that a baby has Down syndrome, she should be careful not to make any definitive statements. Family likeness alone may explain some babies' appearance. Parents themselves may voice their suspicions. If they do not, a sensitive but honest approach should be made by either the midwife or paediatrician to alert them to the possibility and to request permission to conduct further investigations. It is inappropriate to transfer the baby to the special care nursery in order to carry out these investigations under guise of the baby being cold or sleepy.

Down syndrome arising as a result of a non-disjunction process is more likely to be the cause in the case of an older mother, whilst in a younger mother it is more likely to occur as a result of an unbalanced translocation (Figs 41.6 and 41.7). There is no difference between the two in clinical appearance. Parents who have a baby with Down syndrome, therefore, should be offered genetic counselling to establish the risk of recurrence. The overall incidence of Down syndrome is 1 in 700 (Fig. 41.8).

An individual baby's needs will vary depending on whether there are any coexisting abnormalities. Apart from any emotional support the mother may require, the midwife may also offer help with feeding. Problems are likely to be encountered because of the baby's generalised hypotonia. Breast feeding is still possible and should be encouraged if the mother had so planned. Providing a video tape or reading material about Down syndrome for the parents may be helpful, or the address of the local branch of the Down Syndrome Association.

Trisomy 18 (Edwards syndrome)

This condition is found in about 1 in 5000 births. An extra 18th chromosome is responsible for the characteristic features. The lifespan for these children is short and the majority die during their first year. The head is small with a flattened forehead, a receding chin and frequently a cleft palate. The ears are low-set and maldeveloped.

The sternum tends to be short, the fingers often overlap each other and the feet have a characteristic rocker-bottom appearance. Malformations of the cardiovascular and gastrointestinal systems are common.

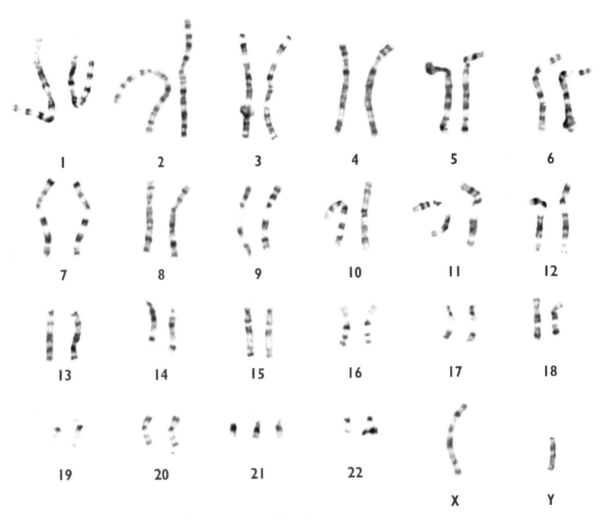

Fig. 41.6 Trisomy 21: nondisjunction (courtesy of Mr J. Colgan).

Trisomy 13 (Patau syndrome)

An extra copy of the 13th chromosome leads to multiple abnormalities. These children have a short life. Only 5% live beyond 3 years. Affected infants are small and are microcephalic. Midline facial abnormalities are common and limb abnormalities are frequently seen. Brain, cardiac and renal abnormalities may coexist with this trisomy.

Potter syndrome

The baby's face will have a flattened appearance, low-set ears, anti-mongoloid slant to the eyes with deep epicanthic folds, and a beaked nose. These babies are usually severely asphyxiated at birth because they have lung hypoplasia. They also have renal agenesis. It is a syndrome incompatible with sustained life.

Turner syndrome (XO)

In this monosomal condition, only one sex chromosome exists, an X. The absent chromosome is indicated by 'O'. The child is a girl with a short, webbed neck, widely spaced nipples and oedematous feet. The genitalia tend to be underdeveloped and the internal reproductive organs do not

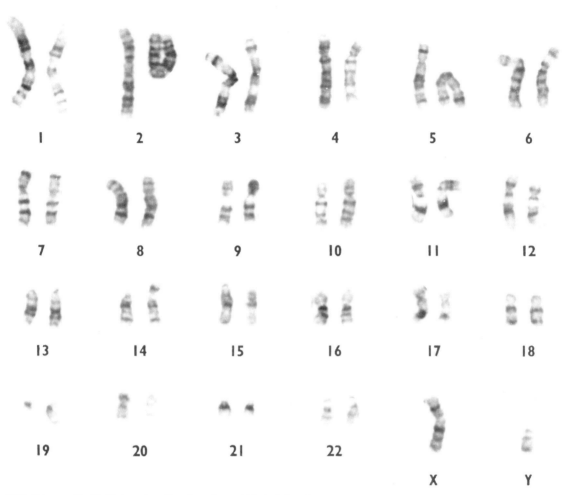

Fig. 41.7 Trisomy 21: 14–21 translocation (courtesy of Mr J. Colgan).

mature. The condition may not be diagnosed until puberty fails to occur. Congenital cardiac defects may also be found. Mental development is usually normal.

Klinefelter syndrome (XXY)

This is an abnormality affecting boys but it is not normally diagnosed until pubertal changes fail to occur.

SUPPORT FOR THE MIDWIFE

Caring for a mother whose baby has some major

congenital abnormality can place extra demands on the midwife. This stress is compounded if the abnormality was not anticipated prior to delivery or if the midwife has not previously encountered the particular problem. The exercising of effective counselling and communication skills is invaluable in helping the family adjust and in facilitating appropriate lines of support. The extra effort expended can be costly not only in terms of time but in the emotional stress the midwife may experience.

It is important that support is available for midwives in these situations. Clinical supervision with 'time out' for reflection and discussion is a management strategy being explored in some areas. One of the benefits claimed is reduction of stress.

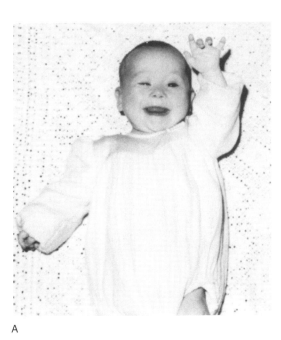
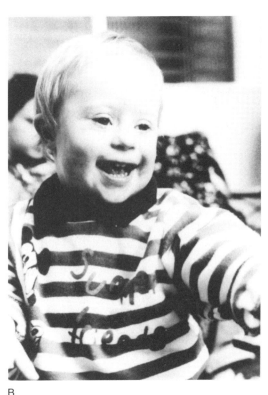

A   B

Fig. 41.8 (A) Baby with Down syndrome: note slant of eyes and incurving little finger. (B) With good parental involvement and stimulus these infants can reach maximum potential. (Photographs courtesy of Scottish Down's Syndrome Association.)

Although not specifically designed for this situation the same principle obtains. Preparatory courses on grief and bereavement counselling may also be of some benefit. Midwives who have acquired experience in this realm should not, however, automatically be targeted as the experts and always be called upon to fulfil this role. Conversely, student midwives ought not to be deliberately shielded from being involved in caring for such families. The provision of quality care for parents who have a child with a congenital abnormality is contingent upon meeting the needs of the carers.

READER ACTIVITY

Arrange to visit a local self-help group for parents of children with a congenital abnormality. (These groups normally welcome professional observers.) When at the group use your skills of communication to ascertain the particular concerns of the parents and whether they feel that they were given sufficient explanation at the time of diagnosis.

The results of this exercise might be useful for class presentation and subsequent discussion with your peers. In discussion, try to determine how you would develop your approach to such parents subsequent to diagnosis.

USEFUL ADDRESSES

Association for Spina Bifida and Hydrocephalus (ASBAH)
ASBAH House
42 Park Road
Peterborough
PE1 2UQ

Cleft Lip and Palate Association (CLAPA)
138 Buckingham Palace Road
London SW1 9SA

Cystic Fibrosis Research Trust (CF)
11 London Road
Bromley, Kent
BR1 1BY

Scottish Down's Syndrome Association (SDSA)
158–160 Balgreen Road
Edinburgh
EH11 3AU

Down's Syndrome Association
155 Mitcham Road
London SW17 9BR

Support around Termination for Abnormality (SATFA)
71–75 Charlotte Street
London W1P 1LB

Reach: The Association for Children with Hand or Arm Deficiency
12 Wilson Way
Earls Barton, Northamptonshire
NN6 0NZ

STEPS (National Association for Children with Lower Limb Abnormalities)
11 Eagle Brow
Lymm, Cheshire
WA13 0LP

REFERENCES

Bagwell C E 1993 Surgical lesions of pediatric airways and lungs. In: Koff P B, Eitzman D, Neu J (eds) Neonatal and pediatric respiratory care, 2nd edn. Mosby Year Book, St Louis, ch 8, p 132

Barr D G D 1992 Disorders of bone. In: Campbell A G M, McIntosh N (eds) Forfar and Arneil's textbook of paediatrics. Churchill Livingstone, Edinburgh, ch 23, p 1628

Butler J 1993 Assessment and management of musculoskeletal dysfunction. In: Kenner C, Brueggemeyer A, Gunderson L P Comprehensive neonatal nursing. W B Saunders, Philadelphia, ch 30, pp 690–705

Carr A J, Lui D T Y 1994 Chorionic villus sampling. Advantages and disadvantages for prenatal diagnosis. Midwives Chronicle 107(1279): 284–287

Danner S C 1992 Breast feeding the infant with a cleft defect. NAACOGs Clinical Issues in Perinatal and Women's Health Nursing 3(4): 634–639

Department of Health 1986 Screening for detection of congenital dislocation of hip. HMSO, London

Habel A, Sell D, Mars M 1996 Management of cleft lip and palate. Archives of Disease in Childhood 74(4): 360–366

Le Maistre G 1991 Ultrasound and dislocation of the hip. Paediatric Nursing 64: 13–16

Levene M I, Tudehope D 1993 Essentials of neonatal medicine, 2nd edn. Blackwell Scientific Publications, Oxford, ch 14, p 195

Modell B, Modell M 1992 Towards a healthy baby. Oxford

University Press, Oxford, ch 1, p 5

Nixon H, O'Donnell B 1992 Essentials of paediatric surgery, 4th edn. Butterworth Heinemann, Oxford, ch 8, pp 57–69

Paul K 1995 Recognition, stabilisation and early management of infants with critical congenital heart disease presenting in the first days of life. Neonatal Network 14(5): 13–25

Raine P 1994 Cleft lip and palate. In: Freeman N V, Burge D M, Griffiths M, Malone P S J (eds) Surgery in the newborn. Churchill Livingstone, Edinburgh, ch 34, p 375

Roberton N R C 1993 Neonatal intensive care, 3rd edn. Edward Arnold, London, ch 16, p 271

Rose V, Clark E 1992 Etiology of congenital heart disease. In: Freedom R M, Benson L N, Smallhorn J F (eds) Neonatal heart disease. Springer Verlag, London, ch 1, p 7

Spohr H L, Wilms J, Sternhausen H C 1993 Prenatal alcohol exposure and longterm developmental consequences. Lancet 341(8850): 907–910

Sullivan G 1996 Parental bonding in cleft lip and palate repair. Paediatric Nursing 8(1): 21–24

Toliss D 1995 Who was Down? Nursing Times 91(5): 61

Wallis S, Harvey D 1979 Disorders in the newborn – 1. Nursing Times 75: 1315–1327

Whyte A 1995 Folic acid fortifying the pregnancy message. Health Visitor 68(10): 397–398

Wirt S, Algren C L, Arnold S L 1992 Cleft lip and palate: a multidisciplinary approach. Plastic Surgical Nursing 12(4): 140–145

FURTHER READING

Beverley M, Nathan S 1995 Diagnosing developmental dysplasia of the hip. Maternal Child Health 20(4): 120–124

Birth Defects Foundation 1997 What next? Birth Defects

Foundation, Cannock

Clark E 1995 Reach: the association for children with hand or arm deficiency. Midwives 108(1295): 392–393

Crawford D, Morris M 1994 Neonatal nursing. Chapman & Hall, London

Gilbert P 1993 The A–Z reference book of syndromes and inherited disorders. Chapman & Hall, London

Greig C 1995 Congenital talipes equinovarus. Professional Nurse 11(1): 30–32

Johnston P G B 1994 Vulliamy's the newborn child. Churchill Livingstone, New York

Kelnar C J H, Harvey D, Simpson C 1995 The sick newborn baby, 3rd edn. Baillière Tindall, London

Lafferty P M, Emmerson A J, Fleming P J, Frank J D, Noblett H R 1989 Anterior abdominal wall defects. Archives of Disease in Childhood 64: 1029–1031

Martin V 1995 Helping parents cope. Nursing Times 91(11): 38–40

Selikowitz M 1990 Down syndrome: the facts. Oxford Medical Publications, Oxford

Syed S, Harper J 1996 Vascular birthmarks and treatment with pulse dye laser. Maternal Child Health 21(2): 44–47

Thomas S 1992 Congenital defects of the heart. Nursing Standard 6(18): 47–49

Jaundice and infection

42

Patricia Percival

Mild jaundice is a common and normal condition in newborn babies. This 'physiological jaundice' appears 48 hours after birth and usually settles within 10–12 days. Jaundice that appears earlier, is persistent or associated with abnormally high bilirubin levels may have one of a number of pathological causes, including increased haemolysis, metabolic and endocrine disorders, and infection.

The newborn baby is very vulnerable to infection; defence mechanisms are immature and the skin is thin and easily damaged. Infections may be acquired before, during or soon after birth and, while some may be minor, others are potentially damaging or life-threatening.

The chapter aims to:

- describe the process of conjugation whereby fat-soluble bilirubin is converted to a water-soluble form which can be excreted

- consider the physiological basis of neonatal jaundice and the causes and consequences of pathological jaundice

- stress the role of the midwife in the prevention of Rhesus iso-immunisation

- discuss the management of jaundice and its treatment by either phototherapy or exchange transfusion

- discuss the role of the midwife in the prevention, assessment, diagnosis and treatment of infection

- review those infections that may be acquired by the neonate before, during and shortly after birth.

CONJUGATION OF BILIRUBIN

Bilirubin is a waste product of the breakdown of haem, most of which is found in red blood cells

(RBCs). RBCs are removed from the circulation and broken down in the reticuloendothelial system using a normal process that destroys ageing, immature or malformed cells. The haemoglobin in the red blood cells breaks down into its by-products of haem, globin and iron. Globin is broken down into amino acids that are re-used by the body to make proteins, while the iron is stored in the body or used for new red blood cells. Enzymes convert the haem to biliverdin and then to unconjugated bilirubin.

Two major forms of bilirubin are found in the body. These are indirect-reacting or unconjugated bilirubin and direct-reacting or conjugated bilirubin:

- Unconjugated bilirubin is fat-soluble, cannot be excreted easily either in bile or urine and can build up in the blood and be deposited in extravascular fatty and nerve tissues, for example under the skin and in the brain. Deposits under the skin lead to jaundice while deposits in the brain can cause bilirubin toxicity or kernicterus.
- Conjugated bilirubin has been rendered water-soluble in the liver and can be excreted either in faeces or urine.

(Blackburn 1995, Schneider 1993, Stephenson 1996, Torres-Torres et al 1994.)

Knowledge of bilirubin conjugation and the processes that surround it is required to understand the underlying aetiology of jaundice. Three stages are involved: transport, conjugation, and excretion of bilirubin (Fig. 42.1).

Transport of bilirubin

Unconjugated bilirubin is transported in the plasma to the liver. It is bound to albumin with an estimated 8.5–10 mg of bilirubin bound by each gram of albumin. This albumin-bound bilirubin does not usually move out from the circulating blood. However, bilirubin not bound to albumin, that is free bilirubin, can move from the circulation into other tissues such as the skin and brain (Blackburn 1995).

Conjugation

Unconjugated plasma bilirubin bound to albumin is taken up by the liver. The bilirubin is then detached from the albumin and transported by intracellular carrier proteins Y and Z to the smooth endoplasmic reticulum of the liver. Here the bilirubin is combined with glucose and *glucuronic acid* and conjugation occurs in the presence of oxygen. *Uridine diphosphoglucuronyl transferase* (UDP-GT or *glucuronyl transferase*) is the major enzyme involved in bilirubin conjugation. Following conjugation, bilirubin is water-soluble (Blackburn 1995, Knudsen 1994, Torres-Torres et al 1994).

Excretion

The conjugated, or direct-reacting, water-soluble bilirubin is excreted via the biliary system into the small intestine where it is catabolised by normal intestinal bacteria to form urobilinogen. This urobilinogen is then oxidised to form orange-coloured urobilin. Most of the conjugated bilirubin is excreted in the faeces but a small amount is excreted in urine (Blackburn 1995).

Following conjugation in the liver, the bilirubin can be unconjugated in the small intestine by an enzyme *β-glucuronidase*. This unconjugated bilirubin can then be absorbed back into the portal circulation, a process known as enterohepatic reabsorption or shunting.

JAUNDICE

Jaundice results from deposition of bilirubin in the skin. Neonatal jaundice becomes apparent at serum bilirubin concentrations of 85–120 µmol/l (5–7 mg/dl). In Caucasian infants jaundice is usually evident in the face and sclera at total bilirubin levels of 100–140 µmol/l (6–8 mg/dl) (normal levels during the first 2–3 days of life). Jaundiced shoulders and trunk indicate a bilirubin level of 140–165 µmol/l (8–10 mg/dl); jaundice of the lower body appears at 165–200 µmol/l (10–12 mg/dl) and jaundice of the entire body usually indicates a bilirubin level of 200–250 µmol/l (12–15 mg/dl).

Asian and Native American babies tend to have higher bilirubin levels than white babies, who in turn have higher levels than black infants. Premature infants are also more likely to develop jaundice.

(Gartner 1994a, Levy 1994, Maisels 1994, Sater 1995, Stephenson 1996.)

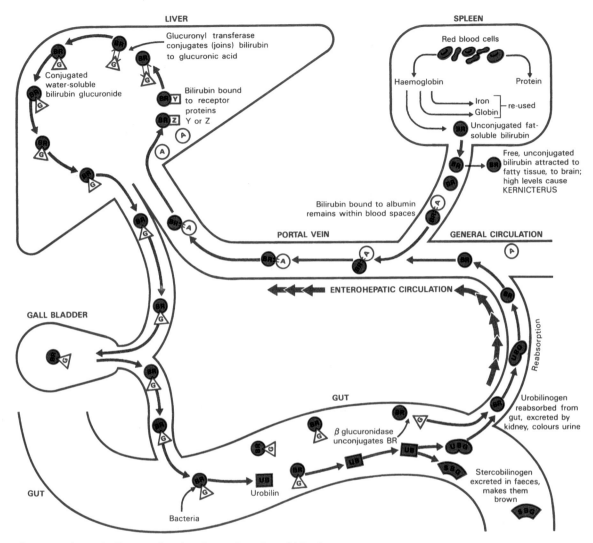

Fig. 42.1 Schematic diagram showing the conjugation of bilirubin.
Key: BR   bilirubin
      =   bound to
      A   albumin
      G   glucuronic acid
      UB   urobilin
      UBG urobilinogen
      SBG stercobilinogen

Physiological jaundice

More than 50% of full-term infants and 80% of preterm infants will have some physiological jaundice. The classic pattern of hyperbilirubinaemia that results in physiological jaundice is that of a regular rise in unconjugated bilirubin from 25 μmol/l (1.5 mg/dl) in the cord serum to 85–120 μmol/l (5–7 mg/dl) on the third day of life. This peak is usually followed by a decline to normal adult levels of bilirubin by the 10th to 12th days of life. In a full-term, well baby physiological jaundice *never* appears before 24 hours of age, *never* exceeds 200–215 μmol/l (12–13 mg/dl) and usually fades by 1 week of age (Gartner 1994a, Hicks & Altman 1993, Lasker & Holzman 1996, Schneider 1993, Stephenson 1996).

Causes of physiological jaundice

Neonatal physiological jaundice is the result of a discrepancy between RBC breakdown and the new infant's ability to transport, conjugate and excrete unconjugated bilirubin. Newborns must deal with the results of increased red cell destruction at a time when they also have decreased albumin-binding capacity, enzyme deficiency and increased enterohepatic reabsorption (Alvarez et al 1993, Rubaltelli 1993).

Increased red cell breakdown. Bilirubin production in the newborn is estimated to be more than twice that of the normal adult per kilogram of weight. In the hypoxic environment of the uterus, the fetus relies on haemoglobin F (fetal haemoglobin); this has a greater affinity for oxygen than haemoglobin A, the primary haemoglobin after birth. This greater affinity ensures that the fetus obtains sufficient oxygen via the placenta from the maternal blood. Following birth, as haemoglobin A replaces fetal haemoglobin, the latter must be broken down into bilirubin and other products. In addition, the newborn's red blood cells have a shorter life span (100 days in term infants and 60–80 days in preterm infants, as opposed to 120 days in adults).

The average concentration of serum conjugated bilirubin in neonates is three to seven times higher than that of adults, whereas the concentration of unconjugated bilirubin is four to 24 times higher. Most of the unconjugated bilirubin produced by healthy newborns, that is 70–75%, is a result of the breakdown of circulating red blood cells. In addition, 20–25% comes from enterohepatic shunting (Alvarez et al 1993, Blackburn 1995, Gartner 1994b).

Decreased albumin-binding capacity. The ability of neonates to effectively transport bilirubin to the liver for conjugation is reduced because of lower albumin concentrations, decreased albumin-binding capacity and possible competition for albumin-binding sites from some drugs (see also below).

Levels of unbound, unconjugated, fat-soluble bilirubin in the blood rise as the binding sites on the albumin are used. Although albumin-bound bilirubin does not usually move out from the circulating blood, bilirubin not bound to albumin can move from the circulation into other tissues such as the skin and brain (Blackburn 1995).

Enzyme deficiency. Bilirubin conjugation is reduced because the newborn infant has low levels of UDP-GT enzyme activity during the first 24 hours after birth. Although levels increase after the first 24 hours, normal adult levels are not reached for 6–14 weeks (Kowardi & Onishi 1981, quoted in Blackburn 1995).

Increased enterohepatic reabsorption. Enterohepatic reabsorption of bilirubin is increased in neonates for several reasons. Newborns lack the normal enteric bacteria that break down bilirubin to urobilinogen. In addition, increased β-glucuronidase activity in the bowel of the newborn (intestinal mucosa enzyme) hydrolyses conjugated bilirubin back into the unconjugated state. This bilirubin can then be absorbed back into the system. Finally, bowel motility is decreased until feeding is established.

Asian newborns have enhanced enterohepatic circulation of bilirubin. They also have a higher peak bilirubin concentration and more prolonged jaundice (Gartner 1994a).

Exaggerated physiological jaundice

Exaggerated physiological jaundice is characterised by bilirubin levels of 165 µmol/l (10 mg/dl) or greater by the third to fourth day of life (Brown et al 1993).

Preterm and breast-fed infants are more prone to exaggerated physiological jaundice.

Jaundice in preterm infants

Preterm infants are more likely than full-term babies to have exaggerated physiological jaundice with peak bilirubin concentrations on the fifth to seventh day that return to normal over several weeks (Lasker & Holzman 1996).

Factors contributing to this exaggerated physiological jaundice include:

- a delay in the expression of the enzyme UDP-GT (more marked in preterm infants)
- shorter red cell life
- complications such as hypoxia, acidosis and hypothermia that can interfere with albumin-binding capacity (Blackburn 1995, Gartner 1994b).

Sater (1995) argued that it is not the prematurity itself that is the problem but the fact that preterm infants frequently experience complications, for example acidosis, sepsis or intracranial haemorrhage, which increase bilirubin levels and may also facilitate bilirubin entry into the central nervous system.

Jaundice in breast-fed infants

Gartner (1994a) considered that few issues in the management of newborn infants have generated as much confusion, uncertainty and anxiety as jaundice in the breast-fed newborn. This jaundice can be either of early or late onset.

Early onset. There is little consensus in research findings about the rates and reasons for early-onset jaundice in breast-fed infants. In a group of 153 term healthy babies, Salariya & Robertson (1993) found 41% of breast-fed babies developed marked to moderately severe jaundice compared to only 18% of artificially fed babies. 36% of babies, initially breast fed but then formula fed, developed jaundice. Conversely, the results of a larger study of 1454 neonates showed no significant difference in serum bilirubin concentration between breast-fed on demand and artificially fed neonates (Rubaltelli & Griffith 1992).

Research in the 1980s linked higher rates of early jaundice in breast-fed infants to a decreased milk intake (DeCarvalho et al 1982, Kuhr & Paneth 1982). However, more recently, Maisels et al (1994) found no relationship between the frequency of breast feeding and serum bilirubin levels in 275 infants who were randomly assigned to either frequent or demand breast-feeding schedules. Sater (1995) argued that during the first 5 days after birth, adequately fed breast-fed babies should not have higher rates than artificially fed babies.

Late onset. Late-onset jaundice occurs in about 1% of breast-fed infants, becoming evident after 5–6 days of feeding. Levels of unconjugated bilirubin do not usually exceed 340 µmol/l (20 mg/dl). Other causes of jaundice must be excluded, but discontinuing breast feeding is not considered necessary.

Several theories have been proposed to explain jaundice in breast-fed infants. A substance in breast milk appears to inhibit the action of UDP-GT or *glucuronyl transferase* thus affecting conjugation. Some breast-fed infants may also have an enhanced enterohepatic reabsorption of unconjugated bilirubin (Arias et al 1964, Gartner & Lee 1993, Kivlahan & James 1984). Demirkol & Bohles (1994) found that taurine concentration was highest in breast milk at the time when breast-milk-induced jaundice developed.

It has also been suggested that bilirubin may be of physiological importance and could possibly be beneficial to the newborn because of its antioxidant properties. Recent research has demonstrated this possible antioxidant effect of bilirubin both before and after the birth (Dennery et al 1992, Stocker et al 1987, Stocker et al 1990).

Management of physiological jaundice

Early, frequent feeding helps newborns to deal with their increased bilirubin load by helping them overcome the factors causing physiological jaundice (particularly decreased albumin-binding capacity, enzyme deficiency and increased enterohepatic reabsorption). With breast-feeding infants, early, frequent, demand feeding (without fluid supplementation) ensures adequate volume and frequency of colostrum and milk in the intestine. Effective feeding supplies glucose to the liver, encourages bowel colonisation with normal flora and increases bowel motility. In turn this helps production of the enzymes needed for conjugation and decreases enterohepatic reabsorption (Gartner 1994b).

Of particular importance to midwifery practice is that breast-fed babies who receive water or dextrose water supplements have higher bilirubin levels than infants not given supplements (DeCarvalho et al 1981). In most cases ceasing breast feeding is not necessary; it deprives the baby of the known advantages of breast milk without any proven benefit.

The management of jaundice in newborns is a challenge for midwives. Careful observation will help to distinguish between healthy babies with a normal physiological response (needing no active treatment) and those where serum bilirubin testing is required.

Pathological jaundice

Pathological jaundice usually appears within 24 hours of birth, and is characterised by a rapid rise in serum bilirubin and prolonged jaundice. Criteria for pathological jaundice in newborns include:

- clinical jaundice within the first 24 hours of life
- increase in total serum bilirubin > 85 µmol/l (5 mg/dl) per day
- total serum bilirubin > 200 µmol/l (12.9 mg/dl)
- conjugated (direct-reacting) bilirubin > 25–35 µmol/l (1.5–2 mg/dl)
- persistence of clinical jaundice for 7–10 days in full-term infants or 2 weeks in preterm infants.

Causes of pathological jaundice

A large number of studies have been undertaken to better understand the relationship between neonatal jaundice and other factors. These factors include maternal smoking or contraceptive use, maternal diet, type of delivery, use of epidural analgesia and oxytocin, delayed cord clamping, infant race and infant gender. A critical review of these studies is provided in Knudsen (1994).

The underlying aetiology of pathological jaundice is some interference with bilirubin *production, transport, conjugation* or *excretion* (Fig. 42.2). Any disease or pathological disorder that increases bilirubin production or that alters the transport or metabolism of bilirubin is superimposed upon normal physiological jaundice (Blackburn 1995, Gartner 1994b, Stephenson 1996).

Production. Alterations during this stage that may lead to pathological jaundice are those that increase haemoglobin destruction, resulting in further elevation of bilirubin levels. A number of conditions can lead to increased haemolysis in the newborn infant, in particular:

- Rhesus (Rh(D)) and ABO blood group incompatibility (these are discussed in more detail later in the chapter)
- abnormalities of the red blood cell membrane, for example spherocytosis and sickle cell disease where the red cells are of an abnormal shape and/or fragility (more likely in African and Mediterranean infants)
- enzyme deficiencies such as *glucose 6-phosphate dehydrogenase* (G6PD) deficiency, where the absence of G6PD increases red cell fragility (more likely in African, Asian and Mediterranean male infants)
- extravasated blood, for example cephalhaematoma and bruising
- sepsis, which can lead to increased haemoglobin breakdown
- polycythaemia, a condition where blood contains too many red cells as in maternofetal or twin-to-twin transfusion, delayed cord clamping or in infants of diabetic mothers.

(Achanna & Monga 1994, Blackburn 1995, Lasker & Holzman 1996, Stephenson 1996.)

Transport. During bilirubin transport, factors that lower blood albumin levels or decrease albumin-binding capacity can lead to pathological jaundice:

- Newborn albumin levels can be further reduced in malnourished or preterm infants, as hypothermia, acidosis or hypoxia interfere with albumin-binding capacity.
- Some drugs may compete with bilirubin for albumin-binding sites, for example aspirin, sulphonomides, ampicillin and benzyl alcohol (Blackburn 1995, Stephenson 1996).

Conjugation. In addition to immaturity of the neonate's enzyme system, other factors can interfere with the conjugation of bilirubin in the liver. These include:

- dehydration, starvation, hypoxia and sepsis, because oxygen and glucose are required for conjugation
- infections, for example TORCH (toxoplasmosis, others, rubella, cytomegalovirus, herpes) where hepatosplenomegaly is usually present

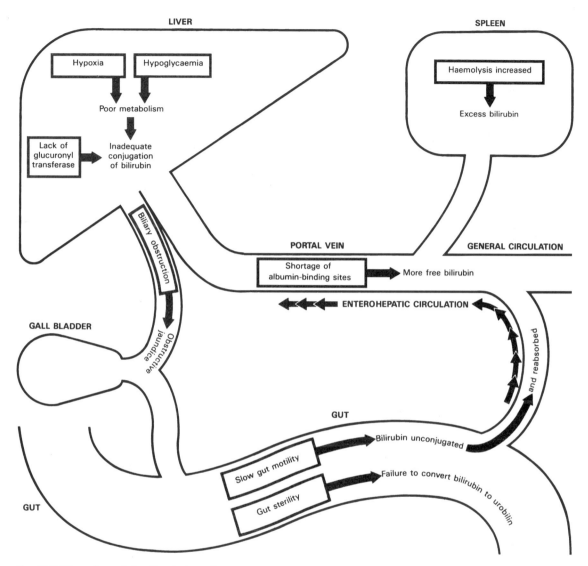

Fig. 42.2 Sites of events leading to jaundice.

- other viral infections, for example neonatal viral hepatitis
- other bacterial infections, particularly those caused by Gram-negative bacteria such as *Escherichia coli*
- metabolic and endocrine disorders that alter UDP-GT enzyme activity, for example, Crigler–Najjar disease and Gilbert's syndrome
- other metabolic disorders such as hypothyroidism and galactosaemia (Blackburn 1995, Lasker & Holzman 1996, Hicks &

Altman 1993, Schneider 1993, Stephenson 1996).

Excretion. In addition to increased enterohepatic reabsorption, other factors can interfere with bilirubin excretion. These include:

• Hepatic obstruction caused by congenital anomalies such as biliary atresia, an obliterative and fibrotic process that may affect the entire intrahepatic or extrahepatic biliary tree or just isolated segments. Extrahepatic biliary atresia, the commonest life-threatening hepatobiliary disorder in childhood, affects between 1 in 14 000 and 1 in 21 000 liveborn infants.

- Obstruction can also be caused by 'bile plugs' in conditions that increase bile viscosity, for example cystic fibrosis, treatment with total parenteral nutrition, haemolytic disorders and dehydration.
- Saturation of the protein carriers required to excrete conjugated bilirubin into the biliary system can increase blood levels.
- An excess of conjugated bilirubin may also be caused by infection, other congenital disorders, and idiopathic neonatal hepatitis.

In hyperbilirubinaemia secondary to interference with the excretion of bilirubin after it has been processed by the liver, most of the elevation in bilirubin is in the conjugated form. As conjugated bilirubin does not readily cross the blood–brain barrier, infants with intrahepatic conditions are at less risk of kernicterus. However, these infants may require urgent treatment for other serious conditions (Blackburn 1995, Stephenson 1996, Tanphaichitr et al 1995).

RHESUS AND ABO INCOMPATIBILITY

An important cause of neonatal jaundice is haemolysis from an incompatibility between maternal and fetal blood. Rhesus and ABO incompatibility are discussed in more detail, the former because of the midwife's role in prevention, and the latter because it is possibly the most frequent cause of haemolysis in newborns.

Rhesus incompatibility

Rhesus or Rh(D) incompatibility can occur when a woman with an Rh(D) negative blood type is carrying a baby with an Rh(D) positive blood type. The situation is more common among Caucasians (about 15% of whom are Rh negative) than it is amongst African Americans or Asians (Fig. 42.3). Rhesus iso-immunisation can occur during the first pregnancy, but usually sensitisation occurs during the first pregnancy and in subsequent pregnancies extensive destruction of fetal red blood cells may occur.

Small amounts of the fetus' Rh positive blood may cross the placenta into the maternal circulation (see Figs 42.4 and 42.5). Here they are treated as a foreign body by the mother's immune system and anti-Rh antibodies are produced (Fig. 42.6). In subsequent pregnancies, these maternal IgG antibodies may cross the placenta and destroy the erythrocytes of the fetus (Fig. 42.7). Sensitisation may also occur following such procedures as amniocentesis, abortion and external cephalic version, or after antepartum haemorrhage. The condition does not occur when a Rh(D) negative mother has a Rh(D) negative baby.

The effect on the fetus depends on the severity of the haemolysis. Lesser degrees of destruction result in haemolytic anaemia, whereas extensive haemolysis of the fetal red blood cells may cause death in utero.

Prevention

Most cases of Rhesus iso-immunisation can be prevented by the administration of anti-D immunoglobulin (anti-D) to Rh(D) negative blood type mothers who have a baby with a Rh(D) positive blood type (Fig. 42.8). Following the birth, the infant's Rh(D) type is confirmed from cord blood testing. In addition, a Kleihauer test is carried out which estimates the number of fetal cells in a sample of maternal blood obtained after the birth.

Midwives play an important preventive role in administering anti-D intramuscularly to the mother within 72 hours of birth or any abortion (see also below); the anti-D immunoglobulin is injected into the deltoid muscle from which absorption is optimal. This destroys any fetal cells in the mother's blood (Fig. 42.9) before her immune system produces antibodies, and thus prevents Rh sensitisation. It is vital that an adequate amount of anti-D is given if Rhesus iso-immunisation is to be avoided in future pregnancies. A second dose is needed if the Kleihauer test indicates that higher levels of fetal cells are present in maternal blood (above 50 fetal cells/50 low-power fields). In such cases a further blood test is also ordered to ensure that an adequate amount of anti-D has been given. In some hospitals or community settings, follow-up Kleihauer and further antibody screens

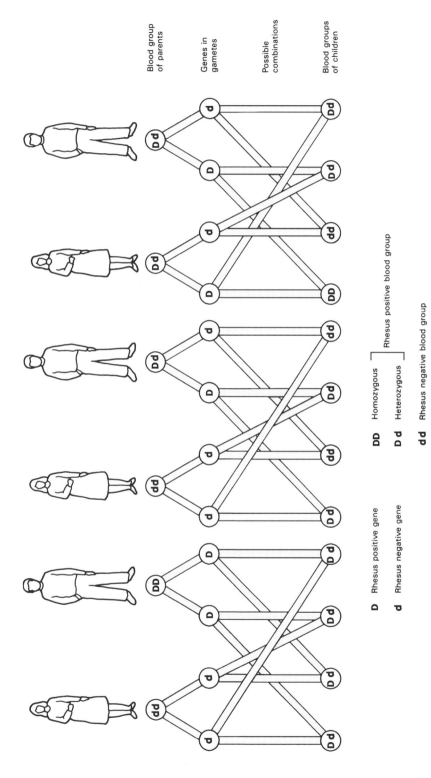

Blood group
of parents

Genes in
gametes

Possible
combinations

Blood groups
of children

D   Rhesus positive gene

d   Rhesus negative gene

DD   Homozygous ⎤
                    ⎥ Rhesus positive blood group
D d   Heterozygous ⎦

d d   Rhesus negative blood group

Fig. 42.3 Patterns of Rhesus factor inheritance.

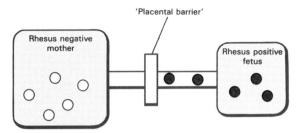

Fig. 42.4 Normal placenta with no communication between maternal and fetal blood.

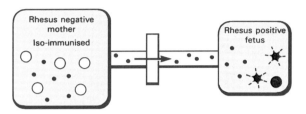

Fig. 42.7 In a subsequent pregnancy maternal Rhesus antibodies cross the placenta, resulting in haemolytic disease of the newborn.

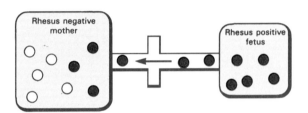

Fig. 42.5 Fetal cells enter maternal circulation through 'break' in 'placenta barrier', e.g. at placental separation.

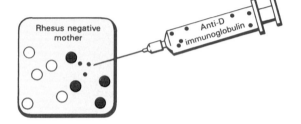

Fig. 42.8 Anti-D immunoglobulin administered within 72 hours of birth or miscarriage.

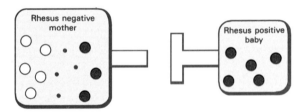

Fig. 42.6 Maternal production of Rhesus antibodies following introduction of Rhesus positive blood.

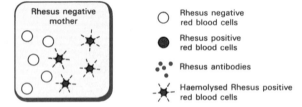

Fig. 42.9 Anti-D immunoglobulin has destroyed fetal Rhesus positive red cells and prevented iso-immunisation.

Figs 42.4–42.9 Rhesus iso-immunisation and its prevention.

are performed 48 hours after injection of anti-D, regardless of the fetal cell count.

Dependent upon hospital and community protocols, anti-D should also be given to the mother before procedures where leakage of maternal blood across the placenta may occur. These include amniocentesis, cordocentesis, chorionic villus-sampling, external cephalic version and termination of pregnancy. Anti-D should also be given to the mother following any other instances where fetomaternal haemorrhage may have occurred, for example after antepartum haemorrhage, fetal death in utero, stillbirth, threatened abortion, incomplete or missed abortion, ectopic pregnancy, motor vehicle acci-

dent, and inadvertent transfusion of Rh(D) positive red blood cells.

Antenatal management

During pregnancy all women have their blood grouped for ABO and Rhesus type. Women who are Rh negative are screened for Rhesus antibodies with an indirect Coombs' test. In the absence of antibodies the blood is retested at 28 and 34 weeks of pregnancy. Antenatal prophylaxis at 28 and 34 weeks is now being advocated for Rh(D) negative women with no living children (Benbow & Wray 1998). If antibodies are found at any stage, antibody titres are measured regularly. In addition, the fetus is monitored closely by ultrasound for any oedema and hepatosplenomegaly.

Amniocentesis may be carried out in the presence of a high maternal antibody titre. Dependent upon the level of bilirubin in the amniotic fluid and the baby's condition, a number of actions are possible:

• The pregnancy may be allowed to continue with ongoing monitoring of bilirubin and antibody levels and fetal status.
• An intrauterine transfusion may be carried out to reduce the effects of the haemolysis until the fetus is capable of survival outside the uterus.
• Delivery of the fetus may be undertaken.

Postnatal management

At birth the following tests are performed on the cord blood:

• ABO blood group and Rhesus type
• a direct Coombs' test to detect the presence of maternal antibodies on fetal red cells
• haemoglobin estimation and serum bilirubin level.

The condition of the baby depends on the severity of the haemolysis: from minimal anaemia and jaundice through to the condition hydrops fetalis. Infants with this latter condition are pale, have oedema and ascites and may be stillborn.

Infants with Rhesus iso-immunisation are usually cared for in intensive care units. Essentially, treatment aims to combat anaemia, reduce bilirubin levels and remove maternal Rh antibodies from the baby's circulation. A packed cell transfusion may be used to restore haemoglobin levels. Phototherapy may be effective but exchange transfusion is often required. Ongoing haemolytic anaemia is also a risk factor for these infants.

(Gartner 1994b, Hicks & Altman 1993, Newman & Maisels 1992, Oski & Naiman 1972, Schneider 1993, Stephenson 1996.)

ABO incompatibility

ABO iso-immunisation occurs usually when the mother is blood group O and the baby is group A, or less often group B. Type O blood contains both anti-A and anti-B antibodies. These antibodies are usually of the IgM class and are too large to cross the placenta. However, some women produce antibodies of the IgG class, which are smaller than the IgM antibodies and can cross the placenta. Once in the fetal circulation, the IgG anti-A and anti-B antibodies attach to fetal red cells and destroy them.

ABO sensitisation can occur from blood transfusion and blood leakage due to pregnancy. However, it may also be caused from other sources including food and bacteria. Both first and subsequent babies are at risk. In subsequent pregnancies the problem may become more severe, because previous exposure to the fetus' type O antigens strengthens the anti-A response. The management of ABO iso-immunisation depends on the severity of the haemolysis. In most cases haemolysis is fairly mild.

(Gartner 1994b, Hicks & Altman 1993, Newman & Maisels 1992, Oski & Naiman 1972, Schneider 1993, Stephenson 1996, Taeusch et al 1991.)

ABO incompatibility protects the fetus from Rhesus incompatibility because any fetal cells leaking into the maternal circulation will be destroyed by her anti-A and anti-B antibodies (Roberton 1993).

BILIRUBIN TOXICITY

The greatest concern in neonatal hyperbilirubinaemia is kernicterus. Infants are at risk from neurotoxicity and the development of kernicterus when there are elevated levels of unbound, unconjugated bilirubin in the serum. Kernicterus is defined as an encephalopathy that is caused by deposits of unconjugated bilirubin in the basal nuclei of the brain (Rubaltelli & Griffith 1992).

The early reversible signs of bilirubin toxicity include lethargy, changes in muscle tone, and a high-pitched cry. Irritability, hypertonic muscles and potential death may follow these early signs. In the longer term, clinical features of chronic bilirubin encephalopathy become apparent soon after the first year. These include extrapyramidal disturbances, for example athetosis, drooling, facial grimace, chewing and swallowing difficulties, hearing loss, cerebral palsy, developmental delay and learning difficulties (Anand & Gupta 1993, Sater 1995).

The blood–brain barrier forms a major defence against kernicterus. Under normal circumstances unbound, unconjugated bilirubin can move into the brain but does not remain there. Significant increases in the levels of unbound, unconjugated bilirubin leads to more bilirubin entering the brain. Although usually associated with serum bilirubin levels greater than 340 µmol/l (20 mg/dl), it is difficult to define the level at which bilirubin is universally toxic. Despite recent advances in the evaluation of the effects of bilirubin on the brain, doubt remains as to the critical threshold of bilirubin for the neonate in terms of long-term morbidity. Kernicterus develops when bilirubin concentration and production rate overwhelm the body's capacity to prevent it reaching the brain at toxic levels (Dennery et al 1995, McFadden 1991).

At the present time no universal screening test is available that predicts which infants are at risk of kernicterus without intervention. Factors such as ongoing haemolysis, sepsis, hypoxia or acidosis may alter bilirubin binding, increasing the amount of unconjugated bilirubin not bound to albumin (Dennery et al 1995). It is also hypothesised that in the presence of anoxia, infection, hypothermia and dehydration the blood–brain barrier is altered to allow both bound and unbound bilirubin to enter the brain (Blackburn 1995).

Changes in neonatal care in more recent years may have reduced the risk of kernicterus, for example better treatment of hypoxia and acidosis (Dodd 1993). Dennery et al (1995) argued that more specific research is needed that investigates whether different populations have different thresholds of bilirubin toxicity depending on such things as gestational age, underlying illness, ethnicity, and so on.

As it is the free or unconjugated bilirubin (not bound to albumin) that causes neurotoxicity, the serum bilirubin itself may not be the most sensitive predictor of the extent of bilirubin toxicity that may occur in an infant. The protein-bound bilirubin or free unconjugated bilirubin may be a more critical factor for assessing neurological risk than total serum bilirubin, and including the bilirubin:

albumin ratio in assessing and managing infants has been suggested (Ahlfors 1994, Gustafson & Boyle 1995, Rubaltelli & Griffith 1992).

It is anticipated that advancements in nuclear magnetic resonance technology will enable more accurate ongoing assessment of bilirubin's influence on the brain stem, cerebellum and basal ganglia areas that are considered vulnerable (Anand & Gupta 1993).

MANAGEMENT OF JAUNDICE

The management of jaundice in term newborns is challenging; there is a need to balance the risks of under- and overtreatment. It is important to differentiate between healthy babies whose jaundice is a normal physiological response and those with an underlying serious illness or liver disease. More than 50% of full-term infants and 80% of preterm infants will have some physiological jaundice. Nevertheless, 1 in 500 newborn babies has some form of liver disease. Diagnosing the latter must be balanced against the risks of needless laboratory tests for the former (Blackburn 1995, Gartner 1994b, Lasker & Holzman 1996).

Moreover, although neonatal jaundice is a very common and minor complication requiring no active treatment in most infants, when severe it can cause bilirubin encephalopathy or kernicterus (Tan 1996). Whilst it is important that neonates are not subjected to repeated bilirubin testing, phototherapy and possibly exchange transfusion if these are not medically indicated, it is vital that bilirubin toxicity be avoided (Beath 1996, Newman & Maisels 1992).

Assessment and diagnosis

In evaluating neonatal jaundice the principal concerns for midwife and medical practitioner are first whether the jaundice results from the physiological breakdown of bilirubin or the presence of another underlying factor, and second whether the infant is at risk of kernicterus. The midwife is referred to the following references that discuss assessment and diagnosis of jaundice: Blackburn (1995), Dodd (1993), Hicks & Altman (1993),

Newman & Maisels (1992), Sater (1995), Schneider (1993), Stephenson (1996).

Assessment includes observation of risk factors that include:

- any birth trauma or evident bruising
- prematurity
- a family history of significant haemolytic disease or jaundiced siblings
- an ethnic predisposition to jaundice or inherited disease
- delayed feeding or meconium passage
- jaundice within the first 24 hours – suggests haemolysis
- prolonged jaundice – may indicate serious disease, for example hypothyroidism or obstructive jaundice
- extent of changes in skin and scleral colour
- presence of lethargy, decreased eagerness to feed, vomiting, irritability, a high-pitched cry, dark urine or light stools
- presence of dehydration, starvation, hypothermia, acidosis or hypoxia.

Laboratory evaluation may include:

- serum bilirubin to determine if the bilirubin is unconjugated or conjugated
- direct Coombs' test to detect the presence of maternal antibodies on fetal RBCs
- indirect Coombs' test to detect the presence of maternal antibodies in serum
- haemoglobin/haematocrit estimation to assess any anaemia
- reticulocyte count – elevated with haemolysis when new RBCs are being produced
- ABO blood group and Rhesus type for possible incompatibility
- peripheral blood smear – red cell structure for abnormal cells
- white cell count to detect any infection
- serum samples for specific immunoglobulins for the TORCH infections
- glucose 6-phosphate dehydrogenase (G6PD) assay
- urine for substances such as galactose.

The midwife is referred to the normal values included in Schneider (1993) *The differential diagnosis of neonatal jaundice*.

Treatment strategies

A number of treatment strategies are available to reduce bilirubin levels. These include phototherapy and exchange transfusion, and possibly some drug treatments (Blackburn 1995).

Phototherapy

Phototherapy can be used in both the hospital and the home setting to prevent the concentration of indirect-reacting or unconjugated bilirubin in the blood from reaching levels where neurotoxicity may occur. During phototherapy the neonate's skin surface is exposed to high-intensity light, which photochemically converts fat-soluble unconjugated bilirubin into water-soluble bilirubin which can be excreted in bile and urine (Behrman & Vaughn 1987, McFadden 1991).

Indications for phototherapy. The golden rule is 'smaller, sicker, sooner, quicker'. That is, with smaller or preterm infants and sick infants (particularly with haemolysis) where jaundice is present sooner (within the first 12–24 hours) phototherapy is started quickly (at lower serum bilirubin levels).

- Healthy term infants jaundiced after 48 hours – between 280 and 365 µmol/l (17 and 22 mg/dl).
- Preterm infants < 1500 g – between 85 and 140 µmol/l (5 and 8 mg/dl).
- Preterm infants > 1500 g, sick infants and those with haemolysis – 140–165 µmol/l (8–10 mg/dl).

The serum bilirubin level at which phototherapy is discontinued also varies. Declining serum bilirubin levels below 215 µmol/l (13 mg/dl) are usually accepted as necessary for stopping phototherapy.

(Lazar et al 1993, Maisels 1994, Newman & Maisels 1992, Schneider 1993, Stephenson 1996.)

Types of phototherapy:

Conventional systems. These rely on high-intensity light delivered by fluorescent lamps. The effectiveness of conventional phototherapy depends on the wavelengths, the distance between the lights and the infant, and the amount of skin exposure. The infant is usually placed at a distance of about 45–60 cm from the phototherapy light with the entire skin exposed (covering the infant's testes and possibly the ovaries with a nappy may be advisable). Turning the neonate frequently ensures maximum skin exposure. Phototherapy treatment may be continuous or intermittent. Continuous therapy is interrupted only for essential care, for example, feeding the infant, whilst intermittent therapy may be given for periods of 6 hours on and 6 hours off.

Fibreoptic light systems.
These are a fairly recent advance in phototherapy. Fibreoptic blankets or woven fibreoptic pads which deliver high-intensity light with no ultraviolet or infrared irradiation are wrapped around the infant under the clothing, thus ensuring that more skin is exposed to light. These pads can be used day and night in hospital or at home with minimal supervision and they also reduce some of the side-effects of phototherapy, for example increased insensible fluid loss. In addition, fibreoptic systems have the advantage of eliminating the need for eye protection.

Researchers have compared fibreoptic phototherapy systems with normal phototherapy. Some have found that the use of a woven fibreoptic pad is as effective as conventional phototherapy. However, others have found fibreoptic systems to be less effective than conventional phototherapy in decreasing serum bilirubin levels, possibly because of decreased irradiance. At the present time fibreoptic phototherapy combined with the standard phototherapy to provide double phototherapy seems to provide optimum results. Nurses in Tan's research found that fibreoptic mats were more comfortable for infants and resulted in less restlessness.
(Costello et al 1995, Peterec 1995, Tan 1994, Torres-Torres et al 1994.)

Management of the baby undergoing phototherapy

Side-effects. The midwife is usually the person responsible for observing any visible side-effects of phototherapy. These can include lethargy or irritability, decreased eagerness to feed, loose stools, hyperthermia, dehydration and fluid losses, skin rashes and skin burns, alterations in state or neurobehavioural organisation, isolation and lack of usual sensory experiences including visual deprivation. Neonates may also experience hypocalcaemia, low platelet counts, increased red cell osmotic fragility, bronze baby syndrome, riboflavin deficiency and DNA damage (Blackburn 1995, Sethi et al 1993).

Eye care. A further and important potential side-effect of phototherapy is the effect of the high-intensity light on the retina (Barrios & Jain 1996). The position of eye shields or patches is closely monitored by the midwife and parent to ensure that they are over the eyes, do not occlude the nose and that the headband is not tight. The infant is also observed for any eye discharge or weeping. Fok et al (1995) conducted a randomised controlled trial of infants whose eyes were either occluded with eye patches or protected by a head box made of lightproof plastic. Of the 102 infants wearing eye patches, pathogens were isolated from 50 eyes of 33 infants. In the control group, pathogens were only detected in 22 eyes of 40 infants. Furthermore, significantly more infants in the eye-patch group had either a purulent eye discharge or clinical conjunctivitis.

Bilirubin levels. Bilirubin levels are usually estimated daily. The reduction in bilirubin levels appears to be greatest in the first 24 hours of phototherapy (James & Williams 1993).

Skin care. The skin is observed frequently for any rashes, dryness and excoriation, and cleaned with warm water when the midwife considers it necessary.

Temperature. The infant is maintained in a warm thermoneutral environment and observed for any hypo- or hyperthermia. If the infant is nursed in an incubator, servocontrol is usually used. Heat loss is minimised as far as possible.

Hydration. Fluid intake and urine output are monitored (including the frequency, amount and colour of urine and stool patterns). Good hydration is maintained with demand feeding if possible, and if breast feeding the mother is encouraged to continue. In a study of 178 term newborns with no underlying haemolysis or birth trauma, James

& Williams (1993) found no significant difference in the rapidity with which serum bilirubin levels dropped when breast feeding was discontinued. Routine supplementation with dextrose water is not indicated. Extra fluids may be required for severely ill or dehydrated infants. Intravenous fluids are not routinely required as they do not stimulate peristalsis or encourage meconium excretion.

Neurobehavioural status. Monitoring the infant's neurobehavioural status is also vital, including sleep and wake states, feeding behaviours, responsiveness, response to stress and interaction with parents and other carers.

Sensory and visual deprivation. To reduce the effects of isolation when feeding, the eye patches are usually taken off and the infant is removed from the lights. Parents can be encouraged by the midwife to hold, feed and also to care for their baby as much as possible.

Parents' needs. The midwife has a particularly important role in providing information, support and reassurance to parents, as well as emphasising the benign nature of jaundice. If the baby is otherwise well, phototherapy may be given at the mother's bedside. This may help reduce any fear and distress in parents and prevent separation from their infant. If all underlying disease has been ruled out, phototherapy can also be given in the home environment; good teaching is essential to ensure parental knowledge and cooperation. If the mother is breast feeding, it is recommended that parents are advised in a positive manner about the possible timescale of the jaundice.

Hypocalcaemia. In neonates, hypocalcaemia is defined as a total serum calcium level of < 1.7 mmol/l (7 mg/dl). Symptoms include jitteriness, irritability, rash, loose stools, fever and dehydration and convulsions. Although hypocalcaemia is a less well-known complication of phototherapy, in a recent study of 60 neonates with hyperbilirubinaemia, Sethi et al (1993) found 90% of preterm neonates and 75% of full-term neonates developed hypocalcaemia following phototherapy. The researchers argued that neonates under phototherapy should be given supplemental calcium. Earlier

research (Romagnoli et al 1979) also noted some incidence of hypocalcaemia in neonates undergoing phototherapy. (Blackburn 1995, Maisels 1995, Mathew 1995, Sater 1995.)

Exchange transfusion

An exchange transfusion process removes bilirubin from the body and, in cases of haemolytic disease, also replaces sensitised erythrocytes with blood that is compatible with both the mother's and the infant's serum (Sater 1995).

Indications for exchange transfusion. As with phototherapy, the golden rule is 'smaller, sicker, sooner, quicker':

- Healthy full-term infants – 400–500 μmol/l (23–29 mg/dl)
- Sick and preterm infants, and infants with haemolysis – 300–400 μmol/l (17–23 mg/dl)
- Small infants weighing < 1500 g – 255 μmol/l (15 mg/dl) (Dennery et al 1995, Newman & Maisels 1992, Stephenson 1996).

Before phototherapy, exchange transfusion was more common for babies with severe jaundice caused by G6PD deficiency and ABO incompatibility. Early research suggested that exchange transfusion was effective in preventing kernicterus in infants with severe haemolysis. More recently, cord blood screening and judicious use of phototherapy has led to a reduction in exchange transfusion for haemolytic and enzyme-deficiency diseases. However, there has been an increase in the number of exchange transfusions carried out on very premature infants because of increased early survival.

Tan (1996) argues that phototherapy has largely replaced exchange transfusion when treating severe neonatal jaundice. Except in Rh incompatibility, exchange transfusion may now be seen as a second treatment of choice that is used only when phototherapy has failed (Maisels 1994). Exchange transfusion would certainly be considered when there is a risk of bilirubin toxicity or kernicterus.

A number of risks are associated with exchange transfusions. These include risks from the transfused blood and from the procedure itself, for example acquired immune deficiency syndrome and hepatitis from the use of blood products, as well as a risk of 3 deaths per 1000 procedures with an experienced practitioner. Exchange transfusion also increases the risk of necrotising enterocolitis (Todd 1995). Newman & Maisels (1992) argued that the mortality and morbidity from this infrequently performed procedure could rise because of inexperienced practitioners (given the decreasing numbers of exchange transfusions).

Management of the baby undergoing exchange transfusion

Exchange transfusion is usually carried out in a neonatal intensive care unit with experienced neonatal nurses caring for the infant before, during and after the procedure. The transfusion is given by the umbilical vein (Fig. 42.10). Removal of blood and replacement is conducted by removing approximately 5 mg/kg at once and replacing this with donor blood. This is usually continued until a total volume of 170 ml/kg of infant blood has been replaced (representing twice the infant's total circulating volume of 85 ml/kg) (Maisels 1994, Poland & Ostrea 1993).

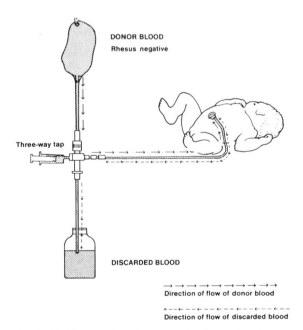

Fig. 42.10 Diagram showing apparatus for performing an exchange transfusion.

Isovolaemic exchange transfusion is an alternative to the traditional exchange transfusion method. This method involves simultaneously removing the baby's blood and administering new blood, thus eliminating fluctuations in blood flow and maintaining a more consistent blood pressure. The baby's blood is removed from one side and the new blood administered by another route at the same time and rate.

As this procedure is becoming less common, the midwife is referred to hospital intensive care protocols. Figure 42.10 shows a traditional exchange transfusion. Todd (1995) also describes the management of the neonate during an isovolaemic exchange transfusion.

NEONATAL INFECTION

Vulnerability to infection

In full-term infants most of the developments in the immune system have occurred within the protective uterine environment. Nevertheless, defence mechanisms are immature during the early weeks of life, and newborns when compared with older children and adults, are immunodeficient. The higher incidence of infection (see Box 42.1 for definitions) during the neonatal period demonstrates this immaturity of the immune system.

The newborn infant is more vulnerable to infection for a number of reasons.

Overall, the immune system's response can be divided into two categories: innate response and acquired immune response. Full immunocompetence requires both innate and acquired immune mechanisms.

Innate immunity. Innate or natural immunity involves responses that do not require previous exposure to microorganisms. These include intact skin and mucous membranes, and gastric acid and digestive enzymes that all act as a first line of defence against infection in the neonate. Immediately after birth, the infant's bowel is not colonised with normal protective flora, and skin is more easily irritated and damaged.

Infection: 'the term infection is used to describe any infectious process caused by bacterial, fungal, protozoal, or viral agents in the fetus or neonate. Infection is present if there is a host response to the invasion of the microorganisms' (Wright Lott & Kenner 1994a, p. 4).

Sepsis or septicaemia: 'Sepsis or septicaemia refers to the presence of microorganisms in the blood and the presence of multiple effects on the body due to these microorganisms and the body's defenses against them' (Wright Lott et al 1994, p. 36). Infection occurring during or after the birth can result in systemic infection. Infants are more vulnerable to systemic infection because of their immature defence mechanisms (this particularly applies to preterm infants).

Septic shock: Septic shock (caused by the release of endotoxic substances by microorganisms) occurs when systemic blood flow and oxygen transport can no longer meet the metabolic demands of the body (Wright Lott et al 1994).

Acquired immunity. Acquired or specific immune responses are responses that develop and improve with ongoing exposure to a pathogen or organism. Although the infant has some immune protection from the mother, to a large extent he must actively acquire this immune response. Immunoglobulins are deficient at birth. Antibody levels are limited by maternal exposure and transfer of IgG across the placenta (this is particularly so in preterm infants as transfer of IgG mainly occurs after 32 weeks' gestation). Breast feeding increases the infant's immune protection through the transmission of secretory IgA in breast milk (see Ch. 36). During the early weeks of life the infant also has deficiencies in both the quantity and the quality of neutrophils.

Preterm infants are particularly vulnerable to infection. They not only have less well-developed defence mechanisms (when compared to term infants) they are also more likely to be exposed to invasive procedures that increase the risk of infection.

(Askin 1995, Behrman 1992, Behrman & Vaughn 1987, Crockett 1995, Greenough 1996, Numazaki et al 1993, Philip 1994, Yancey et al 1996.)

Modes of acquiring infection

Infants may acquire infections through the placenta (transplacental infection), from the amniotic fluid, as they traverse the birth canal, or after birth from such sources as carers' hands, contaminated objects or by droplet infection. The most common routes for neonatal bacterial infection after the birth are the umbilicus, broken skin, the respiratory tract, and via invasive procedures and devices (Askin 1995).

Management of infection

The midwife's role in the management of fetal and neonatal infection includes prevention, assessment, diagnosis and treatment of infection.

Prevention of infection in the baby

Midwives have an important role to play in creating a safe environment that decreases the chances of infants acquiring infections after birth. They can do this by:

- encouraging and assisting the mother with breast feeding, thus increasing the infant's immune protection (see Ch. 36)
- ensuring careful and frequent hand washing by all carers; this simple procedure remains the single most important method of preventing the spread of infection in infants
- where possible, having the infant rooming-in with his or her mother
- adequately spacing cots when infants are in the nursery with other infants
- always using individual equipment for each infant
- avoiding any irritation or trauma to the infant's skin and mucous membranes, as intact skin provides a barrier against infection
- discouraging visitors who have infections, or who have been exposed to communicable disease, from visiting the hospital or early home environment
- isolating infected babies when absolutely essential
- observing for and appropriately treating any infection in the mother prior to the infant's birth

- ensuring the appropriate administration of immunoglobulin and antibiotics to mother or baby if required (prior to and after the birth). However, as midwives are aware the overuse of antibiotics can lead to reduced effectiveness (Askin 1995, Orlando 1995, Polak 1994, Wright Lott 1994).

Prevention of infection in the midwife

As well as decreasing infant infections, protecting midwives from infection is also vital. The underlying assumption of universal precautions is that every patient is presumed to be a potential source of blood-borne infections, for example hepatitis B, hepatitis C and acquired immune deficiency syndrome. Therefore, universal precautions must be used when dealing with any substances or articles that may be contaminated with blood. General infection control measures must also be used with respect to any other body fluids that may be a potential source of other infections.

Assessment and diagnosis

Prompt diagnosis and treatment of infection in an infant is critical in minimising adverse or long-term effects for the neonate. Early signs of infection may be more subtle than in older children and difficult to distinguish from the symptoms of other neonatal problems. Non-specific signs and symptoms can include temperature instability, lethargy, poor feeding, bradycardia or tachycardia and apnoea. The mother or the midwife may simply feel that the baby is 'off colour'. A maternal history of prolonged rupture of membranes, chorioamnionitis, pyrexia during birth, or offensive amniotic fluid increases the risk of infection for the baby (Askin 1995, Yancey et al 1996).

Laboratory evaluation will be guided by the severity and type of signs and symptoms and may include:

- a complete blood cell count
- testing of specimens of urine and meconium for specific organisms
- swabs from the nose, throat and umbilicus
- swabs from any skin rashes, pustules or vesicles to test for specific organisms

- a chest X-ray
- if central nervous system signs are present, a lumbar puncture to enable examination of cerebrospinal fluid (CSF)
- testing of cord blood, amniotic fluid and placental tissue for specific organisms (Askin 1995, Greenough 1996, Wright Lott et al 1994). The midwife is also referred to the specific references under each section.

Treatment of infection

In treating most infections, the aims are essentially the prevention of septicaemia and septic shock, and a reduction in the short- and long-term effects of the infection. The baby is nursed in a warm thermoneutral environment, with the midwife observing for any temperature instability. Maintenance of good hydration and the correction of electrolyte imbalance are vital, with demand feeding if possible and intravenous fluids as required. Systemic antibiotic or other drug therapy is always commenced as soon as possible, as is any local treatment of infection. As with jaundice (see above), monitoring of the infant's neuro-behavioural status is also important (including sleep and wake states, feeding behaviours, responsiveness, response to stress and interaction with parents and other carers).

Septic shock is a life-threatening emergency that requires the baby to be cared for by a team of experienced practitioners in a neonatal intensive care unit.

As with the jaundiced infant, the midwife has a particularly important role in providing information, support and reassurance to parents. Where possible, it is best to avoid separation of the mother and baby; if the baby requires neonatal intensive care then parents could be encouraged to spend time with their baby. Moreover, if the mother is breast feeding, she could be encouraged to continue breast feeding or expressing milk and informed of the important role of her milk in fighting infection.

(Askin 1995, Greenough 1996, Orlando 1995, Wright Lott et al 1994.) For specific treatments of different infections, the midwife is also referred to the references listed under each infection.

Infections acquired before or during birth

Toxoplasmosis

Toxoplasmosis is acquired by swallowing one of the life forms of the protozoan *Toxoplasma gondii*. This protozoan is found in uncooked meat, for example pork and lamb, and also in cat and dog faeces. An immunocompetent person who ingests the protozoan may be asymptomatic or have some malaise and lymphadenopathy. However, *Toxoplasma gondii* may be the cause of intrauterine death of the infected fetus. The mother may also request a termination of pregnancy.

In the neonate, *Toxoplasma gondii* may cause severe disease, including ocular disease and blindness, and developmental delay. If the mother is infected during pregnancy, there is a 50% chance of the fetus being affected by the protozoan. The outcome for the infant is worse if the mother has toxoplasmosis in the first half of the pregnancy. Affected infants may present with low birthweight, enlarged liver and spleen, jaundice and anaemia. 90% of infected neonates may be asymptomatic at birth, but can later develop retinal disease and neurological abnormalities, usually by the age of 20.

Diagnosis is confirmed by the presence of anti-toxoplasma antibodies (IgM) or the persistence of antitoxoplasma IgG in the infant's serum. The organism may also be isolated from cord blood, amniotic fluid and placental tissue.

Once infection has occurred there is no curative treatment. However, research by Roizen et al (1995) showed better neurological and developmental outcomes for infants who had drug treatment (pyrimethamine and sulphadiazine). To date, no randomised controlled trials have compared the outcomes for treated and untreated infants.

Prevention includes advising women about strict hand washing and washing of kitchen surfaces following contact with uncooked meats, and avoiding contact with cat and dog faeces.

(Guerina et al 1994, Holliman 1995, Joynson 1992, Lebech & Petersen 1992, Roizen et al 1995.)

Rubella

The rubella virus causes mild and insignificant illness in the mother but can have serious consequences for the fetus. If primary maternal infection occurs during pregnancy, the virus is transmitted through the placenta to the embryo or fetus. During the first 12 weeks of pregnancy, infection of the fetus occurs in almost 80% of cases, with most having symptoms. Early infections may result in spontaneous abortion. The mother may also request a termination of pregnancy where primary maternal infection occurs during the first 12 weeks of pregnancy.

Fetal infection and damage are less likely with maternal infection later in the pregnancy.

Surviving infants can have cardiac defects, hearing problems, cataracts and very significant developmental delay. Infants born with congenital rubella are highly infectious and should be isolated from other infants and pregnant women for up to 1 year after the birth. The virus can be isolated from the throat, urine and CSF. Infants should always be followed up for problems that may not become apparent until the child is older.

The incidence of rubella in developed countries was reduced following the introduction of routine immunisation programmes in the late 1960s. Although immunisation is usually administered during the first year of life, non-immunised adolescent girls should always be offered this protection (see Ch. 46).

(Miller et al 1982, Preblud & Alford 1990, Ueda et al 1979, Wright Lott et al 1993.)

Cytomegalovirus

Cytomegalovirus (CMV) is a virus of the herpes class that is harboured in leucocytes and transmitted by saliva, semen, urine, cervical secretions and blood. 27% of women giving birth in developed countries have serological evidence of a previous infection with CMV. Although this infection is common, it produces serious illness only in neonates. CMV infects 2.5% of all live neonates, and 10% of these experience serious complications.

Infection in the mother may be primary or recurrent. A primary infection in the mother during the first 20 weeks of pregnancy can result in a spontaneous abortion, intrauterine growth retardation and premature birth of the infant. Infants with CMV can suffer from an enlarged liver and spleen, jaundice, developmental delay, blindness, epilepsy and hearing loss. Most congenitally infected children are asymptomatic at birth, with only 1% showing adverse clinical disease. However, these infants should be followed up for several years because of the possibility of long-term neurological problems. At this time, no specific antiviral treatment is effective against congenital CMV infection.

A study of a set of quadruplets (Schneeberger et al 1994) demonstrated variable outcomes following primary CMV infection of the mother during pregnancy. Of the four infants, one died antenatally, one died of liver failure at 3 months, one had hearing loss and developmental delay, whilst the fourth infant was free of infection and symptoms at 18 months.

It is important for midwives to be aware that CMV can be isolated in children without clinical or laboratory evidence of infection. Infants should be isolated if the virus is present in their saliva or urine.

(Alford et al 1990, Darin et al 1994, Luban 1994, Ricci 1992, Schneeberger et al 1994.)

Herpes simplex

Infection with herpes simplex virus (HSV-2) is associated with genital herpes in the mother. Neonatal infection is more likely with a primary maternal infection during pregnancy and results in high morbidity and mortality. The infection may be acquired through the placenta or from an infected birth canal. The risk of intrapartum transmission is about 50% when the mother has primary genital herpes lesions at the time of the birth and 5% for mothers with recurrent genital herpes infections. Prolonged rupture of the membranes and the use of scalp electrodes both increase the risk of neonatal infection. Therefore, when active maternal infection is present, the baby should be delivered by caesarean section.

Signs of neonatal infection can be non-specific at birth. A herpetic rash (blisters and a papular vesicular rash) is usually, but not always, apparent by the end of the first week of life. Multiple organs may be affected, in particular the brain, liver and adrenal glands. Mortality can be as high as 80%.

Untreated survivors can have long-term neurological damage, in particular microcephaly, blind-ness and severe developmental delay. Encephalitis occurs in a high proportion of children.

The virus is present in vesicles, urine, and CSF. As with other infections, the midwife's role in assisting in the diagnosis of herpes simplex is vital. Diagnosis in the mother and a timely caesarean section may prevent neonatal infection. In addition, following early diagnosis of infected infants, antiviral drugs can be commenced.

(Tarlow 1994, Whitley 1988, Whitley et al 1988.)

Acquired immune deficiency syndrome (AIDS)

AIDS is caused by a retrovirus known as human immunodeficiency virus (HIV). Perinatal infection can occur through the placenta or through exposure to maternal blood in the vaginal secretions during birth. Postnatal transmission can occur through maternal secretions such as breast milk contaminated with maternal blood during feeding. This condition is difficult to diagnose in neonates at birth. As non-specific symptoms may appear at any time in early childhood, infants born of HIV-positive mothers must be closely followed up (Griffith & Booss 1994, Wright Lott & Kenner 1994b; see also Ch. 18).

Varicella zoster virus

In adults and children, primary infection with varicella zoster virus (VZV) causes chickenpox and recurrent infection results in shingles. The baby is mainly affected when primary maternal infection occurs during pregnancy. In the neonate, infection can cause the milder symptoms associated with neonatal varicella or neonatal zoster. Maternal chickenpox from 4 months' gestation up to almost the time of birth usually results in these milder forms of the disease.

However, at different stages of pregnancy the more serious conditions of congenital varicella syndrome (CVS) or disseminated varicella infection can also occur. With maternal chickenpox during the first 20 weeks' gestation, up to 5% of infants will develop CVS, characterised by skin lesions, chorioretinitis and limb hypoplasia. Severe neurological problems can also occur, including encephalitis, microcephaly and significant developmental delay.

24% of infants will develop disseminated infection when the mother is infected from 5 days before the birth to 2 days after. This severe infection develops within days of birth and can result in disseminated skin lesions, viral pneumonia, liver problems, and death in 30% of cases.

Midwives have an important role to play, both antenatally and postnatally, in the prevention of these conditions. Both VZV seronegative pregnant women exposed to VZV and infants with disseminated varicella infection can be given varicella zoster immune globulin (VZIGO).

(Griffith & Booss 1994, Meyers 1974, Tarlow 1994, Weller 1983.)

Chlamydia

Chlamydia infection may be acquired by the infant during birth from a mother with chlamydial cervicitis. The incidence of maternal chlamydia varies in different cultures. Infected infants may develop ophthalmia neonatorum and a small number may have pneumonia (Numazaki et al 1993, Tarlow 1994).

Hepatitis B

Although the most common source of neonatal infection with the hepatitis B virus (HBV) is maternal blood during birth, the virus can be detected in any body secretion, including breast milk. 90% of infected infants will become carriers of the virus; carriers who are at risk of developing hepatocellular carcinoma in the future. Infants of HBV-positive mothers should be given hepatitis B immunoglobulin within 12 hours of birth. This is followed by administration of hepatitis B vaccine during the first week as part of an ongoing vaccination programme. A booster dose at about 5 years of age is given if required (Hallam & Kerlin 1991, Kenner & Wright Lott 1994, Tarlow 1994).

Hepatitis C virus (HCV)

Research into modes and rates of mother-to-infant transmission of HCV is still in the early stages and the findings are not yet conclusive. The primary transmission source of HCV appears to be blood or blood products. In a recent Australian study of 1537 women who gave birth at one public hospital, 17 were HCV seropositive, a prevalence rate of 1.1% (Garner et al 1997). In this latter sample, risk factors for infection were a history of injecting drugs, a sexual partner injecting drugs, having a tattoo or having been in prison.

A higher risk of neonatal infection is reported in the presence of active liver disease in the mother. Zanetti et al (1995) found a higher risk of infant infection with HCV when the mother was also infected with HIV. As with HBV, infected infants are carriers of the virus, who are at later risk of developing hepatocellular carcinoma (Hallam & Kerlin 1991, Kenner & Wright Lott 1994, Kuroki et al 1991, Lam et al 1993, Ohto et al 1994, Zanetti et al 1995).

Syphilis

This infection, caused by the spirochaete *Treponema pallidum*, is transmitted by sexual contact or by maternofetal transmission. While syphilis is now unusual in many countries, infection rates have increased in recent years in the USA. The infant may contract the disease either through the placenta or from the birth canal. There is a 50% chance of a mother with primary or secondary syphilis infecting her fetus during pregnancy. When active lesions are present in the birth canal a caesarean birth is recommended.

Infants with congenital syphilis may be asymptomatic at birth or present with serious abnormalities. Symptoms may include a maculopapular rash, enlarged liver and spleen, jaundice, rhinitis, skin lesions, deformed nails, alopecia, chorioretinitis, iritis and a pseudoparalysis. Late congenital syphilis can also involve the central nervous system, bones, teeth and skin. (See Ch. 18.)

Intravenous or intramuscular antibiotic treatment is commenced immediately on diagnosis, with the infant isolated for the first 24 hours.

(Kenner & Wright Lott 1994, Wright Lott 1994, Wright Lott & Kenner 1994b.)

Gonococcal infections

Although gonococcal infections are now unusual in many countries, infection rates have increased in recent years in the USA. Furthermore, this organism remains an important cause of blindness in developing countries. Neonatal gonococcal infection is acquired during the birth process. It can cause a variety of symptoms including ophthalmia neonatorum, scalp abscesses, vaginitis, proctitis, oropharyngeal infections and systemic infections. These systemic infections can include pneumonia, sepsis, arthritis or rarely meningitis. About 1% of neonates with a local gonococcal infection will develop systemic infections. Diagnosis can be difficult and misdiagnosis may occur, causing enormous stress to families. Early and appropriate antibiotic treatment of both mother and infant is vital (Blanchard & Mabey 1994, Ingram 1994).

Ophthalmia neonatorum

Ophthalmia neonatorum is usually acquired by the infant during vaginal delivery. It is defined in England as any purulent discharge from the eyes of an infant within 21 days of birth, and in Scotland as any inflammation that occurs in the eyes of an infant within 21 days of birth which is accompanied by a discharge. It is notifiable.

It may be caused by a variety of organisms including *Streptococcus pneumoniae*, *Haemophilus influenzae*, *Escherichia coli*, *Klebsiella*, *Pseudomonas*, *Chlamydia trachomatis*, and *Neisseria gonorrhoeae*. The condition usually occurs within 14 days of birth, and presents as an inflammation of the conjunctiva. Oedema and erythema of the eyelids and a purulent discharge can also be present. A swab must be taken for culture and sensitivity testing, and a doctor notified immediately.

Differential diagnosis of the organism is essential, particularly with respect to chlamydial and gonococcal infections. If untreated, these organisms can cause conjunctival scarring, corneal infiltration, blindness and possible systemic spread. Gonococcal ophthalmia neonatorum usually presents as a sudden and severe purulent conjunctivitis. The organism can penetrate the cornea with rapid progression within 24 hours of infection.

When diagnosing ophthalmia neonatorum other causes of conjunctivitis must be considered, for example trauma, foreign bodies, congenital glaucoma and nasolacrimal duct obstruction. Appropriate antibiotic therapy is instituted. With gonorrhoeal

---

Box 42.2　Eye care in cases of infection

The infected eye or eyes are cleaned with sterile swabs moistened with normal saline. Each swab will be used once only, wiping from the inner canthus outwards. If the attendant's hands become contaminated with the discharge, they must be washed again before continuing. The appropriate antibiotic drops or ointment is instilled. If only one eye is affected, the baby should be laid on the side of the affected eye so that the discharge cannot run into the second eye and infect it. Eye care should be repeated at least 4-hourly but in severe cases the treatment must be intensive and may be needed every few minutes as the pus builds up very rapidly.

---

and chlamydial infection, the parent must also be treated. Local cleaning and care of the eyes with normal saline is required in conjunction with appropriate drug therapy (see Box 42.2). Mild eye infections are common in infants and can be treated with routine eye care and antibiotic therapy if required.

Some countries, for example the USA, use routine prophylaxis usually in the form of silver nitrate. However, this is not standard practice in other countries such as the UK and Australia. In countries where prophylactic agents are used, a chemical reaction may occur in the eye that may appear as conjunctivitis. In a large study of 4544 neonates Chen (1992) compared the use of prophylactic silver nitrate, tetracycline, erythromycin or no treatment. No significant difference was found in the group in the incidence of chlamydial conjunctivitis.

(Chen 1992, Datta et al 1994, Hammerschlag 1993, O'Hara 1993.)

Candida

Candida is a Gram-positive yeast fungus. *Candida albicans* is responsible for most fungal infections, including thrush in infants. Infection can affect the mouth (oral candidiasis), the skin (cutaneous candidiasis) and visceral organs (disseminated candidiasis).

Oral candidiasis or thrush presents as white patches on the gums, palate and tongue. It can also affect the skin around the mouth, perineum and anus. It can be acquired during birth or from caregivers' hands or feeding equipment. Oral nystatin is the most effective and least expensive treatment. Removing the lesions is not recommended as this leaves raw areas. Such raw areas on the edge of the tongue (removed by the infant sucking) may be a valuable aid to diagnosis. The breast-feeding mother may also require nystatin if her breasts have become infected. Maternal symptoms include burning, itching or stabbing pain throughout the breast.

Cutaneous candidiasis presents as a moist papular or vesicular rash, usually in the region of the axillae, neck, perineum or umbilicus. The area is kept as dry as possible and topical nystatin applied. Oral nystatin can also be used to reduce the yeast population.

Disseminated candidiasis is usually found only in preterm and ill newborns. Complications can include meningitis, endocarditis, pyelonephritis, pneumonia and osteomyelitis. Appropriate drug therapy is commenced, usually intravenously.

(Barone & Krilov 1995, Chen 1994, Kenner & Wright Lott 1994, Miller 1990.)

Infections acquired after birth

Skin infections

Most neonatal skin infections are caused by *Staphylococcus aureus*. In newborn infants the most likely skin lesions are septic spots or pustules which may be found either as a solitary lesion or clustered in the umbilical and buttock areas. In a well neonate with limited pustules, mild and regular cleansing with an antiseptic solution may be all that is required. More extensive pustules require appropriate antibiotic therapy (Wright Lott 1994).

Infants may also develop paronychia caused by injury of the skin surrounding the finger- or toenails. Again, bathing with an antiseptic solution may be sufficient to treat this problem.

Omphalitis

Symptoms of omphalitis or infection of the umbilicus can include localised inflammation and an offensive discharge. Treatment may include regular cleansing, the administration of an anti-

biotic powder, and appropriate antibiotic therapy. Untreated infection can spread to the liver via the umbilical vein, and cause hepatitis and septicaemia.

Eye infections

Mild eye infections are common in infants and can be treated with routine eye care (see Box 42.2) and antibiotic therapy if required. Other more serious conditions must be excluded, for example ophthalmia neonatorum (see above), trauma, foreign bodies, congenital glaucoma and nasolacrimal duct obstruction (Hammerschlag 1993, O'Hara 1993).

Respiratory infections

These may include such conditions as nasopharyngitis and rhinitis or the more severe neonatal pneumonia.

Nasopharyngitis and rhinitis. These are not severe respiratory infections, but may be distressing for both the infant and mother. Infants with nasal pharyngitis may be isolated with their mothers to prevent the spread of the infection. Both conditions require symptomatic treatment, and antibiotics may be considered appropriate.

Neonatal pneumonia. Pneumonia is the most serious of neonatal respiratory infections. It may be acquired before, during or after birth. In infants, pneumonia is life-threatening and early diagnosis is essential. Non-specific symptoms of infection may also be accompanied by nasal flaring, grunting, substernal and intercostal retraction and cyanosis. In addition to a full blood evaluation, a chest X-ray is important in diagnosing pneumonia. Appropriate antibiotic therapy must be instituted promptly (see Ch. 39).

(Dennehy 1987, Wright Lott et al 1994.)

Gastrointestinal tract infections

These can include gastroenteritis or the more severe necrotising enterocolitis.

Gastroenteritis. Causative organisms include salmonella and shigella and a pathogenic strain of *Escherichia coli*. Rotavirus is the most important cause of viral gastroenteritis in the newborn. The secretory IgA in breast milk offers the infant important protection against gastroenteritis, particularly that caused by rotavirus. Treatment depends upon the severity of symptoms. The correction of fluid and electrolyte imbalance is an urgent priority, as nausea and vomiting can rapidly cause dehydration (Tarlow 1994, Wright Lott 1994).

Necrotising enterocolitis (NEC). NEC is a leading cause of morbidity and mortality in very low birthweight infants under 1550 g. It is characterised by inflammation, ischaemia and necrosis of the gastrointestinal tract. It is the most common and most lethal surgical abdominal emergency in the newborn.

Early signs and symptoms of NEC may be those of a non-specific infection. Stage 1 symptoms can include temperature instability, lethargy, bradycardia, apnoea, decreased appetite, emesis, blood in the stool and abdominal distension. Stage 2 of the disease may be characterised by severe abdominal distension and tenderness, grossly bloodied stools, persistent bowel loops and the presence of hepatic portal venous gas. Diagnosis is confirmed by radiography showing pneumatosis intestinalis (submucosal or subserosal cysts filled with a gaseous mixture of hydrogen, methane and carbon dioxide). In the final stages, gut perforation, peritonitis, septic shock and death can occur. Persistent bowel loops for 24 hours will result in necrosis.

The pathogenesis is not certain. Early theories suggested a reduced blood flow in the gut or gut injury followed by bacterial invasion, and an immature gut. Recent research has implicated two factors: bacteria and a vulnerable host such as a premature infant. Possible risk factors include prematurity, low birthweight, enteral feeding, asphyxia, patent ductus arteriosus and bacterial infection.

Early detection and treatment is critical as non-operative treatment leads to better survival rates in neonates. Treatment depends on the stage and severity of the condition. Non-surgical treatment includes the prevention of shock, the correction of electrolyte imbalance and the administration of broad-spectrum antibiotics. If surgical treatment is needed, only necrotic tissue is resected, with the objective of preserving as much bowel as possible (including the ileocaecal valve).

Breast milk seems to offer protection from NEC. Modification of enteral feeding and oral antibiotics may also be used as a preventive measure.

(Ade-Ajayi et al 1994, Albanese & Rowe 1995, Guritzky & Rudnitsky 1996, Insoft et al 1996, Kabeer et al 1995, Militello & Lim 1995, Parker 1995, Pickler & Terrell 1994, Vasan & Gotoff 1994.)

Urinary tract infections

Urinary tract infections can result from bacterial invasion or less commonly from a congenital anomaly that obstructs urine flow. They are usually caused by Gram-negative bacteria such as *Escherichia coli* but may also be caused by Group B streptococcus and other organisms. The signs and symptoms are usually those of an early non-specific infection, and diagnosis is usually confirmed through laboratory evaluation of a urine sample (Wright Lott 1994).

Meningitis

Meningitis is inflammation of the membranes lining the brain and spinal column. The most common organisms causing neonatal meningitis are *Escherichia coli*, group B streptococci and *Listeria monocytogenes*. More unusually found are candidal meningitis and herpes meningitis. Meningitis usually happens in single cases but outbreaks have occurred.

A number of factors are thought to be associated with neonatal meningitis including neonatal sepsis, a premature birth, prolonged rupture of membranes, prolonged labour and maternal infections. Of these, a proven relationship exists only for maternal infections and pyrexia at birth.

In the early stages the infant may have non-specific signs and symptoms of generalised infection. Specific signs of meningeal irritation may also be present, including increasing irritability, raised intracranial pressure demonstrated by a bulging fontanelle, increasing lethargy, crying, tremors and twitching, severe vomiting, alterations in consciousness and diminished muscle tone. Infants may also present with hemiparesis, horizontal deviation and decreased pupillary reaction of the eye, decreased retinal reflex and an abnormal Moro reflex.

Diagnosis is usually confirmed by lumbar puncture and examination of CSF. Early diagnosis and treatment are vital if collapse and death are to be prevented. Very ill babies will require intensive nursing care, including intravenous fluids and appropriate antibiotic therapy. Blood pressure and head circumference measurements may be recorded daily. Long-term neurological complications of meningitis may occur in about 30–50% of surviving infants. These may include feeding problems and minimal brain damage.

(Adhikari et al 1995, Ali 1995, Barone & Krilov 1995, Chen 1994, de Louvois 1994, Synnott et al 1994, Wright Lott 1994.)

READER ACTIVITIES

1. Link up with the person who is responsible for monitoring neonatal infections. Ask her or him for recent records of microorganisms identified as having caused various infections in babies:

   a. in the maternity unit as a whole
   b. in the neonatal intensive care unit.

Find out to which antibiotics the organisms have been sensitive.

2. Compare the indications for phototherapy and exchange transfusion presented in this chapter with the policies of the neonatologists in your own unit.

3. Talk to one or more mothers whose babies are receiving (or have received) phototherapy. How did the mothers feel about the treatment? Were there particular features of the regimen that gave them cause for anxiety? How can the midwife help the mother overcome such anxieties?

REFERENCES

Achanna S, Monga D 1994 Outcome of forceps delivery versus vacuum extraction – a review of 200 cases. Singapore Medical Journal 35(6): 605–608

Ade-Ajayi N, Kiely E, Drake D, Wheeler R, Spitz L 1994 Resection and primary anastomosis in necrotizing enterocolitis. Journal of the Royal Society of Medicine 890: 385–388

Adhikari M, Coovadia Y M, Singh D 1995 A 4-year study of neonatal meningitis: clinical and microbiological findings. Journal of Tropical Pediatrics 41(2): 81–85

Ahlfors C E 1994 Criteria for exchange transfusion in jaundiced newborns. Pediatrics 93(3): 488–494

Albanese C T, Rowe M I 1995 Necrotizing enterocolitis. Seminars in Pediatric Surgery 4(4): 200–206

Alford C A et al 1990 Congenital and perinatal cytomegalovirus infections. Reviews of Infectious Diseases 12: 745

Ali Z 1995 Neonatal meningitis: a 3-year retrospective study at the Mount Hope Women's Hospital, Trinidad, West Indies. Journal of Tropical Pediatrics 41(2): 109–111

Alvarez J E, Bodani J, Fajardo C A, Kwiatkowki K, Cates D B, Rigatto H 1993 Sighs and their relationship to apnea in the newborn infant. Biology of the Neonate 63: 139–146

Anand N K, Gupta A K 1993 What constitutes a 'safe' level of bilirubin concentration in preterm and full term infants? Indian Journal of Pediatrics 60(4): 475–483

Arias I M, Gartner L M, Seifter S et al 1964 Prolonged neonatal unconjugated hyperbilirubinemia associated with breastfeeding and a steroid, pregnane-3 (alpha) 20 (beta) diol in maternal milk that inhibits glucuronide formation in vitro. Journal of Clinical Investigation 43: 2037

Askin D F 1995 Bacterial and fungal infections in the neonate. Journal of Obstetric, Gynecologic and Neonatal Nursing 24(7): 635–643

Barone S R, Krilov L R 1995 Neonatal candidal meningitis in a full-term infant with congenital cutaneous candidiasis. Clinical Pediatrics 34(4): 217–219

Barrios F, Jain L 1996 Current concepts in neonatal hyperbilirubinemia. Neonatal Intensive Care 9(3): 48–66

Beath S 1996 Detecting paediatric liver disease. Health Visitor 69(6): 238–239

Behrman R E 1992 Nelson: textbook of pediatrics, 2nd edn. W B Saunders, Philadelphia

Behrman R E, Vaughn V C 1987 Nelson: textbook of pediatrics, 2nd edn. W B Saunders, Philadelphia

Bellanti J, Pung Y, Zeligs B 1994 Immunology. In: Avery G B, Fletcher M A, MacDonald G (eds) Neonatology: pathophysiology and management of the newborn, 4th edn. J B Lippincott, Philadelphia

Benbow A, Wray J 1988 Recommendations for the use of anti-D immunoglobulin for RhD prophylaxis. British Journal of Midwifery 6(3): 184–186

Bersman et al 1994 Practice parameter: management of hyperbilirubinemia in the healthy term newborn. Pediatrics 94(4): 558–565

Blackburn S 1995 Hyperbilirubinemia and neonatal jaundice. Neonatal Network 14(7): 15–25

Blanchard T J, Mabey D C W 1994 Chlamydial infections. British Journal of Clinical Practice 48(4): 201–205

Bratlid D 1990 How bilirubin gets into the brain. Clinical Perinatology 17: 449–465

Brown L P 1992 Breastfeeding and jaundice: cause for concern? NAACOG's Clinical Issues 3(4): 613–619

Brown L P, Arnold L, Allison D, Klein M E, Jacobsen B 1993 Incidence and pattern of jaundice in healthy breast-fed infants during the first month of life. Nursing Research 42(2): 106–110

Caglayan S, Candemir H, Aksit S, Kansoy S, Asik S, Yaprak I 1993 Superiority of oral agar and phototherapy combination in the treatment of neonatal hyperbilirubinemia. Pediatrics 92(1): 86–89

Chen J Y 1992 Prophylaxis of ophthalmia neonatorum: comparison of silver nitrate, tetracyline, erythromycin and no prophylaxis. Pediatric Infectious Disease Journal 11(12): 1026–1030

Chen J Y 1994 Neonatal candidiasis associated with meningitis and endophthalmitis. Acta Paediatrica Japonica 36: 261–265

Costello S A, Nyikal J, Yu V Y H, McCloud P 1995 Biliblanket phototherapy system versus conventional phototherapy: a randomized controlled trial in preterm infants. Journal of Paediatric and Child Health 31(1): 11–13

Crockett M 1995 Physiology of the neonatal immune system. Journal of Obstetric, Gynaecologic and Neonatal Nursing Clinical Issues 24(7): 627–634

Darin N, Bergstrom T, Fast A, Kyllerman M 1994 Clinical, serological and PCR evidence of cytomegalovirus infection in the central nervous system in infancy and childhood. Neuropediatrics 25(6): 316–322

Datta P, Frost E, Peeling R, Masinde S, Deslandes S, Echelu C, Wamola I, Brunham R C 1994 Ophthalmia neonatorum in a trachoma endemic area. Sexually Transmitted Diseases 21(1): 1–4

deCarvalho M, Hall M, Harvey D 1981 Effects of water supplementation on physiological jaundice in breast-fed babies. Archives of Disease in Childhood 56: 568–569

deCarvalho M, Klaus M, Merkatz R 1982 Frequency of breastfeeding and serum bilirubin concentration. American Journal of Diseases in Children 136: 737–738

de Louvois J 1994 Acute bacterial meningitis in the newborn. Journal of Antimicrobial Chemotherapy 34: 61–73

Demirkol M, Bohles H 1994 Breast milk taurine and its possible influence on the development of breast milk induced jaundice of the neonate – a hypothesis. Advances in Experimental Medicine and Biology 359: 405–410

Dennehy P H 1987 Respiratory infections in the newborn. Clinics in Perinatology 14(3): 667–683

Dennery P A, McDonagh A F, Stevenson D K 1992 In vivo role of bilirubin in neonatal antioxidant defenses. Pediatric Research 31: A200 (Abstract)

Dennery P A, Rhine W D, Stevenson D K 1995 Neonatal jaundice – what now? Clinical Pediatrics 34(2): 103–107

Dodd K L 1993 Neonatal jaundice – a lighter touch. Archives of Disease in Childhood 68(5): 529–533

El-Nawawy A, Soliman A T, El Azzouni O et al 1996 Maternal and neonatal prevalence of toxoplasma and cytomegalovirus (CMV) antibodies and hepatitis-B antigens in an Egyptian rural area. Journal of Tropical Pediatrics 42(3): 154–157

Fok T F, Wong W, Cheng A F B 1995 Use of eyepatches in phototherapy: effects on conjunctival bacterial pathogens and conjunctivitis. Pediatric Infectious Disease Journal 14(12): 1091–1094

Garner J, Gaughwin M, Willson K 1997 Prevalence of hepatitis C infection in a group of pregnant women in South Australia. Medical Journal of Australia 166: 470–472

Gartner L M 1994a On the question of the relationship between breastfeeding and jaundice in the first 5 days of life. Seminars in Perinatology 18(6): 502–509

Gartner L M 1994b Neonatal jaundice. Pediatrics in Review 15(11): 422–432

Gartner L M, Lee K S 1993 Jaundice in the breast-fed infant: new concepts of pathogenesis. In: Freier S, Eidelman A (eds) Human milk: its biological and social values. Excerpta Medica, Amsterdam, p 153

Greenough A 1996 Neonatal infections. Current Opinions in Pediatrics 8(1): 6–10

Griffith B P, Booss J 1994 Neurologic infections of the fetus and newborn. Neurologic Clinics 12(3): 541–564

Guerina N G et al 1994 Neonatal serologic screening and early treatment for congenital *Toxoplasma gondii* infection. New England Journal of Medicine 330(26): 1858–1863

Guritzky R P, Rudnitsky G 1996 Bloody neonatal diaper. Annals of Emergency Medicine 27(5): 662–664

Gustafson P A, Boyle D W 1995 Bilirubin index: a new standard for intervention? Medical Hypotheses 45(5): 409–416

Hallam A, Kerlin P 1991 Viral hepatitis A to E: an update. Australian Family Physician 20(6): 760–770

Hammerschlag M R 1993 Neonatal conjunctivitis. Pediatric Annals 22(6): 346–351

Hensleigh P A 1994 Undocumented history of maternal genital herpes followed by neonatal herpes meningitis. Journal of Perinatology 14(3): 216–218

Hicks B A, Altman R P 1993 The jaundiced newborn. Pediatric Surgery 40(6): 1161–1175

Holland R M, Lilly J R 1992 Surgical jaundice in infants other than biliary atresia. Seminars in Pediatric Surgery 1: 125–129

Holliman R E 1995 Congenital toxoplasmosis: prevention, screening and treatment. Journal of Hospital Infection 30: 179–190

Ingram D 1994 *Neisseria gonorrhoeae* in children. Pediatric Annals 23(7): 341–345

Insoft R M, Sanderson I R, Walker W A 1996 Development of immune function in the intestine and its role in neonatal diseases. Pediatric Gastroenterology II 43(2): 551–571

James M J, Williams S D 1993 Discontinuation of breast-feeding infrequent among jaundiced neonates treated at home. Pediatrics 92(1): 153–155

Joynson D H 1992 Epidemiology of toxoplasmosis in the UK. Scandinavian Journal of Infectious Diseases 84: 65–69

Kabeer A, Gunnlaugsson S, Coren C 1995 Neonatal necrotizing enterocolitis. Diseases of the Colon and Rectum 38(8): 866–872

Kang J H, Shankaran S 1995 Double phototherapy with high irradiance compared with single phototherapy in neonates with hyperbilirubinemia. American Journal of Perinatology 12(3): 178–180

Kenner C, Wright Lott J 1994 Types of microorganisms. In: Wright Lott J (ed) 1994 Neonatal infection: assessment, diagnosis and management. Nicu Ink, California

Kivlahan C, James E J P 1984 The natural history of neonatal jaundice. Pediatrics 74: 364

Kliegman R M, Walsh M C 1987 Neonatal necrotizing enterocolitis: pathogenesis, classification, and spectrum of illness. Current Problems in Pediatrics 17(4): 213–288

Knudsen A 1994 Prediction, measurement and clinical significance of yellow skin colour in mature healthy neonates. Danish Medical Bulletin 41(4): 386–397

Kuhr M, Paneth N 1982 Feeding practices and early neonatal jaundice. Journal of Pediatric Gastroenterology and Nutrition 1: 485–488

Kuroki T et al 1991 Mother-to-child transmission of hepatitis C virus. Journal of Infectious Diseases 164: 427–428

Lam J P H et al 1993 Infrequent vertical transmission of hepatitis C virus. Journal of Infectious Diseases 167: 572–576

Lasker M R, Holzman I R 1996 Neonatal jaundice. Postgraduate Medicine 99(3): 187–198

Lazar L, Litwin A, Merlob P 1993 Phototherapy for neonatal nonhemolytic hyperbilirubinemia: analysis of rebound and indications for discontinuing therapy. Clinical Pediatrics 32(5): 264–267

Lebech M, Petersen E 1992 Neonatal screening for congenital toxoplasmosis in Denmark: presentation of the design of a prospective study. Scandinavian Journal of Infectious Diseases 84: 75–79

Levy J 1994 Newborn jaundice. Parents Magazine 69(7): 59–60

Luban N L C 1994 Review of neonatal red cell transfusion practices. Blood Reviews 8(3): 148–153

McFadden E A 1991 The Wallaby phototherapy system; a new approach to phototherapy. Journal of Pediatric Nursing 6(3): 206–208

Maisels M J 1994 Jaundice. In: Avery G B, Fletcher M A, MacDonald M G (eds) Neonatology: pathophysiology and management of the newborn, 4th edn. Lippincott, Philadelphia

Maisels M J 1995 Clinical rounds in the well-baby nursery: treating jaundiced newborns. Pediatric Annals 24(10): 547–552

Maisels M J, Vain N, Acquavita A M, de Blanco N V, Cohen A, DiGregorio J 1994 The effect of breast-feeding frequency on serum bilirubin levels. American Journal of Obstetrics and Gynecology 170(3): 880–883

Malpas T 1993 Neonatal jaundice. New Zealand Practice Nurse (Nov): 72

Mathew R 1995 Nursing care of infants on phototherapy. Nursing Journal of India 86(9): 197–198

Meyers J D 1974 Congenital varicella in term infants: risk considered. Journal of Infectious Diseases 129: 215

Militello L, Lim L 1995 Patient assessment skills: assessing early cues of necrotizing enterocolitis. Journal of Perinatal and Neonatal Nursing 9(2): 42–52

Miller E, Cradock-Watson J E, Pollock T M 1982 Consequences of confirmed maternal rubella at successive stages of pregnancy. Lancet 2: 781

Miller M J 1990 Fungal infections. In: Remington J S, Klein J O Infectious diseases of the fetus and newborn infant. Saunders, Philadelphia

Newman T B, Maisels M J 1992 Evaluation and treatment of jaundice in the term newborn: a kinder, gentler approach. Pediatrics 89(5): 809–817

Nicoll A, Ginsburg R, Tripp J H 1982 Supplementary feeding and jaundice in the newborns. Acta Paediatrica Scandinavica 71: 759–761

Numazaki K, Chiba S, Niida Y, Komatsu M, Hashimoto N 1993 Evaluation of diagnostic assays for neonatal and infantile chlamydial infections. Tohoku Journal of Experimental Medicine 170: 123–129

O'Hara M A 1993 Ophthalmia neonatorum. Pediatric Ophthalmology 40(4): 715–725

Ohto H et al 1994 Transmission of hepatitis C virus from mothers to infants. New England Journal of Medicine 330: 744–750

Orlando S 1995 The immunologic significance of breast milk. Journal of Obstetric, Gynaecologic and Neonatal Nursing 24(7): 678–683

Oski F A, Naiman J L 1972 Hematologic problems in the newborn, 2nd edn. W B Saunders, Philadelphia

Parker L A 1995 Necrotizing enterocolitis. Neonatal Network 14(6): 17–27

Peterec S 1995 Management of neonatal Rh disease. Clinical Perinatology 22(3): 561–592

Philip A G S 1994 The changing face of neonatal infection: experience at a regional medical center. Pediatric Infectious Disease Journal 13(12): 1098–1102

Pickler R H, Terrell B V 1994 Nonnutritive sucking and necrotizing enterocolitis. Neonatal Network 13(8): 15–17

Polak J D 1994 Prevention of infection. In: Wright Lott J (ed) Neonatal infection: assessment, diagnosis and management. Nicu Ink, California

Poland R L 1993 Eye prophylaxis in the newborn infant. Pediatrics in Review 14(11): 423

Poland R L, Ostrea E M 1993 Neonatal hyperbilirubinemia. In: Klaus M H, Fanaroff A (eds) Care of the high risk neonate. W B Saunders, Philadelphia

Preblud S R, Alford C A 1990 Rubella. In: Klein J S, Remington J O (eds) Infectious diseases of the fetus and newborn infant, 3rd edn. W B Saunders, Philadelphia

Preutthipan A, Siripoonya P, Ruangkanchanasetr S 1993 Serum bilirubin levels in breast-fed vs formula-fed infants during the first 3–5 days of life. Journal of the Medical Association of Thailand 76(4): 217–221

Ricci J M 1992 AIDS and infectious diseases in pregnancy. In: Hacker N F, Moore I G (eds) Essentials of obstetrics and gynecology, 2nd edn. Saunders, Philadelphia

Roberton N R C 1993 A manual of neonatal intensive care, 3rd edn. Edward Arnold, London

Roizen N et al 1995 Neurologic and developmental outcome in treated congenital toxoplasmosis. Pediatrics 95(1): 11–20

Romagnoli C G, Polidori L, Cataldi G, Tortorlo S G 1979 Phototherapy induced hypocalcemia. Journal of Pediatrics 46: 813–816

Rubaltelli F 1993 Unconjugated and conjugated bilirubin pigments during perinatal development. Biology of the Neonate 64: 104–109

Rubaltelli F F, Griffith P F 1992 Management of neonatal hyperbilirubinaemia and prevention of kernicterus. Practical Therapeutics 43(6): 864–872

Salariya E M 1993 Breast versus bottle feeding. Nutrition and Health 9(1): 33–36

Salariya E M, Robertson C M 1993 Relationships between baby feeding types and patterns, gut transit time of meconium and the incidence of neonatal jaundice. Midwifery 9(4): 235–242

Sater K J 1995 Color me yellow: caring for the infant with hyperbilirubinemia. Journal of Intravenous Nursing 18(6): 317–325

Schneeberger P M, Groenendaal F, de Vries L S, van Loon A M, Vroom T M 1994 Variable outcome of a congenital cytomegalovirus infection in a quadruplet after primary infection of the mother during pregnancy. Acta Paediatrica 83: 986–989

Schneider V 1993 The differential diagnosis of neonatal jaundice. Journal of the American Academy of Physician Assistants 6(8): 533–541

Seidman D S, Stevenson D K, Ergaz Z, Gale R 1995 Hospital readmission due to neonatal hyperbilirubinemia. Pediatrics 96(4): 727–729

Sethi H, Saili A, Dutta A K 1993 Phototherapy induced hypocalcemia. Indian Pediatrics 30(12): 1403–1406

Stephenson K 1996 Neonatal jaundice. Physician Assistant 20(4): 19–38

Stocker R, Yamamoto Y, McDonagh A F et al 1987 Bilirubin is an antioxidant of possible physiological importance. Science 235: 1043–1046

Stocker R, McDonagh A F, Glazer A N, Ames B N 1990 Antioxidant activities of bile pigments: biliverdin and bilirubin. Methods in Enzymology 186: 301–309

Synnott M B, Morse D L, Hall S M 1994 Neonatal meningitis in England and Wales: a review of routine national data. Archives of Disease in Childhood 71(2): 75–80

Taeusch H W, Ballard R A, Avery M E 1991 Schaffer and Avery's diseases of the newborn, 6th edn. Harcourt Brace, Philadelphia

Tan K L 1994 Comparison of the efficacy of fibreoptic and conventional phototherapy for neonatal hyperbilirubinemia. Journal of Pediatrics 125(4): 607–612

Tan K L 1996 Phototherapy for neonatal jaundice. Acta Paediatrica 85(3): 277–279

Tanphaichitr V S, Pung-amritt P, Yodthong S, Soongswang J, Mahasandana C, Suvatte V 1995 Glucose-6-phosphate dehydrogenase deficiency in the newborn: its prevalence and relation to neonatal jaundice. The Southeast Asian Journal of Tropical Medicine and Public Health 26 (suppl 1): 137–141

Tarlow M J 1994 Epidemiology of neonatal infections. Journal of Antimicrobial Chemotherapy 34 SA: 43–52

Todd N A 1995 Isovolemic exchange transfusion of the neonate. Neonatal Network 14(6): 75–77

Torres-Torres M, Tayaba R, Weintraub A, Holzman I 1994 New perspectives on neonatal hyperbilirubinemia. Mount Sinai Journal of Medicine 61: 424–428

Ueda K, Nishida Y, Oshima K et al 1979 Congenital rubella syndrome: correlation of gestational age at time of maternal rubella with type of defect. Journal of Pediatrics 94: 763

Vasan U, Gotoff SP 1994 Prevention of neonatal necrotizing enterocolitis. Clinics in Perinatology 21(2): 425–435

Weller T H 1983 Varicella and herpes zoster: changing concepts of the natural history, control and importance of a not-so-benign virus. New England Journal of Medicine 309: 1362

Whitley R J 1988 Natural history and pathogenesis of neonatal herpes simplex virus infection. Annals of the New York Academy of Science 549: 1103

Whitley R J, Corey L, Arvin A et al 1988 Changing presentation of herpes simplex virus infection in neonates. Journal of Infectious Diseases 158: 109

Wright Lott J (ed) 1994 Neonatal infection: assessment, diagnosis and management. Nicu Ink, California

Wright Lott J, Kenner C 1994a Overview of infection. In: Wright Lott J (ed) 1994 Neonatal infection: assessment, diagnosis and management. Nicu Ink, California

Wright Lott J, Kenner C 1994b Keeping up with neonatal infection: designer bugs, part II. American Journal of Maternal/Child Nursing 19(5): 264–271

Wright Lott J et al 1993 Assessment and management of immunologic dysfunction. In: Kenner C A, Brueggemeyer A, Gunderson L P (eds) Comprehensive neonatal nursing, A physiologic perspective. W B Saunders, Philadelphia, pp 553–581

Wright Lott J, Kenner C Polak J D 1994 Common neonatal infections and complications. In: Wright Lott J (ed) 1994 Neonatal infection: assessment, diagnosis and management. Nicu Ink, California

Yancey M K, Duff P, Kubilis P, Clark P, Frentzen B H 1996 Risk factors for neonatal sepsis. Obstetrics and Gynecology 87(2): 188–194

Yokochi K 1995 Magnetic resonance imaging in children with kernicterus. Acta Paediatrica 84(8): 937–939

Zanetti A R et al 1995 Mother-to-infant transmission of hepatitis C. Lancet 345(8945): 289–291

Metabolic and endocrine disorders and drug withdrawal

Alison Livingston

Metabolic and endocrine disorders in the neonate and the effects of maternal drug and substance abuse all have the potential to cause brain damage, poor growth and development, or even death, unless treatment is initiated promptly. The midwife has an essential role in early recognition of, and screening for, these problems, both antenatally and in the neonatal period.

The chapter aims to:

- review the most common disorders of metabolic and endocrine function

- outline the screening methods available for the early detection of disorders

- describe the effects on the neonate of maternal drug and substance abuse

- consider the management of babies of drug-addicted mothers.

INBORN ERRORS OF METABOLISM

Achievement of metabolic control is part of the neonate's successful transition to extrauterine life. Transient disorders of glucose and electrolyte balance are common in preterm and stressed neonates. Permanent disorders, such as those caused by inborn errors of metabolism (IEM), may also present in the neonatal period. Over 500 known errors of metabolism have been identified. Each condition is rare but as a group IEM contribute significantly to neonatal mortality and morbidity.

Common features of IEM

Most IEM are autosomal recessive inherited conditions. Certain conditions are more common in different populations. In IEM, normal metabolism is disrupted by the absence or deficiency of an enzyme. Metabolites can then accumulate which are toxic to body tissues, including the brain. The fetus is usually not affected as the placenta removes toxins. It is mostly after birth that the neonate will start to show signs of IEM. Many of these signs can be non-specific and could be attributed to other neonatal problems such as sepsis. The signs may become apparent within hours, days or weeks.

Possible indicators of IEM

- History of previous unexplained neonatal death in the family, or parental consanguinity
- Failure of a sick neonate to respond to usual management
- History of a period of apparent health after birth, followed by adverse signs after the introduction of milk feeding
- Severe metabolic acidosis
- Neurological signs: irritability, lethargy, poor feeding, floppy or increased muscle tone, fits
- Respiratory signs: apnoea or respiratory distress secondary to neurological depression and/or severe metabolic acidosis
- Gastrointestinal signs: vomiting, diarrhoea, failure to thrive
- Unusual odour from the baby's skin or urine, discoloration of urine, abnormally coloured or offensive stool
- Prolonged or early jaundice.

Diagnosis of IEM

Antenatal diagnosis for many conditions can be carried out by DNA analysis of fetal cells obtained at amniocentesis or chorionic villus biopsy. After birth mass screening procedures have been developed to detect the commoner conditions. Screening ensures early diagnosis and the prompt initiation of treatment. One of the commonest screening methods is the Guthrie test in which blood dropped onto absorbent filter paper is examined using microbiological techniques. Antibiotics may interfere with the microbiological methods used in this test. If a baby is on antibiotic therapy, or he is breast feeding and his mother is taking antibiotics, the screening laboratory should be notified by including this information in the comments section of the Guthrie test card. The Scriver test involves the chromatographic examination of blood. Conditions screened for will vary throughout the world. In Britain, all newborn babies are screened for phenylketonuria and hypothyroidism.

Common investigations for IEM involve general tests such as blood glucose, blood gases, examination of the urine for reducing substances and ketones, metabolic screening of the blood and urine and enzyme analysis of the blood and urine.

Phenylketonuria (PKU)

This is an autosomal recessive condition with an incidence of about 1 in 10 000 (Roberton 1993) but there is geographical variation. It is due to a deficiency of the enzyme phenylalanine hydroxylase, which converts phenylalanine (an amino acid) to tyrosine in the liver. Because of the failure of conversion, phenylalanine levels rise and although some will be excreted in the urine, most will be converted to phenylpyruvic acid. The raised level of phenylalanine in the blood is found within a few days of birth, after the baby has been subjected to dietary protein. The build-up of phenylpyruvic acid (toxic to the developing brain) takes longer and without treatment mental retardation results.

Clinical features

At birth the baby looks and behaves normally. Signs usually appear after 3 months. These include vomiting, feeding difficulties, eczema, fair skin and hair, blue eyes, and 'musty' smelling urine due to phenylacetic acid.

Diagnosis

Detection is by the routine collection of capillary blood from milk-fed babies between the sixth and eighth postnatal day for either the Guthrie or the Scriver test. A positive screening test is followed up by further assessment of phenylalanine levels to ensure that it is due to genuine PKU and not to some other cause of an elevated serum phenylalanine (Roberton 1993).

Management

A low phenylalanine diet is prescribed. Milk substitutes, such as Lofenalac and Minafen, are available and will be used in conjunction with iron and vitamin supplements. In older children a phenylalanine-free milk, XP Analog, can be used. After puberty the child will graduate to a normal diet but follow-up care is important.

Prognosis

Prognosis is good if parents adhere to the instructions given. In females, a return to the low phenylalanine diet is essential prior to conception and during pregnancy. Fetal damage may be caused by exposure to high concentrations of phenylalanine and its metabolites in the mother.

Galactosaemia

Galactosaemia is the most common disorder of carbohydrate metabolism to appear in the neonatal period. Its incidence is 1 in 60 000–70 000 (Roberton 1993). It is an autosomal recessive condition and can be screened for antenatally and also in the newborn period. The enzyme which aids the conversion of galactose to glucose is absent. Galactose and glucose are the component sugars present in the disaccharide lactose. Signs include vomiting, diarrhoea, failure to gain weight, jaundice, lethargy and hypotonia. An affected baby may also present with septicaemia secondary to damage to intestinal mucosa by high levels of galactose in the gut. In galactosaemia, a Clinitest tablet urine test (detecting all reducing substances, namely sugars) will be positive and a 'dip-stick' urine test (specific to glucose) will be negative. The diagnosis is confirmed by urine and blood enzyme assay. Affected babies need to be fed a lactose-free milk, such as Galactomin.

Other inborn errors of metabolism

Glucose-6-phosphate dehydrogenase (G6PD) deficiency

G6PD deficiency is an inherited disorder of red blood cell metabolism. Haemolysis occurs, resulting in jaundice and anaemia in the neonate. It is especially prevalent in Asian, Middle Eastern and Mediterranean populations. Management is to treat jaundice, which may be severe, to correct anaemia and reduce the baby's exposure to

oxidants which can damage fragile red blood cells. Sometimes vitamin E is prescribed for its antioxidant properties.

Cystic fibrosis

This is an autosomal recessive condition which causes dysfunction of secretory glands. Mucus secretions are thick and may block glands and ducts. The incidence varies in different populations. It is more common in northern European groups and the incidence in the UK is 1 in 2000 (Roberton 1993). It may present in the neonatal period as meconium ileus. The midwife needs to be vigilant in observing for the delayed passage of meconium. Other signs are failure to thrive, prolonged jaundice, bulky pale stools and early respiratory tract infection. Both antenatal and neonatal screening tests are available. Some areas in the UK screen all newborns for cystic fibrosis by measuring serum immunoreactive trypsin in a drop of blood collected on filter paper as for the Guthrie test. Treatment is aimed at preventing complications and optimising growth and development. After diagnosis, parents will need to be referred for genetic counselling and antenatal screening will be possible for future pregnancies.

ENDOCRINE DISORDERS

As a group endocrine disorders are rare. They are usually treatable, and if untreated can lead to significant morbidity. The most common disorders involve the thyroid gland, adrenal cortex and developing sexual organs.

Thyroid problems

Congenital hypothyroidism

The incidence is approximately 1 in 3500 (Roberton 1993). There is often a strong family history of hypothyroidism. Some rare forms of hypothyroidism are autosomal recessive conditions. Hypothyroidism in the neonate can also be caused by the mother taking antithyroid drugs, or by maternal treatment with radioactive iodides in pregnancy. Low circulating levels of thyroid hormone cause impaired intellectual and motor function.

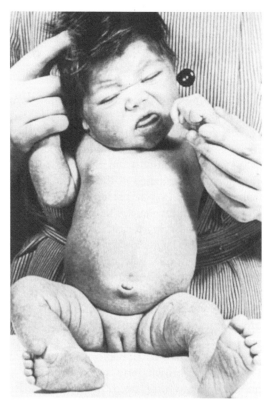

Fig. 43.1 Severe hypothyroidism in 6-week-old baby (reproduced from Forfar & Arneil 1984).

Presentation. There are different degrees of hypothyroidism, depending on the amount of thyroid hormone being produced. Severe hypothyroidism shows a typical appearance of coarse facial expression with a low hairline (Fig. 43.1). The forehead is wrinkled and the nasal bridge flat. The neck is short and thick and may disguise a goitre. Presenting signs include prolonged jaundice, constipation, lethargy, poor feeding and hypothermia.

Diagnosis and treatment. Routine neonatal hypothyroidism screening is well established in many parts of the world, carried out at the same time as the PKU screening. This means that the diagnosis is often established before the baby shows signs and symptoms. A positive screening test will be followed up by thyroid hormone and thyroid-stimulating hormone blood assays, before starting treatment with thyroxine replacement.

Prognosis. Prognosis is good if treatment is in-

stituted quickly, but infants with complete absence of thyroid tissue will have a less favourable outcome. Genetic counselling should be offered to parents. Antenatal detection at present is not possible.

Neonatal thyrotoxicosis

This is a rare complication found in babies delivered to mothers who have hyperthyroidism. The neonate may present with signs of thyrotoxicosis, tachycardia, jittery movements, sweating, vomiting, diarrhoea, poor weight gain and a goitre. There will be high levels of thyroid-stimulating hormone present on blood assay. Treatment is with antithyroid drugs. Once the maternal influence of thyroid-stimulating IgG immunoglobulins has disappeared from the neonate's circulation after 2–3 months, antithyroid drugs can be discontinued (Roberton 1993). The midwife needs to be aware of the importance of noting any maternal thyroid problems when taking an antenatal history.

Congenital adrenal hyperplasia

Adrenal hyperplasia is a rare autosomal recessive condition in which excessive growth of the adrenal cortex occurs. Androgenic hormone production is high and associated adrenal insufficiency can develop with excessive salt and water loss. This can result in dehydration and eventually peripheral vascular collapse in the neonatal period. Abnormal genitalia with a prominent clitoris may be present in the female at birth. Diagnosis is confirmed by biochemical investigation. Correction of fluid and electrolyte balance is the first priority. Once the initial crisis is over, cortisone may be given to suppress the androgenic hormones. Prognosis is poor if untreated, but if corrected, these children will survive on a maintenance dose of cortisone and additional salt to the diet.

ACQUIRED METABOLIC DISORDERS

Hypoglycaemia

This is the commonest acquired metabolic disorder. It is of particular importance to the midwife's management of the neonate, as if it is prolonged or recurrent, it can result in mental retardation and permanent neurological damage (Aynsley-Green & Soltesz 1992).

There is not a universally agreed definition of hypoglycaemia. Most would define it empirically as a blood plasma glucose of less than 2.6 mmol/l (Brown et al 1997).

The fetus stores glucose as glycogen in the liver and muscle and as subcutaneous and body fat, and this occurs largely in the third trimester. After birth, the baby must make metabolic adjustments to maintain a normal blood sugar. The newborn baby's blood glucose is about 80% of the maternal value, falling to its lowest level at 1–3 hours of age. To meet the baby's need for energy in this period, hepatic glycogen is released. Also, hormonal changes following delivery allow the neonate to use ketones and lactate for brain metabolism on the first day of life (Hawdon et al 1992). After the first few hours the neonate is then able to use fatty acids as an alternative energy source.

Normal term babies who have not been stressed have adequate stores of glycogen to be able to meet their energy requirements, provided that they are kept warm and are able to feed.

Infants at risk are:

- hypoxic infants – carbohydrate metabolism is disrupted by lack of oxygen and excessive metabolism of glycogen occurs
- low birthweight infants, especially small for gestational age and preterm babies whose glycogen levels are low
- babies of diabetic mothers who have been subjected in utero to high sugar concentrations from their mothers – insulin production is high and takes some time after birth to return to normal
- hypothermic infants – metabolism is upset because glucose is consumed in order to produce energy for heat production
- sick babies who may have low blood glucose levels
- those with more unusual problems including Rhesus haemolytic disease when the islets of Langerhans in the pancreas are overstimulated to produce insulin, pancreatic tumours, Beckwith–Wiedemann syndrome and inborn errors of metabolism.

Clinical signs of hypoglycaemia

Many infants are asymptomatic, particularly the preterm. Common signs described are:

- tremors and jittery movements
- hypotonia
- lethargy
- poor feeding.

Serious signs due to neuroglycopenia are apnoea and convulsions.

Management of hypoglycaemia

It is of paramount importance for the midwife to recognise the baby who is at risk. Effective management of the baby's feeding and temperature control will help to prevent hypoglycaemia. Blood glucose screening using whole blood obtained by capillary heel stab can be carried out at the bedside. Methods available use enzymatic reagent strips or a reflectance meter. These techniques are limited and may give inaccurate results. The use of whole blood as opposed to plasma may result in underestimation of true blood glucose levels and this is exacerbated by polycythaemic conditions. A cold heel may yield an insufficient sample or the electronic meter may be poorly calibrated. If the estimation of blood glucose in a capillary sample is low, an accurate estimation must be obtained by laboratory analysis of the plasma.

Management of low blood glucose depends on the condition of the baby. Specific guidelines for managing hypoglycaemia will vary in different centres. Generally, if the baby is asymptomatic and otherwise well, hypoglycaemia can be managed by ensuring that the baby receives adequate feeds (by breast if sufficiently alert or by cup and spoon or nasogastric tube if uninterested in sucking). Also, it is important that the baby is kept warm to minimise energy expenditure. In the sick baby, or when oral feeding is not possible, an intravenous infusion of dextrose 10% will be administered until blood glucose levels are stable.

Prognosis

The prognosis is good unless the hypoglycaemia has been severe or has been prolonged over days. One multicentre study of 661 preterm infants suffering moderate hypoglycaemia, with a plasma glucose of less than 2.6 mmol/l on 5 or more separate days, showed a 3.5% increase in the incidence of neurodevelopmental delay (Lucas et al 1988).

Hyperglycaemia

Hyperglycaemia, blood glucose levels greater than 8 mmol/l (Fleming et al 1986), is found most commonly in the preterm infant. It is thought to be a result of the immature infant's inability to handle glucose. It can also occur as a response to infection, dehydration, intravenous glucose, stress, steroids used to treat bronchopulmonary dysplasia, and some surgical procedures (Pildes & Pyati 1986).

Treatment is to reduce the concentration of administered dextrose infusions and give a continuous insulin infusion if necessary. Neonatal diabetes mellitus is rarely seen. The cause is thought to be immaturity of the pancreatic islets with a resultant insulin deficiency. Treatment is with insulin and continues until the condition resolves when the pancreas matures (Roberton 1993).

Electrolyte imbalance

Electrolyte levels will become imbalanced in the neonate when there is not normal hydration. The midwife needs to be aware of the factors that can cause fluid and electrolyte imbalance. Among these are:

- fluid loss through the skin which is increased under radiant heaters and phototherapy
- dehydration from poor feeding.

Sick and preterm infants are most at risk of fluid and electrolyte imbalance.

Hypernatraemia

Hypernatraemia is the condition in which the serum sodium level is greater than 145 mmol/l (Roberton 1993). It may be due to an excessive intake of sodium from incorrectly made up feeds or be a consequence of intravenous therapy and the administration of sodium bicarbonate. Another cause is excessive water loss, which can occur from increased insensible water loss. The baby is usually dehydrated and may present with signs of

cerebral irritation, which if untreated can lead to intraventricular haemorrhage.

Management is to restore fluid and electrolyte balance and treat the underlying cause. It is important that the midwife ensures that a baby under phototherapy receives sufficient fluid to prevent dehydration. Also, it is the midwife's role to ensure that parents are educated to follow the manufacturer's instructions for the reconstitution of artificial milk feeds and are able to cope with the task. Incorrectly made up formula can result in a feed that is too high in sodium.

Hyponatraemia

Hyponatraemia occurs when the serum sodium is less than 130 mmol/l (Roberton 1993). It is the result of water retention or excessive salt loss. Preterm babies are more at risk because of the immaturity of their kidneys, which allow a high salt loss in the urine. The baby may be asymptomatic or present with signs of oedema. If the sodium loss is acute, the baby may present with convulsions.

Management is to replace sodium either orally or intravenously, and correct fluid imbalance.

Hypocalcaemia

This is a condition in which the serum calcium is less than 1.8 mmol/l (Roberton 1993). It occurs most commonly in low birthweight babies, infants of diabetic mothers, babies who have required exchange transfusion or in very sick babies. Other rare causes are lack of maternal and fetal vitamin D (which is most common in ethnic groups more at risk of rickets), infants fed on high-phosphate milks (more common in the past when infants were fed on unmodified cow's milk), renal failure and hypoparathyroidism in the infant.

Signs of hypocalcaemia are irritability, rapid jerky limb movements or even convulsions.

Management is to supplement the baby with either oral or intravenous calcium.

Hypercalcaemia

Neonatal hypercalcaemia, a serum calcium of over 2.8 mmol/l (Roberton 1993), is rare in the newborn. High calcium levels can lead to renal damage and pathological changes in the heart. It may be the result of overtreatment with a calcium infusion or occur when there is insufficient phosphate in the baby's diet. It can also occur when the infant has abnormal vitamin D metabolism. Treatment will depend upon the underlying cause.

Hypomagnesaemia

Hypomagnesaemia is a serum magnesium level of less than 0.7 mmol/l (Roberton 1993). It can occur in the presence of hypocalcaemia. Also, newborn babies who vomit or have diarrhoea may deplete magnesium stores. Treatment is with intramuscular or intravenous magnesium sulphate.

DRUG OR SUBSTANCE WITHDRAWAL

Effects on the baby

A wide range of drugs and substances that have been prescribed or abused in pregnancy have been reported to cause neonatal withdrawal symptoms. Among these are narcotics, alcohol, amphetamines, barbiturates, codeine, benzodiazepines, pentazocine, cocaine, lithium, and tricyclic antidepressants. The drugs and substances that are abused in pregnancy vary according to current trends, availability and geographical location. Multiple drugs and substances may be involved with varying effects on the fetus and baby after birth. Drug and substance abuse is associated with increased fetal and neonatal deaths, prematurity and intrauterine growth restriction. There is an increased risk of sudden infant death syndrome (SIDS). According to Ellwood and others (1987) the risk of SIDS is increased fivefold by maternal narcotic addiction. Pregnant misusers often have chaotic lifestyles with accompanying social, economic and housing problems. This group of women are also more at risk of sexually transmitted diseases such as chlamydia, gonorrhoea, HIV and hepatitis B infection. All of these factors place the mother and baby in this group at risk and this should be taken into account by the midwife and care planned accordingly.

Neonatal abstinence syndrome (NAS)

Many of the clinical features of a baby undergoing drug or substance withdrawal, or what is otherwise known as NAS, are non-specific. The signs that should be observed for by the midwife are:

- tremor
- high-pitched cry
- irritability
- hyperactivity
- hypertonicity
- sweating
- pyrexia
- sneezing
- vomiting
- disorganised suck
- diarrhoea
- convulsions
- respiratory distress.

In opiate misuse, the symptoms of NAS will generally appear within the first 24–48 hours of life but have been reported up to 6 days after birth (Perlmutter 1974). Methadone and barbiturate abstinence signs may not appear for 2 weeks and may go on for a period of several weeks or months.

One of the most important aspects of caring for a baby undergoing withdrawal is the provision of a quiet environment, reducing light and noise stimulus to a minimum. The baby may need to be swaddled, to make him feel secure, and be given small frequent feeds for comfort and adequate nutrition. Convulsions can be controlled with phenobarbitone. If oral feeding is not tolerated, intravenous fluid therapy will be started.

In some centres a scoring system is used for assessment of the presenting withdrawal signs. Drug therapy to control the presenting signs may then be started if the score presents above a fixed figure. There is disagreement about the value of scoring systems, as they are dependent upon the judgement of the observer but they do provide a tool for ongoing assessment of the baby with NAS.

Treatment

The trends for treating NAS will vary in different countries and are also dependent upon the drug of misuse and the severity of presenting signs. Narcotics may be used, giving 0.05 mg/kg of morphine every 3–4 hours or paregoric (4 drops, 4-hourly) increasing the dosage if necessary until the observable signs are controlled (Roberton 1993). In the UK, the sedative chlorpromazine is also used, starting at 3 mg/kg/24 hours split into four to six doses, increasing the dose until presenting signs are controlled (Roberton 1993).

Midwife's management

In managing the baby of a drug-addicted mother, the midwife will need to build up a good working relationship with the parents. This involves the midwife being aware of her own feelings regarding drug misuse and developing the understanding that addiction is a disease. When providing information and guidelines for the parents they should be clearly communicated in a non-judgemental manner.

The midwife needs to explain the baby's presenting signs and emphasise that the behaviour is not a rejection of his parents. Opportunities for the parents to care for their baby should be actively encouraged. The midwife will need to be aware of contraindications to breast feeding with some drugs that are excreted in breast milk which would be harmful to the baby, for example cocaine and heroin (Charnoff 1991). If the midwife is unsure of the advisability of breast feeding she should seek the advice of the paediatrician or pharmacist. In planning discharge of the drug-misusing mother and her baby, the midwife will need to coordinate with the community health and social services to ensure that there is adequate follow-up.

Fetal alcohol syndrome (FAS)

FAS was first described by Jones and Smith in 1973 (Jones 1986). It is characterised by intrauterine growth restriction, failure to thrive, developmental delay and dysmorphic facial features. It is thought that ethanol (a component of alcohol) disrupts cell differentiation and growth in the fetus and also impairs normal placental function.

Characteristics of FAS

These include small eyes with exaggerated epicanthic folds, shallow or absent philtrum with a poorly formed nasal bridge, and ears that appear large. The baby may show signs of alcohol withdrawal and can be fretful and difficult to feed. The baby with FAS may also present with other associated abnormalities of the heart and musculoskeletal system, gut atresias, skin lesions and cleft palate. The baby with FAS will also present with delays in mental and motor development and may have learning and behavioural problems.

Midwife's management

The midwife has a crucial role in the prevention and management of FAS by identifying women at risk and in giving effective antenatal education. In managing the baby suspected of having FAS, the midwife will need to monitor for signs of alcohol withdrawal. Close liaison with community health and social services is essential in coordinating discharge and follow-up.

READER ACTIVITIES

1. Find out what is the policy for managing infants of diabetic mothers in your own unit.

2. What is the appropriate advice to give to a woman with phenylketonuria who is planning a pregnancy?

3. Plan the care of an infant of a diabetic mother and describe the midwife's management of moderate hypoglycaemia, for instance blood sugar levels of 1.5–2.0 mmol/l.

REFERENCES

Aynsley-Green A, Soltesz G 1992 Metabolic and endocrine disorders, Part 1, Disorders of blood glucose homeostasis in the neonate. In: Roberton N (ed) Textbook of neonatology, 2nd edn. Churchill Livingstone, London, ch 22

Brown J, Philips C A, Husain S 1997 Glucose testing in the neonate. Journal of Neonatal Nursing 3(3): 22–23

Charnoff I A (ed) 1991 Chemical dependency in pregnancy. Clinics in Perinatology 18: 1–191

Ellwood D S, Sutherland P, Kent C, O'Connor M 1987 Maternal narcotic addiction: pregnancy outcome in patients managed by a specialised drug dependency antenatal clinic.

Australia and New Zealand Journal of Obstetric Gynaecology 7: 92–98

Fleming P J, Speidel B D, Dunn P M 1986 A neonatal vade-mecum. Lloyd-Luke, London

Forfar J O, Arneil G C (eds) 1984 Textbook of paediatrics, 3rd edn. Churchill Livingstone, London, vol 2

Hawdon J M, Ward Platt M P, Aynsley-Green A 1992 Patterns of metabolic adaptation for preterm and term infants in the first neonatal week. Archives of Disease in Childhood 67: 357–365

Jones K 1986 Fetal alcohol syndrome. Pediatric Review 8(4): 122

Lucas A, Morley R, Cole T J 1988 Adverse neurodevelopmental outcome of moderate neonatal hypoglycaemia. British Journal of Medicine 297: 1304–1308

Perlmutter J 1974 Heroin addiction and pregnancy. Obstetric Gynaecology Survey 29: 439–446

Pildes R S, Pyati S P 1986 Hypoglycaemia and hyperglycaemia in tiny infants. Clinics in Perinatology 13(2): 351–375

Roberton N R C 1993 A manual of neonatal intensive care, 3rd edn. Edward Arnold, London

FURTHER READING

Crawford D, Morris M 1994 Neonatal nursing. Chapman & Hall, London

Hancock J 1997 The passive effects of addiction: how maternal substance abuse affects the health and development of the child. Journal of Neonatal Nursing 3(3): 14–17

Kelnar C J H, Harvey D 1995 The sick newborn baby, 3rd edn. Baillière Tindall, London

Siney C 1995 The pregnant drug addict. Books for Midwives Press, England

Miscellaneous

Complementary therapies in midwifery

44

Helen Stapleton

The sustained interest in complementary therapies
and the growing consumer demand that these
services be made available on the NHS has been an
important challenge to the orthodox medical
model. Many contemporary midwives have much
in common with complementary therapists as both
groups continue their struggle to provide a service
which is responsive to the needs of clients and
respects the autonomy of the practitioner. For
midwives, this has demanded that the
medicalisation of birth be recognised and replaced
with a model of care which is holistic and woman
centred. It is ironic that such a model, the very
cornerstone of complementary therapy, is not
valued by the majority of those responsible for the
purchase of health services locally. It is suggested
that developing an alliance between midwives and
complementary therapists could strengthen the
position of both parties.

The chapter aims to:

• explore a number of the philosophical and
  ideological differences between alternative and
  orthodox medicine

• examine the evolution of an alternative model
  of health care in the UK at a time of rapid
  change within the health service

• illustrate some of the barriers which prevent the
  integration of complementary therapies within
  the NHS

• consider the parallels between midwives and
  practitioners of alternative models of health
  care.

SETTING THE SCENE

People choosing alternative forms of health care
not generally available on the National Health

Service (NHS), nor under the cover of private insurance schemes, are a growing population. This trend, which has been particularly noticeable since the 1970s and has been reflected throughout the industrialised world, can no longer be dismissed as a faddish whim accessed by a fringe minority (Fisher & Ward 1994, Sermeus 1987, Thomas et al 1991, Thomas et al 1995, Wadsworth et al 1971). It echoes other social trends (Wilkinson 1994) and cannot be separated from the focus throughout the 1980s on consumerism and the growing emphasis on personal choice.

In the UK, the movement away from a unitary model of health care, provided free of charge to all, may also be seen as part of an attempt to rationalise that care and make it more acceptable and responsive to changing needs. The rapid growth in both the provision, and the uptake, of alternative models of health care shows no signs of slowing and is prompting a more thorough investigation by practitioners, purchasers and policy makers alike. If the (considerable) amounts of money spent by private individuals is any indicator of potential, then there is much at stake. Figures from the USA (Eisenberg et al 1993) suggest that personal expenditure in this area is around $15 billion per annum. In Australia, it is estimated that the amount of money spent on alternative forms of health care is double that spent on orthodox pharmaceutical products (MacLennan et al 1996).

In tandem with the actual demand for alternative health care within privileged sectors of the industrialised countries, there has also been an explosion in published literature. Contributions have included a range of voices which, at various times, have expressed enthusiasm, indifference or hostility. A selective review of this early literature reveals that complementary therapies, and the therapists who practise them, appear to have been targets for either ridicule or adulation, often without any critical evaluation of the actual claims being made. Although there is now evidence of a shift toward more informed debates, such polarisation of opinion is not unexpected. Indeed, it can be expected to accompany any major change or threat to the established sociocultural norms and, as vested interests are challenged, reactions such as fear and resistance are inevitable.

In the case of orthodox medicine, for example, it is most unlikely that proponents of this model of care will relinquish their clinical supremacy voluntarily. That said, changes in the organisation of health care and demands for a service which is accountable, cost-effective and evidence based, have brought the medical profession under critical scrutiny from a variety of sources (Harrison & Pollitt 1994, Rosenthal 1994, Williamson 1992). It is difficult to say whether this ongoing examination has also been a contributing factor in (successfully) challenging a number of misconceptions held by the medical establishment with regard to alternative medicine. What is apparent, however, is a softening of attitude and a greater willingness to explore ways in which at least some alternative therapies might be incorporated into the NHS. The way in which relationships between all parties providing health care might be improved has been another aspect of this debate (BMA 1993). Many of these issues were reiterated in a more recent study of the use of complementary therapies by a range of health care professionals working within the NHS (NHS Confederation 1997). Midwives contributed a significant voice to this research in which trust management issues were also cited as important factors in determining the acceptance and integration of complementary therapies at a local level.

Rather than focusing on specific therapies, lists of conditions or possible remedies, this chapter is intended to stimulate discussion about the more abstract issues underpinning competing models of health care. Such an overview will inevitably be something of a 'broad sweep', however, as these are complex areas and many of the debates are still at a relatively early stage of development.

TERMINOLOGY

The interchangeable use throughout this chapter of the terms *complementary*, *non-orthodox* or *alternative* as descriptors of practice, is deliberate and not intended merely to confuse the reader. There is currently no consensus as to which term best describes the many different approaches to non-orthodox health care provision, nor indeed the philosophy of the individual practitioner. To complicate things further, the term *traditional medicine* has been adopted by the World Health Organization (WHO) with respect to the indigenous practices of healers working in non-industrialised countries. It is a term which is confusing outside of that context, however, as in western countries, there has been a tendency to associate traditional medicine with mainstream, orthodox medicine. Stephen Fulder (1996), an author who has written extensively on this subject, has opted for the general umbrella term of *complementary medicine* but also notes that the terms *fringe, natural, holistic, unorthodox* or *unconventional* medicine are commonly used to describe what is currently on offer. He has usefully defined complementary medicine as:

> The aggregate of diagnostic and therapeutic practices and systems which are separate from conventional scientific medicine. They are usually less interventionist and technical and make more use of self-healing capacities (Fulder 1966, p. xv).

The term *complementary* medicine has found favour with those practitioners desiring a more equitable relationship with medical colleagues. It is commonly used by those who recognise that patients are better served by a cooperative partnership amongst all health professionals involved in the delivery of care. Other practitioners prefer the term *alternative* as a means of continuing to politicise underlying issues, particularly those concerning the basis of power and control in medicine. This latter group hope that by continuing to be explicit about the fact that other models of health care are available, the domination of the medical model will continue to be diluted.

The confusion surrounding terminology is not restricted to complementary medicine. Neither should this be regarded as an irrelevance to midwifery practice because it underpins allied subjects such as language, information and communication (Stapleton 1997). There are many expressions in current use within midwifery which create misunderstandings because there is usually more than one way of interpreting a word or phrase (see Box 44.1 for some examples). This is a problem which

---

Box 44.1 Examples of words or phrases in midwifery which may have multiple meanings

an active baby
at risk
autonomous practitioner
choice
due date
evidence-based
fetal monitoring
high risk
hospital policy
informed choice
low risk
natural labour/birth
overdue
research-based
screening test
trial of labour
midwifery-led care
team midwifery

---

is amplified by the use of jargon and technical language. It results in maternity service users not only being denied clear and unambiguous information, but also an informed choice and full participation in their care.

The practice of orthodox medicine, then, has varyingly been referred to as *biomedicine, cosmopolitan, allopathic, scientific, rational, mainstream, modern, technical, conventional, orthodox* or *western* medicine. By way of unifying these different terms, Fulder defines this type of medicine as: 'The aggregate of diagnostic and therapeutic concepts and practices which adhere to and employ modern scientific principles and techniques' (Fulder 1996, p. xv).

Unlike complementary medicine, however, these descriptors tend to be more related to the context and the discipline of the author making the reference. Anthropologists and sociologists, for example, might be more likely to use the terms biomedicine or conventional medicine, whilst reference to western, orthodox or conventional medicine is a greater likelihood in the literature of the popular press, public health or policy. The difference here is that these terms do not embrace great differences in epistemological nor philosophical understanding. Furthermore, they are generally used within a universally agreed sociopolitical dimension.

THE CRISIS OF MODERN MEDICINE AND ALTERNATIVES TO THIS MODEL OF HEALTH CARE

Alternatives to the orthodox medical model have always been available. The use of herbs as medicinal agents was, until recently, knowledge which was commonly held and widely applied; homeopathy is at least as old as orthodox medicine in the UK; osteopathy was introduced from America early this century (and has now gained the status of a state-registered profession in the absence of any 'proper' scientific validation); naturopathy has risen steadily in popularity since the 1930s. The post-war years have seen a sustained interest in these existing therapies and the arrival (or revival) of many 'new' ones. Furthermore, sophisticated and highly complex healing systems such as Oriental medicine, Ayurveda (and its offshoot Unani Tibb) have been introduced in conjunction with the settling of ethnic minority groups in the UK. The use of these alternative medical models has not, however, been confined to local, indigenous populations, but has excited a much wider interest and this has led to the establishment of professional organisations and training programmes. (See Box 44.2 for some of the main examples of this.) What is surprising is not so much the fact that the move towards pluralistic medicine has been sustained but the pace at which this has happened.

Things are changing very fast, however, and it is no longer the case that the uptake of non-orthodox medicine is restricted to small groups of gullible enthusiasts. Orthodox medicine is in crisis and is clearly unable to solve the major health issues of the late 20th century. The critique of this predicament, cogently argued more than two decades ago by Rene Dubos (1968), Ivan Illich (1975) and Thomas McKeown (1977), highlighted the inadequacies of the orthodox medical model. The stage was thus set to accommodate a search for an alternative system. It must be noted, however, that the current disaffection with orthodox medicine is not just about a failure to cure modern disease, the escalation of iatrogenic disease or uncommunicative doctors. It is also a reaction to a profession which the public have vilified as being

---

Box 44.2 Examples of alternative therapeutic modalities

Involving the use of medicinal plants:
- Herbal medicine (also known as phytotherapy)
- Homeopathy
- Aromatic medicine (essential oils)
- Bach flower remedies

Involving the mind–body:
- Biofeedback
- Relaxation techniques
- Bioenergetics
- Hypnotherapy
- Autogenics
- Meditation

Involving dietary regulation:
- Naturopathy
- Nutritional therapy
- Veganism
- Fasting
- Macrobiotics

Involving healing:
- Spiritual healing
- Faith healing
- Spirit healing (shamanism/exorcism)

Involving other traditions:
- Ayurvedic, Tibetan, Chinese, Indian, Japanese, etc. medicine

Involving the senses:
- Colour therapy
- Sound therapy
- Flotation therapy

Involving touch:
- Massage
- Reflexology
- Polarity therapy

Involving manipulation:
- Osteopathy
- Chiropractic

Involving posture:
- Alexander technique
- Feldenkrais
- Yoga

---

insufficiently accountable, as self-serving, and as reacting defensively to public criticism. These are issues which should also concern practitioners of alternative health care as it can be anticipated that, in time, they will also be called to account by a critical public. Whilst the fashion to romanticise and idealise products and services which have been deemed 'natural' currently affords some protection, practitioners would be unwise to expect this period of grace to continue indefinitely.

Cultural relativity: explanatory frameworks for alternative medicine

Different models of medicine hold different meanings for what is understood by terms such as health, sickness, illness or misfortune. This is complicated further depending on whether one is considering the issue from the position of patient or practitioner. Every system of healing holds its own explanatory model which accounts for the theories, assumptions, beliefs, values and factual information guiding the delivery of care. There is no one, universal, anatomy, physiology or psychology from which we might generalise and make recommendations which respect all cultural, social, gender and age differences. Cassidy (1996) makes the point that whatever else they might achieve, all health care systems incorporate the notion of trying to alter some aspect of functioning. Changes may be brought about through interventions as diverse as surgery, pharmacological agents (whether biological or botanical), dietary alteration, meditation, massage, manipulation, psychotherapy or prayer.

It may be useful to regard these different modalities as being more, or less, invasive (see Box 44.3

Box 44.3 Degrees of intervention: examples of therapies in different categories

Very invasive
- Surgery
- Electroconvulsive therapy

Moderately invasive
- Acupuncture
- Massage
- Chiropractic
- Herbal medicine

Mildly/not invasive
- Cranial osteopathy
- Spiritual healing
- Dowsing

---

for some examples). At one end of this spectrum then, medical interventions may penetrate the body surfaces through cutting or ingestion; others may only touch the surface of the body, whilst still others work off the body, on the energetic or spiritual dimension. Even within this framework, there are different degrees of potency: synthetic drugs tend to be more toxic and have a greater capacity for producing side-effects than do herbal or homeopathic medicines; colonic irrigation is more forceful on the elimination function than is fasting; encounter groups are more openly confrontational than is meditation.

What needs to be remembered is that force does not equate with effectiveness; healing can be achieved with a 'simple' act of love in the context of a caring environment. Ann Oakley illustrates this with reference to the delivery of maternity care:

> Love is a scientific concept, and its effect on the health of childbearing women can be quantified ... Love-caring is as important as science, technical knowledge, monitoring and intervention in the maternity services today (Oakley 1993, p. 76).

This points to a need for all health care practitioners to be engaged in a constant cycle of self-reflection, particularly with respect to those beliefs we have all been socialised into regarding as 'truths'. Such a commitment eventually makes it more possible to tolerate ambiguity and inconsistency; to even embrace the situations which give rise to them as exciting challenges, rather than as threatening or frightening. This is no easy achievement as it requires that judgement be temporarily suspended to allow for the birth of more radical thought. It also requires a willingness to question personal motivations, to grapple with unfamiliar concepts and to resist the temptation to think that it is others, rather than ourselves, who are ignorant. One writer on this subject has made the following observation:

> Unfortunately, the same derisive tone that labels the interpretation of personal experience as merely superstition is also found in comparisons of medical belief systems. If one is modern then others are, by inference, outmoded; if one is based on fact then others must be laced with

superstition. In this way, biomedicine is seen as somehow more true than any alternative system could possibly be ... Such a view ... fails to consider the internal logic of other explanatory models. But most health systems are logical and rational systems of thought if the underlying assumptions are known; this does not necessarily mean that these assumptions are correct, only that they can be viewed as having been reached by the coherent use of reason (Snow 1993).

Perhaps because this subject is so bewildering and there are now so many therapies from which to choose, various attempts have been made to devise a taxonomy by which they are grouped according to particular characteristics or properties. The arrangement in Box 44.4, comprising three broad divisions, is one such example.

Another approach might be that of dividing therapeutic approaches into those that could be described as 'material' or 'non-material'. Within this framework, biomedicine, with its exclusive focus on the body-physical, would be at one end of a spectrum which locates shamanic and spiritual healers working with dead, dreaming, or otherwise 'absent' bodies, at the other.

The rationale of complementary practice

Despite the diversity of therapeutic modalities, complementary therapists tend to share common

---

Box 44.4 Classification based on specificity of treatment

Treatments which are simple and primarily supportive
• Massage
• Spiritual healing
• Therapeutic touch

Treatments which have specific applications
• Chiropractic
• Osteopathy
• Psychotherapy

Treatments which are complex and applied across the whole spectrum of disease
• Herbal medicine (also known as phytotherapy)
• Homeopathy
• Traditional Chinese or Ayurvedic medicine

---

understandings. One widely held concept is that the body has the capacity to heal itself. The role of the therapist is to find ways in which this (unique) mechanism responds most appropriately to a range of therapeutic interventions. The emphasis is not so much on curing or removing illness, but on restoring maximum function and supporting the individual in making the necessary lifestyle changes needed to maintain this state. Thus, the therapist fulfils an important educative and preventive role and one which is in keeping with an alternative view of nature. In the case of ill health, for example, such a view would see these episodes as meaningful interludes, rather than as random, insignificant events in the individual's life cycle. These are broad principles which have been further elaborated on by Fulder (1996), Miccozzi (1996), Sharma (1992) and Pietroni (1990). Their combined efforts draw together the main issues in this debate and make it possible to categorise these according to the following criteria:

1. *Working with symptoms, not against them.* Symptoms are seen as important way-markers in the journey towards recovery and, as such, are managed rather than suppressed. The accent is on limiting the more debilitating aspects such as pain or nausea, in order that the energy available for healing might be maximised.

2. *Individuality as paramount.* The framework in which most complementary therapies are practised respects that although 10 people may be diagnosed with a peptic ulcer, for example, each one has become ill for different reasons. It is taken for granted that each person has a different constitution and will thus require an individually prescribed treatment package. The details of the treatment regimen are normally determined by the therapist after a full case history has been taken and any physical examination considered appropriate has been carried out.

3. *The human being as an integrated entity.* The individual seeking help is understood to be a unified human being with needs which span the spiritual, intuitive, emotional, physical, mental and psychosocial dimensions. Patients are encouraged to see ill health not simply as an irritating interruption to daily routine, but as having a deeper

significance. In other words, the questions of 'why now?' and 'why me?' are encouraged. On the whole, the influence of anatomy and physiology is less important compared to the emphasis placed on the flow of energy and the strength of the life force.

4. *Health and sickness as having no definitive beginning nor ending.* In contrast to the definition of health described by orthodox medicine – that of an absence of symptoms – practitioners of alternative therapies are more inclined toward the definition offered by the World Health Organization (1946) which stresses states of physical and mental well-being. It would not be considered at all unusual then, for those considered 'well' by the standards of orthodoxy to be receiving treatment from complementary therapists, as there is no fixed point at which either illness, or wellness, would be categorically defined. Conversely, a person with AIDS might seek help to achieve a (relative) state of well-being and adaptation and at that point might decide to terminate treatment although, by orthodox standards, she or he would still be considered as seriously ill.

5. *The importance of safety.* The vast majority of alternative therapies are minimally interventionist when compared with conventional medicine. They could also be described as non-toxic and harmless when practised by a competent person. Treatment cycles are usually considerably longer than those allowed for in conventional medicine as the therapist seeks to help the individual regain normal function. This is achieved by promoting health rather than by simply eliminating symptoms, as is the case with the 'magic bullet' approach of conventional medicine.

6. *Competency in practice.* To date, alternative practitioners have tended to concentrate less on the acute, traumatic, genetic and tropical conditions and more on the chronic, psychosomatic, early-stage, musculoskeletal, immunological and environmentally induced conditions. Whether competence could be gained in the areas which have traditionally been the preserve of conventional medicine, remains to be seen. What will be required of complementary therapists if this is to be achieved, is a willingness to extend their availability beyond the hours of 9 to 5. It would also demand that appointments are always available for the treatment of those with acute illnesses.

7. *The patient as a partner.* In contrast with conventional medicine, the role of the patient in complementary medicine is a very active one and patients are encouraged to help themselves. Specific exercises and/or other lifestyle changes are often recommended and it is expected that these will be undertaken, if only for the duration of the treatment. There is less of a power differential between both parties and consultations tend to be far more informal than is the case in conventional medicine. Thus, the relationship between patient and practitioner may be described as more of a partnership in which an 'equality of esteem' (Williamson 1997) is respected.

8. *An alternative world view.* It is commonplace for practitioners and, to a lesser extent, patients involved in complementary therapies to see patterns of health and illness as inseparable from the relationships they have with the wider environment. These patterns are often quite subtle and describe energetic, rather than physical or material, phenomena. Advocates of complementary therapies may also be described as more likely to be sympathetic to a 'green' philosophy. As such, they are more likely to be vegetarian or vegan, and to be knowledgeable and actively involved with pressure groups concerned with a wide variety of environmental issues. In many cases, this alternative world view demonstrates a shift in values, ranking those of a spiritual nature over those concerned with the material world. As the (negative) environmental impact of contemporary western lifestyles is better appreciated, views which are currently considered as alternative are likely to be incorporated into mainstream philosophy. This has already been demonstrated with the increase in vegetarianism over the past decade as the link between dietary intake of animal fats, cardiovascular disease and certain types of cancer, has been made.

It may be too early to evaluate whether the collective ethos and practice of non-orthodox therapists compares favourably with health promotion experts in reducing selected health risks. What is beginning to be acknowledged is that most complementary therapists routinely offer advice on a range of lifestyle issues including nutrition, smoking, alcohol intake, exercise and stress management. In this way, it could be said that they are instrumental in providing people with 'tools' for self-care, including the need to assume personal autonomy and take some responsibility in health matters.

It is worth noting, however, that non-orthodox practitioners cannot be considered as a homogeneous group sharing a unified belief system. Indeed, they employ a wide range of practices and philosophies which, in some instances, have nothing in common apart from their marginalisation from mainstream medicine. Some therapies, for example, describe a diagnostic and therapeutic model of care within a discrete system which simply cannot be understood within the framework or terminology of the orthodox medical model. Oriental and Ayurvedic medicine both fit this category, therefore practitioners might be more likely to label themselves non-orthodox, or alternative. On the other hand, for practitioners of aromatherapy, reflexology or spiritual healing, the term complementary might be more appropriately applied as these therapies could not be considered as complete systems of health care. This is particularly true with respect to diagnosis and treatment across an extensive range of conditions.

RESEARCH AND THE DEVELOPMENT OF EVIDENCE-BASED PRACTICE

Although the public opinion surveys which generate much of the data informing discussions on alternative models of health care need to be interpreted with some caution, it does appear that complementary medicine is now sufficiently established to warrant a more thorough evaluation of its claims. The problems associated with competing for money to undertake research which is sensitive to, and which accurately reflects, the paradigmatic shift represented by complementary medicine are formidable. In the eagerness to fill the void, however, complementary therapists need to consider what is commonly understood by the term 'evidence'. Similarly, there is a need to decide whether the parameters used to measure

standards in orthodox medicine, are applicable and transferable outside of that domain.

In the hierarchy which dominates western scientific models of research, the physical and biological sciences are prioritised, the social sciences hold an intermediary position and 'indigenous, *unsystematised* or *unprofessional* knowledge (herbal or homeopathic remedies, for example) disappear off the hierarchical ladder altogether' (Walt 1994, p. 179 – italics added). All of this suggests an urgent need to involve more complementary therapists in the research debate in order that they might determine for themselves what is required, rather than have future research circumscribed by orthodox medical standards. A decision taken in 1995 to extend the Cochrane Collaboration data base to include complementary medicine (Wootton 1995) could be seen to support this. In the USA, an Office of Complementary and Alternative Medicine (OCAM) has also been established to fund and promote research on unconventional forms of health care.

Many of these issues are of relevance for contemporary midwifery practice, where there is also a tendency to define research needs in line with the criteria demanded by the terms of the funding agency and other interested parties, in this instance, that of obstetric practice. Such arrangements do little to encourage midwives or complementary therapists to accumulate their own unique, practice-based body of knowledge, nor do they promote ongoing discussion with consumer groups or others who care deeply about developing alternative frameworks for practice. As Barbara Katz-Rothman put it when writing on midwifery as feminist praxis:

> I have come to see that it is not that birth is 'managed' the way it is because of what we know about birth. Rather, what we know about birth has been determined by the way it is managed. And the way childbirth has been managed has been based on the underlying assumptions, beliefs and ideologies that inform medicine as a profession (Katz-Rothman 1990, p. 178).

The current emphasis on evidence-based care and informed client choice does, however, make new demands on all health professionals. It requires, amongst other things, that high quality literature detailing both the pros and cons of different options is available for service users. It could be argued that midwifery has responded well to this challenge as indicated by the production of the Informed Choice series of leaflets (MIDIRS and The NHS Centre for Reviews and Dissemination 1993–1996).

Where once it was good enough simply to do and to say what had always been said and done, there is now an obligation to consider both the process and the outcome in relation to any intervention made during an episode of care. That said, people suffering from backache are currently as likely to visit a chiropractor or osteopath as they are a doctor, despite the fact that the actual basis of skeletal manipulation has never been scientifically investigated nor is it well understood. This holds for the majority of complementary therapies and indeed it is also the case for a great deal of conventional medical practice, as we know from the fields of midwifery and obstetrics.

What is interesting is that osteopaths managed to secure state registration (The Osteopaths Act 1993) without any evidence demonstrating the efficacy of osteopathic treatment, and chiropractors managed to achieve similar status in 1994, on the basis of a single recognised trial. This is particularly odd given the persistent demands from orthodox practitioners for their non-orthodox colleagues to prove themselves on scientific terms, rather than those considered most appropriate within non-orthodox frameworks. Fulder (1996) suggests that possible reasons for this turnabout included a progressive weakening of orthodox medicine's power base, a growing inability to maintain professional boundaries and a failure to successfully exclude competition from opposing systems of thought. The current investigation into the role and function of the statutory body for midwives, nurses and health visitors could provide a similar opportunity for midwives to also make a claim for separate legislation.

Obstacles to commissioning and conducting research in complementary therapies

A variety of issues have impeded the progress of research in complementary medicine, however, and researchers in this field continue to be discriminated against. Practitioners themselves have been reluctant to become involved with research as many have not seen it helping them or their patients in any tangible way. This was possibly exacerbated by ignorance, as this subject has only recently (if at all) been introduced into the educational curriculum of these practitioners. Many were also suspicious of standards and tools which they perceived as belonging to orthodox medicine and, as such, did not want be 'contaminated' by a value system at variance with their own. Some non-orthodox practitioners who were less head-in-the-sand took a more pragmatic approach, however, and this stance was to prove the more successful strategy. The support of many complementary therapy organisations enabled the RCCM (Research Council for Complementary Therapies) to begin work in 1983 with the remit of coordinating all research in this field. Many non-orthodox practitioners have gradually realised that research is not only about proving a point or convincing sceptical orthodox colleagues, but that it can also act as a conduit for improving relationships and this, in itself, aids the development and professionalisation of complementary therapies.

There is still much work to be done to make research attractive to complementary therapists. For example, research proposals which do not pay homage to the 'gold standard' of RCTs (randomised controlled trials, preferably double-blind) or are not written in the reductionist language of scientific medicine are less likely to be funded by mainstream organisations. The need to develop a range of alternative methodologies which are sensitive, needs-specific, and appropriate for use in non-orthodox settings has been addressed by a number of writers in recent years (Fitter & Thomas 1977a,b, Lewith & Aldridge 1993, Mercer et al 1995, St George 1994, Vickers 1995). From these debates, however, there appears to be some question as to whether the need for a separate methodology can still be argued. Research has moved on in the last two decades and is no longer a rarefied activity undertaken by a select minority. Health professionals in all disciplines are now increasingly engaged in the process and this has led to a greater diversity in methodological approaches, particularly those from the qualitative range. What may be more important for complementary therapists in the future is to ensure that the research question(s) and the chosen methodology are well suited. It is this 'fit' which determines the quality of the data and, ultimately, the validity of the study undertaken.

Whilst there is now a growing body of research on outcome measures, there is a need for further work in this area so that the full benefits experienced by users of complementary therapies might be better understood. At present, 'soft' outcome measures such as patient satisfaction and the subjective experience of treatment, are seen as less important than 'hard' data, such as cost-effectiveness or cessation of symptoms. There are similarities here in contemporary midwifery research, where it is not always easy to avoid dancing to the tune of the medical agenda. Further questions need to be asked about the timing of outcome measures and whether these change over time. Methods for measuring outcomes are not always considered important, and therefore are often not given full status as research tools. There are some indications that this attitude may be changing, however, as has been demonstrated recently by the development of new research tools such as the SF 36 (Short Form 36) (Jenkinson et al 1996, Ware & Sherbourne 1992), a validated questionnaire designed specifically to address the current deficit.

Further debate is also necessary with regard to the place of custom and routine in practice, particularly where there is no evidence to support one way of (not) doing things when compared with another. Examples in contemporary midwifery practice include the usefulness of routine uterine palpation in the postnatal period or whether to suture first and second degree tears where apposition of the wound edges is good and there are no other factors which might impede a good healing response. It may well be that the complementary health field generates exciting developments both in the design of research tools and in designing questions which are also of benefit to researchers involved in orthodox medicine.

Despite the enormous amount of available expertise, research journeys for both midwives and complementary therapists could be said to be just beginning. As territories are reframed and senses are opened to all that it is possible to experience, the importance of research to both document and stimulate this process becomes more evident. From her extensive experience as an anthropologist documenting childbirth practices, Brigitte Jordan (1993) cautions against adopting the standards used by the orthodox medical model in determining research priorities for indigenous peoples, as she claims that this invariably leads to a devaluation of indigenous practices. By insisting on the need to compare like with like, or at least to make explicit the terms of comparison, she makes the point that data cannot be obtained from one set of research subjects and the results applied to other populations, in this case western and non-western groups. Her observation applies not only to the Dutch, Swedish, Mexican and American cultures in which her research was undertaken, but also holds true for ethnic minority groups currently accessing maternity services in the UK.

LEGAL, POLICY AND ETHICAL ISSUES

The following section discusses these issues only insofar as they are of relevance to this chapter. Readers wishing to explore these subjects in greater detail with specific reference to complementary medicine are referred to the relevant sections in Fulder (1996), Stone & Matthews (1996) or Budd & Sharma (1994).

The law

With a few exceptions, the operation of common law in the UK affords a right to any member of the public to practise any form of therapy or medicine, subject to the consent of the patient. This therapeutic freedom is the envy of colleagues in Europe and further afield where practice largely tends to conform to the principles of the Napoleonic code. Upholding this code means that activities are restricted to certain professional groups, unless regulations explicitly allow them to be undertaken by others. This compares with the principles of common law, when it is only where restrictions are specifically stated that particular activities are limited. Titles are similarly protected; hence none other than those registered as such may refer to themselves as doctor, nurse or midwife, for example. Only registered practitioners may practise midwifery, dentistry or veterinary surgery, or may diagnose and treat venereal disease. The law also prohibits advertising remedies for cancer; it does not, however, forbid the treatment of it. Other specific diseases for which the advertisement of treatment is not permitted include diabetes, cataracts, glaucoma, epilepsy and tuberculosis. The Companies Act (1982) also prevents any new complementary therapy centre from describing itself as a health centre, unless nurses and doctors are employed on the premises.

Although complementary therapists are somewhat restricted by statute law and the Medical Act of 1956, as far as litigation is concerned, common law right continues to afford them considerable protection. This is primarily because where no case in law has been previously established, 'no-one is in a position to give a definitive legal opinion as to how a court would decide a case against a complementary therapist' (Stone & Matthews 1996, p. 131). The principles of common law, then, act retrospectively, or in other words are precedent-based, and legal principles are established which subsequently provide a basis against which future cases might be compared. Complementary therapists could be said to be in an enviable position at present as, 'where there is no case law, the best that lawyers can do is to try to predict how they think a court would be likely to decide a case' (Stone & Matthews 1996, p. 131). Until such time as cases have been heard and decided against, a court of law can only look to related cases brought against other health professionals and attempt to make a case on the basis of common principles. These might relate to issues concerned with failing in respect to the duty of care expected of any health professional, misrepresentation or professional negligence.

Vicarious liability and perceptions of risk in complementary and orthodox medicine

Actions citing professional negligence against complementary therapists are rare; this is in contrast to the medical profession where cases of litigation are increasing and this is a trend in western countries worldwide. The incidence of litigation is, to a large degree, reflected in the insurance premiums demanded of health professionals and this, in turn, is decided according to the degree of risk and the likelihood of negligence charges. The majority of professional associations to which complementary therapists belong in the UK make insurance a condition for continuing registration. Practitioners currently pay between £40 and approximately £300 p.a. for indemnity cover of £1 million. This figure, which compares very favourably with the average cost incurred by midwives, suggests that the perceived risk of successful prosecution is extremely low. This is in contrast to obstetricians who are currently charged upwards of £11 000 p.a., because their practice is perceived to involve a much higher degree of risk, and because at present they are most likely to be cited as the professional responsible for omissions or negligence in 'successful' legal cases.

Common issues in complementary medicine and midwifery practice

If midwives and complementary therapists are generally perceived as low risk for insurance purposes, it might reasonably be expected that this would be the case across the board. This is not the situation, however, as the perception of risk in midwifery practice is primarily determined by insurance underwriters, assisted by obstetricians and risk managers within local hospital trusts. Thus, definitions of risk vary enormously and are constantly subject to change, reflecting as they do the topical concerns of a select group of senior, primarily male, professionals. As with complementary medicine, the yardstick whereby midwifery practice is measured has not been fashioned by the practitioners themselves, but by those who have an interest in maintaining its (inferior) status.

As the practice of midwifery primarily concerns itself with low-risk women and is regulated by statutory rules and regulations (UKCC 1992a,b, 1993, 1994, 1996), it might be anticipated that midwives as a group would be seen as low to medium risk. This is true, however, only insofar as they conform not only to these statutory requirements, but, increasingly, to the risk management policies of their employing NHS trust. This often necessitates the midwife balancing a formidable range of opposing demands and loyalties. Jilly Rosser has argued in a recent article that it may also frequently require the midwife to 'break the rules' during the course of duty (Rosser 1998). In the wake of *Changing Childbirth* (DH 1993), at a time when midwives are working hard to set up models of care which are midwifery rather than medically orientated, it may seem ironic that their practice is very likely to be circumscribed because risk managers (and insurance underwriters) are more readily persuaded by the pre-existing medical model of care. It appears that midwives, like many complementary therapists, hold an uneasy alliance with the medical profession. Unfortunately for both groups, it is still largely the medical profession who dictate what may be embraced and what can be rejected.

There is another parallel in midwifery practice which reflects the division between complementary and orthodox practitioners. This is with respect to the practice of independent midwives who could be described as providing alternative models of care from that offered by their mainstream colleagues. In the context of this discussion, the current situation regarding indemnity insurance is interesting. The withdrawal of vicarious liability insurance by the Royal College of Midwives in the early 1990s left this group of practitioners no option but to seek alternative cover. Because there is no precedent for midwifery practice outside of the protected conditions of NHS employment, the practice of independent midwives was assessed by the insurance underwriters for the Medical Defence Union (MDU). They were deemed to be of equal risk to obstetricians and consequently they were charged the same £11 000 p.a. fee. Unlike their obstetric colleagues, however, independent midwives have limited earning power and are not in a position to pass this fee on to the women they book. The decision of whether to buy vicarious liability cover from the MDU was not an easy one, but this was all that was on offer. Some independent midwives felt so strongly about the political, moral and financial implications of

purchasing unaffordable indemnity insurance from a *medical* agency, that they opted to inform their clients and to practise without cover. This also meant that they were likely to be refused the honorary contracts necessary for the continuation of care should a client opt for, or at any point require, hospital care.

The timing of all of this was unfortunate in that it occurred at a point when the number of independent practitioners was steadily increasing and the role was beginning to be perceived by mainstream midwives as a feasible career option. The dramatic reduction in the numbers of independent midwives currently in practice – an inevitable result of the removal of vicarious liability cover which was both affordable and easily available – has left remaining practitioners worried about their own futures. It has also raised concerns about the continued viability of the Independent Midwives Association as an organisation which promoted and supported an alternative midwifery model within the UK. Furthermore, the issue of who picks up the bill for vicarious liability cover has not been satisfactorily resolved. It is currently causing concern for midwives crossing trust boundaries and for midwifery lecturers wishing to engage in clinical activities. Both of these groups are currently vulnerable to restrictions on their practice because of unresolved issues with their local employing NHS trusts over arrangements for cover. It would not be altogether unexpected if, at some future date, selected employees were asked to make arrangements for their own insurance cover, particularly if the current escalation in litigation fees for NHS trusts continues. Practitioners working outside of the hospital setting would constitute a vulnerable group in this regard.

Current policy regarding the integration of complementary medicine into the NHS

The current national policy with regard to the provision of complementary therapies on the NHS is best described as conservative, reflecting concerns primarily about efficacy and cost-effectiveness. The impetus to bring about change in service provision

– in this case the availability of complementary therapies on the NHS – has been very similar to recent changes in midwifery practice in that these have also been consumer driven. In 1993 a survey was undertaken which revealed that 38 health authorities and 34 fundholding practices together spent more than £1 million annually on complementary therapies (Cameron-Blackie 1993). If the NHS were to be considered as a whole, this figure is likely to be considerably greater and, as a result, the purchasing authorities of many trusts may need to consider what money could be made available to meet this growing demand. This creates something of a dilemma for risk managers as the majority of complementary therapies have never been scientifically tested nor evaluated and, as illustrated earlier, this requirement might not even be possible to achieve.

If complementary therapies were to be integrated more fully into the NHS, this would not be without major consequences, particularly for the practitioners of these therapies. Regulatory mechanisms at local trust level, such as NHS trust risk management policies (see Ch. 7) and the conveyor system of patient appointments would make care which is tailored to the specific needs of the individual impossible to achieve. Thus, the highly prized patient–practitioner relationship, currently such an important element of complementary medicine, could be jeopardised. It possibly goes without saying that any deterioration in this relationship could be expected to produce similar dissatisfactions which have hitherto been expressed only with respect to conventional medicine. Greater integration might also be expected to lead to practitioners being subject to complaints by dissatisfied consumers and, more seriously perhaps, to an increase in legal charges against them.

Three UKCC documents (1992a,b, 1996) have paved the way for suitably qualified midwives, nurses and health visitors to implement complementary therapies into clinical practice, although one recent study of nurses has found the uptake less than had been previously assumed (Rankin-Box 1997). In effect, therapies which are most commonly used tend to be those which can be learnt within a short period of time, which can be easily accommodated within existing clinical

demands and which do not seriously challenge the dominant biomedical model. Aromatherapy, reflexology, therapeutic touch and massage, for example, are more widely available from these dual-role practitioners than is traditional Chinese medicine or osteopathy. The clinical areas in which complementary medicine is most likely to be practised by nurses are in the relief of pain and stress, oncology, community and palliative care. Midwives, who are also qualified as complementary practitioners, treat a wide range of ailments relating to pregnancy and birth (Tiran & Mack 1995). In one recent study, the therapy stated as most commonly practised (or provided) by this group was aromatherapy (NHS Confederation 1997). As no details were given regarding the referral system, range of conditions treated nor oils most commonly used, however, it was not possible to make any further comments on the midwifery component of this study.

What is unclear at the present time is the extent to which the practice of complementary medicine by qualified midwives and other health professionals occurs exclusively within the private sector, as compared to the NHS. The sustained interest in complementary therapies has, however, led to special interest groups being formed amongst both midwives and nurses. It is intended that these groups will continue to monitor the activities of practitioners, to network with other health care professionals involved with complementary therapies, and to collate information, including statistics, on the number of dual-role practitioners and the formulation of potential research questions.

In response to the demand by some health care professionals, there has been a rapid growth in the number of courses provided by UK universities. In a recent survey of medical training schools in the UK, more than 60% of medical students thought that such training would be helpful and the same survey revealed that only three medical schools were providing such training (Rampes et al 1997). A mapping exercise of midwives' use and perceptions of complementary therapies has yet to be done and it is impossible to predict what such a survey might reveal. If orthodox health professionals continue the trend to learn and practise a complementary therapy, however, those alternatives which appeal to these groups will be medicalised and brought into the mainstream. Such a move could, in theory, lead to complementary practitioners eventually being outlawed.

Ethical concerns

One of the main safeguards by which any profession ensures that it is answerable to concerns about the continued safety and protection of the public is by insisting on registration of its members as a prerequisite to practice. Conditions for membership on professional registers are variable but the majority expect all members to comply with certain regulations. These include codes of ethics and conduct, maintaining adequate indemnity insurance cover, respecting complaints and grievance procedures and, for some professionals, evidence of continual professional updating. None of this holds true, however, for the vast majority of complementary therapists. With the exceptions of the recently state-registered practices of osteopathy and chiropractic, all complementary therapists are voluntarily self-regulated. That is not to say that they operate without professional registers, nor the regulatory mechanisms referred to above, but rather that there is no mandatory requirement for complementary practitioners to conform to these. Complementary medicine is currently organised at a number of different levels, with different schemes operating concurrently, and this makes it difficult to make meaningful observations about practice (Stone & Matthews 1996). For example, the regulatory structures governing osteopathy and chiropractic are quasi-statutory. Those of acupuncturists, herbalists and homeopaths are similar in nature but currently rely heavily on the integrity of the individual to maintain standards. The reputation of yet other groups of complementary therapists is dependent upon the honourable intentions of practitioners to uphold standards which are informally agreed.

Health professionals have a particular knowledge base which is widely perceived to function as an instrument of considerable power and privilege. Traditionally, biomedicine has occupied a position in which monopoly of this power has rarely been challenged. That can no longer be said to be the case as increasing competition from other professional groups, including midwifery, has acted as a diluting agent to this exclusive control. In the struggle for professional equity, it may be worth reiterating that medical knowledge (whether this be of the alternative or conventional variety) should be regarded as a vehicle by which a vulnerable and dependent public are healed of their ailments. It is not a tool for professional or personal self-advancement and that is one of the reasons why a strong ethical code, which is regularly monitored and amended, is an essential requirement for all health care professionals. In order that this remain an effective regulatory tool, it is imperative that consumer involvement is sought throughout the planning and evaluation process. One of the criticisms currently levelled against complementary therapists is that their professional codes are designed for, and used exclusively by, the professional group. Thus, they cannot be said to operate impartially or independently until such time as provision is made for consumer participation.

This issue is especially important with regard to the principle of informed consent, as this is the process whereby patients become actively involved with decisions concerning their health care. Informed choice for all consumers of health care presupposes that informed consent has been given; this results from a dynamic process of constant negotiation between the provider and receiver of health care, rather than something which is tacitly assumed by the former. Informed consent, and the corollary of informed choice, arise from the ethical principle of a respect for autonomy, in this instance that consumers of (complementary) health care have a right to information about the treatment they are receiving. This information should provide the necessary detail concerning the likely outcome and any possible risks; it also acts to protect the patient from the harm of being subjected to unsafe, ineffective, or irrelevant, treatment. The notion of harm is to be understood here in the widest sense 'that it can result from wasted time, money spent on inappropriate care or delayed conventional treatment' (Norton 1995, p. 346). It behoves complementary therapists, then, to ensure that the information provided for patients is adequate and accurate. This will help to ensure that they do not infringe upon their patients' right to self-determination.

CONCLUSION: PARALLELS BETWEEN MIDWIVES AND PRACTITIONERS OF ALTERNATIVE HEALTH CARE

The struggle which many contemporary practising midwives have experienced in attempting to provide a different model of care has many parallels with complementary practitioners. Both groups have encountered considerable opposition to securing professional credibility which is independent of and on separate terms from the medical profession. This has been made all the more difficult as, paradoxically, both rely on the continued support and patronage of this powerful group. A contributing factor is that membership of both groups is relatively small by comparison with the medical profession, and neither is sufficiently resourced to meet the current demands for service provision and ongoing research and development. It has been suggested by one author, referring in this instance to childbirth, that on a global level the economic competition for services can create 'witch-hunts' against innovative and caring practice (Wagner 1995). Whilst compassion can serve to stimulate continued evolution in practice, where power and resources are unevenly distributed (as is currently the case with midwives and practitioners of alternative health care) this is unlikely to happen.

READER ACTIVITIES

1. Assess the extent to which complementary therapies are available in your local area.

   a. Which therapies are the most commonly used?
   b. Why have these particular therapies been chosen by the various practitioners?
   c. How many NHS employees are using complementary therapies?
   d. What training have they received?

2. Evaluate any effects the working environment may have on the delivery of complementary therapies.

   a. Are there differences between institutions such as the NHS and a natural therapy centre?
   b. Does the working environment impose limits on the clinical practice of complementary therapists?
   c. Are the requirements for evidence-based practice the same for orthodox and complementary medicine?

3. Complementary therapists who work within the NHS can only do so by upholding the reductionist model of western medicine. Discuss this, particularly with reference to complementary therapists who are not trained as midwives (or other orthodox health professionals).

4. The difficulties faced by complementary therapists wishing to work in the NHS may be similar to those of direct entrant midwives. Discuss this issue with respect to the socialisation processes absorbed during professional training.

USEFUL ADDRESSES

BHMA (British Holistic Medical Association)
Rowland Thomas House
Royal Shrewsbury Hospital (South)
Shrewsbury
Salop SY3 8XF

Tel: 01743 261155
Fax: 01743 353637

CCAM (Council for Complementary and Alternative Medicine)
Park House
206–208 Latimer Road
London W10 6RE

Tel: 0181 968 3862
Fax: 0181 968 3469

Centre for Complementary Health Studies
Exeter University
Amory Building
Rennes Drive
Exeter EX4 4RJ

Tel: 01932 264498
Fax: 01932 433828
E-mail: chs@ex.ac.uk

Natural Medicines Society
Market Chambers
13a Market Place
Heanor
Derby DE75 7AA

Tel: 01773 710 002
Fax: 01773 533855

RCCM Research Council for Complementary Medicine
60 Great Ormond Street
London WC1N 3JF

Tel: 0171 833 8897
Fax: 0171 278 2412

Special Interest Group for Complementary Therapies in Midwifery
c/o Denise Tiran
Principal Lecturer Complementary Therapies/Midwifery
The University of Greenwich
Elizabeth Raybould Centre
Bow Arrow Lane
Dartford
Kent DA2 6PJ

Tel: 0181 331 8769/8779
Fax: 0181 331 9160

REFERENCES

British Medical Association (BMA) 1993 Complementary medicine; new approaches to good practice. Open University Press, Milton Keynes

Budd S, Sharma U (eds) 1994 The healing bond: the patient–practitioner relationship and therapeutic responsibility. Routledge, London

Cameron-Blackie G 1993 Complementary therapies in the NHS (research paper no 10). Commissioned by NAHAT (National Association of Health Authorities and Trusts). NAHAT, London

Cassidy C M 1996 Cultural context of complementary and alternative medicine systems. In: Micozzi M S (ed) Fundamentals of complementary and alternative medicine. Churchill Livingstone, New York

Companies Act (1982) HMSO, London

Department of Health (DH) 1993 Changing childbirth: report of the expert maternity group. HMSO, London

Dubos R 1968 Man, medicine and environment. Praeger, New York

Eisenberg D M, Kessler R C, Foster C, Norlock F E, Calkins D R, Delbarco T L 1993 Unconventional medicine in the United States: prevalence, costs and patterns of use. New England Journal of Medicine 328(4): 246–252

Fisher P, Ward A 1994 Complementary medicine in Europe. British Medical Journal 309: 107–111

Fitter M, Thomas K 1977a Evaluating complementary therapies for use in the NHS: 'horses for courses' I the design challenge. Journal of Alternative and Complementary Medicine 5(2)

Fitter M, Thomas K 1977b Evaluating complementary therapies for use in the NHS: 'horses for courses' II alternative research strategies. Journal of Alternative and Complementary Medicine 5(2)

Fulder S 1996 The handbook of alternative and complementary medicine. Oxford University Press, Oxford

Harrison S, Pollitt C 1994 Controlling health professionals. Open University Press, Buckingham

Illich I 1975 Medical nemesis. Calder and Boyars, London

Jenkinson C, Layte R, Wright L, Coulter A 1996 The UK SF-36: an analysis and interpretation manual: a guide to health status measurement with particular reference to the short form 36 health survey. Health Services Research Unit

Jordan B 1993 Birth in four cultures: a cross-cultural investigation of childbirth in Yucatan, Holland, Sweden and the United States. Waveland Press, Illinois

Katz-Rothman B 1990 Recreating motherhood: ideology and technology in a patriarchal society. W W Norton, New York

Lewith G, Aldridge D (eds) 1993 Clinical research methodology for complementary therapies. Hodder & Stoughton, London

MacLennan A H, Wilson D H, Taylor A W 1996 Prevalence and cost of alternative medicine in Australia. Lancet 347: 569–573

McKeown T 1977 The role of medicine. Basil Blackwell, Oxford

Medical Act 1956 HMSO, London

Mercer G, Long A, Smith I 1995 Researching and evaluating complementary therapies: the state of the debate. Nuffield Institute for Health, Leeds

Micozzi M S (ed) 1996 Fundamentals of complementary and alternative medicine. Churchill Livingstone, New York

MIDIRS (Midwives Information and Resource Service) and The NHS Centre for Reviews and Dissemination 1993–1996 Informed Choice leaflets 1–10 for professionals and women. MIDIRS, Bristol

NHS Confederation 1997 Complementary medicine in the NHS: managing the issues. Research paper No. 4. The NHS Confederation, Birmingham

Norton L 1995 Complementary therapies in practice: the ethical issues. Journal of Clinical Nursing 4: 343–348

Oakley A 1993 Essays on women, medicine and health. Edinburgh University Press, Edinburgh

Osteopaths Act 1993 HMSO, London

Pietroni P 1990 The greening of medicine. Victor Gollanz, London

Rampes J et al 1997 Introducing complementary medicine into the medical curriculum. Journal of the Royal Society of Medicine 90: 19–21

Rankin-Box D 1997 Therapies in practice: a survey assessing nurses' use of complementary therapies. Complementary Therapies in Nursing and Midwifery 3(4): 92–99

Rosenthal M M 1994 The incompetent doctor: behind closed doors. Open University Press, Buckingham

Rosser J 1998 Breaking the rules. Practising Midwife 1(1): 4

St George D 1994 Towards a research and development strategy for complementary medicine. Homeopath 54: 254–256

Sermeus G 1987 Alternative medicine in Europe: a quantitative comparison of the use and knowledge of alternative medicine and patient profiles in nine European countries. Belgian Consumers' Association, Brussels

Sharma U 1992 Complementary medicine today: practitioners and patients. Routledge, London

Snow L F 1993 Walkin over medicine. Westview Press, Boulder, Colorado. Quoted in: Cassidy C M 1996 Cultural context of complementary and alternative medicine systems. In: Micozzi M S (ed) Fundamentals of complementary and alternative medicine. Churchill Livingstone, New York, p 11

Stapleton H 1997 Choice in the face of uncertainty. In: Kirkham M J, Perkins E R (eds) Reflections on midwifery. Baillière Tindall, London

Stone J, Matthews J 1996 Complementary medicine and the law. Oxford University Press, Oxford

Thomas K, Carr J, Westlake L, Williams B T 1991 Use of non-orthodox and conventional health care in Great Britain. British Medical Journal 302: 207–210

Thomas K, Fall M, Parry G, Nichol J 1995 National survey of access to complementary health care via general practice: a report for the Department of Health. Medical Centre Research Unit, School of Health and Related Research, University of Sheffield, Sheffield

Tiran D, Mack S (eds) 1995 Complementary therapies for pregnancy and childbirth. Baillière Tindall, London

United Kingdom Central Council for Nursing, Midwifery and Health Visiting (UKCC) 1992a The scope of professional practice. UKCC, London

United Kingdom Central Council for Nursing, Midwifery and Health Visiting (UKCC) 1992b Code of professional conduct. UKCC, London

United Kingdom Central Council for Nursing, Midwifery and Health Visiting (UKCC) 1993 Midwives rules. UKCC, London

United Kingdom Central Council for Nursing, Midwifery and Health Visiting (UKCC) 1994 The midwife's code of practice. UKCC, London

United Kingdom Central Council for Nursing, Midwifery and Health Visiting (UKCC) 1996 Guidelines for professional practice. UKCC, London

Vickers A 1995 The NIH Methodology Conference: the methodology debate in the UK during the past ten years. Journal of Alternative and Complementary Medicine 1: 209–212

Wagner M 1995 'A global witch-hunt.' Lancet 346: 1020–1022

Wadsworth M E J, Butterfield W J H, Blaney R 1971 Health and sickness: the choice of treatment. Tavistock, London

Walt G 1994 Health policy: an introduction to process and power. Zed Books, London

Ware J E, Sherbourne C D 1992 The MOF 36-item short-form health survey (SF 36): 1 conceptual framework and item selection. Medical Care 30: 473–483

Wilkinson H 1994 No turning back: generations and the genderquake. Demos Publications, London

Williamson C 1997 Some general principles on partnership. Seminar proceedings, London April 24 1997. Organised by the Primary Care Support Force with the Wells Park Health Project

Williamson C 1992 Whose Standards? Consumer and Professional Standards in Health Care. Open University Press, Buckingham

Wootton J 1995 Establishing a complementary medicine field within the Cochrane collaboration. Journal of Alternative and Complementary Medicine 1: 291–292

World Health Organization (WHO) 1946 Constitution. WHO,

45

Special exercises for pregnancy, labour and the puerperium

Eileen M. Brayshaw

CHAPTER CONTENTS

Specific exercises and postures can help the pregnant woman to adapt to the physical changes in her body during the childbearing year. They will help to ease the minor aches and pains during pregnancy and may also help to prevent longer-term postpartum problems. In addition, coping skills such as relaxation, positioning and breathing awareness will provide the mother and her partner with the practical means of managing labour. If practised during pregnancy, the knowledge of these skills will increase the confidence of both partners.

The chapter aims to:

- give midwives an insight into the teaching of physical skills

- provide practical information about exercise, relaxation and breathing for pregnancy, labour and the puerperium

- discuss the role of exercise in relieving aches and pains

- consider basic back care.

The information given is relevant for group practice or use on a one-to-one basis and includes advice for the whole of the childbearing year.

An obstetric physiotherapist is the ideal choice to teach the physical skills required for parenthood. However, in areas where there is no physiotherapist available, midwives may find themselves responsible for physical preparation as well as parent education in antenatal classes or on a one-to-one basis.

Preparation for parenthood classes provide the opportunity for talks, exercise and discussion sessions with a combined approach from midwives, physiotherapists, health visitors and other health care professionals. They should aim to create a learning environment with a relaxed atmosphere, where parents-to-be can enjoy developing a confidence to cope with pregnancy, labour, delivery and the early postnatal days. Specific therapeutic aims of physical preparation include the prevention or relief of minor discomforts such as backache, the promotion of a speedy postnatal recovery and the prevention of future gynaecological or orthopaedic problems. Exercise sessions should be designed to stimulate interest in the physical changes occurring, to promote body awareness and to facilitate physical and mental relaxation. Classes held early in pregnancy allow for advice and discussion relating to rest, anticipated postural changes and relief of minor discomforts. Sessions covering relaxation, positions for labour and postnatal exercises are probably more appropriate during the third trimester of pregnancy.

Moderate exercise during pregnancy stimulates circulation, helps to keep joints flexible, creates good muscle tone and promotes a general sense of well-being (Jacobson et al 1991). It is also suggested that women who exercise regularly during pregnancy have an improved course of pregnancy and labour compared to those who lead a sedentary lifestyle (Clapp 1990, Huch & Erkkola 1990).

Walking in the fresh air remains the most natural and simplest form of exercise and should be encouraged.

Cycling is another popular form of exercise which allows for good mobility of the lower limbs with the bodyweight supported. It is an easy way to travel, although short distances are preferable. Steep hills should be avoided and it is advisable to stop before feeling tired.

Swimming is excellent exercise as water relieves the effects of gravity on the body and muscles can be strengthened and flexibility of joints retained without undue fatigue. It is important to avoid diving during pregnancy and also the more strenuous strokes such as crawl or butterfly. Breast stroke is usually the most popular but has a tendency to aggravate backache. Leisurely back stroke with gentle supporting arm movements is often the most comfortable.

Aquanatal classes. In many areas local swimming pools hold aquanatal classes. Exercise in water raises the plasma beta endorphin levels significantly (McMurray et al 1990) and has a beneficial effect on the respiratory, cardiovascular and musculoskeletal systems. If the classes are well designed and carefully supervised by a suitably qualified professional following set guidelines (ACPWH 1995), they are an excellent and a very enjoyable way of keeping fit.

Exercise to music. Many midwives have undergone training in exercise-to-music for ante- and postnatal groups. These sessions can be fun as well as providing aerobic exercise.

Energetic and competitive sports activities, such as squash, aerobics, horse riding, jogging and skiing are best avoided during pregnancy and it is not the time to take up new sports. Strenuous keep-fit exercises such as sit-ups and double-leg-lifts should never be performed as these may cause ligamentous strain and consequent back problems. For the same reason, pregnant women should avoid lifting heavy weights or objects.

Postural changes in pregnancy

Accompanying the gradual gain in weight in pregnancy and its centralising redistribution is the hormonal influence on ligamentous structures (see Ch. 11). Both of these factors alter the posture of the pregnant woman (Fig. 45.1) and her self-image. The body's centre of gravity moves forwards and when this is combined with stretching of weak abdominal muscles it often leads to a subsequent hollowing of the lumbar spine with a rounding of the shoulders and poking chin. There is a tendency for the back muscles to shorten as the abdominal muscles stretch, extra strain is placed on the ligaments and the end result is backache, usually of sacroiliac or lumbar origin. Postural re-education, including correction of the 'pelvic tilt', should be taught, preferably with the benefit of a full-length mirror. The theme of back care must be developed with advice relating to comfortable positions in sitting, standing, lying, general mobility and how to lift correctly.

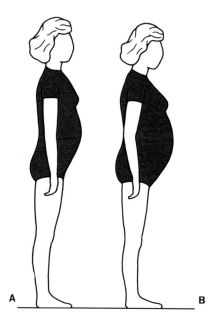

Fig. 45.1 (A) Posture in early pregnancy. (B) Posture in later pregnancy – note increased lordosis.

BACK CARE

Sitting. The pregnant woman should choose a comfortable chair which supports both back and thighs. She should sit well back and if necessary place a small cushion or folded towel behind the lumbar spine for additional comfort. The seat height should allow the feet to rest on the floor, or a small footstool or cushion may be placed under the feet to raise them slightly (Fig. 45.2). If relaxing in an easy chair, the head can be supported and the legs elevated on a stool.

Standing. The posture should be as tall as possible with both the abdomen and buttocks tucked in. Weight must be evenly distributed on both legs, to prevent undue strain on the pelvic ligaments, and spread between the heels and balls of the feet. High heels will throw the balance of the pregnant woman too far forward and are best discarded in favour of a medium- or low-heeled shoe which also gives support. Shoulders which are relaxed and down help to prevent thoracic aches.

Lying. Equal pressures on all parts of the body

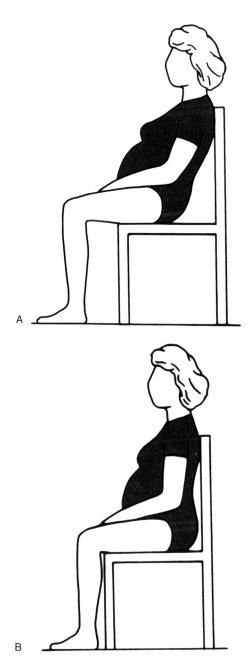

Fig. 45.2 (A) Poor sitting posture. (B) Good sitting posture.

will lead to a good posture in lying with no undue strain on any one area. Lying flat on the back must be discouraged because of the danger of supine hypotension (see Ch. 11): three or four pillows or a wedge or beanbag will raise the head and shoulders

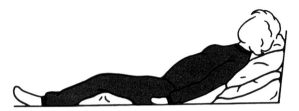

Fig. 45.3 Half back-lying supported with pillows.

sufficiently to avoid that risk (Fig. 45.3). It may be more comfortable with a pillow placed under the thighs to reduce the tension behind the knees. Side-lying (coma position) with pillows under the top forearm and knee is usually a comfortable position in pregnancy (Fig. 45.4).

Getting up from lying by bending the knees, rolling onto one side then using the arms to push up into a sitting or kneeling position will prevent strain on both the back and the abdominal muscles.

Household activities. Discussion needs to take place on the way in which the woman does her housework. Many tasks such as ironing or preparing food can be undertaken in a sitting position instead of standing. Working surfaces at the correct

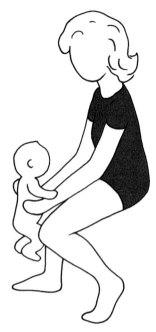

Fig. 45.5 Correct lifting.

height or the use of a high stool will avoid the need to stoop and the subsequent backache which a stooping posture can bring about. Making beds or cleaning the bath in a kneeling position prevents lumbar strain.

Lifting heavy or awkward objects should be avoided during pregnancy if at all possible. If lifting is unavoidable, then the object must be held close to the body with the knees bent and the back kept straight (Fig. 45.5). That way the strain is taken by the thigh muscles, not those of the back. All twisting movements whilst lifting are dangerous and must not be performed.

RELIEF OF ACHES AND PAINS

Back and pelvic pain

This is a common problem during pregnancy. Mantle et al (1977) quoted that 50% of pregnant women surveyed reported significant backache, whilst Bullock et al (1987) found 82% of women experienced back pain at some stage of their pregnancy. Backache can be helped by encouraging good posture and the practice of the pelvic tilting

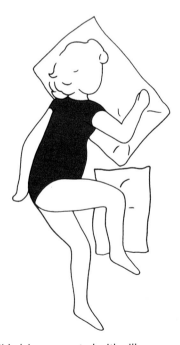

Fig. 45.4 Side-lying supported with pillows.

exercise in standing, sitting and lying positions. Women complaining of severe pain involving more than one area of the pelvis (pelvic arthropathy) should be referred to an obstetric physiotherapist for assessment and possible manipulation. Sciatic-like pain may be relieved by lying on the side away from the discomfort, so that the affected leg is uppermost. Pillows should be placed strategically to support the whole limb.

Cramp

Prevention of cramp is helped by practising foot and leg exercises. To relieve sudden cramp in the calf muscles whilst in the sitting position the woman should hold the knee straight and stretch the calf muscles by pulling the foot upwards (dorsi-flexing) at the same time. Alternatively, standing firmly on the affected leg and striding forwards with the other leg will stretch the calf muscles and solve the problem.

Rib stitch or discomfort

Discomfort around the rib cage can often be relieved by adopting a good posture, or by specifically stretching one or both arms upwards, depending on which side the pain is present.

PREPARING TO TEACH ANTENATAL EXERCISES

Before teaching exercises it is essential to understand the simple anatomy and functions of the muscles involved, in order to be able to select and/or adapt appropriate exercises in different circumstances.

Anatomy of the anterior wall abdominal musculature

The anterior abdominal wall consists of four pairs of muscles, namely: rectus abdominis, obliquus externus (external oblique), obliquus internus (internal oblique) and transversus abdominis.

Rectus abdominis (Fig. 45.6)

This pair of muscles runs vertically one on either

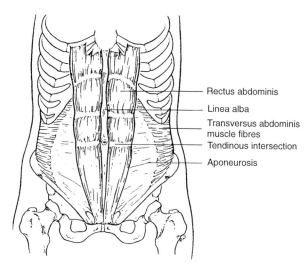

Fig. 45.6 Rectus abdominis (reproduced from Brayshaw & Wright 1994 by kind permission).

- Rectus abdominis
- Linea alba
- Transversus abdominis muscle fibres
- Tendinous intersection
- Aponeurosis

side of the midline from the symphysis pubis to the xiphisternum. Each muscle arises by two tendons; the larger lateral head is attached to the crest of the pubis, the smaller medial head interlaces with fibres from the opposite muscle to be attached to the symphysis and the ligament in front of the joint. The fibres pass upwards to the xiphoid process and the costal cartilages of the fifth, sixth and seventh ribs. Three transverse tendinous intersections are present in the rectus muscles (recti), one at the level of the xiphoid process, one at the level of the umbilicus and the third lying approximately midway between the previous two. The recti are separated in the midline by a tendinous raphe running from the symphysis to the xiphoid process and known as the linea alba. The gap between the two muscle bellies is less than 1 cm below the umbilicus and up to 2 cm above it. Each rectus muscle is enclosed in a fibrous sheath formed by the aponeurosis (see below) of each of the external oblique, internal oblique and transversus abdominis muscles. This sheath is known as the rectus sheath and is described more fully later.

External oblique (Fig. 45.7)

The external oblique muscles are situated on the anterolateral aspect of each side of the abdominal wall and are the most superficial of the flat abdo-

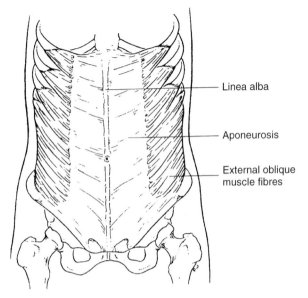

Fig. 45.7 External oblique (reproduced from Brayshaw & Wright 1994 by kind permission).

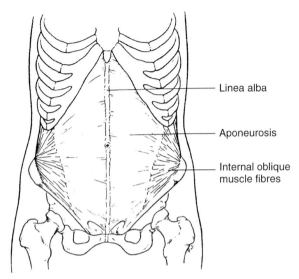

Fig. 45.8 Internal oblique (reproduced from Brayshaw & Wright 1994 by kind permission).

minal muscles. As the name suggests, the main anterior fibres run obliquely in a downwards and medial direction, with the uppermost fibres running in a more medial direction. The anterior fibres arise from the outer borders and costal cartilages of the fifth, sixth, seventh and eighth ribs and insert by an aponeurosis (a flat tendon composed of layers of collagen fibres) into the linea alba. The aponeurosis forms the anterior part of the rectus sheath as it passes anterior to rectus abdominis. The most lateral of the external oblique muscle fibres, which arise from the lower four ribs, pass almost vertically down to insert as the inguinal ligament stretching between the pubic tubercle and the anterior superior iliac spine (ASIS).

Internal oblique (Fig. 45.8)
The internal oblique muscles form the middle layer of the flat abdominals with the majority of fibres running obliquely in an upwards and lateral direction at right angles to those of the external obliques. The lower anterior fibres arise from the lateral two-thirds of the inguinal ligament and the iliac crest near the ASIS and run almost transversely to insert into the crest of the pubis, medial part of the pectineal line and, by an aponeurosis,

into the linea alba. The most posterior fibres run vertically upwards to insert in the inferior borders of the lower four ribs. The upper anterior fibres arise from the anterior one-third of the intermediate line of the iliac crest and travel in an upwards and medial direction to insert into the linea alba via an aponeurosis. The lateral fibres of the internal oblique are attached to the middle one-third of the intermediate line of the iliac crest and from thoracolumbar fascia. These fibres pass upwards and medially (but not as medially as the anterior fibres) to insert into the inferior borders of the 10th, 11th and 12th ribs and, by an aponeurosis, into the linea alba.

Transversus abdominis (Fig. 45.9)
This pair of muscles is the deepest of the abdominal muscle sheets with fibres running transversely from the lateral one-third of the inguinal ligament, the anterior two-thirds of the inner lip of the iliac crest, thoracolumbar fascia and the inner surfaces of the costal cartilages of the lower six ribs. Most of the fibres run transversely to form a broad aponeurosis inserting into the linea alba. The fibres from the inguinal ligament curve down to join with the inferior fibres of the internal oblique to form the conjoint tendon.

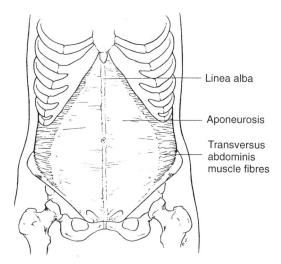

Fig. 45.9 Transversus abdominis (reproduced from Brayshaw & Wright 1994 by kind permission).

Labels in figure:
- Linea alba
- Aponeurosis
- Transversus abdominis muscle fibres

Rectus sheath

The aponeuroses of the oblique and transverse abdominals form the rectus sheath. Anteriorly, the aponeurosis of the external oblique muscle passes in front of the rectus belly. The aponeurosis of the internal oblique muscle divides at the lateral border of the rectus muscle, with the anterior part fusing with the aponeurosis of the external oblique, whilst the posterior part runs behind the rectus belly and fuses with the aponeurosis of the transversus muscle. The aponeuroses from each side fuse in the midline at the linea alba. This arrangement is true from the xiphisternum down to midway between the umbilicus and the sternum, where the posterior wall of the rectus sheath ends in a downwardly curving line called the arcuate line. Below this line, the aponeurosis of the internal oblique muscle passes in front of the rectus belly, leaving only transversalis fascia between the rectus sheath and the peritoneum.

Linea alba

The linea alba lies between the medial borders of the rectus bellies and is formed by the interlacing fibres of the aponeuroses of the external and internal oblique and transversus muscles. As the rectus muscle bellies are closer together below the umbilicus, the linea alba is narrower below and wider above the umbilicus. Above the umbilicus, it may be seen as a shallow groove in fit persons. At its lower end, it is attached to the pubis and the upper end is attached to the xiphisternum and adjacent ribs.

Actions of the abdominal muscles

Rectus abdominis

This flexes the vertebral column by bringing the thorax and pelvis closer together anteriorly. If the pelvis is fixed, the thorax can move towards the pelvis and vice-versa. Flexion of the spine is assisted by the external and internal oblique abdominals, and psoas major and minor. Rectus abdominis also assists in lateral flexion of the spine brought about by the external and internal obliques, plus the appropriate back muscles. Rectus abdominis works with the other abdominal muscles to raise the intra-abdominal pressure. Bilateral weakness of rectus abdominis will cause decreased ability to flex the lumbar spine. Posterior pelvic tilt will be much more difficult to perform, as will head and shoulder raising in the supine position. The difficulty in pelvic tilting posteriorly will result in an increased lumbar lordosis with associated postural problems. Head and shoulder lifting utilise the recti to stabilise the thorax so that the neck flexors can bring about the action of lifting the head.

External oblique

The lateral fibres of the external oblique muscle on one side work with the lateral fibres of the internal oblique muscle on the same side to flex the trunk sideways, approximating the pelvis and thorax laterally at that side. When the anterior fibres of the external obliques of both sides are contracted together with the rectus abdominis, the pelvis is tilted posteriorly. The posterior fibres, working together with the rectus muscles, flex the trunk. Contracting unilaterally, the external oblique muscle works in conjunction with the anterior fibres of the internal oblique muscle of the opposite side to rotate the vertebral column. With the pelvis fixed, the right external oblique and the left internal oblique will rotate the thorax in an anticlockwise direction (to the left) and vice versa.

Internal oblique

The lower anterior fibres of the internal oblique muscles work with transversus to compress and support the lower abdominal viscera. When the upper anterior fibres of the internal obliques of both sides are contracted they flex the vertebral column (approximating the thorax and pelvis anteriorly), support and compress the abdominal viscera, depress the thorax and assist in respiration. Contracting unilaterally, the upper anterior fibres of the oblique muscle work in conjunction with the anterior fibres of the external oblique muscle of the opposite side to rotate the vertebral column. With the pelvis fixed, the right internal oblique and the left external oblique will rotate the thorax in a clockwise direction (to the right) and vice versa. The lateral fibres of the internal oblique muscle on one side work with the lateral fibres of the external oblique muscle on the same side to flex the trunk sideways, approximating the pelvis and thorax laterally at that same side. They also assist in rotation of the spine. Weakness of both the external and internal oblique muscles decreases respiratory efficiency and decreases support of the abdominal viscera. Weakness of the external obliques will decrease the ability to pelvic tilt posteriorly, resulting in an anterior pelvic tilt in standing and an alteration in the relationship between the pelvis and the thorax. Weakness of the internal obliques will result in a decreased ability to flex the vertebral column.

Transversus abdominis

The transversus muscles compress the abdominal viscera, giving support similar to a girdle. They also help to stabilise the linea alba during lateral trunk flexion. Weakness of the transversus muscles contributes to a protruding abdominal wall, increased anterior pelvic tilt and probable backache.

Combined actions

The combined actions of all four pairs of abdominal muscles can be related to the function of raising intra-abdominal pressure. This is achieved by the flat sheet muscles pulling on the rectus sheath via their aponeuroses, so flattening the abdomen and compressing the abdominal viscera.

If the diaphragm is lowered and remains active, the resultant increase in intra-abdominal pressure brings about downward expulsive actions such as defaecation, micturition, and parturition if in conjunction with the relaxation of the pelvic floor. If the diaphragm is relaxed, then the increased intra-abdominal pressure can bring about upward expulsive actions, e.g. sneezing, coughing and vomiting. The combined action of the abdominals and the diaphragm provides a muscular corset keeping the viscera in place.

During pregnancy, the hormones which cause relaxation affect the fascia, aponeuroses and linea alba. It is important to remember the abdominal muscle attachments so that rotation exercises are not encouraged. These could cause a pulling action on the linea alba and separate it and the rectus muscle bellies lying within the rectus sheath.

THE ANTENATAL EXERCISES

The positions pregnant women adopt for exercises should be carefully considered. The women should not be asked to lie flat in the later second and third trimesters because of the danger of supine hypotension (Revelli et al 1992). Instead, a half-lying position with the back raised to an angle of approximately 35° can be used. Foot and leg exercises and pelvic tilting can be performed in sitting or half-lying, whereas abdominal tightening and pelvic floor exercises can be carried out in any position. *Remember, before asking a group to exercise on the floor, that the correct way of getting down and up again must be demonstrated* (see 'Lying' p. 876).

Muscles of good tone are more elastic and will regain their former length more efficiently and more quickly after being stretched than muscles of poor tone. Exercising the abdominal muscles antenatally will ensure a speedy return to normal postnatally, effective pushing in labour and the lessening of backache in pregnancy. An important function of the abdominal muscles is the control of pelvic tilt. As the ligaments around the pelvis stretch and no longer give such firm support to the joints, the muscles become the second line of defence, helping to prevent an exaggerated pelvic tilt and unnecessary strain on the pelvic ligaments.

It must be remembered that overstretched ligaments and weakened abdominal muscles during pregnancy can lead to chronic skeletal problems postnatally (Hodges & Richardson 1995) as well as backache antenatally. To prevent this and to maintain good abdominal tone, abdominal tightening and pelvic tilting exercises are taught.

Exercises which involve the oblique abdominal muscles should be avoided in later pregnancy because these muscles are inserted into the linea alba (see p. 878). If twisting movements are performed, there is the danger that the shearing effect may pull the linea alba and the rectus muscle bellies apart (Noble 1988). If this occurs, the condition is known as diastasis recti and is more often diagnosed postnatally.

Abdominal tightening

- Sit comfortably or kneel on all fours. Breathe in and out, then pull in the lower part of the abdomen below the umbilicus whilst continuing to breathe normally. Hold for up to 10 seconds. Repeat up to 10 times.

This exercise tones the deep transverse abdominal muscles which are the main postural support of the spine and will help to prevent backache in the future (Hodges & Richardson 1995). When mastered, this simple exercise can be practised in any position and whilst doing other activities.

Pelvic tilting or rocking

- In a half-lying position, well supported with pillows, knees bent and feet flat. Place one hand under the small of the back and the other on top of the abdomen. Tighten the abdominals and buttocks, and press the small of the back down onto the underneath hand (Fig. 45.10). Breathe normally, hold for up to 10 seconds then relax. Repeat up to 10 times.

Pelvic tilting can also be performed sitting, standing or kneeling. It plays an important part in good posture.

A great strain is put on the *pelvic floor* during pregnancy because of hormonal influence, the weight of the developing fetus and the altered

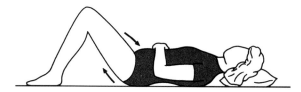

Fig. 45.10 Pelvic tilting exercise.

pelvic posture. It is important, therefore, to teach pregnant women pelvic floor exercises antenatally in order to maintain the tone of the muscles so they retain their functions. They will also relax during parturition and regain their former strength quickly during the puerperium. (For anatomy and functions see Ch. 49.)

All women should be able to perform this simple exercise which can be practised anywhere and at any time.

Pelvic floor exercise

- Sit, stand or half-lie with legs slightly apart. Close and draw up around the back passage as though preventing a bowel action then repeat around the front two passages as though preventing the flow of urine. Hold for as long as possible, up to 10 seconds, breathing normally, then relax. Repeat up to 10 times.

All women should practise this exercise very regularly antenatally, particularly after emptying the bladder. For those with diminished pelvic floor awareness, attempting to 'stop midstream' occasionally or 'gripping' on to an imaginary tampon which is slipping out may assist the ability to contract the correct muscles.

Foot and leg exercises

The *circulation* during pregnancy, particularly the venous return, is sluggish and this can lead to problems such as cramp, varicose veins and oedema. To help to prevent these the following simple exercises and advice will improve the circulation.

- Sit or half-lie with legs supported. Bend and stretch the ankles at least 12 times. Circle both feet at the ankle at least 20 times in each direction. Brace both knees, hold for a count of four, then relax. Repeat 12 times.

These exercises should be performed before getting up from resting, last thing at night and several times during the day. Women should be discouraged from standing unnecessarily and encouraged to put their feet up whenever possible. Crossing the legs at the knee or ankle will impede circulation further. If varicose veins or oedema are present, support tights may be prescribed with the appropriate advice to put them on before allowing the legs to drop over the edge of the bed.

Breathing awareness

It is important to be aware of one's own natural breathing rhythm so variations can be recognised if they occur.

- Sit comfortably with eyes closed. 'Listen in' to your breathing, concentrating especially on the outward breath, recognising the short pause before the inward breath naturally follows. Keep the movement fairly low down in the chest and be aware of your own breathing rate whilst resting.

A few deeper breaths now and again will help the venous return and aid the oxygen supply to both the pregnant woman and her baby but only three or four breaths at a time as hyperventilation is more likely during pregnancy (Bush 1992).

TEACHING EXERCISES

Anyone who is teaching exercises to others must first be proficient at performing those particular exercises herself. Next she must familiarise herself with instructions describing the execution of the exercise and practise teaching two or three colleagues or family members before introducing the teaching to a larger group. It is important to describe or demonstrate fully and to give relevant additional information which makes the topic more interesting and meaningful. When planning to teach specific exercises, such as foot and leg exercises, think in the way shown in Box 45.1.

Box 45.1 Teaching foot and leg exercises

Why the exercise is relevant
- During pregnancy, circulatory changes occur which may lead to cramp, oedema or varicose veins.

What we hope to achieve
- Improvement in circulation and prevention or alleviation of cramp, oedema and varicose veins.

How
- Bend and stretch the ankles.
- Circle feet at the ankles.
- Brace knees and let go.
- Repeat several times.

When
- Several times per day and always before getting up from resting and last thing at night.

Additional information
- Avoid long periods of standing, which may increase oedema, but encourage walking.
- Discourage sitting or lying with legs crossed, which can impede circulation.
- Describe how to relieve cramp.
- Advise on correct use of support tights.
- Stress the importance of supporting footwear of sensible height.
- Advise sitting with feet elevated whenever possible and heels higher than hips if oedema is present.

STRESS, RELAXATION AND RESPIRATION

The normal stresses of everyday life often lead to a build-up of tension within the body. If anxiety, fear or pain are present the body may unconsciously adopt a posture which is extreme. Relaxation is concerned with reducing body tension to a minimum and once learned can be used whenever increased tension is a problem. It can be particularly useful during pregnancy and labour and the early postnatal days. Tension manifests itself with muscle tightening and shows in the following ways:

- frowning face
- tense jaw
- hunched shoulders
- elbows bent and close to sides
- fingers gripping or tapping
- trunk bent forward

- legs crossed
- feet pulled up or tapping.

When tension increases, breathing often becomes shallow and rapid, or when severe, breath-holding may feature. The higher the stress level, the greater the degree of postural change that will be evident. Mental tension often leads to physical tension and a vicious circle is established. Ideas about relaxation have been developed and exchanged over many years but today it is generally recognised that 'Relax' is a negative instruction and does not readily bring results for most individuals. Muscles can work singly but usually they work in groups and when any group of muscles is working, the opposite group relaxes. This is a physiological fact and is known as reciprocal inhibition or reciprocal relaxation. Try the following example:

- Concentrate on your right hand.
- Stretch your fingers really long. Hold for a moment. (This is tightening the muscles on the back of your hand and wrist.)
- Now stop stretching and feel the ease not only in the muscles you were stretching but in the palm of your hand and fingers.

Reciprocal relaxation ensures that when following a series of instructions for the whole body, one will be able to bring release of tension and relaxation to all areas.

Planning a scheme of relaxation

To be effective, relaxation must be practised regularly and it is important to develop a theme running through classes and to encourage daily practice at home. The environment should be relatively peaceful with no irritating distractions such as the telephone. An adequate supply of mats, blankets and pillows is essential. Participants should be encouraged to wear loose, comfortable clothing, to remove shoes and spectacles and then choose a comfortable position in which to relax. This could be side-lying, half-back-lying or sitting with supporting pillows strategically placed.

Physiological relaxation

This technique (see Box 45.2) consists of a series of instructions and movements which help the body to move away from the posture caused by tension and so achieve a position of comfort, ease and relaxation. Following each individual instruction and movement, any tension in that part of the body will disappear.

When group participants are fluent in the practice of relaxation there is no need to go through the whole checklist of instructions every time. Gradually shorten the list of instructions given and work towards the situation where relaxation can be achieved almost spontaneously. The shoulders, arms and hands are usually the first areas to respond to stress and the following can be practised to be used during contractions:

- Shoulders down
- Arms and hands comfortably supported
- Easy breathing and *sigh out slowly*.

This can be practised for the approximate duration of a contraction with concentration on easy breathing which helps to achieve comfort and relaxation.

Respiration

Respiration is affected by stress and adapted breathing is one of the easiest ways of assisting relaxation. Breathing can be used to increase the depth of relaxation by varying its speed; slower breathing leads to deeper relaxation. Natural rhythmic breathing must not be confused with specific unnatural levels or rates of breathing which research has proved to be harmful to both mother and fetus (Bush 1992, Caldeyro-Barcia 1978). Women in labour frequently breathe very rapidly at the peak of a contraction but should be encouraged not to do so. Persistent rapid breathing or breath-holding is usually a sign of panic.

Very slow deep breathing can cause hyperventilation, which produces tingling in the fingers and may proceed to carpopedal spasm and even tetany. Rapid shallow breathing or panting is only tracheal and can lead to hypoventilation with subsequent oxygen deprivation. During pregnancy, labour and delivery, emphasis should be placed on easy, rhythmic breathing and on avoiding very deep breathing, shallow panting or long periods of breath-holding.

Box 45.2 Physiological relaxation technique

For each part of the body where tension manifests itself there is a threefold instruction:

- an order to the reciprocal muscle group to work strongly
- a command to that muscle group to stop working
- a direction to the brain to recognise the new position of ease and to remember it.

As with exercises the teacher of relaxation techniques must first practise them herself and become familiar with the instructions before teaching others.

- Lie down comfortably on a firm surface with pillows supporting your head and thighs (Fig. 45.3) or sit in a suitable chair, with head, shoulders, arms and thighs supported.
- **Shoulders.** Pull your shoulders towards your feet – stop pulling – concentrate on this new position of ease – your shoulders are relaxed and down.
- **Arms.** Push your elbows slightly out from your body as though straightening the elbows – stop pushing, think about this position – your arms are relaxed and comfortably supported.
- **Hands.** Let them rest on your tummy or thighs or the supporting surface – stretch the fingers really long and straight – stop stretching – feel the new position – comfortably supported and relaxed.
- **Hips.** Tighten your buttocks and press your knees out sideways – stop tightening, register this comfortable position – your hips are relaxed.
- **Knees.** Move your knees slightly – stop moving them

– feel the comfort you have created in your knees and thighs.
- **Feet.** Press your feet down – away from your face – stop pressing – you now have comfortably relaxed feet.
- **Body.** Press your body into the support, such as the floor, bed or chair – stop pressing – be aware of comfort and relaxation in your trunk.
- **Head.** Press your head into the support, that is, the pillow or chair – now stop pressing – notice how this movement has relaxed your neck and shoulders.
- **Face.** Close your eyes if you want to. Drop your lower jaw slightly so that your teeth are not touching. Make sure that your tongue is resting comfortably in the lower jaw and not stuck to the roof of your mouth. Imagine that someone is smoothing away the frown lines from your forehead.
- **Breathing.** Give a big sigh out and continue to breathe gently, keeping the movement fairly low down in the chest; be aware of the outward breath. Your body is now in a position of ease and is as relaxed as is possible in that position and you are breathing at your normal resting rate.
- Never get up in a hurry after a spell of relaxation. Instead, gently exercise the hands and feet to stir the circulation and slowly roll over onto one side, getting up in the correct way.
- Relaxation can be adapted and used as labour progresses by combining the most comfortable positions with easy breathing in the lower part of the chest (breathing awareness).

LABOUR

It is important to stress to the parents-to-be the relevance of cooperation with the midwife and a policy of working together. During exercise sessions it is often necessary to give reminders about where contractions are felt, how often they occur and their progression. The need for relaxation and breathing techniques should be stressed together with how and when they can be used. Careful choice of words is essential when describing pain and pain relief. As individuals, we appear to experience discomfort and pain to varying degrees. With good training it is possible to raise the individual's threshold of tolerance. A positive and down-to-earth approach is desirable when explaining the benefits of using breathing and relaxation techniques. It must be remembered

that continual support and reminding will be necessary as labour progresses, if the breathing and relaxation techniques are to achieve their maximum potential.

Early first stage of labour

A woman in labour should be encouraged to keep mobile and active if there are no complications. She should be encouraged to try alternative positions of ease as alteration of position leads to productive uterine contractions (Roberts et al 1983). When discomfort increases, the woman should be encouraged to stay relaxed and concentrate on rhythmical easy breathing during contractions.

Coping with early first stage of labour
The following positions of ease may help during

the early stages of labour and can be discussed and practised in the antenatal period:

- sitting against a table and relaxing forwards so that shoulders, arms and head are supported
- standing, leaning backwards against the wall of the room
- kneeling on all fours
- kneeling on the floor and leaning forwards against a chair
- leaning forward against a partner
- sitting astride an armless chair with arms supported on the chair back and body relaxing forwards.

Pelvic rocking in any of these positions may be helpful. Deep massage of the lower back or gentle stroking of the abdomen soothes many women and can be taught to the partner at couples' classes.

Later first stage of labour

As labour progresses it becomes more difficult to find a comfortable position and frequent changes may be necessary. Many women, however, are content to sit back against pillows on the bed at this stage and concentrate on relaxation and breathing. As each contraction builds up, the speed and depth of breathing sometimes alter but mothers must be encouraged to keep it as natural and easy as possible. They may find that 'sighing out slowly' (SOS) helps to avoid panic breathing and also relaxes physical tension especially in the shoulders.

The emotional aspects of the end of the first stage of labour will be explained to couples antenatally and coping strategies need to be discussed. If there is a premature urge to push, an interrupted outward breath can be introduced (that is, two shorter breaths out followed by a longer breath out). This is often known as 'pant, pant, blow' or 'puff, puff, blow' breathing and it prevents the diaphragm from fixing and the subsequent increase in intra-abdominal pressure. An alteration in position will take away some of the urge to push, for example side-lying or prone kneeling with the forehead resting on the hands.

Second stage of labour

Positions for second stage will depend on individual choice, method of pain relief and obstetric factors but mothers should give some thought to alternatives available in their delivery suite. These may include:

- side-lying
- kneeling and leaning forwards facing the backrest of the bed with pillows placed for comfort
- kneeling on all fours
- squatting on the bed or floor
- supported squatting with partner holding from behind
- sitting fairly upright against the backrest with knees bent and feet resting on the bed.

If there is any pain in the area of the symphysis pubis which may lead to symphysis pubis dysfunction (SPD), abduction of the hips must be avoided. Prone kneeling or side-lying would be the most suitable positions for delivery (Fry 1992).

As the contraction starts, the mother is reminded to breathe in and out gently. When the urge to push becomes overwhelming she will tuck in her chin and bear down, keeping the pelvic floor relaxed. Breath-holding should not be encouraged because of the danger of fetal hypoxia in an already compromised baby (Caldeyro-Barcia 1978). To prevent pushing whilst the head is delivered, deep panting may be useful.

POSTNATAL EXERCISES

These should be started as soon after delivery as possible in order to improve circulation, strengthen pelvic floor and abdominal muscles and prevent transient and long-term problems.

Circulatory exercises

Foot and leg exercises as described in the antenatal section must be performed very frequently in the immediate postnatal period to improve circulation, reduce oedema and prevent deep vein thrombosis (DVT). If oedema is present the foot of the bed may be raised slightly.

Pelvic floor exercises

The pelvic floor muscles have been under strain during pregnancy and stretched during delivery and it may be both difficult and painful to contract these muscles postnatally. Mothers should be encouraged to try the exercise as often as possible in order to regain full bladder control, prevent prolapse and ensure normal sexual satisfaction for both partners in the future. The exercise can be linked to and performed during everyday activities such as feeding, bathing, nappy changing and after each bladder-emptying. The contraction, as described in the antenatal section, should be held for up to 10 seconds if possible before relaxing, and repeated up to 10 times at any one session, breathing normally throughout. When this has been mastered, mothers should follow the 10 slow contractions by 10 quick ones without holding the contraction. This programme will strengthen both the Type I muscle fibres which can contract over a long period of time and the Type II muscle fibres which produce a quick powerful contraction of the pelvic floor (Gilpin et al 1989).

Mothers should be encouraged to test their pelvic floor muscles after 2–3 months. With a full bladder they should be able to jump up and down with legs apart and cough deeply without leaking urine. If there is leakage, then the exercise must be continued several times a day for a further 1 month and the test repeated. If leakage still occurs, the mother should report back to her GP for a physiotherapy or gynaecological referral. Bump et al (1991) showed that only 49% of women who thought they were performing pelvic floor contractions were doing so correctly. Furthermore, 25% were performing the exercise in such a way that could potentially encourage incontinence. Bø (1995) concluded that pelvic floor exercises must be thoroughly taught to be effective. Even if there is no leakage on testing, every woman should exercise her pelvic floor muscles regularly to prevent continence problems.

Abdominal exercises

The straight and deep muscles need to regain tone as soon as possible after delivery in order to protect the spine, prevent back problems and help the mother regain her 'former figure'.

Abdominal tightening

This very easy exercise described on page 881 will strengthen the deep transverse muscles which are the main support for the spine and play a large part in preventing long-term back problems (Richardson & Jull 1995).

Pelvic tilting

Pelvic tilting as described in the antenatal exercise section will tone up the straight abdominal (rectus abdominis) muscles and will ease any postural backache which may occur in the first few days of the puerperium. As the abdominal muscles become stronger, the woman can progress to lifting the head and stretching the hands towards the knees whilst holding the pelvis tilted. This is known as a 'curl-up' but must always be performed with the knees bent (Fig. 45.11).

Rectus check

After 48 hours the rectus muscles (see Fig. 45.12) should be checked for any undue diastasis which may have occurred antenatally or sometimes during labour. A gap of two fingers at this stage is considered normal and the mother may progress to exercising the oblique abdominal muscles. However, if the gap is more than two fingers' width and 'peaking' of the abdominals is visible on head-lifting, then abdominal tightening and pelvic tilting only should be performed very regularly until the gap reduces (Fig. 45.12). An obstetric physiotherapist should assess any woman found to have a gap of more than three fingers' width to advise on a regimen of progressive exercises to avoid

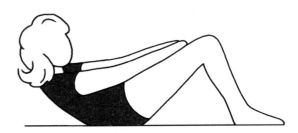

Fig. 45.11 Curl-up exercise.

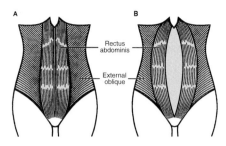

Fig. 45.12 (A) Rectus muscles before pregnancy. (B) Diastasis of rectus muscles after delivery.

future back problems. These women will also require abdominal support.

Knee rolling

This exercise will strengthen the oblique abdominal muscles and may be done if there is no undue separation of the rectus muscles.

- In back-lying with knees bent, pull in the abdomen and roll both knees to one side as far as is comfortable, keeping shoulders flat. Return knees to an upright position and relax the abdomen. Pull in again and roll both knees to the other side. This exercise can be performed up to 10 times.

Hip hitching

Also working the oblique abdominals, hip-hitching or leg-shortening is performed in back-lying with one knee bent and the other knee straight (Fig. 45.13).

- Slide the heel of the straight leg downwards thus lengthening the leg. Shorten the same leg

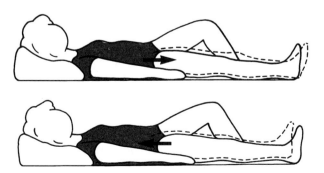

Fig. 45.13 Hip hitching (up-drawing) exercise.

by drawing the hip up towards the ribs on the same side. Repeat up to 10 times, keeping the abdomen pulled in. Change to the opposite side and repeat.

Exercises following caesarean section

Foot and leg exercises as described earlier should be started as soon as possible, especially after epidural anaesthesia, as distal circulation will be especially sluggish. These may be followed by not more than four deep breaths to ensure full expansion of the lungs and pumping action on the inferior vena cava. If a general anaesthetic has been given, the mother may have extra secretions and needs to be taught how to clear them by coughing in a sitting position with the sutures supported by both hands or a pillow. Deep breathing and huffing will help to loosen the secretions.

To ease backache and flatulence the *abdominal tightening*, *pelvic tilting* and *knee rolling* exercises can be practised gently after 24 hours.

Mothers will progress to the *pelvic floor exercise*, *curl-ups* and *hip hitching* when they feel more comfortable, usually after 4–5 days if there is no undue separation of the rectus muscles. Pelvic floor exercises are still important following a caesarean section even though one recent research study has shown that women in this group are less likely to suffer stress incontinence (Wilson 1996).

Adequate rest is essential postnatally to allow the tissues to regain their normal function. After a caesarean section the woman has not only given birth but has also undergone major surgery yet she still has to cope with her baby. The midwife must take every opportunity to remind relatives of the need to help with chores and the organisation of rest periods for the mother.

Care of the back postnatally

It may take up to 6 months before the ligaments completely resume their normal functions (Polden & Mantle 1990) so it is vital that mothers receive advice on back care in relation to everyday activities at this time.

When feeding, the mother should sit back in a chair, well supported, with the baby raised up on pillows to prevent a slouched forward position. Nappy changing and bathing are best carried out at waist level or with the mother kneeling at a surface at coffee-table height.

Lifting should be avoided if at all possible but if unavoidable the object should be as light as possible and kept close to the body. The knees are bent and the back must be kept straight (Fig. 45.5).

Resuming sporting activities

The postnatal exercises shown are safe and effective and need to be practised regularly and increased gradually. Brayshaw & Wright (1996) illustrate further postnatal exercises which are a natural progression before resuming more strenuous prepregnancy activities. Walking, cycling and swimming will increase general fitness but more strenuous keep-fit exercises, aerobics and competitive sports are best left until 10–12 weeks after delivery and then only resumed after ensuring that the pelvic floor muscles are functioning effectively. *Double-leg-lifts* (Fig. 45.14) *and sit-ups should never be performed.*

IMMEDIATE POSTNATAL PHYSICAL PROBLEMS

Diastasis symphysis pubis or symphysis pubis dysfunction

This condition may be present in late pregnancy, occur during labour or appear after delivery (Fry 1992). If the pain is severe, indicating complete separation of the pubic joint, complete bedrest

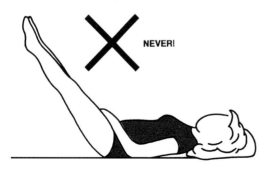

NEVER!

Fig. 45.14 Never attempt double-leg-lifts.

with some support around the level of the pubis is advised. The woman must be instructed to press her knees together when moving in bed. She should be encouraged to perform the abdominal tightening and pelvic tilting exercises plus circulatory exercises whilst she is resting. The obstetric physiotherapist may provide therapeutic ultrasound, TENS or ice to relieve local pain. Mobilisation of the woman should progress gently, only when the acute pain has subsided.

Diastasis recti

If, after performing the rectus check, it is found that the woman's rectus muscles are more than two fingers' width apart, the only exercises which should be prescribed are abdominal tightening and pelvic tilting with head lifting (see p. 881). The latter can be performed with the woman's own hands crossed over the abdomen to support the muscles and draw them towards the midline.

Painful perineum

To reduce pain, advice on positioning should be given plus analgesia and local pain-relieving agencies such as ice, therapeutic ultrasound or pulsed electromagnetic energy. These latter two may only be administered by a physiotherapist. To avoid the possibility of a burn, ice should not be in direct contact with the skin. Instead it may be crushed and placed inside a polythene bag or gauze and positioned against the painful area for no longer than 5–10 minutes. The woman will be most comfortable in side-lying and should be reminded not to sit on the ice-pack as the pressure would impede the circulation. Alternatively the perineum may be massaged for 5–10 minutes by an ice cube held in a disposable cloth. When the pain is less, pelvic floor exercises should be encouraged with the aim of increasing the local circulation and easing the weight off the painful area.

Incontinence

The most common type of postnatal incontinence is stress incontinence. Pelvic floor exercises will help to rehabilitate the pelvic floor, but the woman should be advised to seek a referral to an obstetric physiotherapist if the problem persists.

Backache

Early postnatal backache is usually postural and can be relieved by warmth and pelvic tilting exercises. A woman with persistent and severe back pain should be referred for physiotherapy.

Coccydynia

An acutely painful coccyx is incapacitating for a new mother. Pillows may be placed strategically to give some relief in sitting and advice on alternative positions for feeding should be given. An obstetric physiotherapist can administer therapeutic ultrasound or pulsed electromagnetic energy with beneficial effects or may manipulate a persistently displaced coccyx.

CONCLUSION

During pregnancy, labour and the puerperium, midwives and other health care professionals have many opportunities to influence parents-to-be, incorporating a sensible approach to exercise within the broader sphere of healthy routines for all family members. Relaxation, walking, cycling, swimming and other forms of exercise should be encouraged as part of a general lifestyle. Specific exercises for strengthening pelvic floor and abdominal muscles or relieving aches and pains, e.g. cramp or back-

ache, will have relevance far beyond the months of child bearing. Parents-to-be are an extremely receptive audience. These opportunities to develop both specific and general health care measures should not be missed.

READER ACTIVITIES

1. In any one day, write down all the stressful situations you have experienced.

2. Observe others in stressful situations and note how the stress manifests itself.

3. Practise physiological relaxation, repeating the instructions until you no longer need to read them. Teach your staffroom colleagues the method at lunch-time and explain the theory behind it.

4. Perform each of the exercises in the ante- and postnatal sections. Memorise the instructions until you are ready to teach colleagues or family.

5. Write down why, how, when and how many times each exercise should be performed and also the best position in which to do it.

6. Advise a colleague on the basics of good back care in all positions.

REFERENCES

ACPWH 1995 Aquanatal guidelines. Association of Chartered Physiotherapists in Women's Health, London

Bø K 1995 Pelvic floor muscle exercise for the treatment of stress urinary incontinence: an exercise physiology perspective. International Urogynecology Journal 6: 282–291

Brayshaw E, Wright P 1994 Teaching physical skills for the childbearing year. Books for Midwives Press, Hale

Brayshaw E, Wright P 1996 Relaxation and exercise for the childbearing year. Books for Midwives Press, Hale

Bullock J E, Jull G A, Bullock M I 1987 The relationship of low back pain to postural changes during pregnancy. Australian Journal of Physiotherapy 33(1): 10–17

Bump R C, Hurt W H, Fanti J A, Wyman J F 1991 Assessment of Kegel muscle exercise performance after brief verbal instruction. American Journal of Obstetrics and Gynecology 165: 322–329

Bush A 1992 Cardiopulmonary effects of pregnancy and labour. Journal of the Association of Chartered Physiotherapists in Obstetrics and Gynaecology 71: 3–4

Caldeyro-Barcia R 1978 The influence of maternal position on labour and the influence of maternal bearing-down efforts in the second stage of labour on fetal well-being. In: Simpkin P, Reinke C (eds) Kaleidoscope of childbearing preparation, birth and nurturing. Pennypress, Seattle

Clapp J 1990 The course of labour after endurance exercise during pregnancy. American Journal of Obstetrics and Gynecology 163(6): 1799–1805

Fry D 1992 Diastasis symphysis pubis. Journal of the Association of Chartered Physiotherapists in Obstetrics and Gynaecology 71: 10–13

Gilpin S A, Gosling J A, Smith A R B, Warrell D W 1989 The pathogenesis of genitourinary prolapse and stress incontinence of urine. A histological and histochemical study. British Journal of Obstetrics and Gynaecology 96: 15–23

Hodges P W, Richardson C A 1995 Dysfunction of transversus abdominis associated with chronic low back pain. MPAA Conference Proceedings, Queensland, pp 61–62

Huch R, Erkkola R 1990 Pregnancy and exercise, exercise and pregnancy: a short review. British Journal of Obstetrics and Gynaecology 97: 208–214

Jacobson B, Smith A, Whitehead M 1991 The nation's health: a strategy for the 1990s. King's Fund, London

McMurray R G, Berry M J, Katz V 1990 The beta endorphin responses of pregnant women during aerobic exercise in the water. Medicine and Science in Sports and Exercise 22(3): 298–301

Mantle M J, Greenwood R M, Currey H L F 1977 Backache in pregnancy. Rheumatological Rehabilitation, 16: 95–110

Noble E 1988 Essential exercises for the childbearing year, 3rd edn. Houghton Mifflin, Boston

Polden M, Mantle J 1990 Physiotherapy in obstetrics and gynaecology. Butterworth-Heinemann, London

Revelli A, Durando A, Massobrio M 1992 Exercise and pregnancy: a review of maternal and fetal effects. Obstetrical and Gynecological Survey 47(6): 355–367

Richardson C A, Jull G A 1995 Muscle control – pain control. What exercises would you prescribe? Manual Therapy 1: 2–10

Roberts J E, Mendez-Bauer C, Wodell D A 1983 The effects of maternal position on uterine contractility and efficiency. Birth 10: 243–249

Wilson P D 1996 Obstetric practice and the prevention of urinary incontinence. British Journal of Obstetrics and Gynaecology 103: 154–161

FURTHER READING

Brayshaw E, Wright P 1994 Teaching physical skills for the childbearing year. Books for Midwives Press, Hale

Brayshaw E, Wright P 1996 Relaxation and exercise for the childbearing year. Books for Midwives Press, Hale

Campion M J 1990 The baby challenge: a handbook on pregnancy for women with a physical disability. Routledge, London

Mitchell L 1987 Simple relaxation. John Murray, London

Polden M, Whiteford B 1991 The postnatal exercise book. Frances Lincoln, London

VIDEOTAPES

BBC Pregnancy and Postnatal Exercise Video 1991 (Ashton J, Conley R, Polden M) BBC Publications

Y Plan Before and After Pregnancy Video 1991 (Gaskell J, Jennings M) London Central YMCA

NB: *The books suggested in the further reading list and the videotapes can be obtained from the Association of Chartered Physiotherapists in Women's Health (ACPWH) * Book Secretary, c/o CSP, 14 Bedford Row, London WC1R 4ED.*

*Formerly Association of Chartered Physiotherapists in Obstetrics and Gynaecology (ACPOG).

46

Community health and
social services

Chris McCourt

A midwife needs knowledge of community health and social services for three main reasons: to appreciate better the social context of health and how this impinges on her or his role as a health service provider; to be able to advise a woman appropriately about other services which may be helpful for her; and to refer appropriately to other services when their input would be beneficial.

The chapter aims to:

- discuss community health and social services in the context of a broad theoretical understanding of health and illness

- provide information which will be useful for midwives in key areas of these services

- discuss the principles, structures, policies and practices which influence the character of each

- provide a framework for continuing learning, updating of relevant information and developing local knowledge and networks.

INTRODUCTION

The factors influencing the health of mothers and children are broad and complex. Their impact begins long before pregnancy and will continue long after a woman's discharge from the maternity services. Community health and social services, therefore, play an important role in the cycles of family life in many societies. Social services, community- and hospital-based health services have been through several phases of integration and separation in the UK, since their establishment in the early part of this century. Currently, they are provided under quite separate institutional arrangements but much of recent health policy has focused on developing more 'seamless' models for providing care. To some extent, these policy changes and the structures described in this chapter are products of our tendency to view health within a narrow and mechanistic framework. In consequence, health, social and other personal services, hospital- and community-based services are categorised separately, so that effort is then needed to piece them back together. The boundaries in many of the issues discussed in this chapter are fuzzy and should be so, since that is the way health and illness are influenced and experienced by people, as part of their lives.

The importance of viewing maternal and child health in its social context

It is a common but misplaced assumption that the provision of health care is mainly responsible for our health. Evidence from a range of research disciplines, including epidemiology, social science and natural sciences indicates that health should be viewed much more as an ecological concept; it is a product of many factors including living environment and conditions, nutrition, occupation and education. The health of mothers receiving maternity care, and of their babies, is most likely to be influenced by such issues as their nutritional status, their housing and working conditions and the level of social support they can call on, so that the role of maternity services is additional and relatively short term. Midwives cannot change many of these issues but must work with them and may often be involved in assisting the woman in ameliorating or coping with the effects of social and economic circumstances on her health.

The importance of the social context on women's health is reflected particularly clearly in the different social class patterns of health (Townsend et al 1988, Whitehead 1987). A key example of this is birthweight; this is a useful indicator, since it is readily measurable, and is an important predictor of future health status (Oakley 1992). Although it may at first sight seem to be an indisputably physiological matter, research shows that low birthweight is strongly associated with poverty, inequality and lack of social support. The physical health of the mother will have been influenced by similar factors, which have a very long-term effect. Birthweight is a good example of the multifaceted

nature of health as well as the importance of social context on health.

What is meant by community?

Community is a very broad term which is currently widely used in policy developments in Euro-American societies. It is attractive partly because of its rather open definition which can encompass a range of ideas. Generally, community is identified along three dimensions: place, relationships and sentiment or sense of belonging (Luker & Orr 1985, Turton & Orr 1993). All contribute something to the concept, but the degree of importance attached to each is variable. When discussing health and social services, these aspects of community are all relevant but community tends to be defined by service providers very much in service terms, i.e. the location of a service, the way in which it is delivered and its scale. Popular images of community care often take it to mean care provided at home, rather than in an institution of some type, and provided by family, friends or neighbours rather than professionals or paid workers. To clarify these different concepts of community care – with very different implications for social policy – Bulmer (1987) drew a distinction between care 'in' the community and care 'by' the community, mostly care provided unpaid by friends, kin or neighbours, which is also referred to by service providers as 'informal' care.

The different areas of health services

Historically, the role of medicine has in many respects been peripheral to the concerns of public health, since it is mainly responsive to disease and concerned with the diagnosis and treatment of ill health (McKeown 1979, Stacey 1988). This is reflected in the separation of different health-related activities into the institutional spheres of social services, hospital services and community health services. Before the health service reorganisation of 1974 in the UK, domiciliary midwives were employed by local authorities while hospital midwives (who were gradually increasing in numbers as more and more care took place in hospitals) were employed by health authorities (Robinson

1990). Until this point, domiciliary or community midwives were in closer contact with the Medical Officer of Health, who was responsible for public health in a local area, since community health and social services were combined.

Maternity care, and particularly midwifery, occupies a different role from much of conventional health care, since childbirth is an important life event and transition, and pregnant women are generally understood to be healthy people, requiring care and observation for possible problems, rather than curative treatment. Nonetheless, in the latter half of the 20th century, maternity services in the UK and other industrialised countries have been organised increasingly along the lines of acute medical services, based mainly in hospitals, with women routinely referred to them by their general practitioners (Hunt & Symonds 1995). Women are generally categorised into those deemed high or low risk, on an agreed set of medical indicators. Care for women classified as of 'low risk' is then in many cases referred back to community health services – the GP and midwife – for shared care. Midwives have been divided along similar lines into those working in hospitals and those working mainly in the community. The latter have tended in recent years in the UK to provide mainly antenatal and postnatal care, while also caring for the small proportion of home and 'domino' births. Following the *Changing Childbirth* report (DH 1993a), a number of services in the UK have moved towards greater integration of community- and hospital-based midwifery, for example, through caseload practice (Flint 1993, Page 1995).

The midwife's role in relation to community health and social services

Since midwives specialise in the care of normal pregnancy and birth, they are in a good position to provide general care and support to the woman during a period of great personal and social adjustment as well as physical change. In addition to clinical skills, midwives provide information and advice and, in many cases, social support. Such a role has the potential to provide a positive impact on the general health and well-being of women and their families during a period of change and

development. Midwifery care is relatively short term, and arrangements for care do not always facilitate continuity of carer, but interventions during certain critical periods may have a long-term impact, however small. A good example of this is in the midwife's role in health promotion and in supporting women in feeding their babies (Crafter 1997).

When a woman needs more general sources of advice and social support than those provided through the maternity services, midwives may still play a key role in providing relevant information and advice and in referring her to other professionals and organisations for support. This role is underpinned by:

- developing and updating broad health knowledge
- developing local community knowledge and contacts
- reflection and awareness of one's own impact as a practitioner.

THE STRUCTURE AND ROLE OF COMMUNITY HEALTH AND SOCIAL SERVICES

As indicated in the introduction to this chapter, the structure of these services has been subject to a number of policy changes and varies from one country to another. The structure of the health service is described in more detail in Chapter 47.

The origins of the current system

Prior to 1946 in the UK, health and social services were largely privately paid for or charitable. The Poor Law had been the main instrument for caring for people who were disabled, chronically ill or destitute, and its operation had become punitive over time in order to discourage people from claiming relief. The 19th century, with rapid industrialisation and urbanisation, saw the growth of hospitals as places to provide health care, but it was not until the 20th century that hospitals came to be seen as a desirable option in care for women giving birth (Donnison 1988). The foundations of the current welfare and health system were set down in the years following the Second World War and were in many ways responding to the enormous social changes taking place at that time. The NHS Act 1946 created the National Health Service, with free health care provided according to perceived need, while the National Assistance Act 1948 replaced the Poor Law with a system of means-tested welfare benefits and a duty for local authorities to provide residential care for elderly and disabled people in need and those who were temporarily homeless due to unforeseen circumstances. At this point, the emphasis was very much on creating the institutional structures for welfare and relatively little attention was given to community-based services, that is, supports to people living in their own homes (Clements 1996).

Health services

Between 1974 and 1993 in the UK, health authorities were the main providers of health services, incorporating hospitals and some community services, such as community midwifery. After the NHS and Community Care Act 1990, their role became mainly one of planning and contracting for care on behalf of the local population, although they have maintained responsibility for direct provision of some services, especially those based in community settings. Hospitals, and some community-based services such as those for people with long-term care needs, developed NHS Trust status, working independently within the health service and, in theory at least, competing with other service providers. Until recently, their planning and development role was overseen by a higher layer of Regional Health Authorities. These have been superseded by what are known as NHS Management Executive Regional Offices which are mainly responsible for research and for strategic levels of planning and development. The structures are likely to shift increasingly towards primary care planning and provision of services (DH 1997). For a more detailed account of the development and structure of these services, see Chapter 47.

Local authorities

Local authorities have a key role in planning, monitoring and developing services for the needs of the local community in a range of departments, including education, social services, housing and environmental services. As we have seen, all these areas have an influence on health, giving the Local Authority a potentially powerful role in enhancing the health and welfare of its population. In practice, the different departments have not always worked together effectively in a health-promoting role, partly because the health implications of such public services have been under-recognised.

Since the NHS and Community Care Act 1990, these authorities, like health authorities, have been given a more strategic role in planning services for local needs and purchasing these from independent service providers as well as continuing to provide them where appropriate. Knowledge of local authority social services is the most relevant for midwives, since social services departments have legal duties to assess people's needs for support in the community and to provide or arrange for services which are assessed as being needed.

The Benefits Agency (BA)

The Benefits Agency works at national level on behalf of the UK government's Department of Social Security. It assesses needs for financial support, in line with national legislation, and provides payments, exemption certificates and loans where appropriate. It is responsible for the administration of maternity benefits of various types. Local offices and telephone lines are provided for information and enquiries.

THE LEGAL FRAMEWORK

Community health and social services operate within a legal framework (Acts of Parliament) set out by Government. Local and health authorities are provided with guidance to follow in interpreting and implementing the legislation. Guidance is normally mandatory, for example Executive Letters issued by the Department of Health, while guidelines are advisory (e.g. good practice guides), to assist with the complexities of putting policy into practice. UK legislation also operates within the overarching framework of European (EU) legislation and policy directives and is increasingly expected to develop in line with this framework.

Relevant legislation

The main relevant legislation in the UK is currently as follows:

• the NHS and Community Care Act 1990 – which sets out the framework for community health and social services and duties of local authorities
• the Housing Act 1977 – which established Local Authority Housing Departments with a duty to provide housing for homeless people in certain circumstances (and as amended by subsequent Housing Acts)
• the Disabled Persons Services, Consultation and Representation Act 1986 – which set out the rights of disabled people to receive assessment for community services
• the Disability Discrimination Act 1995
• the Race Relations Act 1976 – which established rights for people of different ethnic groups for protection against discrimination of various forms
• the Children Act 1989 – which replaced the previous confusing array of legislation around the welfare and protection of children
• the Mental Health Act 1983 – which provides a framework for services for people with mental health problems, including community services and the terms under which people in distress can be admitted to hospital or treated without their consent and the rules and procedures for discharge from compulsory admissions.

The central piece of legislation for practitioners is the NHS and Community Care Act 1990, since it sets out a general framework and policy for how health and social services should work. Its key aims were to integrate the different services better and to improve organisation of services for people with care needs, particularly since many services are now community based. Many health problems have long-term consequences and needs for support are not easily divided into health and social care needs. The local authority social services are responsible for assessing the overall community health and care needs of its population and producing regular community care plans.

Care management

Under this Act, anyone who comes to the attention of the local authority as having possible needs for support is entitled to an assessment, followed, where appropriate, by a plan for care, which may include a 'package' of services. This approach is referred to as *care management*. The principle of care assessment is that the needs of the person should be central and services should be sought to respond to these needs, rather than fitting people into the services. In this way, its aims are in line with the *Changing Childbirth* principle of woman-centred care (DH 1993a). This is not always achieved in practice, however, not only because of financial constraints but owing to the difficulties practitioners have in imagining different responses to people's needs and the slow progress in getting used to involving people more in decisions about their care.

A midwife can request or assist a woman or family with care needs in requesting a care assessment. The needs for support – and the possible solutions – can be quite wide ranging, including 'home help' or additional child care. Assessment should involve the woman, her family where appropriate, and all relevant professionals, who may include the community midwife. If she is considered to have care needs, a *care manager* will be appointed to ensure that adequate and suitable support services are arranged. These can be long or short term. Care managers are often social workers but they may be other professionals (including home care organisers, community nurses or midwives) according to the nature of the individual's needs.

A time frame for undertaking assessments is not specified, but some cases are responded to as emergencies and services can be provided on this basis while awaiting a proper assessment. It is important to try to anticipate needs (such as a woman needing home help after birth) well in advance and encourage the woman to make an application. Services may be charged for on a means-tested basis and there is considerable variation in this according to where people live.

Needs for care are not tightly defined because they are meant to be broad, but generally the policy is aimed at people (adults and children) who have disabilities, chronic health problems or mental health problems or who care for people with such problems. Pregnant women and those who have recently given birth are included. Those who are providing regular and substantial care for friends or relatives, informal carers, are entitled to a linked assessment of how they are affected by their caring responsibilities (Clements 1996, Dimond 1997).

Requesting a care assessment: case study
During a routine antenatal visit in the community, a woman who is considered to be 'of high obstetric risk' informs you, as community midwife, that she wants a home birth. After discussion of her request, you learn that the main reason for her preference is concern about the welfare of her older children while she is in hospital. She has no reliable source of support and does not feel able to leave them in the care of their father.

How will you respond to this situation? Consider:

- how you will discuss and consider the woman's needs with her
- what information you need to gather
- which sources will be useful
- which colleagues or other professionals you will contact and why
- how assistance could be obtained to support her.

MATERNITY RIGHTS AND BENEFITS

In most countries, women are entitled to a series of benefits and have particular rights during pregnancy and childbirth regarding employment. Midwives are in an ideal position to advise women of their general rights and entitlements and to respond in a timely fashion to requests for information. Many women will not be familiar with these or they may not know whom to approach for advice. Midwives can offer relevant outline information on rights and benefits and on where to go for further help.

Although the overall framework of rights and benefits is relatively stable, details may change from year to year, so that it is important to stay equipped with up-to-date booklets and leaflets. A checklist of sources of information and advice is important, as is regular renewal of the forms and information leaflets provided by the Benefits Agency. For these reasons, it is crucial not to rely simply on a textbook, but the section below summarises the current system of rights and benefits in the UK.

Maternity rights

Women's rights at work are set out in UK law and in EU directives. Where the two differ, UK law is generally expected to comply with EU directives, unless it provides for greater rights. Maternity rights also operate within the broader framework of employment and discrimination law (Palmer 1996). They include employment protection, health and safety, paid time off for health care and rights to return to work (see Box 46.1). Detailed information on maternity rights is available in the booklet PL958 Maternity Rights available from job centres.

Maternity benefits

These include monetary and non-monetary benefits (benefits in kind or exemptions).

The key monetary benefits related to maternity are set out in Box 46.2. The changes in family circumstances due to childbirth may also mean changes in entitlement for those families which rely on housing benefit, family credit or income support because of low incomes. Generally, each additional child increases entitlement and may sometimes mean the difference between qualifying for a benefit or not. Since women may seek advice on any of these benefits, or general advice about coping with new economic demands, it is important to obtain a full set of advice leaflets (see Box 46.3). Entitlements and benefits are liable to change from one year to another owing to legal and policy changes as well as inflationary

Box 46.1 UK maternity and employment rights 1997 – key points (Palmer 1996)

Protection of employment
A woman with a contract of employment cannot be dismissed from her job for being pregnant or on maternity leave. She maintains general employment rights including protection against discrimination.

Health and safety
Employers are responsible for ensuring health and safety at work for women who are pregnant or breast feeding, or, if not practicable, must provide suitable alternative work or suspension on full pay.

Leave
A woman is entitled to paid leave for antenatal health care, including home visits and parent education or preparation classes. An employer may request verification of appointments. All employees are entitled to *maternity leave* for a minimum of 14 weeks, which can start from the birth or at any time from 29 weeks of pregnancy. Those who have been in continuous employment for a minimum of 2 years are entitled to *extended absence* of up to 29 weeks from the week of actual birth.

Right to return
A woman has a right to return to her previous job, on no less favourable terms, provided she complies with limited conditions of notice and returns within the statutory periods of leave. There are some limited exceptions to this rule.

Box 46.2 Monetary maternity benefits – 1997 (Palmer 1996, Benefits Agency form FB8)

Statutory Maternity Pay (SMP)
This is an allowance payable to women in continuous employment and earning above the statutory limit for National Insurance contributions for 26 weeks before the *qualifying week* (15 weeks before the expected week of confinement (EWC)). Payment is at a level equivalent to 90% of earnings for 6 weeks followed by 12 weeks at a lower rate, set annually, and can commence at any time from 11 weeks before the EWC, or earlier if the baby has been born. It is administered by employers, who must be given 3 weeks' notice of the intended date for taking leave.
  Many employers, especially large organisations, operate more generous schemes than the statutory minimum. The woman should check these terms and whether they apply to her with her employer or personnel department in good time.

Maternity Allowance
This is paid to women not entitled to SMP but who have paid National Insurance contributions during the *qualifying period* (currently 26 of the 66 weeks preceding the qualifying week). It is paid weekly for 18 weeks, at a level comparable to the lower rate of SMP. Application must be made on form MA1 accompanied by forms MATB1 and SMP1 (which is issued by the employer) from 26 weeks of pregnancy and before leaving work.

The Social Fund
Women who receive income support or family credit can claim a single payment to assist in the costs of a new baby. The grant is payable from 29 weeks of pregnancy and must be claimed before the baby is 3 months old. The Social Fund claim form must be accompanied by form MATB1 or B2.

Child Benefit
All primary carers of children under 16 (or in full-time education until 19) are entitled to Child Benefit. It is payable for each child, with a higher rate for the first child and for lone parents. The Child Benefit claim form must be accompanied by the child's birth certificate.

---

increases in benefit levels, so it is important to update all leaflets, and one's own information sources, annually.

Checking entitlements

If in doubt, women should be advised to check their entitlement. Up-to-date details of benefits and entitlements can be obtained by using the relevant Benefits Agency helpline, a freephone number listed in telephone directories, or an independent advice agency. Some local authorities employ welfare rights advisors who have in-depth knowledge of rights and benefits and who can undertake case work where needed.

Pregnant and childbearing women are also entitled to a range of non-monetary benefits, some of which are *universal* (i.e. all are entitled) while others are only available to those who are entitled to income support or family credit. They include:

- for all women: free prescriptions and dental care in pregnancy and for 1 year after birth
- for those receiving income support: free milk (in the form of tokens) and vitamins
- for those receiving family credit: reduced-cost baby milk and vitamins (available from child health clinics).

Forms and certificates to be supplied by the midwife or GP

Midwives or GPs are responsible for providing the certificates that the woman will need to exercise her employment rights and claim relevant benefits. These include:

- proof of *expected date of confinement:* form MATB1, which is issued at 26 weeks of pregnancy
- *certificate of confinement*: form MATB2
- form MA1: for application for statutory maternity pay or maternity allowance
- form FW8: for exemptions from prescription and related charges.

READER ACTIVITY

The checklists given in Boxes 46.3 and 46.4 will help in raising awareness of how to access and update the information a midwife needs for giving advice or referral to specialist advisors. The information is summarised in Form FB8 'Babies and Benefits' which also provides a clear checklist on what to do at each stage of pregnancy and maternity leave, information on where to get advice and help on a wide range of benefits, and an order form for further leaflets. The boxes can be copied for completion as a training exercise for students, for regular review of information sources and as a ready reminder of where to go for information. Key leaflets are now available in a range of languages.

THE COMMUNITY HEALTH SERVICES

Community health services encompass what is generally known as primary health care, which is based on the GP practice. They include community-based services for health promotion, such as child health clinics and school health services and for longer-term health needs, such as mental health centres. Since the 1970s, policy has favoured the development of health centres and primary care teams, based in larger GP practices, to provide these services. Although GP practices may employ professionals such as practice nurses or counsellors, members of primary care teams in many cases practise quite separately, under different

Box 46.3 Benefits leaflet checklist

Form	For:	Obtained from:
FB2		
NI17A		
FB22		
CH1/CH11		
FC1		
CSA2001		
IS1/IS20		
WMV:G1		
SF100		

employing organisations and have limited liaison or knowledge of each other's roles (Bowling 1981). The primary care team, therefore, remains an ideal concept in many areas. Despite these difficulties in developing interprofessional care, the philosophy relates closely to the reality of health needs, which do not fit easily into professional or organisational categories. This is acknowledged in the 1997 Government proposal to introduce primary care groups (DH 1997).

The general practitioner and the GP practice

General practitioners provide much of the everyday health care for families and act as the key gatekeepers for secondary health care. General practitioners are independent professionals, who contracted in to the health service after its inception in 1946, while maintaining much of their independent status. They receive a fee from their local Health Authority based on the number of patients on their list, plus some allowances for

Box 46.4 Advice and information checklist

	Relevant numbers
Benefits Agency helpline	
Benefits Agency local office	
Citizens' Advice Bureau (local office)	
Welfare Rights Officer	
Law Centre	
Community Health Council	
Local authority/neighbourhood office	
Interpreting or language advice service	
Other useful agencies	

ancillary work and for particular areas of work such as health screening, maternity care and contraceptive services. Although their fee structure reflects recent health service emphasis on improving preventive health care, the fact that additional fees are received suggests that historically, this has not been seen as a core part of their work. This structure is likely to change with the advent of primary care groups and more emphasis on designing services around the needs of the local population (DH 1997; see also Ch. 47).

GPs share their basic medical training with other doctors, and undergo 6 months of general obstetric training plus 18 months of general community training before acceptance by the Royal College of General Practitioners, their professional body. The extent of community training they undergo is likely to increase in the future owing to demand for longer and more relevant training from GPs themselves.

General practitioners and maternity care

In the early part of the 20th century GPs had little involvement in maternity care, since birth was largely managed by midwives and regular antenatal care was not established. Many women could not afford a doctor's fees and some doctors, in any case, had arrangements with local midwives, delegating care for uncomplicated births (Leap 1993, Robinson 1990). After increasing in importance during the century, the role of GPs in childbirth in particular has declined since the 1970s, so that GPs now express concern about losing their skills in maternity care. The Peel Report (MoH 1970) and the Short Report (House of Commons 1980) advocated a shift of all maternity services to consultant-led hospital units and the closure of small GP-led units or cottage hospitals, despite lack of research evidence on the relative safety of different places of birth to support this (Tew 1990). Much of current maternity care is offered as 'shared care', shared between the consultant and the general practitioner, but communication between obstetricians and GPs tends to be nominal in this system and much of the hands-on care, in both locations, is given by midwives. Except where GP units remain, or where a GP has a particular interest in birth, GPs are now mainly involved

in antenatal care, which they may share with a practice-linked community or caseload midwife.

Following the NHS and Community Care Act 1990, a number of larger practices were given fundholding status, allowing them to purchase services for their patients directly from health service providers. GP fundholding was not applied to the provision of maternity care, but the Department of Health funded a series of pilot schemes in 1995, following publication of *Changing Childbirth* (DH 1993a), to explore the possibilities for GP practice purchasing of services. The 1996 Government White Paper, *The National Health Service: a service with ambitions* (NHSME 1996), continued the trend indicated by *Changing Childbirth* in its emphasis on primary health care and promised to shift the balance of funding in future away from acute, hospital-based care, to reflect more closely the balance of health care needs. The new strategy for the health services (DH 1997) may provide an opportunity for GPs and midwives to develop community-based services in partnership. This new policy is described in more detail in the next chapter.

Health visitors and child health services

Health visitors specialise in health promotion and advice for families with children under 5 and, sometimes, older people. The health visitor's role can, however, be applied to the positive or preventive health needs of the local community in general. It is distinguished from that of the GP in that it focuses on health education and prevention of ill health rather than responding to illness and so is proactive – looking for health needs – rather than reactive. The health visitor tends to work, therefore, with people who do not define themselves as ill, and who are not actively seeking health care. Four key principles of health visiting were outlined in 1977 and confirmed by the Health Visitors' Association and the Standing Conference on Health Visitor Education in 1992:

* the search for health needs
* stimulation of awareness of health needs
* influence on policies affecting health
* facilitation of health-enhancing activities (Turton & Orr 1993).

According to these principles, health visiting means working with communities and taking political action, in addition to working with individuals and families, but in practice, the collective aspects of their role have been less well developed, perhaps because of their origins, or the general tendency for health to be viewed in a narrow sense and for health education to focus on individual behaviour.

Health visitors are qualified nurses who may have approved maternity care training or a midwifery qualification and who undertake further, college-based, training for 12 months, plus 9 weeks of supervised health visitor practice. Health visiting in the UK had its origins in the 19th century social reform movement which was a response to the problems of rapid industrialisation, urbanisation and poverty (Robertson 1988). Concerns about public health also led to moves to improve general sanitation (especially sewerage and water supply) and housing conditions, so that the most important moves towards improving public health and decreasing the high mortality due to infectious diseases were set in place as a result of careful observation of living conditions, before the precise mechanisms of infection were understood (McKeown 1979). Modern health visitors continue this public health role but since living conditions for many people have improved and mortality has declined, it has focused increasingly on psychosocial care as well as the more traditional concepts of public health. The current framework for health visiting was set out in the Nurses, Midwives and Health Visitors Act 1979. Their role, like that of midwives, is overseen by the United Kingdom Central Council for Nursing, Midwifery and Health Visiting (UKCC). (See also Ch. 9.)

Health visitors visit families to give advice or support and run health clinics which parents can visit for checks on young children's development and progress, general advice with baby and child care and health and immunisations. In some areas, depending on workload, health visitors visit women during pregnancy to offer health advice and preparation for parenthood, or provide parent education classes jointly with community midwives. They may also play a role in care management and assessment, and in providing preventive support or referral for problems such as postnatal depression or parenting problems.

After a baby's birth, the midwife or another professional present at the birth completes a birth notification form which notifies the Registrar of births and deaths and triggers the production of a set of child health records. The health visitor undertakes a primary visit around 10–28 days following the birth (i.e. the point at which local midwifery services discharge most women from their care). The parents are given a child health record book to keep, given general information about community health services and invited to visit the child health clinic regularly.

This broad possible remit of health visitors, including screening, health education and prevention roles for the local population gives them a less clearly defined professional identity than some other health professionals and despite the importance of the social context of health which we have noted, their role has been questioned in recent years (Baker et al 1987). They are increasingly encouraged to work with existing or potential social support networks, rather than to attempt to provide all support themselves or adopt the role of experts. This connects to a wider debate about the nature and effectiveness of health education and promotion programmes. For example, the effectiveness of routine screening programmes such as child development checks has been questioned, and more selective programmes have been suggested with greater attention to parents' observations and knowledge of their children (Hall Report (Hall 1989, 1991) – discussed in Turton & Orr 1993). Like other community health professionals, health visitors have to balance potentially conflicting roles of providing support and monitoring or surveillance of families. Such dilemmas are faced most acutely when considering child protection issues.

Health education and preventive health care

While community health services such as health visiting and midwifery aim to focus on preventive health care, they differ from much of the health services that are provided in industrialised countries, which tend to react to ill health and favour acute care in terms of expenditure. They also encounter the basic problems confronting health professionals in attempting to provide health education and preventive care by anticipating or looking for health needs. While advice is often welcomed and valued, particularly during pregnancy and the early days of child care, it may also be viewed by some women as an unwarranted interference in their lives.

Preventive health care has been described as operating on three levels:

- primary: before a disease process starts, e.g. immunisation or advice on nutrition or accident prevention
- secondary: to alleviate or arrest disease, e.g. screening, early diagnosis and treatment, dental checks
- tertiary: to limit or alleviate the effects of disease or illness, e.g. rehabilitation.

Health education is relevant at all levels of prevention, but is particularly aimed towards preventing the initial development of ill health. Pregnancy and adaptation to parenthood are important life changes and a time when adults are particularly responsive to information and often seek it out actively. Nonetheless, health education, as traditionally conceived, has the important limitation of tending to focus on individual lifestyles and desired behavioural changes, outside the context of the constraints on people's lives and the ways in which such conditions affect health. For example, the 'Health of the Nation' document (DH 1992a) formed the key statement of UK government policy in preventive health care. It set out clear priority areas and targets for reduction of morbidity and mortality, but it has been criticised for its emphasis on altering individuals' behaviour in the absence of structural changes to promote such behaviour or increase individual choices.

Noting this constraint, Crafter (1997) distinguishes *health education*, which largely involves working with individuals or groups to enhance or change knowledge, with the aim of helping people to make informed and positive health choices, from *health promotion*, a broader concept which recognises the importance of social and environ-

mental influences on health. To promote positive health, it is increasingly acknowledged that health education must work hand in hand with efforts to change the structural and environmental factors influencing health, either directly or through the choices people feel able to make. Principles for health education are set out internationally by the World Health Organization and these have shifted since the 1980s towards involving individuals and communities in planning and implementing health care. The *Ottawa Charter* for example, states:

> health promotion works through effective community action in setting priorities, making decisions, planning strategies and implementing them to achieve better health. At the heart of this process is the empowerment of communities, and the ownership and control of their own endeavours and destiny (WHO 1986, p. 1; quoted in Jones & Sidell 1997).

Immunisation

Immunisation is an important aspect of preventive health care globally and will be a topic of concern to many new parents. There are different forms of immunisation, but they all function through stimulation of the immune system in order to enhance resistance to a particular mechanism of infection. Vaccines are available for a range of diseases, some of which have severe symptoms (for example polio) while others are important for protection against congenital defects. Immunisation against rubella (German measles) is a good example of protecting a vulnerable group, namely pregnant women, by means of protecting the general population. While the disease only produces mild symptoms in children and adults, it has severe implications for early fetal development.

Immunisation has a dual role in public health:

- population protection: decreasing the incidence of an infectious disease in the general population
- individual protection: decreasing the individual's likelihood of contracting a disease or the severity of symptoms experienced where protection is not complete.

Although population protection is arguably the most important function of immunisation, epidemiologists have pointed out that, historically, its role in improving public health and decreasing mortality has been overestimated in relation to more general measures such as improved nutrition and sanitation (McKeown 1979).

A series of immunisations focusing on the most common and the most potentially damaging childhood illnesses is offered to all children in the UK from about 8 weeks of age. Since women may ask for advice about immunisation during their postnatal care, it is important to increase one's own knowledge of its benefits and limitations, recommended practice and contraindications for certain individuals. Women can be referred to their health visitor for detailed advice.

Since immunisations can, rarely, have serious side-effects, parents should always be advised about contraindications and precautions when they are encouraged to take up immunisation. Parents are particularly likely to raise questions about vaccinations which have been subject to controversy. The *pertussis* vaccine which protects against whooping cough led to concern regarding severe side-effects during the 1970s, which led to a significant fall in take-up rates. Subsequent studies have failed to confirm the level of risk conclusively, but policy documents emphasise the high level of risk from the disease itself in relation to possible vaccination risks. The combined *measles, mumps and rubella vaccine* (MMR), recently introduced as a mass immunisation programme in children below school age, has also been controversial, with some professionals arguing that the programme was speculative and unnecessary in view of possible side-effects. The complexity of influences on public health mean that definitive evidence on the benefits and risks of immunisation programmes is hard to obtain. Current policy remains that on the balance of evidence, the benefits to public and individual health outweigh possible risks (Charlish 1996, DH 1992c).

SOCIAL SERVICES

The local authority social services departments hold the main responsibility for community care arrangements, liaison with health services and support for specific needs and problems such as child care and protection, although the services arranged to meet such needs may be provided by a range of organisations. Facilities provided or contracted for by social services include home care, respite care and day and residential child care.

Social workers

Social workers play a key role in community care and also have specific statutory duties with respect to mental health and child protection. As care managers, they effectively act as gatekeepers to other services, such as home help or assistance with child care. They also provide direct support to clients, using a casework approach. Most social workers have a generic role which is concerned with a range of client groups and issues which will include children, elders and people with disabilities or mental health problems. Some work as specialists, particularly those working in hospital-based or multidisciplinary teams. This is more common in mental health social work, where some qualify as Approved Social Workers and are obliged to carry out statutory assessments under sections of the Mental Health Act 1983.

Social work, like health visiting, has its origins in social reform movements. Formal training was introduced relatively recently (training for generic work only began in 1964, although training for psychiatric social workers started at the London School of Economics in 1929) and was university-based from the start. The approach of social work in the UK today was laid out when local authority Social Services Departments were created, following the Seebohm Report, in 1970 (Clements 1996). The current social work qualification in the UK is the diploma in social work (DipSW) which is regarded as a degree level qualification. Prior work and life experience is highly valued and many social work students are mature.

The main areas of social work which are likely to be relevant to midwives' work are their child care and protection and their mental health roles. These roles operate within the frameworks of the Children Act 1989 and the Mental Health Act 1983.

Child protection and families needing support

In general, the aim of social services is to provide support to families which will help them to manage their situation and prevent the need for more extensive services or interventions. A good example of this would be the provision of respite care (care for short breaks), home care and aids and adaptations in the home for parents with a disabled child, which may avoid the need for residential care. These aims are not always met in practice owing to funding shortfalls or simply because of problems in coordination of services. Midwives can promote good practice by advising women of

their rights to apply for assessment for services and supporting them in the assessment process.

The Children Act 1989 focused on the needs of the child and emphasised that child care services or proceedings should always consider their welfare and interests as paramount. For example, it states that court orders should only be made where it is in the interests of the child to do so. The policy aims to support families so that they can remain together where possible and provides guidance on appropriate social service responses where this may not be in the interest of the child. It introduced the term *accommodation* (instead of care) where parents voluntarily seek residential care for their children and reformed the procedures for 'involuntary' care. It also replaced the concept of parental rights with that of *parental responsibility*.

The Children Act 1989 has helped to clarify child care policy generally by giving a clear definition of need:

> if he is unlikely to achieve or maintain, or to have the opportunity of achieving or maintaining a reasonable standard of health or development without the provision for him of services by a local authority;
>
> his health or development is likely to be significantly impaired, or further impaired, without the provision for him of such services;
>
> he is disabled (Children Act Section 17(10)).

This definition can help professionals to form a view of what children need to thrive, whatever their social or cultural background. When a child has needs by virtue of disability or other problems, Social Services Departments have a duty to respond. Since midwives have close contact with women and their families in the perinatal period, they may have an important role in identifying where families need additional support and advising those with special needs.

Child protection procedures

Midwives need some awareness of child protection procedures since they are likely to be in contact with families which pose serious concerns about the child's welfare. The distinction between need for support and need for child protection is a difficult one and in many situations, adequate and timely support for a family can prevent the need for child protection measures. The transition to parenthood is an important life event for all parents, and life events, even where they are wanted and viewed positively, can be major sources of stress and emotional distress (Marris 1974). Child care and adjustment to parenthood present a challenge to most parents and there is not a clear and simple line between those who are able or unable to cope with the demands of a new baby.

Care or supervision orders are only sought where there is concern about significant harm to the child. In cases of serious and urgent concern (for example, suspicion of serious non-accidental injury) anyone can apply for an *Emergency Protection Order*, which allows a limited period for the Social Services Department to remove a child from home or to keep him or her in a safe place, to assess the child's situation. In less urgent cases, an *Assessment Order* can be sought where there is concern and the child is repeatedly not produced for assessment. Where appropriate, such assessments will be followed by a strategy meeting and/or a case conference to consider the concerns and plan responses, as set out in the Children Act 1989 (DH 1991a). Case conferences are generally convened by social services child protection teams, who should inform and involve all relevant health professionals including the GP and, where appropriate, midwives.

Basic principles for the effective conduct of child protection procedures have been drawn from inquiries into child protection problems. They include:

- good and clear record-keeping
- communication between professionals
- listening to the child
- taking an open approach
- working with families where possible (DH 1991b).

Midwives may become concerned about potential child abuse antenatally, influenced by factors in the woman's history, her current mental state or her living situation. This may include concerns about domestic violence towards the woman herself. Antenatal care is a good point at which to work with women and to provide support, or assist the woman in obtaining the support she needs, in order to prevent possible problems arising after the baby is born.

When midwives are seriously concerned antenatally, or detect signs of possible abuse after a baby is born, procedures laid down by the local Area Child Protection Committee should be followed. In the first instance, concerns can be raised with the supervisor of midwives or with the named senior midwife with responsibility for child protection, who should ensure that the appropriate Social Services officers are contacted. In emergencies out-of-hours, police Child Protection Teams may be involved and in some areas, specialist child protection teams are provided by the National Society for the Prevention of Cruelty to Children (NSPCC). The midwives' codes of conduct and practice also provides basic guidelines to appropriate conduct (DH 1991b).

Identifying possible child abuse

Although there is no evidence that child abuse has increased over time, or that it is particular to certain cultures or social groups rather than others, public awareness and concern regarding abuse has increased in the recent past. Abuse is difficult to define and even more difficult to judge. It is equally challenging for professionals to define responses which are appropriate and in the best interests of the child, yet health and social services professionals have responsibilities to take action where there is concern (DH 1991a,b).

The incidence of abuse is difficult to measure since it depends on reporting or detection, which is likely to be related to social awareness and policy as much as anything else. Research conducted in the US has suggested that fairly high rates of violence are found throughout society, highlighting the particular social and cultural challenge of judging what constitutes abuse (Parton 1985, discussed in Robertson 1988).

Child abuse can be identified in various forms and although problems tend not to fall into neat categories in practice, these may be of use in assessing possible abuse. The categories used in government policy are listed in Box 46.5.

Signs and symptoms of abuse are not always

> **Box 46.5** Categories of child abuse (DH 1992a)
>
> **Physical abuse**
> Actual or likely physical injury or failure to prevent physical injury (or suffering) including deliberate poisoning, suffocation and Munchausen syndrome by proxy.
>
> **Sexual abuse**
> Actual or likely exploitation of a child or adolescent.
>
> **Emotional abuse**
> Actual or likely severe adverse effect on the emotional or behavioural development of a child caused by severe emotional ill-treatment or rejection. All abuse involves some emotional ill-treatment. This category should be used where it is the main or sole form of abuse.
>
> **Neglect**
> The persistent or severe neglect or failure to protect a child from exposure to any kind of danger, or extreme failure to carry out important aspects of care resulting in significant impairment of the child's health and development, including non-organic failure to thrive.

clear. Bruising, for example, may be the result of a range of causes and suspicion of abuse is more likely if the bruising forms a particular pattern. The signs are more likely to be taken seriously if a number of symptoms are found together or where inconsistent accounts of accidents are given and where there are delays in seeking care (Robertson 1988). Although midwives are not expected to have the expertise of social workers, further reading on signs of abuse and appropriate responses is strongly recommended. In situations of concern it is always important to discuss this with health service colleagues such as the GP, health visitors and with the local social work team.

It is equally important to respond to early signs of stress or distress in pregnant and postnatal mothers and their families, by being ready to listen and to provide advice and information or referrals to other sources of support, including self-help groups. Systems for risk scoring are used by health visitors in some areas as a method of screening. These may be useful if they are used to trigger a positive and constructive response and when support services can be offered. Great care is needed in using such systems to avoid unwarranted label-

ling of families as potential abusers and this risk must be balanced against the possible benefits of positive intervention (Robertson 1988).

A particular area of concern for health professionals is in handling instances of possible or suspected child abuse in a cross-cultural framework. Robertson (1988) argues that health visitors dealing with child protection should work within a framework of cross-cultural and societal violence (by this she means understanding that child abuse is not just an individual issue but takes place within the framework of social and cultural conditions and values) and should maintain a focus on prevention. Professionals should focus on the basic needs of the child and on the child per se and avoid relying on subjective judgements about what constitutes good or appropriate parenting, which are strongly influenced by cultural norms (Cloke & Naish 1992, DH 1991a). It is tempting to believe, particularly as a service provider, that one's own knowledge and values are naturally right or superior. A good example of this is the experience of health professionals' advice on babies' sleeping place and positions. After recent scientific research, which included anthropological, cross-cultural work, health professionals have needed to change the advice given to mothers in earlier years (DH 1993b). The previous advice, to place babies on their stomachs and in a separate bed, ran counter to the beliefs and practices of a range of cultural groups. By taking an open and evidence-informed approach (where evidence is available and using a broad range of sources), it is possible to take a view which avoids culturally biased judgements without avoiding the need to make informed judgements in the interests of the child's well-being (Narducci 1992).

It is important to recognise that child abuse occurs in all types of families, across social class and cultural groups. However, research suggests that problems are clustered in low-income families, those undergoing high levels of stress and families which are socially isolated (Robertson 1988). This evidence lends further weight to the current emphasis in child protection on prevention and efforts to work with families. It is helpful if problems are not seen as resulting from a dichotomy in parenting styles but as occurring on a continuum from calm and confident parenting through the normal range of most parents to those who have great difficulties and potential for abuse. Abuse is also associated in many instances with low self-esteem, mental health problems or substance abuse in parents.

Research evidence suggests that domestic violence (most commonly of men towards female partners) is an important issue in its own right and is also associated with increased risk of child abuse. For both reasons, it is important for health professionals to respond to signs of possible domestic violence. Women may often present problems but in an indirect rather than overt manner, such as repeated visits to health providers complaining of vague illness symptoms, or through self-harm or symptoms of mental distress (NCB 1995, Turton & Orr 1993).

Fostering and adoption

Midwives are often providing care for women whose pregnancy was not planned. This is more common than many professionals may realise and it is important not to make assumptions about the woman's feelings about her pregnancy. For example, in a study of women's experiences of maternity services, between 22% and 40% of women in the groups studied had mixed or negative initial feelings about the pregnancy (McCourt & Page 1996). In many cases women will be happy about an unplanned pregnancy, while others may be ambivalent and need support and possibly counselling to assist them in making decisions and plans for the future. For some women, this may involve relinquishment of the child for adoption. It is important to remember that such women share ordinary needs for information and support in pregnancy and childbirth, as well as having additional needs for support around relinquishing their child. Midwives can make a difference to how women feel in quite simple ways, such as avoiding judgemental or insensitive comments or approaches to care, by offering women a chance to discuss their situation privately, but openly, and by providing advice on where they might find more specialised support.

Adoption procedures were reformed by the Children Act 1989 so that there is now a greater emphasis on open adoption where possible, so that relinquishing mothers may remain in agreed forms of contact with their children. Practice in child care agencies has also developed in recent years so that children who are adopted, fostered or placed in residential care are given more opportunity to understand and talk about their personal history. Fostering (on a short- or long-term basis) may be a consideration for mothers who are unable to care for their babies after birth but who do not wish to relinquish their children for adoption. The Children Act also increases flexibility for family members to care for children or remain in contact with them where mothers are unable to do so.

OTHER COMMUNITY SERVICES

Child care services

Child care services may be valuable for a range of needs, not just when parents are working or studying. They may be important in providing support to families experiencing stress, for example due to poor or temporary housing, caring responsibilities or postnatal depression. Child care services for children under 5 years old are mainly the responsibility of Social Services, although Education Departments may manage Local Authority provision for children aged between 3 and 5. They generally provide a limited number of places but are responsible for the registration and inspection of all other facilities for the under-5s in their local area, including privately owned nurseries and individual childminders. Some services, often run by voluntary agencies, are also geared to the needs of families under stress. These include family centres, where parents and children can attend together and receive parenting support and schemes such as Homestart or Newpin which provide voluntary support and befriending.

Social services departments often provide under-5s' advisors, and health visitors also generally have good knowledge of local facilities. Local authorities often publish guides to local child care facilities, not only day care but those for parents and small children to use together, such as playgroups or toy libraries and for crèche facilities linked to adult education or sports activities. These can be of great value for parents who might otherwise feel isolated.

Interpreting, advocacy and link workers

Women and families from minority ethnic communities have two closely related sets of needs from maternity and other community health and social services. First are the ordinary needs which they share with women of all backgrounds but which are often attended to more poorly owing to language or cultural barriers or because of discrimination. Second are the particular needs resulting from their minority status, which may include language access and more specialised services. In practice, both are likely to be related. For example, women in a small-scale study of a refugee community in West London voiced concerns about lack of information, advice, choices and sensitive personal care. These concerns were widely shared amongst local women but they were experienced as far more severe problems by women from ethnic minorities owing to language and cultural barriers in using the services (Harper-Bulman & McCourt 1997). Women who are refugees may also be socially isolated and need practical support in adjusting to life in a new country.

Studies of the childbearing experiences of women in minority ethnic groups bring out the fundamental importance of good communication. Unfortunately, even where good interpreting services are available, they are often not sufficiently well used, owing to lack of knowledge or lack of professional awareness of the difficulties some women experience. The planning and budgets needed to arrange interpreting services may encourage professionals to rely on informal interpreters, such as family and friends. In many cases, this is inappropriate and rests on assumptions about the availability or suitability of informal interpreters rather than full consultation with the woman.

All health service providers should have access to interpreting facilities, but their quality and availability may vary locally. A national service *Language Line* can provide an immediate telephone interpretation but the costs of such a service are high, and the method is unsatisfactory as a means of communication except for very brief or emergency queries. Many local authorities, particularly in urban areas, have interpreting services available at reasonable notice, usually a minimum of 24 hours, longer for less common community languages. They may be provided by voluntary agencies such as Voluntary Service or Racial Equality Councils.

In areas where there is a sizeable minority community, some health and local authorities provide *link worker* or advocacy schemes. These provide far more than technical interpretation and are valuable since good communication rests on mutual understanding of values and ways of approaching things as much as words. They can also provide the sort of continuity, for example in specialist weekly antenatal clinics, which is difficult for general interpreting services to maintain.

READER ACTIVITY

Talk to local community and health workers and read local publications to inform yourself about local communities and community organisations.

a. Which are the main community languages spoken in your area and what is the range? Which local minority ethnic groups are most likely to have interpreting needs?
b. What services are provided by the Local Authority or voluntary groups and how can they be contacted?
c. Does your local Trust or Health Authority provide training on cultural awareness, antidiscriminatory practice or working with different languages?
d. Does your employing Trust, or the Health Authority, provide or commission any language services and, if so, how can you access them effectively?

Housing

Many women experience housing problems during pregnancy as they are faced with the need for stable and adequate accommodation. Housing is important for both the physical and psychological health of parents and children. Local Authorities have a statutory duty to provide housing for families who are homeless, including pregnant women, but this may involve temporary accommodation which is not well suited to caring for a child. The duty to provide accommodation for those in unsuitable housing is less clear cut and many families join long waiting lists, with priority given to those with the highest 'points' for several categories of need. Local Authorities may also nominate families to the waiting lists of Housing Associations, Trusts and Cooperatives, some of which also operate their own application systems. Midwives may be asked to support applications for housing or improved housing, usually by writing letters.

Accommodation with support may be available or offered for mothers and babies in certain circumstances, including refuges for women experiencing domestic violence and supported accommodation for mothers of school age or those experiencing depression or other mental health problems. Shortage of specialist mother and baby facilities, however, may limit what can be offered to women who need such support. The emphasis is, where possible, on providing care for mothers and babies together, or providing foster care when children need accommodation without their mothers.

Voluntary and independent services

Voluntary organisations have always played an important part in providing community health and social services and have in many cases been a major influence on their development, by showing what can be done and by campaigning for particular interest groups or services. They are linked to a long tradition of charitable work before the advent of the modern welfare state and were traditionally often linked with religious groups, as were the early hospital services in many countries. Voluntary organisations have shifted over time from primarily charitable to a mutual or self-help focus, with many organisations founded by relatives of people in need of long-term services and, more recently, service user organisations. Government policy in the 1980s in the UK strongly encouraged broadening the range of organisations providing services, including private companies. Voluntary and private providers of care are now referred to in policy as 'the independent sector'.

Voluntary organisations have generally combined two rather different roles effectively: that of campaigning or providing information and advice and that of providing community health and social services. Services provided were often innovative, or responded to a gap in provision, which would, if effective, gradually be adopted by the statutory service providers. Since the NHS and Community Care Act 1990, they have been encouraged to take on a far greater role in service provision and in some areas are now key providers of essential services such as residential and day child care.

Voluntary organisations which are particularly relevant for pregnant women and families with young children include:

- informal and mutual support groups – often locally based or focused on a particular issue, e.g. local postnatal support groups facilitated by health visitors or community workers, or developing from formal parent education classes
- parent and baby or toddler groups and clubs – these are generally locally, informally run and play an important part in preventing social isolation
- childbirth groups which combine campaigning with practical and social support, e.g. National Childbirth Trust (NCT)
- breast-feeding support groups which provide practical and moral support to women establishing breast feeding, e.g. La Leche League
- postnatal depression and women and mental health groups
- minority ethnic community groups, refugee organisations and women's groups which play a valuable role for women and families who may need practical and social support, including language services
- groups for people who have suffered pregnancy loss or bereavement including mutual support, advice and counselling organisations, e.g. the Stillbirth and Neonatal Death Society (SANDS)
- groups for families under stress or needing support, e.g. Newpin, Homestart

• groups for parents of children with disabilities or chronic health problems

• support and counselling for relinquishing mothers and those whose children are in residential or foster care – such support is often now provided by voluntary adoption and fostering agencies, e.g. British Association for Adoption and Fostering (BAAF)

• groups for parents with baby crying problems, e.g. Cry-Sis.

A number of directories of local and national organisations are published and will be valuable to keep to hand for reference.

Services for mothers with disabilities

A range of services are provided by Local Authorities and voluntary or mutual-support groups for women with disabilities, including those who are mothers. Although many are informal, and benefit from being so, it is important to remember the framework of rights and procedures provided by the NHS and Community Care Act 1990. In addition to service information, it is important for midwives to enhance their own awareness of disability issues, in order to provide a good service to all women, whatever their needs. Issues for mothers with physical disabilities are considered in Chapter 2. Here, we provide some introductory information on issues for women with learning disabilities and those with mental health problems.

Mental health

The prevalence of mental health problems amongst women is acknowledged to be high, and mental health problems are far more widespread within the population than many people imagine, since mental illness is often associated with distorted media-based images of psychosis or violence. The majority of mental health problems are responded to by the community health and social services, by GPs, community psychiatric nurses, counsellors, health visitors or social workers.

Amongst women, the experience of depression is very widespread and, like other health problems, is strongly associated with stress factors such as poverty, lack of supportive partners, housing prob-

lems and caring for young children without employment outside the home (Brown & Harris 1978, Oakley 1992). Researchers differ in how far they view postnatal depression as one manifestation of depression in women or as a distinct form of depression, and this is partly linked to the continuing lack of clear understanding of causes of depression or other forms of mental illness. Recent research suggests that much postnatal depression begins antenatally and is associated with a range of possible predisposing or precipitating factors, which include personal history and experience of pregnancy and birth (Ball 1994, Cox & Holden 1994). Ball argues that because such depression is likely to be multicausal, midwives should focus their attention on the areas where they might make a difference to women. She identified a range of issues related to social support and the manner in which birth and postnatal care are managed which may help to prevent depression developing in women who are vulnerable.

Screening schedules, such as the Edinburgh Postnatal Depression Scale (Cox & Holden 1994) have been developed which are acceptable to women and which are effective in identifying those who may be experiencing some level of depression. The use of such scales antenatally as well as postnatally may have some value if they can lead to targeting of additional support and advice to the woman. Effective sources of support are not necessarily formal ones, provided by health professionals, but Oakley and colleagues found, in their study of social support and pregnancy, that women offered such support by midwives appeared to be better prepared to seek and obtain support from other people, including their partners (Oakley 1992).

Learning disability

The issues surrounding parents with learning disabilities are particularly sensitive since social policy in the UK and other industrialised societies has historically been strongly influenced by eugenic ideas and focused on preventing people with disabilities from reproduction or parenthood. Many individuals are still sterilised, if not through force, by persuasion, or are encouraged to terminate pregnancies. The category learning disability (formerly called mental handicap and in the US referred to as mental retardation) covers a wide span and includes people who will need particular support in becoming parents and individuals who may cause concerns which will lead to the initiation of child protection proceedings.

Professional knowledge of learning disability, like lay knowledge, is often very limited, partly because of the history, before recent philosophical and policy changes, of keeping people with disabilities socially segregated. Mental handicap hospitals were built in the UK in the early part of the 20th century (rather like the psychiatric asylums built before them) as geographically isolated institutions which functioned rather like self-sufficient communities (Alasewski 1986). It will be valuable to learn more about learning and other disabilities, not only to counter discriminatory practice and

provide education and support for mothers with learning disabilities, but also to be in a better position to advise and counsel parents about antenatal screening and diagnostic tests (Dixon 1997).

SUMMARY

This chapter has highlighted key areas of community health and social services with which midwives need to be familiar. Some are important for general awareness and some for more specific roles such as providing advice, support or referral. A textbook can only provide an introduction and these areas have seen radical and rapid change in recent years. The references, reader activities and further reading suggestions will provide some pointers for developing further knowledge.

REFERENCES

Alasewski A 1986 Institutional care and the mentally handicapped. Croom Helm, London

Baker G, Bevan J M, McDonnell L, Wall B 1987 Community nursing. Research and some recent developments. Croom Helm, London

Ball J 1994 Reactions to motherhood: the role of postnatal care. Cambridge University Press, Cambridge

Bowling A 1981 Delegation in general practice. A study of doctors and nurses. Tavistock, London (*Not up to date but useful for the background to general practice and the working relationships between GPs and nurses*)

Brown G W, Harris T 1978 Social origins of depression. A study of psychiatric disorder in women. Tavistock, London

Bulmer M 1987 The social basis of community care. Allen and Unwin, London

Charlish A 1996 Vaccination and immunisation. What does your child need? Thorsons, London (*A consumer- rather than academically oriented book which sets out all the views expressed in debates about immunisation and focuses on parental concerns*)

Children Act 1989 HMSO, London

Clements L 1996 Community care and the law. Legal Action Group, London

Cloke C, Naish J (eds) 1992 Key issues in child protection for health visitors and nurses. Longman, UK

Cox J, Holden J (eds) 1994 Perinatal psychiatry. Use and misuse of the Edinburgh Postnatal Depression Scale. Gaskell, London

Crafter H 1997 Health promotion in midwifery. Principles and practice. Arnold, London

Department of Health (DH) 1991a Working together under the Children Act 1989 (guidelines). HMSO, London

Department of Health (DH) 1991b An introduction to the Children Act 1989, a new framework for the care and upbringing of children. HMSO, London

Department of Health (DH) 1992a The health of the nation. HMSO, London

Department of Health (DH) 1992b Child protection. Guidance for senior nurses, health visitors and midwives. HMSO, London

Department of Health (DH) 1992c Immunisation against infectious disease. HMSO, London

Department of Health (DH) 1993a Changing childbirth: report of the expert maternity group. HMSO, London

Department of Health (DH) 1993b Report of the Chief Medical Officer's expert group on the sleeping position of infants and cot death. HMSO, London

Department of Health (DH) 1997 The new NHS: modern, dependable. Cm 3807 The Stationery Office, London

Dimond B 1997 Legal aspects of care in the community. Macmillan, London

Disability Discrimination Act 1995 HMSO, London

Disabled Persons Services, Consultation and Representation Act 1986 HMSO, London

Dixon K 1997 Practical tips for supporting pregnant women with learning disabilities. MIDIRS Midwifery Digest 7(1): 40–42

Donnison J 1988 Midwives and medical men. A history of the struggle for the control of childbirth. Historical Publications, Barnet, Herts

Flint C 1993 Midwifery teams and caseloads. Butterworth Heinemann, London

Hall D M B (ed) 1989 Report of the Joint Working Party on Child Health Surveillance: health for all children, 1st edn. Oxford Medical, Oxford

Hall D M B (ed) 1991 Report of the Joint Working Party on Child Health Surveillance: health for all children, 2nd edn. Oxford Medical, Oxford

Harper-Bulman K, McCourt C 1997 Report on Somali

women's experiences of maternity care. Centre for Midwifery Practice, Thames Valley University, London

House of Commons Social Services Committee 1980 Perinatal and neonatal mortality. (The Short Report) HMSO, London

Housing Act 1977 HMSO, London

Hunt S, Symonds S 1995 The social meaning of midwifery. Macmillan, London

Jones L, Sidell M 1997 The challenge of promoting health. Exploration and action. Macmillan/Open University, Basingstoke

Leap N 1993 The midwife's tale: an oral history from handy women to professional midwife. Scarlett Press, London

Luker K, Orr J 1985 Health visiting. Blackwell, Oxford

McCourt C, Page L 1996 Report on the evaluation of one-to-one midwifery. Centre for Midwifery Practice, Thames Valley University, London

McKeown T 1979 The role of medicine: dream, mirage or nemesis? Blackwell, Oxford

Marris P 1974 Loss and change. Routledge and Kegan Paul, London

Mental Health Act 1983 HMSO, London

Ministry of Health (MoH) 1970 Domiciliary midwifery and maternity bed needs: the report of the standing maternity and midwifery advisory committee. (The Peel Report) HMSO, London

Narducci T 1992 Race, culture and child protection. In: Cloke C, Naish J (eds) Key issues in child protection for health visitors and nurses. Longman, UK, ch 2, pp 12–22

National Assistance Act 1948 HMSO, London

National Children's Bureau 1995 Children and domestic violence. NCB, London

National Health Service Management Executive (NHSME) 1996 The National Health Service: a service with ambitions. The Stationery Office, London

NHS Act 1946 HMSO, London

NHS and Community Care Act 1990 HMSO, London

Nurses, Midwives and Health Visitors Act 1979 HMSO, London

Oakley A 1992 Social support and motherhood. The natural history of a research project. Blackwell, Oxford

Page L 1995 Effective group practice in midwifery: working with women. Blackwell Science, Oxford

Palmer C 1996 Maternity rights. Legal Action Group/Maternity Alliance, London

Parton N 1985 The politics of child abuse. Macmillan, London

Race Relations Act 1976 HMSO, London

Robertson C 1988 Health visiting in practice. Longman, Edinburgh

Robinson S 1990 Maintaining the role of the midwife. In: Garcia J, Kilpatrick R, Richards M (eds) The politics of maternity care. Clarendon, Oxford

Stacey M 1988 The sociology of health and healing. Unwin and Hyman, London

Tew M 1990 Safer childbirth? A critical history of maternity care. Chapman & Hall, London

Townsend P, Davidson N, Whitehead M 1988 Inequalities in health. Penguin, London

Turton P, Orr J 1993 Learning to care in the community, 2nd edn. Edward Arnold, London

Whitehead M 1987 The health divide. Inequalities in health in the 1980s: a review. Health Education Authority, London

FURTHER READING

Copies of all the relevant legislation and associated guidelines should be found in a good college library. A number of guides to the legislation, aimed at health professionals, are published. For example:

Department of Health (DH) 1992 The Children Act. What every nurse, health visitor and midwife needs to know. DH/RCN, London

It is important to check their publication dates to ensure that they are up to date.

Introductory texts on health visiting are useful for midwives since they focus on relevant areas of work such as health advice, preventive care and monitoring, and child health and development. Read some introductory texts to increase your understanding of health visitors' aims and ways of working and explore how these relate to the approach of midwives. For example:

Robertson C 1988 Health visiting in practice. Longman, Edinburgh

Introductory social science textbooks will also be useful, as will works which are more directly related to analysis of maternity care, the health of mothers and babies and accounts of research into health beliefs, practices and social conditions. For example:

Cornwell J 1984 Hard earned lives. Tavistock, London

Oakley A 1993 Essays on women, medicine and health. Edinburgh University Press, Edinburgh

It is also important to obtain a good and up-to-date range of local and national directories of organisations and services. For example:

MIDIRS Directory of Maternity Organisations. MIDIRS, Bristol, UK (*Updated regularly by means of the addition of inserts when new information is received*)

Whitfield C (ed) 1992 People who help. A guide to voluntary and other support organisations, 3rd edn. Profile Productions, London

47

Organisation of health care in the United Kingdom

Rosemary Jenkins

The main source of health care in the UK is the National Health Service (NHS), although there is a small independent sector. The Health Service was set up by an Act of Parliament and subsequent changes have also been introduced as a result of new statutes. NHS care is funded out of general taxation so that levels of funding are decided by the parliamentary process.

Not all health-related services, however, are provided by the NHS. Social and environmental services are the responsibility of local government. These include education, environmental health, social services and housing.

The chapter aims to:

- give an overview of the legislation underpinning the organisation of health care in the UK

- describe the structure of the NHS from its inception in 1948 through a series of reorganisations over the last 25 years to the latest proposals for change

- review the functioning of key professionals and groups within the NHS and the contribution made by outside organisations.

CENTRAL GOVERNMENT

The UK has a dicameral parliament. Its two chambers are the House of Commons and the House of Lords.

The House of Commons consists of democratically elected Members of Parliament (MPs) who each represent one constituency. The Prime Minister, chief executive of the Government, is the leader of the largest party in the House of Commons and the legitimate spokesperson for the party's MPs. The Prime Minister of the day determines which of several hundred MPs should serve as cabinet ministers. Some 60 MPs are appointed to junior posts outside the cabinet, either as ministers of state in charge of minor departments or in subordinate posts within departments as parliamentary secretaries or as under-secretaries of state. Collectively, these ministers constitute the front bench of the governing party.

A cabinet minister heads a particular ministry or department. For example the Secretary of State for Health heads the Department of Health, assisted by a team of ministers.

Health matters in Wales are dealt with by the Welsh Office, in Scotland by the Scottish Home and Health Department and in Northern Ireland by four health and social services boards. The respective ministers are the Secretaries of State for Wales, for Scotland and for Northern Ireland.

The House of Lords is made up of bishops, senior judges and peers of the realm who may be life peers or hereditary peers.

Legislation

One of the functions of parliament is to pass legislation. This may be in the form of an Act of Parliament (primary legislation) or a statutory instrument (secondary legislation). The Midwives Rules are a statutory instrument under the Nurses, Midwives and Health Visitors Act 1979.

The actual process of enacting legislation is complex. A bill is introduced to the House of Commons by a minister, given a first reading and published without debate. At the second reading, the general principles of the bill are debated. Major bills are then usually referred to the committee of the whole House; lesser bills are considered by standing committees containing a fraction of the House. The committee reports to the full House (the report stage) and all MPs are given a chance to discuss the bill once again. A third reading debate is the final stage.

The bill can then proceed to the House of Lords, where it goes through the same process. If it is passed it receives the Royal Assent and becomes an Act of Parliament. If the House of Lords makes amendments or votes against a bill, it returns to the Commons for further consideration.

This process does not apply to the enactment of secondary legislation, revisions of which will be placed before the House by a Secretary of State for ratification. Thus many Acts of Parliament contain enabling legislation to allow for subsequent statutory instruments to be revised quickly as circumstances require.

The civil service

The civil service provides the administrative and executive support to the Government. It is staffed by permanent civil servants and is divided into departments and ministries. In serving the Government the civil service follows three guiding principles: impartiality, anonymity and permanence. Although the Department of Health is the main department concerned with 'health' others have a marginal interest. For example, the Department of the Environment, Transport and the Regions is responsible for safe transport policy and the Department for Education and Employment for the provision of sex education in schools.

The Department of Health has three major divisions: the Public Health Group, the Social Care Group and the National Health Service Executive (NHSE). The Public Health Group is concerned with the development of general policy relating to health, for example 'Our Healthier Nation Strategy'. The NHSE is responsible for the development and implementation of policy relating to the NHS. The NHSE has its headquarters in Leeds and also has eight regional offices. Among its other functions, the Social Care Group has responsibility for inspection of local authority social services departments.

Each UK country has a number of chief professional officers including a chief medical officer and a chief nursing officer. Nursing and midwifery officers also work in the civil service.

LOCAL GOVERNMENT

Local government in Britain is the responsibility of elected local authorities which provide local services under specific powers conferred by parliament. The concept of a comprehensive system of councils was first incorporated in statute law in the late 19th century. At that time the local authorities' functions involved public health, highways, the police and regulatory duties. They have since become responsible for education, housing, most of the environmental health services, personal social services, traffic administration, planning, fire services, libraries and many minor functions. Local government in Greater London was reorganised in 1965 and in the rest of England and Wales in 1974. A similar reorganisation was completed in Scotland in 1975. Changes in the structure and function of local government in Northern Ireland were made in 1973.

The Local Government Act 1985 abolished the Greater London Council and the six metropolitan councils. At that time, local authorities consisted of various types of council, at county, district and parish level. Parish councils only exist in small towns and rural areas; in Wales these are known as community councils. Scotland had a two-tier structure while Northern Ireland had a single tier, with fewer functions than those in Great Britain.

In 1992 the Local Government Act set up a local government commission, an independent body, to review and make recommendations for changes to local government structure. Its task was to look at the case for replacing the existing two-tier system with a structure of unitary authorities. There was to be no national framework and the decisions of the commission were to be based on the needs of each locality. The commission reported each of its decisions to the Secretary of State for the Environment who made the final decision on the configuration of each new local authority. Although many unitary systems have been introduced as a result of the review, a few two-tier systems remain.

In 1997 the new Government proposed, subject to a referendum, to set up a Greater London authority with an elected mayor and assembly. If voted for, legislation will be introduced and the mayor and assembly will take office in the year 2000. Its functions are not yet defined but are likely to include London-wide environmental issues.

Financing of local authorities

Services are paid for by three types of revenue:

- council tax or domestic rates (Northern Ireland)
- grants from central government
- exchequer grants for specific projects, e.g. education, housing.

THE NATIONAL HEALTH SERVICE

The Welfare State was set up to overcome the five giant evils of *want*, *squalor*, *poverty*, *ignorance* and *idleness*.

The National Health Service (NHS) came into operation on 5 July 1948 in accordance with the National Health Service Act 1946. It established a system of health care, free at the point of delivery, to combat the 'Giant of Sickness'. The aims of the 1946 Act were:

- that the state should provide health care at the point of delivery for those in need
- that the health service should promote the improvement of the physical and mental health of the people of England and Wales
- that health services should be available without charge upon determination of need by professionals providing the service
- that the service provided should be, as far as possible, of a uniform standard for all.

The Act set up a tripartite system of health care, with hospital services provided by hospital management committees. Some services – notably district nursing and midwifery and ambulances – were to be run by local authorities and general practitioners were contracted to a medical executive committee who paid them fees for services given to the NHS. This system continued until 1973.

From 1973 there have been a series of NHS reorganisations, some introduced through statute and others as a developmental process. Each change has built upon the structures in place before the change. To understand the current structure, therefore, it is useful to see how these developments have evolved.

The National Health Service Reorganisation Act 1973

This Act abolished the tripartite system and

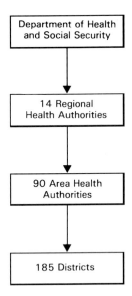

Fig. 47.1 Simplified structure of the National Health Service in England 1974–1982.

integrated all health services under a single management structure (Fig. 47.1). General practitioners continued to be contracted to the health service rather than be employed by it. A committee of the health authority, the Family Practitioner Committee, administered the NHS contracts of GPs, dentists, opticians and pharmacists. Regional health authorities were designated the local supervising authorities in England.

The Health Services Act 1980

The Department of Health and Social Security (DHSS) published *Patients First* in December 1979. This document aimed to encourage decision-making in the locality rather than at the centre and recommended that a tier of administration should be removed.

After consultation, the Health Services Act 1980 was passed and on 1 April 1982 area health authorities and health districts were replaced by district health authorities (DHAs), which would be served by a team of officers. The regional health authorities (RHAs) remained (Fig. 47.2).

The regions were the policy- and strategy-making bodies whereas districts were responsible for operational management. Some large districts were sub-divided into smaller operational units – health districts. Management decisions were reached through consensus agreement of the officer teams working with the health authority.

General management in the NHS: The Griffiths Report 1983 (DHSS 1983)

Sir Roy Griffiths, chairman of a large supermarket chain, was invited to examine the efficiency of the NHS. Following his investigation he recommended the widespread introduction of general management.

To head the management function of the NHS, a Health Services Supervisory Board, chaired by the Secretary of State, and a National Health Service Management Board, chaired by a chief executive, were set up. The latter was to be multidisciplinary, under the direction of and accountable to the Supervisory Board, and its role was to include:

- implementation of policies approved by the supervisory board
- leadership to the managers of the NHS
- control of performance
- achievement of consistency and drive over the long term.

Griffiths also recommended that Regional and District Health Authorities should reorganise their management structures and appoint a general manager at each level.

Regional and district levels
The Health Authority chairman at each level was responsible for the appointment of the general manager. The objective was to extend the accountability process down to unit level. The general manager was charged with the responsibility for achieving the objectives set by the Authority and with initiating and implementing major cost improvement programmes.

Units of Management. Health districts were divided into Units of Management, which could consist of several care groups or sites within the district. A unit had its own Unit General Manager (UGM) whose responsibility was to propose the management structure of the unit and to plan

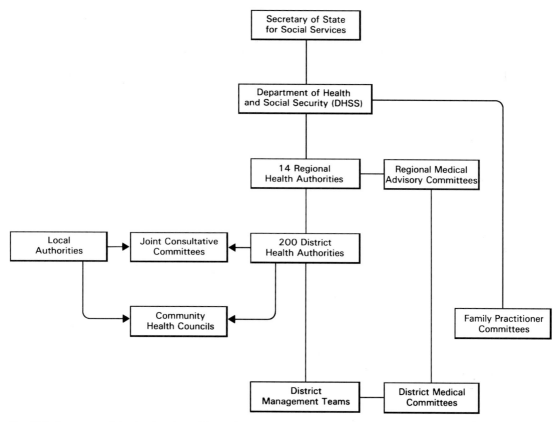

Fig. 47.2 Structure of the National Health Service in England after 1982.

for day-to-day decisions. He or she was to involve clinicians in the management process more closely than was formerly the case. Management budgeting was introduced as a new development.

The implementation of general management in the NHS replaced consensus management by the placing of responsibility upon one identified person at each level. This person was to plan and implement strategies for the efficient running of the service and to monitor and control performance.

The National Health Service and Community Care Act 1990

1987 saw widespread criticism of the level of government spending on health care with stories of bed closures and failure to provide services. A Cabinet-level review of the NHS was announced and the recommendations of this review were

published in 1989 as the White Paper, *Working for Patients* (DH 1989). Also that year, Sir Roy Griffiths was asked to undertake a review of community services for those requiring long-term care. These recommendations were then published as a second White Paper, *Caring for People* (DH 1989). Both these White Papers were incorporated into the National Health Service and Community Care Act 1990. Changes in community care were introduced on 1 April 1993; the NHS changes were introduced in September 1990 and April 1991.

Working for Patients introduced changes in health care that were almost as profound as the original change brought about in 1948. Although the service was to continue to be provided by the State and funded out of general taxation it aimed to bring something of the 'free market economy' to the system. The users of the service would still obtain care along the same lines as envisaged by the 1946 Act, but an 'internal' market would operate inside the NHS with some NHS bodies charged with 'purchasing' health care and others with 'providing' it (Fig. 47.3). Decision-making was to become even more decentralised and systems were introduced to make clinicians – doctors, nurses, midwives and others – more accountable for the resources they used. Paramount to the way health services were to be provided in the future would be patient choice. This was particularly confirmed in the foreword to the White Paper, written by the Prime Minister. The roles of RHAs, DHAs and service providers were also radically changed.

The purchasers of care

District Health Authorities. The 1990 Act changed the composition of DHAs. The old authorities were disbanded on 31 August 1990 and the new took over on 1 September. Each authority consists of:

- a chairman appointed by the Secretary of State
- five non-executive members (i.e. lay members)

appointed by RHAs in England and the Secretary of State in the other countries
- five executive members who are also employees of the health authority: the District General Manager (now the Chief Executive) and District Treasurer are statutory appointments to the DHA; the other three positions are appointed by the eight members already on the authority.

The Authority is advised by a team of officers which includes the Chief Executive, and Director of Public Health. There was no statutory guarantee that the authority would have a Chief Nurse, but all Authorities were charged with ensuring that they obtained the appropriate professional advice.

The new role of the DHA commenced on 1 April 1991. From that date the DHA's prime objectives were:

- to ascertain the health care needs of the population living within its boundaries
- to draw up service specifications for the care it wishes to purchase, taking into account the priorities it has set
- to purchase health care to meet those needs from the providers of care.

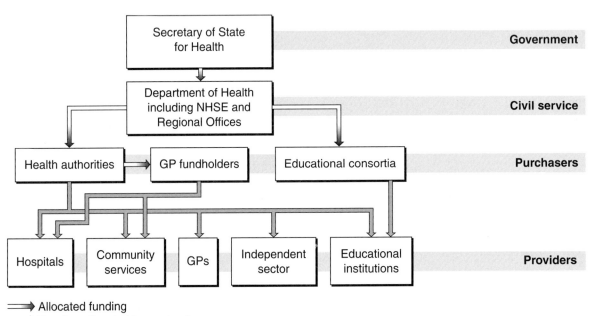

Allocated funding
Funding allocated by contract

Fig. 47.3 Simplified current structure of the National Health Service.

Fundholding general practitioners. When first introduced, practices with over 7000 patients were able to apply to receive a budget with which to buy health care needed by their patients. Since then there have been considerable extensions to the scheme. Currently there are three levels of GP fundholder: community fundholding where the budget held by the GP covers practice staff, diagnostic tests and most community services; standard fundholding where the budget additionally covers elective surgery and outpatient care; total purchasing where all hospital and community services are purchased for the patients on their lists. In 1996 there were about 50 total purchasing schemes operating.

In addition to fundholding, GP commissioning groups have been developing although there is no national blueprint for these. Some were set up by health authorities to ensure a local focus to commissioning of health care whilst others were set up by groups of general practitioners themselves. In general they cover a number of GP practices and purchase services across a 'locality' rather than just for the patients on a practice list. Future plans for primary care commissioning include a strengthening of this locality purchasing approach with additional representation on the 'commissioning team' of other health professionals including nurses and possibly midwives.

The providers of health care

All services offering care are providers of care in the NHS 'internal market'. This includes hospitals, community services, maternity services and ambulance services. Until 1 April 1991 all these services, with the exception of the ambulance services in England, were managed by DHAs. The 1990 Act allowed these services to apply to become NHS trusts. An NHS Trust, which may be based on a single hospital, a community service or a group of services, is a management unit separate from the DHA. It is able to make its own decisions on how to provide a service and what to provide, except for a few facilities, such as accident and emergency, which it will be required to provide if appropriate. Its autonomy and the break from central control is such that it is even able to make decisions on the type of staff it will employ and the terms and conditions for those staff.

To become a Trust, the organisation had to apply to the Secretary of State and to be approved. In 1991 over 50 NHS Trusts came into being and in subsequent years more services made applications. All provider services in the Health Service are now NHS Trusts.

A third, smaller, provider of health care is the independent (private and voluntary) sector, which is able to provide services on behalf of the NHS, under contract.

An NHS contract

The Act set up a system whereby a formal agreement must be reached between a DHA and a provider of care for the amount and level of care needed. The DHA could enter into an agreement with any provider offering the service it wants to buy. Thus there is some element of competition between the providers. Providers and purchasers alike are expected to ascertain consumers' views when entering these contracts. Once the contract is agreed, the DHA will pay the provider unit for the service. These contracts are not enforceable in law but the Secretary of State is ultimately responsible for arbitrating in any dispute arising from a contract.

Audit and resource management. For a contract to work smoothly and efficiently, measures must be introduced to determine the standard of service and the cost. *Working for Patients* stated that a system of medical audit, based on peer review, must be introduced into health care. The Department of Health also encourages the introduction of schemes of nursing and midwifery audit. Pilot projects to introduce computerised costing of care, which is then made available to clinical staff, were also introduced under the title 'resource management'.

Regional Health Authorities after 1991

The composition of the RHAs also changed in September 1990, being the same as for the DHA.

It was envisaged that planning and development of the service would be led by the operation of the NHS contract. The Region's role in planning was therefore diminished. RHAs had a duty to oversee the operation of the contracts to ensure that they work in the interests of the consumer and are efficient. On behalf of the Secretary of State they also arbitrated in any dispute arising from the contract agreement. In England they continued to be the Local Supervising Authorities for midwives. A major new function of RHAs was to determine the manpower needs of the Region and finance the appropriate levels of basic education (for midwives, pre- and post-registration programmes) in order to meet the manpower requirements.

Family Health Service Authorities

The 1990 Act disbanded the Family Practitioner Committees of the DHAs and set up a network of new authorities, Family Health Service Authorities (FHSAs). Each FHSA had a general manager. The main task of these was to administer the family practitioner services. Like the other authorities, the membership consisted of a chairman, five executive and five non-executive members.

The FHSA arranged for family practitioner services to be provided. It issued contracts and investigated any complaints which a person might make against an individual practitioner.

The FHSA issued medical cards. It published lists of practitioners who undertake NHS work including those general practitioners who offer maternity care. These lists are available at local post offices.

Clinical directorates

Although this change was not explicit in the 1990 Act, many services introduced this system of operational management. A Clinical Director, often but not necessarily a senior consultant, heads a clinical specialty. He or she will have the support of a business manager and if appropriate a senior nurse or midwife. He or she, with the others, will be responsible for running the clinical unit, particularly ensuring that care is given within the resources allowed.

The NHS Act 1995

The latest evolutionary change in the overall structure of the NHS introduced changes at region and district level.

On April 1 1996, as a result of the NHS Act 1995 and a 1993 review, Regional Health Authorities were disbanded to be replaced by eight Regional Offices of the National Health Service Executive. These are smaller organisations and are now part of the Civil Service. One of their key roles is to monitor the performance of Health Authorities. They still retain a public health function with a Director of Public Health, a research function with a Regional Director of Research and Development, and a nursing advisory function with a Regional Nurse Director or Advisor. Each Region also has a Regional Education Development Group to advise on overall education and manpower policy.

The Act also merged the District Health Authorities and Family Health Service Authorities into one body, a Health Authority. The functions of the two were merged rather than changed.

Future change in primary care

Following an extensive consultation conducted by the NHSE in 1996, the NHS Primary Care Act was passed. A strong message from the exercise was the need for more flexibility in primary care to encourage innovation. It was felt that the current arrangements for general practitioner fees can militate against this. The Act introduces changes to these arrangements, enabling Health Authorities to contract with practices rather than with individual general practitioners. It also introduced the possibility of salaried general practitioners. The first change could pave the way for partnerships in primary care to be held by professionals other than doctors. The opportunity for doctors to be salaried general practitioners may go some way to relieve the difficulty in recruiting doctors to difficult areas such as inner city areas. The Act also has a clause in it which will enable health authorities to enter NHS contracts with a greater range of professional staff. These changes are not compulsory and practices and other services have been invited to set up pilot schemes for evaluation.

The White Paper – *The New NHS: modern, dependable* (DH 1997)

A new government was elected in May 1997 with a manifesto commitment to abolish the NHS

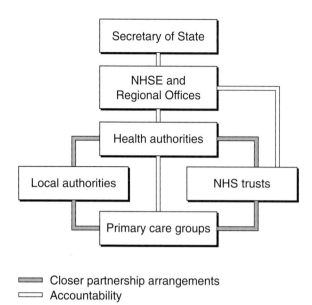

Closer partnership arrangements
Accountability

Fig. 47.4 Proposed NHS structure (DoH 1997).

internal market. In December 1997 it published a White Paper setting out its proposals (Fig. 47.4).

Aspects of the NHS which are seen to be working are to be retained. These include: the separation between planning and purchasing care and the provision of care; the strengthened role of primary care; and decentralised management with NHS Trusts responsible for operational management.

The internal market, including general practitioner fundholding will, however, be abolished. Instead, locality commissioning teams called Primary Care Groups, comprising local GPs and community nurses, will gradually be introduced. The element of competition between providers will go and an ethos of partnership is to be introduced. There will also be a greater emphasis on setting overall national standards for the NHS.

National standards

The White Paper proposes the introduction of National Service Frameworks which will incorporate evidence of clinical and cost effectiveness with the views of service users; a National Institute of Clinical Excellence to give a strong lead on clinical and cost effectiveness by drawing up and disseminating guidelines; a statutory Commission

for Health Improvement to ensure that local systems to monitor and improve clinical quality are in place. The Commission will be able to offer support to local organisations who are experiencing specific clinical problems. Where clinical problems are persistent and unresolved, it will be able to intervene on the direction of the Secretary of State.

There is to be a new national performance framework with six dimensions: health improvement; fair access; effective delivery of appropriate care; efficiency; patient/carer experience; and health outcomes of NHS care.

Local standards

A new concept, clinical governance, is introduced. Although professional and statutory bodies have a vital role in setting and promoting standards, the White Paper will require practitioners to accept responsibility for developing and maintaining standards in their local NHS organisations. This requirement will operate alongside the existing professional self-regulation mechanisms.

Health authorities

It is anticipated that there will be fewer, larger health authorities as some mergers will take place. Over time they will cease to commission health care as this becomes the responsibility of the newly formed Primary Care Groups (see below). The authorities will have a number of key tasks:

- assessing the health needs of the population
- drawing up strategies to meet those needs – to be called Health Improvement Programmes
- deciding the range and location of health care services for the resident population
- deciding local targets and standards
- supporting the development of, allocating resources to and monitoring Primary Care Groups.

Primary Care Groups (PCGs)

These will be introduced throughout the country. They will bring together GPs and community nurses to commission services for local patients. A new form of trust – a Primary Care Trust – will be introduced in legislation for those PCGs which become free-standing. The form of the new groups will be flexible with four options for the way they may function:

- supporting and advising the Health Authority which will continue to commission services
- having devolved responsibility for managing the budget for Health Care in their area
- becoming free-standing bodies accountable to the Health Authority for commissioning care
- becoming free-standing bodies accountable to the Health Authority for commissioning services and with responsibility for the provision of community health services for their population.

Health Improvement Programmes

A Health Improvement Programme will be the local plan for improving health and health care. The Health Authority will have lead responsibility for producing the programme in consultation with other health professionals and agencies (e.g. local authorities). The Programme will cover the most important health and health care needs of the local population and how they will be met either directly by the NHS or in partnership with social services. It will also identify the range, location and investment required in local health services to meet these needs.

Health Services in Scotland, Wales and Northern Ireland

Although most of the structures and changes described above apply across the UK, there are some differences that apply to Scotland, Wales and Northern Ireland.

In Scotland the government body is the Scottish Home and Health Department (SHHD) under the Secretary of State for Scotland. There is a management executive at this level.

There are 15 Health Boards which are directly responsible to the Secretary of State. They have always been the Local Supervising Authorities for midwives working in Scotland.

Overall responsibility for health services in Wales rests with the Secretary of State for Wales. The country is divided into five Health Authorities. These authorities are the Local Supervising Authorities for midwives working in Wales.

Health care services in Northern Ireland are provided by four Health and Social Services Boards and a management executive responsible to the Secretary of State for Northern Ireland. These boards are the Local Supervising Authorities for midwives working in Northern Ireland.

Plans for health service changes in the other UK countries in line with the White Paper will be published in 1998.

The government health strategy

In February 1998 the Government published a Green Paper starting a consultation on the future health strategy for England.

Its key aims are:

- to improve the health of the population as a whole by increasing the length of people's lives and the number of years people spend free from illness
- to improve the health of the worst off in society and to narrow the health gap.

To do this it proposed:

- a national contract for health with action at three levels – government and national, local and community and individual
- four national priority areas – coronary heart disease and stroke, cancers, accidents and mental health
- three healthy settings – schools, workplaces and neighbourhoods
- Health Authorities to set local targets to deal flexibly with local health needs, for example teenage pregnancy, smoking rates.

During 1998 the other UK countries will also be producing their strategies for health.

OTHER RELATED COMMITTEES AND BODIES

Standing advisory committees

These committees advise the Secretary of State on the views of the various professionals. The one which affects midwives is the Standing Nursing and Midwifery Advisory Committee (SNMAC).

Others represent the interests of doctors, dentists and pharmacists.

Local Medical Committees

Local Medical Committees represent the views of medical staff and coordinate the medical aspects of health care at Health Authority level. Members represent the interests of hospital medical staff, GPs, pharmacists, ophthalmologists and the local authority (for public health).

Maternity services liaison committees

The government report, *Maternity Care in Action: Part 1 – antenatal care* (MSAC 1982), suggested that each health authority should consider setting up a Maternity Services Liaison Committee. The membership should include representatives of the professional groups concerned with giving maternity care and preferably a consumer representative. The aim of such committees is to facilitate co-ordination of the services between obstetrician, GP and midwife and between hospital and community services. The way these committees function varies from authority to authority.

Community Health Councils

Community Health Councils (CHCs) are the voice of the people on matters concerning the Health Service. Members come from the local community, local authorities and voluntary organisations.

CHC meetings are held at least once a month and are open to the public. They discuss local policies and can set up enquiries into complaints such as poor hospital food, long waiting lists and lengthy delays at outpatient clinics. They may not investigate clinical aspects of health care but they do inspect NHS premises and have access to NHS policy documents in their own health district.

Each CHC elects its own chairperson and has a full-time paid secretary whose contract of employment since April 1996 has been held by one or two designated Health Authorities in each region. The CHC communicates with the Health Authority and must publish an annual report.

Education Consortia and Regional Education Development Groups

Locally based Education Consortia were introduced in April 1996. They have representatives from the health authority, NHS trusts, local authority social services, the voluntary and independent sectors and GPs. Their role will be to assess the local workforce requirements and contract for appropriate education and training to meet these needs and from April 1998 they will take over training budgets and start commissioning non-medical education and training.

At regional level, each consortium is represented on a Regional Education Development Group, which also includes staff from the Regional Office and representatives from post-graduate medical and dental education. Responsibilities of these groups include advising the Regional Office on the workforce and education plans of the local consortia and creating links between higher education and the NHS.

OTHER PROFESSIONAL PEOPLE AND TEAMS IN THE NHS

Director of Public Health in Health Authorities

Each Health Authority has a Department of Public Health headed by a Director of Public Health who is a doctor of consultant status. The Director is responsible for assessing the health care needs of the population, and the Department collates the epidemiological and demographic statistics needed to assist the health authority to make decisions on the health care it will purchase. The Department is also responsible for communicable disease control. The Consultant in Communicable Disease, who is usually based in the Public Health Department, is also the 'Proper Officer' for the Local Authority, advising that Authority on its obligations in the control of communicable disease. Public health is becoming a multidisciplinary activity and many public health departments now have nurses and midwives working in them.

Primary health care teams

The primary health care team is usually based on a health centre or a general practice surgery. It forms the first line of defence against disease in the community. Much of its work involves prevention, for example child immunisation programmes (see Ch. 46). The team comprises general practitioners, district nurses, practice nurses, a health visitor, a midwife and sometimes a social worker. The practice is supported by administrative and secretarial staff.

Members of the team are responsible for giving care in the community setting, seeing patients at the surgery or health centre or visiting them in their own homes. The midwife who is part of an integrated midwifery service enjoys close liaison with her hospital colleagues as well as with other members of the primary health care team.

General practitioner obstetrician (GPO)

The registered medical practitioner may offer maternity care to any woman on his own list without further training in obstetrics. However, the GP may choose not to offer care, although he is bound not to refuse in cases of emergency. Some GPs offer obstetric care and may give this care to women other than those on their own list. To do so they must be entered onto the local obstetric list. Admission to the list is decided by a local committee of the Health Authority. Although the Diploma of the Royal College of Obstetricians and Gynaecologists is desirable, the minimum requirement is that the GP has completed 6 months' working in a recognised training post in obstetrics. This list is kept by the Health Authority and is available at post offices. The general practitioner obstetrician can give care to women during pregnancy, labour and the puerperium and works in partnership with the community midwife and the hospital obstetric team.

The Health Service Commissioner (the ombudsman)

The Health Service Commissioner is appointed to investigate complaints regarding the Health Service made by members of the public whose complaints have not been satisfactorily resolved at local level. The Commissioner publishes an annual report of his investigations. The Health Commissioner Act 1995 increased the powers of the Commissioner, now allowing the office to investigate complaints about clinical care. To facilitate

this, the office has recently appointed medical and nursing advisors.

OTHER SERVICES PROVIDING CARE

Family planning services (See Ch. 32.)

District Health Authorities assumed responsibility for family planning services in April 1982 and the NHS is still required to provide these services. Couples may obtain free advice and supplies from various sources:

- hospitals – gynaecological wards and clinics, maternity wards and postnatal clinics
- family planning clinics in the community
- a general practitioner
- domiciliary family planning service
- 'one-stop' sexual health services, combining family planning, gynaecology and genitourinary medicine services.

The Family Planning Association can also provide services but these are usually outwith the National Health Service and therefore fees are charged. Certain supplies are also available for purchase at chemists. Brook Advisory Centres provide services for young people. They are frequently contracted to the NHS and therefore provide the services free.

Well woman clinics

Well woman clinics which are run within the NHS mainly provide a service for the early detection of cervical and breast cancer. Some do provide a more extensive service of health advice and screening and also counselling. They are attractive to women who 'just want a check-up' but are not complaining of a specific problem. A few areas have opened well man clinics. Increasingly these clinics are being run by practice nurses.

All mothers attending for maternity care have the benefit of preventive health care. In many areas, well woman facilities are limited and the only opportunity for screening for health – as opposed to sickness – is to attend a private clinic.

Preconception care

Preconception clinics aim to achieve optimum health prior to the onset of a pregnancy in order to reduce the risk of complication for mother and fetus. The advice and counselling which are offered also aim to teach healthy living patterns which will continue into the pregnancy. In this way health can be improved before and during the vital first trimester which is often almost over before the mother attends an antenatal clinic.

Alternatively, preconception advice is frequently given in the GP's surgery and at family planning clinics. Midwives have an opportunity to give this advice during the period of postnatal care in preparation for a subsequent pregnancy.

There are also some preconception clinics in the private sector. (See also Ch. 10.)

READER ACTIVITIES

1. Find out how many NHS Trusts there are in the Region or country where you work.

2. Health Authority meetings have open sessions. Arrange to attend one of these.

3. Attend a meeting of your local Community Health Council and find out the name of the secretary to the Council.

4. Find out who your local MP is and when he or she holds the constituency 'surgery'. These are usually advertised in the local paper.

5. Obtain the latest report by the Health Services Commissioner from your local hospital/medical library

6. Ask to see, if you have not already done so, the main provisions of the contract for maternity services that your service has agreed.

REFERENCES

Department of Health (DH) 1989 Working for patients. HMSO, London
Department of Health (DH) 1989 Caring for people: community care in the next decade and beyond. HMSO, London
Department of Health (DH) 1997 The new NHS: modern, dependable. Cm 3807 The Stationery Office, London
Department of Health and Social Security (DHSS) and Welsh Office 1979 Patients first. DHSS, London
Department of Health and Social Security (DHSS) 1983 National Health Service management inquiry. (Chairman Sir Roy Griffiths) HMSO, London
Health Commissioner Act 1995 HMSO, London

Health Services Act 1980 HMSO, London
Local Government Act 1985 HMSO, London
Local Government Act 1992 HMSO, London
Maternity Services Advisory Committee 1982 Maternity care in action: Part 1 – antenatal care. HMSO, London
National Health Service and Community Care Act 1990 HMSO, London
National Health Service Reorganisation Act 1973 HMSO, London
NHS Act 1995 HMSO, London
NHS Primary Care Act 1996 HMSO, London
Nurses, Midwives and Health Visitors Act 1979 HMSO, London

FURTHER READING

Allsop J 1984 Health policy and the National Health Service. Longman, London
Klein R 1989 The politics of the National Health Service. Longman, London

Merry P (ed) NHS Confederation. NHS handbook, 12th edn. Institute of Health Services Management, London
Rose R 1980 Politics in England, 3rd edn. Faber, London

Vital statistics

48

V. Ruth Bennett   Linda K. Brown   Mary McGowan

Registration of births and deaths is so much taken for granted in the developed world that it may come as a surprise that it was only in the 19th century that it became a requirement in England. Even today a few births and deaths escape registration in the UK and in countries where communication is less easy, many more may be uncounted. The collection of these vital statistics allows for analysis of the rates of birth and death in different population groups. The information is essential for planners at national and local level who must forecast the needs of the community for health facilities, schooling, housing and so on.

The chapter aims to:

- describe the collection of data on births and deaths and the legal requirements for registration

- emphasise the role of the midwife, who, being a person present at virtually every birth, is a key witness who can supply details of births and deaths occurring within her practice and encourage families to discharge their responsibilities

- explain how the various mortality statistics that are of interest to midwives are calculated

- review the causes and trends within each death rate category.

NOTIFICATION OF BIRTH

Legislation

Provision for the early notification of birth was first made in 1907 but it did not become a statutory requirement until 1915. When the early Acts were repealed the legislation was included in The Public Health Act 1936 and slightly amended by The National Health Service Act 1946.

Notification

It is the duty of the father or any other person in attendance or present within 6 hours after the birth to give notice in writing to the appointed medical officer in the district in which the child is born. This must be done within 36 hours of birth for any child born after 24 completed weeks of pregnancy, whether alive or dead. The health authority supplies prepaid addressed envelopes and forms for the notification of birth. It is usual for the midwife to undertake completion of the form. In addition to biographical information about the mother and her baby, the midwife will record the period of gestation, any congenital malformation and factors which may put the baby at risk.

The purpose of notification is to enable the health visitor to call at the home as soon as the midwife ceases to visit. An 'at-risk' register (see Ch. 45) is compiled from the details on the cards and is used for providing appropriate care for the children concerned. The birth information is also made available to the Registrar of Births and Deaths of the district in which the birth took place.

REGISTRATION OF BIRTH

The original Births and Deaths Registration Act was passed in 1837 but updated by the Act of 1953. This Act now governs the registration of births.

Births must be registered within 6 weeks (3 weeks in Scotland) and there is a statutory fine for those who fail to do so.

Place of registration

Every birth must be registered in the district in which it took place. This usually means a visit to the Register Office but some hospitals arrange for Registrars to visit the maternity wards regularly so that the new mothers may register there.

It is possible to make a Declaration of the birth to a Registrar of Births in another Registration District in England or Wales. This will then be sent to the Registrar of the District where the birth occurred and he or she will do the registration and send the certificates to the parent through the post.

Responsibility to register

The primary duty to register a birth rests with the mother of the child, although in the case of a married couple the father may attend to register. If a mother is unmarried and wishes the father's name and details to be included, the couple should attend together to give details to the Registrar. If this is not possible, the couple could re-register the birth later, adding the father's particulars. (It is also a requirement of law for parents who marry after the birth to re-register the child as a married couple.) An unmarried father may also attend alone to register if he takes with him a Statutory Declaration made by the mother that he is the father of the child, or certain other court orders.

There are other people, including a senior administrator at the hospital where the child was born, or someone present at the birth, which could be the midwife, who could attend to register a birth and in the absence of a better informant may be required to do so. However, it is always preferable for the parents to attend as they will give the most accurate information.

Naming a child

Whether or not a couple are married, the same general rules apply to the choosing of their child's names. They may in fact opt for any surname. It could be the same as or different from their own or a double-barrelled combination of their names.

With an unmarried mother, however, the midwife may be in a unique position to give advice, being in touch with the couple so early. If the child of an unmarried couple is given the father's surname and they subsequently part, it is not possible to change that name on the Birth Certificate. If, however, the child has the mother's surname and she later marries the father, it is possible on re-registration to change the child's name to his at that stage. It might be thought prudent therefore to choose the mother's surname. It sometimes happens, however, that the father will put undue pressure on the mother to use his surname but the midwife could make the mother aware that she can side-step the issue by registering the baby on her own. It would have to be without the father's details, but these could be added later on re-registration without legitimation (that is without the marriage of the parents), and the surname could then be changed to that of the father. The extra time for reflection could help to resolve the dispute.

Forenames are of course a free choice as well (although a Registrar may refuse to register an offensive name). There is a facility to add or change the forenames in the registration if a new name is chosen within 1 year. This can either be done by a Certificate of Naming or, if the child has been baptised, with a Certificate of Baptism signed by the Minister. Both these certificates may be obtained from the Register Office.

Statistics

At the time of registration, the Registrar also collects further information which is not entered in the Register but is used for statistical purposes and passed to the Office of National Statistics. This relates to dates of birth and marriage of the parents and previous children born, live or still, and is kept confidential. In addition, brief and simple questions on the employment of the parents may be asked. This further information is not confidential and may be used in an identifiable form.

Birth Certificates

A short Birth Certificate is issued free of charge at the time of registration. It gives the baby's name, sex, date of birth and the Registration District.

A full Birth Certificate may also be obtained for a prescribed fee. This is a copy of the complete entry in the Register.

NHS numbers no longer appear on certificates but on registration the parent or other informant will be given a form for them to register the child on a doctor's list under the NHS. This form is called FORM FP58.

Stillbirths

Definition of stillbirth

The definition of a stillbirth is given in section 41 of the Births and Deaths Registration Act 1953 and the Still-Birth (Definition) Act 1992 in the following terms:

'still-born child' means a child which has issued forth from its mother after the twenty-fourth week of pregnancy and which did not at any time after being completely expelled from its mother breathe or show any other signs of life.

Registration of stillbirths

In order to register a stillborn baby, the mother or other informant must have a Medical Certificate of Stillbirth. A medical practitioner or midwife who is present at the stillbirth or who examines the body of a stillborn child may write and sign this certificate. A midwife would be unwise to offer to complete the stillbirth certificate unless she had personally witnessed the birth.

Informants who have responsibility to register a stillbirth are the same as those in the case of a live birth (see above) and it has been possible since 1997 to make a declaration of the stillbirth to a Registrar in another district.

The Registrar will record the details in a Still-Birth Register and issue an authority for burial or cremation. She will also give a short free Certificate of Still-Birth similar to that for a live birth. The informant can also buy a full certificate which is a copy of the entry in the Register. The chosen names for the child now appear on both these certificates.

In the case of stillbirths the event cannot be re-registered to add the father's name nor to add or change a name for the baby.

Burial of a stillborn baby

Parents may make private arrangements for the baby to be buried or cremated but it is also possible for the hospital to undertake this on their behalf. Midwives who counsel the mother and father should encourage them to think about this carefully and to choose the arrangement which suits their need. Chapter 33 discusses support of the grieving parents.

Duties of a midwife concerning stillbirth

Notification of stillbirth is the same as is required for live birth.

Certificate of Stillbirth. The midwife will ensure

that this has been completed, usually by the doctor (see above).

Registration of stillbirth. The midwife explains to the parents that the birth must be registered and the procedure for burial or cremation.

The Supervisor of Midwives must be notified of the stillbirth by the midwife responsible for the care of the woman and her baby (UKCC 1994, p. 21).

Registration of deaths

This is the responsibility of the family. They should notify the Registrar of any child who has died after having been born alive. (In the rare event of a woman dying in childbirth, they will of course notify her death.)

Funeral arrangements

In the case of a neonatal death (see below) the funeral arrangements are the responsibility of the parents. There is a small death grant payable on the death of a child under 3 years but this will in no way offset the costs incurred. If there is hardship the midwife may refer the family to the social worker. Midwives should be familiar with local policy as in a few cases the hospital administrator may agree to meet some of the cost.

Both a Birth Certificate and a Death Certificate are required. The midwife will need to make sure that the parents are aware of this in order to spare them unnecessary distress.

In the case of a stillbirth where the parents wish to make private arrangements for the funeral, the midwife may need to explain that no death grant is payable.

In the case of a baby born dead before the completion of 24 weeks of pregnancy there is no procedure of notification or registration but if the parents wish the child to have a funeral, they will need a letter from the doctor or midwife stating that the baby was born before the legal age of viability and showed no signs of life.

BIRTH AND DEATH RATES

Vital statistics relate to life and death events, spe-

cifically to the systematic collection of numerical data in order that they may be summarised and studied. In measuring health there are difficulties in finding objective data to quantify, therefore it is pertinent to study the numbers of deaths occurring at different ages and their causes. This helps to explain why there are so many different types of death rate. The statistics of special interest to midwives are:

- birth rate
- stillbirth rate
- perinatal death rate
- neonatal death rate
- postneonatal death rate
- infant death rate
- maternal death rate.

Figure 48.1 shows graphically the periods relating to these different types of death.

Definition of 'rate'

Crude figures give little idea of the real frequency of events. If they are related to a specific number within the population, it becomes possible to compare one year's figures with another. If a particular group is studied, for example women in the fertile years, it is possible to identify the degree of risk in relation to certain events.

To calculate the rate of, for instance, stillbirth, the number of actual stillbirths in a year is compared to the number of total births (both live and still). This ratio is then related to a group of 1000 of those total births. The mathematical formula is as follows:

$$\frac{\text{No. of stillbirths}}{\text{No. of total births}} \times 1000 = \frac{\text{Stillbirth rate per}}{\text{1000 total births}}$$

Perinatal death

Definitions

A perinatal death is either a stillbirth or a death occurring in the first week of life (early neonatal death).

The perinatal death (or mortality) rate is the

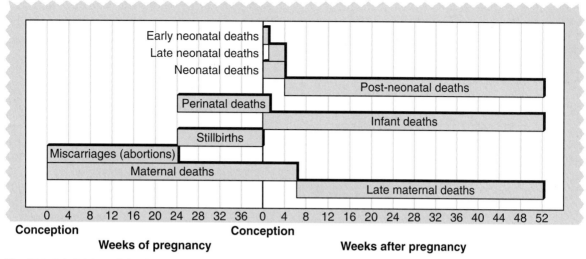

Fig. 48.1 Subdivision of deaths occurring during pregnancy and within 1 year of birth.

number of stillbirths and early neonatal deaths per 1000 total births.

Causes and predisposing factors

The perinatal death rate is often taken as the primary indicator of success or failure in obstetric care. These deaths are those which are closest to the event of birth and some of them are caused by such factors as hypoxia in labour and intracranial trauma during delivery. Others may be the result of genetic factors or of events in pregnancy. The main identifiable causes are:

* low birthweight (preterm and small for gestational age babies)
* intrauterine hypoxia
* respiratory depression at birth
* intracranial injury
* congenital abnormality.

It may be impossible to attribute a perinatal death to any one of the listed causes but a combination of predisposing factors increases the risk of death. These include:

* socioeconomic disadvantage
* poor maternal health (including effects of smoking, alcohol consumption, drug abuse and poor diet)

* multiple pregnancy
* antepartum haemorrhage
* pre-eclampsia
* breech presentation.

Trends

When new figures are published each year, small improvements are welcome but real encouragement is found in viewing the decline in rates over a number of years. These are often plotted in graphical form (Fig. 48.2). In looking for reasons for these trends it is important to take account of a wide range of factors such as the establishment of the National Health Service in 1948. The passing of the Abortion Act 1967 has resulted in the termination of many pregnancies for congenital abnormalities and thus the removal of deaths from these causes from the perinatal mortality statistics. Conversely the redefinition in 1992 of the age of legal viability as being 24 weeks' gestation instead of 28 weeks' gestation has brought numbers of babies into the definition of stillbirth and a consequent increase in perinatal mortality figures.

Rates are consistently higher than average in social classes IV and V as defined by the occupation of a parent, usually the father. Black women, especially those born outside the UK, are generally more likely to lose their babies (OPCS 1992).

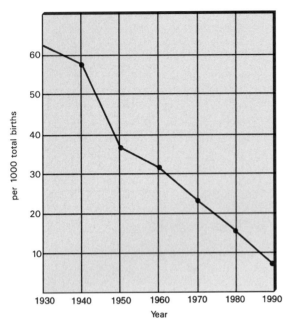

Fig. 48.2 Graph showing the perinatal death rates for England and Wales, 1930–1990.

Reasons for improvement

Improved care in pregnancy identifies the fetus at risk so that it can be monitored and delivered at the optimum time. Mothers receive information about healthy diet, cutting down on smoking and alcohol and care of their own health.

Improved care in labour aims at maintaining the mother and fetus in good condition. Skilled midwifery care aims to minimise intervention and to promote the normal process of labour as far as possible. If assistance becomes needed, medical help may be required and technological aids may become useful.

Improved neonatal care results in more survivors and in a better quality of life for those who do survive. Intensive neonatal care helps babies born after less than 28 weeks of pregnancy to survive, whereas in earlier years little attempt would have been made to prolong life.

Better socioeconomic conditions result in improvement in both survival and health of babies. Health professionals must be wary of assuming,

however, that improvement is continuous. The level of unemployment, for example, may rise and have unhappy effects for families.

Perinatal mortality in the world

Statistics published by WHO (1996) reveal a sharp contrast in rates of perinatal death. Babies in developing countries are five times as likely to die before or just after birth as those in the industrialised world. The rate in Western Africa is almost 10 times that in Northern America. 30% of the world's births occur in south-central Asia and this region accounts for almost 40% of perinatal deaths. Undoubtedly the poorer socioeconomic conditions of these countries contribute to the loss of 7.5 million babies.

Neonatal death

Definitions

A neonatal death is one occurring in the first 28 days of life. Neonatal deaths are divided into early neonatal deaths which occur during the first 7 days of life and later neonatal deaths which occur during the next 21 days. The reason for this is that the causes of early deaths are more similar to those of stillbirth while the causes of later deaths are different. The rates of neonatal deaths are calculated per 1000 live births.

Causes of late neonatal death

Some of the causes are similar to the earlier deaths because babies whose deaths are attributable to birth trauma or perinatal events may survive beyond the first week. After this time there is a greater likelihood of death occurring due to infection, intraventricular haemorrhage, necrotising enterocolitis and iatrogenic disorders.

Infant death

An infant death is one occurring in the first year of life. By definition this includes all neonatal deaths and the remainder are termed postneonatal deaths. The infant mortality rate is calculated per 1000 live births. This rate is taken as one of the best measures of a nation's health.

Causes of postneonatal death

Some of the important causes that a midwife should be aware of are non-accidental injury, infection and, in the older babies, accidents in the home. Sudden infant death also accounts for a significant number; these are unexpected deaths in which no cause is identified.

Trends and reasons for improvement

There has been a dramatic reduction since the beginning of the century in the number of infants who die under the age of 1 year. In 1900 the infant mortality rate was between 140 and 160 per 1000 whereas in 1985 the rate was 9.4 per 1000 in England and Wales. By 1995 this had fallen further to 6.0 per 1000 live births.

Improvement has been due to a number of factors including:

- better housing and standard of living
- immunisation
- antibiotics and chemotherapeutic agents
- prevention of cross-infection
- health education
- intravenous therapy
- appointment of paediatricians, neonatal specialists, health visitors and others.

CESDI

A confidential enquiry into stillbirths and deaths in infancy (CESDI) was established in England, Wales and Northern Ireland in 1992. In the first few years attention has been focused on intrapartum deaths with a separate analysis of sudden, unexplained infant deaths (SIDS). A project has been initiated to study antepartum term stillbirths (SATS) which account for around one-third of perinatal deaths (Persad et al 1995); the proportion of unexplained antepartum stillbirths increased from 1992 to 1995 (MCHRC 1997).

The deaths are examined for instances of suboptimal care. In the 1995 Report (MCHRC 1997) obstetricians and hospital midwives were responsible in over three-quarters of the comments on 'failures to act appropriately, recognise problems or communicate effectively' (p. 27) in those instances where alternative management might or

would reasonably be expected to have made a difference to the outcome. The Report recommends review and regular training and update of relevant professionals.

Some of the important issues highlighted are:

- the failure to recognise problems and act on them swiftly
- failure to identify risk factors for labour
- misinterpretation of cardiotocographs and failure to react to suspicious or abnormal traces
- not believing abnormal fetal blood sample results
- poor quality of record keeping
- inadequate communications:
  - between clinicians and parents
  - between professional groups
- failure by inexperienced people to call for senior help (MCHRC 1997).

Regional reports have also been produced (e.g. South Thames West 1997) and reflect similar matters. The South Thames West Report comments specifically on the importance of not allowing language barriers to prevent adequate communication with parents.

The CESDI Report comments that sudden infant death has fallen substantially since 1992. Robinson (1996a) points out the international success of the 'Back to Sleep' campaign but also stresses the continuing adverse influence of poverty.

Statistics are collected through a rapid reporting system in which midwives may participate. The form should be filled out as soon after the death as possible and sent to the district coordinator (Wallace 1994).

Future reports will include some slightly smaller babies, including legal abortions, and a few other details will be added.

Maternal death

The International Federation of Gynaecologists and Obstetricians (FIGO) defines maternal death as one occurring during pregnancy or labour or as a consequence of pregnancy within 42 days after delivery or abortion. The World Health Organization (WHO) estimates that 585 000 women die every year from pregnancy-related causes, a rate of 430 deaths per 100 000 live births. Whereas the lifetime risk of maternal death for a woman in a developed country is 1 in 1800, in Africa it is 1 in 16, in Asia 1 in 65 and in Latin America 1 in 130 (WHO) 1998).

The Reports on Confidential Enquiries into Maternal Deaths

These triennial reports on maternal deaths in the UK (from 1952 to 1985 they only covered England and Wales) analyse virtually every maternal death. They constitute the longest uninterrupted series of clinical audit in the world. The information is entirely confidential so that contributory factors can be examined without fear of recrimination. Practice in respect of each complication can be assessed and the report makes recommendations which have been most valuable. Any individual obstetrician, midwife or general practitioner is unlikely to see many mothers die in his or her care and cannot therefore rely on personal experience; the availability of a national report shares the knowledge which has been gained.

The UK maternal mortality rate is calculated as the number of deaths occurring per 100 000 or per million *maternities*, that is, pregnancies which resulted in a birth, live or still. The rate includes deaths due to abortion although abortions are not included in 'maternities' since it is impossible to calculate an accurate number. Since October 1992 the definition of stillbirth has been altered from one occurring after 28 weeks of pregnancy to one at 24 weeks or later and this has affected the calculation of the total number of maternities (as well as of stillbirths).

Four groups of deaths are defined:

• 'True' maternal death may be regarded as the *direct maternal death*, which is one 'resulting from obstetric complications of pregnancy, labour and puerperium, from interventions, omissions, incorrect treatment or from a chain of events resulting from any of the above'.
• *Indirect obstetric deaths* are 'those resulting from previous existing disease or disease that developed during pregnancy which was aggravated by pregnancy'.

• Deaths from other causes which happen to occur in pregnancy are defined as *fortuitous deaths*.
• *Late deaths* are those due to direct or indirect causes but which occur between 42 days and 1 year after abortion, miscarriage or delivery. This last category has only been added for the 1991–1993 triennial report (DH et al 1996) and for part of the previous one.

The report identifies the causes of maternal deaths and reveals the trends in incidence. It reveals substandard care and names the disciplines which are responsible. Where shortage of resources has contributed to the death, this is mentioned. The authors of the report are careful to stress that avoiding the elements of substandard care which are discussed would not necessarily have averted the death concerned.

Causes

In the Report relating to the years 1991–1993 (DH et al 1996), the five main causes of direct maternal death were as follows:

• thrombosis and thromboembolism
• hypertensive disorders of pregnancy
• early pregnancy death including abortion
• antepartum and postpartum haemorrhage
• amniotic fluid embolism.

Figure 48.3 illustrates the decline in maternal death since 1952, while Figure 48.4 shows the causes of maternal death in the UK for the triennium from 1991 to 1993.

Trends

Broadly speaking the maternal mortality rate has fallen in each triennium but has levelled off somewhat since 1987. In the 1991–1993 triennium the rate was 55.7 per million maternities.

Deaths from *thrombosis and pulmonary embolism* continue to be the largest group and the rate actually rose in the 1991–1993 triennium. Almost half followed caesarean section and this underlines the fact that caesarean section is not risk-free. Antenatal thrombotic conditions were sometimes unrecognised and caution should be exercised where pregnant women are immobile or on bed rest.

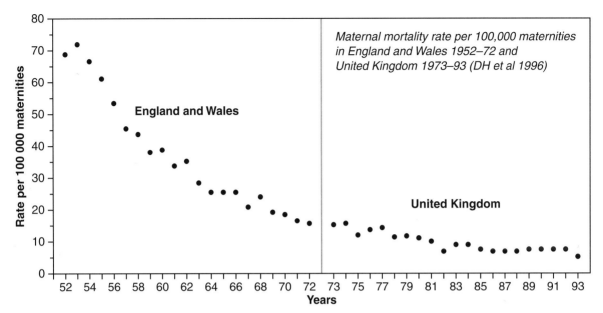

Fig. 48.3 Maternal mortality rate per 100 000 maternities in England and Wales 1952–1972 and UK 1973–1993 (after DH et al 1996).

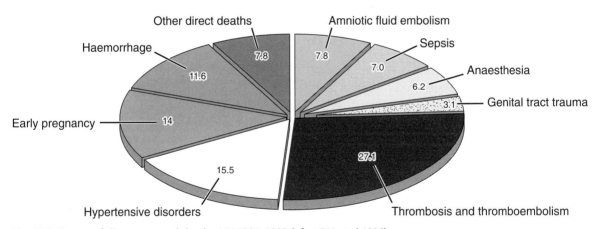

Fig. 48.4 Causes of direct maternal deaths: UK 1991–1993 (after DH et al 1996).

Pre-eclampsia and eclampsia were responsible for fewer deaths in the recent triennium. The use of magnesium sulphate (Eclampsia Trial Collaborative Group 1995) had not yet gained recognition for its effectiveness (see Ch. 17). The report cautions against reduction in the frequency of antenatal visits since five women developed very severe pre-eclampsia in the (conventional) intervals between visits.

While midwives are rarely called upon to deal with *early pregnancy emergencies*, they should note the report's exhortation to refer women early for expert opinion and treatment.

Deaths from *haemorrhage* continue to cause concern particularly in women of over 35 years of age. The report urges obstetricians and midwives to be aware of the speed with which collapse can occur with obstetric haemorrhage. A clear protocol is needed for women who refuse blood transfusion because of religious beliefs.

Other selected problems include the need for careful monitoring during the administration of *drugs affecting uterine action* including prostaglandins, Syntocinon and ritodrine. Robinson (1996b), commenting on a case of uterine rupture in a GP unit following the use of prostaglandins in a highly parous woman, considers that the midwives should have raised their voices in protest and exhorts them to be more assertive. This includes demanding training in any procedures that are not understood and owning up to limitations.

The Confidential Enquiries have had a significant effect in reducing the number of maternal deaths over the second half of the 20th century. Protocols have often been suggested based on lessons learned and these have helped to guide practitioners. The 1991–1993 Report (DH et al 1996) highlights management of haemorrhage where a woman refuses blood transfusion (see above), prophylaxis against thromboembolism in caesarean section and guidance for help for the anaesthetist in obstetric practice. Midwives need to be knowledgeable about these and to play their part in bringing them to the attention of medical colleagues where necessary and in contributing to the formation of local guidelines.

Conclusion

Midwives everywhere are concerned at the loss of a woman's life at or near the time of giving birth.

The WHO Safe Motherhood Initiative (see Ch. 4) has brought this into high profile. Just as tragic is the loss of infant life at the time when the new baby should be welcomed into the family. While the developing world has the greater problem, there is no room for complacency in industrialised countries. Each midwife needs to be aware of local circumstances and seek to apply best practice to the utmost of her ability. This may include initiating research (see Ch. 6) and applying available evidence to ensure that appropriate care is given.

READER ACTIVITIES

1. Investigate the mortality statistics in your local area of midwifery practice. Make a graph of the trends over 10 years.

2. Look up the latest incidence of (a) maternal death (b) neonatal death and (c) stillbirth in your area. Obtain the case records and look at factors that may have contributed to the fatal outcome.

3. Design a simple handout which could guide women as to what they must do to register their babies and which explains the possible alternatives and choices. You may find it helpful to arrange to visit the local Registrar of Births and Deaths.

REFERENCES

Abortion Act 1967 HMSO, London
Births and Deaths Registration Act 1953 HMSO, London
Department of Health, Welsh Office, Scottish Home and Health Department, Department of Health and Social Security, Northern Ireland 1996 Report on confidential enquiries into maternal deaths in the United Kingdom 1991–1993. HMSO, London
Eclampsia Trial Collaborative Group 1995 Which anticonvulsant for women with eclampsia? Evidence from the Collaborative Eclampsia Trial. Lancet 345: 1455–1463
Maternal and Child Health Research Consortium (MCHRC) 1997 Confidential enquiry into stillbirths and deaths in infancy: 4th Annual report 1 January – 31 December 1995. MCHRC, London
Office of Population Censuses and Surveys (OPCS) 1992 Mortality statistics, perinatal and infant: social and biological factors 1989. (Series DH3 no. 23) OPCS, London
Persad P, Hiscock C, Mitchell T 1995 The study of antepartum term stillbirths (SATS). MIDIRS Midwifery Digest 5(4): 479–480

Robinson J 1996a The emperor's new clothes. British Journal of Midwifery 4(11): 609–610
Robinson J 1996b Death of a mother. British Journal of Midwifery 4(7): 381–382
South Thames West Perinatal Audit Team 1997 Perinatal audit report 1994–96: towards improved perinatal outcomes. South Thames West Perinatal Audit Team, London
Still-Birth (Definition) Act 1992 HMSO, London
The National Health Service Act 1946 HMSO, London
The Public Health Act 1936 HMSO, London
United Kingdom Central Council for Nursing, Midwifery and Health Visiting (UKCC) 1994 The midwife's code of practice. UKCC, London
Wallace V 1994 New reporting system for perinatal deaths. MIDIRS Midwifery Digest 4(2): 231
World Health Organization (WHO) 1996 Perinatal mortality. A listing of available information. Maternal health and safe motherhood programme. (WHO/FRH/MSM 96.7) WHO, Geneva
World Health Organization (WHO) 1998 World Health Day 1998 information kit. WHO, Geneva

Basic anatomy and physiology

49

The reproductive organs

V. Ruth Bennett   Linda K. Brown

Woman is first and foremost a person and, when she bears a child, a mother. Many societies define her through her fertility and her body is adapted for this by its shape and function. The midwife needs to be familiar with the anatomical features of the woman and to understand the processes of reproduction but must never forget the social significance of childbearing or that a woman's body is unique, personal and private. It should be approached only with permission and with respect. The physiology of the various organs is described in appropriate chapters throughout the book.

FEMALE PELVIS

Functions

The primary function of the pelvic girdle is to allow movement of the body, especially walking and running.

It permits the person to sit and kneel. The woman's pelvis is adapted for childbearing, and because of its increased width and rounded brim women are less speedy than men.

The pelvis transmits the weight of the trunk to the legs, acting as a bridge between the femurs. This makes it necessary for the sacroiliac joint to be immensely strong and virtually immobile. The pelvis also takes the weight of the sitting body onto the ischial tuberosities.

The pelvis affords protection to the pelvic organs and, to a lesser extent, to the abdominal contents. The sacrum transmits the cauda equina and distributes the nerves to the various parts of the pelvis.

The normal female pelvis

The female pelvis (Fig. 49.1), because of its characteristics, gives rise to no difficulties in childbirth,

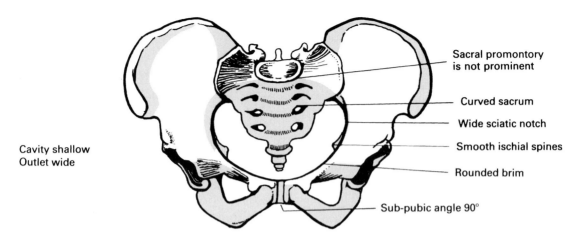

Cavity shallow
Outlet wide

Sacral promontory
is not prominent

Curved sacrum

Wide sciatic notch

Smooth ischial spines

Rounded brim

Sub-pubic angle 90°

Fig. 49.1 Normal female pelvis.

providing the fetus is of normal size. A knowledge of pelvic anatomy is needed for the conduct of labour as one of the ways to estimate the progress made is by assessing the relationship of the fetus to certain pelvic landmarks. A midwife must be competent to recognise a normal pelvis in order to be able to detect deviations from normal and refer them to the doctor.

Pelvic bones

There are four pelvic bones:

- two innominate ('nameless') or hip bones
- one sacrum
- one coccyx.

Innominate bones
Each innominate bone (Fig. 49.2) is composed of three parts:

The ilium is the large flared-out part. When the hand is placed on the hip it rests on the iliac crest which is the upper border. At the front of the iliac crest can be felt a bony prominence known as the anterior superior iliac spine.

A short distance below it is the anterior inferior iliac spine. There are two similar points at the other end of the iliac crest, namely the posterior superior and the posterior inferior iliac spines. The concave anterior surface of the ilium is the iliac fossa.

The ischium is the thick lower part. It has a large prominence known as the ischial tuberosity on which the body rests when sitting. Behind and a little above the tuberosity is an inward projection, the ischial spine. In labour the station of the fetal head is estimated in relation to the ischial spines.

The pubic bone forms the anterior part. It has a body and two oar-like projections, the superior ramus and the inferior ramus. The two pubic bones meet at the symphysis pubis and the two inferior rami form the pubic arch, merging into a similar ramus on the ischium. The space enclosed by the body of the pubic bone, the rami and the ischium is called the obturator foramen.

The innominate bone contains a deep cup to receive the head of the femur. This is termed the acetabulum. All three parts of the bone contribute to the acetabulum in the following proportions: two-fifths ilium, two-fifths ischium and one-fifth pubic bone.

On the lower border of the innominate bone are found two curves. One extends from the posterior inferior iliac spine up to the ischial spine and is called the *greater sciatic notch*. It is wide and rounded. The other lies between the ischial spine and the ischial tuberosity and is the *lesser sciatic notch*.

The sacrum
The sacrum is a wedge-shaped bone consisting

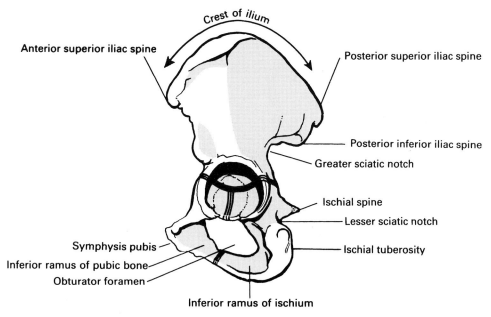

Fig. 49.2 Innominate bone showing important landmarks.

of five fused vertebrae. The upper border of the first sacral vertebra juts forward and is known as the sacral promontory. The anterior surface of the sacrum is concave and is referred to as the *hollow of the sacrum*. Laterally the sacrum extends into a *wing* or *ala*. Four pairs of holes or foramina pierce the sacrum and, through these, nerves from the cauda equina emerge to supply the pelvic organs. The posterior surface is roughened to receive attachments of muscles.

The coccyx

The coccyx is a vestigial tail. It consists of four fused vertebrae, forming a small triangular bone.

Pelvic joints

There are four pelvic joints:

- one symphysis pubis
- two sacroiliac joints
- one sacrococcygeal joint.

The symphysis pubis is formed at the junction of the two pubic bones which are united by a pad of cartilage.

The sacroiliac joints are the strongest joints in the body. They join the sacrum to the ilium and thus connect the spine to the pelvis.

The sacrococcygeal joint is formed where the base of the coccyx articulates with the tip of the sacrum.

In the non-pregnant state there is very little movement in these joints, but during pregnancy endocrine activity causes the ligaments to soften, which allows the joints to give. This may provide more room for the fetal head as it passes through the pelvis. The symphysis pubis may separate slightly in later pregnancy. If it widens appreciably, the degree of movement permitted may give rise to pain on walking. The sacroiliac joints allow a limited backward and forward movement of the tip and promontory of the sacrum, sometimes known as nodding of the sacrum. The sacrococcygeal joint permits the coccyx to be deflected backwards during the birth of the head.

Pelvic ligaments

Each of the pelvic joints is held together by ligaments:

- interpubic ligaments at the symphysis pubis

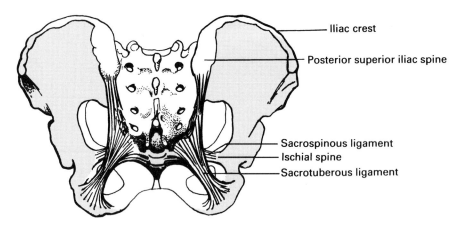

Fig. 49.3 Posterior view of the pelvis to show ligaments.

- sacroiliac ligaments
- sacrococcygeal ligaments.

There are two other ligaments important in midwifery:

- sacrotuberous ligament
- sacrospinous ligament.

The sacrotuberous ligament runs from the sacrum to the ischial tuberosity and the sacrospinous ligament from the sacrum to the ischial spine (Fig. 49.3). These two ligaments cross the sciatic notch and form the posterior wall of the pelvic outlet.

The true pelvis

The true pelvis is the bony canal through which the fetus must pass during birth. It has a brim, a cavity and an outlet.

The pelvic brim

The brim is round except where the sacral promontory projects into it. The promontory and wings of the sacrum form its posterior border, the iliac bones its lateral borders and the pubic bones its anterior border. The midwife needs to be familiar with the fixed points on the pelvic brim which are known as its landmarks. Commencing posteriorly these are (see Fig. 49.4):

- sacral promontory (1)
- sacral ala or wing (2)

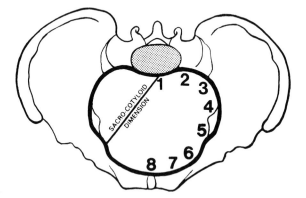

Fig. 49.4 Brim or inlet of female pelvis.

- sacroiliac joint (3)
- iliopectineal line which is the edge formed at the inward aspect of the ilium (4)
- iliopectineal eminence which is a roughened area formed where the superior ramus of the pubic bone meets the ilium (5)
- superior ramus of the pubic bone (6)
- upper inner border of the body of the pubic bone (7)
- upper inner border of the symphysis pubis (8).

Diameters of the brim

Three diameters are measured (Figs 49.5 and 49.8):

The anteroposterior diameter is a line from the sacral promontory to the upper border of the symphysis pubis. When the line is taken to the

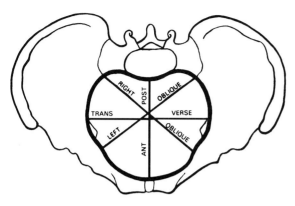

Fig. 49.5 View of pelvic inlet showing diameters.

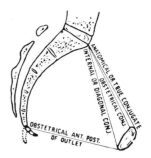

Fig. 49.7 Median section of the pelvis showing anteroposterior diameters.

uppermost point of the symphysis pubis it is called the anatomical conjugate and measures 12 cm; when it is taken to the posterior border of the upper surface, which is about 1.25 cm lower, it is called the obstetrical conjugate and measures 11 cm. The reason for this is that the obstetrical conjugate represents the available space for passage of the fetus (see Fig. 49.6). The term *true conjugate* may be used to refer to either of these measurements and the midwife should take care to establish which is meant.

The diagonal conjugate is also measured anteroposteriorly from the lower border of the symphysis to the sacral promontory. It may be estimated per vaginam as part of a pelvic assessment and should measure 12–13 cm (Fig. 49.7).

The oblique diameter is a line from one sacroiliac joint to the iliopectineal eminence on the opposite

side of the pelvis and measures 12 cm. There are two oblique diameters. Each takes its name from the sacroiliac joint from which it arises, that is, the left oblique diameter arises from the left sacroiliac joint.

The transverse diameter is a line between the points furthest apart on the iliopectineal lines and measures 13 cm.

Certain structures pass through the pelvic brim which may affect the space available for the fetus; for instance, the descending colon enters the pelvis near the left sacroiliac joint.

Another dimension is described, the *sacrocotyloid* (see Fig. 49.4). It passes from the sacral promontory to the iliopectineal eminence on each side and measures 9–9.5 cm. Its importance is concerned with posterior positions of the occiput when the parietal eminences of the fetal head may become caught (see Ch. 27).

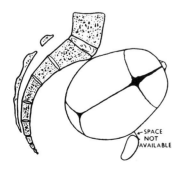

Fig. 49.6 Fetal head negotiating the narrow obstetrical conjugate.

The pelvic cavity

The cavity extends from the brim above to the outlet below. The anterior wall is formed by the pubic bones and symphysis pubis and its depth is 4 cm. The posterior wall is formed by the curve of the sacrum which is 12 cm in length. Because there is such a difference in these measurements the cavity forms a curved canal. Its lateral walls are the sides of the pelvis which are mainly covered by the obturator internus muscle.

The cavity is circular in shape and although it is not possible to measure its diameters exactly, they are all considered to be 12 cm (Fig. 49.8).

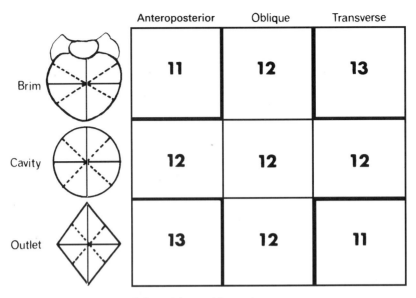

	Anteroposterior	Oblique	Transverse
Brim	11	12	13
Cavity	12	12	12
Outlet	13	12	11

Fig. 49.8 Measurements of the pelvic canal in centimetres.

The pelvic outlet

Two outlets are described: the anatomical and the obstetrical. The anatomical outlet is formed by the lower borders of each of the bones together with the sacrotuberous ligament. The obstetrical outlet is of greater practical significance because it includes the narrow pelvic strait through which the fetus must pass. The narrow pelvic strait lies between the sacrococcygeal joint, the two ischial spines and the lower border of the symphysis pubis. The obstetrical outlet is the space between the narrow pelvic strait and the anatomical outlet. This outlet is diamond-shaped. Its three diameters are as follows (Fig. 49.8):

The anteroposterior diameter is a line from the lower border of the symphysis pubis to the sacrococcygeal joint. It measures 13 cm. As the coccyx may be deflected backwards during labour, this diameter indicates the space available during delivery.

The oblique diameter is said to be between the obturator foramen and the sacrospinous ligament, although there are no fixed points. The measurement is taken as being 12 cm.

The transverse diameter is a line between the two ischial spines and measures 10–11 cm. It is the narrowest diameter in the pelvis.

The false pelvis

This is the part of the pelvis situated above the pelvic brim. It is formed by the upper flared-out portions of the iliac bones and protects the abdominal organs, but is of no significance in obstetrics.

Pelvic inclination

When a woman is standing in the upright position, her pelvis is on an incline. The anterior superior iliac spines are immediately above the symphysis pubis in the same vertical plane. The brim is tilted and if the line joining the sacral promontory and the top of the symphysis pubis were to be extended, it would form an angle of 60° with the horizontal floor. Similarly, if a line joining the centre of the sacrum and the centre of the symphysis pubis were to be extended, the resultant angle with the floor would be 30°. The angle of inclination of the outlet is 15° (see Fig. 49.9). When the woman is in the recumbent position the same angles are made with the vertical, which should be kept in mind when carrying out an abdominal examination.

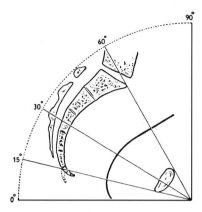

Fig. 49.9 Median section of the pelvis showing the inclination of the planes and the axis of the pelvic canal.

Pelvic planes

These are imaginary flat surfaces at the brim, cavity and outlet of the pelvic canal at the levels of the lines described above (Fig. 49.10).

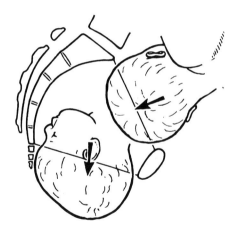

Fig. 49.10 Fetal head entering plane of pelvic brim and leaving plane of pelvic outlet.

Axis of the pelvic canal

A line drawn exactly half-way between the anterior wall and the posterior wall of the pelvic canal would trace a curve known as the curve of Carus. The midwife needs to become familiar with this concept in order to make accurate observations on vaginal examination and to facilitate the birth of the baby.

The four types of pelvis (Table 49.1)

Classically, pelves have been described as falling into four categories according to the shape of the brim (Fig. 49.11). It is unlikely that a woman's pelvis is classified in life unless she encounters difficulties in childbirth. Of much more importance is the individual woman's pelvic capacity and whether it is adequate for the passage of the child she is carrying (Williams et al 1989). It is a common saying that the fetal head is the best pelvimeter. If one of the important measurements is reduced by 1 cm or more from the normal, the pelvis is said to be contracted and may give rise to difficulty in labour (see Chs 26 and 29) or necessitate caesarean section.

The gynaecoid pelvis

As described above, this is the ideal pelvis for childbearing. Its main features are the rounded brim, the generous forepelvis (the part in front of the transverse diameter), straight side walls, a shallow cavity with a broad, well-curved sacrum, blunt ischial spines, a wide sciatic notch and a pubic arch of 90°. It is found in women of average build and height with a shoe size of 4 or larger.

The justo minor pelvis is like a gynaecoid pelvis

Table 49.1 Features of the four types of pelvis

Features	Gynaecoid	Android	Anthropoid	Platypelloid
Brim	Rounded	Heart-shaped	Long oval	Kidney-shaped
Forepelvis	Generous	Narrow	Narrowed	Wide
Side walls	Straight	Convergent	Divergent	Divergent
Ischial spines	Blunt	Prominent	Blunt	Blunt
Sciatic notch	Rounded	Narrow	Wide	Wide
Subpubic angle	90°	< 90°	> 90°	> 90°
Incidence	50%	20%	25%	5%

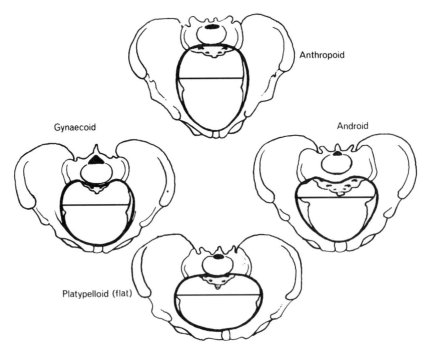

Fig. 49.11 Characteristic inlet of the four types of pelvis.

in miniature. All diameters are reduced but are in proportion. It is normally found in women of small stature, less than 1.5 m in height, with small hands and feet, but is occasionally found in women of normal stature.

The outcome of labour in this situation depends on the fetus. If the fetal size is consistent with the size of the maternal pelvis, normal labour and delivery will take place. Often these women have small babies and the outcome is favourable. However, if the fetus is large, a degree of cephalopelvic disproportion will result. The same is true when a malpresentation or malposition of the fetus exists.

The android pelvis

This is so called because it resembles the male pelvis. Its brim is heart-shaped with a narrow fore-pelvis, and has a transverse diameter which is towards the back. The side walls converge, making it a funnel shape with a deep cavity and a straight sacrum. The ischial spines are prominent and the sciatic notch is narrow. The angle of the pubic arch is less than 90°. It is found in short and heavily built women who have a tendency to be hirsute.

This type of pelvis predisposes to an occipito-posterior position of the fetal head and is the least suited to child bearing.

The heart-shaped brim favours a posterior position of the occiput as a result of insufficient space for the biparietal diameter in the narrow forepelvis, combined with the fact that the greater space lies in the hindpelvis. Funnelling in the cavity may hinder progress in labour. At the pelvic outlet, the prominent ischial spines sometimes prevent complete internal rotation of the head and the anteroposterior diameter becomes caught on them, causing a deep transverse arrest. The narrowed sub-pubic angle cannot easily accommodate the biparietal diameter which displaces the head backwards (Fig. 49.12). (Posterior positions of the occiput are described in Ch. 27.)

The anthropoid pelvis

This has a long, oval brim in which the antero-posterior diameter is longer than the transverse. The side walls diverge and the sacrum is long and deeply concave. The ischial spines are not prominent and the sciatic notch is very wide, as is the

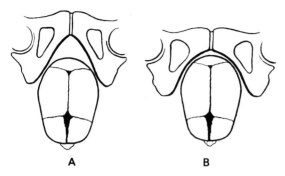

Fig. 49.12 (A) Outlet of android pelvis. The head does not fit into the acute pubic arch and is forced backwards onto the perineum. (B) Outlet of the gynaecoid pelvis. The head fits snugly into the pubic arch.

sub-pubic angle. Women with this type of pelvis tend to be tall, with narrow shoulders. Labour does not usually present any difficulties, but a direct occipitoanterior or direct occipitoposterior position is often a feature and the position adopted for engagement may persist to delivery.

The platypelloid pelvis

This flat pelvis has a kidney-shaped brim in which the anteroposterior diameter is reduced and the transverse increased. The side walls diverge, the sacrum is flat and the cavity shallow. The ischial spines are blunt, and the sciatic notch and the sub-pubic angle are both wide. The head must engage with the sagittal suture in the transverse diameter, but usually descends through the cavity without difficulty. Engagement may necessitate lateral tilting of the head, known as *asynclitism*, in order to allow the biparietal diameter to pass the narrowest anteroposterior diameter of the brim (Box 49.1).

Other pelvic variations

High assimilation pelvis. This occurs when the 5th lumbar vertebra is fused to the sacrum and the angle of inclination of the pelvic brim is increased. Engagement of the head is difficult but, once achieved, labour progresses normally.

Deformed pelvis. Deformation of the pelvis may result from a developmental anomaly, dietary deficiency, injury or disease (Box 49.2).

> **Box 49.1** Negotiating the pelvic brim in asynclitism
>
> **Anterior asynclitism**
> The anterior parietal bone moves down behind the symphysis pubis until the parietal eminence enters the brim. The movement is then reversed and the head tilts in the opposite direction until the posterior parietal bone negotiates the sacral promontory and the head is engaged.
>
> **Posterior asynclitism**
> The movements of anterior asynclitism are reversed. The posterior parietal bone negotiates the sacral promontory prior to the anterior parietal bone moving down behind the symphysis pubis.
>
> Once the pelvic brim has been negotiated, descent progresses normally accompanied by flexion and internal rotation.

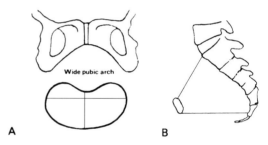

Fig. 49.13 Rachitic flat pelvis. (A) Note wide pubic arch and kidney-shaped brim. (B) The lateral view shows the diminished anteroposterior diameter of the brim and the increased anteroposterior diameter of the outlet.

PELVIC FLOOR

The pelvic floor is formed by the soft tissues which fill the outlet of the pelvis. The most important of these is the strong diaphragm of muscle slung like a hammock from the walls of the pelvis. Through it pass the urethra, the vagina and the anal canal.

Functions

The pelvic floor supports the weight of the abdominal and pelvic organs. Its muscles are responsible for the voluntary control of micturition and defaecation and play an important part in sexual intercourse. During childbirth it influences the passive movements of the fetus through the birth canal and relaxes to allow its exit from the pelvis.

Box 49.2 Deformed pelves

Developmental anomalies

Naegele's and Robert's pelves. Both these rarities are due to failure in development. In the Naegele's pelvis one sacral ala is missing and the sacrum is fused to the ilium, causing a grossly asymmetric brim. The Robert pelvis is similar but bilateral. In both instances the abnormal brim prevents engagement of the fetal head.

Dietary deficiency

Deficiency of vitamins and minerals necessary for the formation of healthy bones is less frequently seen today than in the past but might still complicate pregnancy and labour to some extent. The midwife must be alert for them especially in immigrant or poor populations.

Rachitic pelvis. Rickets in early childhood can lead to gross deformity of the pelvic brim. The weight of the upper body presses downwards onto the softened pelvic bones. The sacral promontory is pushed downwards and forwards and the ilium and ischium are drawn outwards. This results in a flat pelvic brim similar to that of the platypelloid pelvis (see Fig. 49.13). The sacrum tends to be straight with the coccyx bending acutely forward. Because the tuberosities are wide apart, the pubic arch is wide. With the improvements in child care seen throughout the world, this type of pelvis should be infrequently seen. The clinical signs of rickets, bow legs and spinal deformity can occasionally be seen.

If severe contraction is present caesarean section is required to deliver the baby. The fetal head will attempt to enter the pelvis by asynclitism.

Osteomalacic pelvis. The disease osteomalacia is rarely encountered in the UK. It is due to an acquired deficiency of calcium and occurs in adults. All bones of the skeleton soften as a result of gross calcium deficiency. The pelvic canal is squashed together until the brim becomes a Y-shaped slit. Labour is impossible and caesarean section would be performed. In early pregnancy incarceration of the gravid uterus may occur because of the gross deformity.

Injury and disease

Trauma. A pelvis which has been fractured will develop callus formation or may fail to unite correctly. This may lead to reduced measurements and therefore to some degree of contraction. Conditions sustained in childhood such as fractures of the pelvis or lower limbs, congenital dislocation of the hip and poliomyelitis may lead to unequal weightbearing which will also cause deformity. The child puts her weight on the stronger leg and that side of the pelvis is pressed inwards, leading to flattening of the pelvic brim. With the expert orthopaedic care today, this should be less frequently seen.

Spinal deformity. If kyphosis (forward angulation) or scoliosis (lateral curvature) is evident, or suggested by a limp or deformity, the midwife must refer the woman to a doctor. Pelvic contraction is likely in these cases and the outcome of pregnancy is dependent on degree.

Muscle layers

The superficial layer is composed of five muscles (Fig. 49.14):

- *The external anal sphincter* encircles the anus and is attached behind by a few fibres to the coccyx.
- *The transverse perineal muscles* pass from the ischial tuberosities to the centre of the perineum.
- *The bulbocavernosus muscles* pass from the perineum forwards around the vagina to the corpora cavernosa of the clitoris just under the pubic arch.
- *The ischiocavernosus muscles* pass from the ischial tuberosities along the pubic arch to the corpora cavernosa.
- *The membranous sphincter of the urethra* is composed of muscle fibres passing above and below the urethra and attached to the pubic bones. It is not a true sphincter since it is not circular, but it acts to close the urethra.

The deep layer (Fig. 49.15) is composed of three pairs of muscles which together are known as the levator ani muscles. They are so called because they lift or elevate the anus. Each levator ani muscle (left and right) consists of the following:

- *The pubococcygeus muscle* passes from the pubis to the coccyx, with a few fibres crossing over in the perineal body to form its deepest part.
- *The iliococcygeus muscle* passes from the fascia covering the obturator internus muscle (the white line of pelvic fascia) to the coccyx.
- *The ischiococcygeus muscle* passes from the ischial spine to the coccyx, in front of the sacrospinous ligament.

Between the muscle layers, and also above and below them, there are layers of pelvic fascia. This

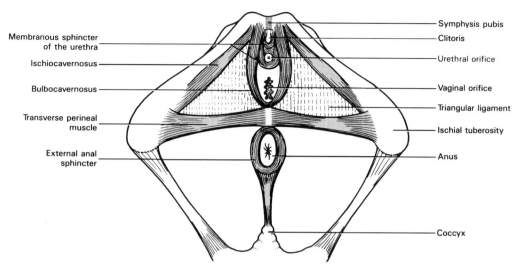

Membranous sphincter of the urethra
Ischiocavernosus
Bulbocavernosus
Transverse perineal muscle
External anal sphincter

Symphysis pubis
Clitoris
Urethral orifice
Vaginal orifice
Triangular ligament
Ischial tuberosity
Anus
Coccyx

Fig. 49.14 Superficial layer of the pelvic floor.

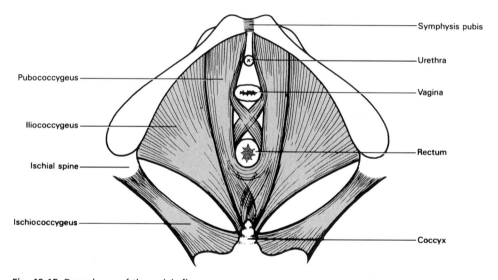

Pubococcygeus
Iliococcygeus
Ischial spine
Ischiococcygeus

Symphysis pubis
Urethra
Vagina
Rectum
Coccyx

Fig. 49.15 Deep layer of the pelvic floor.

is loose areolar tissue which is used like packing material in the spaces. The tissue that fills the triangular space between the bulbocavernosus, the ischiocavernosus and the transverse perineal muscles is known as the *triangular ligament*.

The perineal body

This is a pyramid of muscle and fibrous tissue situated between the vagina and the rectum. It is made up of fibres from muscles described above. The apex, which is the deepest part, is formed from the fibres of the pubococcygeus muscle which cross over at this point; the base is formed from the transverse perineal muscles which meet in the perineum, together with the bulbocavernosus in front and the external anal sphincter behind. The perineal body measures 4 cm in each direction. (See also Chs 24 and 45 for the perineum in labour and for pelvic floor exercises.)

THE VULVA

This term applies to the external female genital organs (Fig. 49.16). It consists of the following structures:

The mons pubis or mons veneris ('mount of Venus') is a pad of fat lying over the symphysis pubis. It is covered with pubic hair from the time of puberty.

The labia majora (greater lips) are two folds of fat and areolar tissue, covered with skin and pubic hair on the outer surface. They arise in the mons veneris and merge into the perineum behind.

The labia minora (lesser lips) are two thin folds of skin lying between the labia majora. Anteriorly they divide to enclose the clitoris; posteriorly they fuse, forming the fourchette.

The clitoris is a small rudimentary organ corresponding to the male penis. It is extremely sensitive and highly vascular and plays a part in the orgasm of sexual intercourse.

The vestibule is the area enclosed by the labia minora in which are situated the openings of the urethra and the vagina.

The urethral orifice lies 2.5 cm posterior to the clitoris. On either side lie the openings of Skene's ducts, two small blind-ended tubules 0.5 cm long running within the urethral wall.

The vaginal orifice is also known as the introitus of the vagina and occupies the posterior two-thirds of the vestibule. The orifice is partially closed by the hymen, a thin membrane which tears during sexual intercourse or during the birth of the first child. The remaining tags of hymen are known as the carunculae myrtiformes because they are thought to resemble myrtle berries.

Bartholin's glands are two small glands which open on either side of the vaginal orifice and lie in the posterior part of the labia majora. They secrete mucus which lubricates the vaginal opening.

The vulval blood supply

This comes from the internal and the external pudendal arteries. The blood drains through corresponding veins.

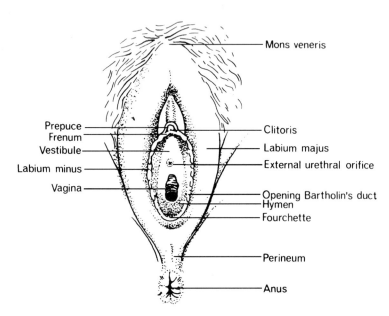

Fig. 49.16 Female external genital organs.

Lymphatic drainage
This is mainly via the inguinal glands.

Nerve supply
This is derived from branches of the pudendal nerve.

THE VAGINA

Functions
The vagina is a passage which allows the escape of the menstrual flow, receives the penis and the ejected sperm during sexual intercourse and provides an exit for the fetus during delivery.

Position
It is a canal running from the vestibule to the cervix, passing upwards and backwards into the pelvis along a line approximately parallel to the plane of the pelvic brim.

Relations (Figs 49.17 and 49.18)
A knowledge of the relations of the vagina is essential for the accurate examination of the pregnant woman and her safe delivery.

Anterior. In front lie the bladder and the urethra which are closely connected to the anterior vaginal wall.

Posterior. Behind, the pouch of Douglas, the rectum and the perineal body each occupy approximately one-third of the posterior vaginal wall.

Lateral. Beside the upper two-thirds are the pelvic fascia and the ureters which pass beside the cervix, while beside the lower third are the muscles of the pelvic floor.

Superior. Above the vagina lies the uterus.

Inferior. Below the vagina lie the external genitalia.

Structure
The posterior wall is 10 cm long while the anterior wall is only 7.5 cm in length because the cervix projects at a right angle into its upper part.

The upper end of the vagina is known as the vault. Where the cervix projects into it, the vault forms a circular recess which is described as four arches or fornices. The posterior fornix is the largest of these because the vagina is attached to the uterus at a higher level behind than in front. The anterior fornix lies in front of the cervix and the lateral fornices lie on either side. The vaginal walls are pink in appearance and thrown into small folds known as rugae. These allow the vaginal walls to stretch during intercourse and childbirth.

Layers
The lining is made of squamous epithelium.

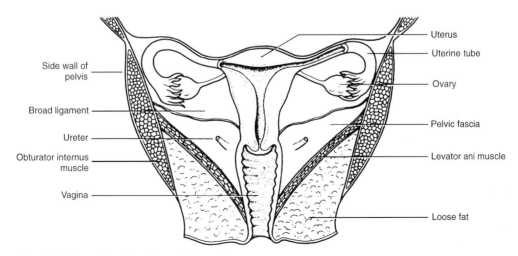

Fig. 49.17 Coronal section through the pelvis.

Side wall of pelvis

Broad ligament

Ureter

Obturator internus muscle

Vagina

Uterus

Uterine tube

Ovary

Pelvic fascia

Levator ani muscle

Loose fat

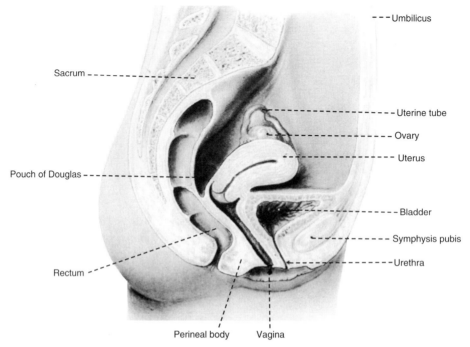

Sacrum

Pouch of Douglas

Rectum

Perineal body

Vagina

Umbilicus

Uterine tube

Ovary

Uterus

Bladder

Symphysis pubis

Urethra

Fig. 49.18 Sagittal section of the pelvis.

Beneath the epithelium lies a layer of vascular connective tissue.

The muscle layer is divided into a weak inner coat of circular fibres and a stronger outer coat of longitudinal fibres.

Pelvic fascia surrounds the vagina, forming a layer of connective tissue.

Contents

There are no glands in the vagina. It is, however, moistened by mucus from the cervix and a transudate which seeps out from the blood vessels of the vaginal wall.

In spite of the alkaline mucus, the vaginal fluid is strongly acid (pH 4.5) due to the presence of lactic acid formed by the action of Döderlein's bacilli on glycogen found in the squamous epithelium of the lining. These lactobacilli are normal inhabitants of the vagina. The acid deters the growth of pathogenic bacteria.

Blood supply

This comes from branches of the internal iliac artery and includes the vaginal artery and a descending branch of the uterine artery. The blood drains through corresponding veins.

Lymphatic drainage

This is via the inguinal, the internal iliac and the sacral glands.

Nerve supply

This is derived from the Lee Frankenhäuser plexus.

THE UTERUS

Functions

The uterus exists to shelter the fetus during pregnancy. It prepares for this possibility each month and following pregnancy it expels the uterine contents.

Position

It is situated in the cavity of the true pelvis, behind the bladder and in front of the rectum. It leans forward, which is known as *anteversion*; it bends forwards on itself, which is known as *anteflexion*. When the woman is standing this results in an almost horizontal position with the fundus resting on the bladder.

Relations (Figs 49.17 and 49.18)

Anterior. In front of the uterus lie the uterovesical pouch and the bladder.

Posterior. Behind the uterus are the rectouterine pouch of Douglas and the rectum.

Lateral. On either side of the uterus are the broad ligaments, the uterine tubes and the ovaries.

Superior. Above the uterus lie the intestines.

Inferior. Below the uterus is the vagina.

Supports (Fig. 49.19)

The uterus is supported by the pelvic floor and maintained in position by several ligaments of which those at the level of the cervix are the most important.

The transverse cervical ligaments fan out from the sides of the cervix to the side walls of the pelvis. They are sometimes known as the cardinal ligaments or Mackenrodt's ligaments.

The uterosacral ligaments pass backwards from the cervix to the sacrum.

The pubocervical ligaments pass forwards from the cervix, under the bladder, to the pubic bones.

The broad ligaments are formed from the folds of peritoneum which are draped over the uterine tubes. They hang down like a curtain and spread from the sides of the uterus to the side walls of the pelvis.

The round ligaments have little value as a support but tend to maintain the anteverted position of the uterus. They arise from the cornua of the uterus in front of and below the insertion of each uterine tube and pass between the folds of the broad ligament, through the inguinal canal, to be inserted into each labium majus.

The ovarian ligaments also begin at the cornua of the uterus but behind the uterine tubes and pass down between the folds of the broad ligament to the ovaries.

It is helpful to note that the round ligament, uterine tube and the ovarian ligament are very similar in appearance and arise from the same area of the uterus. This makes careful identification important when tubal surgery is undertaken.

Structure

The non-pregnant uterus is a hollow, muscular, pear-shaped organ situated in the true pelvis (Fig. 49.20). It is 7.5 cm long, 5 cm wide and

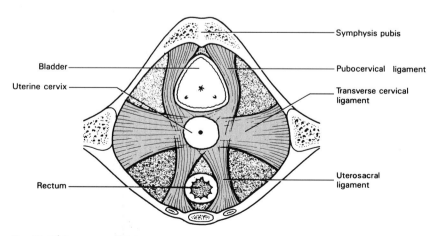

Fig. 49.19 Supports of the uterus.

Symphysis pubis

Bladder

Uterine cervix

Rectum

Pubocervical ligament

Transverse cervical ligament

Uterosacral ligament

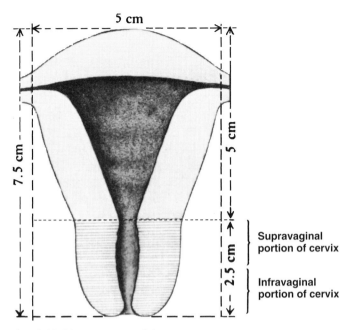

Fig. 49.20 Measurements of the uterus.

2.5 cm in depth, each wall being 1.25 cm thick. The cervix forms the lower third of the uterus and measures 2.5 cm in each direction.

The uterus consists of the following parts:

The body or corpus makes up the upper two-thirds of the uterus and is the greater part.

The fundus is the domed upper wall between the insertions of the uterine tubes.

The cornua are the upper outer angles of the uterus where the uterine tubes join.

The cavity is a potential space between the anterior and posterior walls. It is triangular in shape, the base of the triangle being uppermost.

The isthmus is a narrow area between the cavity and the cervix, which is 7 mm long. It enlarges during pregnancy to form the lower uterine segment.

The cervix or neck protrudes into the vagina. The upper half, being above the vagina, is known as the supravaginal portion while the lower half is the infravaginal portion.

The internal os (mouth) is the narrow opening between the isthmus and the cervix.

The external os is a small round opening at the lower end of the cervix. After childbirth this becomes a transverse slit.

The cervical canal lies between these two ora and is a continuation of the uterine cavity. This canal is shaped like a spindle, narrow at each end and wider in the middle.

Layers

The uterus has three layers, of which the middle muscle layer is by far the thickest.

The endometrium forms a lining of ciliated epithelium (mucous membrane) on a base of connective tissue or stroma.

In the uterine cavity this endometrium is constantly changing in thickness throughout the menstrual cycle (see Ch. 50). The basal layer does not alter, but provides the foundation from which the upper layers regenerate. The epithelial cells are cubical in shape and dip down to form glands which secrete an alkaline mucus.

The cervical endometrium does not respond to the hormonal stimuli of the menstrual cycle to the same extent. Here the epithelial cells are tall and columnar in shape and the mucus-secreting glands are branching racemose glands. The cervical endometrium is thinner than that of the body and is folded into a pattern known as the arbor vitae (tree of life). This is thought to assist the passage of the sperm. (The portion of the cervix which protrudes into the vagina (Fig. 49.20) is covered with squamous epithelium similar to that lining the vagina. The point where the epithelium changes, at the external os, is termed the squamocolumnar junction.)

The myometrium, or muscle coat, is thick in the upper part of the uterus and is more sparse in the isthmus and cervix. Its fibres run in all directions and interlace to surround the blood vessels and lymphatics which pass to and from the endometrium. The outer layer is formed of longitudinal fibres which are continuous with those of the uterine tube, the uterine ligaments and the vagina.

In the cervix the muscle fibres are embedded in collagen fibres which enable it to stretch in labour.

The perimetrium is a double serous membrane, an extension of the peritoneum, which is draped over the uterus, covering all but a narrow strip on either side and the anterior wall of the supravaginal cervix from where it is reflected up over the bladder.

Blood supply (Fig. 49.21)
The uterine artery arrives at the level of the cervix and is a branch of the internal iliac artery. It sends a small branch to the upper vagina, and then runs upwards in a twisted fashion to meet the ovarian artery and form an anastomosis with it near the cornu. The ovarian artery is a branch of the abdominal aorta, leaving near the renal artery. It supplies the ovary and uterine tube before joining the uterine artery. The blood drains through corresponding veins.

Lymphatic drainage
Lymph is drained from the uterine body to the internal iliac glands and also from the cervical area to many other pelvic lymph glands. This provides an effective defence against uterine infection.

Nerve supply
This is mainly from the autonomic nervous system, sympathetic and parasympathetic, via Lee Frankenhäuser's plexus or pelvic plexus.

UTERINE MALFORMATIONS

For pregnancy and labour to be achieved with minimal difficulty, a woman must have normal reproductive anatomy. When structural abnormality of the pelvic organs exists, problems arise which can place an extra burden on mother and

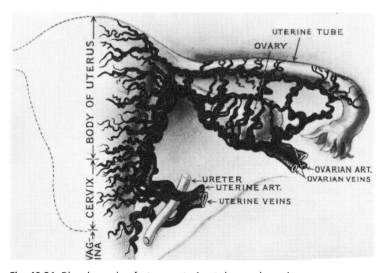

Fig. 49.21 Blood supply of uterus, uterine tubes and ovaries.

Box 49.3 Uterine malformations

Embryological development of the uterus
The female genital tract is formed in early embryonic life when a pair of ducts develop. These paramesonephric or Müllerian ducts come together in the midline and fuse into a Y-shaped canal. The open upper ends of this structure open into the peritoneal cavity and the unfused portions become the uterine tubes. The fused lower portion forms the uterovaginal area which further develops into the uterus and vagina.

Types of uterine malformation
Various types of structural abnormality can result from failure of fusion of the Müllerian ducts. Three of these abnormalities can be seen in Figure 24.1. A double uterus with an associated double vagina will develop where there has been complete failure of fusion. Partial fusion results in various degrees of duplication. A single vagina with a double uterus is the result of fusion at the lower end of the ducts only. A bicornuate uterus (one with two horns) is the result of incomplete fusion at the upper portion of the uterovaginal area. In rare cases, one

Müllerian duct regresses and the end result is a uterus with one horn — termed a unicornuate uterus.

Effect of abnormality on pregnancy
When pregnancy occurs in the woman with an abnormal uterus, the outcome depends on the ability of the uterus to accommodate the growing fetus. A problem only exists if the tissue is insufficient to allow the uterus to enlarge for a full-term fetus lying longitudinally.

If there is insufficient hypertrophy, the possible difficulties are abortion, premature labour and abnormal lie of the fetus. In labour, poor uterine function may be experienced.

Minor defects of structure cause little problem and might pass unnoticed with the woman having a normal outcome to her pregnancy. Occasionally problems arise when a fetus is accommodated in one horn of a double uterus and the empty horn has filled the pelvic cavity. In this situation, the empty horn has grown due to the hormonal influences of the pregnancy, and its size and position will cause obstruction during labour. Caesarean section would be the method of delivery.

---

fetus. The possible effects of such abnormalities are explained in Box 49.3.

THE UTERINE TUBES

Functions
The uterine tube propels the ovum towards the uterus, receives the spermatozoa as they travel upwards and provides a site for fertilisation. It supplies the fertilised ovum with nutrition during its continued journey to the uterus.

Position
The uterine tubes extend laterally from the cornua of the uterus towards the side walls of the pelvis. They arch over the ovaries, the fringed ends hovering near the ovaries in order to receive the ovum.

Relations

Anterior, posterior and superior. The peritoneal cavity and the intestines.

Lateral. The side walls of the pelvis.

Inferior. The broad ligaments and ovaries lie below the tubes.

Medial. The uterus lies between the two uterine tubes.

Supports
The uterine tubes are held in place by their attachment to the uterus. The peritoneum folds over them, draping down below as the broad ligaments and extending at the sides to form the infundibulopelvic ligaments.

Structure
Each tube is 10 cm long. The lumen of the tube provides an open pathway from the outside to the peritoneal cavity. The uterine tube has four portions (Fig. 49.22):

The interstitial portion is 1.25 cm long and lies within the wall of the uterus. Its lumen is 1 mm wide.

The isthmus is another narrow part which extends for 2.5 cm from the uterus.

The ampulla is the wider portion where fertilisation usually occurs. It is 5 cm long.

The infundibulum is the funnel-shaped fringed end which is composed of many processes known

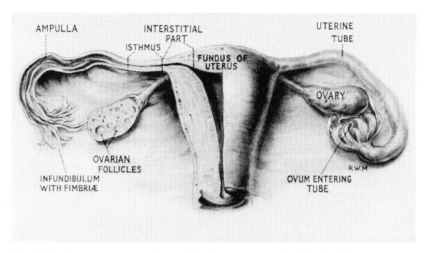

Fig. 49.22 Uterine tube in section. Note the ovum entering the fimbriated end.

as fimbriae. One fimbria is elongated to form the ovarian fimbria which is attached to the ovary.

Layers (Fig. 49.23)

The lining is a mucous membrane of *ciliated cubical epithelium* which is thrown into complicated folds known as plicae. These folds slow the ovum down on its way to the uterus. In this lining are goblet cells which produce a secretion containing glycogen to nourish the ovum.

Beneath the lining is a layer of *vascular connective tissue*.

The muscle coat consists of two layers, an inner circular layer and an outer longitudinal layer, both of smooth muscle. The peristaltic movement of the uterine tube is due to the action of these muscles.

The tube is covered with *peritoneum* but the infundibulum passes through it to open into the peritoneal cavity.

Blood supply
This is via the uterine and ovarian arteries, returning by the corresponding veins.

Lymphatic drainage
This is to the lumbar glands.

Nerve supply
This is from the ovarian plexus.

THE OVARIES

Functions
The ovaries produce ova and the hormones oestrogen and progesterone.

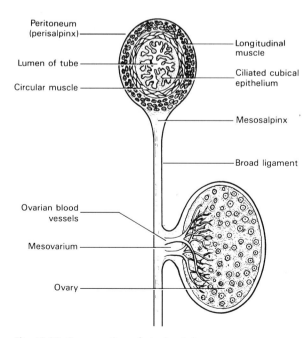

Fig. 49.23 Cross-section of uterine tube.

Position

They are attached to the back of the broad ligament within the peritoneal cavity.

Relations

Anterior. The broad ligaments.

Posterior. The intestines.

Lateral. The infundibulopelvic ligaments and the side walls of the pelvis.

Superior. The uterine tubes.

Medial. The uterus and the ovarian ligament.

Supports

The ovary is attached to the broad ligament but is supported from above by the ovarian ligament medially and the infundibulopelvic ligament laterally.

Structure

The ovary is composed of a medulla and cortex, covered with germinal epithelium.

The medulla. This is the supporting framework which is made of fibrous tissue; the ovarian blood vessels, lymphatics and nerves travel through it. The hilum where these vessels enter lies just where the ovary is attached to the broad ligament and this area is called the mesovarium (Fig. 49.23).

The cortex. This is the functioning part of the ovary. It contains the ovarian follicles in different stages of development, surrounded by stroma. The outer layer is formed of fibrous tissue known as the tunica albuginea. Over this lies the germinal epithelium, which is a modification of the peritoneum.

The cycle of the ovary is described in Chapter 50.

Blood supply

The blood supply is from the ovarian arteries and drains by the ovarian veins. The right ovarian vein joins the inferior vena cava, but the left returns its blood to the left renal vein.

Lymphatic drainage

This is to the lumbar glands.

Nerve supply

This is from the ovarian plexus.

THE BREASTS

The breasts are also linked with the female reproductive system and are described in Chapter 36.

MALE REPRODUCTIVE SYSTEM

(Fig. 49.24)

The scrotum

Function

The scrotum forms a pouch in which the testes are suspended outside the body. It lies below the symphysis pubis and between the upper parts of the thighs behind the penis.

Structure

It is formed of pigmented skin and has two compartments, one for each testis.

The testes

Function

They are the male gonads and produce spermatozoa and testosterone. Testosterone is responsible for the secondary sex characteristics. It also joins with follicle-stimulating hormone (FSH) to promote production of sperm.

Position

The testes are situated in the scrotum. In order to achieve their proper function they must be kept below body temperature, and this is why they are situated outside the body.

Structure

Each testis is 4.5 cm long, 2.5 cm wide and 3 cm thick.

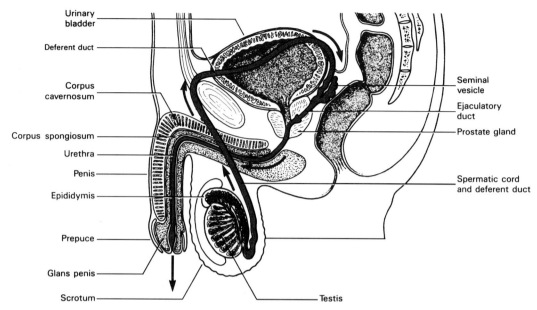

Urinary bladder
Deferent duct
Corpus cavernosum
Corpus spongiosum
Urethra
Penis
Epididymis
Prepuce
Glans penis
Scrotum

Seminal vesicle
Ejaculatory duct
Prostate gland
Spermatic cord and deferent duct
Testis

Fig. 49.24 Male reproductive system.

Layers

Tunica vasculosa. This is an inner layer of connective tissue containing a fine network of capillaries.

Tunica albuginea. This is a fibrous covering, ingrowths of which divide the testis into 200–300 lobules.

Tunica vaginalis. This is the outer layer which is made of peritoneum brought down with the descending testis when it migrated from the lumbar region in fetal life. The duct system is highly intricate:

The seminiferous ('seed-carrying') tubules are where spermatogenesis, or production of sperm, takes place. There are up to three of them in each lobule. Between the tubules there are interstitial cells which secrete testosterone. The tubules join to form a system of channels which lead to the epididymis.

The epididymis is a comma-shaped, coiled tube which lies on the superior surface and travels down the posterior aspect to the lower pole of the testis, where it leads into the deferent duct or vas deferens.

The spermatic cord

Function
The spermatic cord transmits the deferent duct up into the body, along with other structures. The function of the deferent duct is to carry the sperm to the ejaculatory duct.

Position
The cord passes upwards through the inguinal canal, where the different structures diverge. The deferent duct then continues upwards over the symphysis pubis and arches backwards beside the bladder. Behind the bladder it merges with the duct from the seminal vesicle and passes through the prostate gland as the ejaculatory duct to join the urethra.

Structure
The spermatic cord consists of the deferent duct, the testicular blood vessels, lymph vessel and nerves.

Blood supply
The testicular artery, a branch of the abdominal aorta, supplies the testis, scrotum and attachments.

The testicular veins drain in the same manner as the ovarian veins (see above).

Lymphatic drainage
This is to the lymph nodes round the aorta.

Nerve supply
This is from the 10th and 11th thoracic nerves.

The seminal vesicles

Function
The production of a viscous secretion to keep the sperm alive and motile.

Position
The seminal vesicles are two pouches situated posterior to the bladder.

Structure
They are 5 cm long and pyramid shaped. They are composed of columnar epithelium, muscle tissue and fibrous tissue.

The ejaculatory ducts

These small muscular ducts carry the spermatozoa and the seminal fluid to the urethra.

The prostate gland

Function
It produces a thin lubricating fluid which enters the urethra through ducts.

Position
It surrounds the urethra at the base of the bladder, lying between the rectum and the symphysis pubis.

Structure
It is 4 cm long, 3 cm wide and 2 cm deep. It is composed of columnar epithelium, a muscle layer and an outer fibrous layer.

The bulbourethral glands

These are two very small glands which produce yet another lubricating fluid which passes into the urethra just below the prostate gland.

The penis

Functions
It carries the urethra which is a passage for both urine and semen. During sexual excitement it stiffens (an erection) in order to be able to penetrate the vagina and deposit the semen near the woman's cervix.

Position
The root lies in the perineum, from where it passes forward below the symphysis pubis. The lower two-thirds is outside the body in front of the scrotum.

Structure
There are three columns of erectile tissue:

The corpora cavernosa are two lateral columns, one on either side and in front of the urethra.

The corpus spongiosum is a posterior column which contains the urethra. The tip is expanded to form the glans penis.

The lower two-thirds of the penis is covered in skin. At the end, the skin is folded back on itself above the glans penis to form the prepuce, which is a movable double fold. The penis is extremely vascular and during an erection the blood spaces fill and become distended.

The male hormones

The control of the male gonads is similar to the female, but it is not cyclical. The hypothalamus produces gonadotrophin-releasing factors. These stimulate the anterior pituitary gland to produce follicle-stimulating hormone (FSH) and luteinising hormone (LH). FSH acts on the seminiferous tubules to bring about the production of sperm, while LH acts on the interstitial cells which produce testosterone.

Testosterone is responsible for the secondary sex characteristics, namely deepening of the voice, growth of the genitalia and growth of hair on the chest, pubis, axilla and face.

Formation of the spermatozoa

Production of sperm begins at puberty and continues throughout adult life. Spermatogenesis takes place in the seminiferous tubules under the influence of FSH and testosterone. The process of maturation is a lengthy one and takes some weeks. The mature sperm are stored in the epididymis and the deferent duct until ejaculation. If this does not happen, they degenerate and are reabsorbed. At each ejaculation, 2–4 ml of semen is deposited in the vagina. The seminal fluid contains about 100 million sperm per ml, of which 20–25% are likely to be abnormal. The remainder move at a speed of 2–3 mm per minute. The individual spermatozoon has a head, a body and a long, mobile tail which lashes to propel the sperm along (Fig. 49.25). The tip of the head is covered by an acrosome which contains enzymes to dissolve the covering of the ovum in order to penetrate it.

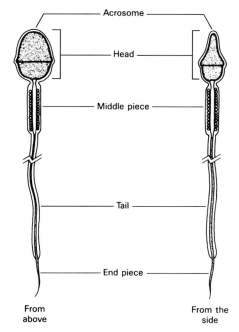

Fig. 49.25 Spermatozoon.

REFERENCE

Williams P L, Warwick R, Dyson M, Bannister L H 1989
    Gray's anatomy, 37th edn. Churchill Livingstone, Edinburgh

---

FURTHER READING

Brayshaw E, Wright P 1994 Teaching physical skills for the childbearing year. Books for Midwives Press, Hale
Burnett C W F 1979 The anatomy and physiology of obstetrics, 6th edn (rev. Anderson M). Faber and Faber, London
Hinchliff S, Montague S, Watson R (eds) 1996 Physiology for nursing practice, 2nd edn. Baillière Tindall, London
Johnson M, Everitt B 1995 Essential reproduction, 4th edn. Blackwell Science, Oxford
Rosevear S K, Stirrat C M 1996 Handbook of obstetric management. Blackwell Science, Oxford
Rutishauser S 1994 Physiology and anatomy: a basis for nursing and health care. Churchill Livingstone, Edinburgh
Smith A 1985 The body. Penguin Books, Harmondsworth
Thibodeaux G A 1987 Anatomy and physiology. Mosby, St Louis
Verralls S 1993 Anatomy and physiology of obstetrics, 3rd edn. Churchill Livingstone, Edinburgh
Williams P L, Warwick R, Dyson M, Bannister L H 1989 Gray's anatomy, 37th edn. Churchill Livingstone, Edinburgh

50

Hormonal cycles: fertilisation and early development

V. Ruth Bennett   Linda K. Brown

The biological cycles of a woman follow a monthly pattern and have a profound influence on her life and behaviour. When a woman is sexually active and no fertility control is used, recurring pregnancies will intervene and may obliterate the pattern for most of her fertile life. These cycles are first described without this interruption.

The hypothalamus is the ultimate source of control and it governs the anterior pituitary gland by hormonal pathways. The anterior pituitary gland in turn governs the ovary by hormones. Finally the ovary produces hormones which control changes in the uterus. All the changes occur simultaneously and in harmony. A woman's moods may change along with the cycle and emotional influences can alter the cycle because of the close relationship between the hypothalamus and the cerebral cortex.

THE OVARIAN CYCLE

The ovarian cortex contains 200 000 primordial follicles at birth. Some of these become cystic and are then known as Graafian follicles. From puberty onwards, certain follicles enlarge and one matures each month to liberate an ovum.

Graafian follicle (Fig. 50.1). The ovum is situated at one end of the Graafian follicle and is encircled by the narrow *perivitelline space*. Surrounding this lies a clump of cells called the *discus proligerus*, the cells of which radiate outwards to form the *corona radiata*. The innermost cells of the corona are very clear and are referred to as the *zona pellucida*. The whole follicle is lined with granulosa cells and contains follicular fluid. The outer coat of the follicle is the *external limiting membrane* and around this lies an area of compressed ovarian stroma known as the *theca*.

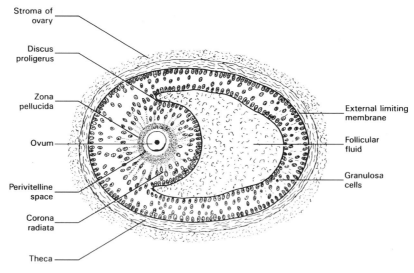

Fig. 50.1 A ripe Graafian follicle.

Under the influence of follicle-stimulating hormone (FSH) and, later, luteinising hormone (LH) the Graafian follicle matures and moves to the surface of the ovary. At the same time it swells and becomes tense, finally rupturing to release the ovum into the fimbriated end of the uterine tube which is cupped underneath the ovary in readiness (Fig. 50.2). This is ovulation. Some women feel pain at this time; this may be related to a small loss of blood into the peritoneal cavity and is termed mittelschmerz. The empty follicle is known as the corpus luteum (yellow body).

Corpus luteum.   After ovulation the follicle collapses, the granulosa cells enlarge and proliferate over the next 14 days and the whole structure becomes irregular in outline and yellow in colour. Unless pregnancy occurs, the corpus luteum will then atrophy and become the *corpus albicans* (white body) (Fig. 50.2). The ovary contains a

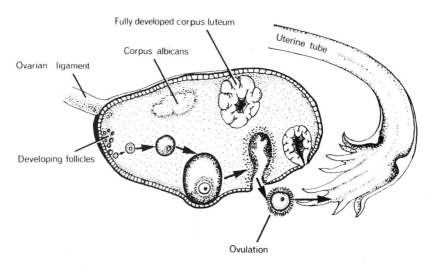

Fig. 50.2 The life cycle of a Graafian follicle.

number of these white bodies in varying stages of degeneration.

Ovarian hormones

Oestrogen. This comprises a number of compounds including oestriol, oestradiol and oestrone. They are produced under the influence of FSH by the granulosa cells and the theca in increasing amounts until the degeneration of the corpus luteum when the level falls.

The effects of oestrogen are widespread. It is responsible for the secondary sex characteristics such as the female shape, the growth of the breasts and the uterus and the female distribution of hair. It influences the production of cervical mucus and the structure of the vaginal epithelium. This in turn encourages the growth of Döderlein's bacilli which are responsible for the acidity of the vaginal fluid. During the cycle, oestrogen causes the proliferation of the uterine endometrium. It inhibits FSH and encourages fluid retention.

Progesterone. This with related compounds is produced by the corpus luteum under the influence of LH. They act only on tissues which have previously been affected by oestrogen.

The effects of progesterone are mainly evident during the second half of the cycle. It causes secretory changes in the lining of the uterus, when the endometrium develops tortuous glands and an enriched blood supply in readiness for the possible arrival of a fertilised ovum. It causes the body temperature to rise by 0.5°C after ovulation and gives rise to tingling and a sense of fullness in the breasts prior to menstruation.

The changes caused by progesterone in pregnancy are listed in Chapter 11.

Relaxin is a hormone which has been measured in human blood and is at its maximum level between weeks 38 and 42 of pregnancy. It originates in the corpus luteum and is thought to relax the pelvic girdle, to soften the cervix and to suppress uterine contractions. Although it reduces oxytocin release it does not affect the increasing number of oxytocin receptors in the myometrium. The presence of these receptors is a more important factor in labour than the actual level of oxytocin (Steer 1990).

PITUITARY CONTROL

Under the influence of the hypothalamus which produces gonadotrophin-releasing hormone (GnRH), the anterior pituitary gland (adenohypophysis) secretes two gonadotrophins, follicle-stimulating hormone (FSH) and luteinising hormone (LH). GnRH is released in a series of pulses about an hour apart and the gonadotrophins likewise are secreted in a pulsatile manner (Johnson & Everitt 1995). This appears to be crucial to the normal pattern of the menstrual cycle. The gonadotrophic activity of the hypothalamus and the pituitary is influenced by positive and negative feedback mechanisms from ovarian hormones.

FSH causes several Graafian follicles to develop and enlarge, one of them more than all the others. FSH stimulates the granulosa cells and theca to secrete oestrogen. The level of FSH rises during the first half of the cycle and when the oestrogen level reaches a certain point its production is stopped.

LH is first produced a few days after the anterior pituitary starts producing FSH. Rising oestrogen causes a surge in both FSH and LH levels, the ripened follicle ruptures and ovulation occurs. Levels of both gonadotrophins then fall rapidly. Progesterone inhibits any new rise in LH in spite of high oestrogen levels but if no pregnancy occurs the corpus luteum degenerates after 14 days. The negative feedback effect of progesterone ceases and FSH and LH levels rise again to begin a new cycle (Johnson & Everitt 1995).

Prolactin is also produced in the anterior pituitary gland, but it does not play a part in the control of the ovary. If produced in excessive amounts, however, it will inhibit ovulation, a phenomenon which occurs naturally during breast feeding (see Ch. 36).

THE UTERINE CYCLE OR MENSTRUAL CYCLE (Fig. 50.3)

Although each woman has an individual cycle which varies in length, the average cycle is taken to

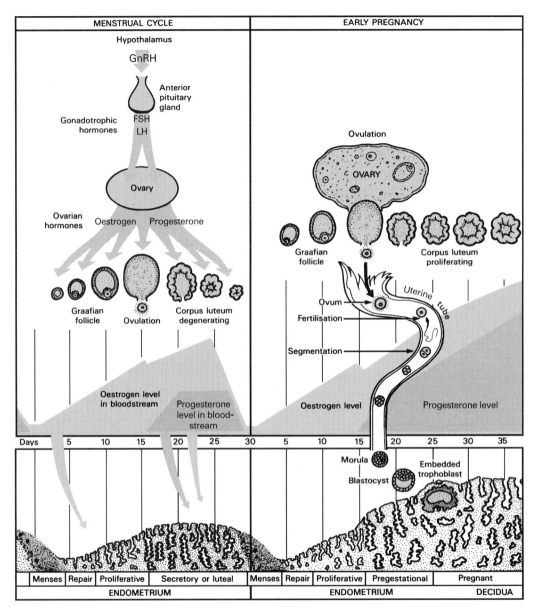

Fig. 50.3 MENSTRUAL CYCLE (*left half*). Diagrammatic representation of the action of the gonadotrophic hormones on the ovary and of the ovarian hormones on the endometrium. EARLY PREGNANCY (*right half*). Diagrammatic representation showing ovulation, fertilisation, decidual reaction and embedding of the fertilised ovum.

be 28 days long and recurs regularly from puberty to the menopause except when pregnancy intervenes. The first day of the cycle is the day on which menstruation begins. There are three main phases and they affect the tissue structure of the endometrium, controlled by the ovarian hormones.

The menstrual phase, characterised by vaginal bleeding, lasts for 3–5 days. Physiologically this is the terminal phase of the menstrual cycle when the endometrium is shed down to the basal layer along with blood from the capillaries and with the unfertilised ovum.

The proliferative phase follows menstruation and lasts until ovulation. Sometimes the first few days while the endometrium is re-forming are described as the *regenerative phase*. This phase is under the control of oestrogen and consists of the regrowth and thickening of the endometrium. At the completion of this phase the endometrium consists of three layers:

A *basal layer* lies immediately above the myometrium, about 1 mm in thickness. This layer never alters during the menstrual cycle. It contains all the necessary rudimentary structures for building up new endometrium.

A *functional layer* which contains tubular glands and is 2.5 mm thick. This layer changes constantly according to the hormonal influences of the ovary.

A *layer of cuboidal ciliated epithelium* covers the functional layer. It dips down to line the tubular glands.

The secretory phase follows ovulation and is under the influence of progesterone and oestrogen from the corpus luteum. The functional layer thickens to 3.5 mm and becomes spongy in appearance because the glands are more tortuous.

Puberty

This is the period in life during which the reproductive organs undergo a surge in development and reach maturity. The first signs are breast development and the appearance of pubic hair. The body grows considerably and takes on the female shape. Puberty culminates in the onset of menstruation, the first period being called the *menarche*. The first few cycles are not usually accompanied by ovulation so that conception is unlikely before a girl has been menstruating for a year or two.

Menopause

The end of a woman's reproductive life is characterised by the gradual cessation of menstruation, the periods first becoming irregular and then ceasing altogether. This is often accompanied by physical symptoms like hot flushes and emotional changes such as mood swings. There is an increased tendency to obesity and in the following years signs of ageing will appear. These changes are due to a fall in the production of oestrogen because the ovary is no longer able to respond to pituitary gonadotrophins. The sexual drive may not be diminished but some women find it difficult to accept that they are no longer fertile. The usual age for the menopause is between 45 and 50 years but it should not be assumed that it is complete until 2 years have elapsed since the last period. In the intervening months the woman should continue to use contraception if appropriate.

FERTILISATION

Following ovulation, the ovum, which is about 0.15 mm in diameter, passes into the uterine tube and is moved along towards the uterus. The ovum, having no power of locomotion, is wafted along by the cilia and by the peristaltic muscular contraction of the tube. At this time the cervix, under the influence of oestrogen, secretes a flow of alkaline mucus that attracts the spermatozoa. At intercourse about 300 million sperm are deposited in the posterior fornix of the vagina. Those that reach the loose cervical mucus survive to propel themselves towards the uterine tubes while the remainder are destroyed by the acid medium of the vagina. More will die on the journey through the uterus and only thousands reach the uterine tube where they meet the ovum, usually in the ampulla. It is only during this journey that the sperm finally become mature and capable of releasing the enzyme, hyaluronidase, which allows penetration of the zona pellucida and the cell membrane surrounding the ovum (Fig. 50.4). Many sperm are needed for this to take place but only one will enter the ovum. After this, the membrane is sealed to prevent entry of any further sperm and the nuclei of the two cells fuse. The sperm and the ovum each contribute half the complement of chromosomes to make a total of 46 (Box 50.1). The sperm and ovum are known as the male and female *gametes*, the fertilised ovum as the *zygote*.

Neither sperm nor ovum can survive for longer than 2 or 3 days and fertilisation is most likely to

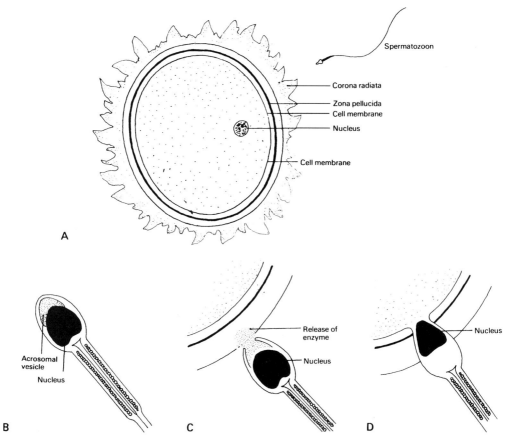

Fig. 50.4 Fertilisation. Diagrammatic representation of the fusion of the ovum and the spermatozoon.

Box 50.1 Chromosomes

Each human cell has a complement of 46 chromosomes arranged in 23 pairs, of which two are sex chromosomes. The remainder are known as *autosomes*. During the process of maturation, both gametes (ovum and spermatozoon) shed half their chromosomes, one of each pair, during a reduction division called *meiosis*. Genetic material is exchanged between the chromosomes before they split up. In the male, meiosis starts at puberty and both halves redivide to form four spermatozoa in all. In the female, meiosis commences during fetal life but the first division is not completed until many years later at ovulation. The division is unequal; the larger part will go on to form the ovum while the remainder forms the first polar body. At fertilisation the second division takes place and results in one large cell, which is the mature ovum, and a

much smaller one, the second polar body. At the same time, division of the first polar body creates a third polar body.

When the gametes combine at fertilisation to form the zygote, the full complement of chromosomes is restored. Subsequent division occurs by *mitosis* where the chromosomes divide to give each new cell a full set.

Sex determination
Females carry two similar sex chromosomes, XX; males carry two dissimilar sex chromosomes, XY. Each spermatozoon will carry either an X or a Y chromosome, whereas the ovum always carries an X chromosome. If the ovum is fertilised by an X-carrying spermatozoon a female is conceived, if by a Y-carrying one, a male.

occur when intercourse takes place not more than 48 hours before or 24 hours after ovulation. It therefore follows that conception will take place about 14 days before the next period is due.

DEVELOPMENT OF THE FERTILISED OVUM (Fig. 50.5)

When the ovum has been fertilised, it continues its passage through the uterine tube and reaches the uterus 3 or 4 days later. During this time segmentation or cell division takes place and the fertilised ovum divides into 2 cells, then into 4, then 8, 16 and so on until a cluster of cells is formed known as the *morula* (mulberry). These divisions occur quite slowly, about once every 12 hours. Next, a fluid-filled cavity or *blastocele* appears in the morula which now becomes known as the *blastocyst*. Around the outside of the blastocyst there is a single layer of cells known as the *trophoblast* while the remaining cells are clumped together at one end forming the *inner cell mass*. The trophoblast will form the placenta and chorion, while the inner cell mass will become the fetus and the amnion. On its journey, the ovum is nourished by glycogen from the goblet cells of the uterine tubes and later the secretory glands of the uterus.

When the blastocyst first tumbles into the uterus, it lies free for 2 or 3 more days. The trophoblast, especially the part which lies over the inner cell mass, then becomes quite sticky and adheres to the endometrium. It begins to secrete substances which digest the endometrial cells, allowing the blastocyst to become embedded in the endometrium. *Embedding*, sometimes known as *nidation* (nesting), is normally complete by the 11th day after ovulation and the endometrium closes over it completely, the only evidence of the presence of the blastocyst being a small bulge on the surface.

The decidua

This is the name given to the endometrium during pregnancy. From the time of conception the increased secretion of oestrogens causes the endometrium to grow to four times its non-pregnant thickness. The corpus luteum also produces large amounts of progesterone which stimulate the secretory activity of the endometrial glands and increase the size of the blood vessels. This accounts for the soft, vascular, spongy bed in which the fertilised ovum implants. Three layers are found:

The basal layer lies immediately above the myometrium. It remains unchanged in itself but regenerates the new endometrium during the puerperium.

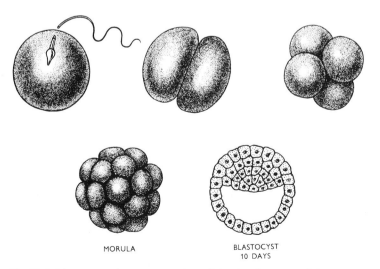

MORULA

BLASTOCYST
10 DAYS

Fig. 50.5 Diagrammatic representation of the development of the fertilised ovum.

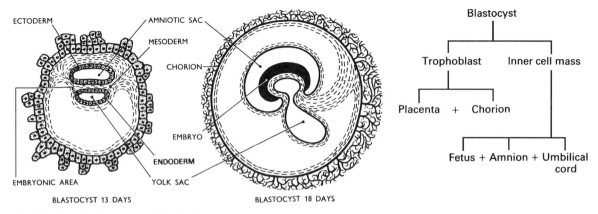

Fig. 50.6 The development of the blastocyst.

The **functional layer** consists of tortuous glands which are rich in secretions. The stroma cells are enlarged in what is known as the decidual reaction. This affords a defence against excessive invasion by the syncytiotrophoblast and limits its advance to this spongy layer. The advantage of this is that it provides a secure anchorage for the placenta and allows it access to nutrition and oxygen but as soon as the baby is born, separation can occur (see Ch. 25).

The **compact layer** forms the surface of the decidua and is composed of closely packed stroma cells and the necks of the glands.

The blastocyst embeds within the spongy layer and different areas of decidua are identified according to their relationship to it.

The decidua underneath the blastocyst is termed the *basal decidua*, that which covers it is the *capsular decidua*, and the remainder is called the *parietal* (or the *true*) *decidua*. Eventually, as the embryo grows and fills the uterine cavity, the capsular decidua meets and fuses with the parietal decidua.

The trophoblast

Small projections begin to appear all over the surface of the blastocyst (Figs 50.6 and 50.7), becoming most prolific at the area of contact. These trophoblastic cells differentiate into layers, the outer syncytiotrophoblast (syncytium), the inner cytotrophoblast and below this a layer of mesoderm or primitive mesenchyme.

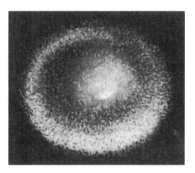

Fig. 50.7 Ovum in early pregnancy covered with chorionic villi (see Ch. 51).

The **syncytiotrophoblast** is composed of nucleated protoplasm which is capable of breaking down tissue as in the process of embedding. It erodes the walls of the blood vessels of the decidua, making the nutrients in the maternal blood accessible to the developing organism.

The **cytotrophoblast** is a well-defined single layer of cells which produces a hormone known as human chorionic gonadotrophin (HCG). This is responsible for informing the corpus luteum that a pregnancy has begun. The corpus luteum continues to produce oestrogen and progesterone. Progesterone maintains the integrity of the decidua so that shedding does not take place. In other words, menstruation is suppressed. The high level of oestrogen suppresses the production of FSH.

The mesoderm consists of loose connective tissue. There is similar tissue in the inner cell mass and the two are continuous at the point where they join in the body stalk.

Further development of the trophoblast is discussed in Chapter 51.

The inner cell mass

While the trophoblast is developing into the placenta, which will nourish the fetus, the inner cell mass is forming the fetus itself. The cells differentiate into three layers, each of which will form particular parts of the fetus.

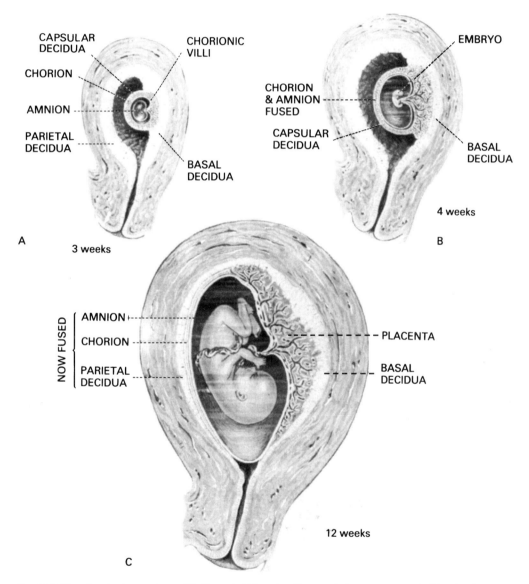

Fig. 50.8 The developing embryo. (A) (3 weeks) Showing the amniotic sac, surrounded by chorion which is covered with capsular decidua. (B) (4 weeks) The amnion is in contact with the chorion. The placenta is seen embedded in the basal decidua. (C) (12 weeks) The capsular decidua has thinned out and atrophied. The chorion is attached to the parietal decidua. (After Williams, *American Journal of Obstetrics and Gynecology*.)

The ectoderm mainly forms the skin and nervous system.

The mesoderm forms bones and muscles and also the heart and blood vessels, including those which are in the placenta. Certain internal organs also originate in the mesoderm.

The endoderm forms mucous membranes and glands. The three layers together are known as the embryonic plate. Two cavities appear in the inner cell mass, one on either side of the embryonic plate.

The amniotic cavity lies on the side of the ectoderm. The cavity, which is filled with fluid, gradually enlarges and folds round the embryo to enclose it. The amnion forms from its lining. It swells out into the chorionic cavity (formerly the blastocele) and eventually obliterates it when the amniotic and chorionic membranes come into contact. Details of the amniotic fluid are found in Chapter 51.

The yolk sac lies on the side of the endoderm and provides nourishment for the embryo until the trophoblast is sufficiently developed to take over. Part of it contributes to the formation of the primitive gut; the remainder resembles a balloon floating in front of the embryo until it atrophies and becomes trapped under the amnion on the surface of the placenta. After birth, all that remains of the yolk sac is a vestigial structure in the base of the umbilical cord, known as the vitelline duct.

The embryo (Fig. 50.8)

This name is applied to the developing offspring after implantation and until 8 weeks after conception. During the embryonic period all the organs and systems of the body are laid down in rudimentary form so that at its completion they have simply to grow and mature for a further 7 months. The conceptus is known as a *fetus* during this time (see Ch. 52).

REFERENCES

Johnson M, Everitt B 1995 Essential reproduction, 4th edn. Blackwell Science, Oxford
Steer P J 1990 Endocrinology of parturition. In: Franks S (ed)

Clinical endocrinology and metabolism. Baillière Tindall, London, vol 4, no 2 (June)

FURTHER READING

Herbert R A 1996 Reproduction. In: Hinchliff S, Montague S, Watson R (eds) Physiology for nursing practice, 2nd edn. Baillière Tindall, London

Rutishauser S 1994 Physiology and anatomy: a basis for nursing and health care. Churchill Livingstone, Edinburgh

The placenta

V. Ruth Bennett   Linda K. Brown

The placenta is a remarkable organ. Originating from the trophoblastic layer of the fertilised ovum itself, it links closely with the mother's circulation to carry out functions which the fetus is unable to perform for itself during intrauterine life. The survival of the fetus depends upon its integrity and efficiency.

DEVELOPMENT

Initially the ovum appears to be covered with a fine, downy hair, which consists of the projections from the trophoblastic layer (see Ch. 50). These proliferate and branch from about 3 weeks after fertilisation, forming the chorionic villi. The villi become most profuse in the area where the blood supply is richest, that is, in the basal decidua. This part of the trophoblast is known as the chorion frondosum and it will eventually develop into the placenta. The villi under the capsular decidua, being less well nourished, gradually degenerate and form the chorion laeve (bald chorion) which is the origin of the chorionic membrane.

The villi erode the walls of maternal blood vessels as they penetrate the decidua, opening them up to form a lake of maternal blood in which they float. The opened blood vessels are known as sinuses, the areas surrounding the villi as blood spaces. The maternal blood circulates slowly, enabling the villi to absorb food and oxygen and excrete waste. These are known as the nutritive villi. A few villi are more deeply attached to the decidua and are called anchoring villi.

Each chorionic villus is a branching structure arising from one stem (Fig. 51.1). Its centre consists of mesoderm and fetal blood vessels, and branches of the umbilical artery and vein. These are covered by a single layer of cytotrophoblast cells and the external layer of the villus is the

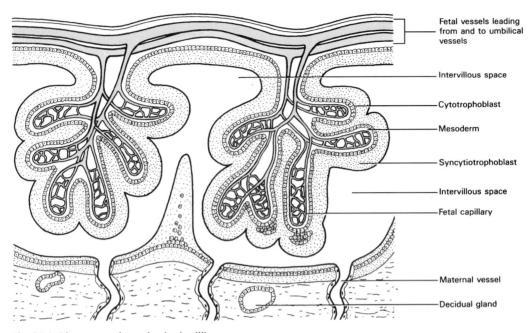

Fetal vessels leading from and to umbilical vessels

Intervillous space

Cytotrophoblast

Mesoderm

Syncytiotrophoblast

Intervillous space

Fetal capillary

Maternal vessel

Decidual gland

Fig. 51.1 Diagram to show chorionic villi.

syncytiotrophoblast. This means that four layers of tissue separate the maternal blood from the fetal blood and make it impossible for the two circulations to mix unless any villi are damaged.

The placenta is completely formed and functioning from 10 weeks after fertilisation. In its early stages it is a relatively loose structure, but becomes more compact as it matures. Between 12 and 20 weeks' gestation the placenta weighs more than the fetus because the fetal organs are insufficiently developed to cope with the metabolic processes of nutrition. Later in pregnancy some of the fetal organs, such as the liver, begin to function, so the cytotrophoblast and the syncytiotrophoblast gradually degenerate and this allows easier exchange of oxygen and carbon dioxide.

Circulation through the placenta

Fetal blood, low in oxygen, is pumped by the fetal heart towards the placenta along the umbilical arteries and transported along their branches to the capillaries of the chorionic villi. Having yielded up carbon dioxide and absorbed oxygen, the blood is returned to the fetus via the umbilical vein.

The maternal blood is delivered to the placental bed in the decidua by spiral arteries and flows into the blood spaces surrounding the villi. It is thought that the direction of flow is similar to a fountain; the blood passes upwards and bathes the villus as it circulates around it and drains back into a branch of the uterine vein (Fig. 51.2). An alternative theory is that it flows in a similar manner to a whirlpool.

THE MATURE PLACENTA

Functions

Respiration. As pulmonary exchange of gases does not take place in the uterus, the fetus must obtain oxygen and excrete carbon dioxide through the placenta. Oxygen from the mother's haemoglobin passes into the fetal blood by simple diffusion and similarly the fetus gives off carbon dioxide into the maternal blood.

Nutrition. The fetus needs the same nutrients as anyone else. Amino acids are required for body building, glucose for energy, calcium and phosphorus for bones and teeth, and iron and other

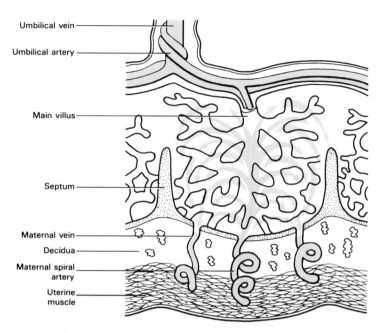

Fig. 51.2 Blood flow around chorionic villi.

minerals for blood formation. Food for the fetus derives from the mother's diet and has already been broken down into simpler forms by the time it reaches the placental site. The placenta is able to select those substances required by the fetus, even depleting the mother's own supply in some instances. It can also break down complex nutrients into compounds which can be used by the fetus. Protein is transferred across the placenta as amino acids, carbohydrate as glucose, and fats as fatty acids. Water, vitamins and minerals also pass to the fetus. Fats and fat-soluble vitamins (A, D and E) only cross the placenta with difficulty and mainly in the later stages of pregnancy. The amino acids are actively transported across the placenta so that the level in the fetal blood is always higher than that in the maternal blood.

Storage. The placenta metabolises glucose, stores it in the form of glycogen and reconverts it to glucose as required. The placenta can also store iron and the fat-soluble vitamins.

Excretion. The main substance excreted from the fetus is carbon dioxide. Bilirubin will also be excreted as red blood cells are replaced relatively frequently. There is very little tissue breakdown

apart from this and the amounts of urea and uric acid excreted are very small.

Protection. The placenta provides a limited barrier to infection. With the exception of the treponema of syphilis and the tubercle bacillus, few bacteria can penetrate. Viruses, however, can cross freely and may cause congenital abnormalities, as in the case of the rubella virus (see Ch. 42). It may be assumed that drugs will cross to the fetus although there are exceptions, for example heparin. Some drugs are known to cause damage, though many will be harmless and others are positively beneficial, such as antibiotics administered to a pregnant woman with syphilis.

Towards the end of pregnancy small antibodies, immunoglobulins G (IgG), will be transferred to the fetus, and these will confer immunity on the baby for the first 3 months after birth. It is important to realise that only those antibodies which the mother herself possesses can be passed on.

Endocrine:

Human chorionic gonadotrophin (HCG). This is produced by the cytotrophoblastic layer of the chorionic villi. Initially it is present in very large

In the figure, the following labels appear:

Umbilical vein
Umbilical artery
Main villus
Septum
Maternal vein
Decidua
Maternal spiral artery
Uterine muscle

quantities, peak levels being achieved between the seventh and tenth weeks, but it gradually reduces as the pregnancy advances. HCG forms the basis of the many pregnancy tests which are available, as it is excreted in the mother's urine. Its function is to stimulate the growth and activity of the corpus luteum.

Oestrogens. As the activity of the corpus luteum declines, the placenta takes over the production of oestrogens, which are secreted in large amounts throughout pregnancy. The fetus provides the placenta with the vital precursors for the production of oestrogens. The amount of oestrogen produced (measured as urinary or serum oestriol) is an index of fetoplacental well-being.

Progesterone. This is made in the syncytial layer of the placenta in increasing quantities until immediately before the onset of labour when its level falls. It may be measured in the urine as pregnanediol.

Human placental lactogen (HPL). HPL has a role in glucose metabolism in pregnancy. It appears to have a connection with the activity of human growth hormone, although it does not itself promote growth. As the level of HCG falls, so the level of HPL rises and continues to do so throughout pregnancy. Monitoring the level of HPL with the intention of assessing placental function has been disappointing in predicting fetal outcome.

Appearance of the placenta at term

The placenta is a round, flat mass about 20 cm in diameter and 2.5 cm thick at its centre. It weighs approximately one-sixth of the baby's weight at term, although this proportion may be affected by the time at which the cord is clamped owing to the varying amounts of fetal blood retained in the vessels.

The maternal surface (Fig. 51.3A). Maternal blood gives this surface a dark red colour and part of the basal decidua will have been separated with it. The surface is arranged in about 20 lobes which are separated by sulci (furrows), into which the decidua dips down to form septa (walls). The lobes are made up of lobules, each of which contains a single villus with its branches. Sometimes deposits of lime salts may be present on the surface, making it slightly gritty. This has no clinical significance.

The fetal surface (Fig. 51.3B). The amnion covering the fetal surface of the placenta gives it a white, shiny appearance. Branches of the umbilical vein and arteries are visible, spreading out from the insertion of the umbilical cord which is normally in the centre. The amnion can be peeled off the surface, leaving the chorionic plate from which the placenta has developed and which is continuous with the chorion.

The fetal sac

The fetal sac consists of a double membrane. The

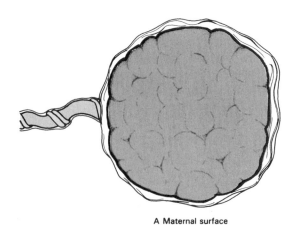

A Maternal surface

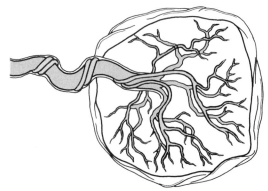

B Fetal surface

Fig. 51.3 The placenta at term.

outer membrane is the chorion which lies under the capsular decidua and becomes closely adherent to the uterine wall. The inner membrane is the amnion which contains the amniotic fluid. As long as it remains intact, the fetal sac protects the fetus against ascending bacterial infection.

Chorion.   This is a thick, opaque, friable membrane derived from the trophoblast. It is continuous with the chorionic plate which forms the base of the placenta.

Amnion.   This is a smooth, tough, translucent membrane derived from the inner cell mass. It is thought to have a role in the formation of the amniotic fluid.

AMNIOTIC FLUID

Functions
The fluid distends the amniotic sac and allows for the growth and free movement of the fetus. It equalises pressure and protects the fetus from jarring and injury. The fluid maintains a constant temperature for the fetus and provides small amounts of nutrients. In labour, as long as the membranes remain intact, the amniotic fluid protects the placenta and umbilical cord from the pressure of uterine contractions. It also aids effacement of the cervix and dilatation of the uterine os, particularly where the presenting part is poorly applied.

Origin
The source of amniotic fluid is thought to be both fetal and maternal. It is secreted by the amnion, especially that which covers the placenta and umbilical cord. Some fluid is exuded from maternal vessels in the decidua and some from fetal vessels in the placenta. Fetal urine also contributes to the volume from the tenth week of gestation onwards. The water in amniotic fluid is exchanged as often as every 3 hours.

Volume
The total amount of amniotic fluid increases throughout pregnancy until 38 weeks' gestation when there is about 1 litre. It then diminishes slightly until term when approximately 800 ml remains. However, there are very wide variations in the amount. If the total amount exceeds 1500 ml, the condition is known as polyhydramnios (often abbreviated to hydramnios), and if less than 300 ml, the term oligohydramnios is applied. Such abnormalities are often associated with congenital malformations of the fetus. The normal fetus swallows amniotic fluid but if anything interferes with swallowing, an excessive amount of fluid will accumulate. Similarly, if the fetus is unable to pass urine, the amount of fluid will be reduced (see Ch. 41).

Constituents
Amniotic fluid (also termed liquor amnii) is a clear, pale straw-coloured fluid consisting of 99% water. The remaining 1% is dissolved solid matter including food substances and waste products. In addition, the fetus sheds skin cells, vernix caseosa and lanugo into the fluid. Abnormal constituents of the liquor, such as meconium in the case of fetal distress, may give valuable diagnostic information about the condition of the fetus. Aspiration of amniotic fluid for examination is termed amniocentesis (see Ch. 20).

THE UMBILICAL CORD

The umbilical cord or *funis* extends from the fetus to the placenta and transmits the umbilical blood vessels, two arteries and one vein (Fig. 51.4). These are enclosed and protected by Wharton's jelly, a gelatinous substance formed from mesoderm. The whole cord is covered in a layer of amnion continuous with that covering the placenta.

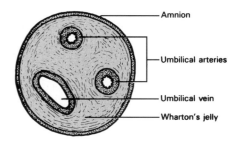

Fig. 51.4 Cross-section through the umbilical cord.

The length of the average cord is about 50 cm. This is sufficient to allow for delivery of the baby without applying any traction to the placenta. A cord is considered to be short when it measures less than 40 cm. There is no specific agreed length for describing a cord as too long, but the disadvantages of a very long cord are that it may become wrapped round the neck or body of the fetus or become knotted; either event could result in occlusion of the blood vessels, especially during labour. True knots should always be noted on examination of the cord, but they must be distinguished from false knots which are lumps of Wharton's jelly on the side of the cord and are not significant.

ANATOMICAL VARIATIONS OF THE PLACENTA AND THE CORD

Succenturiate lobe of placenta (Fig. 51.5). This is the most significant of the variations in conformation of the placenta. A small extra lobe is present, separate from the main placenta, and joined to it by blood vessels which run through the membranes to reach it. The danger is that this small lobe may be retained in utero after delivery, and if it is not removed, it may lead to infection and haemorrhage. The midwife must examine every placenta for evidence of a retained succenturiate lobe – a hole in the membranes with vessels running to it.

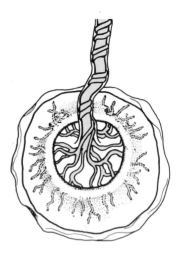

Fig. 51.6 Circumvallate placenta.

Circumvallate placenta (Fig. 51.6). In this situation an opaque ring is seen on the fetal surface of the placenta. It is formed by a doubling back of the chorion and amnion and may result in the membranes leaving the placenta nearer the centre instead of at the edge as usual.

Battledore insertion of the cord (Fig. 51.7). The cord in this case is attached at the very edge of the placenta in the manner of a table tennis bat. It is unimportant unless the attachment is fragile.

Velamentous insertion of the cord (Fig. 51.8). The cord is inserted into the membranes some

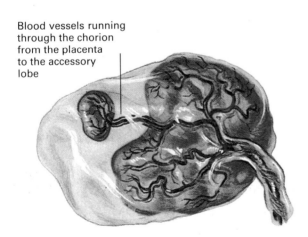

Blood vessels running through the chorion from the placenta to the accessory lobe

Fig. 51.5 Succenturiate lobe of placenta.

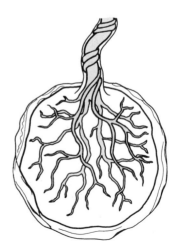

Fig. 51.7 Battledore insertion of the cord.

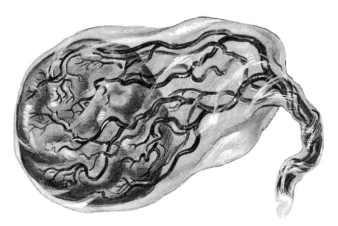

Fig. 51.8 Velamentous insertion of the cord.

distance from the edge of the placenta. The umbilical vessels run through the membranes from the cord to the placenta. If the placenta is normally situated, no harm will result to the fetus, but the cord is likely to become detached upon applying traction during active management of the third stage of labour.

If the placenta is low-lying, the vessels may pass across the uterine os. The term applied to the vessels lying in this position is vasa praevia. In this case there is great danger to the fetus when the membranes rupture and even more so during artificial rupture, as the vessels may be torn, leading to rapid exsanguination of the fetus. If the onset of haemorrhage coincides with rupture of the membranes, fetal haemorrhage should be assumed and delivery expedited. It is possible to distinguish fetal blood from maternal blood by Singer's alkali-denaturation test, although, in practice, time is so short that it may not be possible to save the life of the fetus. If the fetus survives, the baby's haemoglobin should be estimated after birth.

Bipartite placenta (Fig. 51.9). Two complete and separate lobes are present, each with a cord leaving it. The bipartite cord joins a short distance

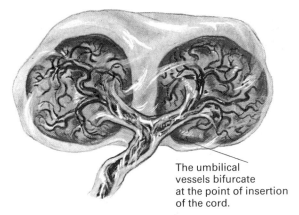

The umbilical vessels bifurcate at the point of insertion of the cord.

Fig. 51.9 Bipartite placenta.

from the two parts of the placenta. This is different from the two placentas in a twin pregnancy, where there are also two umbilical cords, but these do not join at any point. Where there is a succenturiate lobe, the vessels are attached to the placenta directly and never join the cord.

A tripartite placenta is similar but with three distinct lobes.

Except for the dangers noted above these varieties of conformation have no clinical significance.

READER ACTIVITIES

1. Next time you examine a placenta, remove a piece of tissue, for example one lobe. Wash it thoroughly under running water to remove the maternal blood and decidua. Float it in clear water to observe the fronds and delicate structure of the villi.

2. Compare a series of placental weights with the birthweights of the corresponding babies, working out the percentage or fraction in each case. Note whether the cord was clamped immediately or whether pulsation was allowed to cease first or if the placental blood was drained out before expulsion; observe any correlation. You might try weighing placentas before and after blood has been drained out via the cord.

FURTHER READING

Fox H 1978 Pathology of the placenta. Saunders, London
Fox H 1991 A contemporary view of the human placenta. Midwifery 7(1 March): 31–39
Johnson M, Everitt B 1995 Essential reproduction, 4th edn.
Blackwell Science, Oxford
Llewellyn-Jones D 1990 Fundamentals of obstetrics and gynaecology. Vol 1 Obstetrics, 5th edn. Faber, London

52

The fetus

V. Ruth Bennett   Linda K. Brown

The midwife needs to have an understanding of fetal development in order to estimate the approximate age of a baby born before term. It is also helpful to know the outline of organogenesis in order to appreciate the ways in which developmental abnormalities arise. When making reference to the age at which various prenatal events happen, it is important to distinguish between menstrual age (the time since the first day of the last menstrual period) and conceptional age (the interval since fertilisation). Embryologists use the latter while those involved with the pregnant woman tend to use the former.

The time scale of the pregnancy is important. Figure 52.1 illustrates the comparative lengths of the different periods involved. The interval from the beginning of the last menstrual period (LMP) until conception is not strictly part of the pregnancy, although the as yet unfertilised ovum is already being prepared for release. For clinical purposes it is convenient to regard the pregnancy as beginning at the LMP because this is usually the only definitive date available. The midwife should be aware that an individual woman may know the exact date of conception and will rightly consider this as the beginning of her pregnancy.

For the first 3 weeks following conception the term fertilised ovum or zygote is used. From 3–8 weeks after conception it is known as the embryo and following this it is the fetus until birth when it becomes a baby. Although when speaking to mothers the fetus in utero may be referred to as a baby, the midwife should use the correct terminology during professional discussions and in her records.

Development within the uterus is summarised in Box 52.1.

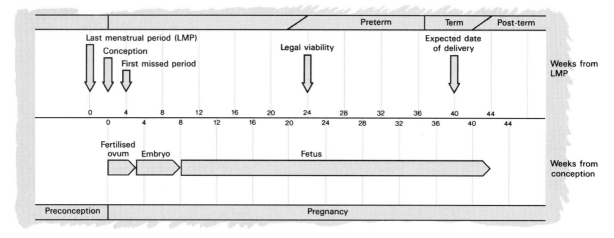

Fig. 52.1 Menstrual age, conceptional age and prenatal events.

Box 52.1 Summary of development (Fig. 52.2)

0–4 weeks after conception
Rapid growth
Formation of the embryonic plate (see Ch. 50)
Primitive central nervous system forms
Heart develops and begins to beat
Limb buds form

4–8 weeks
Very rapid cell division
Head and facial features develop
All major organs laid down in primitive form
External genitalia present but sex not distinguishable
Early movements
Visible on ultrasound from 6 weeks

8–12 weeks
Eyelids fuse
Kidneys begin to function and the fetus passes urine from 10 weeks
Fetal circulation functioning properly
Sucking and swallowing begin
Sex apparent
Moves freely (not felt by mother)
Some primitive reflexes present

12–16 weeks
Rapid skeletal development – visible on X-ray
Meconium present in gut
Lanugo appears
Nasal septum and palate fuse

16–20 weeks
'Quickening' – mother feels fetal movements
Fetal heart heard on auscultation

Vernix caseosa appears
Fingernails can be seen
Skin cells begin to be renewed

20–24 weeks
Most organs become capable of functioning
Periods of sleep and activity
Responds to sound
Skin red and wrinkled

24–28 weeks
Survival may be expected if born
Eyelids reopen
Respiratory movements

28–32 weeks
Begins to store fat and iron
Testes descend into scrotum
Lanugo disappears from face
Skin becomes paler and less wrinkled

32–36 weeks
Increased fat makes the body more rounded
Lanugo disappears from body
Head hair lengthens
Nails reach tips of fingers
Ear cartilage soft
Plantar creases visible

36–40 weeks after conception (38–42 weeks after LMP)
Term is reached and birth is due
Contours rounded
Skull firm

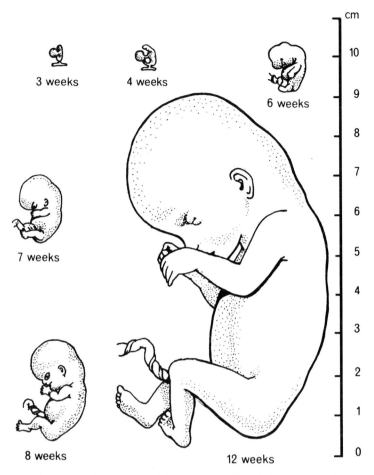

Fig. 52.2 Sizes of embryos and fetus between 3 and 12 weeks' gestation.

FETAL ORGANS

Some aspects of the development of fetal organs and their physiology are of special relevance to the midwife because of their effect on the newborn baby. A brief outline is given of the most important.

Blood

The origin of fetal blood is from the inner cell mass, along with all the other organs of its body. The fetus will inherit the genes which determine its blood group from both its parents and its ABO group and Rhesus factor may therefore be the same or different from those of its mother.

The fetal haemoglobin (Hb) is of a different type from adult haemoglobin and is termed HbF. It has a much greater affinity for oxygen and is found in greater concentration (18–20 g/dl at term). The reason for this is that oxygen must be obtained from the mother's blood in the placental site where the oxygen tension is lower than in the atmosphere. Towards the end of pregnancy the fetus begins to make adult-type haemoglobin (HbA).

In utero the red blood cells have a shorter life span, this being about 90 days by the time the baby is born.

The renal tract

The kidneys begin to function and the fetus passes urine from 10 weeks' gestation. The urine is very dilute and does not constitute a route for excretion, since the mother eliminates waste products which cross the placenta. It is worth noting that the superior vesical arteries arise from the first few centimetres of the hypogastric arteries which lead to the umbilical arteries, so that if a single umbilical artery is found, abnormalities of the renal tract are suspected.

The adrenal glands

The fetal adrenal glands produce the precursors for placental formation of oestriols. They are also thought to play a part in the initiation of labour, although the exact mechanism is not fully understood (see Ch. 21; also Johnson & Everitt 1995).

The liver

The fetal liver is comparatively large in size, taking up much of the abdominal cavity, especially in the early months. From the third to the sixth month of intrauterine life, the liver is responsible for the formation of red blood cells, after which they are mainly produced in the red bone marrow and the spleen.

Towards the end of pregnancy iron stores are laid down in the liver.

The alimentary tract

The digestive tract is mainly non-functional before birth. It forms from the yolk sac as a straight tube, later growing out into the base of the umbilical cord and subsequently rotating back into the abdomen. Sucking and swallowing of amniotic fluid containing shed skin cells and other debris begins about 12 weeks after conception. Most digestive juices are present before birth and they act on the swallowed substances and discarded intestinal cells to form meconium. This is normally retained in the gut until after birth when it is passed as the first stool of the newborn.

The lungs

The lungs originate from a bud growing out of the pharynx, which subdivides again and again to form the branching structure of the bronchial tree. The process continues after birth until about 8 years of age when the full number of bronchioles and alveoli will have developed. It is mainly the immaturity of the lungs which reduces the chance of survival of infants born before 24 weeks' gesta-

tion, owing to the limited alveolar surface area, the immaturity of the capillary system in the lungs and the lack of adequate surfactant. Surfactant is a lipoprotein which reduces the surface tension in the alveoli and assists gaseous exchange. It is first produced from about 20 weeks' gestation and the amount increases until the lungs are mature at about 30–34 weeks. At term the lungs contain about 100 ml of lung fluid. About one-third of this is expelled during delivery and the rest is absorbed and carried away by the lymphatics and blood vessels as air takes its place.

There is some movement of the thorax from the third month of fetal life and more definite diaphragmatic movements from the sixth month. Fetal breathing occurs in episodes of up to half an hour during rapid eye movement sleep (Johnson & Everitt 1995).

The central nervous system

This is derived from the ectoderm. It folds inwards by a complicated process to form the neural tube which is then covered over by skin. This process is occasionally incomplete, leading to open neural tube defects.

The fetus is able to perceive strong light and to hear external sounds. Periods of wakefulness and sleep occur, both deep (slow wave) and rapid eye movement sleep.

The skin

From 18 weeks after conception the fetus is covered with a white, creamy substance called *vernix caseosa*. This protects the skin from the fluid and from any friction against itself. At 20 weeks the fetus will be covered with a fine downy hair called *lanugo* and at the same time the head hair and eyebrows begin to form. Lanugo is shed again from 36 weeks and a full-term infant has little left.

Fingernails develop from about 10 weeks but the toenails not until about 18 weeks. By term the nails usually extend beyond the fingertips but length of the nails is an unreliable guide to maturity.

THE FETAL CIRCULATION (Fig. 52.3)

The key to understanding the fetal circulation is

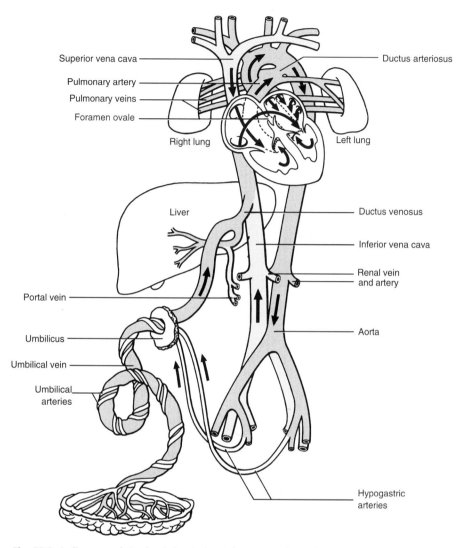

Superior vena cava

Pulmonary artery

Pulmonary veins

Foramen ovale

Right lung

Liver

Portal vein

Umbilicus

Umbilical vein

Umbilical arteries

Ductus arteriosus

Left lung

Ductus venosus

Inferior vena cava

Renal vein and artery

Aorta

Hypogastric arteries

Fig. 52.3 A diagram of the fetal circulation. The arrows show the course taken by the blood. The temporary structures are labelled in colour.

the fact that oxygen is derived from the placenta. In addition, the placenta is the source of nutrition and the site of elimination of waste. At birth there is a dramatic alteration in this situation and an almost instantaneous change must occur. Therefore all the postnatal structures must be in place and ready to take over. There are several temporary structures in addition to the placenta itself and the umbilical cord and these enable the fetal circulation to take place while allowing for the changes at birth.

The umbilical vein leads from the umbilical cord to the underside of the liver and carries blood rich in oxygen and nutrients. It has a branch which joins the portal vein and supplies the liver.

The ductus venosus (from a vein to a vein) connects the umbilical vein to the inferior vena cava. At this point the blood mixes with deoxygenated blood returning from the lower parts of the body. Thus the blood throughout the body is at best partially oxygenated.

The foramen ovale (oval opening) is a temporary opening between the atria which allows the majority of blood entering from the inferior vena cava to pass across into the left atrium. The reason for this diversion is that the blood does not need to pass through the lungs since it is already oxygenated.

The ductus arteriosus (from an artery to an artery) leads from the bifurcation of the pulmonary artery to the descending aorta, entering it just beyond the point where the subclavian and carotid arteries leave.

The hypogastric arteries branch off from the internal iliac arteries and become the umbilical arteries when they enter the umbilical cord. They return blood to the placenta.

The blood takes about half a minute to circulate and takes the following course.

From the placenta, blood passes along the umbilical vein through the abdominal wall to the under surface of the liver. This is the only vessel in the fetus which carries unmixed blood. The ductus venosus carries blood to the inferior vena cava where it mixes with blood from the lower body. From here the blood passes into the right atrium and most of it is directed across through the foramen ovale into the left atrium. Following its normal route it enters the left ventricle and passes into the aorta. The heart and brain each receive a supply of relatively well-oxygenated blood since the coronary and carotid arteries are early branches from the aorta. The arms also benefit via the subclavian arteries which is why they are more developed than the legs at birth.

Blood collected from the upper parts of the body returns to the right atrium in the superior vena cava. This blood is depleted of oxygen and nutrients. This stream of blood crosses the stream entering from the inferior vena cava and passes into the right ventricle. The two streams remain separate because of the shape of the atrium but there is a mixing of 25% of the blood, allowing a little oxygen and food to be taken to the lungs through the pulmonary artery. This is necessary for their development. However, only a small amount of the blood entering the pulmonary artery is required by the lungs. The remainder passes through the ductus arteriosus to the aorta. Blood continues along the aorta and, although low in oxygen, has sufficient to supply the remaining body organs and legs. The internal iliac arteries lead into the hypogastric arteries which return blood to the placenta via the umbilical arteries. The remaining blood supplies the lower limbs and returns to the inferior vena cava.

Adaptation to extrauterine life

At birth the baby takes a breath and blood is drawn to the lungs through the pulmonary arteries. It is then collected and returned to the left atrium via the pulmonary veins resulting in a sudden inflow of blood. The placental circulation ceases soon after birth and so less blood returns to the right side of the heart. In this way the pressure in the left side of the heart is greater while that in the right side of the heart becomes less. This results in the closure of a flap over the foramen ovale, which separates the two sides of the heart and stops the blood flowing from right to left.

With the establishment of pulmonary respiration the oxygen concentration in the bloodstream rises. This causes the ductus arteriosus to constrict and close. For as long as the ductus remains open after birth, blood flows from the high-pressure aorta towards the lungs, in the reverse direction to that in fetal life.

The cessation of the placental circulation results in the collapse of the umbilical vein, the ductus venosus and the hypogastric arteries.

These immediate changes are functional and those related to the heart are reversible in certain circumstances. Later they become permanent and anatomical. The umbilical vein becomes the *ligamentum teres*, the ductus venosus the *ligamentum venosum* and the ductus arteriosus the *ligamentum arteriosum*. The foramen ovale becomes the *fossa ovalis* and the hypogastric arteries are known as the *obliterated hypogastric arteries* except for the first few centimetres which remain open as the superior vesical arteries.

Respiratory and circulatory changes are not the only ones involved. After birth the baby has to obtain nutrition through the establishment of breast feeding or a breast feeding substitute and to eliminate waste via the kidneys and gastrointestinal system. In addition, of course, other complex changes take place including the development of communication and the relationship between parents and child (see Ch. 34). Chapters 34 and 35 discuss further the physiology of the baby at term.

THE FETAL SKULL (Fig. 52.4)

The fetal skull contains the delicate brain which may be subjected to great pressure as the head passes through the birth canal. It is large in relation to the fetal body (Fig. 52.5) and in comparison with the true pelvis; therefore some adaptation between skull and pelvis must take place during labour. The head is the most difficult part to deliver whether it comes first or last.

An understanding of the landmarks and measurements of the fetal skull enables the midwife to recognise normal presentations and positions and to facilitate delivery with the least possible trauma to mother and child. Where malpresentation or disproportion exists she will be able to identify it and alert the medical staff.

Ossification. The bones of the fetal head originate in two different ways. The face is laid down in cartilage and is almost completely ossified at birth, the bones being fused together and firm. The bones of the vault are laid down in membrane and are much flatter and more pliable. They ossify from the centre outwards and this process is incomplete at birth leaving small gaps which form the sutures and fontanelles. The ossification centre on each bone appears as a boss or protuberance.

Bones of the vault (Fig. 52.6)

There are five main bones in the vault of the fetal skull.

The occipital bone lies at the back of the head and forms the region of the occiput. Part of it contributes to the base of the skull as it contains the foramen magnum, which protects the spinal cord as it leaves the skull. At the centre is the *occipital protuberance*.

The two parietal bones lie on either side of the skull. The ossification centre of each is called the *parietal eminence*.

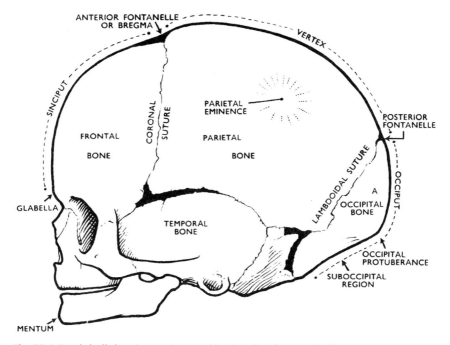

Fig. 52.4 Fetal skull showing regions and landmarks of obstetrical importance.

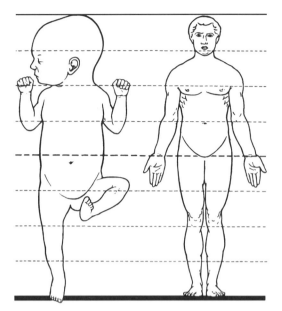

Fig. 52.5 Comparison of a baby's proportions to those of an adult. The baby's head is wider than her shoulders and one-quarter of her length.

The two frontal bones form the forehead or *sinciput*. At the centre of each is a frontal boss or frontal eminence. The frontal bones fuse into a single bone by 8 years of age.

In addition to these five the upper part of *the temporal bone* is also flat and forms a small part of the vault.

Sutures and fontanelles

Sutures are cranial joints and are formed where two bones adjoin. Where two or more sutures meet, a fontanelle is formed. There are several sutures and fontanelles in the fetal skull; those of most obstetrical significance are described below.

The lambdoidal suture is shaped like the Greek letter lambda (λ) and separates the occipital bone from the two parietal bones.

The sagittal suture lies between the two parietal bones.

The coronal suture separates the frontal bones from the parietal bones, passing from one temple to the other.

The frontal suture runs between the two halves of the frontal bone. Whereas the frontal suture becomes obliterated in time, the other sutures eventually become fixed joints. Ossification of the skull is not complete until early adulthood.

The posterior fontanelle or lambda is situated

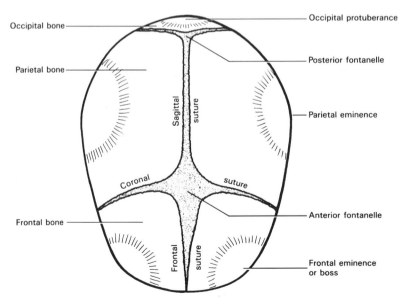

Fig. 52.6 View of fetal head from above (head partly flexed).

at the junction of the lambdoidal and sagittal sutures. It is small, triangular in shape and can be recognised vaginally because a suture leaves from each of the three angles. It normally closes by 6 weeks of age.

The anterior fontanelle or bregma is found at the junction of the sagittal, coronal and frontal sutures. It is broad, kite-shaped and recognisable vaginally because a suture leaves from each of the four corners. It measures 3–4 cm long and 1.5–2 cm wide and normally closes by the time the child is 18 months old. Pulsations of cerebral vessels can be felt through it.

The sutures and fontanelles, because they consist of membranous spaces, allow for a degree of overlapping of the skull bones during labour and delivery.

Regions and landmarks of the fetal skull

The skull is divided into the vault, the base and the face (Fig. 52.7). *The vault* is the large, dome-shaped part above an imaginary line drawn between the orbital ridges and the nape of the neck. In the vault the bones are relatively thin and pliable at birth which allows the skull to alter slightly in shape during birth. *The base* is comprised of bones which are firmly united to protect the vital centres in the medulla. *The face* is composed of 14 small bones

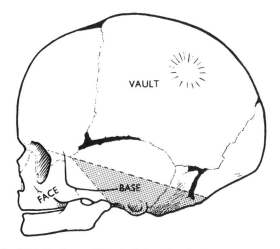

Fig. 52.7 Regions of the skull showing the large, compressible vault and the non-compressible face and base.

which are also firmly united and non-compressible. The regions of the skull are described as follows:

The occiput lies between the foramen magnum and the posterior fontanelle. The part below the occipital protuberance is known as the suboccipital region. The protuberance itself can be seen and felt as a prominent point on the posterior aspect of the skull.

The vertex is bounded by the posterior fontanelle, the two parietal eminences and the anterior fontanelle. Of the 96% of the babies born head first, 95% present by the vertex.

The sinciput or brow extends from the anterior fontanelle and the coronal suture to the orbital ridges.

The face is small in the newborn baby. It extends from the orbital ridges and the root of the nose to the junction of the chin and the neck. The point between the eyebrows is known as *the glabella*. The chin is termed *the mentum* and is an important landmark.

Diameters of the fetal skull

The measurements of the skull are important because the midwife needs a practical understanding of the relationship between the fetal head and the mother's pelvis. It will become clear that some diameters are more favourable for easy passage through the pelvic canal and this will depend on the attitude of the head.

There are two transverse diameters (Fig. 52.8):

Biparietal diameter 9.5 cm – between the two parietal eminences.

Bitemporal diameter 8.2 cm – between the furthest points of the coronal suture at the temples.

The remaining diameters described are anteroposterior or longitudinal (Fig. 52.9):

Suboccipitobregmatic 9.5 cm – from below the occipital protuberance to the centre of the anterior fontanelle or bregma.

Suboccipitofrontal 10 cm – from below the occipital protuberance to the centre of the frontal suture.

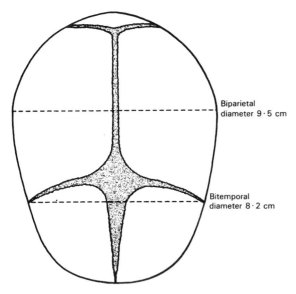

Fig. 52.8 Diagram showing the transverse diameters of the fetal skull.

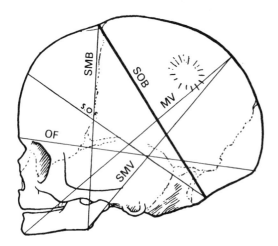

Fig. 52.9 Diagram showing the anteroposterior diameters of the fetal skull.

Diameter			Length
SOB	=	Suboccipitobregmatic	9.5 cm
SOF	=	Suboccipitofrontal	10.0 cm
OF	=	Occipitofrontal	11.5 cm
MV	=	Mentovertical	13.5 cm
SMV	=	Submentovertical	11.5 cm
SMB	=	Submentobregmatic	9.5 cm

Occipitofrontal 11.5 cm – from the occipital protuberance to the glabella.

Mentovertical 13.5 cm – from the point of the chin to the highest point on the vertex, slightly nearer to the posterior than to the anterior fontanelle.

Submentovertical 11.5 cm – from the point where the chin joins the neck to the highest point on the vertex.

Submentobregmatic 9.5 cm – from the point where the chin joins the neck to the centre of the bregma.

Attitude of the fetal head

This term is used to describe the degree of flexion or extension of the head on the neck. The attitude of the head determines which diameters will present in labour and therefore influences the outcome.

Presenting diameters

The diameters of the head which are called the presenting diameters are those which are at right angles to the curve of Carus. There are always two: an anteroposterior or longitudinal diameter and a transverse diameter. The diameters presenting in the individual cephalic or head presentations are as follows:

Vertex presentation. When the head is well flexed, the suboccipitobregmatic diameter and the biparietal diameter present (Fig. 52.10). As these two diameters are the same length, 9.5 cm, the presenting area is circular, which is the most favourable shape for dilating the cervix. The diameter which distends the vaginal orifice is the suboccipitofrontal diameter, 10 cm.

When the head is not flexed but erect, the presenting diameters are the occipitofrontal, 11.5 cm and the biparietal, 9.5 cm. This situation often arises when the occiput is in a posterior position. If it remains so, the diameter distending the vaginal orifice will be the occipitofrontal, 11.5 cm.

Brow presentation. When the head is partially extended, the mentovertical diameter, 13.5 cm, and the bitemporal diameter, 8.2 cm, present. If this presentation persists, vaginal delivery is extremely unlikely.

Face presentation. When the head is com-

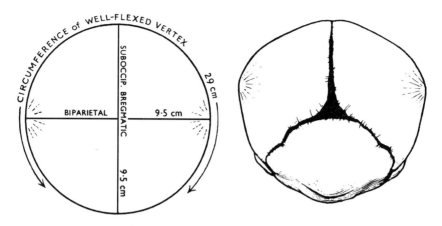

Fig. 52.10 Diagram showing the dimensions presenting when the fetal head is well flexed in a vertex presentation.

pletely extended, the presenting diameters are the submentobregmatic, 9.5 cm, and the bitemporal, 8.2 cm. The submentovertical diameter, 11.5 cm, will distend the vaginal orifice.

Diameters of the fetal trunk are given in Box 52.2.

Moulding

This is the term applied to the change in shape of the fetal head that takes place during its passage through the birth canal. Alteration in shape is possible because the bones of the vault allow a slight degree of bending and the skull bones are able to override at the sutures. This overriding allows a considerable reduction in the size of the presenting diameters while the diameter at right

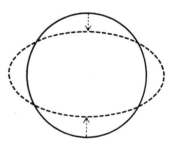

Fig. 52.11 Demonstration of the principle of moulding. The diameter compressed is diminished; the diameter at right-angles to it is elongated.

angles to them is able to lengthen due to the give of the skull bones (Fig. 52.11).

In a normal vertex presentation with the fetal head in a fully flexed attitude the suboccipitobregmatic and the biparietal diameters will be reduced and the mentovertical will be lengthened. The shortening may be by as much as 1.25 cm (Figs 52.12–52.17 illustrate moulding in various presentations).

Moulding is a protective mechanism and prevents the fetal brain from being compressed as long as it is not excessive, too rapid or in an unfavourable direction. The skull of the preterm infant, being softer and having wider sutures, may mould excessively; the skull of the postmature infant does not mould well and its greater hardness tends to make labour more difficult.

Box 52.2 Diameters of the fetal trunk

Bisacromial diameter 12 cm
This is the distance between the acromion processes on the two shoulder blades and is the dimension that needs to pass through the pelvis for the shoulders to be born. The articulation of the clavicles on the sternum allows forward movement of the shoulders which may reduce the diameter slightly.

Bitrochanteric diameter 10 cm
This is measured between the greater trochanters of the femurs and is the presenting diameter in breech presentation.

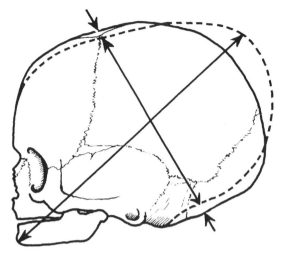

Fig. 52.12 Moulding in a normal vertex presentation with the head well flexed. The suboccipitobregmatic diameter is reduced and the mentovertical elongated.

The intracranial membranes and sinuses (Figs 52.18 and 52.19)

The skull contains delicate structures, some of which may be damaged if the head is subjected to abnormal moulding during delivery. Among the most important are the folds of dura mater and the venous sinuses associated with them. These membranes are continuous with the dura mater which lines the cranium.

The falx cerebri is a sickle-shaped fold of membrane which dips down between the two cerebral hemispheres and runs beneath the frontal and sagittal sutures, from the root of the nose to the internal occipital protuberance.

The tentorium cerebelli is a horizontal fold of dura mater which lies in the posterior part of the skull at right angles to the falx cerebri. It is shaped like a horseshoe and situated between the cerebrum and the cerebellum over which it forms a

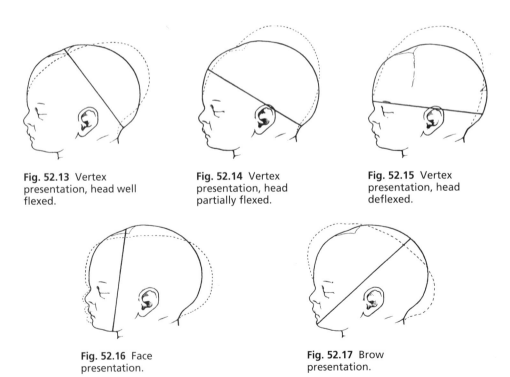

Fig. 52.13 Vertex presentation, head well flexed.

Fig. 52.14 Vertex presentation, head partially flexed.

Fig. 52.15 Vertex presentation, head deflexed.

Fig. 52.16 Face presentation.

Fig. 52.17 Brow presentation.

Figs 52.13–52.17 Series of diagrams showing moulding when the head presents. Moulding is shown by the dotted line.

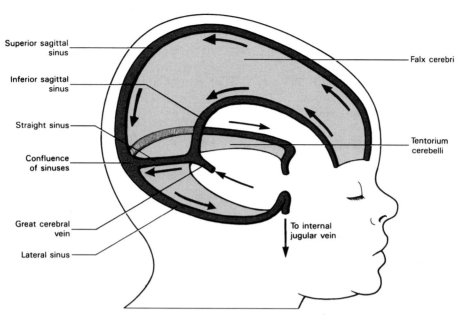

Fig. 52.18 Diagram showing intracranial membranes and venous sinuses. Arrows show direction of blood flow.

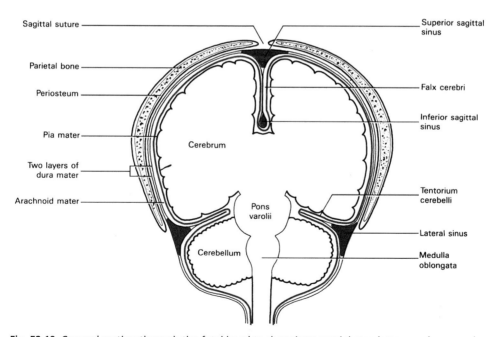

Fig. 52.19 Coronal section through the fetal head to show intracranial membranes and venous sinuses.

sort of tent. The membranes contain large veins or sinuses which drain blood from the brain.

The superior sagittal sinus runs along the upper edge of the falx cerebri from front to back.

The inferior sagittal sinus runs along the lower edge of the falx cerebri in the same direction.

The great cerebral vein of Galen meets the inferior sagittal sinus at the inner end of the junction between the falx and the tentorium.

The straight sinus drains blood from both the great cerebral vein and the inferior sagittal sinus along the junction of the falx and the tentorium. The point where it reaches the skull and receives blood from the superior sagittal sinus is known as the *confluence of sinuses*.

The two lateral sinuses pass from the confluence of sinuses along the outer edge of the tentorium cerebelli and carry blood to the internal jugular veins.

The most vulnerable point of these structures is where the falx is attached to the tentorium. The tentorium is liable to tear and there is a danger of bleeding from the great cerebral vein.

READER ACTIVITIES

1. Examine the head of a baby immediately after birth. From moulding, the position of any caput succedaneum and overlapping of skull bones, calculate the position that the child must have been in during labour. Compare this with the recorded vaginal examinations in labour.

2. Take the skull measurements of a newly born baby. (If calipers are available it is possible to take all measurements; if not, use a tape measure to measure the circumferences.) After 3 days take the same measurements and compare the differences.

REFERENCE

Johnson M, Everitt B 1995 Essential reproduction, 4th edn. Blackwell Science, Oxford

FURTHER READING

Burnett C W F 1979 The anatomy and physiology of obstetrics, 6th edn (rev. Anderson M). Faber and Faber, London
Dryden R 1978 Before birth. Heinemann Educational, London
Moore K L 1998 The developing human, 6th edn. Saunders, London
Moore K L 1998 Before we are born, 5th edn. Saunders, London
Wolpert L 1991 The triumph of the embryo. Oxford University Press, Oxford

The female urinary tract

V. Ruth Bennett   Linda K. Brown

The urinary system is chiefly thought of in connection with its elimination function and the production of urine. It also has important functions in connection with the control of water and electrolyte balance and of blood pressure.

In the female it has an importance associated with its proximity to the reproductive organs. When the woman is not pregnant, her uterus lies just behind and partly over the bladder. When she is pregnant the enlarging uterus affects all the parts of the urinary tract at various times and the hormones of pregnancy have an even greater influence than the mechanical effects. The normal, healthy woman may perceive these changes as a minor nuisance created by frequency of micturition and her kidneys continue to function well. A few may experience complications and those who already have diseased kidneys may undergo deterioration in their condition: some women suffer impairment of the function of part of the urinary tract as a direct result of pregnancy. The midwife may have an important part to play in minimising any ill-effect.

The urinary tract begins at the two kidneys which are linked up to the blood supply by the large renal arteries and veins. It continues as a passage for urine in the two ureters, the bladder and the urethra.

THE KIDNEYS

The kidneys are two bean-shaped glands which have both endocrine and exocrine secretions. Their function is to extract soluble wastes from the blood and to excrete such water and minerals as are surplus to the body's requirements. They also prevent substances which are needed by the body from being lost. They have a part to play in red cell production and in maintaining blood pressure.

Position and supports

The kidneys are positioned at the back of the abdominal cavity, high up under the diaphragm. The right kidney is displaced a little downwards by the liver, so the two kidneys are not quite level. They are maintained in position by a generous packing of perinephric fat and by the closeness of neighbouring organs, particularly parts of the gastrointestinal tract in front and the musculature of the posterior abdominal wall behind (Fig. 53.1).

Appearance

The gland is recognisable by its dark red appearance and typical shape, so that other similarly shaped objects may be called 'kidney-shaped'. It is about 10 cm long, 6.5 cm wide and 3 cm thick. It weighs around 120 g. It is covered with a tough, fibrous capsule.

The inner border of the organ is indented at the hilum; here the large vessels enter and leave and the ureter is attached by its funnel-shaped upper end to channel the urine away.

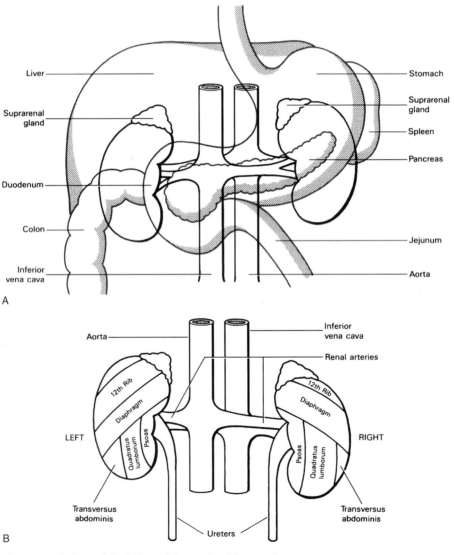

Fig. 53.1 Relations of the kidney: (A) anterior; (B) posterior.

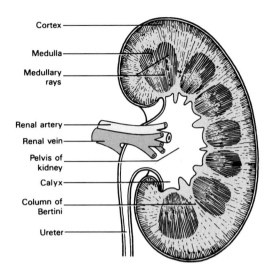

Fig. 53.2 Longitudinal section of the kidney.

Inner structure

The glandular tissue is formed of cortex on the outside and medulla within. The cortex is dark with a rich blood supply while the medulla is paler. A collecting area for urine merges with the upper ureter and is called the pelvis. It is divided into branches or calyces and each calyx cups over a projection from the medulla known as a pyramid. There are some 12 pyramids in all and they contain bundles of tubules leading from the cortex. The tubules create a lined appearance and these are the medullary rays. The base of each pyramid is curved and the cortex arches over it (Fig. 53.2) and projects downwards between the pyramids forming columns of tissue (columns of Bertini).

The nephrons

When the tissue of the kidney is examined under the microscope, it is found to be formed of about 1 million nephrons, which are its functional units.

The manufacture of urine depends on a constant and generous supply of blood. Each nephron starts at a knot of capillaries called a *glomerulus* (Fig. 53.3). It is fed by a branch of the renal artery, the *afferent arteriole*, and the blood is collected up again into the *efferent arteriole*. Afferent means 'carrying towards' and efferent, 'carrying away'. This is the only place in the body where an artery

collects blood from capillaries. The blood vessel continues alongside the nephron.

Surrounding the glomerulus is a cup known as the *glomerular capsule* into which fluid and solutes are exuded from the blood. The glomerulus and capsule together are the *glomerular body* (Fig. 53.3). The pressure within the glomerulus is raised because the afferent arteriole is of a wider bore than the efferent arteriole and this factor forces the filtrate out of the capillaries and into the capsule. At this stage there is no selection; any substance with a small molecular size will filter out.

The cup of the capsule is attached to a tubule as a wine glass to its stem. The tubule initially winds and twists, then forms a straight loop which dips into the medulla, rising up into the cortex again to wind and turn before joining a *straight collecting tubule* which receives urine from several nephrons. The first twisting portion is the *proximal*

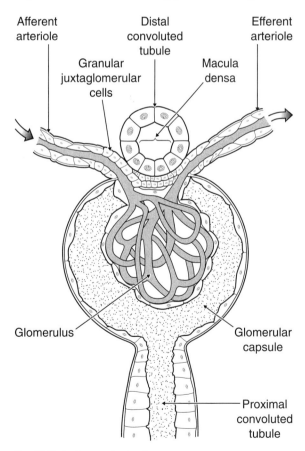

Fig. 53.3 A glomerular body.

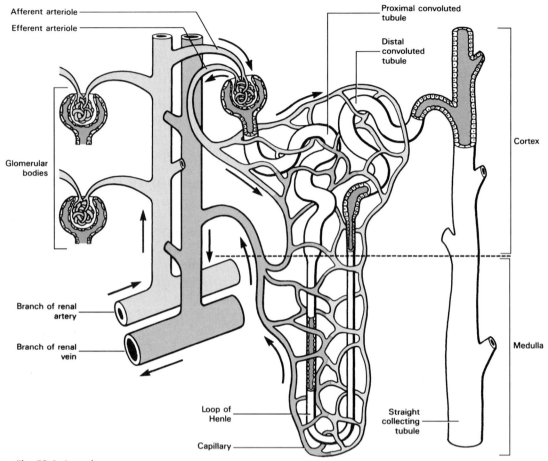

Fig. 53.4 A nephron.

convoluted tubule; the loop is termed the *loop of Henle* and the second twisting portion is the *distal convoluted tubule*. The whole nephron is about 3 cm in length (Fig. 53.4). The straight collecting tubule runs from the cortex to a medullary pyramid: it forms a medullary ray (see above) and receives urine from over 4000 nephrons along its length.

Juxtaglomerular apparatus. The distal convoluted tubule returns to pass alongside granular cells of the afferent arteriole and this part of the tubule is called the macula densa. The two are known as the juxtaglomerular apparatus. The granular cells secrete renin (see below) while the macula densa cells monitor the sodium chloride concentration of fluid passing through.

Blood supply

The renal arteries are early branches of the descending abdominal aorta and divert about a quarter of the cardiac output into the kidneys. The artery enters at the renal hilum between the ureter behind and the renal vein in front. It sends numerous branches into the cortex and forms a glomerulus for each nephron. Blood is collected up and returned via the renal vein (see Fig. 53.1).

Lymphatic drainage

A rich supply of lymph vessels lies under the cortex and around the urine-bearing tubules. It drains into large lymphatic ducts which emerge from the hilum and lead to the aortic lymph glands.

Nerve supply

Nerves enter by the renal hilum and provide a sympathetic and parasympathetic nerve supply.

The making of urine

This takes place in three stages:

- filtration
- reabsorption
- secretion.

Filtration. This is the simple process of water and the substances dissolved in it being passed from the glomerulus into the glomerular capsule as a result of the raised intracapillary pressure. Blood components such as corpuscles and platelets as well as proteins which have a large molecule are kept in the blood vessel; water, salts and glucose escape through the filter as the *filtrate* (Fig. 53.5). A vast amount of fluid passes out in this way, about 2 ml per second or 120 ml per minute. 99% of this must be recovered, or the body would be totally drained of fluid within hours. Filtration is increased in pregnancy as it helps to eliminate the additional wastes created by maternal and fetal metabolism.

Reabsorption. The body selects from the filtrate the substances which it needs: water, salts and glucose.

Normally all the glucose is reabsorbed; only if there is already more than sufficient in the blood, for example after eating sweet or sugary foods, will any be excreted in the urine. The level of blood glucose at which this happens is the *renal threshold* for glucose. In the non-pregnant, the threshold is 10 mmol/l and in the pregnant woman 8.3 mmol/l. It is more likely, therefore, that glucose will appear in the urine during pregnancy.

The water is almost all reabsorbed. If the body has lost fluid by other means, such as sweating, or if fluid intake has been low, more water is conserved, less urine is passed and the urine appears more concentrated. In the opposite circumstances, when the individual has drunk a lot of water and is sweating little, the urine is more copious and dilute. Note that drinking alcohol does not have this effect. The posterior pituitary gland controls the reabsorption of water by producing antidiuretic hormone (ADH). The more ADH produced, the more water is reabsorbed. Newborn babies are poorly able to concentrate and dilute their urine and preterm infants even less so. For this reason they are unable to tolerate wide variations in their fluid intake. Pregnant women pass a greater amount of urine than when non-pregnant.

Minerals are selected according to the body's needs. The reabsorption of sodium is controlled by aldosterone which is produced in the cortex of the adrenal gland. The interaction of aldosterone and ADH maintains water and sodium balance. The pH of the blood must be controlled and if it is tending towards acidity, acids will be excreted. This is commonly the case. However, if the opposite pertains, alkaline urine will be produced. Often this is the result of an intake of an alkaline substance.

Secretion. Certain substances, such as creatinine and toxins, are added directly to the urine in the ascending arm of the loop of Henle.

Endocrine activity

The kidney secretes two hormones. One, renin, is produced in the afferent arteriole and is secreted when the blood supply to the kidneys is reduced and in response to lowered sodium levels. It acts on angiotensinogen, which is present in the blood,

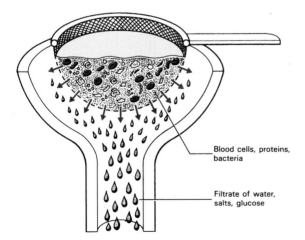

Blood cells, proteins, bacteria

Filtrate of water, salts, glucose

Fig. 53.5 Filtration: larger molecules stay in the sieve (glomerulus) and smaller molecules filter out (into the glomerular capsule).

to form angiotensin which raises blood pressure and encourages sodium reabsorption.

The second hormone, erythropoietin, stimulates the production of red blood cells.

Summary of functions

The kidney functions may be summarised as follows:

- elimination of wastes, particularly the breakdown products of protein, such as urea, urates, uric acid, creatinine, ammonia and sulphates
- elimination of toxins
- regulation of the water content of the blood and indirectly of the tissues
- regulation of the pH of the blood
- regulation of the osmotic pressure of the blood
- secretion of the hormones renin and erythropoietin.

The urine

Urine is a yellow colour ranging from pale straw colour when very dilute to dark brown if very concentrated. In the newborn baby it is almost clear. It has a recognisable smell which in health is not unpleasant when freshly passed. It should never be cloudy.

An adult passes between 1 and 2 litres of urine daily, depending on fluid intake. Less is produced during the night than in the day. Pregnant women secrete large amounts of urine because of the increased glomerular filtration rate and they often have to rise at night to empty the bladder (see Ch. 11). In the first day or two post-partum a major diuresis occurs and urine output is copious.

The specific gravity of urine is 1.010–1.030. It is composed of 96% water, 2% urea and 2% other solutes. Urea and uric acid clearance are increased in pregnancy. Urine is usually acid and contains no glucose or ketones, nor should it carry blood cells or bacteria. Women are susceptible to urinary tract infection but this is usually an ascending infection acquired via the urethra. A low count, less than 100 000 per ml, of bacteria in the urine (bacteriuria) is treated as insignificant.

THE URETERS

The tubes which convey the urine from the kidneys to the bladder are the ureters. They assist the passage of the urine by the muscular peristaltic action of their walls. The upper end is funnel-shaped and merges into the pelvis of the kidney where the urine is received from the renal tubules.

Each tube is about 25–30 cm long and runs from the renal hilum to the posterior wall of the bladder (Fig. 53.6). In the abdomen they pass down the posterior wall, remaining outside the peritoneal cavity. On reaching the pelvic brim, they descend along the side walls of the pelvis to the level of the ischial spines and then turn forwards to pass beside the uterine cervix and enter the bladder from behind. They pass through the bladder wall at an angle (Fig. 53.7) so that when the bladder

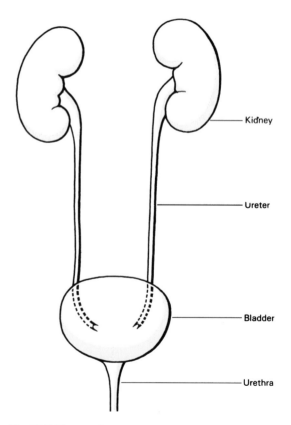

Fig. 53.6 The renal tract.

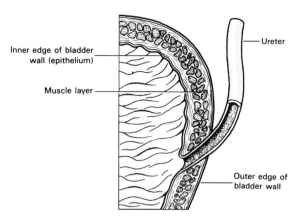

Fig. 53.7 Diagram to show the entry of the ureter into the posterior wall of the bladder.

contracts to expel urine, the ureters are closed off and reflux is prevented.

Structure

The ureters have three main layers:

The lining is formed of transitional epithelium arranged in longitudinal folds. This type of epithelium consists of several layers of pear-shaped cells and makes an elastic and waterproof inner coat.

The muscular layer is arranged as an inner longitudinal layer, a middle circular layer and an outer longitudinal layer. Waves of peristalsis pass along the ureter towards the bladder.

The outer coat is of fibrous connective tissue which is protective. It is continuous with the fibrous capsule of the kidney.

Blood, lymph and nerve supply

The upper part of the ureter is supplied similarly to the kidney. In its pelvic portion it derives blood from the common iliac and internal iliac arteries and from the uterine and vesical arteries, according to its proximity to the different organs. Venous return is along corresponding veins.

Lymph drains into the internal, external and common iliac lymph nodes.

The nerve supply is sympathetic and parasympathetic.

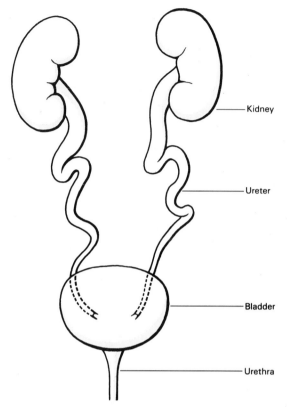

Fig. 53.8 Dilated, kinked ureters in pregnancy.

The ureter in pregnancy

The hormones of pregnancy, particularly progesterone, relax the walls of the ureters and allow dilatation and kinking. In some women this is quite marked and it tends to result in a slowing down or stasis of urinary flow, making infection a greater possibility (Fig. 53.8; see also Ch. 11).

THE BLADDER

The bladder is the urinary reservoir which stores the urine until it is convenient for it to be voided. It is described as being pyramidal; its base is triangular. When it is full, however, it becomes more globular in shape as its walls are distended. Although it is a pelvic organ it may rise into the abdomen when full, and during labour it is certainly abdominal. It is one of the organs which most greatly concern midwives because of its closeness to the uterus.

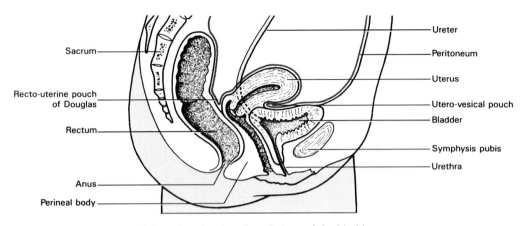

Fig. 53.9 Sagittal section of the pelvis showing the relations of the bladder.

Position

In the non-pregnant female, the bladder lies immediately behind the symphysis pubis and in front of the uterus and vagina (Fig. 53.9). In addition, the anteverted, anteflexed uterus lies partially over the bladder superiorly. The intestines and peritoneal cavity also lie above. The ureters enter the bladder from behind; the urethra leaves it from below. Underneath the bladder is the muscular diaphragm of the pelvic floor which forms its main support and on which its function partly depends.

Structure

The base of the bladder is termed the *trigone*. It is situated at the back of the bladder, resting against the vagina. Its three angles are the exit of the urethra below and the two slit-like openings of the ureters above. The apex of the trigone is thus at its lowest point, which is also termed the neck (Fig. 53.10).

The anterior part of the bladder lies close to the pubic symphysis and is termed the apex of the bladder. From it the urachus runs up the anterior abdominal wall to the umbilicus. In fetal life this is the remains of the yolk sac but in the adult is simply a fibrous band.

The bladder when empty is of similar size to the uterus but when full of urine it becomes, of course, much larger. Its capacity is around 600 ml but it is capable of holding more, particularly under the influence of pregnancy hormones. The midwife

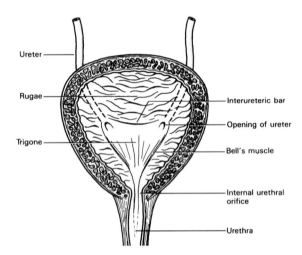

Fig. 53.10 Section through the bladder.

will commonly observe a newly-delivered woman voiding upwards of 1 litre on a single occasion.

Layers

The lining of the bladder, like that of the ureter, is formed of transitional epithelium which helps to allow the distension of the bladder without losing its water-holding effect. The lining, except over the trigone, is thrown into wrinkles or *rugae* which flatten out as the bladder expands and fills.

The mucous membrane lining lies on a sub-mucous layer of areolar tissue which carries blood and lymph vessels and nerves.

The epithelium over the trigone is smooth and firmly attached to the underlying muscle.

The musculature of the bladder consists chiefly of the large detrusor muscle whose function is to expel urine. (To detrude is to thrust down to a lower place.) This muscle has an inner longitudinal, a middle circular and an outer longitudinal layer. Around the neck of the bladder, the circular muscle is thickened to form the *internal urethral sphincter*. It remains constantly contracted except when the individual passes urine.

In the trigone the muscles are somewhat differently arranged. A band of muscle between the ureteric apertures forms the interureteric bar (Mercier's bar). Along the other two sides of the trigone, Bell's muscles run from the entrances of the ureters down through the internal urethral orifice. They are important during voiding of the bladder.

The outer layer of the bladder is formed of visceral pelvic fascia, except on its superior surface which is covered with peritoneum (see Fig. 53.9).

Blood, lymph and nerve supplies

The vesical arteries, superior and inferior, are the main suppliers of blood. A few small branches from the uterine and vaginal arteries also bring blood to the bladder. Corresponding veins return used blood.

Lymph drains into the internal iliac glands and into the obturator glands.

The nerve supply is parasympathetic and sympathetic and comes via the important Lee–Frankenhäuser plexus in the pouch of Douglas. The stimulation of sympathetic nerves causes the internal urethral sphincter to contract and the detrusor muscle to relax, while the parasympathetic nerve fibres cause the bladder to empty and the sphincter to relax.

THE URETHRA

The final passage in the urinary tract is the urethra, 4 cm long in the female and consisting of a narrow tube buried in the outer layers of the anterior vaginal wall. It runs from the neck of the bladder and opens into the vestibule of the vulva as the urethral meatus. During labour the urethra becomes elongated as the bladder is drawn up into the abdomen and may become several centimetres longer.

Structure

The lining. The urethra forms the junction between the urinary tract and the external genitalia. The epithelium of its lining reflects this. The upper half is lined with transitional epithelium while the lower half is lined with squamous epithelium. The lumen is normally closed unless urine is passing down it or a catheter is in situ. When closed, it shows small longitudinal folds. Small blind ducts called urethral crypts open into the urethra of which the two largest are Skene's ducts which open just beside the urethral meatus. Their main significance is in the possibility of infection with an organism such as the gonococcus.

The submucous coat. The epithelium of the urethra lies on a bed of vascular connective tissue.

The musculature. The muscle layers are arranged as an inner longitudinal layer, continuous with the inner muscle fibres of the bladder, and an external circular layer. The inner muscle fibres help to open the internal urethral sphincter during micturition.

The outer layer of the urethra is continuous with the outer layer of the vagina and is formed of connective tissue.

The external sphincter. At the lower end of the urethra, voluntary, striated muscle fibres form the so-called membranous sphincter of the urethra. This is not a true sphincter but it gives some voluntary control to the woman when she desires to resist the urge to urinate. The powerful levator ani muscles which pass on either side of the uterus also assist in controlling continence of urine.

Blood, lymph and nerve supplies

The blood is circulated by the inferior vesical and pudendal arteries and veins. Lymph drains to the internal iliac glands.

The internal urethral sphincter is supplied by sympathetic and parasympathetic nerves but the membranous sphincter is supplied by the pudendal nerve and is under voluntary control.

Micturition

The urge to pass urine is felt when the bladder contains about 200–300 ml of urine but also when psychological stimuli operate such as waking after sleep, arriving or leaving home, and from external stimuli such as the sound and feel of water and the feel of the toilet seat. Helpless laughter or paroxysmal coughing may also trigger a desire to empty the bladder.

In newborn babies there is no resistance to the spontaneous prompting of the bladder that it wishes to be emptied. The sphincters relax, the detrusor muscle contracts and urine is passed.

After about 2 years a child learns to resist the urge to void and by adulthood it is taken for granted. Many women, particularly the pregnant and parous, experience difficulty in maintaining continence under the stress of coughing, laughing, sneezing and other factors which raise intra-abdominal pressure. Regular muscular exercise such as walking, swimming, running and pelvic floor exercises help to raise the tone of the voluntary muscles.

In summary, the bladder fills and then contracts as a reflex response. The internal sphincter opens by the action of Bell's muscles. If the urge is not resisted, the external sphincter relaxes and the bladder empties. The act of emptying may be speeded by raising intra-abdominal pressure either to initiate the process or throughout voiding. The act of micturition can be temporarily postponed but the full bladder becomes progressively more uncomfortable.

FURTHER READING

Beischer N A, Mackay E V 1986 Obstetrics and the newborn, 2nd edn. Baillière Tindall, London
McLaren S M 1996 Renal function. In: Hinchliff S, Montague S, Watson R (eds) Physiology for nursing practice, 2nd edn. Baillière Tindall, London
Rutishauser S 1994 Physiology and anatomy: a basis for nursing and health care. Churchill Livingstone, Edinburgh

Index

Location references in **bold** indicate figures and tables